SPECIAL CONSIDERATIONS

DISORDERS

PROFESSIONAL ISSUES IN THE CARE OF THE AGED

THEORETICAL CONCEPTS RELATED TO AGING

NORMAL AGING CHANGES AND HEALTHY AGING

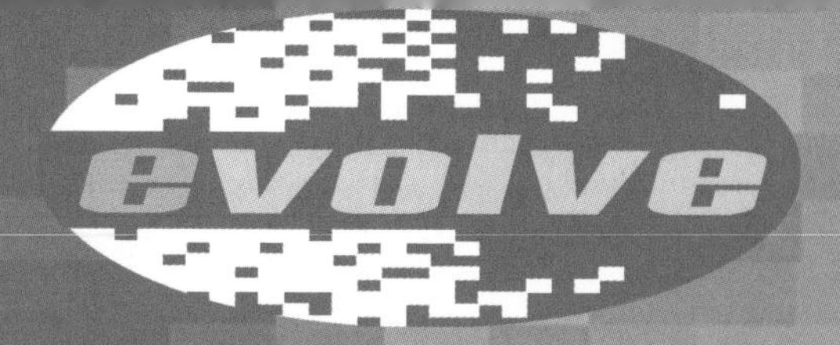

The Latest Evolution in Learning.

Evolve provides online access to free learning resources and activities designed specifically for the textbook you are using in your class. The resources will provide you with information that enhances the material covered in the book and much more.

Visit the Web address listed below to start your learning evolution today!

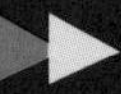

LOGIN: http://evolve.elsevier.com/Ebersole/TwdHlthAging/

Evolve Online Courseware for Ebersole/Hess/Luggen: *Toward Healthy Aging: Human Needs and Nursing Response, 6th Edition* offers the following features:

- **WebLinks**
  Links to places of interest on the Web specific to your classroom needs
- **Review/Critical Thinking Questions**
  Activities designed to help identify important content and test your level of knowledge and understanding

Think outside the book...evolve.

Toward Healthy Aging

Human Needs and Nursing Response

ABOUT THE AUTHORS

Priscilla Ebersole, PhD, RN, FAAN, has been involved in gerontologic nursing for over 30 years. She has conducted nationwide workshops and seminars on aging. Her expertise is in the fields of geropsychiatric nursing, middle age, and aging. She is a graduate of San Francisco State University, the University of California at San Francisco, and Columbia Pacific University, and she has earned a certificate in gerontologic nursing from the University of Southern California at Los Angeles. Dr. Ebersole has held appointments in the Applied Gerontology Certificate Program at San Francisco State University and at the Ethel Percy Andrus Gerontology Center, University of Southern California, and she is professor emerita in the School of Nursing, San Francisco State University. From 1981 to 1984 she was on leave of absence to act as the field director of a gerontologic nurse practitioner project funded by the W.K. Kellogg Foundation and administered by the Mountain States Health Corporation in Boise, Idaho. In 1988 Dr. Ebersole was a visiting professor at Case Western Reserve University and occupied the Florence Cellar endowed gerontologic nursing chair. In 1987 she was named Educator of the Year by the American College of Health Care Administrators. In 1997 Dr. Ebersole was inducted into the Hall of Fame at San Francisco State University. She is currently the editor of *Geriatric Nursing*.

Patricia Hess, PhD, RN, APRN, BC, NAP, has earned certificates in gerontologic nursing from the Ethel Percy Andrus Gerontology Center, University of Southern California at Los Angeles, and Holy Names College in Oakland, California, and she is a graduate of Case Western Reserve University, Francis Payne Bolton School of Nursing, in Cleveland, the University of Colorado at Boulder, and Walden University in Naples, Florida. In 1986 she completed the geriatric nurse practitioner program at the University of California School of Nursing, San Francisco. She is also a member of the National Academies of Practice. She has been involved in gerontologic nursing for over 40 years and has conducted workshops and seminars on aging. Her expertise is in the areas of health promotion and wellness, dying and death, and education of students and staff to the specific needs of the aged in acute care settings. She is a professor in the School of Nursing, San Francisco State University, and she holds an appointment in the Applied Gerontology Certificate Program at San Francisco State University.

Ann Schmidt Luggen PhD, RN, GNP-CS, CNAA, has been involved in gerontologic nursing since she was a research assistant and teaching assistant with the Robert Wood Johnson Teaching-Nursing Home grant at the University of Cincinnati/Maple Knoll Village in the early 1980s. Her MSN is in medical-surgical and oncology nursing and her doctorate is in gerontologic oncology. She has been certified as a gerontology CNS and NP and as an administrator at the advanced level, and she has done a post-doctorate in long-term care nursing administration at University of Kentucky. She has also served as president of the Ohio Gerontological Nurse Practitioners and on the board of the National Gerontological Nursing Association (NGNA) for 10 years. She presently serves on the steering committee of the National Conference of Gerontological Nurse Practitioners. She has presented at conferences nationally, has written and edited ten books (including the first core curriculum for gerontologic nursing), and has published numerous manuscripts. She has been the editor of two national geriatric nursing newsletters, writes a geriatric column for *Advances for Nurse Practitioners,* and has been an editor for *Geriatric Nursing* for more than 10 years. Dr. Luggen teaches in the graduate program at Northern Kentucky University, teaching nursing administration students, as well as teaching geriatrics to nurse practitioner students.

Sixth Edition

Toward Healthy Aging

Human Needs and Nursing Response

Priscilla Ebersole, PhD, RN, FAAN

Professor Emerita
San Francisco State University
San Francisco, California

Patricia Hess, PhD, RN, APRN, BC, NAP

Professor of Nursing
San Francisco State University
San Francisco, California

Ann Schmidt Luggen, PhD, RN, GNP-CS, CNAA

Professor of Nursing
Northern Kentucky University
Highland Heights, Kentucky

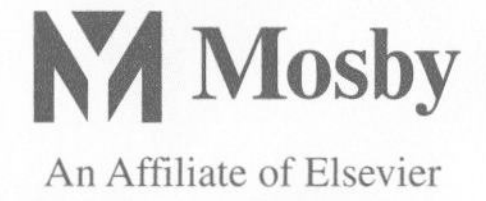

An Affiliate of Elsevier

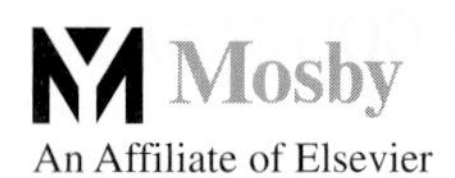
Mosby
An Affiliate of Elsevier

11830 Westline Industrial Drive
St. Louis, MO 63146

Toward Healthy Aging: Human Needs and Nursing Response, sixth edition ISBN 0-323-02012-7

NOTICE

Nursing is an ever-changing field. Standard safety precautions must be followed, but as new research and clinical experience broaden our knowledge, changes in treatment and drug therapy may become necessary or appropriate. Readers are advised to check the most current product information provided by the manufacturer of each drug to be administered to verify the recommended dose, the method and duration of administration, and contraindications. It is the responsibility of the licensed prescriber, relying on experience and knowledge of the patient, to determine dosages and the best treatment for each individual patient. Neither the publisher nor the author assumes any liability for any injury and/or damage to persons or property arising from this publication.

Library of Congress Cataloging-in-Publication Data

Ebersole, Priscilla.
Toward healthy aging: human needs and nursing response / Priscilla Ebersole, Patricia Hess, Ann Schmidt Luggen. – 6th ed.
p. cm.
Includes bibliographical references and index.
ISBN 0-323-02012-7
1. Geriatric nursing. 2. Aging. I. Hess, Patricia A., 1938– II. Luggen, Ann Schmidt. III. Title.

RC954.E23 2004
618.97′0231–dc22

2003060222

Executive Editor: Michael S. Ledbetter
Senior Developmental Editor: Laurie K. Gower
Publishing Services Manager: Catherine Jackson
Project Manager: Clay S. Broeker
Designer: Teresa McBryan Breckwoldt
Cover Design: Studio Montage

Printed in the United States of America

Last digit is the print number: 9 8 7 6 5 4 3 2 1

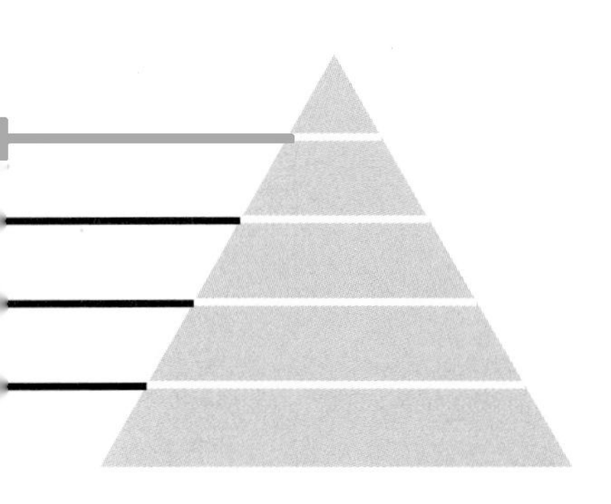

Contributors

John C. Buffum, PharmD, BCPP
Associate Clinical Professor of Pharmacy
University of California at San Francisco
San Francisco, California

Martha Buffum, DNSc, APRN, BC, CS
Associate Chief, Nursing Service for Research
Veterans Affairs Medical Center;
Assistant Clinical Professor, School of Nursing
University of California at San Francisco
San Francisco, California

JoAnn G. Congdon, PhD, RN, CNS
Associate Professor, School of Nursing
University of Colorado Health Sciences Center
Denver, Colorado

Catherine Hill, RN, MSN, CS
Gerontologic Nurse Practitioner
Practitioner Faculty
University of Phoenix
Tampa, Florida

Barbara J. Holtzclaw, RN, PhD, FAAN
Professor Emerita
University of Texas Health Science Center at San Antonio
San Antonio, Texas;
Adjunct Professor, College of Nursing
University of Oklahoma Health Science Center
Norman, Oklahoma

Alice G. Rini, JD, MS, RN
Adjunct Professor of Nursing
Northern Kentucky University
Highland Heights, Kentucky;
Private Consultant
Alexandria, Kentucky

Dianne Thames, DNS, RN
Associate Dean, Academic Affairs
Charity School of Nursing
Delgado Community College
New Orleans, Louisiana

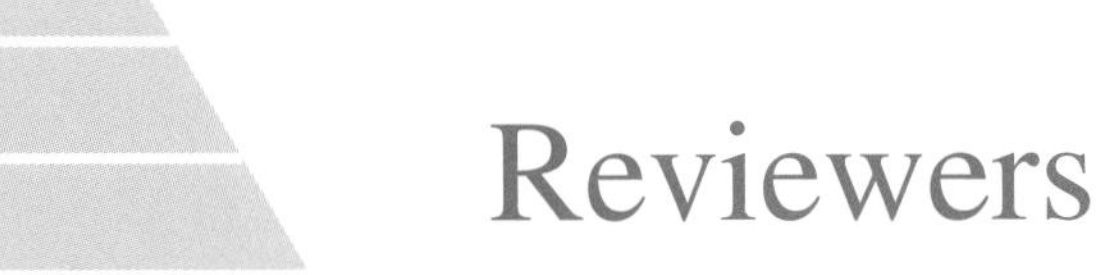

Reviewers

Diana Ballard, RN, MBA, JD
Vice President, Professional Services
Holy Cross Hospital
Fort Lauderdale, Florida

Angeline Bushy, PhD, RN, CS, FAAN
Professor and Bert Fish Chair, School of Nursing
University of Central Florida
Orlando, Florida

Richard W. Conn, BA, MS, PhD, RN, MSN, ANP, aannC
Adult Nurse Practitioner
Pittsburg, California

Dedication

For my children and grandchildren who center my existence: Lorraine and Jerry O'Brien; Jason and Laura Kester; Raymond and Janet Ebersole; Priscilla and Anna Ebersole; Randolph and Valerie Ebersole; CaraLynn Ruth Ebersole; Elisabeth and Ralph Beierly; Paul and Ruby Tanti; and Raymond, Benjamin, Ashley, and great grandson Ethan Paul Tanti.

PE

To Seymour Mann, whose intellect and kinetic energy was exhibited in his prefessional pursuits and his many talents, which touched the lives of family, colleagues, and friends.

PH

To my coauthors, Dr. Priscilla Ebersole and Dr. Patricia Hess, who have so kindly invited me to work with them on the sixth edition of this fine book, and who I proudly join.

ASL

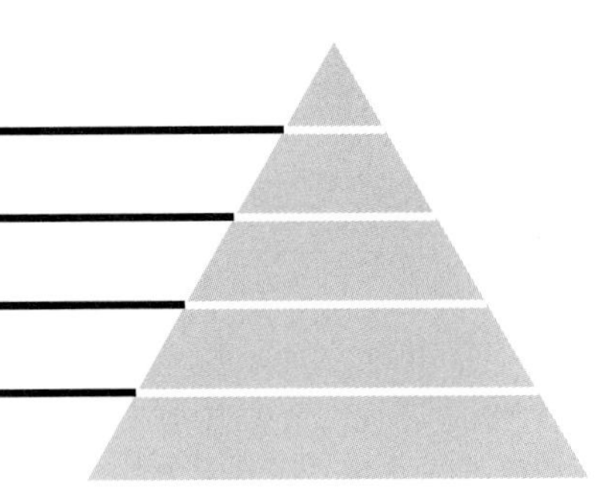

Preface

This text is designed primarily for nursing students in baccalaureate and Master's programs, but it is equally necessary for nurses who daily confront the care of elders in their practice. We believe that professionals in other disciplines will recognize the scope of its breadth and depth and use it as a resource and reference.

Nursing curricula must now include geriatric care as a recognizable aspect of basic nursing education. This is a national and state mandate. It is no longer sufficient to declare the geriatric content "integrated" or to opine that one understands geriatrics because elders happen to be in the care milieu. We continue to favor using *elders* as the correct term for older persons as they have authority by virtue of age and experience. We contend throughout the text that the aged are our guides and teachers in the process of aging.

Our text has grown and developed for more than 21 years and has come of age just as a child does and as geriatric nursing has. Catherine Frey, our 104-year-old friend and exemplar of healthy adaptation, provided innumerable examples for the first edition *of Toward Healthy Aging: Human Needs and Nursing Response.* At that time there were few studies of healthy aging, particularly of the very old. Now there is a glut of information, some important, some that directly influences the quality of life of an elder, and some that seems superfluous. It is no small task to sort through the information overload, but that is the mission of a useful text; content must be current, relevant, practical and add to existing knowledge.

The reader will find more sophistication in the tools, protocols, and guidelines included. As advanced nurse practitioners have increasingly taken their place as primary care providers, particularly in the care of elders, we have included more content tailored to their needs and those of all nurses who are invested in the most current geriatric clinical care and research.

Our basic premise that healthy aging is a right and possibility for every elder has not changed. We believe our stance on this fundamental issue of human potential is the cornerstone of this text. Wellness is possible regardless of situations or conditions. Humans are more than DNA directives, cells, genes, enzymes, and environmental reactors. People have potential we have not yet imagined, much less touched. In continuing the use of the Maslovian hierarchy as an organizing principle, we acknowledge that nurses are best equipped to assist elders in finding sources of fundamental need fulfillment in order to reach the most gratifying levels of their existence. In the last two decades our position on this aspect of aging has been reinforced throughout the specialty. Examples of transcending seemingly impossible situations abound. We have tried throughout to include cameos and anecdotes to elaborate this point.

The current emphasis in elder care on pain management, palliative care, gender differences, caregiver supports, incontinence management, diet and exercise, and *Healthy People 2010* have given support and substance to our beliefs. Expected changes in Medicare and the current delivery modes of the best HMOs have further moved us toward a healthier aging. We can no longer afford, nor desire, to allow conditions to fulminate to become medical emergencies. We are at last forced by policy and economics to proactively preserve health and intervene at the earliest possible time when problems and disorders are subclinical or just emerging.

ACKNOWLEDGMENTS

Through their expert guidance and patience, Michael Ledbetter and Laurie Gower have brought this work to fruition despite the numerous challenges thrown at them. Michael has been responsible for the embryonic stages, labor, and birth of the last three editions of this text as well as the present one. His constancy and down-to-earth approach have made him a joy with whom to affiliate. Laurie is a gift from heaven and is aware of all the details that make a text a delight to read. Our few contributors were selected with great care to be sure they believed in health and wellness as do we. The reviewers have given thoughtful feedback that has clarified and enhanced the content.

Ann Luggen, the third author on this sixth edition of *Toward Healthy Aging*, has provided her special expertise, enrichment of the content, and a unique perspective. We are grateful for her participation.

To you, our readers, who have followed with us through the rocky and rewarding last two decades as the geriatric specialties have flourished, we give our thanks and gratitude.

Priscilla Ebersole
Patricia Hess

Contents

PART I
FOUNDATIONS OF HEALTHY AGING

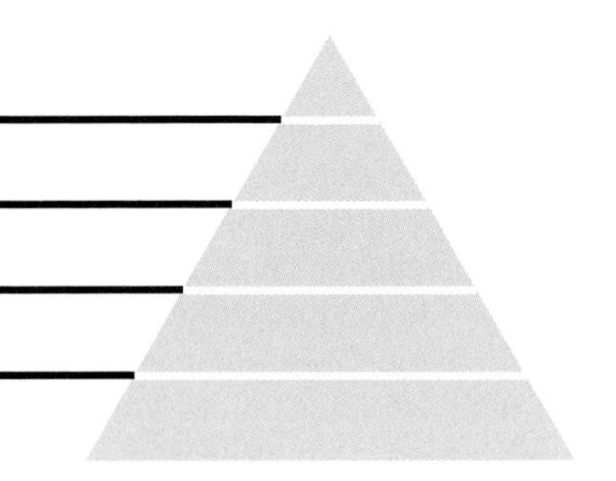

CHAPTER 1

Geriatric Nursing and an Aging Society

Priscilla Ebersole

A youth speaks

Until my grandmother became ill and needed our help, I really didn't know her well. Now I can look at her in an entirely different light. She is frail and tough, fearful and courageous, demanding and delightful, bitter and humorous, needy and needed. I'm beginning to think that old age is the culmination of all the aspects of living a long life.

Jenine, 28 years old

A middle-ager speaks

Nursing care of the aged brings one in touch with the most basic and profound questions of human existence: the meanings of life and death; sources of strength and survival skills; beginnings, ending, and reasons for being. It is a commitment to discovery of the self—and of the self I am becoming as I age.

Stephanie, middle-aged faculty

An elder speaks

I'm 95 years old and have no family or friends that still survive. I wonder if anyone will be there for me when I leave the planet, which will be very soon I am sure. Mothers deliver, but who will deliver me into the hand of God?

Name withheld

LEARNING OBJECTIVES

On completion of this chapter, the reader will be able to:

1. Identify several viewpoints that influence the way aging is perceived.
2. Specify several demographic changes related to the aging experience in the twenty-first century.
3. Develop the beginnings of a personal philosophy of aging.
4. Recognize the great diversity of aged individuals.
5. Better understand the many factors that facilitate or hinder the aging process.
6. Compare variousărontic nursing roles and requirements.
7. Discuss nursing research studies and the role of nurses in their development.
8. Discuss several formal geriatric organizations and their significance to nurses.
9. Identify several factors that have influenced the progress of gerontologic nursing as a specialty practice.

THE STUDY OF AGING

In the past, both religious and secular movements have affected the way individuals viewed aging. Puritans thought the process of aging was a sacred pilgrimage to God, and as such the righteous aged were revered. During the Victorian age it was believed that youth was the symbol of growth and expansion. Later, when the need to provide for an expanding population became more pressing, youthful energy, westward migration, and enormous material progress made the aged seem out of touch, and they were sometimes viewed with sentimental indulgence or irritation. The traditions of the elders seemed cumbersome and a hindrance to progress. In the scientific search for longevity, it was thought that mountain-climbing tribes high in the Andes and the Georgian Alps held the secret, lending a picture of reaching ever upward. Now space rockets silhouetted against the sky before launch represent not only phallic symbols of generativity but emblems of our belief in our potential for an ever-expanding universe of possibilities throughout the life course. There seem to be infinite variations on the metaphors of aging all over the world. What we make of aging, it seems, depends on how we see it. Bernice Neugarten, died in October of 2001, was the foremost gerontologic theorist and editor of the first comprehensive theoretic text, *Middle Age and Aging,* published by the University of Chicago Press in 1968. Dr Neugarten predicted that we are rapidly moving into an age-irrelevant society. It seems so as we are less and less concerned about chronologic age but rather the fiscal, functional, and caregiver burdens of individuals at whatever age. Our society cherishes productivity, monetary success, and accomplishment.

Attitudes toward the aged have shifted along with societal changes. A "reverse ageism" is apparent, largely attributable to gerontology professionals of the "baby boom" confronting their own aging and desperately hoping they will be a part of the elite and vigorous older survivors: sexy, active, involved, and simply amazing. Some are. Many are simply gradually growing older and confronting the changes that can normally be expected. That is what this textbook is all about. How does one maximize the experience of aging and enrich the later years regardless of the physical and psychologic changes that commonly occur?

Several recent occurrences have changed the literal and figurative landscape forever. As we have entered the twenty-first century, we have become painfully aware of the damage a few terrorists can inflict on whole populations materially and psychologically. We are no longer an adolescent nation but have shouldered the burdens of full adulthood and taken on the wariness and questioning posture of individuals who have seen their beliefs and political foundations eroded. We have as a nation grown up and are much older than we were 20 or 30 years ago. We have lost our innocence. Our maturation has been costly. Never have the older generations been more important. They have survived the rigors of wars and the depths of the Great Depression. The most significant learning regarding the intricacies and challenges of aging and survival strategies comes from discussions with elders themselves. These are our role models, and their diversity makes it possible for us to develop greater understanding of life if we only listen to what they say and that which is unsaid.

GERONTOLOGY

Gerontology is the scientific study of the effects of time on human development, specifically the study of older persons. It is at the opposite end of the spectrum from embryology and often includes several decades before death. Gerontology, by virtue of the Greek origin of the word *geron* (old man), should mean the study of old men, but many more women than men grow old. Healthy older men and women frequently elude the attention of gerontologists; thus study samples of elders, most likely taken from institutionalized subjects, have often been extrapolated to the healthier population. In fact, it is not yet certain what healthy old age can be; this will not be known until optimum social and biologic conditions exist for the aged. A large part of the study of aging comes from attending to the aged and the aging person in ourselves, and how we perceive our own aging. These are fundamentally important to gerontology. Inquisitions into and curiosity about aging are as old as curiosity about life and death itself. Much that was thought to have been correct about aging has been shown through research to be half-truth, myth, or supposition. In developing a science and philosophy of aging, one essentially builds on personal experience; ultimately we all do this. How else can we measure the impact of dreams, fantasies, meditation, courage, love, grief, and the phenomena of living?

Gerontology began as an inquiry into the characteristics of long-lived people, and we are still intrigued by them. In 1000 BC the average life span was 18 years, and people who lived to old age were curiosities, stimulating reverence, speculation and myth.

Anecdotal evidence was used in the past to illustrate issues assumed to be universal. It is only in the last 40 years that serious and carefully controlled research studies have flourished. Theoreticians and researchers most commonly interested in the study of aging are sociologists, psychologists, and biologists. Their conceptual bases underlie their perspective regarding survival issues. Nursing draws from all of these disciplines to describe, monitor, protect, and evaluate the quality of life experienced by the old.

An individual ages biologically, psychologically, sociologically, and spiritually as a unitary being. A disciplinary rather than a humanistic perspective sometimes makes it appear that these are separate components of existence. There is such overlap that disciplinary lines are no longer appropriate in planning care. Multidisciplinary approaches and care programs are essential and are rapidly becoming the method of providing health care.

The Biomedicalization of Aging

The term *geriatrics* was coined by an American physician, Ignatz Nascher, around 1900 because he recognized that the medical care of the aged involved special considerations, much as did the field of pediatrics. In fact, he saw many similarities.

Aging, along with technologic progress, has been seen as a biomedical problem that must be reversed, eradicated, or held at bay as long as possible. Therefore the impact of disease, morbidity, and impending death on the quality of life and the experience of aging has provided the impetus for much of the study by gerontologists. In this way, aging has inevitably been seen through the distorted lens of disease. Nevertheless, it is difficult to study such a complex and elusive condition as "healthy aging" without looking at the physical manifestations of function and lifestyle. Chronic disorders, not amenable to cure but requiring long-term adaptation and management, have not been attractive to medicine and nursing until recently. However, we are finally recognizing that aging and disease are separate entities although frequent companions. One of the dilemmas is a lack of clear understanding of normal aging processes. We may never know which changes occur over time because of assaults of the environment and which changes occur because the vital life centers are running out of resources.

The trend toward medicalization of the study of aging has influenced the general public as well. The biomedical view of the "problem" of aging is reinforced on all sides. However, the unquestioning public acceptance of medical authority has been considerably diminished as more and more individuals seek alternative health care methods, as well as diagnose and manage their own care through the Internet.

Even though older adults account for 60% of all ambulatory care, 48% of hospital admissions, 80% of home care visits, and 85% of nursing home care (Rosenfeld et al, 1999), in medicine there is no stand-alone specialty in geriatrics. Subspecialists exist in family medicine, internal medicine, and psychiatry, although it is not known exactly how many of these are certified or simply claim geriatrics as their primary specialty. In some ways this lack has opened more opportunities for advanced practice geriatric nurses (APGNs), who are increasingly being relied on as primary care providers. The APGNs may or may not be adequately compensated, depending on the level of independence their state laws support. At present they may obtain a Medicare provider number and independent billing. My advice to all nurses is to continue on to become certified as an APGN. The need for them will only grow and the opportunities abound. Recently, while being attended at my health maintenance organization (HMO), the young female physician said, "If I had it to do again, I would become an NP."

Organizations Devoted to Gerontologic Research and Practice

The Gerontological Society of America (GSA) demonstrates the need for interdisciplinary collaboration in research and practice. The divisions of Biological Sciences, Clinical Medicine, Behavioral and Social Sciences, Social Research, and Policy and Practice include individuals from myriad backgrounds and many disciplines who affiliate with a section based on their particular function rather than their educational or professional credentials. Nurses can be found in all sections and occupy important positions as officers and committee chairs in the GSA. The nurses' special interest group, which, 30 years ago, met informally in a small hotel suite, now attracts 150 to 200 members and is the most rapidly growing membership contingent. Some nurses argue that the profession should have an established section in GSA. We think not. One of the major benefits of organizations such as GSA is the interdisciplinary contact and multidisciplinary sharing. This mingling of the disciplines based on practice interests is also characteristic of the American Society on Aging (ASA). Other interdisciplinary organizations have joined forces to strengthen the field. The Association for Gerontology in Higher Education (AGHE) has partnered with GSA, and the National Council on Aging (NCOA) is affiliated with ASA. These organizations and others have encouraged the blending of ideas and functions, furthering our understanding of old age and of the integration necessary for optimum care. Organizations specific to geriatric nursing include the National Gerontological Nursing Association (NGNA), the National Conference of Geriatric Nurse Practitioners (NCGNP), the National Association of Directors of Nursing in Long Term Care (NADONA/LTC), and the Canadian Gerontological Nursing Association (CGNA).

DEVELOPMENT OF GERIATRIC NURSING

Efforts to determine the appropriate term for nurses caring for the aged have included *erontic nurses, gerontological nurses,* and *geriatric nurses.* None of these terms is restrictive. We presently prefer the use of the term *geriatric care nurse.*

The origins of geriatric nursing are rooted in England and began with Florence Nightingale as she accepted a position in the Institution for the Care of Sick Gentlewomen in Distressed Circumstances. "Nightingale's concern for the frail and sick aged was continued by Agnes Jones, a wealthy Nightingale trained nurse, who in 1864 was sent to Liverpool Infirmary, a large Poor Law institution" (Touhy, 2003). The care in the institution had been poor, diet meager, and nurses often drunk. But Miss Jones, under the tutelage of Nightingale, improved the care dramatically, as well as reduced the costs.

In the United States almshouses were the destination of the destitute aged. In 1912 the almshouses were still insufferable places, poorly staffed, and controlled by petty politicians. Though Dock and other early leaders in nursing deplored the conditions, the First World War distracted them from attention to these needs. But in 1925 the *American Journal of Nursing* advanced the idea of a specialty in the nursing care of the aged. When the almshouses were dismantled in the mid-1930s, retired and widowed nurses often converted their homes into board and care for elders. This move is thought to have been the genesis of commercial nursing homes. Two nursing journals in the 1940s described centers of excellence for geriatric care: the Cuyahoga County Nursing Home in Ohio and the Hebrew Home for the Aged in New York. An article in the *American Journal of Nursing* by Sarah Gelbach (1943) recommended that nurses should have not only an aptitude for working with the elderly but specific geriatric education (Touhy, 2003).

As early as 1904 the *American Journal of Nursing* published an article on old age and disease. By the 1920s a few visionary nurses called for the development of gerontologic nursing practice as they recognized that a body of nursing knowledge and skills related to nursing care for older persons was distinguishable within the full scope of nursing practice. These nurses also recognized that institutional settings such as old age homes or boardinghouses—all predecessors of today's nursing homes—were settings in which nurses could best provide homelike nursing services for older persons who did not need the acute care services of a hospital. The best of these were truly homes.

In 1962 a focus group was formed to discuss gerontologic nursing, and in 1966 a gerontologic practice group was convened. However, it was not until 1966 that the American Nurses Association (ANA) formed a Division of Geriatric Nursing. The first geriatric standards were published by the ANA in 1968, and soon after geriatric nursing certification was offered. In 1976 the Division of Geriatric Nursing changed its name to the Gerontological Nursing Division to reflect the broad role nurses play in the management of the elderly. In 1984 the Council of Gerontological Nursing was formed and certification for GNPs and clinical specialists became available (Box 1-1). Since that time certification has become available in geriatric nursing specialties and numerous subspecialties. Although most working nurses are heavily involved in the care of the aged in some manner, only a small proportion are certified in geriatric nursing or as advanced practice geriatric nurses (APGNs).

Long-term care and custodial care have historically been neglected by medicine and nursing. Elders with complex chronic conditions and acutely painful problems were largely ignored by the professions and society at large. Visionaries such as Barbara Lee of the W.K. Kellogg Foundation, Robert Butler, first Director of the Institute on Aging, and Linda Aiken of the Robert Woods Johnson Foundation recognized the need and opportunities for improving the situation. Teaching nursing homes were developed, as were numerous other nursing home sites that made the commitment to staff the facility with an APGN on a full-time basis. Immediacy of care improved, transfers to hospitals decreased, and staff morale was enhanced as more knowledge was brought to bear on the problems and conditions of elder residents.

For 40 years the ANA and others have been attempting to make geriatric nursing visible and integral to nursing education. In 1990 the John A. Hartford Foundation began investing in geriatric nursing and in the past decade has granted $35 million in various educational and clinical demonstrations of effective programmatic changes in the provision of geriatric care (Mezey and Fulmer, 2002). This large investment has resulted in major movements toward excellence in education, research, and practice in geriatric nursing.

There is still much to do in ensuring that geriatric curricula will receive the attention needed and become essential to all basic nursing programs. The John A. Hartford initiatives have produced geriatric curriculum materials and competency guidelines that can be obtained by undergraduate nursing programs and institutions so that best practices can be defined and centers of excellence evaluated and publicized. They have also developed clinical models in hospitals that include acute care of the elderly (ACE) units and the placement of a geriatric resource nurse (GRN) on units that care for the elderly (Mezey and Fulmer, 2002). Other encouraging signs include an award of $5 million to enhance the competence of nurses caring for older adults. The grant was funded by Atlantic Philanthropies and is being implemented through a strategic alliance between ANA and the Hartford Institute for Geriatric Nursing. They work together to create permanent structures for geriatric activities in specialty nursing organizations. There are 78 nursing specialty organizations representing 400,000 nurses. Ensuring geriatric competence in the various specialties that care for older adults (about 60 of them) will greatly affect the systems of care (*American Nurse,* 2002; Mezey and Fulmer, 2002).

Gerontic Nurse Pioneers and Leaders*

The foundation of gerontic nursing (we use the term "gerontic" in this section in honor of Laurie Gunter, who first worked with ANA to certify geriatric nurses) as we know it today was largely built by a small cadre of nurse-explorers between 30 and 50 years ago, many of whom are now gone. Gerontic nursing was defined and shaped by these few nurse-pioneers who saw, early on, that the aged individual had special needs and required the most subtle, holistic, and complex nursing care.

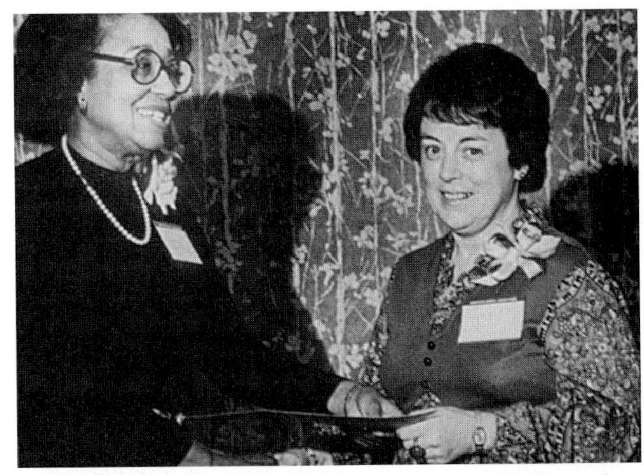

Laurie Gunter issuing first ANA certificate in geriatric nursing.

These gerontic nurse pioneers presented seminal thought and investigated new ideas related to the care of the aged; refuted mythical tales and fantasies of aging; and found realities through investigation, clinical observation, practice, and

*Interview data collected by Priscilla Ebersole between 1990 and 2001.

Box 1-1 Professionalization of Gerontic Nursing

1904	First article published in *American Journal of Nursing* (AJN) on care of the aged.
1925	AJN considers geriatric nursing as a possible specialty in nursing.
1950	Newton and Anderson publish first geriatric nursing textbook.
	Geriatrics becomes a specialization in nursing.
1962	ANA forms a national geriatric nursing group.
1966	ANA creates the Division of Geriatric Nursing.
1970	ANA establishes Standards of Practice for Geriatric Nursing; Committee chaired by Dorothy Moses, included Lois Knowles and Mary Shaunnessey.
1973	Revised Standards of Practice for Geriatric Nursing.
1974	Certification in geriatric nursing practice offered through ANA; process implemented by Laurie Gunter and Virginia Stone.
1975	*Journal of Gerontological Nursing* published by Slack; first editor, Edna Stilwell.
1976	ANA renames Geriatric Division, "Gerontological" ANA publishes Standards for Gerontological Nursing Practice, committee chaired by Barbara Allen Davis.
	ANA begins certifying Geriatric Nurse Practitioners *Nursing and the Aged* edited by Burnside and published by McGraw-Hill.
1977	First Gerontological Nursing Tract funded by Division of Nursing and established by Sr. Rose Therese Bahr at University of Kansas School of Nursing.
1979	*Education for Gerontic Nursing* written by Gunter and Estes; suggested curricula for all levels of nursing education
	ANA Council of Long Term Care Nurses established, group first chaired by Ella Kick.
1980	*Geriatric Nursing* first published by AJN; Cynthia Kelly, editor.
1981	ANA Division of Gerontological Nursing issues statement regarding scope of practice.
1983	Florence Cellar Endowed Gerontological Nursing Chair established at Case Western Reserve University, first in the nation; Doreen Norton first scholar to occupy chair.
1984	National Gerontological Nurses Association established.
	Division of Gerontological Nursing Practice becomes Council on Gerontological Nursing (councils established for all practice specialties).
1986	ANA publishes *Survey of Gerontological Nurses in Clinical Practice.*
1987	ANA revises and issues *Standards and Scope of Gerontological Nursing Practice.*
1989	ANA certifies Gerontological Clinical Nurse Specialists.
1990	ANA establishes a Division of Long Term Care within the Council of Gerontological Nursing.
1992	ANA redefines *long-term care* to include life span approach.
1994	ANA forms strong Political Action Committee (ANPAC).
1996	ANA officials advise President Clinton regarding Health Care Reforms.
	ANA celebrates centennial in Washington, D.C.; President Clinton gives keynote address.
1998	ANA certification available for GNPs and GCSs as advanced practice geriatric nurses (APGNs).
2000	ANA collective bargaining and appropriate staffing for nurses becomes strong focus.
2001	ANA Board of Directors adopts the Bill of Rights for Registered Nurses.
2002	ANA partners with the Hartford Institute for Geriatric Nursing to promote geriatrics in basic nursing curricula.

documentation, setting in motion activities that markedly influenced the course of the aging experience. They saw new possibilities and a better future for the aged.

When interviewed, most were quite matter-of-fact and had not thought of themselves as pioneers. "It was there to be done." "Someone needed to do it." "Well, I wouldn't say I was really a pioneer . . . have you spoken to . . .?" They saw something that others had not seen before, but because it was self-evident to them it did not seem at all remarkable. One said, "You asked why I established the [gerontology academic] chair and I haven't yet given you a precise answer; I must give that some more thought" (Florence Cellar).

Some demonstrated a very personal connection to the aged that involved a certain view of humanity from a more universal or spiritual perspective than is commonly held; a stark awareness of the interdependence of generations and individuals. With humor, grace, and dignity they tell what old age means to them.

Who were these individuals that paved the way to the future of gerontic care? There are many to whom we owe the origins of gerontic nursing as a specialty, many unnamed or presently unrecognized. To name only a few and some of their outstanding accomplishments: Sister Rose Therese Bahr (vitally involved in the development of the National Gerontological Nurses Association); Terri Brower (generated gerontology curricula and the first relevant nursing research); Irene Burnside (mentored numerous nurses interested in geriatric nursing); Florence Cellar (donated funds to establish first gerontologic nursing chair in the nation); Barbara Allen Davis (generated gerontologic interest and foci at ANA); Laurie Gunter (established geriatric certification requirements at ANA); Mary Harper (developed dynamic programs for aged veterans; instrumental in guiding development of geropsychiatric programs); Cynthia Kelly (first editor of *Geriatric Nursing Journal*); Ella Kick (developed humanistic care strategies in long-term care); Lois Knowles (instrumental in developing first geriatric nursing standards); Barbara Lee (sponsored development of geriatric nurse practitioner programs through Kellogg Foundation funding); Mathy Mezey (director of the National Teaching Nursing Home Project and presently director of the nationally influential John A. Hartford Foundation Institute for Geriatric Nursing); Terry Fulmer (codirector of the John A. Hartford Foundation Institute of Geriatric Nursing; has generated seminal research on elder abuse); Mary Quinn (has generated seminal research on elder abuse and undue influence); Dorothy Moses (developed first gerontology radio and television programs for lay public in San Diego); Sister Marilyn Schwab (conceived, developed, and administered national model nursing home); Doris Schwartz (coauthored the first textbook related to geriatric nursing care; developed interdisciplinary alliances); Eldonna Shields-Kyle (created staff development curricula for nursing homes); Bernita Steffl (political advocate for aged in Arizona; contributed to understanding of sexuality and aging); Edna Stilwell (first editor of *Journal of Gerontological Nursing*); Kathleen Buckwalter (present editor of the *Journal of Gerontological Nursing;* for more than 30 years has consistently studied the care of demented elders and mentored numerous students interested in these disorders); Virginia Stone (developed first graduate program in gerontologic nursing); Thelma Wells (numerous research projects and publications relevant to understanding the aged; particular expertise in study and care of urinary incontinence); Mary Opal Wolanin (research, mentorship, and seminal work in understanding confusion and aging); and Neville Strumpf and Lois Evans (researched the dangers of restraints and led the way to the decreased use of restraints throughout the United States). Some characteristics apparent in this select group are independence and innovation, interpersonal investment, persistence, practicality, assertiveness, strong will, and ability to earn the respect of others both within and outside the nursing profession (Box 1-2). Additionally, they expended incredible amounts of energy.

Mary Opal Wolanin particularly remembers the "pneumonia nurse" as one of the first in the genre of the geriatric nurse (interview, San Antonio, September 1995). "These nurses, by sheer nursing skill and devoted care, literally held the life of the pneumonia-stricken elder in their hands. This was in the days before penicillin . . . much less third- and fourth-generation antibiotics." We are presently relearning respect for the virulence, morbidity, and mortality of many diseases we thought had all but disappeared but have now adapted to the best antibiotics available. We continue to need adventurous nurses who can find new and better ways to care for the aged and the young and who can facilitate self-care in the most efficacious manner.

Box 1-2 Wisdom from Gerontic Nurse Pioneers

We need to remind ourselves constantly that the purpose of gerontic nursing is to prevent untimely death and needless suffering, always with the focus of doing with as well as doing for, and in every instance to attempt to preserve personhood as long as life continues. (Doris Schwartz)

Aging individuals are persons, not burdens or problems, and nurses can be educated to a more positive attitude about the older adult and can aid in implementation of professional behaviors to upgrade care of older citizens in America. (Sr. Rose Therese Bahr)

What a fortunate teenager I was!! On September 15, 1946, when I was almost 16, I took a job in a small (25 beds) hospital in a small Ohio community. I was always assigned to the older patients because we got along so well. (Ella Kick)

There is always an interesting person there, sometimes locked in the cage of age. I think I have helped at least a few of my students with this approach, "You see me as I am now, but I see myself as I've always been and all the things I've been—not just an old lady." (Bernita Steffl)

I am less fearful of medical afflictions that befall me in my old age than I am of the system and the professionals to whom my care may be entrusted. (Bernita Steffl)

Among the first lessons that I learned from working with older patients was of patience and perseverance. I found that if they were treated as normal human beings and one took the time to talk to them, and above all listen to what they had to say, they responded normally. (Dorothy Moses)

I believe that one of the most valuable lessons I have learned from those who are older is that I must start with looking inside at my own thinking. I was very guilty of ageism. I believed every myth in the book, was sure that I would never live past my seventieth birthday, and made no plan for my seventies. Probably the most productive years of my career have been since that dreaded birthday, and I now realize that it is very difficult, if not impossible, to think of our own aging. (Mary Opal Wolanin)

I am opposed to anyone going into the field of geriatric nursing until she has experienced the human condition at many points—vicariously through literature and our culture or by close observation. This field demands maturity since recognizing the diversity of aging people is very important in caring for the elderly during acute illness, chronic illness, and wellness. We need a broad knowledge base and a broader mind. (Mary Opal Wolanin)

Geriatric Nursing Education

Traditional nursing curricula included maternity, pediatrics, medical-surgical care, and public health nursing. This formula, based on agency and institutional staffing needs, has been slow to change, but with shifts in population, clientele, and service venues, changes have been gradually incorporated.

The influence of state and national organizations and requirements regarding geriatric content have had some impact, but the largest has been through the John A. Hartford Foundation's multipronged approach as developed by Mezey and Fulmer (2002) to support individuals, groups, and institutions to move toward appropriate geriatric knowledge integration. Often the content has been difficult to promote because faculty may not have the expertise or enthusiasm, it is regarded as an extra requirement that overloads the already extensive informational requirements of the accrediting organizations, it is thought to be "integrated" throughout the program, and students tend to be most interested in critical care and maternity care. Some of this is because of age identification and some because the highly technical care is intriguing and challenging in a specific and concrete way that is not true of the subtle complexities of geriatric care. Yet, many educational institutions have incorporated dynamic courses in aging into their curricula.

Geriatric Nursing Roles

Geriatric nursing roles encompass every imaginable venue and circumstance. Many nurses have created their own roles, some in ghettos, on cruise ships, in industrial health care, in neighborhood clinics, in national organizations, in retirement centers, in mobile clinics, and in entrepreneurial ventures. The more traditional institutionalized nursing roles in critical care, acute care, postacute care, long-term care, and community centers are in dire need of individuals with geriatric nursing expertise. The opportunities are limitless because we are in a rapidly aging society. One of the most promising developments has been the emergence of GNPs as major service providers. The educational and training programs arose from evident need, particularly in long-term care settings. These midlevel medical practitioners were trained in certificate and graduate nursing programs, varying in length from 1 to 2 years of intensive didactic and clinical practice experiences. Basic nursing concepts undergirded the medical aspects of their practice in a manner that brought forth particularly comprehensive care. Early on, management of individual cases was aided by protocols, physician supervision, and algorithmic decision-making trees. With further educational program development and recognition of GNPs' abilities, more independent practice has developed. States proposed various laws to regulate practice, some allowing far more independence than others. This often reflected the population needs and the density of medical practitioners in a given area. With the advent of HMOs, cost-cutting care, increased surveillance by government agencies, Medicare demonstration project initiatives, and the mass retreat of physicians from private practice, the roles of nurse practitioners, and particularly of GNPs, has expanded and become integral to the provision of care. Advanced nurse practitioners (ANPs) with geriatric expertise have become primary care providers in health care organizations, particularly HMOs. Entering the mammoth and varied field of professional geriatrics and gerontology has never been more resonant with opportunity.

Advanced practice geriatric nurses (APGNs) include geriatric nurse practitioners (GNPs), geriatric clinical nurse specialists (GCNs), and geropsychiatric nurses (Box 1-3). These are nurses who have completed a master's program in geriatric nursing and have been certified by the ANA. Practice privileges vary from state to state, but the federal Medicaid and Medicare programs allow for individual provider numbers and direct reimbursement. There are presently 63 educational programs that prepare APGNs, and 4200 nurses have been certified by the American Nurses Credentialing Center (ANCC); however, there are 12,500 adult nurse practitioners and 24,400 family nurse practitioners (Smolensky, 2002), many of whom are caring for the aged. Some have had intensive attention in their curricula to geriatric care, but some have not and must learn on the job. Major problems are the lack of faculty with the necessary level of geriatric expertise, sparse attention to geriatrics in basic nursing programs, and the routing of federal grants for education in medicine and nursing to family practice.

Geriatric nurses care for the aged in homes, clinics, hospitals, long-term and chronic care institutions, and community centers. They are practitioners, educators, managers, researchers, consultants, politicians, inventors, entrepreneurs, and social advocates. Wherever geriatric nurses are found their mission is to preserve function, enhance health, and enhance the quality of life and dying (Figure 1-1). Some anecdotes provide a look at poignant moments in the lives of these nurses (Hudacek, 2000).

Caring Moments in Geriatric Nursing. Quentin was 89 years old, blind and lived in a county nursing home. When his body began filling with fluid, Martha Debbie Dixon, RN, asked him what he would most like to do. His response, "One more time before I die, I want to feel the grass under my feet." Martha got Quentin dressed except for shoes and stockings, then took off her own shoes and stockings and both walked out into the warm summer evening. When she asked how he felt, his response was, "(the grass) Soft and moist with dew and oh, so good, I'm almost in heaven." A woman who had been married 58 years was dying of lung cancer. Her husband was at her bedside most of the time trying to help with her care and keep her comfortable. When she became comatose and near death he seemed lost. The nurse (name withheld) suggested he sit by her side and reminisce with her as dying persons often can hear even when they cannot respond. He spent 3 hours talking and reminiscing with her. After she died he said, "You can't know what a great gift you gave us. I talked all about our life together. You helped us to die in love" (Hudacek, 2000, p. 77).

Linda Wessel, a wound, ostomy and continence nurse, was sent on a home visit to check a patient who had undergone surgery for carcinoma of the common bile duct. She was terminal and had fluid and bile pouring from her long chest and abdominal incision. The bedding was soaked and the family had tried unsuccessfully to keep her dry with rolled up towels. Ms. Wessel "applied a large wound drainage collector over

Box 1-3

Acute Care Model 2—HOPE (Hospital Outcomes Project for the Elderly)

A cluster of five models that focus primarily on nursing care.

Geriatric Resource Nurse (GRN)—Integrating Expertise

A team composed of primary nurses, trained geriatric resource nurse, gerontologic nurse specialist, and geriatric physicians helps staff with specific problems of the elderly, such as delirium, physical functioning, incontinence, etc. Implemented nationally. Originated in New England area, 1980s.

Acute Care of the Elderly (ACE)—Designed Environments

A 29-bed specialty unit designed for acutely ill older patients with attention to physical needs of older patients; appropriate colors, carpeting, art, music, activity room, and recliners in patient rooms.
Team of nurses, gerontologic nurse specialist, social workers, nutritionists, and physical therapist to prevent functional decline and multiple clinical problems.
Developed by University Hospitals of Cleveland conjointly with Frances Payne Bolton School of Nursing at Case Western Reserve University. An innovative though expensive model that has demonstrated rapid implementation, which is accomplished easily because of the interdisciplinary team.

Geriatric Nurse Specialist (GNS)—Targeting Common Problems

Clinical specialist who consults and educates staff about specific problems of the aged. NICHE project used this inexpensive way to focus on nursing care and issues of delirium.
Developed by University of Chicago hospitals. Disadvantage: immediate access to GNS not available.

Comprehensive Discharge Planning (CDP)—Planning Ahead

Focus of GNS is on high-risk older patients and caregivers. Assessment occurs at admission and every 48 hours thereafter. Available to family members and patients 7 days a week. Continuity of care continues after discharge. Developed by University of Pennsylvania Hospital for continuity of care while minimizing readmissions. Findings concur success; extended time between discharge and readmission.

Case Management: Multidisciplinary Approach

A multidisciplinary case management model for patients with complex conditions, high acuity, and increased potential for complications, noncompliance, and absence of a support system. Developed at Beth Israel Medical Center, New York.

Compiled from Strumpf NE: Innovative gerontological practices as models for health care delivery, *Nurs Health Care* 15(10):522, 1994; NICHE Project Faculty: Geriatric models of care: which one's right for your institution? *Am J Nurs* 94(7):21, 1994; and Mezey M, Fulmer T, Fletcher K: A perfect NICHE for gerontology nurses, *Geriatr Nurs* 23(3):118, 2002 (entire issue devoted to models of geriatric practice).

the extensive incision and taught the family how to change it. The lady lived two more days dry and comfortable surrounded by her family. I know I made a difference in the last days of her life" (Hudacek, 2000, p. 92).

Paul was a 55-year-old veteran of the Korean War; anxious and asthmatic, he was frequently hospitalized with the diagnosis of "status asthmaticus." During the course of one episode, Bob Gaudreau, his nurse, saw the same look of absolute terror that Paul had shown on other hospitalizations. Bob went through the usual care protocol for Paul but was able to make some sense out of his nightmarish ramblings. Paul had been a prisoner of war for 18 months. Bob then sat and encouraged him to talk of some of the physical and psychological traumas he had endured, "I started focusing on his mental condition. With calmness and reassurance on my part, Paul slowly calmed down and his breathing became less labored." I know my interactions with Paul "were significant in turning around the physical manifestations of his relived torture sessions. As I look back now and try to address what I did for Paul, I would have to say that not only was it the drugs that worked, but more importantly it was the human contact and understanding of his needs during those times that was most important" (Hudacek, 2000, p. 87).

AGING TODAY

A revolution is occurring in geriatric nursing as the aged are gaining full status and recognition in society. The "baby boomer" generation (the parents of the present young adults and most nursing students) are entering the ranks of the "young-old" (those 50 to 70 years old). The very old and the elite-old (those 90 years and above) are the fastest growing segment of the aging population as technologic advances have facilitated their survival.

Demographics of Aging

Demographics, the statistical study of the size and distribution of population, is extremely significant in gerontology.

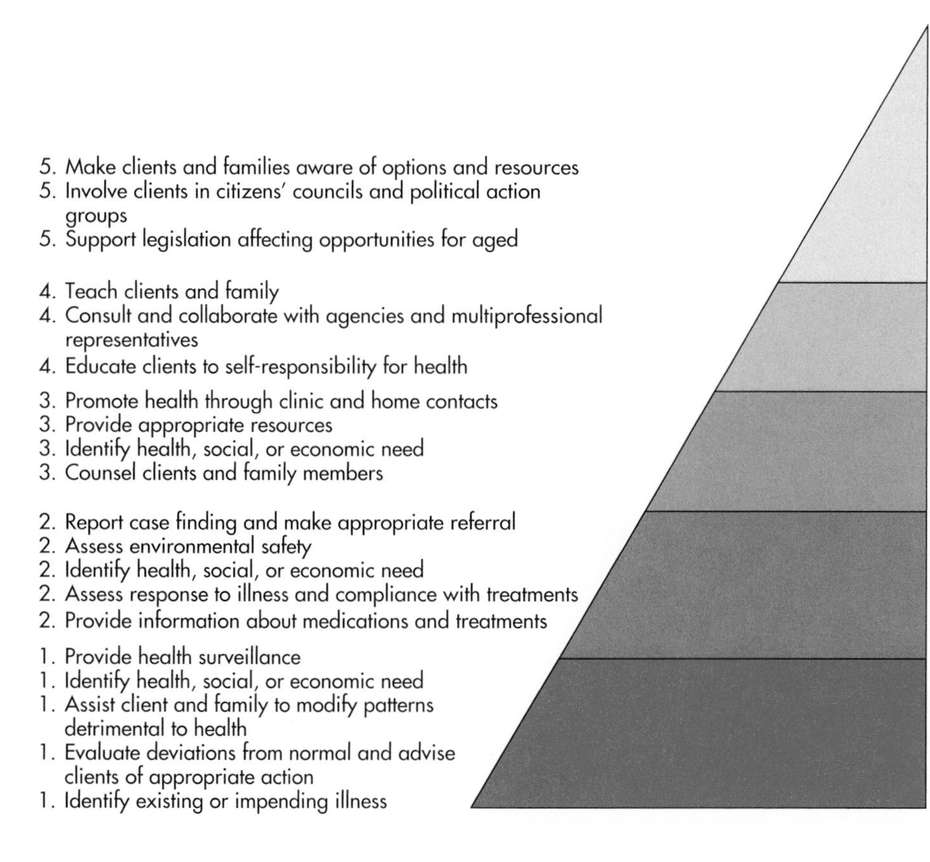

Figure 1-1. Nursing functions: caring for elders in the community.

The decennial census occurs every 10 years, and thus the 2000 census was especially important because it will dictate national concerns and policies regarding aging, as well as future directions.

Aging in the United States. The total population of the United States, according to latest figures in the U.S. Statistical Abstract (U.S. Bureau of the Census, 2001) is 281,421,906, a 13% increase over the 1990 census; of these, 35.1 million persons are over age 65, making up 12.4% of the population. About 20.5 million of these are older women, and 14.4 million are older men. The average life expectancy for infant girls in the United States is now 79.7 years, whereas for boys it is 74.1 years. In the United States, more than 36% of people over 65 live alone. However, for men over 75 years old, 69.3% live with a spouse, whereas only 31% of women over 75 live with a spouse (U.S. Bureau of the Census, 2001) (Figure 1-2).

In 2000 about half (52%) of persons 65 and older lived in nine states: California (3.6 million); Florida (2.8 million); New York (2.4 million); and Ohio, Illinois, Michigan, and New Jersey (well over 1 million each). About 77% of persons over 65 lived in metropolitan areas (50% in suburbs, 27% in central cities), and 23% lived in nonmetropolitan areas. In the comparatively mobile population of the United States, the experience of aging is greatly influenced by where one lives (Table 1-1).

Diversity of the aged in the United States. Peak immigration to the United States occurred between 1901 and 1910 when nearly 9 million people, mostly European immigrants, were admitted to the country. In the following 10 years another 5 million were attracted to this "land of opportunity." Most are now dead, and their descendants are well assimilated and have produced four and sometimes five generations of descendants—all with varying degrees of attachment to their roots. In 1998 emigration to the United States from numerous countries exceeded 856,000. Mexico, China, India, and the Philippines sent almost 300,000 individuals to the United States. Most settled in California and New York (U.S. Bureau of the Census, 2001). The various wars throughout the world have also brought further mingling of people whose lives would not have otherwise touched.

Old folk have been catapulted through socioscientific periods too numerous to mention. The shifts in human thought, technical capacities, and modes of life that have occurred within the single lifetime of the very old are stunning. These include the agrarian age, the industrial age, the atomic age, the space age, the microelectronic age, and the cyberspace age as we are all connected by the World Wide Web.

A large, unstudied group of older folk, released from the need to keep a work schedule, make up the majority of cruise travelers, organized tour groups, and globe-trotters. Many explore the wonders of the world through educational programs, guided by the Elderhostel organizers. Exposure to lands and peoples previously unknown has had profound effects on the perspectives of these elders. Such experiences affect the present aged, whose values and attitudes range from radical

American Perceptions of Aging in the 21st Century

- Throughout this report, patterns of perceptions and attitudes **within** the older sample are separately described by gender, by age (65-74 vs. 75+), and by education as a general indicator of socioeconomic status (categorized as less than high school versus high school graduation or more education). The distribution of these three variables within the age 65+ sample is:

TOTAL AGE 65+ SAMPLE N = 1,155

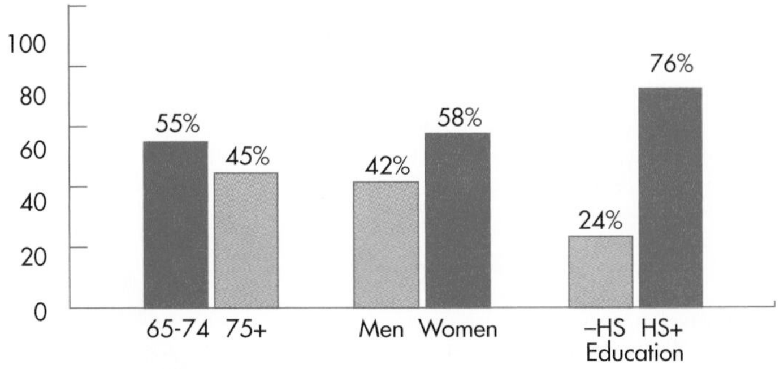

65-74	75+	Men	Women	–HS Education	HS+ Education
55%	45%	42%	58%	24%	76%

SELECTED CHARACTERISTICS OF THE AGE 65+ SAMPLE

Married 58%
Widowed 34%

Own Home 87%
With Paid Mortgage 74%

Children
0 ....8%
1-2 ....37%
3+ 56%
(average age of oldest child: 49)

Grandchildren
0 ....13%
3+ 72%

White 86%
Black 8%

Protestant 45%
Catholic 25%
Jewish 2%
Other 28%

Figure 1-2. Characteristics of men and women age 65 and over, 2000. (Source: National Council on the Aging, Inc., *American perceptions of aging in the 21st century,* telephone survey, Jan-Feb 2000. Available at *www.ncoa.org.*)

to anachronistic. Most amazing is the ability of elders to survive, adapt, and cope with extreme changes, yet retain a fundamental sense of self.

As the world shrinks and awareness of planetary vulnerabilities increases, understanding of the aging processes and experience must necessarily be expanded. Our consciousness has been raised to the recognition that we are not only of the world but inextricably linked to all that happens in the world.

Global Aging. The world population, now totaling over 6 billion people, is getting older. Japan (81.5 years) and Sweden (80.1 years) continue to have the longest life expectancy (United Nations Population Division, 2002). Of course, these statistics are influenced by the infant mortality rates, which are lowest in Sweden (3.4 deaths per 1000 live births) and Japan (3.3 deaths per 1000 live births). The life expectancy at birth in the United States is 77.5 years, and the infant mortality rate at birth is 6.8 per 1000 live births. Germany, Greece, Italy, and Japan have the greatest number of elders over 60 years of age, 23.2%, 23.4%, 24.1%, and 23.2%, respectively. In the more developed areas of the world the population 65 years and older rose from 8% in 1950 to 14% of the total population in 2000. It is expected to rise to 29% by 2050. The aged dependency, or support ratio, is presently almost 4 to 1 in developed countries and projected to be 2 to 1 by 2050 (AARP, 2001) (Figures 1-3 and 1-4).

The number of old and very old is increasing dramatically worldwide, and there are startling predictions for the future. In 2050 it is expected that the population of India will be over 1.5 billion, and the population of China will be 1.4 billion; the United States will have the third largest population at nearly 400 million persons. Gender imbalances exist in many countries, most notably in China (m106:f100), Kuwait (m139:f100), Qatar (m184:f100), Russia (m88:f100), and the United Arab Emirates (m195:f100). In the United States, though we hear much about the gender imbalance, it is less drastic (m97:f100). One must remember that this is a comparison of gender at all ages and does not indicate the ratio

Table 1-1 The 65+ Population by State (2000)

	Number of persons	Percent of all ages	Percent increase 1990-2000	Percent below poverty 1998-2000
U.S. Total	34,991,753	12.4	12.0%	10.1%
Alabama	579,798	13.0	10.9%	15.3%
Alaska	35,699	5.7	59.6%	6.0%
Arizona	667,839	13.0	39.5%	8.8%
Arkansas	374,019	14.0	6.8%	15.2%
California	3,595,658	10.6	14.7%	8.4%
Colorado	416,073	9.7	26.3%	5.0%
Connecticut	470,183	13.8	5.4%	6.9%
Delaware	101,726	13.0	26.0%	6.8%
District of Columbia	69,898	12.2	−10.2%	16.7%
Florida	2,807,597	17.6	18.5%	8.4%
Georgia	785,275	9.6	20.0%	10.3%
Hawaii	160,601	13.3	28.5%	7.3%
Idaho	145,916	11.3	20.3%	7.5%
Illinois	1,500,025	12.1	4.4%	10.0%
Indiana	752,831	12.4	8.1%	9.3%
Iowa	436,213	14.9	2.4%	6.7%
Kansas	356,229	13.3	4.0%	7.9%
Kentucky	504,793	12.5	8.1%	13.3%
Louisiana	516,929	11.6	10.2%	16.8%
Maine	183,402	14.4	12.3%	10.3%
Maryland	599,307	11.3	15.8%	12.1%
Massachusetts	860,162	13.5	5.0%	9.0%
Michigan	1,219,018	12.3	10.0%	8.5%
Minnesota	594,266	12.1	8.7%	10.7%
Mississippi	343,523	12.1	6.9%	17.7%
Missouri	755,379	13.5	5.3%	8.7%
Montana	120,949	13.4	13.6%	7.6%
Nebraska	232,195	13.6	4.1%	10.1%
Nevada	218,929	11.0	71.5%	8.5%
New Hampshire	147,970	12.0	18.3%	8.2%
New Jersey	1,113,136	13.2	7.9%	7.3%
New Mexico	212,225	11.7	30.1%	14.5%
New York	2,448,352	12.9	3.6%	13.1%
North Carolina	969,048	12.0	20.5%	12.7%
North Dakota	94,478	14.7	3.8%	11.5%
Ohio	1,507,757	13.3	7.2%	7.6%
Oklahoma	455,950	13.2	7.5%	10.7%
Oregon	438,177	12.8	12.0%	8.3%
Pennsylvania	1,919,165	15.6	4.9%	7.8%
Rhode Island	152,402	14.5	1.2%	10.4%
South Carolina	485,333	12.1	22.3%	12.6%
South Dakota	108,131	14.3	5.7%	9.8%
Tennessee	703,311	12.4	13.7%	15.2%
Texas	2,072,532	9.9	20.7%	13.0%
Utah	190,222	8.5	26.9%	7.3%
Vermont	77,510	12.7	17.2%	9.0%
Virginia	792,333	11.2	19.2%	11.5%
Washington	662,148	11.2	15.1%	6.9%
West Virginia	276,895	15.3	3.0%	13.2%
Wisconsin	702,553	13.1	7.9%	8.3%
Wyoming	57,693	11.7	22.2%	9.8%

Source: Administration on Aging, 2001.

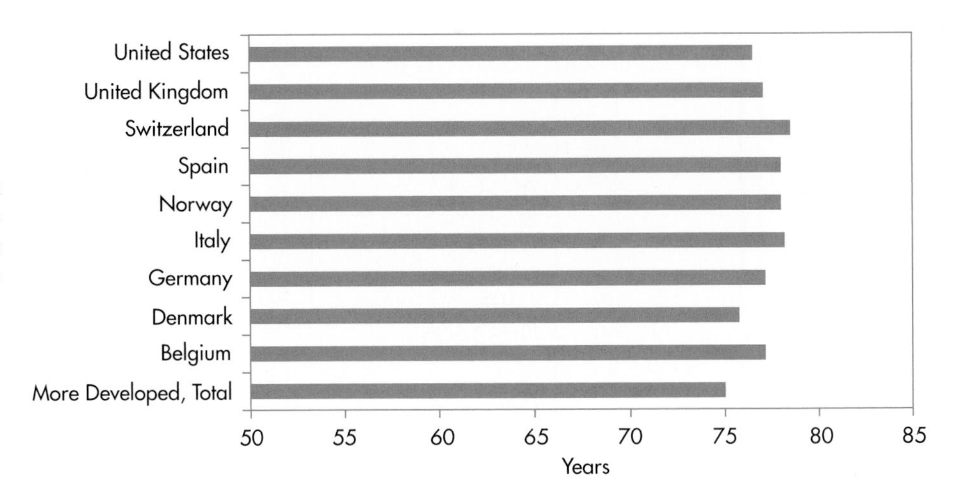

Figure 1-3. Life expectancy at birth, both sexes, selected developed countries, for the period 1995-2000. (Source: United Nations Population Division, *World population highlights,* Nov 2002. Available at *www.un.org/esa/population/unpop.htm.*)

of very old males to females (United Nations Population Division, 2002).

Chronologic Age

Chronology is becoming a less significant factor to consider in aging. "Old" is a relative concept based on how one acts and feels physically, mentally, socially, and culturally. One can feel old when competing with younger folk or feel young when much healthier or younger looking than age contemporaries. In the United States, the chronologic age of 65 years is the standard by which one is awarded the status of senior citizen, whether or not it is desired. Discounts on goods, services, and opportunities may begin as early as age 50, although many more begin at age 60 or 65. In other words, the category of old is arbitrary and varies with time, place, cohort, and perception. Special recognition because of one's advancing age is given in many ways, some desirable and some not so welcome. Throughout life there are marker events—physical, social, and psychologic—that measure our path through time. However, when these events begin to include more losses than gains, aging may become an onerous burden, particularly for those who have few social and spiritual resources. From the geriatric nursing perspective, functional age, or the ability to perform activities of daily living (ADLs), is a more essential measure of age than chronologic age. "Old age," categorically, is likely to last for 25 additional years if one is healthy at age 65 (Figure 1-5).

The Old. The parents of the "baby boomers," the children of the Great Depression, make up the majority of the present old numerically. Some immunizations became available in their childhood, but many parents feared them and most children had all of the "childhood" diseases, such as measles, mumps, chicken pox, and whooping cough. Some had tuberculosis, poliomyelitis, and smallpox. There was rampant malnutrition among the poorer people. Dental care was neglected. In areas where the water was "soft," lacking minerals, teeth were soft and cavity prone. "Pigeon chest," a malformation of the rib-cage caused by lack of vitamin D, was common. Goiter and myxedema were less common but were present regionally because of unrecognized iodine deficiencies. These problems were identified and almost eradicated before the next generation, the baby boomers, came along. The survivors in this generation are called the "notch" babies; few in number at birth, even fewer survived childhood, adolescence, and World War II. War and patriotism molded their young adulthood. Posttraumatic stress disorder (PTSD), only recently named, is now

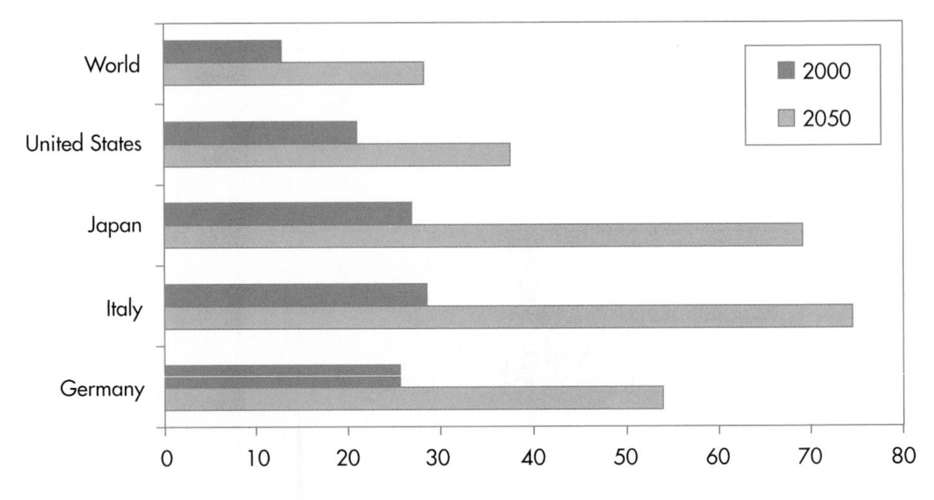

Figure 1-4. Aged dependency ratios, world total, and selected countries, 2000 and 2050. (These ratios include the number of persons ages 65+ per every 100 persons ages 20 to 64.) (Source: U.S. Bureau of the Census, International Data Base, 2001.)

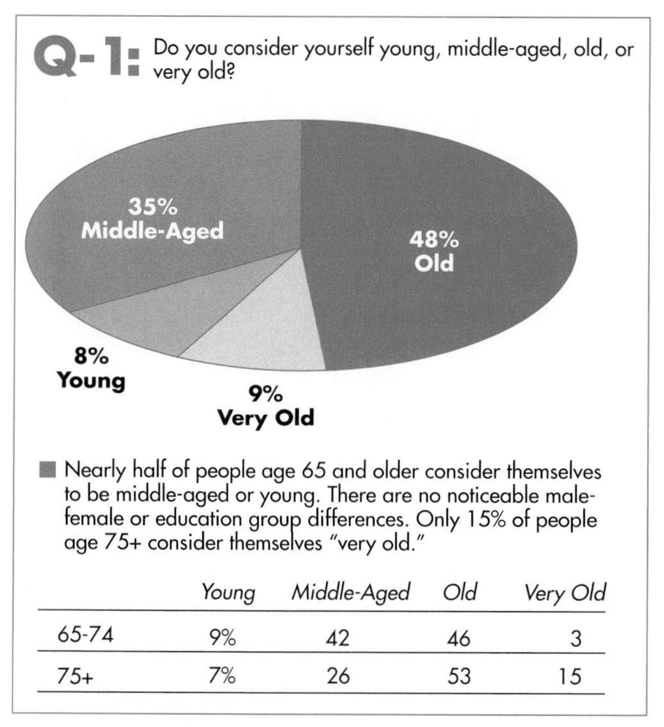

	Young	Middle-Aged	Old	Very Old
65-74	9%	42	46	3
75+	7%	26	53	15

Figure 1-5. Age self-identification. (Source: National Council on the Aging, Inc., *American perceptions of aging in the 21st century,* telephone survey, Jan-Feb 2000. Available at *www.ncoa.org.*)

being recognized among aged veterans who never fully recovered from the traumas of World War II (Buffum and Wolfe, 1995). Most of these elders are fairly sturdy, but their adolescent and young adult lifestyles contributed to many problems that are now evident. The use and abuse of cigarettes and alcohol were considered sophisticated. A double standard prevailed in the expectations of men and women. Exercise was not valued by most because desirable work was steadily becoming less physically strenuous, and physical exertion was still associated with hard work. Remote memories of poverty and deprivation haunted many of them and propelled them into excesses when such were available and affordable. Few gave much thought to their own aging when in their middle years because most were preoccupied with providing for their children the things they had missed. Saving for children's college education was a high priority.

Nonagenarians and Centenarians. There is an expanding group of the very old, those now over 90, who remain mobile and active. They are genetically hardy. These are an extraordinarily select group of individuals who have managed to survive the numerous dangers and diseases of childhood and, with the advancement of medical science, have overcome disorders that would have killed their parents. Some remember the influenza pandemic of 1918 in which numerous young and vital individuals died within a few hours of developing influenza (Cantor, 2002). Many of these present elders, because of the rigorous conditions of survival in their youth, are now living well into their nineties. Yet there are an equal number who are frail and vulnerable; they are discussed more fully in Chapter 16. This generation raised their families during the depths of the Great Depression. Desperation was prevalent in the country at the time. Few were able to achieve a higher education, and many did not even complete grade school. The bulk of the working population were farmers, agricultural workers, factory workers, miners, and clerks. Unemployment was rampant. Individuals worked very hard for the essentials of existence and felt fortunate if they were employed. Henry Ford became famous for offering wages of $5 a day and producing assembly-line cars that made automobiles available to the common person. With the availability of automobiles, the trek to find a better life began. Often it was an ongoing search that lasted a decade or more. These individuals, who are the last to remember traveling by horse and wagon, have also flown across the nation in supersonic jet airplanes. This generation has experienced more hardship and more lifestyle disruption and change than any of which we are aware. Federal aid, Social Security, the Works Progress Administration, and numerous other New Deal programs were instituted as survival measures during the depths of the Depression. Few of these individuals thought much about old age, and many say they are surprised to have lived so long. These elders rarely throw anything away because every scrap has potential value when one has known early deprivation. Many of them arrived in the United States in early childhood as steerage passengers, emigrating with their parents from Europe.

Centenarians, the "elite-old," are approached with some awe as our society seeks routes to longevity. About 1 in 10,000 people in developed countries lives to be a hundred or more (Christensen, 2001). A select few of these expert survivors have experienced the turning of two centuries. Many are bright, alert, and have an unequaled personal history. The number of centenarians in the United States has doubled every decade since 1970. In 1970 the U.S. Census revealed 4475 people age 100 or over; the 2000 U.S. Census estimated that there were between 69,000 and 81,000 (U.S. Bureau of the Census, 2001). About 30% have no children or siblings still living. Most centenarians are female and come from families in which longevity is common. Though there are fewer men, they are less likely than women to have significant mental or physical disabilities at that age (Christensen, 2001). They are often sought for their opinions on the key to longevity. There is the supposition that because they have lived so long they know the secrets to learning, growing, and thriving. Various centenarians have recommended such things as a daily highball, hard work, church attendance, healthy diets, or the continuation of sexual activity. Unfortunately, few agree and the myths abound. Lifestyle factors that do seem significant include diet, exercise, social connections, and how well a person handles stress (Christensen, 2001).

Belle Boone Beard, who died in 1984, conducted several thousand interviews with centenarians during 40 years of study. Elsner and colleagues (1999) carry on her work and are concerned that little thought is being given to the ethical and policy considerations for this fastest growing segment of the population. There are still many questions and conflicting findings regarding both the physiologic and psychologic adaptation of centenarians. Most centenarians are likely to be extremely frail and vulnerable both mentally and physically. Frailty is dealt with more completely in Chapter 16.

Attitudes toward Aging

Attitudes toward aging are inextricably tied to history and culture. Views of aging in any era or ethnic group are influenced by expected life span, economic conditions, social expectations, and the way these are dealt with in the media, arts, and literature of the time. A unique situation presently exists in our society. Rapid change and cataclysmic shifts in lifestyles, universal threats to survival, a shrinking world and an expanding universe, and previously undreamed of possibilities and opportunities have created remarkable differences in the life experience of each generation.

Ageist attitudes may be excessively positive or negative, depending on one's tendency to stereotype individuals based on their age. The aged, collectively, have often been seen in negative terms; however, a most striking change in attitudes toward the aged has occurred in the past 20 years. The impact of media presentation is enormous, and we are gratified to see robust images of aging; fewer aged are portrayed as victims or those to be pitied, shunned, or ridiculed by virtue of achieving old age. The image of aging has shifted from pity to envy of the "greedy geezers."

Attitudes of Elders. Attitudes of the aged toward other elders are often far more rejecting than those of younger persons. The aged with mental disabilities are particularly vulnerable because they represent the fears of their healthier contemporaries. In senior centers and retirement centers the cliques of highly functioning elders are quite noticeable.

Attitudes of Children. Children are able to identify with old persons and feel comfortable with them in direct proportion to their frequency of contact. Those who see elders frequently are more aware of the reality of aging persons. Closeness with grandparents is highly correlated with attitudes young people hold toward older persons. Attitudes of school-age children and adolescents are generally positive regarding the aged. These tendencies could be sustained and cultivated by giving more attention to aging in public school curricula. To decrease stereotypic notions, students in some schools are given opportunities to work with the elderly. Generally, persons who are younger and who have had extensive contact with the well elderly have the most positive regard for the aged.

Attitudes of Nurses. Few students or professionals set out early on to be gerontology specialists. They enter the field most often by accident, by job opportunity, or through a revered mentor. Often, in nursing, an early serendipitous experience of a student caring for a physically debilitated or dependent elder who had amazing fortitude and courage was the impression that fostered an interest in the field. For many others it was intimate contact with grandparents, often in a caregiving capacity, that instilled the desire to care for elders. For those inspired, it is usually a combination of events. When nurses do become involved in caring for elders, they are most often very positive in their attitudes.

Research and Aging

In the nearly four decades since the institution of Medicare and Medicaid, there has been colossal growth in gerontology as a scientific pursuit. Federal and foundation dollars in support of research and research training attracted many to the field of aging.

Some of the major problems in aging research are that the "aged," although statistically ranging from 65 to 115 years old, are often lumped into a single category. We would no more think of categorically comparing the experience of a 3-year-old and a 13-year-old than we would compare apples and oranges. Studies of the aged often include those 50 years old, eligible for certain memberships and discounts based on age deference, and the 104-year-old residing in a nursing home. These are considered as a group, though they have few if any similar characteristics. Some researchers extrapolate from studies of young adults or institutionalized elders, and conclusions are attributed to the aged in general. A great deal of cross-sequential research and small samples are also suspect.

Research and gerontologic knowledge are strongly influenced by federal bulletins that are distributed nationwide to indicate the type of research that is most likely to receive federal funding. These are published in requests for proposals (RFPs). In a very real way, the "alzheimerization" of aging has come about because, since the establishment of the National Institute on Aging (NIA) in 1971, the study of Alzheimer's disease has been awarded the largest share of research dollars for aging. Since the last edition of this textbook was published in 1998, there have been a plethora of studies, some significant and some not. Alzheimer's disease remains a primary area of research concentration, with a considerable focus on etiology, prevention, and medications that may halt or slow progress of the disease.

The investigators of the Baltimore Longitudinal Studies of the Aged have been collecting data and periodically publishing findings for almost 40 years. These studies were initially restricted to males, but more recently studies of females have been included as well. Several substantial longitudinal studies of the aged are now presenting current evidence about elders from several cohorts.

The Harvard Women's Health Study, begun in 1976, has now accumulated more than 25 years of data regarding nurses' health (available at *www.nurseshealthstudy.org*). Although not specifically focused on aging, the Harvard Women's Health Study is providing needed data on the women who have grown old with the study. Of course, this is a problem because a specific population group has been targeted: nurses.

Several pharmaceutical companies, in consort with universities, are currently conducting long-range studies of medications and their potential for alleviating some of the problems that tend to develop in the aged, such as osteoporosis, benign prostatic hypertrophy, coronary artery ischemia, atherosclerosis, and the effects of hormonal depletion. The National Institute on Aging, the National Center for Nursing Research, the National Institute of Mental Health, and the Agency for Health Care Policy and Research continue to make significant research contributions to our understanding of the aged. Some recent research focuses on the study of the subtle, progressive diseases that frequently accompany aging, such as hypertension and cardiovascular disease. Of particular interest is the study of non–insulin-dependent diabetes mellitus (type 2). There is speculation that type 2 diabetes mellitus represents a form of accelerated aging and thus may yield important information related to the aging process. Meneilly and Tessier (2001) found evidence to suggest that normally shifting hormonal levels and age-related changes in carbohydrate metabolism in both men and women may contribute to the development of type 2 diabetes mellitus. Studies of older women have also assumed greater importance because the preponderance of the very old are females. Their special needs and capacities are slowly being recognized. The studies referred to here are too numerous to summarize, but a few of the interesting findings include those noted in Box 1-4. All of these studies are examples of findings that need further exploration and replication. The meaning and experience of aging remain elusive, complex, and highly individualistic. Phenomenologic studies, therefore, will continue to provide some of the richest information, though they are subject to variable interpretation. Also, in both quantitative and qualitative research, the study of the ethnic aged is most lacking. Federal statistics often include general categories of black and white but seldom more discrete statistics.

Box 1-4 Focus of Geriatric Nursing Research Studies: United States

- Quality of care
- Chronic illness: coping and symptom management
- Cognitive impairment
- Depression
- Pain management
- Informal caregivers
- Wandering
- Safety, falls, restraints
- Factors related to independence in ADLs
- Exercise programs

International Nursing Research Priorities

- Health promotion
- Care of the elderly
- Chronic illness care
- Patient self-care
- Health care systems
- Quality/cost of care
- Symptom management

Adapted from Hinshaw AS: Nursing knowledge for the 21st century: opportunities and challenges, *J Nurs Sch* 32(2):117, 2000; Fitzpatrick JJ, editor: *Annu Rev Nurs Res* 20, 2002 (entire issue devoted to geriatric nursing research).
ADLs, Activities of daily living.

Nursing Research

Geriatric nursing research and practice have evolved to the point where best practice standards are being published and distributed through several organizations. Nurses have generated significant research in the care of the aged. The 2002 issue of the *Annual Review of Nursing Research* (volume 20) is entirely devoted to geriatric nursing (Fitzpatrick, 2002). Numerous nursing research studies over the past two decades are cited, described, and analyzed. Issues most relevant to present concerns in geriatric care include end-of-life care, diversity of the aged, telehealth management, pain management (especially in dementia), and caregivers' burden. Neglected areas of research include the dyadic experience of hearing impairment, cultural influences on the experience of hearing loss, the long-term impact of oxytocic medications, and strategies to assist elders in coping with hearing loss (Wallhagen, 2002). Fulmer (2002) addresses the need for more studies of elder mistreatment, particularly on interventions that have shown effectiveness. Even though $20 million is spent annually on adult protective services for elder mistreatment, there are no good data to explain how it was spent and if the results were satisfactory (Fulmer, 2002). There are also other volumes in this series relevant to geriatric nurses, such as volume 18 (focused on chronic illness) and volume 19 (focused on women's health). International nursing research priorities vary from one country to the next, depending on the organization of their services to the aged. Hinshaw (2000, p. 122) presents a comparative table of several of these.

Nursing research that has significantly affected the quality of life of older persons gains more prominence each decade. Some of the most important studies have investigated methods of caring for individuals with dementia (Buckwalter et al, 1999), reducing falls and the use of restraints (Strumpf and Evans, 2003; Strumpf et al, 1998), pain management (Ferrell, 1999), and humane end-of-life care (Matzo and Sherman, 2003). These are discussed later in the text. Hinshaw (2000) notes that most research regarding health and illness of older adults has been in the following areas: ADLs and maintaining independence, managing cognitive impairment and depression, and providing supportive care environments for the aged. She suggests that we need research that will identify those at risk of losing function, interventions for enhancing and maintaining memory, and interventions to enhance optimism and self-esteem. She sees a need for a stronger emphasis on intervention research and more interdisciplinary collaboration to ensure relevance of nursing research to practice.

The Politics of Aging

The actual development of gerontology has probably been more influenced by political expediency than by any other factor, but politics and economics are so intermeshed that they can rarely be untangled. In the United States the first real interest in the aged emerged in the 1930s, when a population of aged persons, who were largely impoverished, became demographically significant. Under the Roosevelt administration and the National Recovery Act (NRA) in the mid-1930s, the United States began moving toward a socialistic political control that still persists today, although it is often assailed by conservative policy makers. During the 1940s the study of aging was set aside to devote attention to the more pressing problems of national defense and developments in weaponry. However, interest in aging rose rapidly after World War II.

Today funding for social services is often tied to stringent governmental requirements. Although we hear about shifting the funding responsibility from federal agencies to state agencies, we have yet to see the full effects of this in action. One of the paradoxes that hinders the delivery of services to the aged in the United States is that America is both a capitalistic and a socialistic society, with health care moving rapidly into a highly competitive marketing mode. Therefore life-sustaining services are now designed for profit, although we simultaneously federally subsidize them. See Box 1-5 for a summary of important political developments in the field of aging.

White House Conferences on Aging. The first White House Conference on Aging (WHCOA), in 1961, paved the way for the establishment of the Older Americans Act, the Administration on Aging, and the Medicare program. Following the second WHCOA, the National Institute on Aging was established in 1971 with Robert Butler as the first director. The commitment to sustain these programs sometimes seems tenuous, although politicians are well aware of the strength of elders' votes and therefore are likely to enact laws that will accrue votes. The aged, although a large part of the voting population, are highly individualistic and as yet have not formed a political power block except on issues such as erosion of Social Security or reduction of Medicare and Medicaid. The greatest congressional threats to these programs, as they vie for the defense dollars, will demonstrate the strength of elders, their diverse opinions, and their collective power on certain issues. The 1995 WHCOA (thus far the most recent) concurred with the 60th anniversary of Social Security and was focused on four main issues:

- Ensuring comprehensive health care, including long-term care
- Promoting economic security
- Increasing housing and supportive services
- Maximizing options for quality of life

At this time we have heard of no plans for another WHCOA. There have been and will continue to be necessary modifications to ensure the viability and continuation of the programs. The late Maggie Kuhn, founder of the Gray Panthers, was an eloquent voice for the aged and the necessity of intergenerational support toward health and social services (Box 1-6).

Older Americans Act. The Older Americans Act (OAA), instituted following the 1961 WHCOA, established a vehicle for delivering community-based services through state Area Agencies on Aging (AAAs). AAAs have some flexibility in services provided, but they generally include senior centers, nutrition sites, in-home services for frail elderly, elder abuse prevention programs, long-term care ombudsmen, employment services, legal assistance, preretirement counseling, health promotion, and respite care. Federal appropriations and services have historically increased markedly each year as the numbers of aged have increased. Now seniors fear that these may not continue. The current political agenda is to transfer much of the responsibility for provision of services to the states, the cities, and the individual. This could mean more individual autonomy in the future. At present the transferring of responsibility has greatly increased the burdens to families. Recently the Administration on Aging (AOA) has given considerably more attention to the needs of caregivers of the aged (Greene, 2002).

The Business of Aging

Aging is not only a phase of life, a philosophy, or an experience—it is big business. Major marketing attention has been extended to the aged as businesses grasp the market potential of the upcoming young-old. Presently, individuals between ages 35 and 54 number 83 million (U.S. Bureau of the Census, 2001). The American Society on Aging published an entire issue of Generations entitled "Developing and Marketing New Products for Older People" (ASA, 1995). Even the revered American Association of Retired Persons (AARP) is primarily designed to provide services, education, and conveniences to the well-heeled, well-educated young-old. The AARP offers insurance for every purpose, travel and cruise packages, luxurious retirement facilities, and art objects all marketed to the anticipated tastes and needs of vital and prosperous elders.

The revival of 1940s and 1950s memorabilia, music, and nostalgia all reflect market trends that stir memories of childhood in active young-elders. In addition to a large market of well elders, there is an enormous market for those needing assistive devices, supplies, and equipment for management of chronic disorders. Herbs and supplements claim an increasing share of the market, but the greatest of all is in the pharmacologic market. Annual expenditures for prescription drugs exceeded all other health care costs except hospitals and doctors. The advertising and business world is beginning to create niches for gerontologists as they realize the benefits of their special skills as applied to marketing. However, there are growing concerns that elders are prime targets for anti-aging scams (U.S. Senate Special Committee on Aging, 2001).

GERIATRIC NURSING AND AGING: THE FUTURE

Baby boomers are looming on the horizon. A healthier old age seems to be within reach for the population in general and

Box 1-5

Political Events Influencing Aging

1935	Social Security Act signed by Franklin D. Roosevelt.
1937	National Institute of Health established first of the special institutes to study diseases common to older people.
1948	Hospital Construction and Facilities Act (Hill-Burton) provided funds for construction of long-term care facilities.
1950	First National Conference on Aging held in Washington, D.C.
1951	Federal Committee on Aging and Geriatrics created to coordinate federal programs for the aging.
1952	First Federal-State Conference on Aging held in Washington.
1956	Special Staff on Aging established within U.S. Department of Health, Education, and Welfare. Federal Council on Aging replaced Intradepartmental Working Group on Aging.
1959	Senate subcommittee authorized to consider problems of the aged and aging. Federal Council on Aging reconstituted at Cabinet level.
1960	First appropriation passed for Section 202, Housing Act of 1959, authorizing direct loans for housing for the elderly.
1961	First White House Conference on Aging held in Washington. Senate Special Committee on Aging established as advocate for older Americans. First Annual Conference of State Executives held in Washington.
1962	Federal Council on Aging became President's Council on Aging.
1963	John F. Kennedy sent Congress the first presidential message on elderly citizens; designated May as Senior Citizens Month. Special Staff on Aging became Office of Aging in HEW's new Welfare Administration.
1965	President Johnson signed Older Americans Act, creating Adminstration on Aging (AOA). Amendments to the Social Security Act established Medicare program. Foster Grandparent Program initiated by Office of Economic Opportunity and Administration on Aging.
1967	Age Discrimination in Employment Act brightened job outlook for Americans 40 to 65 years old.
1970	Older Americans White House Forums held across the nation to identify problems and issues for upcoming White House Conference on Aging.
1971	Second White House Conference on Aging held in Washington. Cabinet-level Domestic Council Committee on Aging created. ACTION—the federal volunteer agency—established and given responsibility for senior volunteer programs previously administered by AOA.
1972	New act passed establishing Nutrition Program for the Elderly to be administered by AOA.
1973	Amendments to Older Americans Act called for State agencies on aging to establish area agencies on aging to plan for comprehensive, coordinated service delivery systems for older people at the local level. Establishment of a National Clearinghouse on Aging and a Federal Council on the Aging with members appointed by the President. Amendments included a separate Older Americans Community Employment Act with responsibility for administering given to Department of Labor. Federal Aid Highway Act of 1973 provided funds for a demonstration program of public transportation in rural areas with an emphasis on the needs of the elderly and handicapped.
1974	Research on Aging Act established National Institute on Aging within National Institute of Health, Robert N. Butler appointed Director. Amendments to Urban Mass Transportation Act of 1964 made funds available to nonprofit private organizations and corporations for transportation vehicles and equipment for the elderly and handicapped. National Mass Transportation Act mandated reduced fares for the elderly and handicapped on all public transportation systems assisted by the Act.
1975	House of Representatives Special Committee on Aging established. Amendments to the Older Americans Act establish four new priority areas under Title IV: a. Transportation b. Home Services c. Legal Services d. Residential Repair and Renovation
1976	Title V of the Older Americans Act received an appropriation for the first time since inception of the Act in 1965. Five million dollars was appropriated "to pay part of the cost of acquisition, alteration, or renovation of community facilities that will serve as multipurpose Senior Centers."
1977	Title V re-funded at rate of $20 million annually.
1981	Third White House Conference on Aging held in Washington, D.C. Mandatory retirement laws revised.
1982	T. Franklin Williams appointed director of National Institute of Aging.
1983	Diagnostic Related Groups (DRGs) instituted by the Health Care Financing Administration to control costs of Medicare.
1984	Sexual discrimination in pension benefit payments outlawed by U.S. Supreme Court.
1988	Medicare Catastrophic Coverage Act.
1989	Medicare Catastrophic Coverage Act repealed.
1991	Fourth White House Conference on Aging stalled. AOA Funds cut drastically.
1992	Proposals from multiple sources for rescue of health care system.
1995	Fourth WHCOA. Focused on preservation of Medicare, Medicaid, Social Security, and the Older Americans Act (OAA).
1996	Majority of elders moved through Medicare changes to managed care systems.
1998	Congress considers privatizing Social Security.
2000	Numerous methods of reducing drug costs are proposed.

Box 1-6 History of the White House Conferences on Aging

1950	The National Conference on Aging, the precursor of the White House Conference on Aging, was called under the Truman Administration. It was followed by two Conferences of State Councils on Aging and Federal Agencies, one in 1952 and the other in 1956.
1958	Legislation calling for the first White House Conference on Aging (WHCOA) was introduced in Congress.
1961	Initiated by President Dwight Eisenhower, the first WHCOA focused on the problem of providing health care to the nation's older citizens. The eventual result was the Medicare program.
1971	By the time the second WHCOA took place, the Older Americans Act (OAA) had been enacted. The Conference examined ways of expanding social services and benefits for older people, including the nutrition program and transportation services.
1981	The third WHCOA took place. When the OAA was reauthorized that year, the emphasis was on developing supportive services that could help older people stay independent and in their own homes.
1991	The White House called for a WHCOA to take place in 1993, but the conference never materialized.
1992	Amendments to the OAA authorized the fourth WHCOA. In the legislation, Congress recommended that the conference's primary focus be on fostering public awareness of the interdependence of all generations.
1994	President Bill Clinton called for the fourth conference. Describing the conference as a way of "keeping faith with the senior citizens of this country," the president pledged that the conference would take place no later than May of 1995.
1995	The fourth WHCOA took place on May 2 to 5. This conference was the first to focus on how to meet the challenges posed by the aging of the "baby boom" generation.

Note: As of this writing, no fifth WHCOA has been proposed.

particularly for the segment dubbed "baby boomers." They are informed, educated, and have been alerted to the importance of beginning to prepare early for a good old age. Most have grown up in a health-conscious environment with the best of medical care and social and recreational services, yet wars and nuclear threats have undergirded and overshadowed their whole lives. They have assiduously cultivated diversity and ethnic integration throughout their lives. They are the "Spock" babies and the "duck-and-cover" children. They blossomed in adolescence, searching for causes and hoping for a peaceful world as the space age dawned. They are now the mature suppliers and consumers of goods and services. Marketing forces are reaching out to them with "adult living" communities and numerous products and services geared especially to their later middle years. More and more of them find that they are caregivers to the older members of their family, sometimes as many as two generations, and have a very personal understanding of the needs of elders. These almost-elders are giving us new perspectives on the aging process. They and the numerous longitudinal studies of aging now in progress are changing the concepts of aging and the field of gerontology. Yet much depends on world economics, and there is unrest among these individuals as they contemplate the possibility of insufficient resources in their final years.

There is no typical baby boomer. Although it has been fashionable to consider the baby boomers en masse, they are extremely diverse, differing by as much as 19 birth years, separated by race, culture, and socioeconomic status. To plan well for their retirement years, we must consider the following:

- Their diversity
- The uncertain political and economic future
- Potential major shifts in lifestyle expectations
- Radical differences in health care delivery systems
- Progress in technology and medical management of some disorders and an increase in iatrogenic disorders
- Shifts in values and ethics that will profoundly affect daily life

Articles about menopause proliferate, midlife crises abound, and anxiety about the future is rampant. Will there be income support, adequate retirement, available health care, disability benefits, and all the things the present generation of the old have relied on? At present the major concerns of baby boomers are health, finances, job security, sending children to college, and caring for parents. They have been called the "sandwich generation," as they try to meet the needs of "boomerang" children (those young adults who repeatedly return home as they cannot generate sufficient incomes to live independently) and elderly parents. Often they are also the primary caretakers of grandchildren. Shirley Chater (a nurse and recent director of Social Security) called them the "double whopper" generation. Gerontologists, marketing strategists, and the age industry are attempting to predict anticipated challenges.

Adult children (offspring of the World War II generation) are of increasing significance in gerontology. This segment of the population is characterized by its affluence, relative good health, and vitality. The most potent influences on their development are the almost universal opportunities for higher education, inflationary economics, political participation, urban and suburban lifestyles, assimilation of myriad cultures into the mainstream of American life, technologic innovations, youth-centered family life, and now the increasing responsibility for elderly parents. Migratory tendencies and travel opportunities throughout their working lives have led to sophistication and a world focus.

These space-age children can only wonder what the future holds for their own later years. They seem more concerned about healthful lifestyles than previous generations, are better educated, have higher expectations of themselves (and others), and formed the core of the "moral majority" (though disillusionment is setting in). Although formal religion seems to have been supplanted by a sense of personal responsibility, many have sought leadership or inspiration among gurus, charismatic personalities, cults, and mystics.

Many uncertainties remain about the conditions, status, and benefits baby boomers will experience. Some of the major concerns are based in the shift of lifestyles away from the traditional family. Single parents, blended families, limited parenthood, unmarried parents, and gay and lesbian parents all represent lifestyles that may or may not produce children willing or available to assist parents as they age.

The parents of these baby boomers continue to plan for their needs in a generational reciprocity mode. The greatest transfer of assets in history is taking place right now, from elders to their middle-aged children. Children of the 1940s and 1950s, the golden children, have increasingly had to face the issues of aging parents and are strongly aware of the need for redirection of a system that, for all its extravagances, is not serving them or their parents well.

The Nursing Shortage

The much publicized shortage of nurses is, in my opinion, related to the absence of satisfaction, enormous increases in the technologically sophisticated aspects of care, and inadequate compensation for the level of responsibility expected of nurses. In addition, registered nurses (RNs) are so sparsely represented in many institutions that their legal responsibilities and presence in truly nursing roles conflict and are impossible to achieve. The recent shortage of nurses is felt most keenly in the long-term care industry and Veterans Administration (VA) medical centers. Testimony from the nursing profession (American Nurse, 2002) before the Senate Veterans Affairs Committee in 2001 provided the following information: the average age of nurses in the United States providing inpatient care is 45 and in the VA it is 48. Within 4 years 35% of these will be eligible to retire. Too few nurses are caring for too many patients now, and the prospects for nursing home staffing does not appear hopeful (Larson Long Term Care Group, 2001).

A study published by the American Health Care Association (AHCA, 2001), the national organization of for-profit-nursing homes, warned of the increasing demand for skilled nursing care in the United States and the decreasing supply of nurses in these settings. The AHCA recommended to congress and the president that 60,000 new licensed practical nurses (LPNs) and RNs were needed by January 1, 2002. Some congressional efforts have been visible in that respect.

Box 1-7 The American Nurses Association's Bill of Rights for Registered Nurses

Registered nurses promote and restore health, prevent illness and protect the people entrusted to their case. They work to alleviate the suffering experienced by individuals, families, groups, and communities. In so doing, nurses provide services that maintain respect for human dignity and embrace the uniqueness of each patient and the nature of his or her health problems, without restriction with regard to social or economic status. To maximize the contributions nurses make to society, it is necessary to protect the dignity and autonomy of nurses in the workplace. To that end, the following rights must be afforded:

1. Nurses have the right to practice in a manner that fulfills their obligations to society and to those who receive nursing care.
2. Nurses have the right to practice in environments that allow them to act in accordance with professional standards and legally authorized scopes of practice.
3. Nurses have the right to a work environment that supports and facilitates ethical practice, in accordance with the *Code of Ethics for Nurses* and its interpretive statements.
4. Nurses have the right to freely and openly advocate for themselves and their patients, without fear of retribution.
5. Nurses have the right to fair compensation for their work, consistent with their knowledge, experience, and professional responsibilities.
6. Nurses have the right to a work environment that is safe for themselves and their patients.
7. Nurses have the right to negotiate the conditions of their employment, either as individuals or collectively, in all practice settings.

Disclaimer: The American Nurses Association (ANA) is a national professional association. ANA policies reflect the thinking of the nursing profession on various issues and should be reviewed in conjunction with state association policies and state board of nursing policies and practices. State law, rules and regulation govern the practice of nursing. The ANA's "Bill of Rights for Registered Nurses" contains policy statements and does not necessarily reflect rights embodied in state and federal law. ANA policies may be used by the state to interpret or provide guidance on the profession's position on nursing.

This Bill of Rights was adopted by the ANA Board of Directors on June 26, 2001.

From The American Nurses Association: The American Nurses Association's bill of rights for registered nurses, *Am Nurse* 34(6):16, 2002.

The entire study can be accessed at *www.ahca.org/news/staff-02-2001.htm*.

The current approach to collective bargaining has stunted professional growth in nursing. Anderson (1999) suggests that collective bargaining in nursing should refocus on professional issues such as workplace climate, differentiated practice, continuing formal educational requirements for various positions, family-friendly policies, and a structure and process for systematic advancement and compensation. Even more exciting, she writes that doctors and nurses face similar areas of disgruntlement, such as loss of autonomy over practice, eroding incomes and increasing workloads, and a sense of helplessness within the health care system. She asks, "Why not have a union whose membership would be comprised of physicians and nurses, and the focus of collective bargaining would be the ensuring of high-quality patient care?"

The present dilemmas in the care of the aged are summarized by Fulmer et al (2001). The following issues will have substantial influence on the future quality of the aging experience:

- Who should receive advanced technologic care?
- How old is old?
- Who should pay for care?
- When should care stop?
- How should care be stopped?
- Who determines viability?

With the attention shifting to reassessment of where the health care dollar should be spent, geriatric nurses are increasingly focused on pain management and palliative care. Other dilemmas that must be addressed are:

- How can we begin now to deal with the greatly increased dependency ratio expected by 2050?
- What assistance can realistically be given to caregivers?

Global challenges must be considered as well. Policies are needed that will adequately meet income, health, and long-term care needs for women as well as men throughout the world. The following are some of the issues and strategies that have been proposed to be considered by the international community (AOA International Division, 2002). First and foremost, especially in some of the less developed countries, is that women and men should have equal access to resources, the right of inheritance, and ownership of land. Others include the following:

- Adapt economic security systems that protect young and old and remove gender biases.
- Provide access to basic education and lifelong learning opportunities.
- Teach the continuity of life to children at very young ages.
- Promote healthy lifestyles and avoidance of risk behaviors.
- Ensure universal and affordable access to adequate health care.
- Support age-integrated environments using universal design principles.
- Provide training, counseling, financial assistance, and social service supports to adapt to the changing needs of families and their vulnerable members.

Many other suggestions can be retrieved from *www.ban-gate.aoa.dhhs.gov*. The message is that a much better distribution of resources and opportunities to all ages and cultures worldwide is essential if civilization is to endure.

Nurse Leaders and Followers

Clearly there is a great need for strong leaders and loyal followers and individuals who can comfortably occupy both roles as necessary within their bailiwick. To transform geriatric nursing we will need "transformational" leaders and followers.

In an investigation of the leadership principles held by eight transformational nursing leaders, Ward (2002) found that transformational leaders strive for excellence and integrity, mold the environment toward successful outcomes, persevere, support and inspire those around them, and have a vision of the future. Characteristics of these unnamed leaders included expertise, credibility, resilience, honesty, sense of humor, energetic, innovative, patience, and strong interpersonal skills. Transformational leadership implies a change in focus to "create supportive environments of shared responsibility that lead to new ways of knowing" (Ward, 2002, p. 121).

Travis (2002), the president of the National Gerontological Nursing Association, asks this question of leaders: "Can you be an effective leader if you always end up on the leadership end?" She points out some of the advantages of being a good follower even though a leader: Do you listen to others? Can you let someone else take responsibility for bringing a group to consensus? Are you noting the different leadership styles? Travis also advises that followers who have never taken a leadership position find a mentor who is working toward a goal they find attractive and do one thing every day that challenges. She emphasizes that every organization must have leaders and followers, but each must move out of a single role if they are to grow.

Nursing's obligation to the next generation of nurses was articulated very clearly in an editorial by Anderson (2000). Especially in this time of shortage, she admonishes nurses to step back from the difficulties and instill in students the intrinsic rewards of nursing. She challenges *every* practicing nurse with the obligation to teach students. The inspiration to focus on the half-full rather than half-empty profession is clearly in the hands of practicing nurses. The shape of the future of geriatric nursing and the baby boomers is on us now.

LONG-TERM CARE	ACUTE CARE	COMMUNITY CARE
Provide a milieu for living and holistic support in illness and dying	Support patient in achieving highest level of autonomy possible in situation	Make clients and families aware of options and resources Involve clients in citizens' councils and political action groups Support legislation affecting opportunities for the aged
Teach resident and families Counsel resident and families Learn about and use community resources, advise family and patient of same Establish short-term and long-term goals: evaluate progress toward both periodically Secure and maintain health, recreation, and social history	Provide appropriate information to patient and families about treatment plan, medications,and diagnosis in collaboration with physician	Teach clients and families Cousult and collaborate with agencies and multiprofessional representatives Educate clients to self-responsiblity for health
Plan and coordinate care Teach ancillary personnel Communicate resident's needs in written and verbal form	Collaborate with multiprofessionals, patient, and family to develop a comprehensive care plan Supervise ancillary personnel	Promote health through clinic and home contact Provide appropriate resources Identify health, social, or economic needs Counsel clients and family members
Give treatments, medications, and rehabilitative exercises Observe and evaluate patient response to treatment, medication, and care plan Teach health care maintenance to staff and residents	Recognize implications of syndromes for patient care (e.g., renal failure, coronary disease, emphysema) Protect patient from injury or iatrogenic disease Perform physical and psychologic assessment and integrate in nursing care plan Initiate action as outlined in nursing protocols regarding various conditions	Report care finding and make appropriate referral Assess environmental safety Assess response to illness and compliance with treatment Provide information about medications and treatments
Keep physician aware of changes in residents' conditions Institute life-saving measures in the absence of a physician Perform physical assessment of residents Ensure adequate medical, dental, and podiatric care for residents Maintain hydration, nutrition, aeration, and comfort	Provide emergency treatment as needed for cardiopulmonary crisis, amelioration of shock, hemorrhage, convulsions, poisoning Alert physician to changes in patient status and abnormal findings of tests Maintain hydration, nutrition, aeration, and comfort	Provide health surveillance Identify health, social, and economic need Assist client and family to modify patterns detrimental to health Evaluate deviations from normal and advise clients of appropriate action Identify existing or impending illness

Nursing function in caring for the aged in institutions and in the community.

Human Needs and Wellness Diagnoses for Nurses

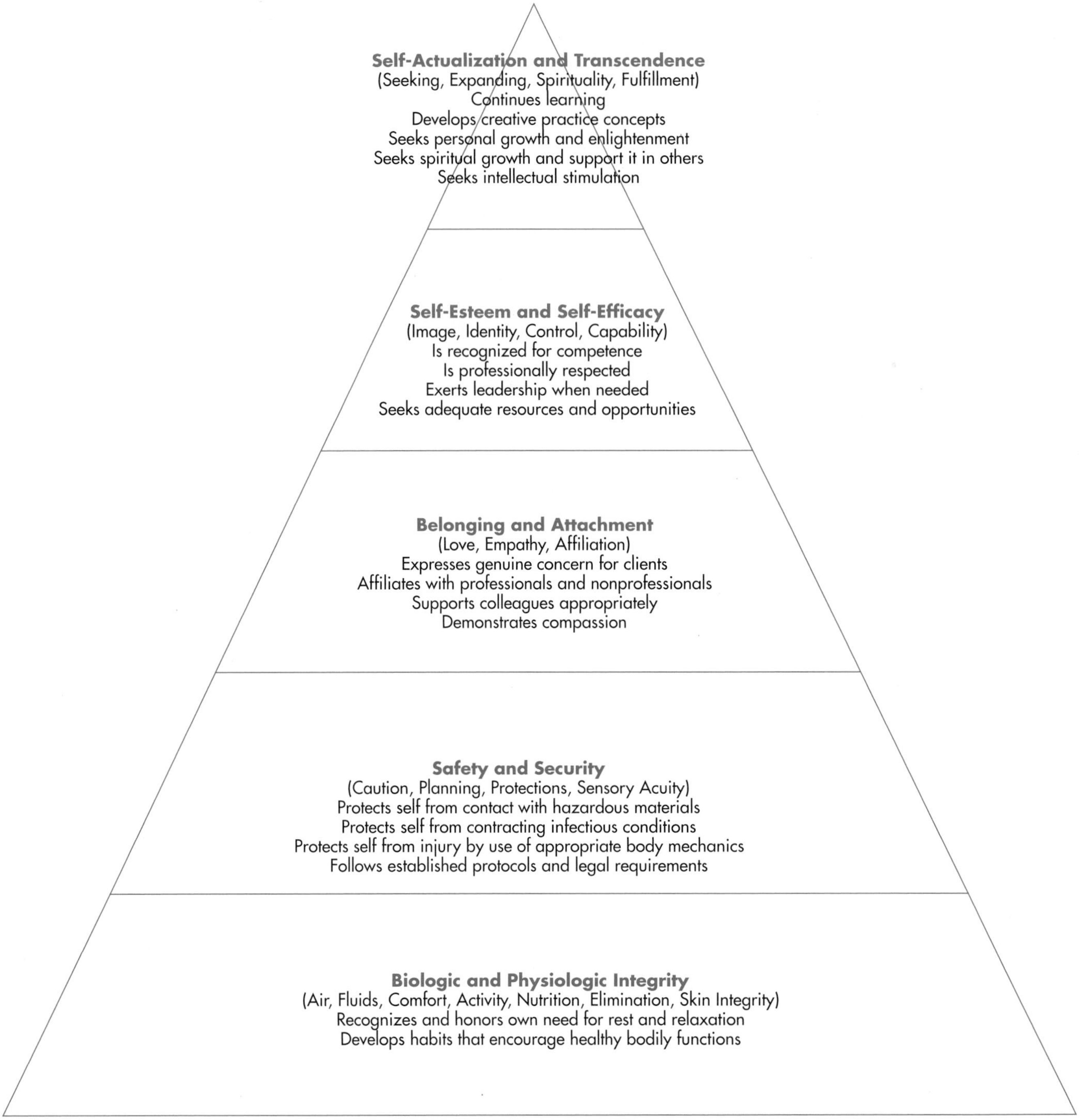

Self-Actualization and Transcendence
(Seeking, Expanding, Spirituality, Fulfillment)
Continues learning
Develops creative practice concepts
Seeks personal growth and enlightenment
Seeks spiritual growth and support it in others
Seeks intellectual stimulation

Self-Esteem and Self-Efficacy
(Image, Identity, Control, Capability)
Is recognized for competence
Is professionally respected
Exerts leadership when needed
Seeks adequate resources and opportunities

Belonging and Attachment
(Love, Empathy, Affiliation)
Expresses genuine concern for clients
Affiliates with professionals and nonprofessionals
Supports colleagues appropriately
Demonstrates compassion

Safety and Security
(Caution, Planning, Protections, Sensory Acuity)
Protects self from contact with hazardous materials
Protects self from contracting infectious conditions
Protects self from injury by use of appropriate body mechanics
Follows established protocols and legal requirements

Biologic and Physiologic Integrity
(Air, Fluids, Comfort, Activity, Nutrition, Elimination, Skin Integrity)
Recognizes and honors own need for rest and relaxation
Develops habits that encourage healthy bodily functions

These are not all the possible wellness diagnoses that may be identified. The above are examples of nursing diagnoses that should be considered when planning care for the older adult.

KEY CONCEPTS

- Although the population as a whole is aging, the greatest categorical increase by group percentage is occurring among those 85 years old and over.
- Old age must be studied as a complex phenomenon with biopsychosocial and spiritual aspects affecting the manner in which an individual ages.
- Each aged cohort is in some ways distinctly different from others, and individual aged persons become more unique the longer they live. Thus one must be careful in attributing any specific characteristics to "old age."
- Normal old age cannot be easily measured as compared with young or middle adulthood.
- It is expected that as the majority of baby boomers become categorically old, in about the year 2010, there will be many changes in the experience of aging in the United States.
- The serious study of gerontology in the United States is comparatively new, reaching back only about 50 years.
- The number of centenarians is increasing rapidly, and the study of their lives holds fascination for many scientists and laypersons.
- Political actions and appropriations have had far-reaching influence on the individual experience of aging, chiefly through Medicare, Medicaid, and Social Security.
- With the advance of medical science, there has been a tendency to prolong the lives of the old and to consider their medical needs predominant.
- Nursing has led the field in gerontology because nurses were the first professionals in the nation to be certified as geriatric specialists.
- Certification assures the public of nurses' commitment to specialized education and qualification for the care of the aged.
- Requirements for accreditation of nursing programs should include solid evidence of special study in the care of the aged.
- The major U.S. organizations devoted exclusively to nurses caring for the aged are the National Gerontological Nursing Association, the National Conference of Gerontological Nurse Practitioners, and the National Association of Directors of Nursing Administration in Long Term Care.
- Clinical research in gerontic nursing is becoming more prevalent because nurses are better prepared and more confident in conducting research.
- The major changes in health care delivery have resulted in numerous revised, refined, and emergent roles for nurses in the field of gerontology.
- Advanced practice nurses have either nurse practitioner qualifications or clinical nurse specialist education. Advanced practice role opportunities for nurses are numerous and are seen as potentially saving money in health care delivery while facilitating more holistic health care.
- Geriatric nurses who desire to do so have found many opportunities for independent practice.
- Geriatric nursing at its best requires specialized education, maturity, commitment, and sensitivity.

▲ CASE STUDY

Joe was 55 years old and had just completed an accelerated program in nursing because he already had academic degrees in physics and biology before entering the program. He had not really been interested in nursing until working in hospice brought him in contact with people at their most vulnerable and he knew that he was helpful in their passage. It was a very gratifying experience. He thought more expertise in nursing would augment his natural caring capacities and sensitivities. His one concern was that his age might be a limiting factor in getting employment. However, he was aware of the nursing shortage and did not worry much about it. When he began looking into the job market he discovered that the beginning wages were not sufficient to support his established lifestyle and the positions that were open demanded he be responsible for numerous individuals on a critical care unit that was poorly staffed. As a new graduate and a mature individual, he realized that the situation would be much too demanding, as well as dangerous, but he gave it a try for a couple of months. He soon realized that there was no time for the nursing activities he had expected to find most fulfilling. He knew he needed to make a change. When he saw one of his classmates in the supermarket he learned that she had taken a position in a long-term care facility. "Why?" was his only comment. When she responded that she was also in an advanced geriatric nurse practitioner program, he again asked, "Why?"

Based on the case study of Joe, this newly graduated nurse, develop a plan for the counseling and discussion you might have given if you were his classmate, using the following procedure:

List his comments that provide subjective data.
List information that provides objective data.
From these data, identify the nurse's present needs.
Discuss the options that are open to Joe.
Speculate on the outcome criteria that you would anticipate.
How would you evaluate the success of his nursing education as it influenced his early career in nursing?

▲ CASE STUDY

Karen began to be aware of her own aging just as she approached menopause. At 47, she occasionally felt stiffness in her joints on arising in the morning. She found herself wishing her grown children would leave the nest, which they showed little inclination to do. Her husband was concerned about his job security because there were numerous companies "downsizing." Karen realized that she was depressed and yet continued in the same pattern as she had for a number of years: work as office manager for a small firm 40 hours each week, go to the gym two nights each week after work to exercise, clean house on Saturday, loll about on Sunday and perhaps work in her garden. Then she began to worry about her widowed mother as she saw some of her friends overwhelmed with caretaking responsibilities for parents and adult children. There seemed no end in sight. She was beginning to look forward to a time when she could retire but realistically knew that was a long way off. She became aware that her life offered little adventure and had become routine; that she was rapidly entering the ranks of the "older Americans." She read numerous ads about hormone replacement therapy for older women. She questioned herself—was she fearful of aging? What was it she feared? What did she want from the remainder of her life? Alarmed, she realized she was thinking of "remainder" rather than "future." She found herself saying, "Is this all there is? Is life just one day after another filled with small and large problems?" "Is there anything I should be doing in preparation for my old age?"

Based on the case study, develop a nursing care plan using the following procedure:

List Karen's comments that provide subjective data.

List information that provides objective data. From these data identify and state, using accepted format, two nursing diagnoses you determine are most significant to Karen at this time.

List two of Karen's strengths.

Determine and state outcome criteria for each diagnosis. These must reflect some alleviation of the problem identified in the nursing diagnosis and must be stated in concrete and measurable terms.

Plan and state one or more interventions for each diagnosed problem. Provide specific documentation of source used to determine appropriate intervention. Incorporate Karen's strengths into at least one intervention.

Evaluate success of intervention. Interventions must correlate directly with the stated outcome criteria in order to measure the outcome success.

STUDY QUESTIONS/ACTIVITIES

What do you think are the triggering events that have increased your interest in aging persons?

Name five beliefs you have that are based on your experience with aging people. Discuss these and locate references within the text that either support or refute your belief.

What are some of the sociocultural factors that have influenced our present views of the aged?

Complete the Expectations Regarding Aging survey and discuss.

How has the history of aging influenced our present concerns about aging?

Discuss how an individual's personal needs should influence the direction of her or his studies.

Discuss your thoughts about the relevance of the nursing educational system to the actual care of the aged.

Discuss your expectations of and obligations toward professional organizations that relate to nursing and gerontology.

Survey your community for available positions in nursing and summarize the areas of need and those that are being neglected.

Interview a supervising nurse in each of the following settings: hospital, emergency department, home care, hospice, and nursing home. Ask the supervising nurses what they consider to be the greatest needs in the care of the aged within their settings. Ask what they consider to be the advantages of their setting in the care of the aged.

Compare variations in institutional and community roles in geriatric nursing and discuss some of the underlying differences.

Prioritize some of the immediate needs in the field of geriatric nursing and how these might best be addressed.

Discuss some of the pioneers in geriatric nursing and how their contributions and thoughts have affected your feelings about gerontic nursing.

Write a short essay (two or three pages) about the old person you have enjoyed or most respected in your lifetime.

Develop a collage depicting themes of aging.

Explore literature and identify attitudes toward aging conveyed in the literature.

Carefully examine the photograph of an unknown elder. Make up a story about him or her.

RESEARCH QUESTIONS

What aspects of geriatric nursing roles do nurses find most gratifying?

Why do nursing home nurses stay and why do they leave?

What is the actual time spent in baccalaureate nursing programs on clinical experiences caring for the aged?

What is the actual time in the curriculum of baccalaureate nursing schools spent on content related only to the care of the aged?

At what age or in which circumstances are individuals most likely to begin considering their own aging?

What are the most frequently held assumptions related to the experience of aging?

What effect has the changing intergenerational structure had on attitudes toward aging?

The field of historic investigation is ripe for further studies, and there are pioneering gerontic nurses that need to be interviewed regarding their perceptions of the specialty. Some who need to be studied: Doreen Norton, Irene Burnside, Margaret Dimond, Neville Strumpf, Lois Evans, Lois Knowles, Barbara Lee, and Loretta Ford. What are the perspectives of gerontic nurse-pioneers on the future of nursing the aged?

REFERENCES

Administration on Aging (AOA): Geographic distribution—a profiles of older Americans, 2001. Available at *www.aoa.gov/aoa/stats/profile/2001/6.html*

Administration on Aging (AOA), International Division, Department of Health and Human Services: Strategies for a society for all ages, Oct 2002. Available at *www.aoa.dhhs.gov/international/soc-allage-eng.html*

American Association of Retired Persons (AARP): *Global aging: achieving its potential,* Washington, DC, 2001, AARP.

American Health Care Association (AHCA): New study on skilled nursing care in America: strong demand for nurses far exceeds supply. Available at *www.ahca.org/news/staff-02-2001.htm*

American Nurse 34(4):4, July/Aug 2002. Available at *www.NursingWorld.org*

American Nurses Association (ANA): The American Nurses Association's bill of rights for registered nurses, *Am Nurse* 34(6):16, Nov/Dec 2002. Available at *www.NursingWorld.org*

American Society on Aging: Developing and marketing new products for older people, *Generations* 19(1): whole issue, Spring 1995.

Anderson CA: From the editor: a new vision for collective bargaining, *Nurs Outlook* 47(5):197, 1999.

Anderson CA: From the editor: our obligation to the next generation, *Nurs Outlook* 48(4):149, 2000.

Atchley RC: Gerontology and business: getting the right people for the job, *Generations* 19(2):42, 1995.

Buckwalter KC, Stolley JM, Farran CJ: Managing cognitive impairment in the elderly: conceptual, intervention and methodological issues, *On Line Journal of Nursing Synthesis* 6(10), 1999. Available at *www.stti.iupui.edu/library/ojksn*

Buffum MD, Wolfe NS: Post-traumatic stress disorder and the World War II veteran, *Geriatr Nurs* 16(6):264, 1995.

Cantor N: *In the wake of the plague,* New York, 2002, Harper Collins.

Christensen D: Making sense of centenarians: genes and life style help people live through a century, *Science News Online* 159(10), 2001. Available at *www.sciencenews.org*

Elsner RJF et al: Ethical and policy considerations for centenarians—the oldest-old, *Image J Nurs Sch* 31(3):263, 1999.

Ferrell BR: The marriage: geriatric and oncology, *Geriatric Nursing* 20(5):238-240, 1999.

Fitzpatrick JJ, editor: *Annu Rev Nurs Res* 20, 2002 (entire issue devoted to geriatric nursing research).

Fulmer TT: Elder mistreatment, *Annu Rev Nurs Res* 20:369, 2002.

Fulmer TT et al: *Critical care nursing of the elderly,* ed 2, New York, 2001, Springer.

Gelbach S: Nursing care of the aged, *Am J Nurs* 43(12):1113, 1943.

Greene R, Administration on Aging (AOA): American Society on Aging (ASA) CAREPro Project report, ANA, Philadelphia, July 1, 2002.

Hinshaw AS: Nursing knowledge for the 21st century: opportunities and challenges, *J Nurs Sch* 32(2):117, 2000.

Hudacek S: *Making a difference: stories from the point of care,* Indianapolis, IN, 2000, Center Nursing Press, Sigma Theta Tau International Society of Nursing.

Larson Long Term Care Group: LTC-alert, June 20, 2001. Available at *gsherman@iris.net*

Matzo ML, Sherman DW: *Quality nursing care for the older adult at the end of their life,* St. Louis, 2003, Mosby/Elsevier.

Meneilly GS, Tessier D: Diabetes in elderly adults, *J Gerontol* 56A(1):M5, 2001.

Mezey M, Fulmer T: The future history of gerontological nursing, *J Gerontol* 57A(7):M438, 2002.

Mezey M, Fulmer T, Fletcher K: A perfect NICHE for gerontology nurses, *Geriatr Nurs* 23(3):118, 2002 (entire issue devoted to models of geriatric nursing practice).

Neugarten BL: *Middle age and aging: a reader in social psychology,* Chicago, 1968, University of Chicago Press.

Rosenfeld P et al: Gerontological nursing content in baccalaureate nursing programs: findings from a national survey, *J Prof Nurs* 15(2):84, 1999.

Sarkisian CA et al: Development, reliability and validity of the Expectations Regarding Aging (ERA-38) survey, *Gerontologist* 42(4):542, 2002.

Smolensky M (executive director, the American Nurses Credentialing Center): Personal communication, Washington, DC, Jan 2002.

Strumpf N, Evans L: Leaders in geriatric nursing: Strumpf and Evans, *Geriatr Nurs,* 2003.

Strumpf NE et al: *Restraint-free care: individualized approached for frail elders,* New York, 1998, Springer.

Touhy T: A history of geriatric nursing. In Dunphy C, editor: *Gerontological nursing: caring for and about older adults,* 2003, Delmar.

Travis S: President's message: leadership and followership, NGNA president's message, Sept 2002. Available at *www.ngna.org/html/presmsg.htm*

United Nations Population Division: World population highlights, Nov 2002. Available at *www.un.org/esa/population/unpop.htm*

U.S. Bureau of the Census: *Statistical abstract of the United States: 2002,* ed 122, Washington, DC, 2001, U.S. Government Printing Office.

U.S. Senate Special Committee on Aging: *Swindlers, hucksters and snake oil salesmen: hype and hope marketing anti-aging products to seniors,* serial no 107-114, Washington, DC, 2001, U.S. Government Printing Office. Available at *www.bookstoregpr.gov* and *www.frwebgate.access.gpo.gov/ cgi-bin/ getdoc.cgi?*

Wallhagen MI: Hearing impairment, *Annu Rev Nurs Res* 20:341, 2002.

Ward K: A vision of tomorrow: transformational nursing leaders, *Nurs Outlook* 50(3):121, 2002.

Wolanin MO: Personal communication, San Antonio, TX, 1995.

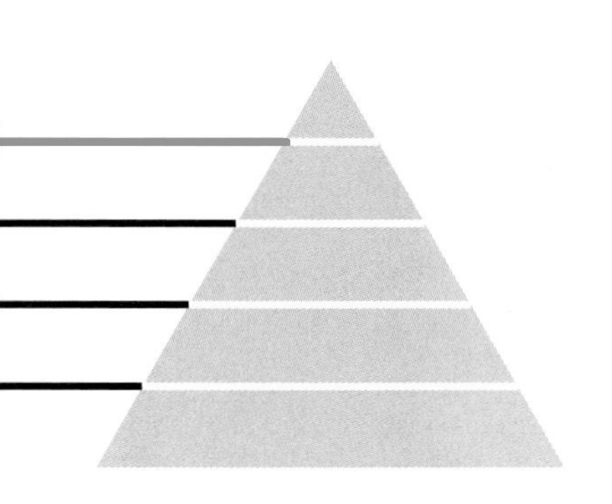

CHAPTER 2

Theories of Aging

Patricia Hess

A student learns

Due to the fact that some periods of life are set apart by certain events, it is generally assumed that a period labeled "Old Age" begins with a definite entrance at a certain year or following some outward event which manifests its beginning. However, unless there is a sudden onset of one of the chronic bodily disorders associated with age, we cannot detect an external symbol of entrance into old age.

Tatyana Urisman, age 30

An elder speaks

When I was a young girl Einstein was proposing the molecular theory of matter, and we still believed there were some truths that were beyond dispute. We had never heard of DNA or RNA and only knew of genes in the most rudimentary theoretical sense. Now truth is the greatest of all the theories of relativity, and I hear that scientists believe there is a gene that is controlling my life span. I really hope they find it before I die.

Bessie, age 72

LEARNING OBJECTIVES

On completion of this chapter, the reader will be be able to:

1. Name the major theorists who have contributed to theories of aging.
2. Identify some of the historic beliefs about aging that have influenced present-day theorists.
3. Discuss longevity and the beliefs about it that have changed over time.
4. Compare several major theories of aging.
5. Relate some of the problems encountered in attempting to explain aging within one consistent, all-encompassing theory.
6. State a definition of aging that is comprehensive and present it for discussion.
7. Contrast several personality types and how these may influence the aging process.
8. Explain the major biologic, psychologic, and sociologic theories of aging.

EARLY THEORIES OF AGING

This chapter is meant to provide the reader with background on the most prominent and accepted theories of aging—biologic, psychologic, and sociologic. None of the theories are treated in depth, but all should be investigated in cited original works for a more thorough understanding. The student must keep in mind that there are no core theories that all people accept. Ultimately one must consider all aspects of development and attempt to combine them into a holistic view of the individual—personally unique as he or she deals with problems common in the history of the human race.

Buhler (1964) was one of the first humanistic psychologists who saw the uniqueness and potential in each life span. Buhler began in the 1930s to collect biographic and autobiographic material, production and performance records, and biologic and psychologic studies to define three distinct types of adult developmental progression: (1) a type dominated by biophysical performance, (2) a type dominated by production and achievement, and (3) a type dominated by contemplative integration. Her approach, followed by Lehman (1953) and Kuhlen (1968), gave a clearer picture of the multifaceted nature of adult development. This approach might be useful in understanding the varied developmental patterns of individuals of different personality types—for example, Jung's introverts and extroverts (1971). The important notion is that individuals may be genetically or socially endowed to follow a unique developmental style within their historic and cultural framework. Newer works, such as Benner's "interpretive phenomenology" (1994), are adding further dimensions of understanding to the phenomenon of aging. As she indicates, the study of humans cannot be reduced to a set of procedures or characteristics but must provide an interpretation of the lived experience that is plausible and auditable, and one that offers understanding of practices, meanings, and concerns.

Theories have for the most part emerged from studies of vulnerable populations being served by professionals of one sort or another. The aged are prime targets for medicine and nursing care—thus the biomedicalization of aging. Theories that arise from the study of elderly male veterans or individuals in nursing homes have often been extrapolated, in all sincerity, to explain aging. Some theorists have even speculated that corollaries of the stages of early childhood may be seen in reverse order as one ages. Of course, these presumptions and assumptions have led to gross errors in understanding the mass of aging individuals; in fact, the silent majority of the aged are not available for study. Only recently has serious attention been given to the fact that the aged are composed of two distinctly different genders; this has come about in large part because of pharmaceutical interest in the huge market potential of postmenopausal women. Further discussion of gender issues can be found in Chapter 19.

Many questions about development in old age remain unanswered. How do people change in the later years? What is the reason for and purpose of aging? What is one meant to accomplish in the last half of the life span? What are the tasks? What are the expected internal and external resources? What is the meaning of this last part of the life span? These are not new questions. Theories about them have been debated since the early Greeks; Plato, Aristotle, Cicero, and Montaigne sought the answers (Box 2-1).

Box 2-1 Historic Figures and Their Beliefs about Aging

Aristotle	Disengagement, interiority
Cicero and Montaigne	Self-discovery, pursuit of gentility and complexity
Plato	Development of wisdom Metamorphosis of the soul
Galen	Statesmanship and responsibility
Villanova	Moderation and humoral balance critical to vitality
Leonardo da Vinci	Coping with reality of physical decline
Cornaro	Restricted diet and moderation for long life
Sanctorius	Decay of body "spirits" leading to "universal hardness of fibres"
Fothergill	Effects of mind on body Positive attitudes recommended
Rush	Importance of heredity
Charcot	Latency periods of disease that only appear in old age

LIFE SPAN THEORY DEVELOPMENT

Life span development refers to an individual's progress through time and implies an expected pattern of change. Traditionally, it has been seen as a composite of three elements: biologic, sociologic, and psychologic, expressed through a combination of many variable and some predictable processes.

Although linear time and causal relationships are largely a scientifically cultivated and Eurocentric cultural preoccupation, we are aware that many human and biologic processes are time dependent. Some of the conceptual hurdles in determining developmental issues and phases in adult life are the lack of a clear definition of aging and the overreliance on culturally embedded expectations. Most definitions focus on the gradual decline of cellular replication and function based on either stochastic or nonstochastic theories as discussed later in this chapter. Stochastic theories propose error catastrophes in control mechanisms such as RNA that cannot be predicted but occur randomly. Nonstochastic theories propose changes biologically "intrinsic" to human beings and genetically programmed. "Usual aging" refers to changes in the elderly that are determined by a combination of disease and adverse environmental and lifestyle factors. "Successful aging" refers to those elderly individuals demonstrating only physiologic decrements uncomplicated by disease, environmental exposures, and lifestyle factors (Rowe and Schneider, 1990). As usual, it is apparent that bodily functions are deemed most significant. We have yet to find a clear definition of biopsychosocial aging that does not involve excessive reliance on the nature of cellular and systemic changes. We believe that an integrated understanding of aging remains elusive. However, life span theorists provide some useful ideas.

Two opposing metatheoretic issues have formed the foundations for life span developmental theorists. One is the belief that over time predominant personality characteristics become enlarged and are maintained at the expense of more complex characteristics that simply require energy the aging individual no longer has. The organism eventually runs down and at last becomes chaotic. The contrasting view is that living organisms tend to differentiate and acquire increasing complexity, but ultimately the differentiation becomes disorganization. Birren and Cunningham (1985) suggest that ultimate disorganization begins when the central nervous system control mechanisms lose their effectiveness in maintaining the dynamic equilibrium necessary to adapt to changes in the internal and external environment.

We believe that aging is an energy process beginning at conception that is directed by genetic endowment and impelled by perceived phenomenologic events that sustain the process until the biologic mechanism ceases to function. The course of behavior throughout the life span appears to have three major forces: heredity, culture, and individual choice (Birren and Cunningham, 1985). In addition, the totality of influences that impinge on any one individual, conceptualized by Kurt Lewin (1951) as "life-space," must be considered. To determine the manner in which these influences form patterns that intermingle in some loosely predictable way is the quest of the developmental gerontologist.

Biologic age is the individual's present position with respect to potential life span. Vital organ and functional capacities are as important as elapsed time in applying such a definition. Pure chronologic measure of time since birth tells us little about the vigor of an individual, but it is usually the primary measure of aging. Although we have been aware of the ebb and flow of vitality in individuals and the significance of biorhythms for several decades, these have stirred renewed interest and study only recently. Circadian rhythms, or day/night shifts in capacity and function, are time and light dependent and regulate many hormonal and enzymatic processes. There is some evidence that biorhythms are altered and become less consistently rhythmic during the aging process. Van Gool and Mirmiran (1986) reviewed the literature on the subject of aging, circadian rhythms, and the metabolic clock. They believe that the human organism can be visualized as a complex of clocks in a clock shop that is located in the suprachiasmatic nucleus of the brain. These numerous "clocks" under ideal circumstances are synchronized but may be desynchronized in the process of aging by some unknown factors. This conceptualization suggests that metabolic age may be a more accurate measure of aging status than chronologic age (Schroots and Birren, 1990). The search for psychosocial rhythms, on the other hand, has never been made explicit because these defy measurement and seem purely conjecture, yet we suspect there are psychosocial waves lapping at the shores of each lifetime that are just as predictable as the more measurable biologic ebb and flow of physiologic juices. We would like to know how behavior becomes organized over the life course in response to intrinsic biologic changes and which psychologic patterns might be common enough to allow some predictablity.

Psychologic age is expressed through the efficiency and control with which one exhibits memory, learning capacity, skills, emotions, and judgment. Maturity and efficacy are indices of the manner in which one is able to adapt psychologically over time to the requirements of the physical and social environment. To complicate this, the satisfactory and effective psychologic adjustment to one's life-space may be excellent but totally inappropriate for another place and time. For example, a healthy psychologic adaptation to a nursing home would be entirely different than that of psychologic adaptation to community living; such adaptations may have little chronologic correlation. Thus individuals may demonstrate the psychologic characteristics of maturity or immaturity at any age, totally incongruent with chronologic age. Psychologic time is nonlinear; it is past, present, or future oriented; and it may be regressed or progressed by internal and external events. One may be older or younger biologically, functionally, and psychologically than his or her chronologic age.

Social age is measured by age-graded behaviors carrying an expected status and role within a particular culture or society. Transitions are often marked by ritual in stable societies. Type of dress, language, institutional and role participation, and status are all indices of social age that become less distinct or predictable in the course of chronologic aging.

In a divergent, rapidly changing society such as ours where diversity is encouraged, there is less tendency toward age-graded behaviors. Often, it is only wrinkles and gray hair that may provide age categorization because activities, dress, and living situations are not usually predictably based on age in the United States.

Biologically, humans have some influence on their destiny, although we have tended to give this undue emphasis in our present era; sociologically, they have considerably more. On a psychologic level human potential for adaptation is most clearly apparent. The intimate relationship between biologic, social, and psychologic development that exists through childhood and adolescence does not remain as closely intermeshed in adulthood.

ANTHROPOLOGY AND ETHNOGRAPHY OF AGING

Anthropologic studies of the aged in remote places have emerged intermittently since the early nineteenth century as exotic curiosities. They are rarely exclusive studies of the aged but rather are a part of a general cultural study. Tidbits of information about how the aged have been treated in other societies, cultures, and subcultures have sometimes filled us with guilt or wonder. It is easy to believe that historically less industrialized societies somehow treated their aged better than we, but we must remember that there were usually fewer aged and by virtue of attrition only the very hardy and unusual lived to be very old.

It is also important to be aware that anthropologists must cultivate sources in whatever society they study, and these sources are often the aged. These culture bearers will share what they wish and keep secret what they do not care to reveal. There may also be problems with the subtleties of language in translation. Anthropologists often live within a culture for a period of time and win friends and confidants; it is likely that their presence will influence the actions around them, just as our families are usually much different when visitors are present than when alone. There is currently great interest in the care and treatment of the aged in remote times and places as we ferret out the intricacies, meanings, and mysteries of the aged. Geographic pockets of remarkably long-lived people are of particular interest, although documentation of births may be unreliable. Additional discussion of longevity is found later in this chapter.

Presently we have the unsound inclination to study blacks and whites as separate ethnographic groups. Federal statistics are often presented in this manner (U.S. Bureau of the Census, 2001) as if these were the major and basic ethnographic categories. Clearly, these categories are inaccurate, are exclusionary, and perpetuate stereotypic thinking. Divisiveness is promoted when groups are labeled as Mexican American, African American, Native American, or any of the various other contractions that have no implicit meaning except that of distant geography. To understand our aged, it is important to inquire about origins and customs while fully recognizing that socioeconomic status and educational opportunities have had much more to do with present lifestyle than origins of forebears. Chapter 19 deals more fully with cultural issues.

EVOLUTIONARY BASIS FOR AGING

An evolutionary perspective of old age implies the emergence of certain characteristics best fitting the individual for survival in changing social and environmental conditions. From that perspective, survival is an end in itself. However, evolutionary theorists tend to view old age as an addendum to the life of sexual maturation and propagation. People usually have raised their children to maturity by the time they are 50 years old. In such cases, seemingly, the last 30 years of life appear meaningless from a species survival perspective. Rosenfeld (1985) postulated a reason for those years of existence unnecessary to species reproduction and nurturance. He proposed the concept of "nature's redundancy," the overassurance that an individual will survive to reproduce and raise progeny to the point of propagation. From a species propagation model, old age has seemed to have little meaning until recently. Now it is becoming more apparent that "nature" has been wise in keeping people alive and vigorous long enough to care for grandchildren. In an increasingly complex, dangerous, and demanding society, many parents simply cannot cope and their capacities for parenting are eroded. Grandparents have become the primary caretakers of 20% of the children in the United States today (Fuller-Thomson et al, 1997). This role will be discussed more completely in Chapter 18.

PERSPECTIVES ON AGING

All theories and perspectives of aging emerge from underlying premises of the researcher, philosopher, culture, and historic era. A factor of supreme importance in examining old age as a phenomenon is the human inability to be objective about being human and most especially about aging. We are all aging, and, depending on our exposure to and involvement with old persons, we may have a negative, moderate, or positive view of that stage of life. It must be accepted at the outset that we cannot extricate ourselves from the fabric of our own physical, social, cultural, and personal experience. Since the last edition of this textbook was published, we have observed heightened interest in ethnographic, phenomenologic, and spiritual aspects of aging. The questions reflect a growing interest in the experience of aging, as well as its functional parameters. Questions are now being raised more insistently about the meaning of the life experience.

BIOLOGIC THEORIES OF AGING

Scientifically, the architectural basis of a person begins with the cell and cell division. Cell division (meiosis and mitosis) continues to shape the human organism with its varied systems at different rates of generation and regeneration throughout the life span.

Theories of biologic and physiologic aging attempt to explain three in vivo biocomponents: (1) cells that multiply clonally (meiosis) throughout life, such as white blood cells and epithelial cells; (2) cells that are incapable of division and renewal, such as neurons; and (3) noncellular material with little turnover that comes under integrated physiologic control, such as collagen and intercellular substances. These cellular characteristics result in mechanical failure of nonreplaceable parts in organ systems, accumulation of metabolites, depletion or exhaustion of body reserves, and morphologic problems of cell development, which give organs size, shape, and structure.

Various biologic theories of aging have been more persuasive than others at various times. A unifying theory does not yet exist that explains the mechanics and causes underlying the biologic phenomenon of aging. Theories of aging can be addressed from a molecular, cellular, or systems level point of view. It will become apparent that some theories emerge from others and that one or more theories could be superimposed on others. Each theory in its own right provides a clue to the aging process. However, many unanswered questions remain. Scientists in their continual search for truth persist in piecing together the puzzle of aging. New and exciting data concerning biologic theories of aging have emerged recently through the application of more sophisticated methods of unlocking the secrets of the cell. We are beginning to confirm some of the previous suppositions and to develop a more thorough understanding of the genetic, molecular, and biochemical basis of cellular changes of aging. In time, the student will begin to discriminate and develop an eclectic approach to theories of aging as he or she becomes familiar with the many facets of the aging process.

Stochastic Theories

Stochastic theories suggest that aging events occur randomly and accumulate with time. These theories include the gene theory, the error theory, the somatic mutation theory, the free radical theory, the cross-link theory, the clinker theory, and the wear-and-tear theory.

Gene Theory. The gene theory suggests that one or more harmful genes in the organism become active in later life, causing failure of the organism to survive. Two variations on this theme exist. One postulates that there are two types of genes: those that mediate youthful vigor and mature adult well-being (juvenescent genes) and those that promote functional decline and structural deterioration (senescent genes). The second variation infers that genes play a dual role: The juvenescent aspects of genes function in early life, and senescent aspects of genes are activated in middle age and thereafter. The second concept is exemplified in female menopause. During the reproductive years estrogen facilitates the normal reproductive cycle. At the point of perimenopause and menopause, the estrogen level declines, increasing the risk of arteriosclerosis and hypertension in women (Hayflick, 1987).

The most important recent discovery in genetics has come from the lowly worm *Caenorhabditis elegans.* One might say the worm has turned and shown one identifiable gene that controls its life span. Researchers are systematically mapping the involved genome with the expectation that it may serve to point the way to a gene controlling the life span in humans (Makinodan, 1990; Recer, 2000).

Error Theory. The error theory of aging (sometimes called the Orgel theory or the error catastrophe theory) proposes an accumulation of errors in protein synthesis over time resulting in impaired cellular function. Weakening of organic synthesis produces defective cells. Successive generations of these faulty cells develop and eventually interfere with the ability to maintain biologic function. Two steps are important in normal protein synthesis: (1) An amino acid must be selected by an activating enzyme and then must attach to an appropriate RNA molecule, and (2) an RNA codon must pair with an anticodon. Errors may occur in the RNA synthesis; if great enough, these errors will impair cell function. The greater the number of errors accumulated in the macromolecule of the cell, the faster the accumulation of further error. Errors of ribonucleic acid (RNA) and deoxyribonucleic acid (DNA) synthesis are indistinguishable from each other. The error catastrophe theory, although no longer widely accepted, has spurred a great deal of research.

In fact, some research has shown that the amino acid sequence does not change in young and old animals, nor is there an increase in defective RNA with aging. Age-related changes have not been found in the accuracy of Poly (V)–directed protein synthesis either. Errors have been found to occur more readily in the posttranscription of proteins (Schneider, 1995).

Normal somatic cells may become aberrant through spontaneous and innocent error or through radiation, permitting an undefined life span and errant cell propagation. Similar behavior is seen in cancer cell activity.

Somatic Mutation Theory. The somatic mutation theory is similar to the error theory, but it suggests that when cells are exposed to x-ray radiation or chemicals a cell-by-cell alteration of DNA occurs, increasing the incidence of chromosomal abnormalities. These mutations are a time-dependent accumulation of chromosome aberrations thought to be more frequent in youth. Subsequently, replicated cells are perpetuated and harbored, with the deleterious effects appearing in later life. The ultimate result is a decrease in cellular function and organ efficiency. Those somatic cells that are of the non-dividing type and possess a limited life span such as brain and muscle cells are not replaced when injured or dead.

Free Radical Theory. Free radicals contain unpaired ions that exist momentarily and are highly reactive molecules that can damage protein membranes, enzymes, and DNA. Their molecular structure differs from ordinary molecules in that they possess an extra electric charge (free electron). This charge instigates a one-time, irreversible, and energy-wasteful reaction that damages or alters the original structure or function of the cell membrane.

The free radical theory, proposed by Harmen (1956), emphasizes the importance of the mechanism of oxygen use by the cell (Hayflick, 1987). The greatest source of free radicals is the metabolism of oxygen, which produces the superoxide radical O_2^-. Oxygen is a highly reactive gas both inside and outside the human body. Internally, the mitochondria, the energy generator of cells, emits destructive oxidizing molecules of proteins, fats, and carbohydrates, resulting in free radical formation and unstable end products or compounds. For example, oxidation of polyunsaturated fats forms lipid peroxides that cross-link proteins, lipids, and DNA (Hampton, 1991; Olshansky et al, 2002).

In the course of normal living, oxidation is continually causing cell destruction and a biologic dichotomy: the need for oxygen for metabolic survival opposed to the gradual self-destruction through the release of free radicals from peroxidation referred to by some as the "oxygen paradox" (Sohal and Weindruch, 1996). Although body cells possess the capacity to eliminate unwanted waste and materials, neutralize by-products, and repair damage, free radical accumulation is thought to be faster than the repair process of the organism.

Scientists who favor the free radical theory consider the cell membrane the key to survival and think that the greatest damage is perpetuated by free radicals at this level. Within the cell, metallic ions, enzymes, and cellular materials combine with oxygen to form free radicals and compounds. Oxidation of cellular waste provides an additional source of radicals and electrons. In arterial walls, oxygen interacts with lipoprotein (a substance in the artery wall), forming free radicals. When DNA, the genetic component of the cell, is irradiated, it responds with free radical formation and establishes aberrant cellular growth and development, which affect aging. Copper, iron, and magnesium in the body increase free radical activity by catalytic action in the oxidation process.

Free radical activity is also introduced into the body from the environment. The best-known source is smog. Other environmental sources thought to cause harmful cumulative breakdown effects in cells are oxidation of gasoline in automobile engines, by-products in the plastic industry, drying linseed oil paints, and atmospheric ozone (Hampton, 1991; Sharma, 1988).

The mitochondria, major site of cellular oxidation, are thought to be protected from the hazards of free radical activity by vitamin E and coenzyme Q or Q10. It is thought that vitamin E provides protection through its antioxidant behavior (Walford, 1983; Hampton, 1991; Scheer, 1996). Studies exploring vitamin E's effectiveness as an antioxidant demonstrate that vitamin E deficiencies increase excessive lipid oxidation. At normal cellular levels of vitamin E, a slower oxidation rate occurs. The drug COQ (ubiquinone), also known as coenzyme Q, Q10, or COQ10 (Kidd et al, 1988; Scheer, 1996), is an essential energy carrier and antioxidant that sparks mitochondrial energy production and easily gives up its electrons to neutralize oxidants. Q10 exists in many foods, but the ability of an individual to synthesize the nutrient from diet begins to wane in middle age (Scheer, 1996).

Certain enzymes function to degrade, neutralize, or detoxify free radicals that attack the cell membrane. These free radical scavengers include superoxide mutanase, catalase, and glutathione peroxidase. Research at the National Institute of Aging has found that the enzyme dismutase increases proportionally to metabolic rate with increased life span of various species. Individuals who enjoy high levels of protection against oxygen metabolism by-products (free radicals) should live longer than those with lower levels of protection (Walford, 1983). Vitamin A and C and niacin have also been considered to be free radical scavengers because they possess similar properties to mercaptans (free radicals) (Hampton, 1991). Older people generally have decreased blood levels of vitamin A and C. It is thought that these two easily oxidized vitamins form free radical scavengers, binding and neutralizing free radicals in a manner similar to the antioxidant behavior of vitamin E.

The body is thought to be bombarded by both internal and external sources of free radicals (oxidative stress). Injection or daily intake of antioxidants, such as vitamin E, selenium, vitamin C, and various food additives (BHT, BHA, and others), has been found to produce a free radical scavenger effect. If the free radical theory is fundamental to aging, as its proponents believe, monitoring the kind of food consumed and the environment lived in should play an important role toward healthier aging in the future. Food selection might be directed toward intake of items with high antioxidant properties and low potential for stimulating free radical activity (Walford, 1986; Sawada and Carlson, 1987; Agarwal and Sohal, 1996).

Advocates of the free radical theory point to the fundamental microscopic nature of the theory and its relationship to cross-link and chromosomal mutation theories (Hayflick, 1987). Agarwal and Sohal (1996) suggest that susceptibility of living animals to experimentally induced O_2 stress increases with age. Research also continues to determine the significance of age pigment, lipofusin, which accumulates in aging tissue (predominantly in heart and brain cells). Lipofusin is thought to be a by-product of lipid and protein fragmentation from perioxidation of the cell membrane. The significance of lipofusin and the role of free radical scavengers and antioxidants continues to be explored in their relationship to the aging process. Many of today's proported anti-aging therapies by longevity clinics consider this the way to eradicate aging. However, to date, there is no "cure" for aging (Olshansky et al, 2002).

Cross-Link or Connective Tissue Theory. The cross-link theory is based on the internal and external behavior of collagen, elastin, and ground substance in cells, tissues, and extracellular substances. These materials are widespread and involved in the transport and exchange of material for cell function. The theory is thought to explain some of the age-dependent diseases and disorders (Schneider, 1995).

The theory suggests that chemical reactions create strong bonds between molecular structures that are normally separate. Cross-link agents are so numerous and varied in the diet and in the environment that they are impossible to avoid. Aldehydes, minerals (copper and magnesium), and oxidizing fats serve as biologic reservoirs of cross-link–inducing agents. Lipids, proteins, nucleic acid, and carbohydrates are major body chemicals that exist in repetitive, linear structural patterns and are capable of cross-linking.

Saccharides are important ingredients in collagen, elastin, and DNA. Collagen makes up about 25% to 30% of body protein and is important in physiologic function and in some pathologic processes (Sharma, 1988). Collagen forms the gelatinous cell matrix that is responsible for maintaining structural form, support, and strength of tissues. High concentrations of collagen appear in the skin, tendons, bones, muscle, blood vessels, and heart. Discovering the relationship between cross-linkage and aging remains a scientific challenge. Cross-linkage is most rapid between 30 and 50 years of age, but it is not yet known how to prevent cross-links from occurring.

The concept of cross-linkage can best be defined in terms of behavior and characteristics of collagen and elastin, components of connective tissue. Changes in connective tissue indicate that cross-linkage has occurred. Synthesis of new collagen reveals minimum signs of cross-linkage. With age, collagen develops an increased number of cross-links in both intracellular and intercellular structures (Sharma, 1988). Aging collagen becomes increasingly insoluble, chemically stable, and progressively rigid as a result of the cross-link phenomenon. Consider agar or gelatin as an example of cross-linkage. Gelatin, like collagen, loses its sheen, becomes firmer, cracks, and dries out when exposed to air, heat, or sunlight for several days. Its original resilience and rebound disappear. The sheen turns cloudy and dull. Likewise, collagen molecules dehydrate and develop a bonding pattern that links the molecules together.

Elastin in connective tissue mirrors collagen behavior and is equally prone to cross-linkage. Old elastin is frayed, fragmented, and brittle. Extracellular water diminishes and produces a concentration of calcium, sodium, and chloride. Deposits of calcium salts are found throughout the cardiovascular system: in the epicardium and endocardium, in the valves of the heart, and in the major blood vessels. Amino acids are considered to be part of elastin and also cross-link agents. Skin is one of the best examples of what happens in the cross-linkage of elastin. One cannot help but notice the gross change in skin texture and response with age. Skin that was once smooth, silky, firm, and soft becomes drier, saggy, and less elastic.

Cross-linkage of skin tissue has been compared to the changes that occur in the tanning process of animal hides; chemicals applied to hides cause cells or molecules to stick together and transform soft, stretchy skin into a shiny, stiff leather. The importance of connective tissue cross-linkage in the body with age has numerous implications affecting cell permeability, fibril flexibility of muscles, and heart contractility. The passage of gases, nutrients, metabolites, antibiotics, and toxins throughout the vessels are all affected. Tendons become dry and fibrous, teeth may loosen, arterial walls decline in tensile strength, and the lining of the lungs and gastrointestinal tract decreases in efficiency. Glycolated immunoglobulins, glomerular basement membrane proteins, and glycolate lipoproteins and arterial wall proteins are important in development of age-related kidney and arterial diseases (Schneider, 1995). Glycolated proteins are thought to play a major role in age-dependent opacification of crystalline lens protein, leading to eventual cataract development. Elastin, prominent in connective tissue morbidity and distensibility, affects the function of muscle contraction and all types of tissue pulsation that occur in the matrix of connective tissue. DNA also is capable of cross-linkage (Hayflick, 1987). Linkage is attributed to free radicals that bind DNA molecules together somewhere in their chemical makeup. This raises the question of the possible relationship between the free radical and cross-link theories.

Research continues into what stimulates, depresses, and blocks cross-linkage. Caloric restriction has been found to increase life expectancy and decrease cross-linkage in protein and DNA experiments with rats. Prednisolone, too, has been found to decrease the number of cross-links and prolong life (Walford, 1983). Research has identified chemicals known as lathyrogens that inhibit cross-link formation in collagen (Balazs, 1977). Studies have shown that β-aminopropionotrile (BAPN) and penicillamine produce this antilinkage effect. BAPN, however, causes retardation in the development of young collagen. Penicillamine does not seem to disturb young collagen synthesis but instead affects only mature insoluble collagen (Sacher, 1977).

Clinker Theory. The clinker theory can be considered an independent theory or a variation of the somatic, cross-link, or free radical theories. It assumes that there is an accumulation of time-related deleterious substances in the cells of the body. As chemical by-products of metabolism (lipofusin hystones, aldehydes, free radicals) accumulate in the cell cytoplasm, there is interference with the normal cell function by displacement. Free radicals denature protein, and lipofuscin accumulates in the heart, skeletal muscle, the brain, and the nervous system.

Wear-and-Tear Theory. A programmed process is the concept considered in the wear-and-tear theory. Cells are aggravated by the harmful effects of internal and external stressors, which include injurious metabolic by-products and increased failure of DNA to repair the organism or replace vital cellular components. These may cause a progressive decline in cellular function or the death of an increasing number of cells. Striated muscle, heart muscle, muscle fibers, nerve cells, and the brain are nonreplaceable when destroyed by wear and tear or by mechanical or chemical injury.

Nonstochastic Theories

The nonstochastic theories consider aging to be predetermined. These theories include the intrinsic pacemaker theories; immune and neuroendocrine theories, suggesting genetic programming of a specific time for the life span of an organism; and programmed senescence, which implies aging of the entire organism.

Programmed Aging Theory. The initial premise of the programmed aging theory, or biologic or genetic clock, begins with an original pool of genetic information that is played out in an orderly manner. Time correlations with this intrinsic process and the development, maturation, and cessation of activity have been made between the beginning of menopause, thymic atrophy, graying of hair, and myriad other changes, all of which are considered normal aging decrements in physical function over time but not pathologic.

In vitro studies of programmed aging (Hayflick, 1968, 1975, 1977, 1983) are still widely discussed. Experiments with human diploid cell strains have demonstrated that cells double a limited number of times before dying. The number of cell divisions is proportional to the life span of the species. Human cells double 40 to 60 times before the ability to replicate is lost. This in vitro behavior, termed *phase III phenomenon* by Hayflick, is a gradual and sequential degeneration of cell tissue; the precise moment of its occurrence remains elusive.

Preservation of the cells and subsequent extension of the duration of their existence were achieved by keeping the cells at subzero temperatures for long periods. When thawed years later, the cells continued to double from the point at which doubling action had been interrupted. The total number of doublings remained constant. Continued experimentation showed that cells from embryonic donors underwent more population doublings than those acquired from adult donors. Proponents of the programmed aging theory support the inverse relationship between donor age and number of doublings. Cell death or destruction is a normal part of the morphologic and developmental sequence in animals, particularly mammals. It is one way to shed or eliminate those organs necessary only in the embryonic state of development.

Lockshin and Zakeri (1990) added new thoughts to programmed cell death. They theorized that programmed cell death demonstrates (1) that the capacity to self-destruct is common and may be universal among both mitotic cells (lymph system) and postmitotic cells (neurons and muscle fibers), both of which lead to the mechanisms of senescence; (2) that cell death is a response to many factors, including stress, changing developmental states, and trophic support with the resultant effect of rapid fragmentation of the cell DNA, also known as physiologic death (apoptosis) (Pollack and Leeuwenburgh, 2001); and (3) that initiation of the program can involve the activities of only a handful of genes.

Run-Out-of-Program Theory. A variation of the theory of programmed aging, the run-out-of-program theory, suggests that at the time of ovum fertilization a certain amount of genetic material is allocated. When this material is used up, the cells, tissues, and organs fail. This is reflected in the gradual age-related diminution of activity of certain enzymes and organ functions, such as those in the liver and the brain.

Neuroendocrine Control Theory (Pacemaker). The neuroendocrine control theory focuses on aging as part of the life span program regulated by neurohormonal signals that begin at the time of fertilization and continue until death. Common neurons in the high brain centers act as pacemakers that regulate the biologic clock during development and aging.

Aging is manifested in a slowing down or activity imbalance of the pacemaker neurons, affecting neural, muscular, and secretory function as evidenced in involution, reproduction, loss of fertility, menopause, decreased muscle strength, less ability to recover from stress, and impaired cardiovascular and respiratory activity. Specifically, the performance of an organism is linked to a variety of control mechanisms that regulate the interplay between different organs and tissues. Homeostatic adjustment declines, with consequent failure to adapt, and is followed by aging and death. These results may be considered homeostatic failure. Rudman (1992) demonstrated that there was more than one biologic clock (genetic) for aging. Along with other scientists, Rudman looked for chemicals that directly affect the length of life. Adaptation to stress, both internal (emotions, hormones, immunity, metabolism) and external, depends on control mechanisms of nervous and hormonal systems. The pituitary gland is considered to be in direct control of the thyroid, adrenals, and gonads through the indirect signals of the nervous center, the hypothalamus (Wise et al, 1996). With age, some signal efficiency of the pituitary-hypothalamus connection is lost or changed, leading to desynchronization and decreased function of the hypothalamus (or the biologic clock) and an increase in pathology of most organ and tissue systems (Wise et al, 1996). Current thinking suggests that understanding the aging of the reproductive cycle may help us better understand the process of biologic aging because of the interconnectedness of so many neurotransmitters (Wise et al, 1996).

Immunologic Theory. Studies of cell division in numerous vertebrate animals suggest that the cells of the immune system become increasingly more diversified with age and demonstrate a progressive loss of a self-regulatory pattern between the body and the cell (Strehler, 1960; Walford, 1983; Miller, 1996). The result is an autoaggressive phenomenon in which (1) cells normal to the body are misidentified as alien and are attacked by the body's immune system or (2) there is impaired surveillance by antibody cells.

Control of immunity is shared by humoral (B-cell) and cellular (T-cell) systems. In brief, the humoral (B-cell) system provides protection for the body against bacterial and viral reinfection. This function occurs through activity of the plasma cells, tonsillar tissue, abdominal mesentery Peyer patches, and the peripheral lymph system. Cellular immunity (T-cell system) delays hypersensitivity and rejection of foreign tissue cells and organ grafts and provides protection against tumor formation through the activity of the thymus gland and its associated organs (Hershey, 1974). The primary organs in cell-mediated immunity are the bone marrow and the thymus. The spleen and lymph nodes are also important but play a secondary role in cellular immunity. Lymphocytes produced by the thymus and bone marrow serve as precursor cells because they evolve through embryonic development in the organ tissue. Figure 2-1 illustrates the sources and movement of the thymic-independent (B-cell) humoral system and the thymic-dependent (T-cell) cellular immune system. There is presently great interest in the involution of thymic hormonal activity and its relation to aging. Current research suggests that previously thought thymic involution early in adult life may be key in T-cell immune senescence. However, although thymic activity declines by 90% during the first quarter of one's life span, T-cell emigration, proliferation, and removal now strongly indicate the need to look for more evidence to account for the T-cell population changes in adults.

Autoaggression. Lymphocytes generated and released by the lymph nodes are considered to be sensitized to specific antigens. These white blood cells are thought to develop a programmed self-recognition by the time an individual is 1 year old (Hershey, 1974). It has been hypothesized that regulatory cells, particularly the suppressor cells, diminish with age, allowing "previously suppressed clones of autoactive cells to respond" (Birnbaum and Swick, 1981). Any antibodies that are not programmed by this time are identified by the body as foreign and adjudged as invading organisms. Antibodies of the cell-mediated (T-cell) immune system are dispatched from the lymph nodes to surround and devour the invasive antigens by phagocytosis. B and T cells are able to regulate the differential events of humoral and cell-mediated responses. However, the immune response of the cell-mediated system, although major, does receive immune assistance from the

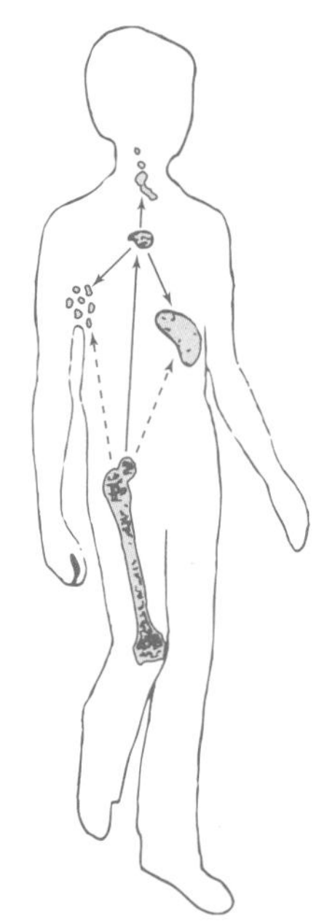

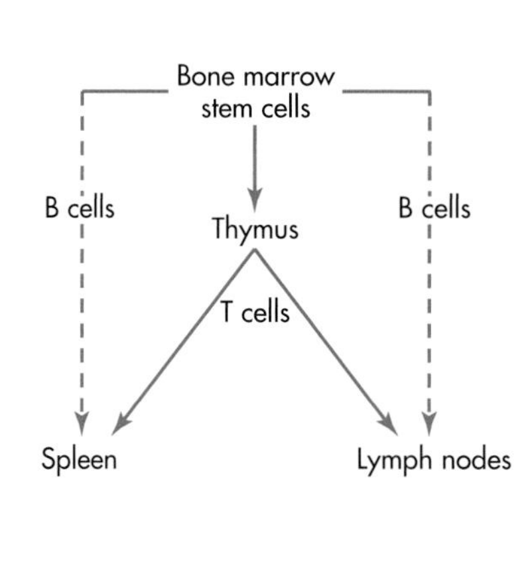

Figure 2-1. Cellular traffic of the immune system. (From Finch C, Hayflick L, editors: *Handbook of the biology of aging,* New York, 1977, Van Nostrand Reinhold.)

humoral system. Nevertheless, cell-mediated reactions take place before humoral ones. Antibodies of the humoral system (B cells) circulate in the blood and attach themselves to antigens in sufficient numbers to dilute the antigens in a neutralizing effect. Specific B and T cells respond to specific antigenic stimulation by generating functional effector cells (antibodies) or by developing a tolerance so that reexposure does not elicit a destructive reaction. Imbalance of B- and T-cell activity gives rise to an increased production of autoantibodies. Cytotoxic (cellular toxicity) effects occur in host tissue when thymic-deprived lymphoid cells are transferred to the peripheral lymphoid circulation. B- and T-cell imbalance results in a compromise of the humoral mechanism, decreasing the body's immune surveillance capability and causing hypersensitivity to the autoimmune phenomenon. The cell-mediated T cells are responsible for hastening the age-related changes attributed to autoimmune reactions; the body battles against itself. The demonstration of chromosome fragility in T cells provides better understanding of the genetic basis of cellular aging (Makinodan, 1990; Miller, 1996). T cells also pinpoint early deficiencies in transduction that influence the transcription of cellular information and may result in identification of metabolic events that create vulnerability (Makinodan, 1990). Box 2-2 outlines key cell changes that occur in old age.

Haptens (low-molecular-weight compounds) in combination with natural body proteins form hapten-protein units. Antibodies mistake these hapten units for antigen and thus attack their own body protein (Guyton and Hall, 1994). The release of abnormal protein products during infectious processes or the release in later life of particular antibodies, which have been dormant or sequestered in various immune system organs from the early development of the individual, is an additional cause for autoimmune responses. Research has shown instances of age-related autoimmune and immune-deficient responses.

Graft-versus-host reaction experiments with mice have demonstrated significantly higher rejection rates of tissue grafts in older mice than in younger mice. This has led to the postulation that greater cell aberration occurs with age and that cell self-regulation is greatly lacking (Makinodan, 1990). This might be one reason why wound healing and generation of

Box 2-2 Important Areas of Immunologic Change in Old Age

Germinal Center
↓ Processing of immune complexes
↓ Dendritic cell traffic
↓ Ig hypermutation

B Lymphocytes
↓ Affinity maturation
↑ Repertoire degeneracy
↓ Idiotype focusing

T Lymphocytes
↑ Memory cells
↓ Naive T cells
↓ IL-2 production
↓ IL-2 receptors
↓ Calcium signals
↓ Protein kinase signals

Modified from Miller RA: The aging immune system: primer and prospectus, *Science* 273:71, 1996.
IL-2, Interleukin-2.

healthy tissue seem to progress more slowly in the aged, despite proper diet, rest, and care.

Immunoglobins, which contain two or more antigen-binding sites and other unique structures, are part of the humoral system and are responsible for antibody activity of globins. There is evidence that gamma globulin, Rh factor, and antithyroid and antiinsulin antibody activity accelerates with increasing age (Rowe and Schneider, 1990). The possibility of immune system exhaustion as a cause of aging has been considered and may eventually explain the number of cases of adult-onset diabetes mellitus and rheumatoid arthritis exacerbations, as well as the development of other conditions among older individuals. Miller (1996) points out that it is not clear from current in vivo findings whether or not immunodeficiencies are due to expansion of others that diminish the functional repertoire of the immune system in old age, thus limiting the ability to respond to new immunogens.

Depletion. Immunodeficient conditions such as infection, autoimmunity, and cancer have been thought to be the body's response to several types of events (Hayflick, 1987; Macieira-Coelho, 1987). Studies of newborn mice with slow virus infections showed a suppression of normal immune function.

Mice infected with leukenogenic virus also responded with suppression of the immune system. In long-lived mice the onset of the decline of immune function began early in life (Makinodan and Yunis, 1977). Correlations can be made with human responses in similar situations because the responses of laboratory animals generally reflect what might occur in human tissue. The question arises whether all vertebrates harbor slow viruses that can induce the gradual decline in the immune system with advancing age. It would seem reasonable to assume that a decline in immune system function would occur because the function of all systems seems to diminish with age and that age-dependent anatomic and physiologic changes, such as decreased secretions, dry skin, and collagen changes, would add to the disruption of the host's defense mechanisms. The simultaneous decline in the immune system and increase in the autoimmune response would seem to constitute an important consideration. A decline in immunity would allow malfunctioning immune cells to surface or exert themselves. Decreased efficiency of the immune system certainly increases vulnerability to disease and malignancy (Kent, 1977; Makinodan, 1990). Figure 2-2 depicts the immune system process of aging.

Immune system, disease, and aging. Viruses or their antigens and corresponding antibodies make up some of the antigen-antibody complexes. When these lodge in specific body sites, such as kidneys and arteries, factors injurious to the tissue are released and initiate the onset of deterioration. This may be instrumental in triggering or causing normal aging and disease.

Autoimmune disorders and aging may be correlated, as evidenced by several shared characteristics. Both processes exhibit lymphoid depletion and hypoplasia, thymic atrophy, and increased plasma cells in lymphoid organs. The most relevant pathologic change that can be evidenced in the immune system with age is thymic atrophy. T-cell–dependent immunity is probably related to decreased circulating thymic hormone levels (see Figure 2-5). As early as 1969 (Quinti et al, 1981), thymic transplants, as well as the administration of young thymocytes or thymic extract to patients, were shown to be able to correct several age-dependent immunologic impairments, such as antibody formation. In the aged, if hypergammaglobulinemia is present, the tests for antibodies are positive. However, the alloantigen response (which requires B- and T-cell cooperation) is decreased. Two types of autoimmune and immunodeficient diseases exist: those that affect the young person and those that affect the older adult. Autoimmune and immunodeficient diseases in older adults illustrate the impact of the immunologic theory on aging. Cell-mediated immunity decreases in older persons and may be responsible for decreased survival (Wayne et al, 1990).

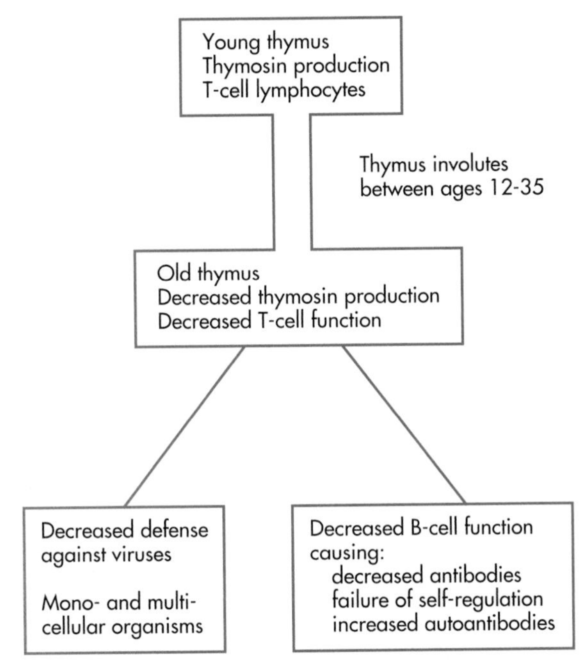

Figure 2-2. Immune system process of aging.

Decline in the immunologic state is conducive to the development of infections, autoimmunities, and cancer. Amyloidosis, cancer, and adult-onset diabetes mellitus have been considered diseases of aging that emanate from immunodeficiencies. Fibers that appear in amyloidosis are identified as chains of immunoglobulins and are present in various body organs of the aged individual. The islets of Langerhans, for instance, in the pancreas show signs of amyloidosis and complement-fixing antiinsulin antibodies with aging. Cancer appears to be strongly influenced by immunodeficiencies, particularly those associated with immunosuppressant drugs. Individuals who require immunosuppressants are 80 times more vulnerable to cancer than those who do not receive such therapy (Makinodan, 1990). Autoimmune mechanisms also contribute to atherosclerosis, hypertension, and thromboembolism in certain susceptible people. Cardiovascular disease, allergic angitis, and rheumatic heart disease are considered partially the result of immune system dysfunction. Senile plaque, found in aging degenerating human brain tissue, contains a large quantity of amyloid fiber. Studies of aging mice suggest that the cause of neuronal degeneration may lie in the neuron-reactive antibodies in the sera of old mice (Nandy et al, 1983).

There is a growing interest in the effects of aging on the mucosal immune system. Evidence suggests that the secretory immune system may be affected by the aging process. It is known that secretory antibodies play an important role in protection of mucosal surfaces from a variety of pathogens. The complexity of the aging regional immune system suggests that a number of factors (e.g., immunoglobulin A [IgA] antibody production) in local ocular, salivary, nasal, and intestinal sites play a pivotal role in the larger immune response (Makinodan, 1990; Michel, 2000).

The acute antibody response to extrinsic antigens, such as pneumococcal and influenza vaccines, is considerably reduced in the elderly. It is thought possible that lowered circulating immunoglobin levels reflect increased response to intrinsic antigens (autoantibodies) (Nicoletti et al, 1993).

Cellular immunity most clearly exhibits an age-related decrease in functional ability. The decline of cell-mediated immunity with increasing age correlates with an increasing frequency of reactivation tuberculosis. However, although reduction in the levels of thymic hormones is clearly age related, it is unclear if thymic involution is associated with increased susceptibility to infection (Tockman, 1990).

Challenging the immunologic theory of aging. No theory is without counter arguments. Studies at Duke University have shown through cross-analysis and longitudinal analysis of immune changes that immunoglobins increased with age in about two thirds of the study population (Makinodan and Yunis, 1977; Michel, 2000).

A correlation was made between low immunoglobin levels in the blood and failure to survive. However, normal to high levels of immunoglobins were noted in the blood of long-lived individuals with various immunodeficiencies. This raised the question, "To what extent do immunoglobins affect aging?" Cell-mediated immunity, presented earlier as a primary factor in immunity, was found to remain relatively intact for the whole life span in long-lived strains of experimental mice (Makinodan and Yunis, 1977).

Early studies suggested a relationship between the immune system and mortality. Researchers continue to attempt to demonstrate the relationship between immune status as an indicator of general health or biologic aging to provide a prognosticator for survival and disease risk. A decline in peripheral blood lymphocyte count has been shown to correlate with diminished 1-year survival in old mice (Bender et al, 1986). Correlation between survival and the pace or extent of immune changes has been demonstrated in three studies of immunity in mice. One study illustrated the relatively short life span of mice with high levels of CD8 T cells (Boersma and Steinmeier, 1985). Another study found a long life span and low tumor generation in a certain type of mouse with high concentrations of induced antibody production (Covelli et al, 1989).

Current research suggests a combination of immune status indices: High T-cell proliferation, high B-cell numbers, and low CD8 to CD4 cell ratio can predict survival over a 2-year follow-up interval in the very old (ages 86 to 92) (Ferguson et al, 1995). Wayne and associates (1990) suggest that the lack of immunity, anergy, in skin tests for delayed hypersensitivity may also prove a good indicator for subsequent mortality.

Miller (1996) found an associated high risk of early mortality when there was a high number of memory T cells at 6 months of age. Confounding the analysis of age-related changes in immune competency from a clinical perspective is the comparatively long human life span.

Biologists are looking at the field of immunoengineering for possible approaches to control the decline of the immune system and to retard the aging process. Immunoengineering, the manipulation of some conditions in organ transplants, and the attempt to find a cure for acquired immunodeficiency syndrome (AIDS) have opened avenues for exploring aging and the benefits of aging. A number of years ago, it was shown that the complicated immune system was regulated by an aggregate of genes on a single chromosome. Like a super blood grouping system with numerous different types, the cluster of genes was called the *major histocompatibility chromosome* (MHC). Part of the responsibility of the MHC is self-antiself recognition. Susceptibility to many diseases of aging, such as Alzheimer's disease, is influenced by the MHC type of the affected person, and organ graft survival rate is noted to be better when both donor and recipient have the same MHC type (Walford, 1983). Some of the first evidence that MHC was influential in extending the life span of different mice strains was provided by the research of Smith and Walford (1977) and later confirmed by Williams and coworkers (1981). Two approaches on which immunoengineering is focused are (1) selective alteration by diet, temperature regulation, and drugs in conjunction with surgery and (2) replenishment or rejuvenation.

Selective alteration is an attempt to suppress abnormal immune function through such actions as moderate protein restriction. This restriction would depress the humoral system while leaving the cellular system intact. Severe diet restriction (undernutrition) can delay or extend maturation of both humoral and cellular immune activity. High-fat diets have produced an increase in autoimmunity, a propensity for autoimmune diseases, and a decrease in cell-mediated immunity and life span (Makinodan, 1990; Walford, 1986).

Immune factors have also been found to be temperature dependent. Diet restriction and mild hypothermia appear to enhance survival and alter patterns of immunity in test animals. Immunosuppressants have at this point provided marginal effectiveness in life span extension because of loss of autoimmune reactions. Surgical removal of the spleen in test animals before manifestation of immunodeficiencies occurred has shown limited results.

Replenishment of rejuvenation of the human immune system is based on the idea of injecting immune cells of a compatible young donor into older recipients. The intent is to return the immune system of the aging individual to its normal effective state.

In summary, the immune system responses are thought to produce age-related changes. Accurate accumulated data show that the immune system begins to decline (1) when thymic atrophy occurs and possibly as soon as there is a decrease of thymic hormone (thymosin) in the blood, (2) when there is a significant increase in plasma cell activity, (3) when circulating lymphocytes with an abnormal number of chromosomes are increased, and (4) when there is an increase in immunoglobins in the blood. Research has identified various diseases that may be linked to immunity and aging. Selective alteration and replenishment or rejuvenation are immunoengineering challenges for exerting control and moderating or eliminating the effects of autoimmunity, immunodeficiencies, and perhaps, one day, the aging process.

Although all of these theories provide possible clues to aging, they also raise many questions and stimulate continuing research (Table 2-1). Many symptoms that are attributed to failing circulation in the aged may actually be the effects of nondividing cell death. The frequency of mutations in mammalian aging is influenced by genetic mutation of autoimmune reactions, metabolic rate, genetic background, and environmental factors. In the past few years, the investigation of cellular senescence has expanded to additional cell types, such as endothelial cells and T lymphocytes. These cells have been combined with immortal cells, which has indicated that many or all cell types may have similar pathways. Conversely, as more cell types are studied, the expression or repression of specific genes is appearing. It is hoped that more research will lead to the discovery of other pathways and key changes in gene expression used by other cells to establish senescence (Smith and Pereira-Smith, 1996; Pereira-Smith and Bertram, 2000). Biogerontologic research has demonstrated that longevity is frequently considered to be related to enhanced metabolic capacity and the response to stress, as well as multiple mechanisms of aging (Jazwinski, 1996).

The biogerontologist has long considered that genes play a part in the aging process, while acknowledging that

Table 2-1 Summary of Biologic Theories of Aging

Theory	Dynamics	Retardants
Stochastic theories		
Error	Faulty synthesis of DNA and/or RNA	
Somatic	Alteration in RNA/DNA; protein or enzyme synthesis causes defective structure or function	
Transcription	Failure of transcription or translation between cells; malfunctions of RNA or related enzymes	
Free radical	Oxidation of fats, proteins, carbohydrates, and elements creates free electrons that attach to other molecules, altering cellular function	Improve environmental monitoring; decrease intake of free radical-stimulating foods; increase vitamin A and C intake (mercaptans; increase vitamin E; use of coenzyme Q10)
Cross-link	Lipids, proteins, carbohydrates, and nucleic acid react with chemicals or radiation to form bonds that cause an increase in cell rigidity and instability	Caloric restrictions, lathyrogen-antilink agents
Clinker	Mix of somatic, free radical, and cross-link theories	
Wear and tear	Repeated injury or overuse of cells, tissue, organs, or systems	
Nonstochastic theories		
Programmed	Biologic clock triggers specific cell behavior at specific time	Hypothermia and diet can delay cell division but not number of divisions
Run-out-of-program	Organism capable of specific number of cell divisions and specific life span	
Neuroendocrine	Control mechanism (pituitary and hypothalamus) regulate interplay between various organs and tissues; efficiency of signals between mechanisms is altered or lost	Treatment with potent hormones such as DHEA (dehydroepiandrosterone) and RU486
Immunologic/autoimmune	Alteration of B and T cells leads to loss of capacity for self-regulation; normal or age-related cells recognized as foreign matter; system reacts by forming antibodies to destroy these cells	Immunoengineering, selective alteration, and replacement or rejuvenation of immune system

environmental influences are also important. It is important, however, to realize that life span is not the same as the action of a genetic program. Aging, according to the biogerontologists, is determined by genetic construction.

More thought is being directed toward the immune function of the body, multigene interaction, environmental effects, and longevity in nearly one half of the chromosomes tested. Life span correlates positively with a high immune responsiveness, both of which were controlled by a small number of gene loci. The inference is that low antibody response has a detrimental effect.

PSYCHOLOGIC ASPECTS OF AGING

Healthy psychologic aging refers to the age-related adaptive capacity of the individual to experience and interpret events in such a way that coping is ensured as one continually seeks greater understanding and higher levels of adaptation. Gerontology has emerged as a subspecialty of psychology within the last quarter century. The first journal devoted exclusively to psychology and aging was published in 1985 by the American Psychological Association. Before that, the psychology of the old was primarily focused on studying cognitive losses or impairments or slowing of various responses.

The psychology of aging is the study of changes in behavior that characteristically occur after young adulthood. Behavior in this sense includes sensation, perception, learning, memory, intellect, motivation, emotion, personality, attitudes, motor movement, and social relationships (Birren and Birren, 1990). The psychology of aging attempts to "discern laws governing the way humankind grows up and grows old" (Birren and Birren, 1990, p. 12) (Box 2-3). Quite naturally, aging psychologists often give more attention to the psychologic development of the aged. Dr. James Birren has been one of the true leaders in the field for 30 years and has with his own aging become increasingly interested in the psychology and metaphysics of aging. His contributions have been broad, but his focus on the importance of a developmental autobiography has generated considerable interest in the field. Nursing leaders who have helped us understand the psychologic components of aging include Mary Opal Wolanin and Virginia Stone, as they studied the experience and memories of nonagenarians, and May Wykle and Kathleen Buckwalter, who established academic programs in psychogeriatric care.

Essential to the concept of psychologic development are the following ideas: (1) the organism is a dynamic system, (2) time is a quantifying element, (3) movement in time is toward complexity of organization, (4) parts are incorporated into the whole, and (5) the highest state of organization is self-regulatory. Little is known about intrinsic psychologic needs and changes that occur as a result of primary aging processes, because we have no such sample of aged persons. All persons are embedded in a cultural matrix that influences every aspect of their lives and that cannot be extricated from the primary and essential components of aging. This is the basis for our firm conviction that we do not yet know the potential of the aged—possibilities are limitless given an enhancing milieu. We therefore caution against attributing any particular psychologic change to age alone.

Morality

Obviously, morality must be personally defined within a value context. When values are shaken, the crisis threatens self-view and psychologic distress occurs. Questions about fundamental changes in behavior that occur with age are exceedingly difficult to answer. The classic theory of Kohlberg (1973) proposes that crises and turning points of adult life are moral dilemmas that form structural stage changes analogous to

Box 2-3 Theories of Development

Maturational	The biologic unfolding according to genetic programming determines development (White, mastery)
Personality	Early formation of responses caused by family and peer influences determines behaviors (Sullivan, interpersonal)
Behaviorist	Learning determines the organization of behavior (tabula rasa)
Cognitive	Development of cognitive capacities provides the basis for differentiation and increasing complexity of goals and behavior (Piaget)
Ecologic	The nature of adult development is quite different from that of children and has yet to be thoroughly articulated (Lewin)
Instinctual	Development of controls of instinctual responses through feedback, based in psychoanalytic thought (Freud)
Psychobiologic	Progress in neuroscience has shown that the balance of 50 or more neurotransmitters may, to a large extent, modulate behaviors, emotions, and thoughts
Dialectic	Crises and transitions release positive and negative forces that lead to developmental progression (Riegel)

Piaget's cognitive operations in youth. The last stage of moral development is defined as "universal ethical principle orientation." This stage fits nicely into the Eriksonian model of development because integrity is built on morality and ethics. Moral reasoning in later life may take on a pragmatic function, corresponding to changes associated with one's position in the life span. The nature of moral decisions in old age may be characterized by a shift from purely logical justification to a dialectic resolution between justice and personal caring. Much discussion about the nature of moral aging has been centered around the obligations of adults and the old toward future generations (Moody, 1988). We believe these discussions will become ever more pressing as world populations grow and as economic and environmental debts increase. Some writers believe that such moral dilemmas can only be effectively dealt with by the aged because the very complexity of situations relies on the wisdom of long experience (Fjelland and Gjengedal, 1994).

Competence

The founders of ego psychology recognize the importance of stimulating experiences and mastery of new situations. According to them, the ego is continually striving for more challenges rather than a state of rest or satisfaction. An invigorating environment is needed to maintain an energized level of stress. Accordingly, individuals do not seek homeostasis (a steady state) but rather stimulation. This has important implications for the elderly. Most old people have had many experiences, and new situations occur with less frequency. Some elders are isolated from the mainstream of life and may deteriorate from boredom and lack of stimulation (see Chapter 18). Experiments with sensory deprivation seem to confirm this notion. Perhaps the most challenging stimuli for the aged are maintaining autonomy and independence. Commitment to mastery or competence is critically linked to motivating drives, incentives, needs, and the degree of control one feels. Satisfaction can arise from several channels, although opportunity for mastery relates to social class, health, life stage, and sex. In old age the sense of control is thought to be an important precursor of successful coping.

Self-View

Retaining dignity and self-respect in the face of the catastrophes accompanying aging are the poorly understood psychologic components of successful aging (Lenker and Polivka, 1996). Self-efficacy has received some attention as the mediator of behavior (Bandura, 1977). A longitudinal study has shown that social network supports and the availability of financial resources were the strongest factors in maintaining feelings of self-efficacy (McAvay et al, 1996). The existential dimensions of "self" reside within the boundaries of a personal moral stance and perceived competence and as such may be vulnerable to internal and external changes. Yet some individuals maintain a strong sense of self. These are the psychologically "hardy" persons (Bowsher and Keep, 1995). The hardy ones are capable of enduring physical and emotional stressors because they maintain a sense of control and challenge. Each event is seen as an open door on new experience and one that allows for choice (Kobasa, 1979; Ebersole, 1996). As we work with the aged it is important to keep in mind the three cornerstones of hardiness: control, competence, and challenge. Some also add a fourth—compassion. Indeed, it seems that those who manage effectively against all odds are those whose central concerns go beyond self to include others. This presupposes some underlying altruism, as well as a sense of humor. These topics are considered later in the text. Banks (1996) believes that it is also essential to psychologic health in later life to be capable of imagining oneself as old. It is a revealing exercise to ask students to imagine themselves as old. Our readers will recognize, among the student quotes at the beginning of each chapter in this edition of the textbook, that some students are very capable of imagining being old and assigning meaning to old age.

Psychologic Tasks of Aging

Theories are the organizing framework from which tasks quite naturally will arise (Box 2-4). Some of the theories give little recognition or attention to the unique characteristics and potential of the aged. The exchange model is one we particularly favor. It implies that with the waning of physical energy one is less inclined to seek more of anything and is more inclined to seek less, but with more emphasis on quality than quantity. According to Lewin (1951), all developmental theories are faulty because childhood development, from which they all arose, is undoubtedly distinctively different in all respects from adult development. In 1922 G. Stanley Hall's work, although largely descriptive, was the first to suggest a science of gerontic development. Jung and Erikson have both written of needs that emerge in the "last half of life." We still rely on their original thought as a starting point for understanding the tasks of the aged. Clark and Anderson (1967) were among the first to identify specific adaptive tasks. These primarily focus on the need to overcome decrements in function and to seize opportunity by substitution, redefinition, acceptance, and reassessment. These all imply that adulthood is the stage of maximum adaptation.

Developmental Tasks and Status

Cynthia Kelly has identified the three *R*s that define the tasks of aging as (1) accepting reality, (2) fulfilling responsibility, and (3) exercising rights (Kelly, 1990). Realities have to do with accepting one's capacities in the health, social, and financial realms; responsibilities include planning for one's survivors and for making the best choices regarding the remainder of life; and rights include exercising the right to move at one's own pace, the right to privacy, the right to respect, the right to refuse what one does not desire, and the right to participate in plans and decisions related to one's own life. Developmental tasks, as defined by several theorists, are included in Figure 2-3.

Box 2-4 Summary of Theories of Human Development

I. Life stages model
  A. Jungian (popular)
    1. Anchored in psychoanalytic theory
      a. Midlife shift—second stage of development
        (1) Anima—female; emergence of in men
        (2) Animus—male; emergence of in women
    2. Issues
      a. Masculinity-femininity
      b. Creativity-destructiveness
      c. Attachment-loss
  B. Eriksonian—psychosexual stages
    1. Organized in sequences of life structures and transitions (6- to 10-year average)
      a. Stability-disruption (1- to 3-year average)
      b. Equilibrium-imbalance
      c. Denial, rebirth (Kübler-Ross)
      d. Socially and personally motivated with genetic and chronologic influence
  C. Levinsonian—mentors (7 to 10 years older) to guide
    1. 35- to 45-year shift
      a. Guided by a dream
      b. Midlife crises
      c. End of dream
      d. Death of youth

II. Adaptational model (Valliant)
  A. Basic premises
    1. Gradual shifting of self and understanding
    2. Incremental-decremental shifts
    3. Trade-offs
    4. Holding on and letting go—critical
  B. Examples
    1. Sensory decrease/quality of perception increase
    2. Excitement decrease/experience increase
    3. Physical decrease/wisdom increase
  C. Quantity versus quality
    1. What are you willing to let go of or diminish?
    2. What is not worth pursuing?
    3. What are your best assets?
    4. What is possible?
      a. Undiscovered self
      b. New births of self
    5. Stay with growing edge of self
    6. Bargaining is the essence

III. Life structure and transitions (Lowenthal) (based on organizational life cycles)
  A. Family life cycles
  B. Transitions
    1. College
    2. Marriage
    3. Retirement
  C. Premises
    1. Significant others may not be in the same sequence
    2. Evidence from clinical world
    3. Accelerated life structure transitions
      a. Toffler—Future Shock
    4. Choice—intolerance of change or creative change

IV. Dialectic/ecologic/systems (Riegel)
  A. Premises
    1. Based on social psychology
    2. No life span approach
    3. Intersection of events produces change by breaking equilibrium
      a. Triggering event
      b. Turning point
      c. Timing of events (Rossi)
    4. Discover self by reaction
    5. Perspective on development by looking backward
    6. Metaphoric conceptualizations
    7. Restoration of balance
    8. Essence in energy exchanges with impact
  B. Examples
    1. World events, trends, culture, milieu
      a. Geography
      b. Ideational
      c. Situational
      d. Micro and macro systems
      e. Health evolution

V. Fielding model—Roger Gould—psychoanalytic consultation
  A. Premises
    1. Become finest self
      a. Give up safety
      b. Creativity reaches beyond myth of safety
      c. Self-actualizing
        (1) Maslow
        (2) Bueler
      d. Past life, future self
      e. Autonomy/control/taking charge
      f. Pilgrimage of the self
        (1) Teleologic
        (2) Future oriented
        (3) Proactive
        (4) Goal oriented
        (5) Shaping one's own world
  B. Agenda for mature adulthood
    1. Individualization
    2. Recreation
    3. Undo the boring—trigger a transition, renewal
    4. Endings and beginnings—the essence of development

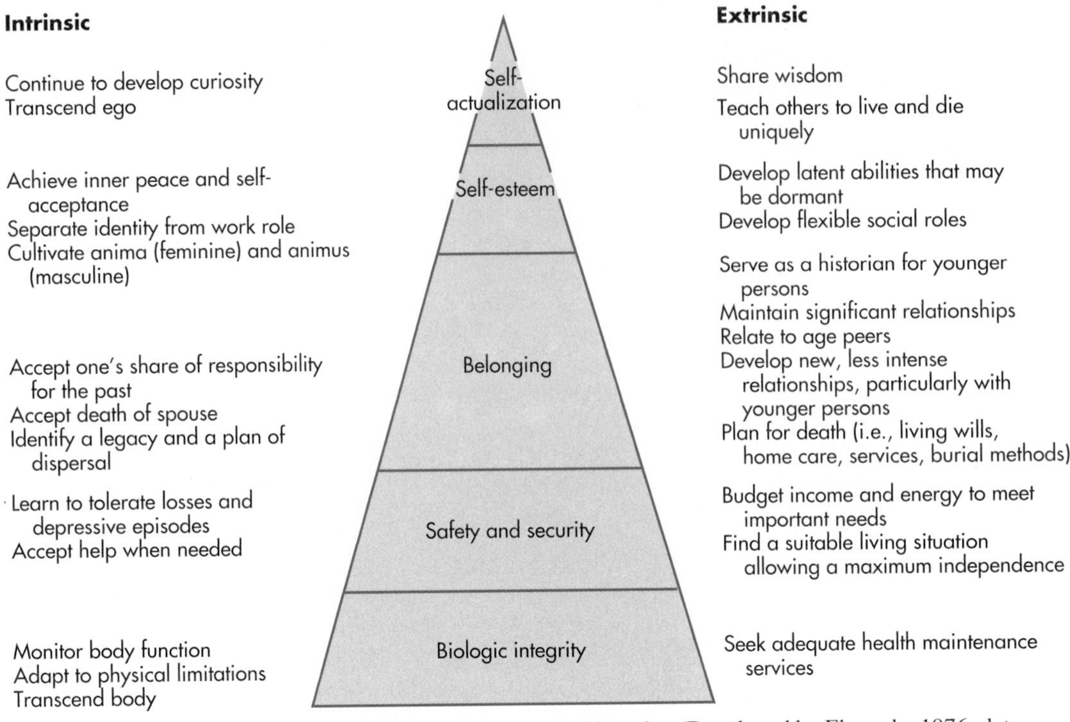

Figure 2-3. Developmental tasks of late life in hierarchic order. (Developed by Ebersole, 1976; data from Peck, 1968; Havighurst, 1972; and Butler and Lewis, 1977.)

We remain convinced that old age is valid in and of itself and that adaptation is toward maximizing and making events meaningful in the last stage of life. Birren and Birren (1990) believe that as more theorists and investigators mature who have their primary training in the field of gerontology we can expect more theories to emerge that are seminal rather than borrowed from other life stages or disciplines.

Establishing Integrity. Erikson is to human development as Maslow is to motivation. Each has framed the depth and clarity of concepts that provide an organizational framework for students and practitioners to categorize behaviors and understand dynamics of individuals. Erikson (1963) described the specific developmental stages and tasks of each age. He saw the last stage of life as a vantage point from which one could look back with integrity or despair on one's life. Erikson believed in a predetermined order of development that proceeded by critical steps, all dependent on timing and sequence. However, he also theorized that individuals return again and again to the stages that have been poorly resolved. His theory does not clearly explain why the organism moves from one state to the next; it is assumed that certain inner biologic and outer sociologic conditions are required. These concepts are cultural and class bound, and the centrality of identity achievement reflects Erikson's own need to establish his identity sans any knowledge of his biologic father.

Acknowledging the necessary stages of development proposed by Erikson, Peck (1968) identified discrete tasks of old age that must be addressed in order to establish integrity:

- *Ego differentiation versus work role preoccupation:* The individual is no longer defined by his or her work.
- *Body transcendence versus body preoccupation:* The body is cared for but does not consume the interest and attention of the individual.
- *Ego transcendence versus ego preoccupation:* The "I" becomes less central and one becomes a felt part of the mass of humanity, their struggles, and their destiny.

It is clear that to achieve integrity by Peck's model one must develop the ability to redefine self, to let go of occupational identity, to rise above body discomforts, and to establish meanings that go beyond the scope of self-centeredness. Although these are admirable and idealistic goals, they place a considerable burden on the aged individual. Everyone may not have the courage or energy to laugh in the face of adversity or surmount all the assaults of old age. There are traces of Aristotelian thought in both Peck's and Erikson's theories.

Interestingly, questions have been raised as to whether integrity is indeed the highest development in old age. Erikson's concept of integrity in old age and the concomitant ego attribute, wisdom, may not be attainable by many elders. The wisdom of old age is an adaptive perception of reality to elicit new meanings from prior experience, but paradoxically this means a mode of knowledge beyond time or age. Unlike ordinary knowledge, wisdom leads to an apprehension of reality in its fullest. The wisdom of old age becomes a crisis of explanation in which the ordinary structures are shaken and the meaning of life is reexamined. It may include the wisdom of questioning assumptions in the search for meaning in the last stage of life.

In later years, Erikson and his wife, Joan (Erikson et al, 1986) reconsidered his seminal work from the perspective of their own aging (they were both octogenarians at the time) and from the experience of a select group of their cohort, 29 surviving parents of the children studied in the guidance study of the Institute of Human Development at the University of California in Berkeley. They reframed their presentation of the theoretic framework to focus on a dialectic process of achieving balance at each stage of life. Thus ego integrity is tinged with some regrets, wisdom is balanced with frivolity, and letting go is balanced with hanging on. The Eriksons define wisdom as "detached concern with life itself, in the face of death itself. It maintains and learns to convey the integrity of experience, in spite of the decline of bodily and mental functions" (Erikson et al, 1986, p. 38).

Caring and Continuity. In 1927 Dr. Herbert Stolz established the Institute of Child Welfare under the aegis of the Institute of Human Development and began a longitudinal study of the health and development of every third child born in Berkeley for the ensuing 18 months. The original sample totaled 248 infants. Although they were randomly selected, they nevertheless represented a very select population because Berkeley at that time was an "ivory tower" town. The children are now septuagenarians. Their parents, now mostly nonagenarians, were interviewed by the Eriksons. Their preoccupation at this last stage of life was caring. For many, caring remained focused on children and grandchildren and seemed a vicarious way of continuing vital involvement in living. Others had grown beyond the central focus of the family, and their caring had more universal and altruistic components. For most of these very old, concern for their septuagenarian children dominated their thoughts. Reflecting on the successes of their children seemed to confirm their own parenting. The aspect of caring, so predominant during the generative stages in the adult years, is the quality that provides the greatest sense of continuity. As individuals nurture their young and watch their descendants nurture their young, they experience a connectedness with the repetitious cycles of life and at times an opportunity to redo their youth. As the dialectic around caring is cultivated, the elder is challenged "to accept from others that caring which is required and to do so in a way that is itself caring" (Erikson et al, 1986, p. 74).

Continuity and vicarious fulfillment are experienced as one sees qualities in grandchildren that were identified in the self, parents, or grandparents. As many as six generations may be viewed in continuous progression.

My great-grandmother (Ebersole) left me a watercolor of wildflowers. I am obsessed with the beauty of spring flowers and walk for hours admiring them. Recently my granddaughter bought a field guide to flowers and asked to accompany me on the "flower walks." Although the sixth generation is yet to appear, my granddaughter is in her twenties and I in my seventh decade. I expect to see a great-granddaughter before I die, and I will eagerly wait to see where her interests lie. Although the life history data at the disposal of the Eriksons was rare and of an exceptional longitudinal nature, they did not explore the dynamics of individual lives over time but rather used the collective themes to support conclusions regarding old age, which in their view reiterated the issues of development earlier identified and continued to provide the essence and meaning of life in the later years. They believed that achieving each of the eight stages of psychosocial development produces the necessary strength for extension of one's self in vital involvement with an ever-increasing concern beyond self.

Intimacy and Isolation. The balance between the capacity for intimacy and the need for isolation allows for individual and mutual development in relationships. The elder must reconfirm the joy of being alone with the closeness of supportive and intimate relationships. The capacity for aloneness, the ability to revel in one's own company, may be a developmental requirement of late life. This is not to the exclusion of significant others but only in preparation for the aloneness of loss and the ultimate aloneness of death. Developing the capacity to enjoy being alone has not been identified by developmental theorists as a significant aspect of adaptation in old age, but it seems clear that it may be. In fact, reminiscence may allow one to joyfully relive the past and may be a tool for achieving satisfaction in being alone. This is not to negate the reality of loss and the pain of loneliness, but, just as a child must learn to reach out to others, the aged must learn to value interiority. May Sarton said, "Solitude is the wealth of spirit and loneliness is poverty of spirit" (Sarton, 1989).

Relationships, the most intimate and the most distant, change over time, and the vital older individual learns to adapt to the changes. Although the Eriksons (1986) say that it may be easier to think with "fond longing" about friends who are deceased, we think it may be more important to rekindle ties that have lain dormant and unattended. It is also important to reach beyond one's generation to develop intergenerational supports that will tend to be sustaining during the loss of peers and cohorts. Yet Wolanin (1996) says, "I didn't believe that people in their mid-eighties could develop such new and intimate relationships as I have experienced in the last few years." This ability has disproved the myth that the old no longer develop new and close relationships with each other.

Achieving a Balance. Erikson and co-workers propose that each of the major stages of development involves a balance of the "syntonic" and "dystonic" modes of coping if one is to remain vitally involved (Erikson et al, 1986). In other words, trust must be balanced with mistrust to achieve a vital adjustment that proceeds toward higher levels of development. Too much trust results in maladaptation, which is considered neurotic, and too much mistrust results in malignant adaptation, which has the potential for psychoses. Trust is mandatory for development, but it can exist positively only in juxtaposition with a sensible mistrust. The balance of trust versus mistrust results in a sense of hope. The notion of too much and too little is vague and variable, but the contention is that if an appropriate individual balance has been achieved the individual is hopeful. Likewise, for each of the other stage dichotomies the balance must be achieved. "The process of bringing into balance feelings of integrity and despair involves a review of and a coming to terms with the life one has lived thus far" (Erikson et al, 1986, p. 70). All individuals have a central mental tendency to organize experience, a function of the ego. Erikson and associates found that many informants refrained from mentioning any former discontent with their lives, although the data indicated periods of profound discontent. The researchers speculate that the omissions may result from a desire to construct a satisfactory life view by "pseudo-integration," from the need to maintain privacy, from a lifelong process of recasting and finding new meanings in events, from denial, or from putting traumatic events over the years into perspective. Those who seemed most well adapted were able to draw sustenance from the past but remained vitally involved in the present (Erikson et al, 1986).

Reviewing and Transmitting. Fitch (1992) points out that when we visit our elder relatives we see the same old house, same old furniture, and sometimes believe the people are as unchanging as their surroundings. Little is known about the developmental issues and phases of the very old. With encouragement old people will share their understanding of life and forge additional links in the chain of understanding that grows with each generation. Some contend that our materialism is a natural outgrowth of our separation from aging and death. We avoid the intimate knowledge and heroism that confrontation with aging and death can cultivate. Fitch says the psychologic tasks of old age are slowing, life review, transmission, and letting go. However, these describe activities rather than issues of development. Developmental tasks certainly include arrival at a personally acceptable philosophy of existence that transcends the limitations of the aging body and its systems. Butler (1963) described the growth potential for aged individuals through the "life-review" process. This process of review and integration of events throughout the mature years is the catalyst for personal growth, integration, and evolving identity. Regrets and disappointments are fuel for reflection and deeper self-awareness. Butler's observations have confirmed Jung's views that reflective activity is intense and healing for many elders. Butler (1975, p. 412) wrote, "the old are not only taking stock of themselves as they review their lives, they are trying to think and feel through what they will do with the time that is left and with whatever emotional and material legacies they may have to give others." The task of transmission may be made more urgent in the presence of vulnerability or recent trauma (Fitch, 1992).

Letting Go and Hanging On. The task of letting go initially sounds deteriorative. We believe it means letting go of the nonessentials, the facades and charades, the need to conform and please, of long-held hurts and slights, of the need to brood over injustice. In addition, while letting go, the elder must simultaneously hang on to ideas and objects that are laden with meaning. The pace of this process is unique to each individual and frequently misunderstood by others. Fitch says that the last phase of life involves a shift from conceptual thought to a more intuitive, emotional mode. Choices may reflect this in extraordinary ways. She suggests that "there is an organic, evolutionary dynamic in the elderly that happens even in the midst of confusion and which is tremendously potent and valid. There is some real victory and celebration possible even in the midst of existential decrepitude. We must do all that we can to see that everyone has that final and crowning opportunity" (Fitch, 1992, p. 106). Facilitating an atmosphere that allows letting go and hanging on in whatever way is significant to the individual can be extremely important. We can support or undermine these developments by the attitudes we hold and the environment we create (Fitch, 1992).

Personality Styles and Phases

The concepts of personality are based on several theoretic viewpoints: (1) neopsychoanalytic, (2) psychometric, (3) behaviorist, and (4) environmental. These viewpoints determine the expectations of personality in old age. From the neopsychoanalytic viewpoint, childhood forms lifelong personality traits. The psychometric view involves testing in order to develop a profile of specific personality traits such as extroversion-introversion, neuroticism, and psychoticism that can be traced through the life cycle; such traits may be genetic, environmental, or nurtured. Descriptive studies of these personality traits at various ages are of considerable interest to psychometricians. The behaviorists' concern is focused on that which can be observed and measured in old age, often with the desire to modify. Motivation is not of major interest to behaviorists. The environmentalists contend that traits and situations are both potent predictors of adaptation in later life, and that in some persons personality traits predominate and for others situations are more influential to development. It is difficult to sort out personality traits that are developed or suppressed because of experience rather than age. To further complicate the issue, certain personality traits tend to emerge strongly in particular situations and with particular persons. Personality under ordinary conditions is assumed to remain stable across the adult life span. Such personality traits as stability, sociability, imaginativeness, neuroticism, extroversion, and openness to experience do not seem to change when studied longitudinally and cross-sequentially.

Empirically, it would seem that all of these components of personality exist in each individual. Some are nurtured by families and various societies, and some are squelched. Studies confirm that even minor personality characteristics may be genetically predetermined or are at least strongly dispositional (McClearn et al, 1990). Personality stability is a central belief of most life span psychologists.

Interiority. Jung (1971), a contemporary of Freud, was one of the first psychologists to define the last half of life as having a purpose of its own, quite apart from species survival—the development of self-awareness through reflective activity. He strongly believed in the importance of the last half of life, which is characterized by inner discovery, as opposed to the first half, which is oriented to biologic and social issues. Jung's theories contain elements of those of Cicero. The development of the psyche and the inner person is accompanied by a search for personal meaning and the spiritual self. Jung believed that a person who denies the validity of unconscious experience and the existence of the psyche is in self-conflict, consciously denying the relevance of the psyche because it reaches into obscurities beyond understanding. This denial of an aspect of one's nature results in restlessness, uprootedness, disorientation, and meaninglessness. However, many old persons may not be inclined to value psychologic exploration. Nevertheless, spirituality is an important aspect of development in later life and the means by which one becomes whole and develops the integrity described by Erikson. Jung also supports this view of the mature religious sentiment carrying one forward to holistic development in late life. Neugarten (1968) believes that increased "interiority" is characteristic of aged persons and also indicates a growing interest in inner development.

Inherent and accumulated personality characteristics influence the adaptation of the individual at any given stage. The following questions must be investigated in regard to the adaptation of the aged:

- How do the lives of introverts differ from the lives of extroverts?
- Do neuroticism and poor coping styles interfere with an orderly life plan?
- What personality dispositions influence adaptation to stressful life events?

The question that has not been addressed by gerontologists is, What happens to persons who have unstable personalities as they age? Stability of personality over time is in itself a personality characteristic. In other words, some persons will act in very predictable ways throughout their life, whereas others seem to have a thread of inconsistency in their life patterns and actions. Age as a developmental variable does not appear to be strongly related to most personality traits in healthy, community residents, although serious disease states, brain pathologic conditions, and institutional living may bring about major personality changes. Personality factors, cultural age norms, and expectations interact in undetermined ways to affect the individual life course. In short, the uniqueness, the highly prized fruit of a long life well lived, is the very factor that belies our efforts to predict norms for the later years.

PSYCHOSOCIAL THEORIES OF AGING

The three classic psychosocial theories of aging are essentially behavioristic and examine how one most successfully experiences late life: by disengaging, by maintaining activities of middle age, or by reinforcing personal continuity. These three theories view the processes of aging quite differently, and, because of the controversy arising from the different viewpoints, much research has been stimulated.

Disengagement

The disengagement theory of Cumming and Henry (1961) states that "aging is an inevitable, mutual withdrawal or disengagement, resulting in decreased interaction between the aging person and others in the social system he belongs to" (Cumming and Henry, 1961, p. 2). They contend that when the disengagement is complete a new equilibrium is established between the individual and society that is characterized by increased distance between the individual and society and that the relationship between the two is different than in middle age but mutually satisfactory. High morale is evident at the completion of the process, but the transition is characterized by low morale. The measures of disengagement are based on age, work, and decreased interest or investment. The theory is seen as universal and applicable to the aged in all cultures, although there are expected variations in timing and style. Hultsch and Deutsch (1981) note that when disengagement occurs, it proceeds at variable rates and patterns in various persons with unpredictable psychologic outcomes.

Activity

Activity theory supports the maintenance of regular actions, roles (formal and informal), and solitary as well as social pursuits for a satisfactory old age. Activists began to champion the notion that old age was only an extension of the middle years and could be abolished by keeping active (Maddox, 1963). Longino and Kart (1982) attempted to replicate many of the assumptions of activity theory based on the concepts of Lemon and associates (1972), who articulated an interactionist model of activity, promoting the concept that intimacy and frequency of activity reinforce one's self-concept. Formal activity was deemed less useful than informal activity because it tended to segregate by age, reinforcing a lower self-concept. Longino and associates (1980) found that even average activity levels in retirement community residents resulted in a more positive self-concept than among their counterparts in the general population. The activity theory may make sense when individuals live in a stable society, have access to positive influence and significant others, and have opportunities to participate meaningfully in the broader society if they continue to desire to do so. Attempts at clarifying activity theory as a general concept of satisfactory aging have not been supported.

Continuity

The continuity theory proposed by Havighurst and coworkers (1968) in reaction to the disengagement theory and activity theory more realistically focuses on the relationship between life satisfaction and activity as an expression of enduring personality traits. Personality is considered the important factor in determining the relationship between role activity and life satisfaction, and personality is seen to be not only enduring but becoming more entrenched and pronounced as one ages. Three ideas important to this perspective, inferred from Neugarten and associates (1968), remain fundamental to beliefs about the aged individual:

- In normal aging personality remains consistent in men and women.
- Personality influences role activity and investment in role activity.
- Personality influences life satisfaction regardless of role activity.

Criticisms of the three major theories focus on the obscurities in *life satisfaction* and *morale* and the value-laden term *successful*. In addition, it has been found in many studies that self-report is likely to convey a more positive picture than might be reported by an observer and that the aged tend to express dissatisfaction through the "generalized other." For instance, "I am very happy with my life, but other people my age are miserable and complaining all the time." The scales, of which there are many, to measure success, life satisfaction, attitude adjustment, and morale have been questioned in terms of both reliability and validity. None of the three theories can be clearly supported with data. In addition, they have little to do with personal meaning and motivation.

SOCIOLOGIC AGING

Social Gerontology

Social gerontology is a subfield of gerontology that deals with the nonphysical aspects of aging. It focuses on role development and group behaviors of older people, the impact of social phenomena on them, and the impact of older persons on the social system. Essentially, it is the study of how the individual and society adapt to each other. Occasionally a giant in the field, with astute perception, articulates a phenomenon that strikes a responsive chord in enough people to be accepted as a contemporary truth. Social gerontologists tend to see aging as a social problem because our society is not prepared to absorb the ever-increasing number of aged persons into meaningful social roles, particularly those of power and influence. Sociologists often study the disenfranchised members of the population or subcultures: stigmatized individuals and their social status. Some knowledge gaps recognized by social gerontologists include the scant comparisons of cross-national data and the dearth of data on older members of minority groups—particularly of those who are not black. The tendency to study "white and black" is indeed unfortunate because the blending of races and cultures negates the validity of these divisions.

Sociologic aging is a composite of the performance of expected social roles appropriate to one's chronologic age, culture, and capacity. Terms that are associated with sociologic aging are *age norms, social time clocks, age grading,* and *social time*. All of these are descriptive of the place individuals should occupy in a society at any given time in their lives. Socioeconomic status is intrinsically woven into the social roles occupied. Birren and Schroots (1984) developed the concept of "eldering," the process by which elders begin to fill the roles expected of them in their society. Sociologic aging is problematic in societies that have diversified traditional backgrounds, such as the United States, and in which flexibility in roles and age-related expectations have become the norm. Age-graded activities were far more reliable in primitive societies from which anthropologists derived these notions. Again, many of the developmental theories are far more applicable to schoolchildren or traditional societies than to mature, individualized adults in our era of highly diversified populations. Social scientists have, in the last decade, focused considerably more attention on the interaction of age, period, and cohort in attempts to study the social aspects of aging from a life span perspective. Each issue must be seen as a complex interaction of personal and social variables over time and in culture and subculture. Psychologists often focus on life span development, whereas sociologists speak of life course.

A social psychology of the life course is built on the following assumptions:

- Age structures are necessary for social organization, providing rights and responsibilities and governing rules and expectations.
- Biologic models of the life span are inadequate to account for aging without consideration of social dimensions.
- Continuities and changes in social expectation occur over the entire life course.
- Transformation of identity occurs with each new constellation of social expectation and behaviors.

Life Course

Life course is composed of elements that make up the overall structure and timing of events in one's life from cradle to grave. It must be examined and taken into account to understand the aged individual. This is the basis for longitudinal studies. Life structure is composed of roles (occupational, social, and family), relationships (intimate, personal, and professional), and inner structure (goals, values, motives, and memories). The progress of all these aspects of life can be considered a life course. Change and continuity are the elements that must be examined to understand the progression. Lenker and Polivka (1996) focus on the richness and uniqueness of elders' life course. Helping elders understand the story of their lives preserves identity and feelings of self-worth.

Life Transitions. Transitional periods are a major focus of understanding aging from a sociologic perspective. The transitions throughout the life course include major shifts attributed to age, role, occupation, family, and economics (Cunningham and Brookbank, 1988).

Changes are stressful but often provide opportunities for growth because they require development and application of distinctly different adaptive skills. For many of the major transitions in life, which may be especially traumatic, we receive little preparation. In cases of role accumulation, such as that of grandparent, some previous development will be applicable, with modification, to the new role. Likewise, the shifts in filial relationships are often gradual and do not require complete role deletion or role reversal. Those transitions that make use of past skills and adaptations may be least stressful. Some shifts, such as from functional independence to functional dependence, cut across many aspects of life and require several transitional shifts. Chapters 16 and 18 address some of these issues. From a life course perspective, the transitions and adaptations required produce both stability and change in individual preferences, capacities, expectations, and behavior. Age-related transitions are socially created, shared, and recognized. A transition is socially recognized and entails a reorientation of perceptions and expectations of and by the individual. It is also important to remember that cohort and gender differences are inherent in all of life's major transitions.

Age Norms. Norms are socially shared expectations that present "shoulds" or "oughts" for behavior. Age norms and age constraints are concepts that underscore the need for persons of a given age to conduct their lives in a manner that is socially expected and acceptable at that age. When individuals do not do so it is expected that they will feel stressed and perhaps stigmatized. In reality, much depends on the particular social expectation, status of the individual, circumstances, and whether one acts older or younger than one's age. In late life, there are few socially structured expectations and few studies of late life transitions. Some of the difficulty lies in how recently large numbers of cohort members have survived to be extremely old. No investigator seems to have seriously examined the nature of predictable transitions, sequencing of events, or spacing after age 70. Age-graded behaviors at that point are lacking. Issues on which social gerontologists focus most assiduously are (1) social integration, (2) successful adaptation, (3) age variables in social scientific research, (4) society as a succession of cohorts, (5) environment as a variable in understanding behavior, and (6) the search for a unified perspective of aging (Maddox and Campbell, 1985). "The study of the life course is a search for systematic regularities in events of unique meaning" (Back, 1980, p. 2).

Status and Role Changes. Status and role are the concepts around which norms, relationships, conformity and deviance, and stability and change are organized. Rosow (1985) considers four problems involved in applying role concepts to the aged: (1) is there a role, (2) what are the boundaries, (3) what are the interactions with other roles, and (4) what are the levels of the role performance? When considering the role of the aged in our society, we might examine the regard in which they are held as a measure of role relevance, boundaries, and performance. Rosow refers to an earlier publication (Rosow, 1973) to identify the major issues in role theory as applied to the aged:

- Loss of roles excludes the aged from significant social participation and devalues their contribution.
- Old age is the first stage of life with systematic status loss for the entire cohort.
- Persons in our society are not socialized to the fate of aging.
- Because there is no specified role for the aged, their lives may become unstructured.

Informal and tenuous roles are identified by Rosow (1985) as those lacking structure and stability and not linked to social status. In late life it is expected that institutionalized roles will decrease in number and significance while the tenuous roles will increase in significance if not in number. Tenuous roles are those that embody a definite social position but with vague or insubstantial role expectations (Rosow, 1985).

Social Supports

Social support is derived from the assurance of love, esteem, and belonging to a network involving common and mutual concerns. This certainly sounds like the ideal social support one would wish from intimates and family. However, the social support derived from informal ties may be much less intense but every bit as vital in old age. Friendships, neighbors, and spontaneous social ties may increase in later life. Sociogerontologists are interested in these types of social supports and how such interpersonal ties contribute to the health and well-being of older individuals. See Chapter 18 for further discussion.

Reciprocity

Attitudes of autonomy and independence are highly prized and cultivated within our society and seem to be clung to more ferociously as we see them ebbing away. A single power outage or gas war and we are immediately confronted with our dependency. Unusual lifestyles, weddings conducted in hot air balloons, bizarre clothing and haircuts, and the need to be especially assertive about the small details of our lives seem to assume more importance in direct proportion to our increasing dependence on technology for survival. In quite the opposite fashion, our elders, many of whom grew up in a self-sufficient style, were not so in need of symbols of independence but were succored by tradition and other symbols of continuity and collective thought. Undergirding all this is the deep awareness that as humans we must depend on others and be depended on if we are to survive individually and culturally. The concept of reciprocity in relationships and society is basic to survival. In old age, as one becomes physically and functionally dependent in various ways, it is important to cultivate the exchange process, reciprocal activities, and interpersonal reliance to avoid erosion of self-esteem. Elders often receive retroactive earnings in the human exchange system. See Chapters 16 and 18 for additional discussion of this concept.

Longevity

The mean life expectancy, or age of survivors within a group born near the same date, has risen almost 40 years in the twentieth century (Begley et al, 1990). A child born in 1994 can now expect to live 25 years longer than his or her counterpart of 1900. However, a person age 65 today can only expect to live 5 years longer than his or her 1900 counterpart (Downs, 1994). Through postponement of major chronic disorders, we may eventually expect to markedly shorten the period of senescence (Fries, 1980, 1992). However, the attainable maximum life span in the very best of circumstances will remain unchanged.

There is the popular presumption that elders will live longer and be healthier and happier and that, given continuing advances in technology, we will in the future almost totally conquer mortality. This sort of thinking is stimulated by popular articles such as appeared in *Insight* (1987) purporting to extend life to 180 years by dietary restriction or the scenario offered in *Life* magazine titled "The War on Aging," which describes living 700 years (Darrach, 1992). Cowley (2001) indicated that our bodies are designed to last only so long; however, if cared for and maintained, "they would live out their warranties in style."

Some theorists delving into the processes of aging now contend that perhaps there is no such thing as primary aging. However, most gerontologists today agree that 115 years is a realistic maximum life span (Downs, 1994). Studies of life extension through food restriction have been conducted on rats. Not only do such rats live almost twice as long as the projected life span, but also they do not develop the disorders common to aging rats. The theory is that life is prolonged by restricting food and thus increasing metabolic efficiency. Walford (1986; Cowley, 2001), a renowned and respected gerontologist and theorist in aging research, addresses this approach to life extension in *The 120-Year Diet.* Walford and seven other scientists lived in Biosphere 2, located in the Arizona desert, for 2 years and found themselves unexpectedly having to live on limited but nutrient-rich food and enforced caloric restrictions. The results were a positive effect on their hematologic, hormonal, and other biochemical parameters. Despite the drastic weight loss by all, both physical and mental activity remained at a high level. The situation was similar to the effect on caloric restrictions on experimental monkeys (Walford et al, 2002).

Others believe that humans may extend their physical and mental capacity in later years by continued use and stimulation (Begley, 2001). Brain dendrites grow when the brain is stimulated; muscles remain strong and resilient when used. Extensive research into mental function and aging by Schaie (1965) indicates that mental decline is less in people who learn new things, have a flexible attitude in middle age, adapt to change, and continue to pursue keen mental interests when they retire. Gradual physical decline begins early in youth but remains gradual if the lifestyle is not abusive. Better diet, more exercise, and better medical care are usually given credit for elders being in better condition than those of a generation ago.

Even if heart disease, cancer, stroke, and other diseases were eradicated, humans would still be subject to accidents. Cunningham and Brookbank (1988; Olshansky et al, 2002) indicate that after 35 years of age the probability of death doubles every 5 to 8 years. Gompertz mathematically described this phenomenon in 1825. Accidents among those who are 85 years and older, the fastest growing group of elders, are four times more frequent than in other age-groups (Darrach, 1992). However, Carry and Judge (2000) show that age-specific mortality patterns of contemporary humans in developed societies vary with life cycle phases (Figure 2-4). Jazwinski (1996) illustrates the physical determinents of aging and longevity in Figure 2-5.

Rudman (1990), in a 6-month experiment, was able to reverse some symptoms of aging in a group of men in their sixties and seventies. A comparable control group was also used. The experimental group injected themselves three times a week for 6 months with a synthetic version of human growth hormone, a potent secretion of the pituitary gland. The dosage used remained within the limits of that naturally secreted in younger men. The variance between the two groups was significant. Those taking the hormone therapy regained 10% of their muscle mass and 9% of their skin thickness, and lost 14% of their body fat. Although there were some side effects, Rudman indicated that "the treatment reversed body composition changes that would occur in 10 to 20 years of aging" (Darrach, 1992). Rejuvenation and longevity clinics outside the United States are enticing individuals with the same or similar human growth hormone injections (Humatrope) (Foote, 1994). This "treatment for aging" has not been approved by the Food and Drug Administration for use in the United States on the basis that the dosage is not known for healthy adults. The doses of Humatrope being used by these rejuvenation and longevity clinics are at levels used for children who have growth defects. Yen (1996), at University of California, San Diego, found that in a group of elders who received DHEA (growth hormone), 75% felt better. The question remains, What is the role of this steroid hormone in the maintenance of healthy aging? Longevity clinics in the United States and elsewhere are luring gullible individuals into investing in anti-aging products. The two biologic theories that seem to help in this sham are the free radical theory (antioxidant reversal) and the cross-link theory. Hormone replacement (melatonin, estrogen, testosterone, DHEA [growth hormone]) is also included in the anti-aging pitch. Although DHEA (growth hormone) has been shown to ease some age changes, it does not reverse the aging process. No product intervention has yet been proven to slow or reverse the human aging process (Olshansky et al, 2002).

Eventually, however, we may be able to slow the aging process. Biologists are beginning to locate genes that govern cellular mortality, and they are attempting to identify genes that are responsible for the "on-off switch" (Darrach, 1992; Recer, 2000; Schlessinger, 2000). A gene responsible for premature aging (Werner's syndrome) has been identified (King, 1996), causing excitement in biogerontologic circles.

Exceptional Longevity. Data gathered from these groups have been important in pursuit of maximum life span.

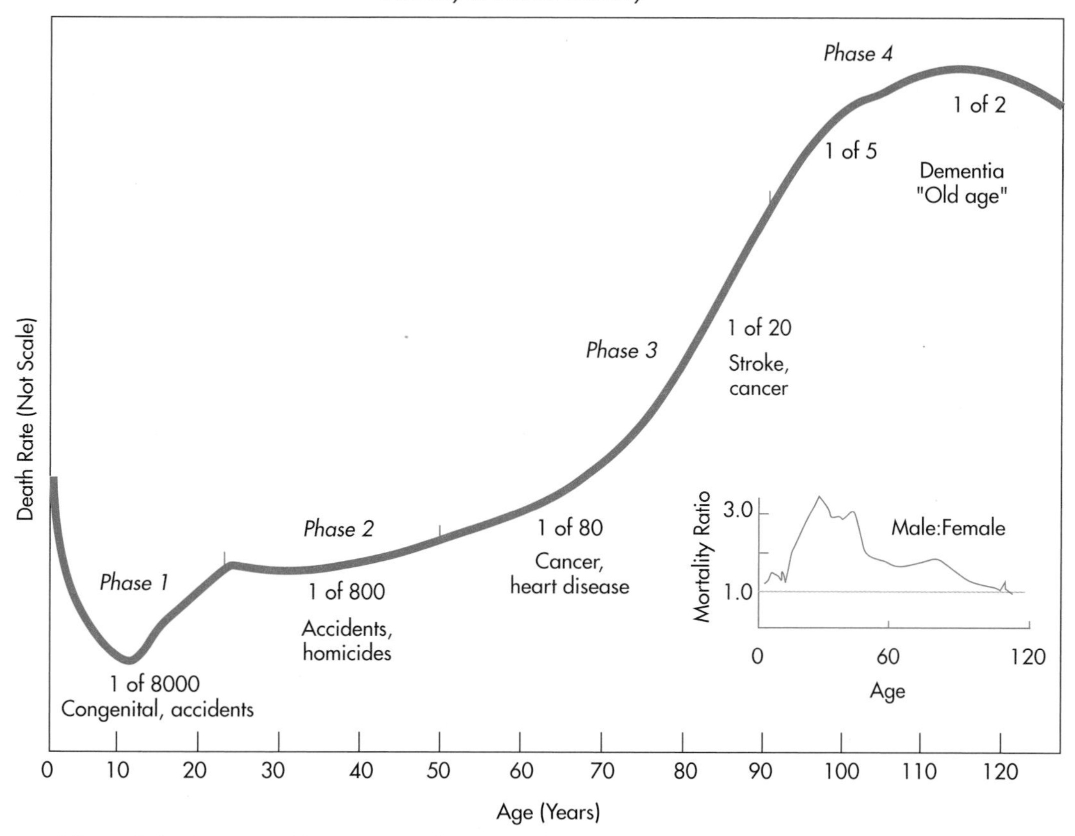

Figure 2-4. Anatomy of human mortality. (From Carry JR, Judge DS: Mortality dynamics of aging, *Generations* 24[1]:19, 2000.)

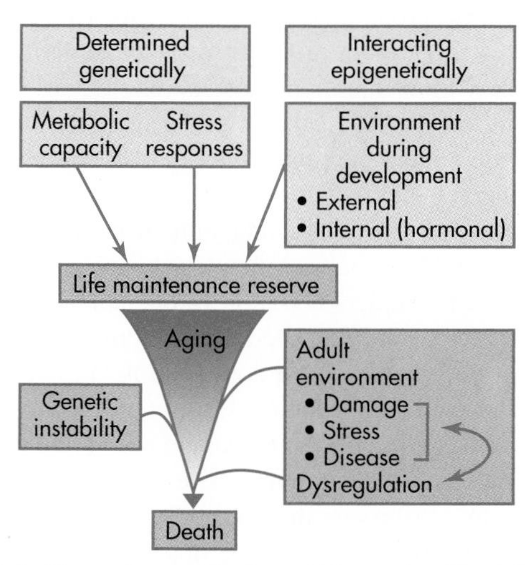

Figure 2-5. Determinants of aging and longevity. Physiologic relations, not molecular mechanisms, are shown. Metabolic capacity, stress responses, and environment during development all contribute to the life maintenance reserve, where they interact. Genetic instability is genetically determined, results in genetic alterations, and is influenced by environmental factors. Aging plays itself out at all levels of biologic organization; it is not possible to separate cellular changes from organismal aging. (From Miller RA: The aging immune system: primer and prospectus, *Science* 273:70, 1996, and Jazwinski SM: Longevity, genes, and aging, *Science* 273(5271):54, 1996.)

Common factors influential to longevity were dietary restrictions (low fat, high vegetable protein, high fiber, and limited caloric intake), exercise, and sociability. The value of undernourishment as a means of extending life span seems to arise from lifelong patterns of minimum intake. High altitudes and decreased temperature may also be important factors (Walford et al, 2002).

Rosenfeld (1985) indicated that animal studies have shown that a decrease of a few degrees centigrade in body temperature could add approximately 15 to 25 years to human life. One must be careful not to assume that a decrease in measured temperature means a decrease in metabolic rate. It is the core temperature that makes the difference. If the substance that triggers hibernation in animals could be isolated and transferred, researchers might seek ways to trick the human body into periods of torpor or hibernation, thus extending the life span. Drugs, biofeedback, and yoga are other means that are also being explored as methods of lowering body temperature to extend life span.

Heredity. The most provocative studies of the influence of genetics on aging adaptation come from Kallman and Sander (1948; 1949) and the Swedish Adoption/Twin Study of Aging (McClearn et al, 1990). The Kallman-Sander study surveyed cognitive similarities of 1000 pairs of twins over 60 years old residing in the state of New York. Similarities for disease, life span, and time of death were significant for identical twins, more so than for fraternal twins. The authors concluded that genetic influences are primarily responsible for individual differences in aging. The Swedish Adoption/Twin Study on Aging includes a comparison of identical twins reared apart, which has added a strong component to the study of genetics and behavior in late life. This ongoing longitudinal study indicates at this time that, although remaining strong, the significance of genetics on behavior in late life is probably less than in earlier life. However, there is a high correlation of similar life experiences that seems to exist and that may have a genetic basis (Plomin and McClearn, 1990). A replication of the Swedish twin study concluded that increased environmental effects were responsible for the major variants after age 70 (Pederson, 2000).

Heredity, once thought to have a great influence on life span, is not considered as important today. An individual born of long-lived relatives may live a very long life, but heredity is only partially influential in this process. The major developmental theorists of aging (Baltes et al, 1980) propose that the older one gets the more influenced one is by nonnormative life events. The last third of life requires very different adaptive capacities than the first two thirds. Ordinarily, one is consumed with and measured by performance until the later years. In older age, existential issues move to the forefront: losses, transitions to roles not yet understood by society, living in the moment, defining meanings in existence, and learning the measure of one's mettle. In addition, it has always been a problem to sort cohort variances and their influence on adaptation to given situations and life stages (Schaie, 1965).

Nutrition. Nutrition is receiving considerable attention as a major influence on longevity. Americans have become increasingly conscious of the implications and consequences of nutritional status on disease processes and on life span. Even the government now supports nutritional research. Studies as far back as Davis (1975), Benet (1976), and others show distinct differences in the dietary patterns of long-lived populations as compared with the dietary regimens of short-lived populations. Vegetables form the major portion in diets of long-lived people. These foods are high in nutrients and essential trace elements, the latter having been washed into the soil from mineral deposits at higher elevations. Little beef is consumed: mutton and other meats are eaten. Refined sugar does not exist in the diets, nor is obesity evident. The overall caloric intake is estimated to be approximately half that of a typical American diet. Walford (1986), from his ongoing research, advocates the "high/low" diet, a diet that provides the greatest concentration of nutrients with the least amount of calories. In the laboratory, Walford began restricted diets on rats at the time of weaning and found significant extension of life span. Restricted diets at weaning are not feasible for humans because they tend to decrease ultimate body size. However, studies conducted on adolescent rats found that restricting diets at this point in time was just as effective on life span extension as was weaning-initiated restriction. Calorie-restricted diets for rats have received considerable attention in research (Masoro et al, 1989; Weraarchakul et al, 1990). The National Institute on Aging (NIA), which began a study on monkeys in 1987 (monkeys being closer to man than rats), so far has shown that reducing caloric intake by 30% leads to lower body temperature in the monkeys. Speculation is that lower body temperature slows body biochemical reactions and lowers levels of pentosidine. Pentosidine has been found to strongly correlate with onset of age-related diseases. Cutting calories may increase monkey life span by 30% to 50% (Ciabattari, 1996). Walford and colleagues (2002) found similar results in themselves in the 2 years that they lived in Biosphere 2.

Findings show that dietary restriction hastens DNA repair. The theory of aging based on the accumulation of DNA damage in somatic cells is an old one, but it was unknown whether repair of DNA was gradually diminished in the aging process. These studies have shown that DNA repair processes are involved in aging and, not only does restricted caloric intake slow DNA error accumulation during aging, but it also facilitates the repair process, resulting in longer-lived mice. The success of caloric restrictions on life extension of mice dates back to Cornero, who in 1507, because of illness at age 40, limited his food intake to 12 ounces a day and lived another 60 years. Dr. M. Lane of NIA suggests that average life span may be 100 to 110 years with a maximum of a 150-year possibility in the years ahead. He theorizes that if men can reduce daily calorie intake from 3000 to 2100 calories per day and women reduce their intake from 2500 to 1800 calories per day, life could be prolonged (Ciabattari, 1996). Currently, there have been a few exceptions with individuals living to 120 years of age without intentional dietary restrictions. However, it is known from the physical changes in aging that the elderly in general do not eat the same quantity of food that they did when younger.

Environment. Environmental influences affect longevity of an individual in certain obvious ways and many obscure ways not yet fully understood. Environmental factors include the physical, chemical, and thermal environments, humidity, solar radiation, soil and water composition, altitude, various pollutants, and ionizing radiation. Persons living in urban areas are exposed to more pollutants, have more varied economic capacity, and are exposed to more life-threatening situations and psychologic stressors than those living in rural settings. Urban mobility is hazardous. The opportunity for exercise, although improved in the past 15 years, is often hampered by one's lifestyle or chosen work. Hubert and colleagues (2002) believe that a healthy lifestyle and attention to other preventive measures will exert a great influence on postponing debilitating morbidity while increasing life span. There would be a compression of morbidity and a decrease of overall lifetime disability. Disability would be limited to the very last few years of life if this compression of morbidity hypothesis is correct.

Socioeconomic Status. Education, health, and marital status have been considered to have a direct or indirect influence on longevity. Education affects and is affected by social standing, income, occupation, and other factors. The higher the education, the fewer physical hazardous job risks. Individuals who complete college and graduate studies are more often able to select high-paying, low-risk jobs. Higher-paying positions afford the individual better opportunity for health care, with health maintenance being a universally recognized important longevity factor. Intelligence, too, is thought to be related to life span. Some researchers believe that those who are intelligent find better ways to survive, and others believe that greater intelligence is an obvious index of generalized superior endowment. Intelligence is genetically and environmentally determined. The potential of each of us will be able to surface and be cultivated to its optimum level, given a conducive environment, proper nutrition, and socioeconomic advantages.

Statistics have shown that marital status influences longevity, particularly for men. Whether it is the result of mutual caring by the spouse that occurs in the relationship or because of a more regulated lifestyle has not been definitely established, but those who are married have a longer life expectancy than those who are single. Social interaction, which is one component of a marital relationship, may reinforce the meaning of life, and attention to the maintenance of self for one's spouse may be a psychologic advantage toward longevity.

The 25-year follow-up of the first Duke University longitudinal study on aging (Palmore, 1982) reaffirms the variables stressed in Woodruff (1977) for the attainment of longevity. Palmore noted that intelligence, health, activities, sexual relations, and life satisfaction were all factors that contributed directly to longevity of the study group.

Jensen and Bellecci (1983) studied a group of nonagenarians in a state veterans' home and found that those very old persons measured up favorably against a group of noninstitutionalized 65- to 75-year-olds. The nonagenarians had few mental health problems or chronic illnesses, took few medications, and were more socially and physically active than their younger counterparts. Their longevity indicates an interplay of many factors as yet poorly defined. Today, increasing numbers of nonagenarians and centenarians provide an ever-increasing group for longevity research. However, biologic theories of aging, which are thought to be more sophisticated than other aspects of longevity research, are still rudimentary. Questions yet to be answered thoroughly in order to understand factors influencing longevity include the following:

- What factors account for individual longevity?
- How can predisposition to diseases be determined?
- What accounts for the increasing longevity of women as compared with men?
- What are the effects of social class?
- What are the ultimate differences caused by habits of smoking, exercise, and diet?
- How are wisdom and creativity cultivated and demonstrated in old age?

The most critical questions do not concern how long we live, but for what reasons and in what conditions. Human progress can be measured by the total percentage of individuals who achieve longevity while maintaining a life of meaning and purpose. An integrative matrix, drawing from psychologists, biologists, and sociologists, to organize the voluminous outpouring of data and fragmented bits of information is needed.

In summary, the complexities of aging and the numerous predictable and unpredictable events that occur in an individual lifetime have made many theorists conclude that aging in adulthood is a random process of change with no discernible pattern or undergirding theory. From this viewpoint, the individual organism progresses through the ordered state of programmed development to the chaotic state of later life in which patterns are no longer discernible; when the undefined, and perhaps individually developed, critical thresholds of function are exceeded and incapacity results. However, even though at this time there is not sufficient conceptual sophistication to embrace the intricacies of adult development, we continue to try to organize our expectations of the aging process into predictable, or at least expectable, patterns. There are still many areas of adult development and aging that have been minimally explored and may be the essence of development in maturity and old age. The development of love, compassion, creativity, and wisdom are areas that need considerably more attention and may in the future yield specific patterns in the aged. Tentative theories of aging recognize changes in conception of time, self-concept, hope, and future orientation as one grows old. The sense of inner control has important ramifications in terms of how one ages. Being old is an art, a science, and a challenge.

We have attempted to introduce the reader to an overview of oldness as it is seen in our society today. The body of the text will consider the relevance of all these views to health care provision and explore them in depth in further chapters. *Life* magazine featured aging in the October 1992 issue with the question, "Can we stop aging?" The next question, of course, is, "Do we want to?" The notion of a prolonged and perhaps endless life span as a possibility is one that reemerges in gerontology periodically—just as fads and fashions discipline. Frequently we hear that only 100 years ago life expectancy was 48 years and now it is in the eighties. The implication seems to be that in another 100 years most of us will live to be over 100 years old. However, the figures really mean that far fewer people are dying young, not that the human life span has increased significantly. In 1850, 50% of all deaths occurred in children under age 15. Less than 15% of people lived 60 years or longer. The actual extension of average life span has increased only approximately 0.4% per decade for a century. However, as scientists unlock the genetic code and the secrets of DNA, the next challenge is to confront the master control of death. The question is whether the maximum life span can be extended much beyond the 120 years that has been the scientifically accepted outer limit of individual human survival.

KEY CONCEPTS

- Aging is a gradual process of change over the course of time. Each species has an expected life span, and that of the human species as presently understood is limited to approximately 120 years.
- It is unknown at this time what changes over time are due specifically to aging, disease, lifestyle, or environmental impact. In other words, the changes due purely to the aging process are unknown.
- Studies of the aged in other times and places often lend interest and insight into the present study of the aged.
- There are eight or nine accepted theories of biologic aging, and they are all believed to be true to one extent or another. However, none can stand alone as the explanation of the aging process and why it occurs.
- The immunologic theory of biologic aging is one of the most coherent and widely accepted.
- Psychologic theories of aging are particularly culture and cohort bound and must be studied with that in mind. Jung and Erikson have made major contributions to our understanding of aging from the psychologic perspective.
- Life span developmental theorists tend to study the total life course of cohort groups to determine major influences on their development.
- It is becoming more generally accepted that personality characteristics, as well as biologic characteristics, are to some degree inherent in the individual.
- Studies of exceptional longevity in various geographic pockets have shown the importance of diet, exercise, environment, and, most important, adequate documentation of age. Those studies of individuals thought to be over 150 years old have proved to be questionable because of unverified birth records.
- It is expected that within the coming century we will see further "rectangularization" of aging—meaning there will be increased years of healthy aging and a more abrupt and rapid deterioration before death.

▲ CASE STUDY

Jennie attained the remarkable age of 100 the day before Christmas. There were numerous celebrations of her birthday by friends and family. She was delighted and surprised because little had been made of her birthday in previous years. She always explained it away by the fact it was so near Christmas. Aside from rheumatic aches, difficulty in breathing at times (even though she had never smoked), frequent falls, and limited energy, she considered herself healthy, had rarely been ill enough to see a doctor, and had only recently begun taking digitalis. Jennie sometimes woke during the night with urinary urgency and then had difficulty falling asleep again. At those times she would sip a shot of brandy and read until she fell asleep. During the day she wore a protective pad because she tended to leak urine when she coughed or laughed. Jennie said, "This getting old is like the one-hoss shay: everything falls apart."* Jennie had a large network of friends and an attentive family, though she was well acquainted with grief and loss. Her husband of 75 years had died 3 years before, and she had left her lovely home and beloved dog when she moved into the retirement center at age 97. She was deeply spiritual but not religious in a ritualized sense. Her granddaughter was majoring in gerontology at the local university and often talked to Jennie about her old age and remarkable adaptation in an attempt to find the key to her longevity.

Based on the case study, develop a nursing care plan using the following procedure:

List comments of client that provide subjective data.

List information that provides objective data.

List two client strengths you have identified from data.

From these data, identify and state, using accepted format, two nursing diagnoses you determine are most significant to this client's needs and strengths at this time.

Determine and state outcome criteria for each diagnosis. These must reflect some alleviation of the problem identified in the nursing diagnosis and must be stated in concrete and measurable terms.

Plan and state one or more interventions for each diagnosed problem. Provide specific documentation of source used to determine appropriate intervention. Plan at least one intervention that incorporates the client's existing strengths.

Evaluate success of intervention. Interventions must correlate directly with the stated outcome criteria in order to measure the outcome success.

STUDY QUESTIONS/ACTIVITIES

What factors would you consider important in determining Jennie's longevity?

Discuss Jennie's physical changes as they relate to theories of aging.

Discuss the factors in longevity that have presently been identified and whether these are evident in the cases of individuals you know, or have heard of, who have attained great old age.

Which of the psychologic or sociologic (or both) theories of aging seem most relevant in Jennie's case?

What theories of aging seem most plausible to you? Compare the outstanding characteristics of each.

Imagine you are Jennie and discuss with your granddaughter your thoughts about your own aging.

Discuss the meanings and the thoughts triggered by the student's and elder's viewpoints as expressed at the

*A "one-hoss shay" was a cart drawn by a horse, popular around 1910.

beginning of the chapter. How do these vary from your own experience?

Imagine yourself at 90 years old and describe the lifestyle you will have and the factors that you believe account for your long life.

Organize a debate in which each individual attempts to convince others of the logic of one particular concept of aging.

List and discuss the psychologic tasks of aging that you believe will be most difficult for you to accomplish.

Describe in a brief essay the characteristics of the oldest person you have known.

RESEARCH QUESTIONS

What physical changes can be attributed strictly to the aging of an organism?

What environmental factors in our present sociocultural milieu are clearly sources of early mortality?

What factors in relationships contribute to survival?

What variables may affect cell replication patterns?

What are the identifiable factors in extreme longevity?

What caloric distribution of carbohydrates, proteins, and fats contributes to longevity?

REFERENCES

Agarwal S, Sohal RS: Relationship between susceptibility to protein oxidation, aging, and maximum life span potential of different species, *Exp Gerontol* 31:387, 1996.

Back K: *Life course: integrative theories and exemplary populations,* Boulder, CO, 1980, Westview Press.

Balazs EA: Intercellular matrix of connective tissue. In Finch CE, Hayflick L, editors: *Handbook of the biology of aging,* New York, 1977, Van Nostrand Reinhold.

Baltes PB, Reese HW, Lipsitt LP: Non-normative developmental events, *Annu Rev Psychol* 31:65, 1980.

Bandura A: Self-efficacy: toward a unifying theory of behavioral change, *Psychol Rev* 84:191, 1977.

Banks JT: The sad but instructive case of Virginia Woolf, *J Ident Aging* 1(1):23, 1996.

Begley S: The brain in winter, *Newsweek* special edition, *Health for Life, Science and Aging,* Fall/Winter 2001, pp 24-29.

Begley S, Hagar M, Murr A: The search for the fountain of youth, *Newsweek* 115(10):44, Mar 5, 1990.

Bender BS et al: Absolute peripheral blood lymphocyte count and subsequent mortality of elderly men, *J Am Geriatr Soc* 34:649, 1986.

Benet S: *How to live to be 100,* New York, 1976, Dial Press.

Benner P, editor: *Interperative phenomenology: embodiment, caring and ethics in health and illness,* Thousand Oaks, CA, 1994, Sage Publications.

Birnbaum B, Swick L: Human suppressor lymphocyte II: changes in condanava lin A–induced suppressor cells with age, *J Gerontol* 36:410, 1981.

Birren J, Birren B: The concepts, models, and history of the psychology of aging. In Birren J, Schaie K, editors: *Handbook of the psychology of aging,* ed 3, San Diego, 1990, Academic Press.

Birren J, Cunningham W: Research on the psychology of aging: principles, concepts, and theory. In Birren J, Schaie K, editors: *Handbook of the psychology of aging,* ed 2, New York, 1985, Van Nostrand Reinhold.

Birren J, Schroots JJF: Steps to an ontogenetic psychology, *Acad Psychol Bull* 6:177, 1984.

Boersma WJA, Steinmeier FA: Age-related changes in the relative number of THy-1 and LyT-2 bearing peripheral blood lymphocytes in mice: a longitudinal approach, *Cell Immunol* 93:417, 1985.

Bowsher JE, Keep D: Toward an understanding of three control constructs: personal control, self-efficacy, and hardiness, *Issues Mental Health Nurs* 16:33, 1995.

Buhler C: The human course of life in its goal aspects, *J Hum Psychol* 4:1, 1964.

Butler R: Why survive? *Being old in America,* New York, 1975, Harper & Row.

Butler R, Lewis M: *Aging and mental health positive psychosocial approaches,* ed 2, St. Louis, 1977, Mosby.

Butler RI: Life review: an interpretation of reminiscence in the aged, *Psychiatry* 26:65, 1963.

Carry JR, Judge DS: Mortality dynamics of aging, *Generations* 24(1):19, 2000.

Ciabattari J: Parade's special intelligence report: another reason to diet, *Parade Magazine,* Aug 4, 1996, p 8.

Clark M, Anderson PB: *Culture and aging,* Springfield, IL, 1967, Charles C Thomas.

Covelli V et al: Inheritance of immune responsiveness, life span, and disease incidence in interline crosses of mice selected for high and low multispecific antibody production, *J Immunol* 142:1224, 1989.

Cowley G: The biology of aging: the body, the brain, hormones, *Newsweek* special edition, *Health for Life, Science and Aging,* Fall/Winter 2001, pp 12-19.

Cumming E, Henry W: *Growing old,* New York, 1961, Basic Books.

Cunningham W, Brookbank J: *Gerontology: the physiology, biology and sociology of aging,* New York, 1988, Harper & Row.

Darrach B: The war on aging, *Life* 15(10), Oct 1992.

Davis D: *The centenarians of the Andes,* New York, 1975, Doubleday.

Downs H: Must we age? *Parade Magazine,* Aug 21, 1994, p 21.

Ebersole PR: May your goals never be fully accomplished, *Geriatr Nurs* 17(5):258, 1996.

Erikson E: *Childhood and society,* New York, 1963, WW Norton.

Erikson EH, Erikson JM, Kivnick HQ: *Vital involvement in old age: the experience of old age in our time,* New York, 1986, Norton.

Ferguson FG et al: Immune parameters in a longitudinal study of a very old population of Swedish people: a comparison between survivors and nonsurvivors, *J Gerontol* 50:B378, 1995.

Fitch V: The psychological tasks of old age, *Naropa Inst J* 8:91, 1992.

Fjelland R, Gjengedal E: The theoretic foundation for nursing as a science. In Benner P, editor: *Interpretive phenomenology: embodiment, caring and ethics in health and illness,* Thousand Oaks, CA, 1994, Sage.

Foote J: Mexico resorts take shot at eternal youth, *San Francisco Examiner,* March 1, 1994, p. B-1.

Fries JF: Aging, natural death, and the compression of morbidity, *N Engl J Med* 303:130, 1980.

Fries JF: Healthy aging. Conference sponsored by Institute for Advancement of Human Behavior (IAHB), San Francisco, Oct 1-4, 1992.

Fuller-Thomson E, Minkler M, Driver D: Grandparents raising grandchildren, *Gerontologist* 37(3):386, 1997.

Guyton AC, Hall JE: *Textbook of medical physiology,* ed 9, Philadelphia, 1994, WB Saunders.

Hall GS: *Senescence: the second half of life,* New York, 1922, Appleton.

Hampton J: *The biology of human aging,* Dubuque, IA, 1991, William C Brown.

Harmen D: Aging: a theory based on free radical and radiation chemistry, *J Gerontol* 11:298, 1956.

Havighurst R: *Developmental tasks and education,* New York, 1972, David McKay.

Havinghurst RJ, Munnichs JMA, Neugarten BL, Thomas H: *Adjustment to retirement,* The Netherlands, Van Goreum and Company, N.V., 1969.

Havighurst RL, Neugarten BL, Tobin SS: Disengagement and patterns of aging. In Neugarten BL, editor: *Middle age and aging,* Chicago, 1968, University of Chicago Press.

Hayflick L: Human cells and aging, *Sci Am* 218:32, 1968.

Hayflick L: Why grow old? *Stanford Mag* 3:36, 1975.

Hayflick L: The cellular basis for biological aging. In Finch CE, Hayflick L, editors: *Handbook of the biology of aging,* New York, 1977, Van Nostrand Reinhold.

Hayflick L: Theories of aging. In Cape R, Coe R, Rossman I, editors: *Fundamentals of geriatric medicine,* New York, 1983, Raven Press.

Hayflick L: Biologic aging theories. In Maddox G, editor-in-chief: *The encyclopedia of aging,* New York, 1987, Springer.

Hedrick M: Immune cells. In Maddox G, editor-in-chief: *The encyclopedia of aging,* New York, 1987, Springer.

Hershey D: *Lifespan and factors affecting it,* Springfield, IL, 1974, Charles C Thomas.

Hubert HB et al: Lifestyle habits and compression of morbidity, *J Gerontol Med Sci* 57A(6):M347, 2002.

Hultsch DF, Deutsch F: *Adult development and aging: a life span perspective,* New York, 1981, McGraw-Hill.

Insight: prolonging lives in the lab, *Insight* 3:15, Mar 2, 1987.

Jazwinski SM: Longevity, genes, and aging, *Science* 273(5721):54, July 5, 1996.

Jensen GD, Bellecci P: The physical and mental health of nonagenerians (abstract), *Gerontologist* 23:290, 1983 (special issue).

Jung C: The stages of life. In Campbell J, editor: *The portable Jung,* New York, 1971, Viking Press (translated by RFC Hull).

Kallman FJ, Sander G: Twin studies on aging and longevity, *J Heredity* 39:349, 1948.

Kallman FJ, Sander G: Swedish twin studies, *Am J Psych* 106:29, 1949.

Kelly C: Personal communication, Gwynedd, PA, 1990.

Kent S: Can normal aging be explained by the immunologic theory? *Geriatrics* 32:111, 1977.

Kidd PM et al: Coenzyme Q10: essential energy carrier and antioxidant, *HK Biomedical Consultants,* Aug 1988 (monograph).

King W: Scientists find gene link to aging: landmark discovery made in patients suffering from Werner's syndrome, *San Francisco Examiner,* Apr 12, 1996, p A-18.

Kobasa SC: Stressful life events, personality, and health: an inquiry into hardiness, *J Pers Soc Psychol* 37(1):1, 1979.

Kohlberg L: Continuities in childhood and adult moral development revisited. In Boltes P, Schaie K, editors: *Life span developmental psychology: personality and socialization,* New York, 1973, Academic Press.

Kuhlen R: Developmental changes in motivation during the adult years. In Neugarten B, editor: *Middle age and aging,* Chicago, 1968, University of Chicago Press.

Lehman H: *Age and achievement,* Princeton NJ, 1953, Princeton University Press.

Lemon BW, Bengtson VL, Peterson JA: An exploration of the activity theory of aging: activity types and life satisfaction among inmovers to a retirement community, *J Gerontol* 27:511, 1972.

Lenker LT, Polivka L: Project rationale and history, *J Aging Identity* 1(1):3, 1996.

Lewin K: *Field theory in social science,* New York, 1951, Harper (theoretical paper selected and edited by Cartwright).

Lockshin RA, Zakeri ZF: Programmed cell death: new thought and relevance to aging, *J Gerontol* 45(5):B135, 1990.

Longino CF, Kart CS: Explicating activity theory: a formal replication, *J Gerontol* 35:758, 1982.

Longino CF, McClelland KA, Peterson WA: The aged subculture hypothesis: social integration, gerontophilia and self-conception, *J Gerontol* 35:758, 1980.

Macieira-Coelho A: Cancer. In Maddox G, editor-in-chief: *The encyclopedia of aging,* New York, 1987, Springer.

Maddox G: Activity and morale: a longitudinal study of selected elderly subjects, *Soc Forces* 42:195, 1963.

Maddox G, Campbell R: Scope, concepts and methods in the study of aging. In Binstock R, Shanas E, editors: *Handbook of aging and the social sciences,* ed 2, New York, 1985, Van Nostrand Reinhold.

Makinodan T: Immunity and aging. In Finch CE, Hayflick L, editors: *Handbook of the biology of aging,* New York, 1977, Van Nostrand Reinhold.

Makinodan T: Gerontologic research. In Beck J, editor: *The year book of geriatrics and gerontology, 1990,* St Louis, 1990, Mosby.

Makinodan T, Yunis E, editors: *Immunology and aging,* New York, 1977, Plenum.

Masoro EF, Katz MS, McMahan CA: Evidence for the glycation hypothesis of aging from the food-restricted rodent model, *J Gerontol* 44(6):B20, 1989.

McAvay GJ, Seeman TE, Rodin J: A longitudinal study of change in domain-specific self-efficacy among older adults, *J Gerontol* 51B(5):P243, 1996.

McClearn GE et al: The Swedish adoption/twin study on aging (submitted). Cited in Birren J, Schaie K, editors: *Handbook of the psychology of aging,* ed 3, San Diego, 1990, Academic Press.

Michel JP: Aging and the immune system. In Beers MH, Berkow R, editors: *The manual of geriatrics,* ed 3, Whitehous Station, NJ, 2000, Merck Research Laboratories.

Miller RA: The aging immune system: primer and prospectus, *Science* 273(5721):70, July 5, 1996.

Moody HR: *The abundance of life: human developmental policies for an aging society,* New York, 1988, Columbia University Press.

Nandy K, Lal H, Bennett M: Brain reactive antibodies in aging NZB mice. Paper presented at annual meeting of Gerontological Society of America, San Antonio, TX, Nov 21, 1983.

Neugarten B: Adult personality: toward a psychology of the life cycle. In Neugarten G, editor: *Middle age and aging,* Chicago, 1968, University of Chicago Press.

Neugarten B, Havighurst R, Tobin S: Personality and patterns of aging. In Neugarten B, editor: *Middle age and aging,* Chicago, 1968, University of Chicago Press.

Nicoletti C, Yang J, Cerney J: Repertoire diversity of antibody response to bacterial antigens in aged mice, *J Immunol* 150:543, 1993.

Olshansky SJ, Hayflick L, Carnes BA: No truth to the fountain of youth, *Sci Am,* June 2002, pp 92-95 (essay).

Palmore E: Predictors of the longevity difference: a 25-year follow-up, *Gerontologist* 22:513, 1982.

Peck R: Psychological developments in the second half of life. In Neugarten B, editor: *Middle age and aging,* Chicago, 1968, University of Chicago Press.

Pedersen NL: Genetics of human aging: Swedish twin studies, *Generations* 24(1):31, 2000.

Pereira-Smith OM, Bertram MJ: Replicative senescence, *Generations,* 24(1), Spring 2000.

Plomin R, McClearn GE: Human behavioral genetics of aging. In Birren J, Schaie K, editors: *Handbook of the psychology of aging,* ed 3, San Diego, 1990, Academic Press.

Pollack M, Leeuwenburgh C: Apoptosis and aging: role of the mitochondia, *J Gerontol Bio Sci* 56(11):B475, 2001.

Quinti I et al: T-dependent immunity in aged humans: evaluation of T-cell subpopulations before and after short-term administration of thymic extract, *J Gerontol* 36:6, 1981.

Recer P: Showing your age? Quality-control genes at fault, study finds, *San Francisco Examiner,* Mar 31, 2000, p A-11.

Rosenfeld A: *Prolongevity,* New York, 1985, Alfred A Knopf.

Rosow I: Status and role change through the life cycle. In Binstock R, Shanas E, editors: *Handbook of aging and the social sciences,* ed 2, New York, 1985, Van Nostrand Reinhold.

Rosow I: The social context of the aging self, *Gerontologist* 12:82, 1973.

Rowe J, Schneider E: Aging processes. In Abrams W, Berkow R, editors: *The Merck manual of geriatrics,* Rahway, NJ, 1990, Merck Sharp and Dohme Research Laboratories.

Rudman D: 1990 (cited in Darrach B: The war on aging, *Life* 15[10]:38, Oct 1992).

Sacher GA: Life table modification and life prolongation. In Finch CE, Hayflick L, editors: *Handbook of the biology of aging,* New York, 1977, Van Nostrand Reinhold.

Sarton M: Poetry reading sponsored by Women's Lecture Series, San Francisco, 1989.

Sawada M, Carlson JC: Association between lipid perioxidation and life: modified factors in rotifers, *J Gerontol* 42:451, 1987.

Schaie KW: A general model for the study of developmental problems, *Psychol Bull* 64:92, 1965.

Scheer JF: Jack of all nutrients: coenzyme Q19, *Better Nutrition* 58(8):48, Aug 1996.

Schlessinger D: Alleles and aging: the effects of different forms of genes on aging and longevity, *Generations* 24(1):36, Fall/Winter 2000.

Schneider EL: Organ systems: introduction. In *The Merck manual of geriatric medicine,* ed 2, Whitehouse Station, NJ, 1995, Merck Research Laboratories.

Schroots JJF: In growing, formative change and aging. In Birren JE, Bengtson VL, editors: *Emergent theories of aging,* New York, 1988, Springer.

Schroots JJF, Birren JE: Concepts of time and aging in science. In Birren J, Schaie K, editors: *Handbook of the psychology of aging,* ed 3, San Diego, 1990, Academic Press.

Sharma R: Theories of aging. In Timiras PS, editor: *Physiologic basis of geriatrics,* New York, 1988, Macmillan.

Smith GS, Walford RL: Influence of the main histocompatibility complex on aging in mice, *Nature* 270:727, 1977.

Smith JR, Pereira-Smith OM: Replicative senecence: Implications for in vitro aging and tumor suppression. *Science* 273:63-67, 1996.

Sohal RS, Weindruch R: Oxidative stress, caloric restriction, and aging, *Science* 273(5721):59, July 5, 1996.

Strehler B, editor: *The biology of aging, symposium, no 6,* Washington, DC, 1960, American Institute of Biological Science.

Tockman M: Effects of age on the lung. In Abrams W, Berkow R, editors: *The Merck manual of geriatrics,* Rahway, NJ, 1990, Merck Sharp and Dohme Research Laboratories.

U.S. Bureau of the Census: *Statistical abstract of the United States, 2001,* ed 211, Washington, DC, 2001, U.S. Government Printing Office.

Van Gool WA, Mirmiran M: Aging and circadian rhythms, *Prog Brain Res* 70:255, 1986.

Walford RL: *Maximum life-span,* New York, 1983, Norton.

Walford RL: *The 120-year diet: how to double your vital years,* New York, 1986, Pocket Books.

Walford RL et al: Caloric restriction in Biosphere 2: alterations in physiologic, hematologic, hormonal, and biochemical parameters in humans restricted for a 2-year period, *J Gerontol Bio Sci* 57A(6):B211, 2002.

Wayne SJ et al: Cell-mediated immunity as a predictor of morbidity and mortality in subjects over 60, *J Gerontol* 45(2):M45, 1990.

Weraarchakul N et al: The effect of aging and dietary restriction on DNA repair. In Beck J et al, editors: *Yearbook of geriatrics and gerontology,* Chicago, 1990, Mosby.

Williams RM et al: Genetics of survival in mice: localization of dominant effects to sub-regions of the major histocompatibility complex. In Serge D, Smith L, editors: *Immunological aspects of aging,* New York, 1981, Marcel Dekker.

Wise PM, Krajnak KM, Kashon ML: Menopause: the aging of multiple pacemakers, *Science* 273(5721):67, July 5, 1996.

Wolanin MO: Personal communication, San Antonio, TX, Sept 28, 1996, Air Force Village II.

Woodruff D: *Can you live to be 100?* New York, 1977, Chatham Square Press.

Yates FE: The dynamics of aging and time: how physical action implies social action. In Birren JE, Bengtson VL, editors: *Emergent theories of aging,* New York, 1988, Springer.

Yen S: Newsclip, NBC News, Sunday, June 18, 1996.

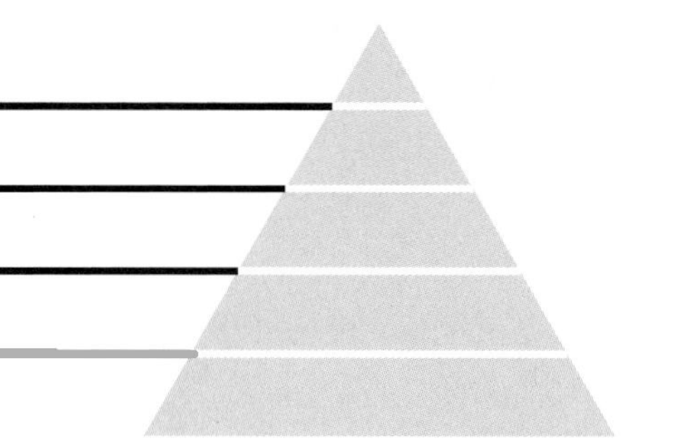

CHAPTER 3

Health and Wellness

Patricia Hess
Priscilla Ebersole

A student speaks

I was so surprised when I went to the senior center and saw all those old folks doing Tai Chi! I feel a bit ashamed that I don't take better care of my body.

Maggie, age 24

An elder speaks

Just a change in perspective! I can choose to be well or ill under all conditions. I think, too often we feel like victims of circumstance. I refuse to be a victim. It is my choice and I have control.

Maria, age 86

LEARNING OBJECTIVES

On completion of this chapter, the reader will be able to:

1. Define *health* and *wellness.*
2. Compare the difference between the health/wellness concept offered in the health and wellness and medical models.
3. Discuss the five dimensions of wellness.
4. Explain wellness in the context of chronic illness.
5. Identify gender differences that affect health/wellness and chronic illness.
6. Explain how and if the goals of wellness for elders can be accomplished.

HEALTH

Health and wellness are vague concepts; we do not fully understand either health or wellness. Our concepts and beliefs about healthy living habits are in constant flux. Jog until you develop a shin splint, run for euphoria, bike to exhaustion, ski, and exercise. For some time now the focus has been on eliminating fat from the diet, attending to cholesterol, at other times sugar, then the salt intake, and there are also the organic food enthusiasts. A recent example from *Science* magazine (Taubes, 2001) tells us that nutritional science has demonized fat but that they have not yet proved that eating a low-fat diet will help you live longer. In fact, they say, the low-fat emphasis has run parallel with increased carbohydrate intake and the epidemic obesity since 1980. Temporary fashions have merit when done moderately, but, rather than bounding from one craze to the next, one must listen carefully to one's own body and to the source and quality of research. Elders in particular must be fine-tuned to the messages the body gives them and take responsibility for maintaining its function at the best level possible (see Chapter 6 for a discussion of nutrition).

As society moves into the twenty-first century, the long-existing but ignored concept of illness prevention and health promotion has emerged as individuals recognize that the present "health care" system does not meet their needs. Only recently have aging persons been considering health in a proactive manner. Elderly individuals are now being strongly encouraged through media and health care systems to take personal responsibility for their own health through knowledge and behavioral change. Terms increasingly heard in the health arena now are *empowerment of the individual, prevention,* and *health promotion.* The U.S. Department of Health and Human Services publications *Healthy People 2000* (1991) and *Healthy People 2010* (2000) offer direction for the achievement of a better quality of life across the life span in the United States through measures that are directed at the reduction and prevention of health risks, unnecessary disease, disability, and death. The goals set forth by *Healthy People 2000* include

Box 3-1 Summary Objectives for Adults Age 65 and Older *(Healthy People 2000)*

Health Status

Reduce:

- Suicide among white males
- Death by motor vehicle accidents (age 70+)
- Death from falls and fall-related injury, particularly age 85+
- Death from residential fires
- Hip fractures
- Number of persons who have difficulty performing two or more personal care activities so as to enhance independence
- Significant visual impairment
- Epidemic-related pneumonia and influenza deaths
- Pneumonia-related days of restricted activity

Increase:

- Years of healthy life to at least 65 for blacks and Hispanics

Risk Reduction

Increase:

- The percentage of individuals who regularly participate in light-to-moderate activity for at least 30 minutes a day
- Immunization levels for pneumococcal influenza among the chronically ill older population
- The percentage of older persons who receive, within appropriate intervals, screening and immunization services and at least one counseling service

Services and Protection

Increase:

- Percentage of recipients of home food service
- Percentage of older adults who have the opportunity to participate yearly in at least one organized health promotion program through senior centers, life care facilities, or community-based settings serving the older adult
- Percentage of states in the United States that have design standards for signs, signals, markings and lighting, and other roadway environmental improvements to enhance visual stimuli and protect the safety of older drivers and pedestrians
- The proportion of primary care providers who routinely review with their patients prescribed and over-the-counter medications each time a new medication is prescribed
- The usage of the oral care system
- The proportion who receive clinical breast examinations and mammograms
- The number of women age 70+ with uterine cervix who receive Pap tests

Extend:

- Long-term institutional facilities, the requirement for oral examinations, and service provided to new admissions no later than 90 days after entering a facility

From *Healthy People 2000,* 1991, US Department of Health and Human Services, US Government Printing Office, Washington, DC, pub no (PHS) 91-50212.

the following: (1) increasing the span of healthy life for Americans, (2) reducing health disparity among Americans, and (3) achieving access to preventive services for all Americans through health promotion, protection, and preventive services. A summary of the *Healthy People 2000* objectives for adults 65 years of age and older appears in Box 3-1. Box 3-2 shows the leading health indicators. The intent of these proposals is not only to lengthen life but, more important, to improve quality of life and functional independence of the aged. Many of those 85 years of age and older are not independent in their physical function, thus affecting their day-to-day living. The ultimate goal for the elderly is to delay illness, prevent the ill from becoming disabled, and assist those who are disabled to function and prevent further disability. Largely, the *Healthy People 2010* goals do not comprehensively address the health of individual elders but address

Box 3-2 Leading Health Concerns from the *Healthy People 2010* Database

- Physical activity
- Overweight and obesity
- Tobacco use
- Substance abuse
- Responsible sexual behavior
- Mental health
- Injury and violence
- Environmental quality
- Immunization
- Access to health care

From National Center for Health Statistics: *Data 2010: the Healthy People 2010 database,* Washington, DC, 2002, Centers for Disease Control and Prevention.

Box 3-3 ***Healthy People 2010* Objectives for the Public Health Infrastructure**

Increase access to information systems to apply data and information to public health practice.
Increase public awareness of leading health indicators, health status indicators, and priority needs.
Increase nationwide use of geographic information systems.
Increase proportion of population-based *Healthy People 2010* objectives for which national data are available for all population groups identified for the objective.
Increase availability of leading health indicators for select populations.
Increase proportion of *Healthy People 2010* objectives that are tracked regularly at the national level.
Increase proportion of *Healthy People 2010* objectives that are released within 1 year of data collection.
Increase incorporation of specific competencies in essential public health systems and personnel systems.
Increase integration of curricula specific to competency in public health services.
Increase proportion of agencies that provide continuing education to develop competency in essential public health services for all their employees.

From U.S. Department of Health and Human Services: *Healthy People 2010,* Washington, DC, 2000, U.S. Government Printing Office.

the public health system in response to the 2002 Institute of Medicine study (U.S. Department of Health and Human Services, 2000; Institute of Medicine, 2002) (Box 3-3).

In the medical arena, health is considered to be the absence of disease. Conformity to physical and mental capacity norms indicates one's health status. Therefore the more observable the evidence, the more definite the degree of health that can be declared or the diagnosis that can be affixed. Those biologic and physiologic capacities not considered essential for the performance of *well* activity are less likely to be considered significant.

The emergence of a strong holistic health movement has refocused on a clear definition and operational approach to health and wellness. The holistic approach has long been in existence but has received little attention. Dunn (1961) saw health in a holistic context and defined it as an integrated method of functioning that is oriented toward maximizing the potential of which the individual is capable within the environment where he or she is functioning. Maslow recognized this as self-actualization. The holistic definition does not limit health to just its physical or mental or even social aspects but rather incorporates all of these facets in the total picture.

Sometimes health, per se, seems to be a limiting term that does not encompass the breadth that the terms *wellness* or *well-being* suggest. Spector (1996) indicates that we find it difficult to define health without the use of some form of medical jargon, whereas "well is a state of being, an attitude . . . it is more than the absence of illness . . . it is an ongoing adaptational process" (Travis, 1977). Wellness involves one's whole being, physical, emotional, mental, and spiritual, all of which are vital components. Spector (1985) and Markides and Mindel (1987) add the dimension of culture to the holistic health approach. Accordingly, what is considered wellness to the individual must include his or her cultural orientation. Culture cannot be relegated to a subposition under any other health component. It must stand equally so that health care providers can realize and more adequately respond to the significance of culture in the attainment of well-being. Perhaps Pender and colleagues (2002) have synthesized this most difficult concept from all the preceding definitions by defining health as "the actualization of inherent and acquired human potential through satisfactory relationships with others, goal-directed behavior and com-petent personal care while adjustments are made as needed to maintain stability and structural integrity." And yet, no specific definition of health can really convey the entirety of it (Spector, 1996; Pender et al, 2002).

The meaning that we attribute to health is continuing to change, and now the increasing focus is on prevention. Health is also being seen as a more expansive phenomenon with multiple dimensions: biopsychosocial, spiritual, environmental, and cultural (Pender, 2002). Change in any of these dimensions affects the health of an individual in a positive or negative manner. A change initiates (triggers) a behavioral change that can lead to empowerment. Empowerment may open many options for improving one's health. A positive approach to health emphasizes *strengths, resilience, resources, and capabilities*, rather than existing pathology.

Confusion often arises when the definitions of health, wellness, and well-being are used interchangeably by the general public and medical practitioners when discussing an individual's condition. The wellness model refers to health as one aspect in the achievement of wellness. The wellness approach suggests that every person has an optimum level of functioning for each position on the wellness continuum to achieve a good and satisfactory existence (well-being) (Figure 3-1). Even in chronic illness and dying there is an optimum level of wellness and well-being attainable for each individual. Lawton (1983) offers the "good life" concept as useful in considering health of the aged in its broadest context. Well-being in the Lawton model consists of four intersecting yet autonomous segments of life: psychologic well-being, perceived quality of life, objective environment, and behavioral competence. Nurses have been among those caregivers who have attempted to provide care using the holistic philosophy, but they continue to struggle to make it integral to patient care. In an attempt to meld the broader health-wellness concepts and initiate a more positive approach to the capacities of the aged, we offer this working definition for the care of the aged individual: Wellness is the best achievable balance between one's environment, internal and external, and one's emotional, spiritual, social, cultural, and physical processes. Figure 3-2 attempts to illustrate the interrelationship of the facets that compose health and successful aging.

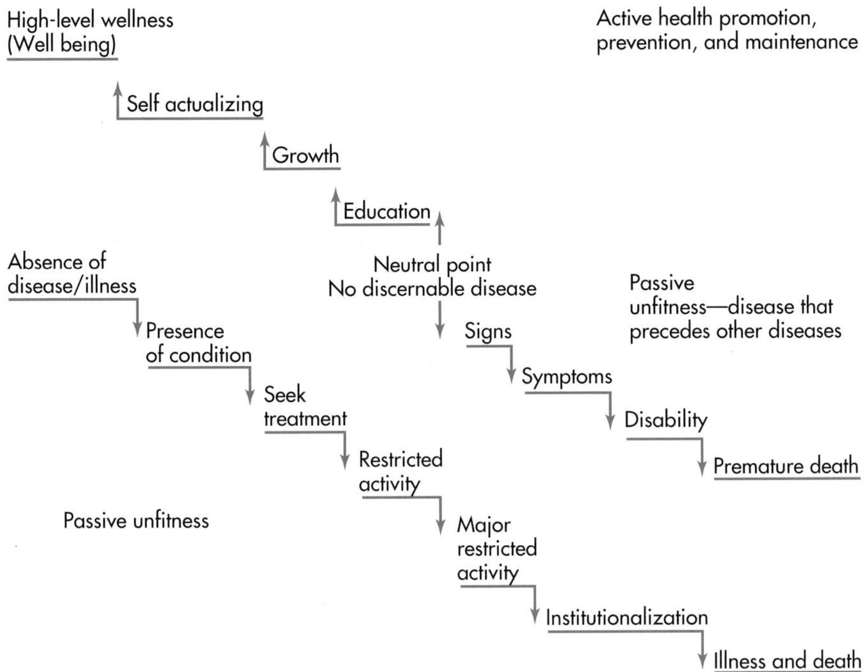

Figure 3-1. Comparisons of wellness/health and traditional medical continuum.

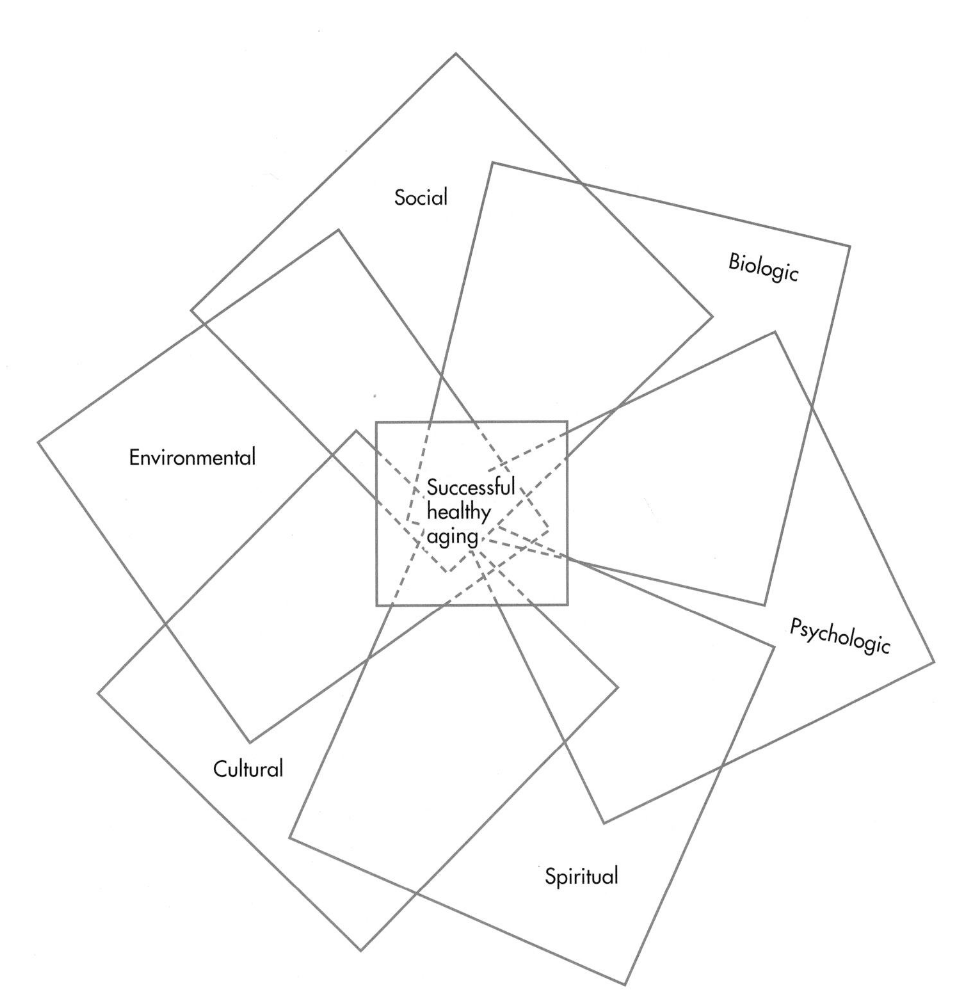

Figure 3-2. Healthy aging. (Developed by Patricia Hess.)

Each aspect is like a petal, anchored to the center and overlapping the other petals, each affecting the whole. Alterations in or loss of a petal can change the overall effect or appearance and its wholeness.

To achieve wellness or assist an individual to attain wellness potential, one needs to consider the dimensions of wellness: self-responsibility, nutritional awareness, physical fitness, stress management, and environmental sensitivity (Pender et al, 2002, pp. 20-22). Each of these is discussed later in this chapter.

Measurements of a population's health status rely on life expectancy, morbidity, and death tables. These figures provide information on illness but do not reveal the extent to which the living are affected by these conditions. They do not indicate the health status, only the illness. For example, in morbidity tables people who are actually functioning at a high level of wellness are assigned to illness categories. Persons compiling these tables do not consider that the person with health disorders, malignancies, and other conditions may be able to attain and function at a high level of wellness and be a contributing member of the community. The wellness approach is perhaps the most equitable in the evaluation of the aged individual's potential for maximum functioning. Thus the individual who has acute and chronic conditions and those with disabilities may all seek wellness.

What are health and wellness for the aged? Are they determined by an individual's health history, a comparison with peers, the population at large, previous generations, or none of these? Worrying excessively about health is often more disabling than incurable illness. When individuals or clients acknowledge disease processes that cannot be cured they are then able to take up their lives and feel better because they are able to cope. With the onslaught of medication ads on television, we have learned to take minor symptoms too seriously and are in danger of becoming a nation of hypochondriacs. In other words, those who believe that they are ill, act ill, even in the absence of clinical signs, and those who perceive themselves well will act well.

Cousins (1983) presents a case demonstrating how expectations can induce illness or promote health. Larry went for his annual checkup. After seeing his cardiogram, the physician asked when he had had his heart attack. Larry responded that he had never had one. The doctor convinced him he had previously suffered a silent coronary of massive proportions. That night Larry experienced severe chest pain, was admitted to the hospital, and collapsed during a treadmill test. An angiogram showed blockage of the major coronary arteries, and he was scheduled for coronary bypass surgery. He was so emotionally devastated, the surgeon called Norman Cousins in to talk with him. Cousins reviewed his chart and suspected he had been frightened into his symptoms. After a week of reassurance, support, making a game of the treadmill exercise, laughing and joking about the machine, and playing music, he exhibited no symptoms at all and the surgery was canceled. Additional evidence that mind influences physiologic responses in an appreciable and measurable way comes from recent endocrinologic studies. A corollary can be drawn to describe interactions between the nurse or other caregivers and aged clients; treat the aged as if they are ill and dependent and they will respond with illness and dependence.

The assumption that old age is a downhill course may be realistic from a physiologic point of view. It is also recognized that the overall physical functioning of the body is mainly determined by the available energy and adaptive capacities. The conviction by nurses and other caregivers that the aged are individuals with declining health generates responses that includes treating the aged as ill and feeble, or potentially so. It is therefore expected by some that attempts to reverse conditions or situations, maintain a level of ability, or institute preventive health measures are useless for the aged. Nothing could be further from the truth; all old people are improvable (Bortz, 1991). Rehabilitation becomes a major part of care of the aged. It may be the key to returning the aged person to his or her best or highest level of independence and functioning on the wellness continuum. Once there, maintenance of health becomes of prime importance.

Rehabilitation involves strengthening weakened muscles, improving endurance, increasing range of motion, improving coordination of movements and skills, restoring a functional gait, and reestablishing activities of daily living that will enable aged persons to regain control over their lives and achieve their own concept of good and satisfactory existence: the attainment of well-being. Rehabilitation is a dynamic process that engenders all of the aforementioned components.

In some instances this may be the total return of body function; in other circumstances the individual may not completely recover but is at an acceptable level for himself or herself and others involved. The individual must be allowed to use his or her resources and capacities.

Statistics show that despite the fact that approximately 86% of the aged experience chronic conditions, 95% of these people are able to live in the community (Farquhar, 1992). The image of the poor and sick old has been continuously emphasized by the mass media, despite the fact that it reflects neither the real world of the aged nor the findings of social scientists. Maggie Kuhn, founder of the Gray Panthers and advocate for the aged, in an open letter to the Gerontologic Society of America, pointed out that social gerontology tends to focus on the individual, to the neglect of the socioeconomic structure and forces that segregate, stereotype, and victimize old people. She went on to state that, as the objects of research, the old, poor, and stigmatized persons are viewed as problems to society, not the victims of that society. The end result is that these aged are then directed to adjust to the situation rather than the society seeking ways to be more humane and making changes that meet the needs of the aging. Well-being for those over 60 years old is strongly related to health but is also affected by socioeconomic factors, degree of social interaction, marital status, and aspects of one's living situation and environment. Needs of the old and the very old differ in kind and degree, just as health behavior differs from one country to another, reflecting a different cultural style and physical and social environment. The aged attempt to be active and

Box 3-4 Traits of a Healthy Person

Attuned to mind-body signals of pain and pleasure as well as fatigue, anger, and sadness.
Can confide own secrets, traumas, and feelings to others instead of keeping them locked inside.
Exhibits control over health and quality of life.
Exhibits a strong commitment to work, creative activities, or relationships.
Able to see stress as a challenge rather than a threat.
Demonstrates appropriate assertiveness concerning needs and feelings.
Forms relationships based on unconditional love rather than power.
Is altruistically committed to helping others.
Is willing to explore many different facets of own personality, which provides strength to fall back on if he or she fails.

Modified from Dreher H: *The immune power personality: seven traits you can develop to stay healthy,* New York, 1995, Dutton.

self-sufficient in nearly every cultural group. The key words seem to be *productive* and *useful.* Admission of illness or incapacity is, to the aged person, a sign of weakness, and to others of that society, it is a sign that the individual cannot carry his or her own weight or be helpful to the goals of the group. The aged are cognizant that illness leads to dependency and that illness with all its ramifications does not mesh well with modern society and its youth and productivity orientation. Only recently have the aged begun to break out of this mold of illness and dependency. It bears repeating here that every aged person has an attainable optimum level of wellness, which can be achieved independently or with the aid and support of caregivers. Hey (1996) contends that the aged can achieve high-level wellness through the promotion of productivity, self-actualization, self-respect, self-determination, and continued personal growth. In essence, the aged need to make themselves necessary (Bortz, 1991). With limited disability, the aged can still achieve a high level of wellness if the emphasis of care is placed on prevention of the loss of independence and the promotion of function in the least restrictive environment, in other words, aging in place. Box 3-4 presents traits of a healthy person.

HEALTH CONTINUUM

The medical interpretation of the health continuum is that if the individual is in good health or is well, there is an absence of disease or impairment. Figure 3-1 indicates the progression along the traditional health continuum. When an individual develops a condition, it is expected that treatment will be sought to resolve the ailment. The individual, at this point, begins the descent to dependency and despondency, either temporarily or for an extended period. The role of the individual is more passive than active. This dilemma is common in the aged. The individual becomes reliant on the caregiver for wellness; the caregiver, in turn, tends to foster that dependent position; and as a result, "the more help older people are given the more help they will come to need . . . well-meaning practitioners undermine autonomy" (Bortz, 1991).

Health care continues to be based on acute cause and cure, the traditional medical model. In the early 1900s, this was an appropriate approach to health care: Individuals contracted diseases that medical science could hope to cure (smallpox, diphtheria, syphilis, tuberculosis, polio, appendicitis, etc.). Today, however, chronic diseases and illnesses are the predominant conditions. Chronic disease or illness does not have a single cause, nor does it have a cure (Fries, 1992). Instead it has a universal progression based on risk factors that may begin and remain unseen for decades before the condition surfaces in a pathologic state. Examples include heart disease, diabetes mellitus, arthritis, and cancer. Another issue in the medical model is that if the aged person's malady does not fit an already existing disease entity or diagnostic category, it is generally written off as a "sign of old age."

When one uses the wellness or holistic approach, which has been suggested as a more appropriate model for the aged, one regards the health and wellness continuum from a more positive direction and the role of the individual is more active.

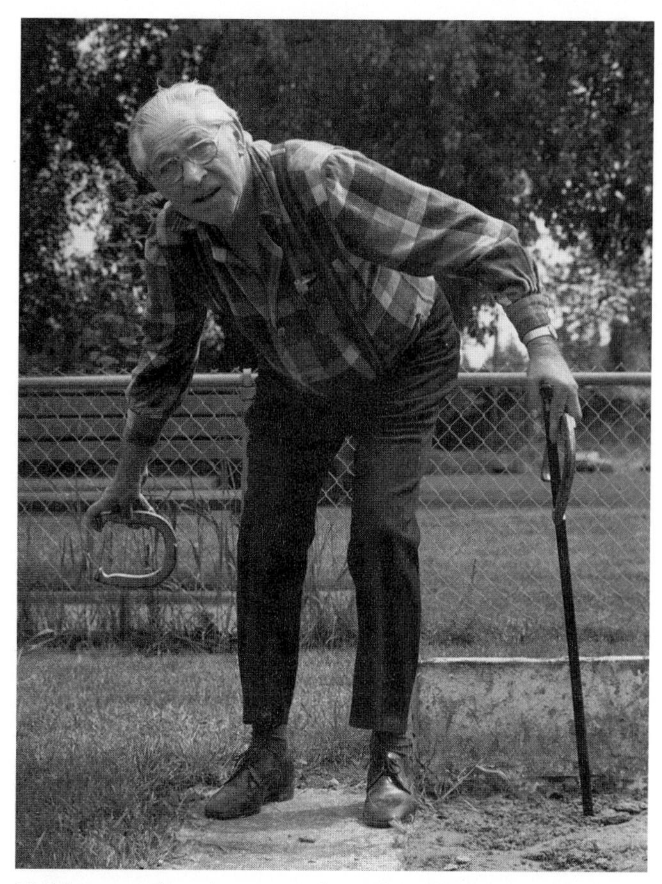

Nothing stops the enjoyment and exercise of horseshoes. (Courtesy Rod Schmall.)

The traditional or medical model of health questions whether everyone is capable of reaching or maintaining a high level of wellness. The wellness model places wellness within the grasp of all persons, regardless of age. The significance for the aged is a new and positive approach to what the nurse and other caregivers call "healthy." Wellness begins with the individual and stimulates the desire for growth and change. This means nurturing the physical self, expressing emotions more freely, improving personal decision making, becoming more creative with others, staying in touch with the environment despite physical incapacities, and improving health practices (Hey, 1996). The wellness continuum picks up where the traditional medical model leaves off. Instead of a downward negative trajectory for the health of the aged, focused on deterioration, the wellness model rises and moves in a positive direction (see Figure 3-1). The individual may reach plateaus in his or her ascension to higher-level wellness. The person may also regress because of an illness event, but the event can be a stimulus for growth potential and a return to moving up the wellness/health continuum (Figure 3-3). The division between the traditional and wellness continuums is a neutral point, where no discernible illness or weakness exists. Wellness is not given to a person; rather it is a state of being and feeling that one strives to achieve through motivation and health practices. An individual must work hard to achieve wellness just as he or she must work hard to perform competently at a job.

It is encouraging to note that some physicians are recognizing the limitations of the traditional medical model for most of the aged within our health care system and are assuming a primary care mode that includes diagnosis and treatment of acute episodic disease, monitoring chronic illness, controlling the rate of established disease, promoting wellness through vaccination programs, offering behavior modification to decrease health risk factors, and encouraging regular visits to obtain psychologic support, counseling, education, and monitoring (Rowe, 1991; Kotthoff-Burrell, 1992; Schmidt, 1994). In addition, some practitioners acknowledge and incorporate alternative therapies such as body work (massage, touch therapy), herbal and nutritional therapies, psychoneuroimmunology, and acupuncture into their practice (Gillespie, 1996).

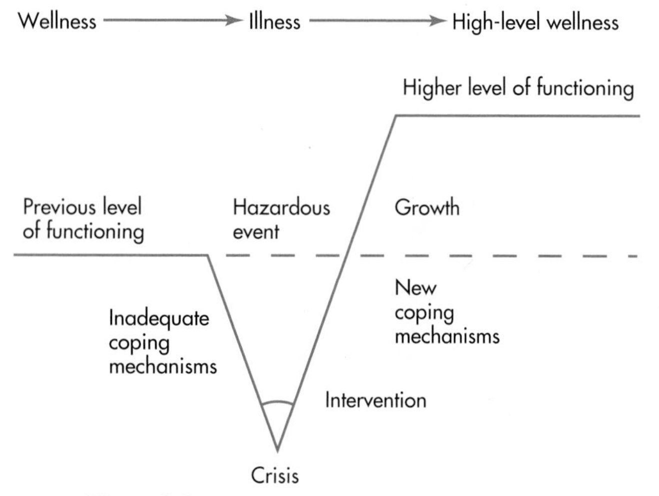

Figure 3-3. Growth potential: crisis as a challenge.

Wellness and self-actualization develop through learning and growth. Education for wellness concerns the pursuit of the five dimensions of wellness mentioned earlier in this chapter: self-responsibility, nutritional awareness, physical fitness, stress management, and sensitivity to the environment. All of these dimensions are crucial to one's wellness. Incorporation of these five dimensions into a lifestyle facilitates individual growth and attainment of Maslow's self-actualization and Erikson's eighth stage of growth and development, integrity. Growth and self-actualization are one's ultimate reward.

Wellness means more than preventive medicine. Preventive medicine is largely offensive in its approach to illness, employing vaccinations and screenings to avoid illness. Whereas, wellness is a collaborative effort between an individual and the primary care provider to maximize the quality of life. Wellness encourages health promotion and life enhancement, as well as addressing risk factors that can lead to disease and chronic illness if ignored.

DIMENSIONS OF WELLNESS

Self-Responsibility

Self-responsibility, or self-efficacy, implies control and places one's wellness in one's own hands. It says to the individual, "Your body is your house; how you maintain your body is your choice." It has a strong effect on one's health behavior. Many aged are not attuned to their body messages and have little or no knowledge about their health status, while others are attuned to negative rather than positive messages. Often the aged have placed the responsibility for keeping well in the hands of the nurse or others who give care. As a result of abdicating control over their own wellness, dependent behavioral expectations and roles evolve among the family, the caregiver, and the client.

Times are changing. The self-help movement for taking care of one's health needs has expanded enormously in the past few years. Governmental agencies have changed their focus to health promotion and disease prevention, necessitating client involvement in health outcomes. Elders and retired workers are teaching each other self-help strategies (Weinrich et al, 1993; Uzelac, 1994). People are responding to these approaches and taking control of their lives. People are learning how to be in touch with their body signals and to take and seek action accordingly. People are now cognizant of wellness through health education and the publicity holistic health has received, but many aged are still functioning within the earlier framework, which is reinforced by Medicare. For the aged to be exposed to new ideas and provided with options or choice, we must have changes in the politics of health care delivery—positive changes rather than an interpretation of self-care as a political solution to the health care problem and an answer to the distribution of resources. Nor should self-care or management be considered a social remedy to the redistribution of power away from the medical profession. Early on, Senator Inouye (Hawaii) and others promoted legislation to establish nurse-managed community clinics for the express purpose of serving individuals vulnerable to institutionalization. These have been piloted successfully at several sites throughout the nation, and nurse-managed community clinics have been established but still are too few in number. In such clinics, the client is a partner in maintaining maximum levels of health and independence in the community.

There is always a significant time lag between change and acceptance of new ideas. The aged today are taking control of their lives and bodies and are taking initiative and becoming empowered to educate themselves by actively seeking out those who can provide the particular information about their physical and mental needs, nutrition, and management of stress. Media blitzes and the Internet have made enormous differences in their ability to obtain desired information. Efforts that are most successful build group responsibility and social processes that are intrinsic to the self-health focus of the movement. Early publications such as *Take Care of Your Self* (Fries and Vickery, 1990) and *Healthwise for Life* (Kemper and Mettler, 1992) provide the aged with information to make decisions for themselves about health care and teach them how to get their questions answered by physicians. Recent offerings through the National Institutes of Health (NIH), health insurance companies, for-profit companies, and health maintenance organizations (HMOs) make numerous publications available to interested parties. In addition to self-help books, the aged are learning to more clearly communicate with their health care providers.

Consumer readiness and willingness to adapt new behaviors and learn self-care skills will not lead to increased health or economic benefit unless providers of care simultaneously make adjustments in their own attitudes and responses to the active consumer role. It is becoming essential as better prepared consumers bring their ideas to their health care providers for discussion (Walker, 1994).

Hirschfeld (1985) cites basic behaviors that must be fulfilled for self-care and responsibility. The individual must initiate the definition of a health care need, define a plan of action, and decide what actual health-related activity steps to take, as well as assume responsibility and accountability for the actions. Another important point made by Hirschfeld is that the individual can act on his or her own behalf or can have a family member or friend act on his or her behalf. The same behaviors apply to groups of elders in the community. Self-care activities can respond to needs along the entire health continuum of promotion, prevention, acute care, chronic conditions, maintenance, and terminal care.

Change of health care behaviors is difficult for both the aged and the caregiver. Dr. James O. Prochaska (1994) outlines five steps toward change: *precontemplation, contemplation, preparation, action,* and *maintenance.* An individual may spend months in precontemplation and contemplation before he or she considers the benefits of action. Once the action occurs, maintenance begins about 6 months later. It is not uncommon and should not be considered failure if an individual has to make several cycles through the stages before the desired effect is achieved. Behavioral researchers have shown that, in the example of smoking, 85% of smokers who eventually quit recycled back through precontemplation and contemplation stages. However, each relapse taught them something new to try in the next cycle. Box 3-5 outlines the steps in health behavior change.

The nurse can empower, enhance, and support the aged person's movement toward self-responsibility by exploring with the aged the underlying situations that may be creating a wellness imbalance and discussing with the aged the alternatives available to them. Given sufficient unbiased information, the aged can, in most instances, make meaningful decisions. Nevertheless, some aged persons choose not to be responsible for their wellness. At times people prefer illness because it offers an escape from unpleasantness and responsibility, a means of gaining needed attention, a way of masking

Box 3-5 Steps for Health Behavior Change

Precontemplation

Extended time period

Negative aspects of undesirable behavior stay in the periphery of the mind

Contemplation

Toy with ideas of change

Examine behavior problem

Consider balance between cost and benefit

May take a long time

Preparation

Intention to change unites with plan of action

Concrete steps to be taken within the next month

Action

Actual steps taken to modify behavior

Person feels empowered and in control of life

Frequently relies on support from others

Takes 1 day at a time

Maintenance

Begins 6 months after action

Prevention of relapse

Lasts a lifetime

From Prochaska JO et al: *John Hopkins medical health letter: health after 50,* Baltimore, 1996, John Hopkins Medical Institutions.

inadequacies, and a legitimate role for the aged person in society. That choice, although contrary to the wellness concept, is a choice made by the individual. Many very old persons are imbued with the idea that the doctor always knows best and would feel very insecure taking charge of their own care. Given the choice of wellness or not, however, most aged will opt to be in control of their bodies, minds, and spirits. Self-responsibility includes developing a personal health guide for maintaining good health by seeking important health examinations. There is general agreement about what examinations are important for persons 50 years and over, as well as a timetable for such examinations and tests. Table 3-1 lists the suggested preventive examinations that should be sought to maintain good health for those over 50 years old, according to the group involved and the frequency of testing. In addition, self-responsibility incorporates universal self-care requirements (Box 3-6).

Nutritional Awareness

The nation as a whole is obese and remains undernourished because of an imbalanced diet. The nutrition of the elderly reflects this current dietary practice of food intake and use. Nutritional awareness involves learning about the foods that will make the body respond in a physically and emotionally healthy way. Heightened awareness is learning about "live" foods (fresh food, not canned or frozen) and nutrient-dense foods. Economic considerations, mobility, and other factors may place the aged in nutritional jeopardy. Eating habits evolve from childhood, and specific dietary preferences and ethnic diets, although favored by an individual, may not provide the best nutrition. The aged frequently depend on fast foods, prepared foods, and soft foods because of their convenience and the ease with which they can be carried and consumed. However, those foods are more expensive and contain many empty calories in addition to high amounts of salt, fats, and sugar. In the aged, caloric needs decrease, but the need for nutrients does not change. Selection of food should be directed toward the highest nutritional density. The problem with nutritional awareness among the aged is the lack of nutritional education. Through reading, counseling, and classes, the aged can learn to select and use "live" food in endless ways. Nutritional education might stimulate creative meal planning and bring to light both the economic benefits and the joy of new discoveries. The aged can be made more cognizant that good nutrition can prevent some of the chronic conditions that occur during old age. Problems such as constipation need not occur if the diet includes sufficient quantities of raw fruits and vegetables and whole wheat grains. Caloric intake for most aged

Table 3-1 Suggested Examinations for Preventive Health Maintenance for Persons 50 Years Old and Older

Examinations and tests	Population group	Frequency
Complete physical, including cholesterol check every 5 years	All persons	Every 1-3 years until age 75; then every year thereafter
Pelvic examination and Pap smear	Women	Annually if sexually active; every 3 years otherwise
Breast self-examination	Women	Monthly
Clinical breast examination	Women	Yearly
Mammogram	Women	Annually after age 50
Digital rectal examination	All persons	Annually for women with pelvic examination; every 2 years for men
Sigmoidoscopy	All persons	Every 3-5 years after age 50
Stool for occult blood	All persons	Annually
Prostate examination	Men	Yearly
Blood pressure	All persons	Every office visit
Eye examination	All persons	Annually after age 50
Glaucoma test	All persons	Every 3 years after 55; every year if family history
Dental examination and cleaning	All persons	Yearly for those with teeth; cleaning every 6 months, every 2 years for denture wearers
Hearing test	All persons	Every 2-5 years
Immunizations		
Flu vaccine	All persons (well and with chronic conditions)	Annually for age 65 and over
Pneumonia vaccine	All persons (well and with chronic conditions)	Once after age 65 or over; ask physician about booster
Tetanus booster	All persons	Every 10 years
Hepatitis B	Those at risk	Complete series

Compiled from AARP strategies for good health; *Healthy People 2000*, Washington, DC, 1991, U.S. Government Printing Office; Schmidt RM: Preventive health care for older adults, societal and individual services, *Generations* 18(1), 1994; *Healthwise*, Kaiser Permanente, 1994; St. Mary's Medical Center, San Francisco, 1995; *Mayo Clinic Health Letter* 14(1), 1996; and Burke MM, Laramie JA: *Primary care of the older adult: a multidisciplinary approach*, St Louis, 2000, Mosby.

Box 3-6

Universal Self-Care Requirements

1. Maintaining sufficient intakes of air, water, food
   a. Taking in that quantity required for normal functioning with adjustments for internal and external factors that can affect the requirement, or, under conditions of scarcity, adjusting consumption to bring the most advantageous return to integrated functioning
   b. Preserving the integrity of associated anatomic structures and physiologic processes
   c. Enjoying the pleasurable experiences of breathing, drinking, and eating without abuses
2. Provision of care associated with eliminative processes and excrements
   a. Bringing about and maintaining internal and external conditions necessary for the regulation of eliminative processes
   b. Managing the processes of elimination (including protection of the structures and processes involved) and disposal of excrements
   c. Providing subsequent hygienic care of body surfaces and parts
   d. Caring for the environment as needed to maintain sanitary conditions
3. Maintenance of body temperature and personal hygiene
   a. Bringing about and/or maintaining internal and external conditions necessary for regulating body temperature processes
   b. Using personal capabilities and values as well as culturally prescribed norms as bases for maintaining personal hygiene
   c. Caring for the environment to maintain a healthy living condition
4. Maintenance of a balance between activity and rest
   a. Selecting activities that simulate, engage, and keep in balance physical movement, affective responses, intellectual effort, and social interaction
   b. Recognizing and attending to manifestations of needs for rest and activity
   c. Using personal capabilities, interests, and values as well as culturally prescribed norms as bases for development of a rest-activity pattern
5. Maintenance of a balance between solitude and social interaction
   a. Maintaining that quality and balance necessary for the development of personal autonomy and enduring social relations that foster effective functioning of individuals
   b. Fostering bonds of affection, love, and friendship; effectively managing impulses to use others for selfish purposes, disregarding their individuality, integrity, and rights
   c. Providing conditions of social warmth and closeness essential for continuing development and adjustment
   d. Promoting individual autonomy as well as group membership

From Department of Health and Human Services: *Toward a plan for the chronically mentally ill,* report to the Secretary of Health and Human Services, Washington, DC, 1980, Department of Health and Human Services.

individuals is uncertain; many do not eat the recommended 1200 to 1400 calories per day, whereas others eat well over this amount. In general, though, elders' appetites seem to diminish as they age. The aged may need to take a vitamin supplement. If aged individuals are insecure about their nutrient intake from food, taking a daily supplement that supplies no more than 100% of the recommended amount of any nutrient will suffice. Beyond that, however, they risk distorting the body's nutrient requirements and suffering toxic effects from nutrient excess. Those who do not get exposure to sunshine may need vitamin D supplementation.

We are what we eat, and if the aged are to take control of their mind, body, and spirit to provide themselves with the highest level of wellness possible, it is essential that they become active in their nutritional intake. Aged persons who are institutionalized and capable of making food selections should be allowed to do so, not only from the menu offered but also by perhaps forming a dietary selection group to plan menus with the dietitian or the institution's administration.

In summary, few aged individuals eat an adequate diet. Nutrition is discussed in more depth in Chapter 6.

Physical Fitness

Almost ¾ of older adults are sedentary. By age 75, 33% of men and 50% of women are inactive in their leisure time (Buckner, 2002; Pender et al, 2002). Inactivity poses serious health hazards to young and old alike. It can lead to hypertension, coronary artery disease, obesity, tension, chronic fatigue, premature aging, poor musculature, and inadequate flexibility. Many people do not exercise often, but, when they do, it is usually a crash program that ends in injury, failure, or death. Many aged believe that they are too old to begin or participate in an active fitness program, but, even with chronic conditions, a fitness program is possible. The fundamental issue often overlooked is that each individual requires a program of activity that will work best for him or her. No matter how nutritionally aware, practiced in self-responsibility, or able to cope with stress, without physical fitness, one will not be fit or well.

Fitness involves aerobic capacity, body structure, body composition, balance, muscle flexibility, and muscle strength. The rewards are a better self-concept, the ability to cope with stress, decreased depression, improved eating habits, less joint stiffness, a better overall ability to relate to people, and improved balance. The most well-known type of fitness program is aerobic activity. The goal of aerobic activity is to fortify the body against stress. Aerobic activity such as jogging, swimming, and tennis is not out of reach for many aged. Doing the activity fast is not so important as is sustaining the endeavor long enough to accelerate the respiratory and cardiac rate sufficiently to reap benefits. Regular sustained aerobic exercise of the type and duration that will benefit the heart and blood vessels has been found to produce higher levels of high-density lipoproteins (HDLs) and lower blood triglyceride and cholesterol levels. Exercise also affords more efficient use of carbohydrates and a decreased resistance to insulin. Activity is discussed in greater depth in Chapters 6 and 13. Those aged persons who have continued activity and exercise because as a part of their everyday lifestyle continue to feel happier and healthier and look younger than those who were active but have now abandoned fitness. Those aged who begin physical fitness regimens need to be aware of the benefits but should also seek medical guidance when embarking on an exercise program.

Those who are capable of walking and being relatively active have a number of fitness activities open to them. Brisk walking for a sustained period of 10 to 15 minutes will tone the leg and arm muscles, provide improved oxygen exchange, and increase heart function. Some aged enjoy dancing, which can be as strenuous as programmed exercise; others who enjoy gardening can benefit from this as well (Bortz, 1996; Ulene, 1996). For those aged who are limited in ability or confined to a chair, exercises can be done from a sitting position, which will accomplish many of the same benefits as if the individual were ambulatory.

Body balance is important to prevent falling. Muscle flexibility facilitates full range of motion for life's many activities that require stretching, bending, and reaching (Figure 3-4 demonstrates stretching exercises to maintain and increase flexibility). Muscle strength should be such that one can exert force and control over movement of the body. MacRae (Steinberg, 1994) took 60 residents from 10 California nursing homes who ranged in age from 80 to 106 (average age 90 years) and put them through a 5-month exercise program. Each of the participants had four chronic conditions and took at least four medications daily. After 5 months the elders were found to regain lost abilities as well as retain what they already had. A study conducted by the Hebrew Rehabilitation Center for the Aged in Roslindale, Massachusetts, used 100 residents ages 72 to 98 for an exercise program that included lifting weights. Each person received an individually designed program of regular 45-minute exercise periods. Some in the program needed canes, walkers, and wheelchairs, and more than 60% had fallen in the past year. The results of this physical activity produced a 113% increase in muscle strength and an 11% increase in walking speed. Four participants who had used walkers were now able to use only canes (Steinberg, 1994). Easily accessible household objects, such as 1-pound bags of rice or beans or unopened half-pound or one-pound cans, or partially filled quart or half-gallon water bottles, can be used for weight lifting in sustained continuous repetitions to strengthen arm muscles. It is also possible to purchase variable wrist and ankle weights in sporting goods stores. Ginsberg (1994) reports that weights increased older women's muscle strength and bone density and decreased the risk of falls. Individuals who are weak or have poor balance should begin balance exercises, walking and strength training programs before attempting aerobic-type programs (*Harvard Health Letter,* 1999, 2000). Figure 3-5 illustrates a progression for strengthening the upper body with dumbbells.

Regardless of age or situation there is some activity the older person may find that will be suitable to his or her condition. Following are examples of the myriad ways in which elders keep fit:

- Em, an 84-year-old nursing home resident, jogged every morning in place for about 5 minutes and then briskly walked around the outside of the facility. Although she occasionally had lapses of memory, she was vital, erect, and interested in life around her.
- Nellie, 83 years old, began swimming to ease the discomfort of a short left arm, the residual effect of poliomyelitis, and for a frozen shoulder. She became an award-winning synchronized swimmer with 20 gold medals, 12 blue ribbons, and 13 trophies to her credit. Nellie continued to exercise this way despite the need to wear cataract goggles.
- At 64 years old, Dick became an avid wind surfer.
- In 1977, 91-year-old Madame Alexandra Baldina-Kasloff, prima ballerina in the early 1900s with the Bolshoi Theater, Moscow, was still participating in 90-minute workouts with her dance students.
- Hans Selye was known to swim for 30 minutes in the morning and ride his bicycle through the McGill University campus and then swim another 30 minutes in the evening and lift weights until his death in 1982 at 75 years old.
- Ada, age 82, still runs daily.
- Anabel, age 70, just completed her one-hundredth marathon.
- Woody, age 83, is a surfer.
- The Sun City Aqua Suns, synchronized swimmers, range in age from 68 to 88.
- Catherine, who died at 106 years old, walked to the bathroom three times each day; this was her activity. It was difficult for her to do this, but without it she would have no longer walked or been able to sustain herself.

Many programs are designed to reduce premature institutionalization of the elderly and alter the sedentary lifestyle of the aged by acquainting them with the health benefits of regular physical activity. Table 3-2 compares sedentary and active approaches to daily living. Nursing homes need to consider

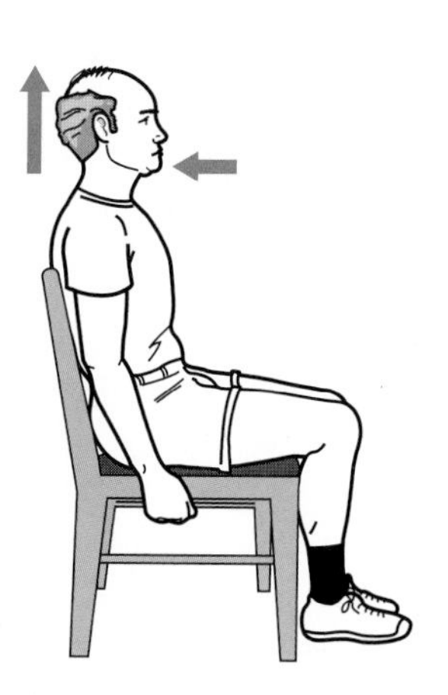

A Gently pull chin in while lengthening back of neck. Hold 10 seconds.

Repeat: ______Times
______Times a day

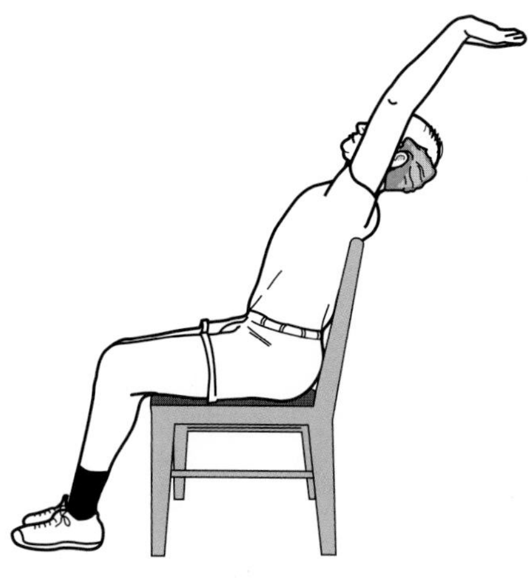

B Bring arms straight up over head and back as far as possible, causing back to arch gently. Hold 10 seconds.

Repeat: ______Times
______Times a day

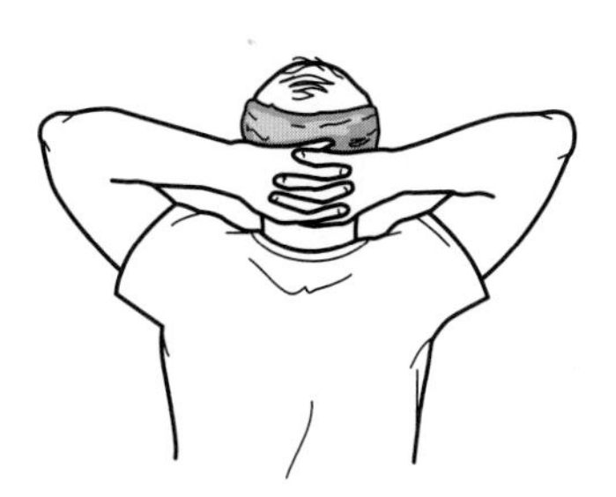

C Place hands behind your head and pull elbows back as far as possible. Hold 10 seconds.

Repeat: ______Times
______Times a day

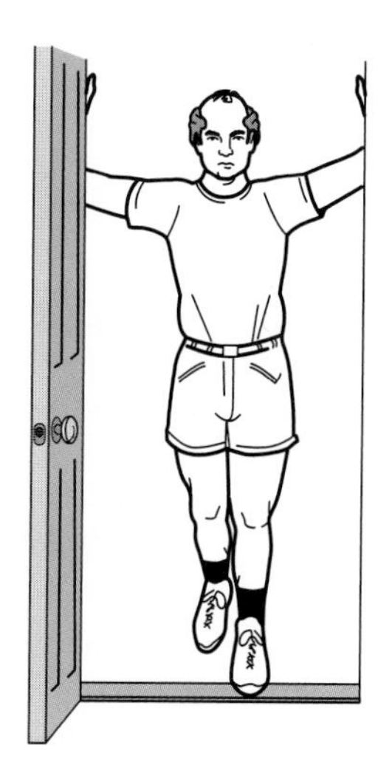

D With arms behind doorjamb, gently lean forward. Hold for ____ seconds. Stretch is felt across chest.

Repeat: ______Times
______Times a day

Figure 3-4. Examples of stretching exercises. (From Burke MM, Laramie JA: *Primary care of the older adult: a multi-disciplinary approach*, St Louis, 2000, Mosby.)

exercise programs, such as walking, for their residents even if they are frail. A walking program for frail elders was instituted to promote functional mobility. The outcome was a decrease in falls (Koroknay et al, 1995). The basic theory behind the fitness emphasis is that the better a person's condition, the more oxygen the person can inhale from the air. Although the individual may not need this extra oxygen most of the time, in stress situations he or she will; it is at these times that oxygen reserve can make a difference between health and disease or even life and death.

The nurse who is knowledgeable in aging, age changes, health risk factors, and exercise science can develop and lead exercise programs for older adults. This was demonstrated by Gillett and colleagues (1993) when they worked with

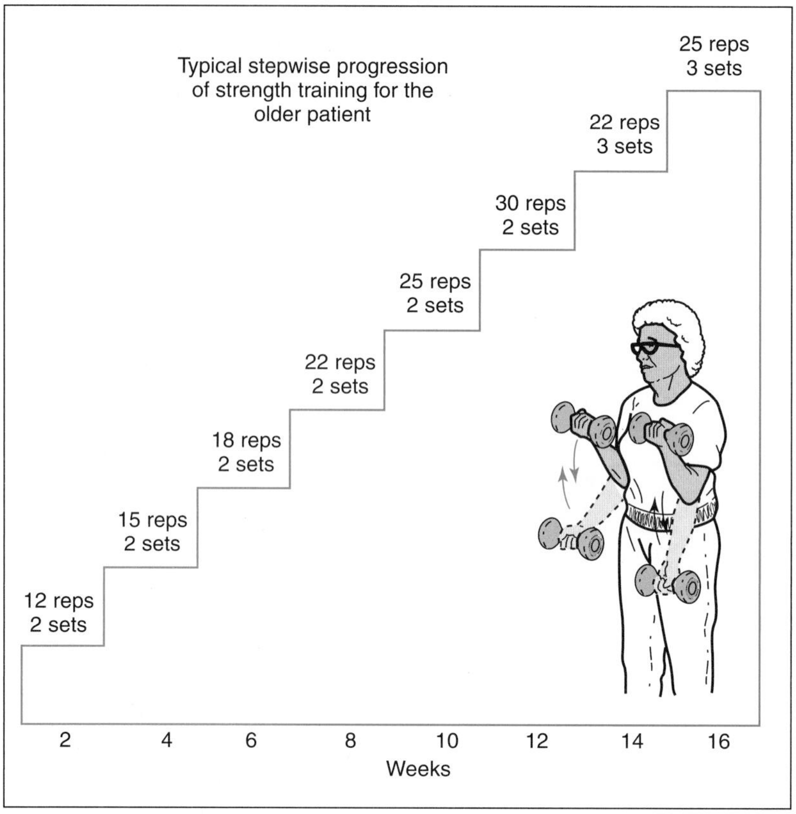

Figure 3-5. An approach used in progressing an older person's dumbbell exercise program. The approach can be applied to other forms of strengthening programs. (Reproduced with permission from *Geriatrics* 47(8):34, 1992. Copyright 1992 by Advanstar Communications, Inc. Advanstar Communications, Inc. retains all rights to this article.)

overweight women ages 50 to 70 in a health, fitness education, and aerobic training program for a period of 16 weeks. Nurses who were 50 to 60 years of age and not athletically inclined were chosen and educated to lead the women. The outcomes proved to be positive. The study suggests that nurses who work with the aged obtain knowledge of exercise science.

Table 3-2 Sedentary and Active Approaches to Daily Living

Sedentary	Active
Take the elevator or escalator.	Climb the stairs.
Call on the phone.	Walk down the hall or walk next door.
Drive to lunch.	Walk to lunch.
Sit in a chair throughout a meeting.	Get up quietly and walk about the room.
Park right next to your destination.	Park some distance away from your destination.
Use the TV remote control.	Get up and walk to the TV when you want to change the channel.
Remain sedentary at your desk.	Take several minutes to do arm and leg exercises.
Visit with your colleagues in the "break room."	Take a walking break while you visit.

From Pender NJ, Murdaugh CL, Parsons MA: *Health promotion in nursing practice*, ed 4, Upper Saddle River, NJ, 2002, Prentice Hall.

The aged population would benefit greatly from nurse-led programs designed specifically for the aged, which deal with their health conditions such as arthritis, diabetes, obesity, hypertension, and low self-esteem.

Stress Management

Attitudes toward various life events determine one's perceptions of pleasure or displeasure. Uncontrollable events in daily life are responsible for many of the stresses experienced by the individual, but the individual also creates many stress situations. Selye (1974) defined *stress* as the body's response to any nonspecific demand placed on it, whether pleasant or not.

Any stressor will initiate stimulation and elevation of the enzymes in the adrenal glands to produce the major stress hormones: epinephrine, norepinephrine, and adrenal corticoids. These hormones are responsible for activating biochemical changes in the nervous, endocrine, and immune systems, which in turn affect all organ systems. Stein (1982) and Lazarus and Folkman (1984) investigated the association among psychosocial phenomena, stress, and alterations in the immune system. The findings revealed a significant depression of lymphocyte response following the loss of a spouse, particularly during the first 2 months. The lymphocyte response returned to prebereavement levels by 5 months after the death. These findings support a biologic basis for a link among psychosocial processes, immune function, and health and illness. Sustained stress can lead to such physical consequences as heart disease, hypertension, bowel irritation, and skin disorders (Eliot, 1992). These conditions, when identified with stress as a major factor, are called *stress-related diseases.*

Dubos (1965) stated that the mind influences the body and vice versa. Dubos cited the following points: Scientific experimentation shows that immunologic and physiologic processes can affect the course or perception of disease. The course of infection depends on the humoral and cellular immunity mechanisms, but these are influenced by the mental state. Digestion can be accelerated or slowed by mental processes. Mental states have long been known to affect secretion of certain hormones, for example, those of the thyroid and adrenal glands. It has been shown that the brain and the pituitary gland contain a class of hormones that are chemically related and collectively called endorphins. Their physiologic activity is similar to morphine, heroin, and other opiate substances that relieve pain. Acupuncture can trigger the release of these pituitary hormones that somehow gain access to the cells of the spinal cord and affect the perception of pain. The neuropsychoimmunologic link is associated with both acute and chronic infections, as well as cancer (Cacioppo, 1994).

Most people recognize visible manifestations of stress such as increased body movement or language, irritability, sweaty or clammy hands, insomnia, and accelerated heart rate. The body responds to stress through the general adaptation syndrome (fight or flight). Fight or flight is an inborn response and part of the human character. It is frequently referred to as that "extra squeeze of adrenaline." At times it provides the individual with what seems to be superhuman power to escape from danger or the necessary stamina to complete essential detailed information by a deadline.

The general adaptation syndrome (Selye, 1956) is composed of the alarm reaction, the stage of resistance, and the stage of exhaustion. Most stressors produce change only in the first two stages; more serious stressors lead to the exhaustion stage and thus death. However, exhaustion does not always terminate in death; when only part of the body is involved, the exhaustion stage may be reversible. For example, this frequently is the situation in exercise or local or regional infections. The hormonal activity initiated by the alarm reaction triggers the sympathetic nervous system to respond by elevating the blood pressure, pulse, and respirations and increasing metabolism and blood flow to the muscles. Biochemical changes begin, and the varied defense mechanisms of the body attempt to organize as a united front. At this point, while the body is mobilizing its forces, the individual's resistance is lowered. Once mobilization of defenses is completed, resistance rises to meet the threat. Adaptive capacity of the body is used to establish the individual at a new level of functioning or return the person to the prestress level; in other words, a return to a balanced state.

Adaptive energies are finite. When an individual is stressed over long periods, adaptive capacity is taxed and adaptive reserves are depleted. Minor happenings become major events, causing the body to remain mobilized in a ready state. Bortz (1991) refers to this as "too much energy." When stressed again, one is forced to deal with or handle the stress at a lower threshold. Homeostasis remains tenuous and terminates eventually in illness or an irreversible state of exhaustion: death.

The aged are more frequently in a position of decreased ability to cope with daily hassles, cumulative life events, and other stressors because of their waning adaptive capacity. The deficits in adaptability are most evident in neuroendocrine interaction and in the separate responsiveness of the nervous and endocrine systems. It does not make a difference whether stress is physical or emotional; the aged require more time to recover or return to prestress levels than when they were younger. In other words, the rate of recovery decreases with increasing age (Pender et al, 2002). Stress inventories are helpful in determining areas and degrees of stress, but it is wise to keep in mind that these tests have flaws. Stress inventories do not weigh individual differences; they relate to generalized stresses. What is stressful to one individual may not be perceived as such by another. It is also important to note that some individuals thrive on stress, whereas others require peace, quiet, and tranquillity. Further discussion of stress can be found in Chapter 22.

Various means of stress reduction exist. Some individuals use one; others use a combination of methods. Most people believe relaxation is best achieved by being in tune with one's feelings. Four basic emotions (anger, fear, enthusiasm, grief) are common to all people. Some cultures place more emphasis on expression of one emotion than on another. Americans have great difficulty expressing anger. Instead of releasing feelings and thoughts, these are internalized, with such manifestations as muscle tension, voice changes to high tones, cold hands, posturing, and a general feeling of tightness. With an understanding of one's feelings and thoughts, the individual is more able to deal with these emotions and direct them positively to minimize the frequency of stress-involved responses. Exercise is one of the best antistress activities. Other methods include 10 to 20 minutes each day of deep relaxation, yoga, prayer, deep breathing, or fantasizing or daydreaming to remove oneself from stressful situations.

Meditation. Meditation is a form of relaxation and coping with stress. It is an experimental exercise involving the individual's actual attention. There are many forms of meditation. In Eastern tradition, meditation involves working toward a psychologic state termed *transcendental awareness* that restricts the focus or attention to an object of meditation, a physiologic process, or an internal sensation. Mastery over attention develops an awareness that allows every stimulus to enter into consciousness devoid of our natural selection process; the ordinary cognitive process is stopped. To truly quiet the mind, practice and perseverance are necessary. Dramatic changes in lifestyle are not necessarily inherent in effective meditation. Two forms of meditation practiced in Western culture are Zen meditation and transcendental meditation. Both of these induce a state of relaxation.

Biofeedback. Biofeedback is a technique of getting feedback from the body's internal processes. By observing monitoring devices, persons can learn to influence heart rate, circulation, and muscle tension. Biofeedback is a learned skill in stress control and explores the body-mind connection. Biofeedback can be used to treat about 50 different psychosomatic disorders. It is particularly useful in conjunction with a wide variety of relaxation techniques. Machines show the individual the body-mind connection by providing visual or auditory signals to help the person develop awareness and then gain control of a specific autonomic function such as heart rate, blood pressure, muscle tension, or body temperature. Once learned, feelings that evoke the desired responses on the machine are applied by the person to everyday stresses without the aid of the machine. If the skill has been well learned and practiced, the results will be helpful to the person in stressful situations. Pioneer work at the Menninger Foundation demonstrates that individuals can be taught to control such body responses as vascular dilation and constriction to counteract migraine headaches, to lower blood pressure associated with hypertension, and to regulate heart rate in certain cardiac arrhythmias such as premature ventricular contractions.

Autogenic Training. Autogenic training is a system of total body biofeedback or self-regulation without machinery; it is a combination of yoga and autosuggestion. Anyone without excessive hearing impairment or inability to concentrate can learn to regulate involuntary psychologic and physiologic processes through autogenics. Autogenics has been found to be effective in treatment of disorders of the gastrointestinal, circulatory, and endocrine systems, as well as anxiety, irritability, and fatigue. It can be used to increase resistance to stressors, reduce or eliminate sleep disorders, and modify pain. Autogenic training requires motivation. Those without motivation or with severe emotional disorders should not consider autogenics as a means of stress reduction.

Additional Methods of Stress Reduction

Progressive relaxation. Relaxation decreases muscle activity and activity in the sympathetic and parasympathetic nervous systems. Relaxation results in decreases in oxygen consumption of the body, metabolic rate, respiratory rate, heart rate, premature ventricular contractions, both systolic and diastolic blood pressure, and muscle tension, and an increase in alpha brain waves.

Progressive relaxation, a method developed by Edmund Jacobson in 1938, can be achieved through tension-relaxation techniques of specific muscles or muscle groups or, without tension, through the countdown method, imagery, or recall of pleasant events or experiences.

Arranging one's environment. Arranging one's environment to reduce the potential for stress is also possible. Designing a quiet environment, a place where one can take a momentary break to reenergize, is a way to reduce stress. For the aged, the proximity of familiar belongings and environment can do much to reduce stress. Stress arises not only from worry, anger, expectations, and demands but also from loneliness, noise, and lighting. One should preplan to prevent stress from occurring or, if it does occur, to be ready for it. Application of what one has learned from a previous situation can help dissipate the intensity of stress. Occasionally getting lost in some creative pursuit is an excellent means of dealing with stress. For some, knitting is helpful, whereas others find that painting a pastoral scene or the side of the house works well. Just stroking a pet or watching fish swim in an aquarium can serve as a tranquilizer to stress. Others enjoy fishing, a game of golf, reading a book, or listening to music. Still others find writing poetry a means of releasing frustration and stress. Physical activity is an appropriate means of handling stress for some individuals. It provides time to revitalize after a stressful incident.

Developing selfishness. It is important to clearly understand what the aged person's goals are and to make sure that those goals are really expressive of self and are not goals that someone else wants fulfilled. Acceptance of someone else's goals can create much stress. Frequently the aged are caught in this situation, when an individual trying to help imposes expectations on the aged person.

Perhaps one of the better ways of handling stress was expressed by Selye in an interview (Cherry, 1978) in which he recommends the practice of altruistic egotism; that is, look out for oneself first and give pleasure to self and others. *Eustress,* a term coined by Selye, is a balance of selfishness and altruism (altruistic egotism) that facilitates self-care and through which an individual has the desire and energy to care about others. Most individuals who exhibit stress-linked disease tend to be either too selfish or too self-sacrificing.

All methods and means to achieve stress management are open to all ages. Stress management requires education and change, which in itself can be stressful. In this technologic society, stress reduction includes changing the environment, avoiding excessive change, time control, and time management. However, if stress management is taught in the context of eustress, that is, taking stress and making it work positively for you, the individual will gain in ability to control the stress in life.

Environmental Sensitivity

More attention is beginning to be focused on physical, social, and personal environmental spaces and their relationship to stress and health. The physical components of environmental sensitivity (air, water, and land mass) and the social components (government, economics, and culture) are avenues through which the individual's health and wellness can be enhanced or limited. For example, the personal component of environmental sensitivity, one's immediate environs, affects the individual's ability to pursue health and wellness. In midlife, one creates much of his or her own personal environment by career, job, friends, and lifestyle choices. However, the individual's influence on physical and social environment

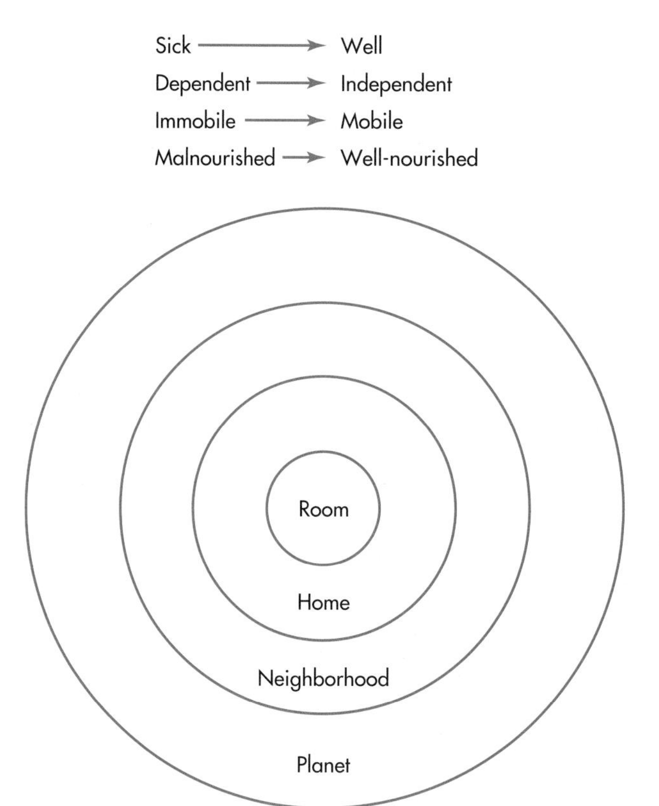

Figure 3-6. Environmental sensitivity. (From States D: Personal conversation, San Francisco, 1986.)

is more limited than in the personal sphere. One can consider where to live based on pollution, energy conservation measures, and food sources available, but, if a work situation or a relocation is mandated, there is little one can do. The aged are confronted with social and economic issues that force environmental changes against their wishes.

Energy conservation is an important environmental issue that influences one's health and wellness. Nations would be healthier by economizing their fuel resources. Body heat can adequately be maintained by wearing additional clothing and using extra blankets at night rather than turning the thermostat up. The aged would not find this too difficult despite the concern about their inability to tolerate temperature variations. The variations of temperature that would be of concern would be extreme temperature alterations rather than several degrees one way or other.

Personal space should be designed to include the opportunity for increasing self-development and experience, for receiving helpful feedback, and for establishing roles that are judged important. Personal environment should also facilitate time to be with friends, provide a supportive network, allow for enjoyment of beauty and nature, and provide abundant opportunities to give and receive affection and reinforce wellness behavior. The personal environment of many aged persons living in the community and in institutions is devoid of the ingredients that make and reinforce a state of wellness. Again, instead of watching the aged languish or by chance discover means of improving their personal spaces, it should be the role of the caregiver to help the individual learn about opportunities and ways to design a better, happier, and healthier personal environment. Within confines, this is done in nursing care facilities that allow the aged individual in residential care to bring a limited number of meaningful items.

The sights and sounds confronting the aged person and the opportunities to socialize, to make friends, and to feel wanted and perhaps loved should be important to the caregiver. Directly or indirectly, all of one's senses are affected by and affect the environment. Without this fifth dimension, wellness will not be of a high level. All dimensions are interrelated and influence one's state of health and wellness.

States (1986) uses the environmental components of the individual's room, the home, the neighborhood, and the planet at large as a basis of environmental sensitivity. Figure 3-6 provides a graphic view of the interrelation between environment and the four dichotomous elements: sick-well; dependent-independent; immobile-mobile; and malnourished –well-nourished. Environmental sensitivity, or *crush,* at any one of these levels may determine the individual's response to wellness or illness.

Self-efficacy affects all dimensions of health and wellness. Measurement of self-efficacy is a potential predictor of an aged person's ability to create and recover from new challenges of failure and loss, and it should concur with individuals' estimate of their ability to deal with complex ambiguous and pressure-filled situations (Bortz, 1991).

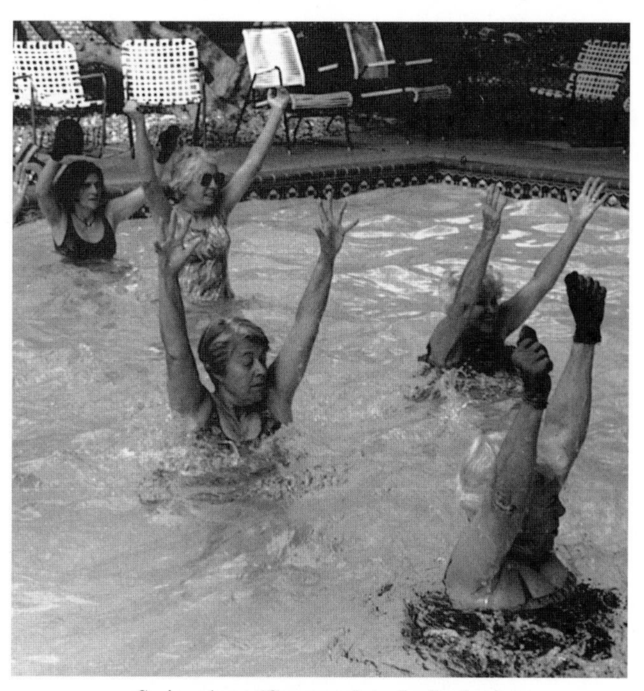

Swim class. (Courtesy Loy Ledbetter.)

CHRONICITY AND WELLNESS

Chronicity

Chronic illness is the hallmark of aging and the number one health problem for the elderly in the United States. Chronic disorders are difficult to delimit because so many acute disorders have chronic sequelae and, too often, the results of treating acute disorders is a chronic residual disability. Chronic conditions are the accrual of life's earnings, sometimes self-generated, often inherited, or occurring as the result of imposed lifestyle and environmental hazards. Lubkin and Larsen (2002, p. 8) define chronicity as "the irreversible presence, accumulation, or latency of disease states or impairments that involve the total human environment for supportive care and self-care, maintenance of function, and prevention of further disability."

The prevalence of chronic conditions continues to rise with the decline in mortality rates, the lengthening of the frail aged life span, and highly technical medical care. The incidence of chronic illness triples after age 45 but decreases markedly in relation to higher socioeconomic status. Although limited in scope, a study of a northern California socioeconomically advantaged community revealed that the individuals in that community lived longer without chronic illness but spent a longer portion of late life in a state of debilitating health (Reed et al, 1995). At times the aggressive treatment of one disorder results in the emergence of additional disabilities iatrogenically induced (Reed et al, 1995).

Certain terms describing the accompaniments of chronic disorders, such as *handicap, impairment,* and *physical limitation,* are used rather indiscriminately. Decreased function without incapacitation also needs to be stated consistently because these and other terms are often used interchangeably. Available statistics may be easily misinterpreted if one does not question how these terms are being used.

The explosion of chronic illness is a catalyst for change. Presently two thirds to three fourths of disabled elders are cared for at home with few or no formal services. Because the present approach to health care and health emphasizes symptoms and symptom reduction, society is becoming more malignant in terms of environment, diet, and stress inducers, and health care is becoming economically unavailable to more and more of our population. Estimates now exceed 40 million. Great changes are needed in our philosophy about health and health care. There is a noticeable revival of the American ideal of individualism and self-responsibility with considerable focus on "self-care." It is suggestive of a system failure and adoption of whatever devices one can muster for self-extrication. We believe deeply in self-responsibility, but, as in every situation, if a similar level of responsibility is not exerted in the metasystem one can hardly be successful within the microsystem. For example, an individual intent on a healthy diet may find it difficult to find vegetables and fruits free of pesticides, prepared foods free of preservatives, fish free of toxic waste products, and meat and poultry free of hormones and antibiotics. How, then, can one take appropriate self-care? In addition, without adequate information one cannot make responsible decisions or choices to facilitate self-care.

The appropriate approach is highly individualistic and may involve changing the situation, modifying treatment, or retraining the individual to compensate for the pathophysiologic changes. The impact of chronic illness is also highly individual and may include identity erosion, expectations of death, dependency conflicts, and feelings of failure or fatalism, or it may mobilize the individual to live life to its fullest.

Wellness in Chronic Illness

A state of wellness may be achieved and maintained consistently during chronic illness if the individual feels capable of and motivated to manage the problems with or without assistance. The aged can be supported toward the achievement of wellness and maximizing their life satisfaction when caregivers ascribe to a holistic philosophy that incorporates efforts directed toward the maintenance of the aged person's self-care and self-esteem.

Figure 3-7 shows how the wellness continuum and Maslow's hierarchy of needs can complement each other in the attainment of wellness and self-actualization. Also Orem's self-care model has increased awareness of the individual's direct impact on disease and the impotence of nursing and medicine to effect positive change in a depressed, declining individual who no longer cares.

It is clear that a reorganization of this nihilistic thinking is needed by the aged and those associated with them: kin, friends, and caregivers. Physical manifestations of chronic illness should not be the sole determinative factor in the establishment of the elder's state of health or wellness. A study by Markides and colleagues (1993), although limited, suggested that one should not always assume that physician assessments represent an objective "gold standard" for validating self-reported measures of health. The greatest factor in establishing wellness is adaptation. To achieve maximization of life satisfaction, adaptation of lifestyle is necessary whether it is through environmental manipulation, modification of treatment, or retraining the individual to compensate for pathophysiologic changes. Positive coping or adapting to chronic conditions is contingent on the accomplishment of the following tasks:

- Ability to neutralize harmful environmental conditions
- Adjustment to negative events consequent to the illness
- Maintenance of self-image and self-sufficiency
- Maintenance of social relationships
- Coping with emotional reactions of anxiety and depression.

What is wellness in the face of chronic illness? This question produced a lively discussion from the contentious voices of an assertive group of elders, with responses such as the following: "Let's get real!" "I'm like the old one-hoss shay . . . losing a little something every day. Someday, I'll wake up and find that nothing works."

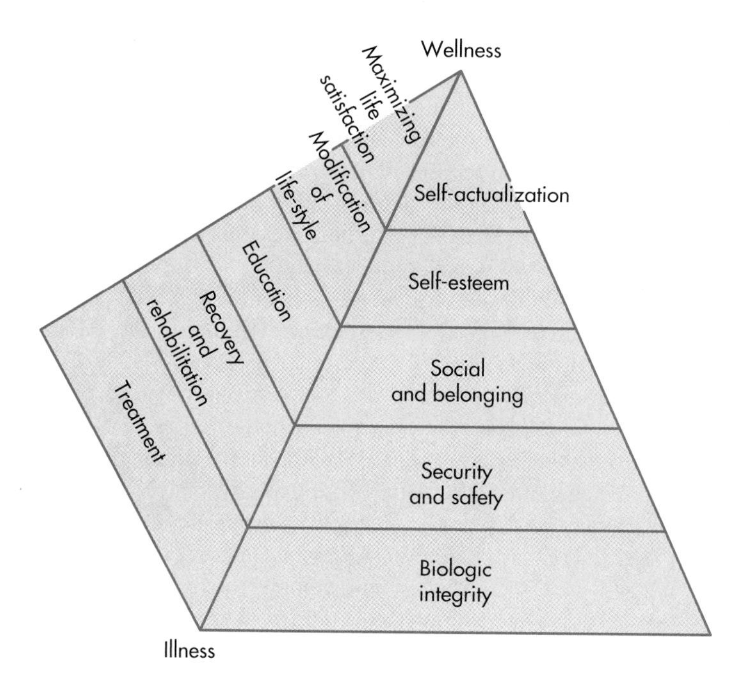

Figure 3-7. Correlation between illness-wellness continuum and Maslow's hierarchy of needs. (Developed by Patricia Hess.)

Most elders do not graciously accept their chronic disorders; they mourn their losses. They talk about them, but not to the exclusion of other events and interests in their lives. They believe that competition and conviction undergird their remarkable survival capacity and will always remain important. They also believe in being responsible and responsive to their community.

Nurses can assist and empower the aged toward an enriched capacity for living in the shadow of chronic conditions through the role of resource person, advisor, teacher, advocate, and at times assistant to the aged person. It is essential, however, to remember that the aged individual is in control of his or her own adaptation.

Nurses can assist by doing the following:

- Identifying and stating strengths the individual demonstrates
- Discussing healthy lifestyle modifications
- Encouraging the reduction of risk factors in the environment
- Assisting the individual to devise methods of improving function, halting disabilities, and adapting lifestyle to reasonable expectations of self
- Providing access to resources when possible
- Referring appropriately and when needed

It bears repeating that a state of wellness, regardless of physical condition, may be achieved and maintained consistently if the individual believes that he or she is capable of and motivated to manage problems, whether it is with or without assistance from others.

Gender and Wellness

The recent upsurge in attention to women's health has brought to the fore differences in health and health care of men and women. There appears to be an innate or philosophical difference in the perception of health between the genders. Implicit in this gender perception of health are cultural and regional factors (Boys, 1994). Differences in health and mortality for men and women are rooted in alterable and unalterable biologic and psychosocial components. Biologic elements include genetics, hormones, and physiologic structure, and acquired risk factors are based on lifestyle, work hazards, and environmental exposures. Psychosocial factors include how symptoms are perceived, health-reporting behavior, and previous health care (Verbrugge, 1994).

Because women typically live longer than men and more frequently live alone, the issues of management of chronic disorders have a large female gender component. The Rand Corporation (Shoben, 1992) released findings from a large study (sample: 11,242) of elders hospitalized with congestive heart failure (CHF), heart attack, pneumonia, and stroke. The study indicated that elderly men receive more care and more expensive, highly technical services than do women. Whether these findings would be true as the individuals are discharged to home care is unknown and certainly remains a question for further research. Although this study relates only to in-hospital service, one must wonder if there are differences in rehabilitation and chronic care management based on overt or covert attitudes toward older men and women. Much is yet to be done in this potentially fruitful area of research.

Since 1990, the immense knowledge gap related to women's health care is being closed. Under the guidance of Bernadine Healy, the Women's Health Initiative, a longitudinal study of women's health needs, was launched several years ago.

The most prevalent chronic conditions in individuals over 75 years of age are (in order) arthritis, twice as common in women; hypertension, about a third more common in women;

heart conditions, about a third more prevalent in women; and cataracts, nearly twice as common in women. Of course one must consider the population predominance of women over age 75 and the possibility that only the hardier men survive beyond age 75.

Women generally suffer more sickness and dysfunction at any given time and over their whole lifetime. Men, on the other hand, incur life-threatening diseases and, because of them, die sooner. Nevertheless, men universally see themselves as healthy despite serious problems. It takes a trip to the hospital or the terror of the possibility of dying to motivate most men to do something about their health. Most of the time it is a wife or a significant woman (sister, mother, girlfriend) in the man's life who prods him to seek care and keep physician appointments. Even with an overseer, there is little or no follow-through by the man (Boys, 1994). There is no difference in what is considered good health among white collar and blue collar men and ethnic men. Fear is the cause of the inability of men to care for themselves. Fear slows action, and illness is too upsetting to be considered (Doheny, 1993; Boys, 1994).

Men consider good health to be the following (Boys, 1994):

- The ability to take care of self
- Energy
- Healthy attitude
- Good sex, healthy sex life, good loving
- Having fun in life
- Keep on dreaming, hope
- In good physical condition

Barriers to men seeking health care should be considered if nurses wish to intervene in promoting better health care for men. These include the fear of seeing a physician, the perception of good health when medically this may not be the case, intellectual versus practical outlook (the awareness of poor health but not doing anything about it), and frustration about the mixed messages most men get from the health community (Boys, 1994).

There are many issues to consider in wellness and chronicity. How these issues apply to the aged is similar yet different from how they apply to the young. It must be remembered that the aged are a population with many chronic conditions, which may only have been thought of in terms of decrements rather than looking at potential positive aspects and promoting self-care, self-efficacy, and empowerment. Nurses must learn to guide and support rather than to take over for the aged. Care of the chronically ill is a national issue that deserves a high priority. As the health system changes, nurses are carving out their role as it relates to supporting the aged and maintaining their highest level of wellness with or without underlying chronic conditions.

Human Needs and Wellness Diagnoses

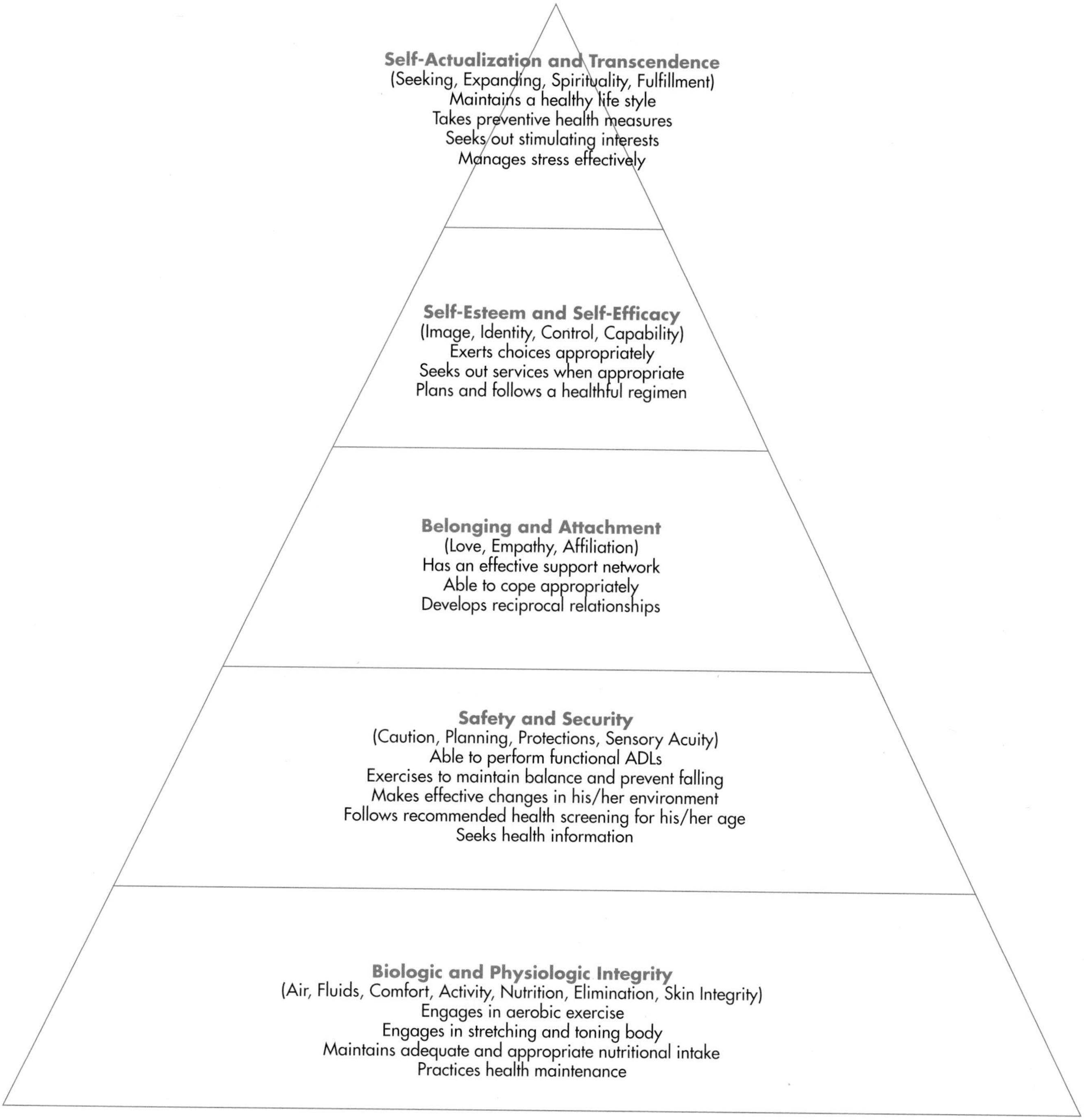

Self-Actualization and Transcendence
(Seeking, Expanding, Spirituality, Fulfillment)
Maintains a healthy life style
Takes preventive health measures
Seeks out stimulating interests
Manages stress effectively

Self-Esteem and Self-Efficacy
(Image, Identity, Control, Capability)
Exerts choices appropriately
Seeks out services when appropriate
Plans and follows a healthful regimen

Belonging and Attachment
(Love, Empathy, Affiliation)
Has an effective support network
Able to cope appropriately
Develops reciprocal relationships

Safety and Security
(Caution, Planning, Protections, Sensory Acuity)
Able to perform functional ADLs
Exercises to maintain balance and prevent falling
Makes effective changes in his/her environment
Follows recommended health screening for his/her age
Seeks health information

Biologic and Physiologic Integrity
(Air, Fluids, Comfort, Activity, Nutrition, Elimination, Skin Integrity)
Engages in aerobic exercise
Engages in stretching and toning body
Maintains adequate and appropriate nutritional intake
Practices health maintenance

These are not all the possible wellness diagnoses that may be identified. The above are examples of nursing diagnoses that should be considered when planning care for the older adult.

KEY CONCEPTS

- Wellness is a concept, not a condition. It is human adaptation at the most individually satisfying level in response to internal and external existing conditions.
- Wellness incorporates the holistic health movement, which assumes that health involves biopsychosocial and spiritual components of existence.
- Even in chronic illness and the dying process, there is an optimum level of wellness and well-being attainable for each individual.
- *Health* is a term that is subsumed under *wellness* and indicates behaviors that are preventive of biopsychosocial problems.
- Pender (1987; 1996; Pender et al, 2002) states that health is "the actualization of inherent and acquired human potential through satisfactory relationships with others, goal-directed behavior, and competent personal care while adjustments are made as needed to maintain stability and structural integrity."
- *Healthy People 2000,* a document developed by the U.S. government, provides measurable goals by which to indicate our population's progress toward health.
- The goal of *Healthy People 2010* for the elderly is to prevent disability, delay illness, and modify its disabling effects as much and for as long as possible.
- Wellness includes behaviors fundamental to healthy adaptation, such as self-responsibility, physical fitness, stress management, nutritional awareness, and environmental sensitivity.
- The "medicalization" of our society has brought about the common belief that the absence of disease is health.
- The wellness model reinforces the belief that self-care and satisfactory adaptation are uniquely and individually defined.

▲ CASE STUDY

Rhonda recently celebrated her ninetieth birthday with a large number of family and friends attending from far and near. She said, "That was the best day of my life! I was married three times but none of the weddings were as exciting as this. I have attained what I would never have thought possible when I was 50. Yes, life has been a struggle. One husband died in the second World War, one was abusive and we were divorced, and the last husband, a wonderful man, developed Alzheimer's and I cared for him for 6 years. My children sometimes wonder how I have managed to keep such a positive outlook. I believe my purpose in living so long is to be an example of aging well."

Rhonda is frail and thin, and she has advanced osteoarthritis for which she routinely takes ibuprofen and calcium tablets. She does not tolerate dairy products, so she uses lactose-free products. She eats sparingly but likes almost all foods and is concerned about good nutrition. She daily rides the stationary bike in her apartment and last year walked a mile each day but has not regained her full function since a broken hip last June. While she was immobilized she developed pressure wounds on her heels and coccyx but recently went to a wound center at a nearby hospital and is being treated effectively. She religiously follows the routine. As for religion, she says, "The closer I get to dying, the more I wonder what it is all about but I really just enjoy every day. Of course, I got depressed when I fell and broke my hip and I don't enjoy using the walker when I go out of the apartment but I feel blessed to have so many good people in my life."

Based on the case study, develop a nursing care plan using the following procedure:

List comments of client that provide subjective data.

List information that provides objective data.

From these data identify and state, using accepted format, two nursing diagnoses you determine are most significant to this client at this time. List two client strengths that you have identified from the data.

Determine and state outcome criteria for each diagnosis. These must reflect some alleviation of the problem identified in the nursing diagnosis and must be stated in concrete and measurable terms.

Plan and state one or more interventions for each diagnosed problem. Provide specific documentation of source used to determine appropriate intervention. Plan at least one intervention that incorporates the client's existing strengths.

Evaluate success of intervention. Interventions must correlate directly with the stated outcome criteria in order to measure the outcome success.

STUDY QUESTIONS/ACTIVITIES

What lifestyle changes might you suggest for Rhonda, and what would be your reason for doing so?

Where would you place Rhonda in the continuum of wellness? Explain your reasons for doing so.

Construct a definition of health that seems to you to incorporate the essential elements of a holistic perspective.

Discuss your thoughts about wellness as it relates to the medical concerns about old age.

Define *wellness* for yourself. What would you want to change in your life to achieve a sense of wellness?

Discuss the concept of wellness while dying and your thoughts about this issue.

RESEARCH QUESTIONS

Which physical conditions are most likely to impede the capacity for wellness?

Do most elders believe there is a state of wellness in spite of physical illness?

What are the factors that indicate one is in a state of "wellness"?

Is the physical deteriorative mode of defining old age related to the medical model or individual perceptions?
What are the variables that indicate a dying person is in a state of "wellness"?
How many people over 50 years old can explain wellness?
What do elders believe about the concept of "wellness"?

REFERENCES

Bortz WM: *We live too short and die too long,* New York, 1991, Bantam Books.
Bortz WM: *Dare to be 100,* New York, 1996, Fireside.
Boys J: Staying strong. Presentation at the American Society on Aging annual meeting, San Francisco, March 1994.
Buchner DM: *CDC's initiative on physical activity targets the 65-75% of older persons who are sedentary*, Atlanta, 2002, Centers for Disease Control and Prevention. Available at *www.cdc.gov/nccdphp/dnpa*
Cacioppo JT: Social neuroscience: autonomic, neuroendocrine, and immune response to stress, *Psychophysiology* 31:113, 1994.
Cherry L: On the real benefits of eustress, *Psychol Today* 11(10):60, 1978.
Cousins N: How doctors cause disease, *Medical Self-Care,* Winter 1983.
Doheny K: Real men don't see doctors, *Modern Maturity* 36(1):57, 1993.
Dubos R: *Man adapting,* New Haven, CT, 1965, Yale University Press.
Dunn HL: High-level wellness, Arlington, VA, 1961, RW Beatty Ltd.
Eliot SR: Stress and the heart: mechanisms, measurement and management, *Postgrad Med* 92(5):237, 1992.
Farquhar JW: The future of illness care and health promotion. Healthy Aging: Challenges and Choices for Health Professionals, conference, San Francisco, Oct 1-4, 1992.
Fries JF: Where in health are we going? Healthy Aging: Challenges and Choices for Health Professionals, conference, San Francisco, Oct 1-4, 1992.
Fries JF, Vickery DM: *Take care of yourself,* ed 4, Menlo Park, CA, 1990, Addison-Wesley.
Gillespie L, editor: *Health connection,* St Mary's Medical Center (community newsletter), San Francisco, Summer 1996, p 7.
Gillett PA et al: The nurse as exercise leader, *Geriatr Nurs* 14(3):133, 1993.
Ginsberg M: Weights strengthen older women's bones, *San Francisco Examiner,* Dec 28, 1994, p A1.
Harvard Health Letter: Vigilance pays off in preventing falls, *Harvard Health Letter* 24(6):6, 1999.
Harvard Health Letter: Walk this way to health, *Harvard Health Letter* 26(2):3, 2000.
Hey RP: Healthy, wealthy, and wise, *Bull AARP* 37(7):6, July/Aug 1996.
Hirschfeld M: Self-care potential: is it present? *J Gerontol Nurs* 11(8):28, 1985.
Institute of Medicine: *The future of the public's health in the 21st century,* Washington, DC, 2002, National Academy Press.
Kemper D, Mettler M: *Healthwise for life: medical self-care for healthy aging,* Boise, ID, 1992, Healthwise Inc.
Koroknay VJ et al: Maintaining ambulation in the frail nursing home resident, *J Gerontol Nurs* 21(11):18, 1995.
Kotthoff-Burrell E: Health promotion and disease prevention for the older adult: an overview of current recommendations and a practical approach, *Nurs Pract Forum* 3(4):195, 1992.
Lawton MP: Environment and other determinants of well-being in older people, *Gerontologist* 23:350, 1983.
Lazarus RS, Folkman S: *Stress, appraisal, and coping,* New York, 1984, Springer.
Lubkin IM, Larsen PD: *Chronic illness: impact and interventions,* ed 5, Boston, MA, 2002, Jones & Bartlett.
Markides KS, Mindel CH: *Aging and ethnicity,* vol 163, Newbury Park, CA, 1987, Sage Library of Social Research.
Markides KS et al: Physician's rating of health in middle and old age: a cautionary note, *J Gerontol Soc Sci* 48(1):24, 1993.
National Center for Health Statistics: *Healthy people: tracking the nation's health,* 2002, Centers for Disease Control. Available at *www.cdc.gov/nchs/about/otheract/hpdata2010/2010 indicators.htm*
Pender N: *Health promotion in nursing practice,* Norwalk, CT, 1987, Appleton-Century-Crofts.
Pender N: *Health promotion in nursing practice,* ed 3, Stamford, CT, 1996, Appleton & Lange.
Pender N, Murdaugh CL, Parson MA: *Health promotion in nursing practice,* ed 4, Stamford, CT, 2002, Appleton & Lange.
Prochaska JO: *Changing for good,* New York, 1994, Avon Books.
Reed D, Satariano WA, Gildengorin G, McMahon K: Health and functioning among elderly of Marin County, California: a glimpse of the future, *J Gerontol Med Sci* 50A(2):M61, 1995.
Rowe JW: Reducing the risk of usual aging, *Generations* 15(1):25, 1991.
Schmidt RM: Preventive health care for older adults: societal and individual services, *Generations* 18(2):33, 1994.
Selye H: *The stress of life,* New York, 1956, McGraw-Hill.
Selye H: *Stress and distress,* New York, 1974, JB Lippincott.
Shoben A: *Hospitals provide similar care to elderly women, men: Rand study finds differences in quality very small,* Rand News Release, October 14, 1992.
Spector RE: *Cultural diversity in health and illness,* Norwalk, CT, 1985, Appleton-Century-Crofts.
Spector RE: *Cultural diversity in health and illness,* ed 4, Stamford, CT, 1996, Appleton & Lange.
States D: Personal conversation, San Francisco, 1986.
Statistical abstract of the United States, ed 115, Washington, DC, 1995, US Department of Commerce, Economic and Statistics Administration, Bureau of Census.
Stein M: *Stress, brain, and immune function.* Paper presented at the meeting of the Gerontological Society of America, Boston, Nov 1982.
Steinberg D: Senorities: best way to stay young is to stay fit with exercise, *San Francisco Examiner,* July 23, 1994, p B-5.
Strategies for successful change, *Johns Hopkins Med Lett Health After 50* 8(5):1, 1996.
Taubes G: The soft science of dietary fat, *Science* 291(3):2536, 2001. Available at *www.sciencemag.org*
Travis J: *Wellness workbook: a guide to high level wellness,* Mill Valley, CA, 1977, Wellness Resource Center.
Ulene A: *Forever young series,* NBC Today, July 12, 1996.

U.S. Department of Health and Human Services: *Healthy people 2010,* ed 2, Washington, DC, 2000, U.S. Government Printing Office.

U.S. Department of Health and Human Services: *Tracking healthy people 2010,* Washington, DC, 2000, U.S. Government Printing Office.

U.S. Department of Health and Human Services: *Healthy people 2000*, pub no (PHS) 91-50212, 1-8; 22-27, 587-591, Washington, DC, 1991, U.S. Government Printing Office.

Uzelac DG: Keeping fit: put yourself in control, *Golden Age Monthly,* July 1994, p 16.

Verbrugge LM: *Pathways of health for women and men.* Healthcare for the Older Woman: New Approaches to Old Problems, conference, UCSF/Mount Zion Center on Aging, San Francisco, April 1994.

Walker SN: Health promotion and prevention of disease and disability among older adults: who is responsible? *Generations* 18(1):45, 1994.

Weinrich SP et al: Using elderly educators to increase colorectal cancer screening, *Gerontologist* 33(4):491, 1993.

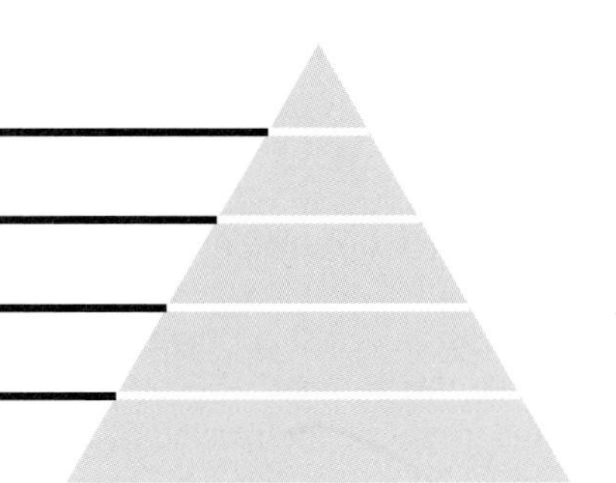

CHAPTER 4

Age-Related Changes

Patricia Hess

An elder speaks

Strange how these things creep up on you. I really was surprised and upset when I first realized it was not the headlights on my car that were dim but only my aging night vision. Then I remembered other bits of awareness that forced me to recognize that I, that 16-year-old inside me, was experiencing normal changes that go along with getting old.

Sally, age 60

LEARNING OBJECTIVES

On completion of this chapter, the reader will be able to:

1. Identify and discuss the common age-related changes that occur in the following systems: musculoskeletal, integumentary, cardiovascular, respiratory, gastrointestinal, genitourinary, nervous and special senses, and endocrine.
2. Describe the importance and objective of assessing basic activities of daily living (BADLs) and instrumental activities of daily living (IADLs).
3. Discuss the place of home visits in assessment.
4. Explain what is necessary to consider when obtaining assessment data from an elder of another cultural background.
5. List the essential components in obtaining a health assessment from an elderly person.

PHYSIOLOGIC CHANGES

Goldman (1979) indicates four characteristics of physiologic aging: it is universal, progressive, decremental, and intrinsic. The universality of aging places it outside the realm of pathologic study. The changes that occur are normal for all people but take place at different rates and depend on accompanying circumstances in an individual's life. Physiologic changes have a cumulative effect in the continuum of biologic, psychologic, social, and environmental processes of aging. This cumulative effect suppresses the body's ability to repair damaged tissue. The eventual wearing down of essential organs and systems leads to signs and symptoms of aging such as decreased muscle mass, decreased bone density, decreased vision and hearing, and increased susceptibility to disease (Pope, 2002). Normal age changes have usually been studied in concert with pathologic or disease conditions, which has led to the misconception that age changes indicate illness or disease. Progressive and decremental alterations of the whole body often interfere with an aged individual's ability to interact successfully with the environment and increase the risk of death. Bodily aging as a whole is a matter of gradual awareness. Most of these changes are intrinsic, that is, unmodifiable, whereas other alterations are the result of extrinsic influences specific to one's way of life. Extrinsic factors that affect intrinsic factors are discussed in the biologic theories of aging in Chapter 2.

Interesting approaches to the aging process and age-related changes are proffered by Sloane (1992) and Lakatta (1995). Sloane suggests the "rule of thirds," which postulates that one third of age-related changes occur as the result of functional decline resulting from disease, one third are due to inactivity or disuse, and one third are caused by aging itself. Lakatta places age-related changes into two categories: usual (average) aging and successful (pure) aging. Usual aging refers to the "combined effects of the aging process, disease and adverse environmental and lifestyle factors" (Lakatta, 1995, p. 422). Successful aging refers to "the changes due solely to the aging process uncomplicated by damage from environment, lifestyle, or disease" (Lakatta, 1995, p. 422).

To illustrate this, oxygen consumption by sedentary elderly is usually low (usual aging); however, take the sedentary elder and place him or her on a regular aerobic exercise regimen and he or she can achieve oxygen levels equal to those of sedentary young adults (successful aging). In essence, normal (usual) age-dependent reductions in biofunction reduce compensatory reserve, but with successful aging the age-related changes may not result in clinical symptoms or disease.

Individual variations are enormous at every age and in every part of the body. For many years most research studies of the physical and biologic age changes have based conclusions on the comparison of different age-groups in cross-sectional and random samples rather than on groups using the longitudinal study approach. This method may result in changes caused by cohort and environmental differences (Goldman, 1979). The Baltimore Longitudinal Study (1984), which began in 1958, followed a group of 1000 men as they aged, with the objective of identifying normal changes of aging not associated with disease. The Baltimore Longitudinal Study of women began in the 1980s. Table 4-1 provides a summary of selected anatomic and physiologic changes with age of healthy adults.

Changes in body structure and function are lifelong alterations that begin to take on significance internally and externally in the fourth and fifth decades of life. External signs are the clues by which most people judge aging. However, these signs can be deceptive. Skin can become deeply wrinkled or hair become gray early in adult life, even though these features are considered signs of aging. Today individuals have at their disposal cosmetic surgery, hair coloring, makeup, and clothing choices that can make a person look younger than his or her chronologic age.

A study conducted by the National Institute on Aging (*Special Report on Aging,* 1981) found that people who appear older than their chronologic age may indeed share the characteristics of an older biologic age. Many internal changes mimic disease manifestations and might be interpreted as a pathologic state in need of medical attention. On the other hand, normal changes can mask early signs of disease processes. This dichotomous situation makes it important for those who care for the aged to carefully explore the changes that do occur rather than immediately categorizing them as pathologic or normal. The individual must be evaluated as a whole being for a correct interpretation of the changes that are occurring.

Common denominators emerge when one looks at age-related changes. Many changes are effected by a decrease in blood supply to tissues because of the natural deposition of fat and calcium in the vessel intima. Reduced circulation perfusion is also thought to produce the diminished endocrine secretion commonly noted in old age (Costa and Andres, 1986). Finally, lifelong use and abuse of the body through diet, accidents, athletic injuries, and other physical trauma are responsible for some of the changes thought of as wear and tear. When one is young, it is difficult to realize that neglect of skin, teeth, or nutrition will not necessarily produce visible or significant changes until one moves into old age and compensatory reserve becomes limited. At that time the effects

Table 4-1 Summary of Selected Anatomic and Physiologic Changes with Aging in Healthy Adults

System affected	Change noted	Age span (years)
Height	Average loss 2 inches	40-80
Weight:		
Men	Peaks in midfifties, then declines	
Women	Peaks in midsixties, then declines	
Total body water:		
Men	Declines from 60% to 54%	20-80
Women	Declines from 54% to 46%	20-80
Muscle mass	30% decrease	30-70
Taste buds	70% decrease	30-70
Cardiac reserve	Decrease from 4.6 to 3.3 times resting cardiac output	25-70
Maximum heart rate	195-155 beats/min	25-70
Lung vital capacity	17% decrease	30-70
Renal perfusion	Reduced by 50%	30-80
Cerebral blood flow	Reduced by 20%	30-70
Bone mineral content	Reduced by 25%-30% in women; 10%-15% in men	40-80
Brain weight	Reduced by 10%	20-80
Amount of light reaching retina	Diminished by 70%	20-65
Plasma glucocorticoid levels	No change	30-70

Modified from Kenney PA: *Physiology of aging: a symposis,* Chicago, 1982, Year Book Medical Publishers; Shock NW et al: *Normal human aging: the Baltimore study of aging,* NIH pub no 84-2450, Washington, DC, 1984, US Government Printing Office; Timiras P: *Physiological basis of aging and geriatrics,* Boca Raton, FL, 1994, CRC Press; and Beers MH, Berkow R, editors: *The Merck manual of geriatrics,* ed 3, Whitehouse Station, NJ, 2000, Merck Research Laboratories.

of earlier laxness become more apparent and important to a person's health.

Significant changes in structure, function, and biochemistry, as well as genetic endowment and lifestyle, are responsible for the alterations in tissue elasticity, subcutaneous fat, gastrointestinal function and motility, muscle, bone, immunity, and the sensorium. These changes are not mutually exclusive but rather are synergistic and contribute to alterations in each system and the general evidence of advanced age.

Structure and Posture

The average person loses 1.5 to 3 inches of height in his or her lifetime or 1 cm every 20 years as aging occurs (Jacobs, 1981; Cunningham and Brookbank, 1988; Lamb, 1996). Obvious manifestations, which are an interaction of many factors such as age, sex, race, and environment, begin to occur in the fifth decade of life. Long bones take on the appearance of disproportionate size (long arms and legs) because stature decreases. Vertebral disks become thin as a result of dehydration, causing a shortening of the trunk. Many aged persons assume a stooped, forward-bent posture with a kyphotic curvature of the dorsal spine, with hips and knees somewhat flexed and arms bent at the elbows, raising the level of the arms. To maintain eye contact, the head is tilted backward, which makes it appear that the elderly individual is jutting forward. In addition, shoulder width decreases because of shrinkage of the deltoid muscles and acromions, chest width and pelvis width increase, and abdominal length decreases while its girth increases, giving the overall picture of a disproportionate individual who needs to be stretched out a bit. These changes involve multiple developmental factors: skeletal, muscular, subcutaneous tissue, fat, and dermal changes.

Bone mass is constantly undergoing cyclic resorption and renewal. Disequilibrium of this process with greater resorption and less calcium deposition is characteristic of aging bone. Aging bone is composed of about two thirds minerals and one third connective tissue, the reverse of childhood bone development (Timiras, 1994). Posture and structural changes occur primarily because of calcium loss from bone and as a result of atrophic processes of cartilage and muscle. This type of degeneration begins in both sexes in the fifth decade, with women more vulnerable than men as estrogen levels decline (Manolagas, 2000). This type of degeneration is four times more prevalent in women because of the rapid loss of bone density in the first 5 to 10 years after menopause and less accumulation of skeletal mass during early pubescent growth (Lindsay, 1985). The skeletal mass then results in smaller, narrower, and more fragile bone with thinner cortices. Maintaining muscle use and bone stress, for example, by walking, can slow the process (see Chapter 8). Excessive leaching of calcium from the bone matrix creates the condition called *osteoporosis*. Progressive bone loss affects the trabicular and cortical skeleton. Trabicular changes include thinning and total destruction of the trabiculae (the network that makes up the core of bone). Reduced thickness and porosity are changes in the cortical component of bone. The loss of bone density is responsible for kyphosis and osteoporosis, two factors that contribute to the shorter stature of the aged. Bone demineralization affects the jaw or alveolar bone of the lower jaw, especially in individuals who are edentulous. In addition, resorption of the bone leads to poorly fitting dentures and painful sensations when chewing or biting (Coni et al, 1984).

Skeletal muscle atrophy and a reduction in the number and size of muscle fibers (sarcopenia) occur because of physical inactivity, a change in the central and peripheral nervous system that decreases the motor units to muscle cells, and reduced skeletal protein synthesis. By age 75, muscle composes only 50% of lean mass and 15% of body weight. Half of muscle mass loss is due to sarcopenia.

Muscles are of two types. Type I maintains posture and rhythmic endurance exercise. Type II consists of muscle fibers associated with sudden powerful and fast contractions. Loss of muscle mass is associated with loss of maximum isometric contractile force, which decreases 20% in the sixth decade and 50% by the eighth decade (Manolagas, 2000). Abdominal muscles decrease in size and number of fibers, in part because of disuse. Why this occurs remains unknown. Strength and stamina decrease from 65% to 85% of the maximum strength an individual had at 25 years of age. Muscle function is important to increase functional ability of the aged: To maintain specific task training and muscle strength, exercise is necessary regardless of health condition. The frequency, intensity, duration, and type of exercise that will maintain desired fitness are not known. This remains an area for further research in geriatrics.

Cartilage, ligaments, and *tendons* (articular and nonarticular) undergo age-related changes. Nonarticular cartilage (ears, nose) grow throughout life; thus one observes elongation of ears and nose. Articular cartilage changes result from biochemical changes: increases in transglutaminase and possibly calcium pyrophosphates. These changes do not necessarily correlate with joint disease. Knee cartilage decreases in thickness a quarter of a millimeter per year, most likely because of wear and tear (Manolagas, 2000). Degeneration of underlying cartilage appears to decrease intervertebral distance. Worn-down cartilage around joints produced by continuous flexing over the years coupled with stray pieces of cartilage and diminished lubricating fluid in the joints can lead to slower and painful movement at times. The forward-leaning posture is attributed to muscle shrinkage, and breasts that were full and firm begin to sag and become pendulous as the glandular envelope of fat atrophies. Nipples may also invert because of shrinkage and fibrotic changes.

Ligaments, tendons, and joints show the result of cellular cross-linkage over time, resulting in hardened, more rigid, less flexible movement and predisposing these structures to tears. The *subcutaneous fat layer* around the orbit of the eye disappears, creating a sunken appearance of the eyes. Landmarks become more prominent, and muscle contours are easily identified. Skinfold thickness, a measure of subcutaneous fat content, is markedly reduced in the forearm with age. Women over 45 years of age begin to see the skinfolds on the back of their hands rapidly diminish, even if there is a substantial weight gain. Such areas as the pubis, umbilicus, and waist do not change appreciably.

Subcutaneous tissue plays a significant role in the body's adjustment to temperature change. The natural insulation that subcutaneous fat affords is lost, and it is not uncommon to hear aged people mention that they are cold, nor is it unusual to see them wearing a sweater or sitting with a lap blanket. Windy, dry winter weather can accelerate loss of body heat by evaporation, and subsequent hypothermia may lead to death by decreasing core body temperature (Cunningham and Brookbank, 1988). Although subcutaneous tissue does not markedly affect the aged person's tolerance of heat, it is important to mention that problems exist. The efficiency of sweat glands is reduced through diminished size, number, and activity. Eccrine glands become fibrotic, and surrounding connective tissue becomes avascular. The remainder of the eccrine glands may function improperly. These changes cause a decline in the efficiency of the body's cooling mechanism. The aged person is no longer able to perspire freely and becomes highly susceptible to heat exhaustion and heat stroke, common causes of death during the summer.

Education of the aged about the natural phenomenon of the loss of subcutaneous fat will help them realize why they respond to hot and cold temperature fluctuations so dramatically. In cool or cold weather most elders compensate with sweaters, lap blankets, or other pieces of apparel. In hot weather, shade, sufficient fluids, an air-conditioned or cool environment, or wet cloths to the head and neck should be considered. It is important for the nurse in the institutional setting to be aware of the temperature discomforts of the aged when bathing, dressing, or examining them and to be cognizant of the need for shade, cool temperature, and sufficient fluids and a cool environment in hot weather.

Stengel (1983) studied oral temperature norms in well old persons and found that they were significantly lower in women over 80 years than in younger women. Older men consistently had an even lower temperature than women of comparable age. The old-old may have a temperature of 96.8° F with an average range of 95° to 97° F. By tympanic membrane thermometer the temperature may be 96° F (Hogstel, 1994). These findings emphasize the need to carefully evaluate the basal temperature of aged individuals and recognize that even low-grade fevers (98.6° F) in the elderly may signify illness.

Skin, Hair, and Nails

Skin-related changes can either be due to true aging (intrinsic) or the result of photoaging. Intrinsic changes occur gradually over time. Characteristic dryness, roughness, wrinkles, laxity of the skin, and increase of benign and malignant neoplasms are to be expected at the epidermal level. All of the functional activities of the skin—cell replacement, barrier action, wound healing, immunologic response, thermo-regulation, and vitamin D synthesis—decrease in the older adult (Timiras, 1994).

Epidermis. After 50 years of age epidermal cell renewal time increases by one third. The normal young adult renews epithelium every 20 days, whereas an older person requires 30 or more days because of diminished mitotic epidermal activity. This slow cell replacement affects wound healing, which is approximately 50% slower than at 35 years of age (Leyden et al, 1978). The amount of collagen decreases approximately 1% per year, causing the skin to "give" less under stress and tear more easily (Richey, Richey et al, 1988). Fewer melanocytes are identifiable in the epidermis as skin ages. However, in some areas of aged skin, melanin synthesis is increased. Pigment spots (freckles and nevi) enlarge and can become more numerous with increased exposure to natural and artificial light.

Dermis. Dermis loses about 20% of its thickness, becoming thinner in the absence of subcutaneous fat (Grove and Kingman, 1983; Chiu, 2000; Gilchrest, 2000). Loss is greater when the skin is photodamaged. In unprotected areas ultraviolet rays cause hyperplastic changes followed by atrophic changes. There is a reduction in dermal blood vessels, which accounts for resultant skin pallor and cooler skin temperature (Timiras, 1994). Vascular hyperplasia causes more pronounced varicosities, benign cherry angiomas, and venous stars. Collagen synthesis decreases, slowing the rate of wound healing. Elastin fibers diminish in number and diameter, leading to loss of stretch and resilience. Fragmentation and progressive cross-linkage affect skin turgor. In normal aging, the vascular supply to hair bulbs and eccrine, apocrine, and sebaceous glands decreases in size and function. The eccrine gland efficiency diminishes, causing a decrease in spontaneous sweating in heat. This, combined with a decrease in vascularity, can lead to altered thermoregulation such as heat stroke in hot weather. Sebaceous glands secrete 23% less sebum each decade (Chiu, 2000; Gilchrest, 2000). This begins soon after puberty in relation to a concomitant decrease of gonadal and adrenal androgens, to which sebaceous glands are extremely sensitive. This however, does not contribute to the roughness or dryness of aged skin (Timiras, 1994). Nerve density decreases in cutaneous tissue. Sensory and end-organ activity is gradually diminished beginning at age 10, and by 90 years of age one third of sensory function is altered. Light touch, vibratory, and corneal sensitivity and two-point discrimination are diminished (Chiu, 2000; Gilchrest, 2000).

Subcutaneous Fat. Subcutaneous fat serves both as a shock absorber of trauma and as a thermoregulator. The amount of subcutaneous fat decreases with age, yet the proportion of body fat increases until age 70. The distribution of fat decreases on the hands and face, decreases over bony prominences such as the ilial tuberosities, and increases on the thighs and abdomen, thus affecting the diffusion of pressure.

Hair. Hair becomes gray as melanin production in the hair bulbs decreases. Regardless of sex, 50% of the population over 50 years of age has gray or partly gray scalp hair. At times the hair color may turn shades of yellow or yellow-green. Vertex and frontal and temporal hair loss in some men is prominent beginning in the late teens or early twenties, and by 60 years of age 80% of men are substantially bald. Women may experience the same pattern of hair loss as men, but it is less pronounced. Alopecia, however, is diffuse in both sexes with old age and can result from factors such as iron deficiency, hypothyroidism, certain drugs, and renal failure, to mention a few. As a result of the altered balance of estrogen and androgens in women after menopause, excessive unwanted terminal hair can occur in the chin area. Overall body hair diminishes with advanced age. Race, sex, sex-linked genes, and hormonal influences determine the maximum amount of hair that one has and the changes that will occur with it throughout life. In both sexes, hair distribution becomes more sparse; hair on the head thins, and leg hair frequently is lacking. This latter finding is often interpreted as a sign of peripheral vascular disease. Other, more conclusive, signs and symptoms should be observed to validate the diagnosis of abnormal hair loss. Asians and blacks are less hairy than whites, and Native Americans have little or no hair on their bodies (Rossman, 1986). Axillary and pubic hair diminishes in quantity and thickness of the hair fibers.

Nails. Nails of the fingers and toes thicken and change shape, color, and growth rate. Nails become brittle, flat, or concave (rather than convex) with longitudinal striations and, in blacks, pigmented bands. Nails may yellow or appear grayish with poorly defined lunulae. Nail growth is at a slower rate than in youth. Toenails grow at a 15% slower rate than fingernails in the aged (Jacobs, 1981; Cornell, 1986). The nail plate may thicken and distort (onychogryphosis) or separate from the distal part of the nail plate (onycholysis or fungal infection). Brittle nails with splitting ends or layers occur commonly in middle-aged women and elders of both sexes. With age the cuticle becomes less thick and wide. Vigorous manipulation of the cuticle may lead to retardation of the already slowed nail growth.

Photoaging

Skin protected from sun damage looks younger. Exposed skin areas differ clinically, histologically, and physiologically from intrinsic or true aging. Skin cancers in elders occur almost entirely in photo-aged skin. Common manifestations are exaggerations of the normal changes: fine and coarse wrinkles, irregular mottled pigmentation, liver spots (lentigines), roughness, sallowness, and telangiectasis. Depigmented areas called *stellate pseudoscars* may be on the extremities. Cigarette smoking exacerbates wrinkles of photoaging. At the cellular level, epidermal dysplasia occurs. Langerhans' cells decrease and dermal elastosis develops, as well as a greater decrease in the immune and inflammatory response of the skin.

Facial Changes

Facial changes occur as a result of altered subcutaneous fat, altered dermal thickness, decreased elasticity, and lateral surface compression of underlying muscle contractions. Loss of bone mass, particularly the mandibular bone, accentuates the size of the upper mouth, nose, and forehead. Indented "loss of lip" appearance of the mouth occurs with tooth loss when uncorrected by dentures or other oral prostheses. Eyelids appear swollen as a result of the redistribution of fat deposits. Conversely, eyes that look sunken are the result of the loss of orbital subcutaneous fat. Loss of elasticity accentuates jowls and elongated ears and contributes to the formation of a "double" chin.

Loss of Tissue Elasticity

The aged skin loses resilience and moisture, taking on a characteristic dryness. The epithelial layer thins, and elastic collagen fibers shrink and become rigid. The face and neck wrinkles reflect life patterns of muscle activity in facial expressions, the pull of gravity on tissue, and diminished elasticity in general. Sun and heat exposure affects collagen flexibility and accelerates fiber alterations. The influence of sun and heat on tissue is discussed in the cross-link theory in Chapter 2.

Elasticity affects blood vessel integrity, particularly the arteries. Elastic fibers fray, split, straighten, and fragment. Calcium that leaves the bone is deposited in the vessels. This chemical and anatomic alteration decreases the lumen size of the vessels and causes the blood flow to various organs to become uneven. There is little flow change to the coronary arteries and the brain, but perfusion of the liver and kidneys shows significant changes in the amount of blood brought to these two organs (Wardell, 1979; Cunningham and Brookbank, 1988; Malasanos et al, 1989). Peripheral resistance in the vessels, which increases both the systolic and diastolic pressures with advancing age, is a reflection of the elastic changes and calcium deposits. (See the section on cardiovascular changes later in this chapter.)

Lung elasticity declines, causing a rigidity in lung tissue. This alone is not responsible for the decrease in oxygen capacity, but it is a contributing factor (Tichy and Malasanos, 1979). (See the discussion of respiratory system changes later in this chapter.)

Nursing interventions are limited where tissue elasticity of internal structures is concerned, but retention of tissue moisture can be assisted through the use of body lotion and judicious use of soap in bathing, as well as teaching the aged that overexposure to the sun, heat, and other elements is detrimental to skin. Chapter 7 discusses skin integrity and maintenance in more detail.

Body Composition

Alteration in body weight occurs as lean body mass declines and body water is lost: 54% to 60% in men; 46% to 52% in women (Kee and Paulanka, 2000) (Figure 4-1). Fat tissue increases until 60 years of age; therefore body density is higher in youth because of the density of muscle versus the lightness of fat. From 25 to 75 years of age fat content of the body increases by 16%. Cellular solids and bone mass decline;

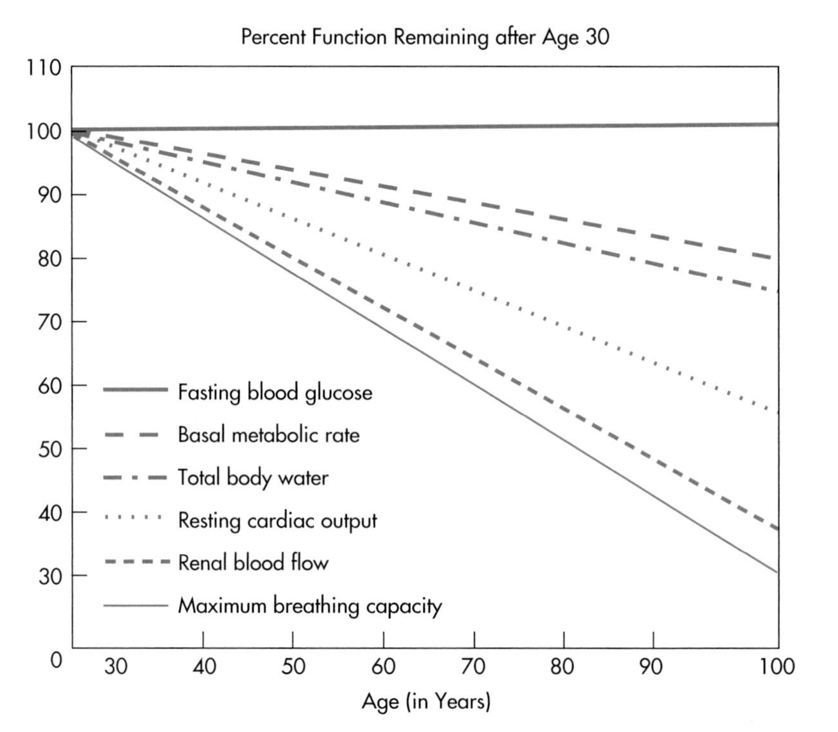

Figure 4-1. Changes in biologic function with age. (Modified from Shock NW: In Carlston LA, editor: *Nutrition in old age*, Tenth Symposium of the Swedish Nutrition Federation, Uppsala, 1972, Almquist & Wiksell.)

extracellular water, however, remains relatively constant. Cellular sodium increases 20% from 30 to 70 years of age, and there is a need to increase the proportion of protein, calcium, and vitamin D nutritional intake (Gugoz and Munro, 1985; Lakatta, 1995). The intercellular matrix (collagen and elastin) cross-link, reducing resilience. Intracellular concentrations of structural proteins, enzymes, and chromosomal components, including deoxyribonucleic acid (DNA) and ribonucleic acid (RNA), change. Lipofuscin, or "aging pigment," increases in the nervous system and other non-renewing tissues (e.g., the heart).

Cardiovascular Changes

Heart. For centuries the heart, which must function continuously to maintain life as we know it, was considered the center of life until the technologic redefinition of death included the cessation of brain activity as well as heart function. Cardiovascular disease is a major cause of death worldwide in people age 60 and over. In the United States, one half of all cardiovascular disease occurs in those 65 years of age and older (*Johns Hopkins Medical Letter,* 1994). One of every two persons age 60 and over may have some severe narrowing of the coronary arteries, but only about 50% of those have clinical signs of coronary artery dysfunction. Screening for this occult manifestation can now be done with magnetic resonance imaging (MRI) (*Johns Hopkins Medical Letter,* 1994). It is difficult to know whether widespread disease exaggerates functional decline presently considered to be the result of age-related change.

Health care professionals are accustomed to caring for aged persons with cardiac-related conditions such as congestive heart failure and hypertension and may be inclined to assume that all aged individuals have enlarged hearts; however, the aged heart can atrophy from wasting diseases, remain unchanged, or hypertrophy (Lakatta, 2000). Generally, the atrium increases about 20% in size between 18 and 93 years of age, which may give rise to a fourth heart sound in a healthy aged person (Lakatta, 1993). Studies suggest that the left ventricle wall thickens about 30% between ages 25 and 80 as a result of the increase in myocyte size, but an exaggerated increase occurs when persistent hypertension is present. Ventricular adaptation enhances filling of the ventricle. In the healthy adult, heart size remains relatively unchanged. Cardiac mass is estimated to increase 1.5 g in women and 1 g in men per year after age 30 (Lakatta, 1993). Radiologic silhouette of cardiac size shows a slight increase but remains within a clinically normal range (Gerstenblith et al, 1977; Gardin et al, 1979; Lakatta, 2000).

By age 60, the maximum coronary artery blood flow provides the cardiovascular system with 35% less blood than in earlier years. The decline in work response of the left ventricle at rest is a reflection of decreased stroke volume and cardiac output and a delay in heart muscle irritability and contractile recovery. Contraction of the older heart is prolonged, most likely because of the slow release of calcium into the myoplasm during systole. Reduced efficiency and contractile strength of the heart muscle are reflected in (1) a reduced cardiac output that decreases by 1% per year from the average baseline of 5 L/min and (2) a stroke volume decline of 0.7% per year (Jacobs, 1981; Kenney, 1982) (see Figure 4-1).

Under normal conditions the aged heart is able to sustain adequate function to maintain an average active life. Under nonstressful conditions the smaller cardiac output is adequate because the mechanisms that determine cardiovascular function depend on the interaction of intrinsic cell performance, heart rate, coronary flow, cardiac filling (preload), and cardiac afterload. All of these are governed by autonomic tone and a negative feedback system. Decreased overall energy demands and a moderate degree of body atrophy place less demand on cardiac function. Diminished cardiac output becomes significant when the aged person is physically or mentally stressed by illness, worry, or excitement. Sudden demands for more oxygen and energy brought on by various physiologic, psychologic, social, and environmental stress result in poor response of heart function, attributed to the limited cardiac reserve, or presbycardia. It takes longer for the heart to accelerate to meet the demands placed on it and to return to a normal level. Tachycardia is not as great in the older person, but, when it occurs, the heart requires a longer time to return to its baseline rate. The expected increase in the heart rate when the patient is anxious, is in pain, hemorrhages, or demonstrates the presence of an infectious process is not as evident in the aged as in the young. Heart rate in a resting supine position does not change in older men but does increase slightly for both sexes when in a sitting position. Although it is known that the intrinsic sinus rate decreases significantly with age, no data are available for individuals who are over 55 years of age (Lakatta, 2000).

General risk factors that can cause stress and strain on the heart include the following:

- Continued intake of high amounts of dietary animal fat, salt, and calories
- Obesity and excessive weight
- Long-term cigarette smoking
- Lack of regular exercise
- Internalization of emotions
- Air pollution
- Existing chronic conditions

Other physical conditions that impose added demand on the aged heart or aggravate existing cardiac conditions include infection, anemia, pneumonia, cardiac arrhythmias, surgery, fever, diarrhea, hypoglycemia, malnutrition, avitaminosis, circulatory overload, and drug-induced and noncardiac illnesses such as renal disease and prostatic obstruction.

Circulation time for the adult averages 15 seconds. Diettert (1963) found an average circulation time of 27 seconds to be normal for men in the seventh decade of life. Electrocardiogram changes with age under normal circumstances are minimum. There is a slight lengthening of the PR, QRS, and QT intervals. Catecholamines and other enzymes that influence the effect of the force and speed of heart contractions diminish in amount, producing a long interval between contractions, a weakened cardiac force, and a greater energy demand on heart muscle. Lower contractile strength, smaller cardiac output, and reduced enzymatic stimulation together cause the heart to respond to the work demand with less efficient performance and greater energy expenditure than would be required when the individual was younger.

Valves. Valves may be thicker and stiffer as a result of lipid deposits, collagen degeneration, and fibrosis. Valvular conditions in the aged are considered residual effects of earlier rheumatic infections and arteriosclerosis. Aortic and mitral valves are most commonly affected and result in slight to moderate regurgitation of blood. Valvular disease in the aged is often misdiagnosed because it is assumed that murmurs are the result of the arteriosclerotic process. Some aged individuals have aortic and mitral murmurs that were chronicled from childhood, others from the stiffening of the valve leaflets. Generally those murmurs are not as prominent as murmurs that occur in later life. At least 50% of elders have a systolic ejection type of murmur that is a grade 1 or 2 without radiation. Murmurs that are diastolic, however, should always be considered significant because these indicate important alteration in cardiac hemodynamics (Lakatta, 2000).

Conductivity. Sinus rhythm is the expected norm of the aged person's heartbeat. During the third and fourth decades of life, pacemaker cells decrease in number as myocardial fat, collagen, and elastin fibers increase. This change affects the sinoatrial (SA) node, which shows evidence of causing an acceleration through the sixth decade. The number of SA cells at age 75 is only 10% of that which existed at age 20 (Wei, 1988; Gawlinski and Jensen, 1991; Morgan, 1993). Similarly, the atrioventricular (AV) node and the bundle of His lose a number of conductive cells into the fourth decade and the left bundle between the fifth and seventh decade (Fujino et al, 1982; Miller, 1990). Alteration in the excitation and contraction mechanism is an adaptive rather than a degenerative change because it maintains contractile function of the aged heart. The mean resting rate remains unchanged with age, but the maximum heart rate is achieved with decreased activity.

Sinus rates of less than 50 beats per minute are common in the elderly and do not necessarily indicate SA node disease. Significant interference with the blood flow to the SA node, either by occlusion or by narrowed arteriosclerotic vessels, can produce arrhythmias.

Arrhythmias may be primary or secondary, but the majority of heart rate irregularities in the aged are attributed to myocardial damage. The heart muscle is damaged directly by interference with the coronary circulation or indirectly by valvular insufficiency and concomitant interference with circulation to the responsible neurologic mechanisms essential to heart action.

Baroreceptor sensitivity declines, resulting in a decreased ability for compensatory response to hypertensive or hypotensive stimuli. Stiffening of the arteries and a reduced cardiovascular responsiveness to adrenergic stimulation is responsible for the decreased baroreflex (Banaski, 1995; Lakatta, 2000).

Accumulation of collagen, mononuclear cells, and smooth muscle cells increases the subintimal areas, and vessel walls thicken as a result of reorganization of the cellular and extracellular matrix (Cooper et al, 1994).

Vessels. "Atherosclerosis is universal in almost all animal species and throughout all populations within a species" (Timiras, 1994). It is progressive and culminates in overt manifestations in old age. Decreased elasticity of arteries and arterioles is responsible for changes that affect blood flow to body organs such as the heart, liver, kidneys, and pituitary gland. The aorta dilates and elongates as collagen and elastin changes occur, and calcium deposition from degenerating elastin occurs (Lakatta, 1995). Circulation in the coronary arteries diminishes by approximately 35% after the sixth decade; increased resistance to peripheral blood flow occurs at a rate of about 1% per year. Weakness of vessel walls and varicosities can lead to abnormal swelling when subjected to increased pressure. With normal aging, some atherosclerosis is normal, but it can be exacerbated to a pathologic state by a diet high in saturated fat (see Appendix 4-A).

Peripheral Vascular Changes

Both arteries and veins exhibit changes as the intima becomes fibrotic and endothelial cell variation increases. The amount of elastin and smooth muscle diminishes as the amount of collagen and fibrotic tissue increases. The result is loss of flexibility and recoil, an increase in systemic peripheral resistance, and a reduced perfusion to tissues and organs. The stiffening and more rigid structure of the vascular system may lead to the elevation of blood pressure in addition to influencing cardiac and renal changes. Veins lose their elasticity and become less able to store blood volume. Pooling of blood increases the venous pressure, diminishing the effectiveness of peripheral valves and creating tortuous varicosities (Beare and Myers, 1994).

Not more than 20 years ago, it was thought that systolic blood pressure of an aged person should be 100 plus the person's age. Thus an individual age 70 was thought to have a normal systolic pressure of 170 mm Hg. Another accepted approach to normal blood pressure was to consider 160/90 as the upper limits of normal for the aged adult. However, the *Special Report* (1998) states that both young and old should have similar blood pressure. The Joint National Committee on Prevention, Detection, Evaluation, and Treatment of High Blood Pressure (*Special Report,* 1998) defines *hypertension* as systolic pressure at or above 140 mm Hg and diastolic pressure at or above 90 mm Hg for those who are not acutely ill or on antihypertensive medications. It is estimated that 50% of persons over age 65 in industrialized society have blood pressure at or greater than 140/90 mm Hg (Frohlich, 1995). Isolated systolic hypertension (ISH) occurs when the systolic pressure is high and the diastolic pressure is within the normal range. This form of hypertension is often seen in elderly persons.

The importance of the redefinition of normal blood pressure and hypertension points out the impact that elevated blood pressure has as a risk for cardiovascular disease. Both essential hypertension and ISH increase during the eighth and ninth decades of life; elderly women are more likely to experience such increases than are elderly men.

The incidence of hypertension is higher in the African American population than in the white population. The National Health and Nutrition Examination Survey (NHANES III), which occurred between 1988 and 1991, confirmed this. The survey found that 40% of white men and over 30% of white women ages 50 to 59 had hypertension. The rate was higher for African Americans: over one half of the African American men ages 50 to 59 were hypertensive and almost half of the African American women in that age-group were also hypertensive. By ages 60 to 69, the rates increased to over 50% for both white men and women, over 60% for African American men, and nearly 80% for African American women (*Johns Hopkins Medical Letter,* 1996).

Gardner and Poehlman (1995) looked at age-related increases in blood pressure of men and women. They found a relationship between systolic pressure and age that was stronger in women than in men by age 50 to 60 years. This was primarily due to an accelerated increase in systolic pressure that occurred at a greater rate in women. Reasons are unclear. The age-related increase in men was thought to be related to an increase in body fat as opposed to a shift in body fat in women. The greater increase in blood pressure in women older than age 62 suggested that the years after menopause might influence this rise. The acceleration was also thought to be related to a reduction in estrogen, but blood pressure changes did not occur until 5 to 10 years later, which is the time required to manifest its effects on blood pressure. It was concluded that the amounts of subcutaneous fat deposition and alcohol intake of men were predictors for elevated systolic pressure for men and that the waist-to-hip ratio and aerobic fitness were predictors for systolic and diastolic pressure, respectively, for women. The highly complex phenomenon of the blood pressure mechanism within an aging individual is influenced in many ways (Box 4-1).

Weber, Barnard, and Ray (1983) studied older individuals who were on a high–complex carbohydrate, low-fat

Box 4-1 Some Factors Affecting Normotensive/Hypertensive Blood Pressure

Increased action of adrenergic nervous system
and/or
Catecholamines (norepinephrine is elevated in elders)
Increase in renin-angiotensin systemically or autocrine of arteries and other organs (there is a decrease of this in elders with hypertension)
Distensibility of great vessels (affected by atherosclerosis)
Altered fluid and electrolyte balance caused by renal, hormonal, and humoral factors

diet and daily exercise, which involved walking approximately 3.1 miles (5 km) daily, for 26 days. Following this closely monitored program, half of the individuals were able to reduce hypertension, discontinue hypertensive medication, and reduce cholesterol intake. Their work capacity and health status were significantly improved with this dietary program and daily walking. Exercise and diet control remain the mainstay of therapy today.

Even though the death rate from heart and vascular disease is declining, *the aged of today still are a reflection of previous health practices.* Some damage can be lessened by modifying behavior with continuing education regarding self-care issues such as diet, smoking, exercise, activity, and weight control. The multiple origins of cardiovascular conditions, which include disruptions in the heart muscle, the valves, the vessels, or the conductive system, as well as congenital defects, can cause problems in the function of other structures dependent on cardiovascular performance.

Respiratory Changes

The respiratory system includes the nose, pharynx, larynx, trachea, bronchi, bronchioles, alveolar ducts, and alveoli. In addition, an interplay exists with the musculoskeletal and nervous systems. The respiratory muscles begin to weaken and the chest wall gradually becomes stiffer as a result of calcification of intercostal cartilage, kyphoscoliosis, and arthritic costovertebral joints. The outer muscle force and chest wall stiffness are counterbalanced by loss of the elastic recoil of the lungs (Anderson, 2000; Tockman, 2000). Other deficits occur from circulatory alterations and lifelong exposure to environmental pollutants (Sheahan and Musialowski, 2001).

The respiratory system matures by age 20 and begins to decline in healthy individuals after 25 years of age (Timiras, 1994). Changes occur in the lungs, thoracic cage, respiratory muscles, and respiratory centers in the central nervous system. These changes are small when compared with the constant bombardment of environmental and other insults to the respiratory system. Elders continue to breathe effortlessly in the absence of pathologic states.

The prominent age-related changes in the respiratory system are reduced efficiency in ventilation and gas exchange. It is accepted that exercise tolerance declines and that breathlessness leads to varying degrees of fatigue, but under usual or resting conditions the aged have little difficulty accomplishing and participating in customary life activities. However, when the aged are confronted with unusual and stressful circumstances, the demand for oxygen surpasses the available supply and establishes a significant respiratory deficit, which must be resolved. A lower resistance to infection is engendered by a diminished immune system response and less effective self-cleansing action of the respiratory cilia. Respiratory changes that do occur in structure and function are greatly affected by acute illness and chronicity that can be sufficiently debilitating to limit life enjoyment.

Upper Airway

Nose. With age, the nose elongates downward as support of the upper and lower lateral cartilage weakens. The subsequent droop of the end of the nose can restrict airflow at the nasal valve junction. Narrowing of this valve in the presence of minor septal deviations that were no problem in one's younger years can cause breathing problems in one's later years (Sheahan and Musialowski, 2001).

Trachea and larynx. Stiffening of the larynx and tracheal cartilage occurs as a result of calcification. The cilia that line the trachea and help to push up mucus, debris, and dust into the pharynx are less effective. Cilia decrease in number with a resultant decrease in respiratory epithelium and an increase in bronchial mucous gland hypertrophy (Schumann, 1995). Tockman (2000) and Anderson (2000) suggest that the importance of age to mucociliary transport is not fully established but may be clinically significant in the recurrence of respiratory infections. Voice pitch increases for men and decreases for women, but substantially more so for elders who are in poor health. Breathlessness in speech is the result of less air passing through and incomplete closure of the glottis. Limited mobility of the jaw may also contribute to this.

Chest wall and lungs. During one's youth, the chest wall and lungs grow in proportion to the body and correlate with height (Tockmann, 1995). Around age 55, respiratory muscles begin to weaken, chest wall compliance begins to decrease, and there is a loss of elastic recoil. The results of these changes affect ventilation and gas exchange. Normal physiologic changes can resemble pathologic entities. The lungs of healthy elders who are nonsmokers show evidence of small, scattered areas of lung destruction similar to the manifestations identified in emphysema (Timiras, 1994). This reduced efficiency of air expulsion found in the aged population resembles emphysema but is considered normal and is referred to as "senile emphysema" (Anderson, 2000; Tockman, 2000). The extent of change is the critical factor in differentiating normal from pathologic conditions.

Ossification or rigidity of the costal cartilage and the downward slant of the ribs creates a less compliant, more rigid rib cage, which limits chest expansion. Intercostal and accessory muscles and the diaphragm become more compliant, or "floppier," as a consequence of muscle weakness. The potential for greater lung expansion exists but cannot be realized because of the structural limitations that develop in the thoracic walls. Skeletal defects such as kyphosis and scoliosis and the generally stooped posture of the aged also contribute to restricting chest expansion by further reducing the size of the chest cavity area in which the lungs can expand. These changes increase dead space, decrease vital capacity, and decrease expiratory flow (Anderson, 2000; Tockman, 2000). Collagen remains relatively constant, yet there seems to be an increased amount of vascular collagen as a compensatory response to the decreased number and size of the alveoli (see Appendix 4-A).

Lungs do not shrink in size but do become flabbier and decrease in weight by 20% (Krumpe et al, 1985). The elastin and collagen changes that are due to cross-linkage and deterioration result in a decrease of outward movement and an inward pull with the end result of slightly smaller total lung capacity, increased residual capacity and residual volume, and early airway closure.

After age 30, the alveoli progressively enlarge and thus structurally resemble air sac changes associated with emphysema. The elastin fibers in the alveolar walls are bound to the respiratory and terminal bronchioles, which help maintain the small airway patency at low lung volumes. The loss of the elastin attachment causes an increase in compliance, collapse of the small airways, and uneven alveolar ventilation, trapping air and increasing dead space (Schumann, 1995; Anderson, 2000; Tockman, 2000). The alveolar dilation with the loss of alveolar attachments and the increase in the number of collapsed small airways, a physiologic change, is called *ductectasis* (Campbell and Lefrak, 1978) or *senile lung* (Tockman, 1995) and is seen in some individuals over age 60. This creates an increase in lung resonance with percussion.

Total lung capacity is not significantly altered, but rather it is redistributed. Residual capacity increases with the diminished inspiratory and expiratory muscle strength of the thorax. Incomplete lung expansion does not provide for inflation of the lung bases and leads to basilar lung collapse and hyperinflation of the lung apices. Greater diaphragmatic motion is needed because of the restriction of the costal structures and the general overall change in muscle strength of the body. This is evidenced in the shallow breathing of the elderly. The changes that have occurred in the anatomic structures of the chest and the altered muscle strength do not lend themselves to the forcefulness needed to expel material that accumulates or causes an obstruction in the airway. Therefore the aged individual has a less effective cough response or cough reflex. However, when other clearing mechanisms are intact, the cough reflex is not essential for respiratory clearance. When there is impairment such as dysphagia or decreased esophageal motility, an intact cough reflex is a necessity to prevent aspiration (Anderson, 2000; Tockman, 2000). The lack of basilar inflation, ineffective cough response, and a less efficient immune system pose potential problems for the aged who are sedentary, bedridden, or limited in activity.

Oxygen exchange. The aged blood oxygen (Po_2) level is approximately 75 mm Hg, whereas the Po_2 level for younger adults ranges from 90 to 95 mm Hg (Timiras, 1994). Pierson (1992) suggested that Po_2 falls 4 mm Hg per decade. The blood carbon dioxide (Pco_2) level remains constant for both the young and older adult. The blood oxygen (Po_2) tension also remains constant, but the distribution of inspired air to dependent parts of the lung is less sufficient (Timiras, 1994). The absolute lowest normal Po_2 level for an elder is 70 mm Hg.

The transmural gradient that is responsible for holding open airways is diminished. Airway collapse limits the ability of the lungs to empty and decreases the exhalation of Pco_2. This places a greater demand on cardiac function to increase cardiac output to compensate for less oxygen delivery to body tissue. Diminished elastic recoil of the lungs makes gaseous exchange across alveolar membranes more difficult. Aged individuals with Po_2 levels as low as 40 mm Hg have little or no immediate compensatory response in cardiac function. Younger persons with the same blood gas level show a marked increase in cardiac rate as an attempt to compensate and deliver more oxygen to body tissues.

Chemoreceptor function is altered or blunted at the peripheral and central chemoreceptor sites or in the integrating central nervous system pathways. In healthy men ages 64 to 73, response to hypoxia is 51% less and to hypercapnia is 41% less than in younger adults. This response is independent of mechanical lung changes and is attributed to the neuromuscular drive to breathe. Maximum inspiration and expiration pressures, which have declined as a result of chest wall inflexibility, reduce functional respiratory reserve and increase risk for respiratory failure. Compensatory responses are significantly hindered when the aged person is experiencing moderate amounts of stress. Decreased physical fitness further limits the availability of adequate gaseous exchange.

Reliable pulmonary function values that depict normal respiratory function of the aged are difficult to obtain. There are few published values on respiratory function tests for the elderly, particularly test values for aged women. Many values considered normal for old people have been derived from studies using small numbers of patients, often highly selected, under specific testing conditions. The absence of reliable pulmonary function values on which to evaluate the respiratory status of the aged requires that the nurse use other methods to assess the aged person's respiratory ability and needs through such means as attention to respiratory rate, evidence of shortness of breath with routine activities, and fatigability.

Respiratory problems. It is suggested that airway problems with age are due to repeated inflammatory injuries, disruption of inflammatory mediators and humoral protection (elastase-antielastase, oxidants-antioxidants), neutrophil aggregation, and tissue repair (Timiras, 1994; Anderson, 2000; Tockman, 2000; Sheahan and Musialowski, 2001). Diminished immune response, environmental factors, and structural changes are all factors that predispose the aged to respiratory problems. Conditions that affect the respiratory system are among the most common life-threatening disorders experienced by the aged and are considered to be among the leading causes of death.

Pneumonias are the fourth leading cause of death by disease in the United States and the leading cause of death in the elderly (Anderson, 2000; Tockman, 2000). The old-old (85 years and older) are five times more likely to die of pneumonia than young-old or old adults. The organisms responsible for causing pneumonia in the elderly include *Streptococcus pneumoniae,* gram-negative bacilli, anaerobic bacteria, *Haemophilus influenzae, Legionella* species, and viruses. *Streptococcus pneumoniae* is the most common bacteria in community-acquired pneumonia in the elderly. Gram-negative bacilli such as *Klebsiella, Pseudomonas,* and *Escherichia coli* are generally nosocomial (acquired in the institutional setting) (Anderson, 2000; Tockman, 2000). Signs and symptoms of pneumonia manifested in the young are not commonly seen in the aged. The tendency toward atypical responses can easily lead to an incorrect diagnosis or a diagnosis made too late in the progress of the pneumonia. Aspiration pneumonia is a high-risk condition for the obtunded client who is force fed, a client with swallowing difficulties or esophageal disease, a client who regurgitates food, a client with an endotracheal tube or tracheostomy, and a client who is heavily sedated.

Chronic obstructive pulmonary disease (COPD) includes bronchitis, asthma, emphysema, and bronchiectasis. COPD and lung cancer constitute the medical conditions from which many of the elderly's respiratory problems develop.

Renal Changes

All aspects of kidney function are affected by old age. The rate at which this occurs varies (Timiras, 1994). However, under physiologic or pathologic stress, the ability of the kidney to function adequately is greatly decreased. Kidneys are the primary organs responsible for regulation of the chemical composition of the body and blood and fluid volume. The age-related loss of as many as 50% of the millions of nephrons (each kidney has at least 1 million) leads to little change in the body's ability to regulate its body fluids and the ability to maintain adequate fluid homeostasis in old age under usual circumstances. Renal blood flow decreases 50% by the time one is 80 years of age. This is due to the changes in the renovascular bed (Horowitz, 2000).

The size and function of the kidney begin to decrease in the fourth decade and significantly decrease by the middle of the sixth decade; the kidney is 20% to 30% smaller by the eighth decade. The kidney contour remains relatively smooth. Kidney mass and weight decrease mainly in the cortical portion where the number of glomeruli correspond to the weight loss of the organ. This decline in size parallels the general decrease in size and weight of other body organs.

Glomeruli. By the eighth decade, 30% of the glomeruli are lost and there is evidence of age-related glomerular sclerosis, which is in proportion to that found elsewhere in the body. Microscopically the renal tubules develop diverticula in the distal portion of the nephron. These may become retention cystic, common to the elderly; however, the clinical significance of this is unknown. The cause of sclerosis of the glomeruli is unclear, but it is thought that a high-protein diet or glomerular ischemia may be responsible (Rowe, 1995). In general, these changes pose little threat to the well-being of the aged unless there is an abrupt reduction in nephron function by an acquired renal disease (Richard, 1995; Rowe, 1995).

Renal Vessels. The large renal vessels show evidence of sclerosis with age but do not narrow the vessel lumen. Smaller vessels do not show this change. Only 15% of elders who are normotensive have sclerotic changes in the renal arterioles.

Changes occur in the arterioglomerular units affecting the cortical area (hyalinization and collapse of the glomerular tufts). Preglomerular arterioles become obliterated, resulting in loss of blood flow. The medullary area of the kidney demonstrates sclerosis of the glomeruli and shrinking between the afferent and efferent arterioles with a loss of glomeruli. The arteriolae rectae verae preserve blood flow to the medullary area. Age does not decrease the number of arterioles in this area.

Glomerular Filtration. Blood flow through the kidney decreases from 1200 ml/min in young adults to 600 ml/min by age 80 as a result of the vascular and fixed anatomic and structural changes described previously. Figure 4-1 illustrates the altered renal blood flow. In view of these changes, the glomerular filtration rate (GFR), dependent on the number of glomeruli, steadily declines. The GFR is measured by the creatinine clearance, which also changes with age. It is directly related to muscle mass and is a product of muscle metabolism. By age 80, the creatinine clearance is decreased to 100 ml/min. Urine creatinine, secondary to loss of muscle mass, alters the expected relationship of serum creatinine to the creatinine clearance. A linear decline begins at about age 40 with a rate of 8 ml/min/1.73 m^2/decade (Lindeman, 2000). Approximately one third of the elderly do not exhibit a decline in GFR, suggesting that factors other than age-related change may be responsible for altered renal function (Lindeman, 2000). Plasma creatinine clearance is constant throughout life. The decline in urine creatinine clearance is an important indicator for appropriate drug therapy in the aged (see Chapter 10).

Renin-Angiotensin. Basal renin is reduced by 30% to 50% even with normal levels of renin substrate (Rowe, 1995). The lower renin levels are associated with a parallel reduction of the same proportions in aldosterone. However, after corticotropin stimulation, aldosterone and corticol responses are not impaired with age. This decreases the kidneys' ability to conserve sodium and delay the response of the acid/base loading.

There is a slight shift in the antidiuretic hormone (ADH). A reduced ability to concentrate urine and conserve water, due to medullary loss, makes the collecting ducts less responsive to ADH. The importance of the age-related kidney changes is that elders are more susceptible to fluid and electrolyte imbalance and renal damage from medications and contrast media of diagnostic tests. Under normal circumstances, kidney function is sufficient to meet the regulation and excretion demands of the body. However, with stress of disease, surgery, or fever, the kidneys have reduced capacity to respond.

Endocrine Changes

Hormones are responsible for and control reproduction, growth and development, maintenance of homeostasis, and energy production. Two principles must be kept in mind when considering hormonal control and effects: (1) A particular hormone may have an effect on many body systems and functions, and (2) one body function may require the coordinated action of many hormones (Bartz, 1995). It is suggested here that backup and fine-tuning mechanisms and natural adjustments are made to maintain homeostasis or close-to-normal limits. Changes may produce hypoactivity from disease or physiologic down regulating. Serum hormone levels are reflective of changes. Most glands atrophy and decrease their rate of secretion. There is no uniform direction of change; some are less active, slightly active, or not at all active (Solomon, 1995).

Pancreas. The pancreas possesses both endocrine and exocrine functions. The exocrine function is concerned with digestion. Endocrine function is mainly the secretion of insulin and glucagon, which is responsible for the regulation of carbohydrates, protein, and lipid metabolism. Few changes occur in the pancreas with age; changes may include atrophy, an increased incidence of tumors, and deposits of amyloid material and lipofuscin granules (Timiras, 1994, 2003b).

Insulin. Insulin is an anabolic hormone that increases the storage of glucose, fatty acids, and amino acids in cells and tissues. There is little difference in insulin secretion from the beta cells and glucose metabolism throughout life. The age-related change is in the tissue sensitivity to insulin, thought to be due to a change in the molecular makeup of insulin (Bartz, 1995). In addition, higher levels of circulating proinsulin are found in older adults than in younger adults. Alteration of insulin receptor sites by the aging process is also thought to render insulin less effective because of factors at the pancreas level; secretion of insulin may be depressed at the peripheral level, or target tissue may have an increased resistance to insulin (Timiras, 1994, 2003b). When the pancreas is stressed with sudden concentrations of glucose, blood levels are higher and prolonged (see Figure 4-1). Because of this intolerance, increased levels of glucose in the blood make it difficult for physicians to determine if it is a physiologic decline or a genetic trait for which a treatment plan is needed.

Thyroid Gland. The thyroid's ability to maintain euthyroid (normal) function with age continues throughout aging even with changes in production. secretion, and action. The thyroid gland decreases in mass and becomes fibrotic with an increasing number of colloid nodules. There is also slowing of the metabolic rate and oxygen use by the body. Secretions of thyroid-stimulating hormone (TSH) continue unchanged even with a decrease of 50% between youth and advanced old age. The decrease correlates with a decrease in lean body mass and a decrease in metabolic activity and protein-rich tissue. The serum concentration of T4 (thyroxin) also remains unchanged (Timiras, 1994, 2003b; Bartz, 1995; Solomon, 1995). A significant decline in triiodothyronine (T3) occurs with age, which is thought to reflect reduced conversion of T4 to T3 in extrathyroidal locations. Collective signs, such as a slowed basal metabolic rate, thinning of the hair, and dry skin, are characteristic of hypothyroidism in the young but are normal manifestations in the aged who have no history of thyroid deficiencies (see Appendix 4-A). Some of the aged do develop hypothyroidism and should be evaluated. This is one instance in which it is difficult, on the surface, to establish the presence or absence of disease.

Adrenal Gland. Cortisol, an important glucocorticoid of the adrenal cortex, although diminished by 25%, does not seem to have an adverse effect. Likewise, the effect of decreased adrenocorticotropic hormone production has not been evaluated. Epinephrine, norepinephrine, and dopamine produced by the adrenal medulla decrease with age, but again the significance is unclear.

Pituitary Gland. The pituitary gland, with its diverse functions and central role in the complex hormone feedback system, decreases in volume by 20%. The significance of this is unclear in light of the maintenance of adequate hormonal secretions.

Adrenogenic, estrogenic, and gonadotropic hormones undergo secretory and stimulatory changes. Diminished hormone levels lead to atrophy of the ovaries, uterus, and vaginal tissue in aged women. Aged men develop firmer testes and a tendency for prostatic hypertrophy, which is a benign condition in most instances. Women lose the ability to procreate. Sexual capacity may diminish as the tissues change and physical and mental health changes occur, but libido usually remains present in both sexes. Intercourse may be less frequent and take longer to accomplish, but this does not mean that it is less satisfying to the couple involved.

There tends to be a subliminal belief on the part of nurses and other caregivers that persons (at an arbitrary age) in general no longer are sexually active or possess sexuality. It is true that when one is seriously ill or in poor mental or physical health, the body does not require sexual activity as one of the primary responses. Most institutional care neglects the genital sexual need and the touch, intimacy, and sexuality needs of persons of any age. It behooves the nurse and others to view and care for the aged individual as a total being. Chapter 16 addresses touch, intimacy, and sexual needs in greater detail.

Gastrointestinal Changes

The digestive system handles age-related changes better than most systems of the body. The primary functions of the gastrointestinal tract are digestion and absorption, which are accomplished by gastrointestinal secretions and motility. Changes in other organ systems affect gastrointestinal structure and function. Studies have determined that extraintestinal causes, such as diabetes and vascular and neurologic changes, previously may have been mistaken for age-related changes in the gastrointestinal system.

Mouth and Teeth. Dentition is an important adjunct to the gastrointestinal system and can affect digestive activity. Poor dentition is a major factor that contributes to impaired chewing and reduced caloric intake. The chewing surfaces of the teeth wear down from chewing and bruxism (grinding of teeth), which occurs during rapid eye movement (REM) sleep with some individuals. Food entering the mouth is prepared for digestion by the action of saliva, which contains ptyalin to break down starch, and mastication by the teeth. Many aged are edentulous or dependent on dentures. A number of aged who have dentures choose not to wear them; others are unable to afford them.

Normally food is well masticated in the mouth. As a result of systemic disorders and their treatment, the saliva level may decline. Some medications are notorious for causing "dry mouth." Normally there is a slight decline in saliva production in the aged (Schuster, 1995; Horowitz, 2000). In addition, in the presence of few teeth or ill-fitting dentures, the process of preparing the food for swallowing is incomplete with food morsels improperly chewed. The inclination is to place many aged on a pureed diet even though this type of diet lacks the appeal, taste, texture, and appearance needed to stimulate appetite, gastrointestinal motility, eating enjoyment, and the maintenance of adequate nutrition.

In the future, as an effect of better dental hygiene and fluoride in water systems and in dental preparations, the aged may retain their own teeth for the full extent of their lives. The primary problem that will remain and be responsible for tooth loss is periodontal disorders. Gum disease threatens tooth structure and compromises healthy teeth, requiring removal. Many gum conditions can be prevented with proper toothbrushing and oral hygiene. Chapter 7 discusses dental health.

Esophagus. Gastrointestinal muscle strength and motility decrease with a resultant decrease in peristalsis. The esophagus increases the number of muscle movements but does not effectively propel its contents. Decreased peristaltic action and the relaxation of the lower esophageal sphincter slow the emptying of the esophagus. Improperly masticated food antagonizes this situation and in part is responsible for the forceful, emphatic, propulsive contractions that propel the food on its way to further digestion. The sluggish emptying of the esophagus also forces the lower end to dilate, sustaining greater stress in this area and causing digestive discomfort to the aged (referred to as *presbyesophagus*). Gastroesophageal reflux disease is common among the elderly, even those who are asymptomatic. Horowitz (2000) suggests that this may be due to the reduction in the intraabdominal length of the lower esophageal sphincter and an increased incidence of hiatal hernias.

Stomach. Aging has no significant effect on secretion of acid and pepsin; however, conditions that reduce acid production are common (Horowitz, 2000). It is now acknowledged that reductions in basal and stimulated gastric acid secretions are the result of atrophic gastritis. When there is no atrophy, the number of parietal cells increases with age. Age is a major factor in the diminished capacity of the gastric mucosa to resist damage even when the older adult is healthy.

The protective alkaline viscous mucus of the stomach is lost because of the increase in stomach pH. This makes the aged more susceptible to peptic ulcer disease, particularly with the use of nonsteroidal antiinflammatory drugs. Loss of smooth muscle in the stomach delays emptying time, which may lead to anorexia or weight loss as a result of distention, meal-induced fullness, and the feeling of satiety.

Liver, Gallbladder, and Pancreas. The glandular secretions of the digestive system come from the liver, gallbladder, and pancreas. The liver is a sturdy organ and continues to function throughout life even with a decrease in volume and weight (mass) by about 17% to 28% between ages 40 and 65. The weight decreases by 25% between ages 20 and 70 in both men and women. The decrease in mass brings with it a concomitant decrease in liver blood flow. The age-related changes are macroscopic in nature. Increased lipofuscin (brown pigment) in the hepatocytes turns the liver brown. This pigment is the remnant of a lifelong buildup of unexcreted metabolic residue of lipids and proteins, but it is not clinically significant (Horowitz, 2000). The increased fibrotic changes in the capsular and parenchymal tissues do not represent cirrhosis. Protein synthesis and the rate of degradation result in the accumulation of abnormal protein with a corresponding inability to break down protein. Liver regeneration is slow but not greatly impaired. Liver function tests remain unaltered with age.

Bile manufactured by the liver to emulsify fat is stored in the gallbladder. There does not seem to be a specific change in the gallbladder, but the aged 70 years of age and older account for one third of gallbladder surgeries (Tompkins, 1995; Welch, 1995). This is possibly due to the increased lipogenic composition of bile from biliary cholesterol. The decrease in bile salt synthesis increases the incidence of cholelithiasis and cholecystitis (Altman, 1990; Cassmeyer and Blevin, 1993). In addition, the decrease in bile acid synthesis causes a reduction in hydroxylation of cholesterol. This, in conjunction with a decrease in hepatic extraction of low-density lipoprotein cholesterol from the blood, increases the level of serum cholesterol in the aged. The pancreas becomes more fibrotic and shows evidence of ductal hyperplasia, but these changes do not necessarily lead to physiologic dysfunction. There is a decline in pancreatic secretions and enzyme output after age 40. This affects fat digestion and may be the reason for increased intolerance of fatty foods with age.

Small Intestine. Smooth muscle, Peyer's patches, and lymphatic follicles decrease with age. No major changes occur to the motility, transit, permeability, or absorption in the small intestine. Bacterial overgrowth in the small intestine is a common problem with the aged and is usually associated with malnutrition. It may be nonspecific in symptomatology but affects the absorption of micronutrients such as iron, calcium, folate, and vitamins K and B_6. The tendency toward vitamin and mineral deficiency is also caused by inadequate dietary intake of the aged. Vitamins K, B_1, and B_{12} and minerals such as iron and calcium are the most frequently deficient. Protein consumption may be lower than in early life as a result of difficulty chewing and digesting meat or the cost of obtaining dentures. For some aged it would be judicious to take a daily vitamin to ensure at least a minimum ingestion and availability of the necessary vitamins and minerals. It might be prudent for the nurse to assist the aged person to learn about inexpensive sources of protein nutrients and to suggest that better absorption and digestion might be promoted by eating small snack-size meals throughout the day rather than the typical three meals per day. Chapter 6 discusses nutrition for the aged in depth.

Large Intestine. No major changes occur in the large intestine. There is a reduction in the perception of anorectal distention. The internal sphincter of the large intestine loses its muscle tone and can create problems in bowel evacuation. The external sphincter, which retains much of its original tone, cannot by itself control the bowels. Slower transmission of neural impulses lessens the awareness of sensations of a forthcoming bowel evacuation. The outcome of this may be either fecal incontinence or constipation. There is structural atrophy of the layers and glands and a decrease in mucous secretions. Weakness of the intestinal walls may also lead to outpouching of small segments of the colon (diverticula), which may or may not be symptomatic. The implication for the nurse is to routinely evaluate the elimination pattern of the aged person, which may help avoid embarrassment and provide a positive frame of mind for the aged person. Elimination needs are presented in Chapters 6 and 8.

Nervous System Changes

Mental Performance. In general, intellectual performance of the elder without brain dysfunction remains constant into and beyond the eighties. Verbal skills remain intact until age 70, after which some healthy elders gradually experience a reduced vocabulary and a tendency toward semantic errors. Other subtle mentation changes occur, such as learning difficulties and forgetfulness (not to be confused with dementia). The performance of tasks may take longer, an indication that central processing is slowed (Joynt, 2000; Timiras, 2003a). Mental health and cognition are discussed in Chapters 21 and 23.

Brain. Nerve cell loss is minimal in the brainstem but more profound in the hippocampus. Brain weight decreases by approximately 10% between the second and ninth decades. The cerebral ventricles enlarge three to four times from the third to the ninth decades. Lipofuscin, an aging pigment, is deposited in nerve cells, and amyloid deposition occurs in the blood vessels and cells. Senile plaque and, less frequently, neurofibrillary tangles are also found. The latter are usually associated with Alzheimer's disease, but they also appear in the brain of elders without evidence of dementia (Joynt, 2000).

Neurotransmitters. Changes in neurotransmitter systems of dopaminergic and cholinergic systems occur with levels of choline acetylase, serotonin, and catecholamines decreasing. Other enzymes such as monoamine oxidase (MAO) increase. Redundancy of brain cells may forestall some changes, but the exact number of cells required for certain functions is not clear.

Nerve Cells. The brain has the ability to compensate for areas of injury or destruction, with compensation more effective in the higher centers. The spinal cord has less ability to do so. Peripheral nerves remain relatively unchanged and will regenerate slowly; however, conduction time of the peripheral nerves decreases in the aged.

As nerve cells gradually deteriorate and die, there is a compensatory lengthening of and an increase in the number of dendrites of the remaining nerve cells. The new connections in the dendrite tree may make up for the lower number of cells. This phenomenon is a normal age change, even though this may be seen to occur extensively with Alzheimer's disease.

External factors affect the positive and negative age-related changes. Medical or psychologic stress may result in the elder exhibiting confusion, delirium, or depression. Sleep medication may also affect the elder by creating a confused or delirious state.

Sensory Changes

A number of sensory changes occur with age as a result of the intrinsic aging process in sensory organs and their association with the nervous system. Other changes are extrinsic and linked to the environment (see Appendix 4-A). One cannot totally escape diminution of taste, smell, sight, sound, and touch.

Taste Perception. Elders lose some of their ability to identify food by taste (Horowitz, 2000) and require a greater taste threshold for sodium chloride than for sucrose, although the threshold of both rises (Meisami, 1994). Taste buds atrophy, lose efficiency in relaying flavor, and decline in number. The threshold necessary to relay flavors rises for the four primary taste qualities: sweet, salty, bitter, and sour.

Crude taste (sweet and sour) is mediated by the taste buds; fine taste is olfactory mediated. Both taste and smell receptors are diminished. Taste bud receptor cells are in the papillae of the tongue and have a short life span of days. Loss of taste buds begins in the sixth decade and gradually progresses as a result of neural degeneration (Wilson, 1995). In crude taste there is a decrease in the number of nerve endings, papillae, and taste buds. This is, however, more pronounced when there are estrogen and protein deficiencies (Wilson, 1995). Smoking may also accelerate the loss. Changes may also be due to dental problems, medications, or illnesses that create background taste and weaken stimuli and a decreased sense of smell.

Fine taste mediated by olfactory apparatus is associated with cognition and linguistics. A decrease in this aspect of taste may be due to loss of interest in food and maintaining a proper diet in addition to excess use of sugar and salt. Taste changes in the healthy aged are modest and not considered to be significant. The quality of taste may vary, but taste remains robust in the aged.

Smell Perception. Changes in smell are attributed to loss of cells in the olfactory bulb of the brain and a decrease in the number of sensory cells in the nasal lining. In addition, numerous upper respiratory infections and long-term exposure to tobacco smoke and other toxic agents interfere with adequate olfactory function. Of all the senses, age takes the greatest toll on smell perception. There is strong evidence that smell perception declines markedly. Studies have found that women are better than men at determining 10 odorants. Nonsmokers are also able to smell better than smokers. Smell deteriorates in about half of the aged in their sixth decade and affects those age 80 and older (Eliopoulos, 1997; Williams, 2000).

Pain Perception. At times caregivers have been amazed by the aged person's lack of response to pain. Conditions that are normally painful occur with an absence of pain or create only minor discomfort or a sense of pressure. Life-threatening myocardial and abdominal infarctions are often experienced this way. Another condition that has been missed because of the lack of expected pain response is appendicitis (Anderson, 1976; Rossman, 1986). *This does not mean that elders do not experience postoperative pain or pain from arthritis or other conditions.* The diminution of normal pain signals creates some potentially dangerous situations for the aged and their state of wellness. Persons with limited activity, such as those confined to a wheelchair or to bed, may not feel the pressure on bony prominences or the body messages to change position. Transmission of hot and cold impulses may be delayed long enough for the aged individual to sustain significant tissue damage to some part of the body. Contact with such items as heating pads, hot water bags, radiators, and iced items can result in serious consequences and lengthy hospitalizations for the aged. Issues related to pain and thermal perception are not yet definitive (Timiras, 1994).

Somatesthesia and Tactile Perception. Somatesthesia, or tactile sensitivity, decreases with age because of skin changes and the loss of a large number of nerve endings. This is particularly striking in the fingertips, palms of the hands, and lower extremities (Meisami, 1995).

Kinesthetic Sense. The kinesthetic sense, or proprioception (one's position in space), is altered with age because of the changes in the central nervous system and muscles. Elders have more difficulty orienting their body in space when externally induced changes in body position are made. Slowed movements and altered position in space can lead to considerable difficulty with balance and spatial orientation. The aged cannot avoid obstacles as quickly in ordinary situations such as those that occur on a crowded street, nor are the aged as able as they once were to prevent an accident from happening to themselves or to others when fast movement might be essential. The automatic response to protect and brace oneself when falling is slower, and one can observe the aged making more precise and deliberate movements, such as placement of the feet when walking. Conditions such as arthritis, stroke, some cardiac disorders, or damage to the structures of the inner ear may affect peripheral and central mechanisms of mobility. Further discussion of sensory alterations appears in Chapter 12.

Eye and Vision Changes

Decline in visual acuity is a progressive change that occurs in the optic compartment (cornea, lens, pupil, aqueous and vitreous humor, retina) of the eye. All persons will eventually experience some decline in visual capacity with age.

Extraocular. *Eyelids* droop (senile ptosis) as a result of the loss of elasticity, and skin atrophy can interfere with vision if the lids sag far enough over the lower lid margin. Decrease in the orbicular muscle strength of the eyes may result in ectropion or entropion. Ectropion may cause the lower lid not to close completely with sleep and lead to corneal dryness. Spasms of the orbicular muscle may cause the eyelashes, particularly of the lower lid, to turn inward (entropion), irritating the eyeball with each blink (Jarvis, 1996).

The *conjunctiva* is the thin membrane over the sclera with goblet cells that provide mucin, essential for eye lubrication and movement. Mucin slows the evaporation of tear film. The number of goblet cells decreases, resulting in a deficiency of lubrication for the eye. Lack of tear secretions or nonspecific causes contribute to dry eye syndrome (Tumosa, 2000).

Ocular. The *cornea,* which is responsible for refraction of light, is among the first eye structures to be affected by aging. A flatter, less smooth, and thicker cornea is noticeable by its lackluster appearance or loss of sparkling transparency and leaves the aged individual more susceptible to astigmatism. A gray-white ring or partial ring, known as arcus senilis, forms 1 to 2 mm inside the limbus. It does not affect vision and is composed of deposits of calcium and cholesterol salts. This nonsignificant finding has at times been linked to systemic hyperlipidemia. Almost everyone over age 65 will exhibit some degree of arcus senilis, which gives credence to an age correlation of this specific change.

There is some degeneration of endothelial cells lining the inner surface of the cornea. Major changes that become progressive can lead to failure to keep the cornea free of extracellular fluid, causing corneal edema. This situation requires immediate treatment by a physician.

Two sets of *iris* muscles regulate pupil size, affecting the amount of light that reaches the retina and limiting the efficiency of pupillary constriction and dilation. Pupil size is smaller in older adults, creating the problem of being dazzled in bright light by sluggish constriction. Slowness to dilate to the dark creates moments when elders cannot see where they are going. Because of the slow ability of the pupils to accommodate to changes in light, glare is a major problem for the aged. Glare is a problem created not only by sunlight outdoors, but also by the reflection of light on any shiny object and especially light striking polished or linoleum floors (Meisami, Brown, and Emerle, 2003).

The inability of the eyes to accommodate to close and detailed work (presbyopia) begins in the fourth decade and continues throughout the rest of one's life. *Presbyopia* occurs earlier in individuals who live in warm climates and later in individuals who are nearsighted (myopic). Suspensory ligaments, ciliary muscles, and parasympathetic nerves contribute to the decreased accommodation that occurs.

Pupil diameter and the speed of direct and consensual responses decreases. If the pupil response is sluggish or absent, it may be that medication to dilate or constrict the pupils is being taken. Older people require three times more light to see things than younger adults. It is more effective to place high-intensity light on the object or surface that is involved than to increase the intensity of the light in the entire area or room—for example, it is more effective to focus a light directly on the newspaper a person is reading than to turn on an overhead room light.

The extent of the visual field begins to wane, affecting the breadth of vision that is possible. No longer can the aged view things panoramically, but the peripheral vision is not as discrete and may be missed (Kupfer, 1995; Tumosa, 2000). The decreased ability to respond to rapid eye movement in front of the eyes presents problems for the aged. Rapid blinking or flickering lights or motion cannot be accommodated as well as in youth.

The *anterior chamber* of the eye decreases due to the thickness of the lens. The iris becomes paler in color as a result of pigment loss and increases in the density of collagen fibers. Resorption of the intraocular fluid becomes less efficient with age and may lead to eventual breakdown in the absorption process. This creates the potential for the pathologic condition known as glaucoma.

The constant compression of *lens* fibers with age, the yellowing effect, and the inefficiency of the aqueous humor, which provides the lens with nutrition, all have a role in altered lens transparency. Lens cells continue to grow but at a slower rate than previously. The cells on the periphery of the lens regenerate very slowly, whereas those toward the center are more active. Nearly everyone between ages 40 and 45 begins to discover the need for assistive lenses for reading and accommodation. Those who are nearsighted (myopic) tend to experience reading and accommodation difficulties in their fifties and sixties.

Lens opacity (cataracts) begin to develop around the fifth decade of life. The origins are not fully understood, although ultraviolet rays of the sun contribute, with cross-linkage of collagen creating a more rigid and thickened lens structure.

Intraocular. The *vitreous humor,* which gives the eye globe its shape and support, loses some of its water and fibrous skeletal support with age. Opacities other than cataracts can be lines, webs, spots, or clusters of dots moving rapidly across the visual field with each movement of the eye. These opacities (floaters) are bits of coalesced vitreous that have broken off from the peripheral or central part of the retina. Mostly they are harmless and annoying until they dissipate or one gets used to them. If, however, the person sees a shower of these and a flash of light, immediate medical attention is required because it might indicate retinal problems (Tumosa, 2000; Meisami, Brown, and Emerle, 2003).

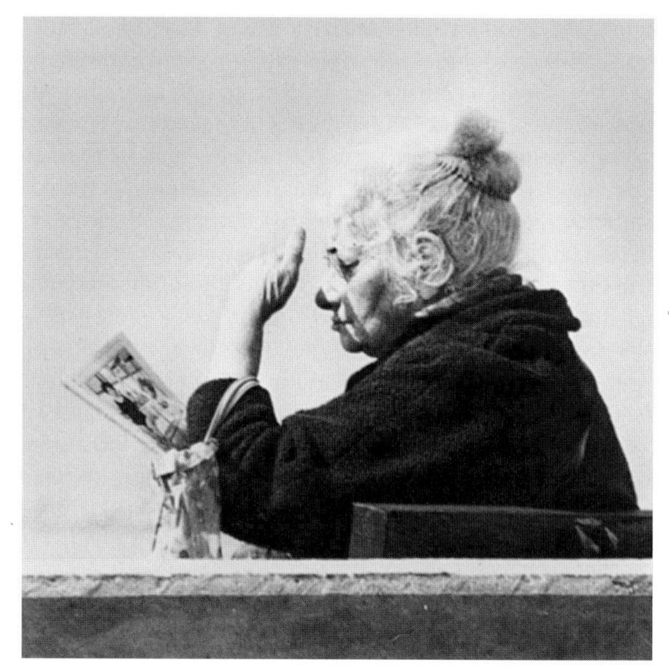

Glare.

The *retina* has less distinct margins and is duller in appearance than in younger adults. Fidelity of color is less accurate with blues, violets, and greens of the spectrum; light colors such as reds, oranges, and yellows are more easily seen. Color clarity diminishes by 25% in the sixth decade and by 59% in the eighth decade. Some of this difficulty is linked to the yellowing of the lens and impaired transmission of light through the retina, and the macula may not have as bright a fovea reflective light either. Drusen (yellow-white) spots may appear in the area of the macula (Tumosa, 2000). As long as these changes are not accompanied by distortion of objects or a decrease in vision, some pigment deposition is not clinically significant.

Arteries may show atherosclerosis and slight narrowing. *Veins* may show indentations (nicking) at the arteriovenous crossings.

The lubricating and cleansing actions of the lacrimal secretions diminish. Eyes take on a dull appearance, and there is a sensation of dryness, scratchiness, or tightness, which, if uncomfortable, may respond to artificial tears as a lubricant.

Auditory Changes

External Ear. The *auricle,* or *pinna,* loses flexibility and becomes longer and wider as a result of diminished elasticity with the appearance of tophi. The lobule sags, elongates, and develops wrinkles. Together these changes make the ear appear larger. The periphery of the auricle develops coarse, wiry, stiff hair in men. The tragus also becomes larger in men.

The *auditory canal* narrows, causing inward collapsing. Stiffer and coarser hair lines the ear canal. Cerumen glands atrophy, causing thicker and dryer cerumen, which is more difficult to remove and a substantial cause for hearing impairment.

Middle Ear. The *tympanic membrane* becomes dull, less flexible, retracted, and gray in appearance. The ossicle joints between the malleus and stapes develop calcification, causing joint fixation or reduced vibration of these bones and reduced sound transmission.

Inner Ear. Vestibular sensitivity decreases as a result of degeneration of the *organ of Corti* in the cochlea and otic nerve loss. Changes in the efficiency of the cochlea and hair cells of the organ of Corti are responsible for the impaired transmission of sound waves along the nerve pathways of the brain and are considered to be the most common cause of presbycusis. Atrophy of the organ of Corti begins in middle age and causes sensory hearing loss. Loss of cochlear neurons that occurs in late life, even with the preservation of the organ of Corti, is a neural hearing loss and is considered to be related to genetic factors. Familial tendencies in middle life associated with electrophysiologic function of the organ of Corti are the basis of metabolic hearing loss (Gulya, 1995). Altered motion of the cochlear ducts occurs in middle age and is considered to be cochlear conductive hearing loss. The role of *basilar membrane* stiffening as a possible cause of this type of hearing loss is speculated. All of these types of loss are presbycusis. Many elders have a combination of causes for their hearing deficit.

Constant or recurring high-pitched *tinnitus* (clicking, buzzing, roaring, ringing, or other sounds in the ear) unilaterally or bilaterally is usually caused by impairment of the *otic nerve* accompanying the aging process. Medications, infection, cerumen accumulation, or a blow to the head may also cause tinnitus (Gulya, 1995). Tinnitus becomes most acute at night or in quiet surroundings. It is a nuisance that is difficult to combat or treat. The most helpful strategy is to use "masking" techniques that introduce another competing sound. "White noise" (soft static between FM radio stations) on low volume can be soothing (*Harvard Medical School Health Letter,* 1983).

Auditory changes occur subtly. Normal decrements in hearing acuity, speech intelligibility, level of auditory threshold, and discrimination of pitch, especially in the speech frequencies, is referred to as presbycusis. *Presbycusis,* "hearing loss of aging," describes the type of loss, not the cause, and can be classified according to the structural source of impairment (Table 4-2). It is a bilateral and symmetric sensorineural hearing loss associated with age. Accumulated wax in the ear canal also intensifies presbycusis. Men seem to experience more severe presbycusis than women of the same age. High frequency is not interfered with in understandable speech; however, it does begin to affect high-frequency sibilant consonant discrimination, with "z," "s," "sh," "f," "p," "k," "t," and "g" being the most difficult in conversation. Vowels that have a low pitch are more easily heard. Without consonants, the high-frequency–pitched language becomes disjointed and misunderstood. Consider the simple sentence "How are you today?" To the individual with presbycusis it might sound like "hOw arE yOU tOdAy?" The older adult might complain of having difficulty understanding women and children, conversations in large groups, or when there is background noise as in restaurants. Loud music or intercom or paging systems, such as those used in hospitals or airports, mask conversation with noise. Rapid speech when conversing with an older adult will make words sound garbled and unintelligible. Even though this latter problem is related to presbycusis, it is one that can be easily remedied by hearing aides.

Environmental noise, genetic disease, ototoxic agents, and a circulatory deficit to the vital structures of the inner ear are additional factors that contribute to the extent of hearing loss.

Some hearing loss affects about one third of all adults between ages 65 and 74 and about one half of those ages 75 to 79. More than 10 million elders have hearing impairments (Williams, 2000). Hearing loss is not only frustrating to the aged individual, but also threatens security and self-esteem. The nurse and others often respond with impatience and anger to the aged person's inability to hear clearly, a response that only compounds the hearing problem. Unless there is an injury or a genetic defect, individuals can usually hear well enough in the absence of the problems that arise from noise, rapid speech, or varied voice modulation.

Table 4-2 Types and Causes of Presbycusis

Types	Description	Cause
Sensory	A sharp hearing loss at high frequencies, with little effect on speech understanding	Degeneration of hair cells and atrophy of the organ of Corti
Neural	Hearing loss reduces speech discrimination	Widespread degeneration of cochlea nerve fibers and spiral ganglia
Metabolic or strial	Hearing loss that initially reduces sensitivity to all sound frequencies; it later interferes with speech discrimination	Degeneration of the stria vascularis and interruption in essential nutrients
Mechanical	Hearing loss that gradually increases from low to high frequencies and affects speech discrimination when high-frequency hearing loss occurs	Mechanical changes in the inner ear

Immunologic Changes

"Immune senescence," the lapse of time between exposure and rechallenging by pathogens, decreases, as does the strength of response with advanced age (Miller, 1990; Hirsh, 1995; Yehuda, 1995). Immunologic responses are mediated by natural immunity (innate immunity), consisting of dendritic cells, macrophages, natural killer cells, and the complement system, and adaptive immunity (acquired immunity), composed of T cells and B cells (Michel, 2000; Proust, 2000).

Innate Immunity. Innate immunity provides a rapid but incomplete first cell interaction with an invading microbe or pathogen, creating the environment for the slower adaptive immune system to respond. The CD4+ T helper cells recognize the antigen on the surface of invading cells. Macrophages support the T-cell response. Natural killer cells can spontaneously kill target cells and are involved in the host's resistance. The complement system initiates cytolysis and activates the inflammatory process to defend against microorganisms. With aging there are fewer dendritic cells; the rate of macrophage clearance of antigens decreases, but natural killer cells increase. The complement system functions only slightly less well than in younger persons.

Adaptive Immunity. Cell-mediated activities involve the thymus and T-cell function. The thymus is the organ where T-cell maturation and differentiation occur (CD8+ T lymphocytes and CD4+ T lymphocytes). Beginning about age 30, there is a loss of gland mass that continues until age 50. At this time there is approximately 5% to 10% thymus gland function. Whether there is complete involution of the thymus at age 60 remains unclear (Michel, 2000; Proust, 2000). T cells remain relatively unchanged with age except in the substrate, where CD4+ T helper cells increase and CD8+ T suppressor cells decrease in number. The thymus loses the ability to differentiate T-cell precursors and T-cell–related B-cell differentiation. The result is that 25% of healthy adults show evidence of a marked decline in cell-mediated immunity, 50% show a moderate decline, and 25% have no decline (Hirsh, 1995; Yehuda, 1995).

The loss of functional capacity of the cell-mediated system is demonstrated by a decreased hypersensitivity response to such common skin tests as the tuberculin test. The implications are that the aged are more susceptible to reactivation of latent herpes zoster and mycobacterium. Opportunistic infections such as those associated with *Pneumocystis* or *Aspergillus,* seen in severely immunosuppressed individuals, are not generally seen in the aged. Humoral change is reflected in the impairment in T cells. Serum immunoglobulins (IGs) change little with age, but the distribution changes with increases in IgA and IgG and decreases in IgM and IgD. The decrease in antibody response suggests that to achieve a maximum antibody response, a larger dose of antigen is necessary. The effect, however, lasts a shorter period of time because of the decreased IgG production from altered function of cytokine stimulation, a response that still is unclear (Miller, 1990).

The decrease in self-recognition of autoantibodies to foreign antigens shows the dysregulation of the immune system. The decreases in T-cell–related B-cell differentiation and B-cell receptors are blocked by specific antigens that cap or patch the receptors, preventing their normal function (Michel, 2000; Proust, 2000).

In summary, old age brings a decrease in T-cell function resulting from a decrease in innate immunity, adaptive immunity, and self-tolerance. The response to foreign antigens decreases, but immunoglobulins increase, creating an autoimmune response not associated with autoimmune diseases, which usually occur before middle age (Michel, 2000; Proust, 2000). (See Chapter 2, Figure 2-4, for a diagram of immunologic changes.)

Biochemical and Genetic Changes

Much interest has been directed at the molecular structure and function of the aging human organism. Investigations designed to reveal the biochemical changes that underlie aging are often directed toward substances that will suppress the phenomenon of aging. Evidence of this emerges from the biologic theories of aging discussed in Chapter 2.

Chromatin, which is involved in the transfer of genetic information, is central in the elaboration of protein and enzymes and thus has become the focus of interest. Changes in chromatin reflect DNA and associated translation mechanisms in aging. Life-span variations among different species of animals and the uncertainty of life span in humans are examples of issues considered in the biochemical and genetic arena.

In summary, many of the age changes that occur have been discussed here and will be elaborated further in subsequent chapters. Biologic age changes are universal, progressive, decremental, and intrinsic. It can be concluded that complex functions of the body decline more than simple body processes; that coordinated activity, which relies on interacting systems such as nerves, muscles, and glands, has a greater decremental loss than single-system activity; and that a uniform and predictable loss of cell function occurs in all vital organs. Yet most aged individuals are able to function effectively within the physical dictates of their body and continue to live to a healthy old age, capable of wisdom, judgment, and satisfaction.

HEALTH ASSESSMENT

Health assessment, physical examination, and health screening, regardless of the nomenclature, is a process of collecting and analyzing data. This approach is the initial step in the nursing process. Assessment provides information critical to the development of a plan of action that can enhance personal health status, decrease the potential for or the severity of chronic conditions, and assist the individual to gain control over health through self-care.

A comprehensive geriatric assessment requires not only physical data, but also an integration of the biologic, psychosocial, spiritual, and functional aspects of the aged person. Inquiries into physiologic and anatomic function, growth and development, family relationships, group involvement, and religious and occupational pursuits are essential in a health assessment interview. Genetic background information, although important, is less significant for the aged because genetic consequences usually appear in earlier phases of life. However, genetic inheritance must be considered because latent changes do occur and affect physical and mental well-being.

As part of the health assessment it is most important to include appraisal of basic activities of daily living (BADLs), also referred to as functional assessment (life necessities—BADLs); instrumental activities of daily living (IADLs); and advanced activities of daily living (AADLs), which refer to occupational, recreational, and leisure activities that are based on choice rather than necessity. A functional assessment consists of the fundamental tasks and demands of daily life. It is generally agreed that functional assessment is divided into those abilities that are fundamental to independent living, such as bathing, dressing, toileting, transferring from bed or chair, feeding, and continence (Katz Index, Appendix 4-C). IADLs are more complex daily activities that include using the telephone, preparing meals, and managing money (Barthel Index, Appendix 4-C). An evaluation of mental ability is also essential. Questions directed at mental intactness are often incorporated into assessment of BADLs and IADLs. Specific tools are addressed later in this chapter. Psychologic status can be appraised by using such questions as appear in Box 4-2. Many books provide essential discussions of examination tools, techniques, and methods, and these are not presented here.

Health assessment data allow health care providers to develop and implement primary, secondary, and tertiary care regimens. Primary care addresses disease prevention and health promotion and maintenance. Care is directed toward limiting health risks and avoidance of sequelae from common health problems, uncomplicated illness, chronic illness, or mental states induced by a stressful environment. The individual is usually able to receive the benefits of such care either at home or on an outpatient basis. Secondary care focuses on specific illness or pathologic conditions and places its efforts on the retardation or termination of physical, mental, social, or environmental situations that have induced the condition or situation. Care is provided in a health care setting by professionals who have specific knowledge and skill in the area of concern. Tertiary care involves restorative measures that will enable the aged individual to achieve an optimum level of function, whatever that might be. Appropriate care requires professionals with specialized knowledge and skill either in an institutional health care setting or in the home or outpatient environment.

Aged persons do not usually seek assistance from health care professionals until there is obvious physical or emotional difficulty. Some aged individuals have had adverse experiences with the health care system; others assume that their problems are age related and do not realize that relief and assistance are possible.

Box 4-2 Questions to Elicit Information Significant to Health Status*

1. What is the first health problem you can remember? What happened and how was it taken care of? (traumatic expectations)
2. When you were young, what did you think about old people? What did you expect to be like when you were old? (ageist attitudes)
3. How old do you feel now? (health status, grief, depression)
4. What was your most gratifying experience? (expression, elaboration, imagination exhibited in description)
5. How did your mother describe you as a child? How did your father describe you as a child? (incorporation, self-evaluation, self-fulfilling prophecies)
6. How would you describe yourself as a child? (identity, self-concept)
7. What is the most important thing that you have done? (values)
8. What is the most difficult thing that you have done? (strength, integrity, endurance, courage)
9. How did you manage to do that? (coping style and patterns)
10. What would you change if you could? (life satisfaction, integrity, acceptance)

*These are only a few thoughts that can be modified or expanded on in any particular situation.

The initiation of the health history marks the beginning of the nurse-client relationship and ushers the aged person into the health care system. The interview requires skill in establishing client trust and confidence and in avoiding offending the individual. A considerable amount of time is required to complete a health assessment of the aged client, often because of a lack of schooling, the use of English as a second language, impaired communication skills from previous illness, or elder fatigue. It may be difficult for the interviewer to proceed slowly, one question at a time, and wait for the slow response, a result of perceptive and receptive changes that occur in the nervous system of the aged. The client may find giving certain types of health information stressful and may even decline to discuss changes or problems that might confirm fears of illness, limitations, or old age. Any illness is seen as a threat to independence and viewed as leading to eventual institutionalization. Sometimes an initial health questionnaire can be completed by the client (if vision and intellectual ability are not problems) before an office visit or while waiting to see the practitioner. The client often feels freer to respond to the printed question, it reduces time needed, and it provides a background from which the interview can develop. In addition, if the aged client can do the questionnaire at home before the visit, it often provides time to remember or find the requested information about his or her health. The health care provider can clarify questionnaire answers, and the client can elaborate with details.

Many of our present assessment tools do not provide for the attainment of accurate data with the rapidly changing ethnic mix of elders. Assessment must utilize ways to elicit health care beliefs from the ethnogeriatric groups. Cultural/ethnic sensitivity of the care provider is important in order to disentangle cultural normative behavior from behavior that mimics pathology. Available tools that can facilitate this type of assessment data are limited. Pfeifferling and Kleinman have developed tools that assist a caregiver in gleaning pertinent assessment information to provide appropriate health promotion, prevention, maintenance, and interventions. (See Chapter 19 for the health inquiry tool.)

Assessment of the aged requires special abilities of the nurse: ability to listen patiently, to allow for pauses, to ask questions that are not often asked, to observe the minute details, to obtain data from all available sources, and to recognize normalities of late life that would be abnormal in one who is younger. The quality and speed of the assessment are an art born of experience. The novice nurse should not be expected to do this. According to Benner (1984), it is a task for the expert. Preferably, all initial assessments when an aged individual enters the health care system would be conducted by the most knowledgeable and experienced person available. When this is not possible, it would be useful to have a checklist format that would alert even the novice to pressing concerns.

Guidelines for the components of a complete health history can be found in any health assessment text and are not presented here. However, it is important to include areas or problems not frequently addressed by health care providers or mentioned voluntarily by the aged when the history is taken. These include sexual dysfunction, depression, incontinence, musculoskeletal stiffness, alcoholism, and hearing loss (Ham, 1997). Much of the information obtained in the assessment is oral, but it can also be gotten by observation of personal grooming, facial expression, responsiveness to the interview, and physical examination. Information about involvement with the surrounding community and group participation should reveal additional information about the emotional state and feelings of self-worth. The comprehensive geriatric assessment differs from the standard medical evaluation. It includes nonmedical areas and places emphasis on functional ability and quality of life. The geriatric assessment includes the following:

- Diagnosis of health-related problems
- Treatment planning
- Follow-up
- Coordination of care
- Determination of the need for long-term-care placement
- Optimal use of health care resources

Geriatric assessment of the frail and chronically ill elderly can improve care by addressing the elder's functional and mental status, decreasing use of long-term care and acute care facilities, and decreasing mortality rates (Boult, 2000). A comprehensive geriatric assessment must include functional, physical, social, and mental assessment of the aged and the caregiver (if used) and assessment of the environment in order to plan care and prevent problems.

Home visit assessment complements or provides information that is difficult to gauge in a clinic, physician's office, or other formal setting. Especially difficult to ascertain are such areas as nutrition, alcoholism, actual level of function on a daily basis, and suitability and safety of the environment. Even when the individual is relatively independent, an appreciation for the difficulty encountered in food preparation, use of the bathroom, showering, and heating and cooling the house is important (Boxes 4-3 and 4-4).

The nurse must be cognizant of inherent obstacles and benefits of the health assessment, particularly the potential for developing a stereotyped view of the aged and perceiving the elderly as objects rather than persons. This is especially true

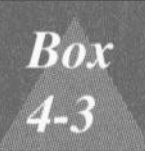

Indications for Home Visits

Lives alone (especially if recently bereaved)
Mental impairment
Major mobility problems
Several risk factors for dependency
History of falls or accidents
Recent hospital discharge (especially if recovery incomplete)
Imminent institutionalization

From Ham RJ: *Geriatrics: I. AAFP home study of self-assessment monograph 89,* Kansas City, MO, 1986, American Academy of Family Physicians.

Necessary Home Visit Information

1. Suitability and safety of home for client's functional level
2. Attitudes and presence of other persons at home
3. Proximity and helpfulness of neighbors and relatives
4. Emergency assistance arrangements
5. Nutritional and alcohol habits
6. Actual and required daily living skills
7. Hygiene habits
8. Safety and convenience modifications needed
9. Problems in getting to local community stores and services

From Ham RJ: *Geriatrics: I. AAFP home study of self-assessment monograph 89,* Kansas City, MO, 1986, American Academy of Family Physicians.

when assessment is viewed in terms of potentially meeting the nurse's need for data instead of meeting the needs of the aged person and as a task rather than the basis of care.

The comprehensive assessment is most successful when there is a team approach, generally, a physician, nurse, social worker, and pharmacist. Geriatric assessment programs attempt to target high-risk elders to combine their assessment with an individually tailored program of rehabilitation, education, counseling, and support services. The cost of these programs has been a deterrent and has limited their use; however, Boult (2000) outlines a less extensive assessment for office, clinic, and emergency room use (see Appendix 4-B).

ASSESSMENT TOOLS

An abundance of assessment tools exist that can broadly categorize motor capacity, manual ability, self-care ability, and more complex or instrumental abilities. Some community agencies and nursing care facilities routinely use health assessment tools designed to obtain specific information needed. Other institutions have developed or modified available tools because the available assessment tools are too complex or too time consuming to be of practical value. Regardless of the method used (established or self-developed), most health forms contain variants of the same basic information (see Appendix 4-B).

Physical Assessment

One assessment tool uses a survival-needs framework with an emphasis on function. The acronym FANCAPES represents fluids, aeration, nutrition, communication, activity, pain, elimination, and socialization and social skills. The information provided is helpful in the appraisal of the aged person's ability to meet his or her needs and the extent to which assistance is necessary. FANCAPES is applicable to all types of care environments in which the aged are found, may be used in part or total (depending on the need), and is easily adaptable to the functional pattern grouping of nursing diagnosis. Assessment data obtained from this method are based on the following considerations in each area.

Fluids. Evaluation of fluids includes assessment of the client's state of hydration and those physiologic, situational, and mental factors that contribute to the maintenance of adequate hydration: the ability of the client to obtain adequate fluids on his or her own, to express feelings of thirst, to effectively swallow, and to evaluate medications that affect intake and output.

Aeration. Aeration looks at the adequacy of oxygen exchange and includes observations of respiratory rate and depth at rest and during activity, talking, walking, and situations requiring added exertion; the presence or absence of edema in the extremities or abdomen; auscultation of breath sounds; and a medication review to evaluate the effects of medication on aeration.

Nutrition. Assessment of mechanical and psychologic factors in eating include the type and amount of food consumed; making sure the client can bite, chew, and swallow adequately; and proper fit and condition of dentures and that they are worn for meals. Alteration in diet because of culture, medical restrictions, available economic resources, and living conditions should be considered. Visual and neurologic impairment, which might interfere with the elder's ability to prepare a meal or feed himself or herself, should be noted.

Communication. The sending and receiving of verbal and nonverbal information in the external world and signals in the internal environment of the body require mechanical function of body parts and psychosocial responses from others in the environment. Assessment includes sight and sound acuity; voice quality; adequate function of the tongue, teeth, pharynx, and larynx; and appraisal of the client's ability to read, write, and understand the spoken language. Undetected disability in these skills can lead to erroneous conclusions.

Activity. Ability to perform activities of daily living should be assessed: the ability to feed, toilet, dress, and groom oneself; to prepare meals; to dial the telephone; and to move around with or without assistive devices. Coordination and balance, finger dexterity, grip strength, and other actions necessary to daily life and independence should also be assessed. Ambulation, a major component of activity, should be tested with the timed "get up and go," in which the elder rises from a chair, walks 9 feet, returns to the chair, and sits down; this test indicates the degree of mobility dysfunction (Podsiadlo and Richardson, 1991).

Pain. The presence of both physical and mental pain should be assessed. The presence or absence of pressure and discomfort, information about recent losses, or visible symptoms of anxiety may also help determine manifestations of pain. The manner by which pain or discomfort is customarily relieved provides further information.

Elimination. Bladder and bowel elimination should be investigated for mechanical factors: evidence of dribbling or incontinence, use of assistive devices or altered body structures resulting from surgical intervention, and medications that affect voiding and intestinal peristalsis.

Bowel function can be helped or hindered by what the client uses to purge himself or herself, by how concerned the client seems to be about bowel function, and by the amount of privacy needed for excretory functions. Colloquialisms used by the client must be recognized and used to accommodate obtaining reliable data.

Socialization and Social Skills. The individual's ability to negotiate in society, to give and receive love and friendship, and to feel self-worth are discussed in Chapter 18 (see the section on the Apgar score). Responses to such influences as hearing and visual losses and approved gestures of friendship are considered under this category. Attention should focus on the individual's ability to deal with loss and to interact with other people in give-and-take situations. Behavioral responses not previously observed may become evident by discussion of the client's feelings of self-worth.

Functional Assessment

The goal of *Healthy People 2000* (1991) was to increase the healthy life span of all Americans. Rather than delay mortality, focus was directed at the preservation of function and extending active life expectancy. Functional assessment speaks to the "quality of life" in ways medical diagnoses do not (Gallo et al, 1995).

Functional assessment is the evaluation of a person's ability to carry out basic tasks of self-care and tasks needed to support independent living. It is based on physical and psychosocial evaluation with the assumption that any clinical condition can be diagnosed and properly treated (Williams, 1995). Additional reasons why functional assessment is so important are that the objective data obtained in a functional assessment accomplish the following:

- Define elder's concerns
- May indicate a manifestation of disease
- Assist in determining a need for service(s)
- Assist in determining the type of placement
- Assist in determining cost/benefit of treatment/intervention
- Assist in realistic goal setting for those with chronic conditions
- Decrease fragmentation of care by reviewing goals according to functional status
- Assist in ethical/quality-of-life issues
- Help track untreated conditions (e.g., effects of arthritis)

As can be seen from the value of functional assessment, tools that assess ability in BADLs and IADLs should provide numerically qualified data regarding an individual's capacity to be or remain independent. The BADLs (eating, toileting, ambulation, bathing, dressing, and grooming) are tasks needed for self-care and are international and cross-cultural in nature. Three of these tasks (grooming, dressing, and bathing) require cognitive function. When the BADLs are vertically listed, it is not unusual for the individual who performs an activity to be able to do the activities above it but not below it. Change in or loss of ability occurs in the reverse order of acquisition. The IADLs are tasks needed for independent living (see Appendix 4-C). The progression of loss of IADLs begins with cognitive functions, especially finances and shopping. Cooking is least important to community-dwelling elders, even when adjusted for gender differences (Williams, 1995). When the IADLs are arranged in vertical order, performance by a person of one type of activity indicates that the person can probably do all the activities below it but not above it (Gallo et al, 1995).

Numerous tools are available that describe, screen, assess, monitor, and predict functional ability. Generally the assessment does not break down a task into its component parts, such as picking up a spoon or cup or swallowing water when assessment of eating is done; instead, eating is seen as a total task. Functional assessment also shows the result, not the cause, of an altered task. This is particularly true with persons who have varying degrees of dementia (Tappan, 1994). The Katz Index (Katz et al, 1963; see Appendix 4-C) provides a basic framework to evaluate a person's ability to live independently and serves as a focal point to provide remedies. Scoring of the Katz Index is based on a three-point scale and allows one to score client performance abilities as independent, assistive (or semidependent), or dependent.

The value of the Katz Index is that it can be administered by anyone, with minimum training, and it can provide data that identify the abilities of an aged person and the kind of services that might be needed. The physical self-maintenance scale (PSMS) developed by the Philadelphia Geriatric Institute includes the six functional areas of BADLs and can also be administered by any health care person without prior training.

Another tool used to assess self-care of the elderly is the Barthel Index (1981). This instrument was devised to evaluate the amount of physical assistance required when a person can no longer carry out BADLs. Because it is so detailed, a modified Barthel Index was developed that has proved useful in any setting. It is particularly useful in the home care setting. The index is divided into two categories: independent and dependent. Under each of these headings activities are rated as independent (intact and limited ability) or dependent (requiring a helper or unable to do an activity or activities at all) (see Appendix 4-C).

The Barthel Index provides data to determine the type of support that is needed in BADLs and can serve in rehabilitation settings as a method to document patient improvement. The IADLs are considered to be more complex activities: abilities such as traveling, shopping, preparing meals, doing housework, dialing a telephone, and handling money. Although some of these tasks may seem more specific to one gender or the other, these activities are required of most individuals in modern society today (see Appendix 4-C).

Functional performance tests for balance, walking ability, and upper and lower extremity strength are also important . These can provide valuable information on mobility issues, as well as independence and risk of falls (see Appendix 4-C).

Mental Assessment

Many times questionnaires that evaluate mental capacity are combined with BADL and IADL instruments. One such tool is the Functional Dementia Scale (Moore et al, 1993), which can be administered in written or oral form. This brief assessment tool provides quantification of the presence of dementia and changes in the review of physiologic systems. Whether this tool provides data, over time, of diminished capacity is not evident (Gallo et al, 1995).

The Folstein Mini Mental State Examination (MMSE) is a short, convenient mental function test composed of two parts: One part requires verbal response and assesses orientation, memory, and attention, and the other component requires the ability to write a sentence, draw a complex design, respond to written and oral commands, and name objects. As with other assessment tools, there is a rating scale to quantify ability or disability. Further discussion appears in Chapter 21.

The Short Portable Mental Status Questionnaire (SPMSQ) (Pfeiffer, 1979) is a frequently used mental status examination. Its effectiveness as a method for clarifying cognitive function is still undetermined. The 10 questions are asked to assess the person's orientation, remote memory, and calculation ability; however, there is no question to evaluate short-term memory. Its value as an assessment tool is the ease of administration and the fact that it requires no equipment (Gallo et al, 1995).

The clock-drawing task, which has been used since 1992 (Mendez et al, 1992; Tuokko, 1992), is a screening tool that differentiates normal cognition from cognitive impairment. It is particularly sensitive for constructional apraxia but also can reflect general deficits in conception of time (Mendez et al, 1992; Tuokko, 1992; Nolan and Mohs, 1994). The results correlate with MMSE findings. Less threatening than the MMSE, the clock-drawing task can be administered as sort of a game. The clock-drawing task requires manual dexterity, and individuals with severe arthritis, parkinsonism, or stroke affecting the dominant hand are at a disadvantage using this test. If the test indicates a possible impairment, further evaluation is warranted and the MMSE should be considered.

Integrated Assessments

The Multidimensional Functional Assessment of the Older American's Resources and Services (OARS) organization is a lengthy and comprehensive tool designed to evaluate ability, disability, and the capacity level at which the aged person is able to function. Five dimensions are considered for assessment: social resources, economic resources, physical health, mental health, and activities of daily living. Each component uses a quantitative rating scale: 1—excellent, 2—good, 3—mildly impaired, 4—moderately impaired, 5—severely impaired, and 6—completely impaired. At the conclusion of the assessment a cumulative impairment score (CIS) is established, which can range from the most fit (5) to total disability (30). This aids in establishing the degree of need. Information considered in each domain includes the following.

Social Resources. This part of the OARS evaluates the social skills, availability of assistance, and the degree of ability to negotiate and make friends (the number of times friends are seen, the number of telephone conversations). Is the person able to ask for things from friends, family, and strangers? Is a caregiver around if needed (if yes, who and how long available)? Is there a social network or group?

Economic Resources. Data about monthly and other sources of income (Social Security, Supplemental Security Income, pensions, and income generated from capital) to determine the adequacy of income compared with the cost of living and food, shelter, clothing, medications, and small luxury items provide insight into the client's relative standard of living and point out areas of need that might be alleviated by use of additional resources unknown to the aged person.

Mental Health. Consideration is given to intellectual function, the presence or absence of psychiatric symptoms, and the amount of enjoyment and interaction the aged person gets from life.

Physical Health. Diagnosis of major and common diseases of older persons, the type of prescribed and over-the-counter medications the person is taking, and the elder's perception of his or her health status are the basis of evaluation.

Activities of Daily Living. Assessment of activities of daily living involves assessment of BADLs and IADLs. The OARS assessment tool is designed so that each component can be used individually. This enables it to be added to or integrated into self-designed tools. Other comprehensive assessment instruments include the Patient Appraisal and Care Evaluation (PACE) and the Comprehensive Assessment and Referral Evaluation (CARE). Both of these methods of appraisal are lengthy.

Recording of Data

Problem-oriented medical recording (POMR) was designed primarily by a physician for use by physicians, but it has been adapted to the needs of nurses who care for geriatric clients. The database can be broadened to encompass a multidimensional assessment of a client. The components of the problem-oriented system are database, problem list, initial plan, and progress notes, which assume the SOAP format (subjective data, objective data, assessment or nursing diagnosis, and plan).

The database is usually derived from patient complaints. To obtain an initial database from well elders, however, the nurse should consider obtaining information from the physical, psychologic, social, and economic realms. A database can be obtained through various assessment tools presented in this chapter or from those designed by the agency with which the nurse is affiliated. When no tool is available, the nurse will need to create one geared to assessment of functional ability or disability in the physical, mental, social, economic, and daily activity spheres of the aged person's life.

Once data are collected, a problem list (including potential problems) can be generated that reflects more than the physical arena and will serve as a reference in future encounters with the elder. The initial plan includes diagnosis (if appropriate), treatment (if appropriate), education, and follow-up, as well as progress notes that emanate from the problem list.

The assessment formats in this chapter attempt to provide direction in the development of one's own assessment tool or modification of existing tools that may not fully evaluate the needs of the aged client being assessed. Feeling comfortable with an assessment method requires practice using the tool

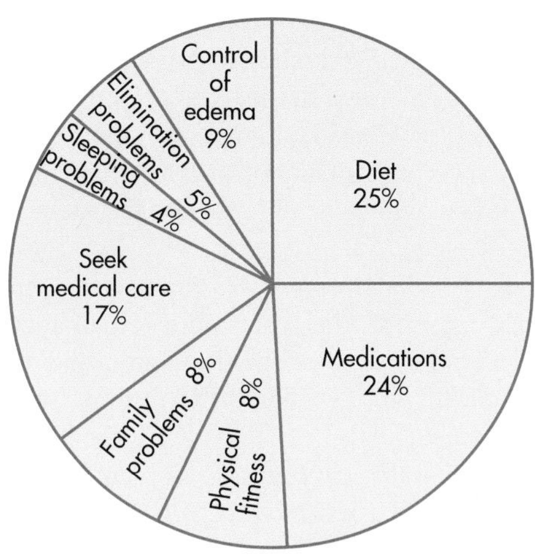

Figure 4-2. Frequency of health counseling topics. (From Furukawa C: In Wells T, editor: *Aging and health promotion*, Rockville, MD, 1982, Aspen.)

and refining it so that it will be appropriate to the aged person and the particular setting of the nurse.

Findings and conclusions from the assessment should be discussed with the aged client so that responsibility for the health program can be appropriately delegated. This connotes that the client is an active participant in health care and is encouraged to apply wellness concepts presented in Chapter 3. Given sufficient information, the aged client should be capable of making decisions about his or her health status and needed resources. One must keep in mind that the goal is preventive health care that is aimed at maintenance of the present health status and maximizing function.

Furukawa (1982) found certain recurrent topics requested by the elderly in health counseling sessions that remain appropriate today (Figure 4-2). If assessment findings indicate that the client is able to monitor his or her own physical health condition, the client should be taught to do so. Taking one's own blood pressure, cooperation with medications, and conscientious adherence to an exercise program or a nutritional regimen are all examples of self-responsibility and the beginning of wellness, rather than disease, orientation.

Health assessment is appraisal of health status in an attempt to identify latent and obscure conditions, to serve as a screening process, as a follow-up on health care plans, and as the initial establishment of a health baseline. The aim is to help the aged person remain independent and functional at his or her highest level of wellness regardless of place of residence: in acute or long-term institutional settings or in one's own home.

NURSING DIAGNOSIS AND THE AGED

The North American Nursing Diagnosis Association (NANDA) has developed a system of nursing diagnoses by which nurses can formulate a nursing care plan and initiate interventions based on client assessment. Gordon (1987) organized the NANDA diagnostic categories into 11 functional health patterns that are easily learned, can be used as a basis of a holistic assessment, and lead to the identification of possible nursing diagnoses.

Maslow's hierarchy of needs and Gordon's functional health patterns are complementary when used with the elderly who have health problems. The Gordon format provides the nurse with the nursing diagnosis, and Maslow's hierarchy provides a means by which the diagnoses can be prioritized (Figure 4-3).

Many older adults have at least one chronic condition that is amenable to NANDA diagnoses. These diagnoses are oriented to dysfunction rather than to both functional and dysfunctional health. Although the elderly will usually have some degree of dysfunction, the NANDA guidelines create the mind-set that the aged are always dysfunctional and do not recognize that the aged can be highly functional but still need to be monitored to prevent illness and disease, maintain their present state of wellness, and improve on an existing state of wellness.

Nursing diagnoses for older adults should include wellness, to reflect individual responses that are actually or potentially unhealthy. Interventions must reinforce those that are healthy. A pioneer group of nurses has tenaciously advocated for nursing wellness diagnoses because they describe human responses to levels of wellness in an individual that have the potential for enhancement to a higher state of wellness despite the presence or absence of a chronic condition or an acute illness. Stolte (1994) believes that well nursing diagnoses should focus on wellness patterns, client responses, and strengths that can be accomplished by focusing on progressive attainment of health behaviors or developmental tasks. Houldin and co-workers (1987) produced a manual of wellness diagnoses using functional health patterns.

Stolte (1996) offers a strong argument for the inclusion of wellness nursing diagnoses in all types of health settings. These settings apply not only to elders but to all ages. By using wellness nursing diagnoses in addition to NANDA diagnoses, the approach becomes holistic, not dysfunction oriented, and provides the opportunity to draw on strengths and coping abilities inherent in the individual.

Some individuals may argue that these wellness diagnoses are more prescriptive than behavioral, but wellness focuses on prevention, maintenance, and improvement of behavior or physical status from a state of wellness or health. The task of nurses then is to consider wellness diagnoses along with the established dysfunctional diagnoses to generate categories that apply to the practice of gerontic nursing. This is not to imply that gerontic nursing is elitist and must have separate categories, but it is intended to point out that the aged cannot be measured by the norms of health that are attributed to those who are young and middle aged. Pathologic states in

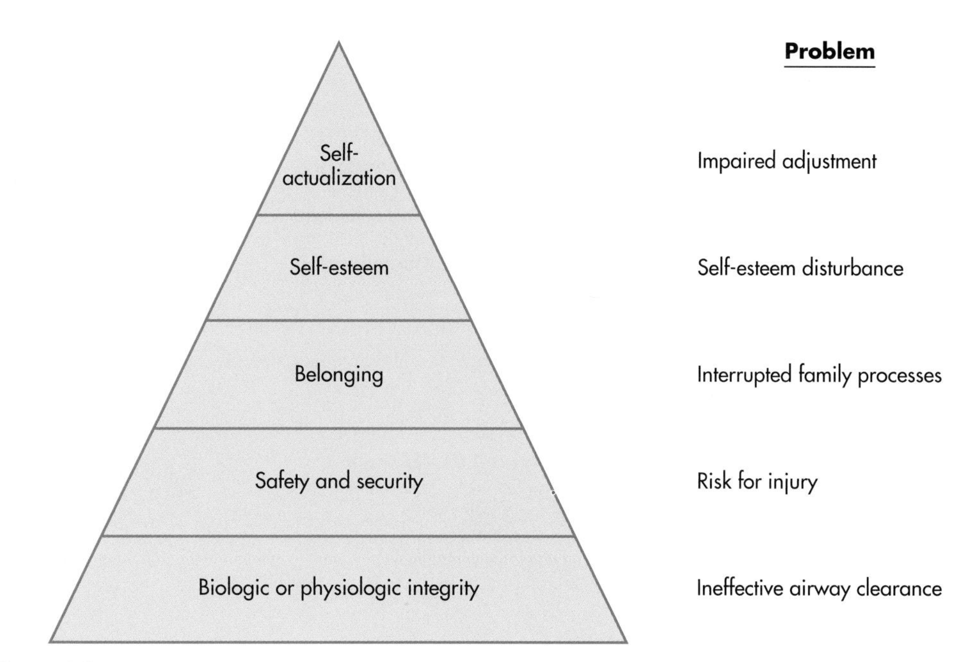

Figure 4-3. Correlation between Maslow's hierarchy and Gordon's functional pattern of nursing diagnosis.

these age-groups are not always pathologic states for the elderly.

When it is considered that a person does not have a "problem," a health-oriented focus could provide encouragement to successfully move through the normal developmental and maturational tasks.

The formulation of wellness nursing diagnoses should reflect positive behaviors (based on the client's strengths), using such action responses as adapting to, reestablishing, adjustment to, assumes responsibility for, participation in, developing a pattern, involvement in, increasing recognition of, improving, and maintaining, which indicate progression and allow the nurse to use interventions that reinforce client response and achieve goals. Goals should facilitate task achievement, provide information, teach or reinforce new skills, foster role attainment, or enhance strengths. Appropriate qualifiers for goals include terms such as attainment, continued, increased, sustained, completion, and acceptance, to mention a few.

For example, an aged individual may be at the optimum level of mobility and activity based on normal cardiac output and respiratory exchange for the person's physiologic age. The wellness diagnosis might be adapting to the present mobility level (if optimal level is now different than before) with the goal of sustaining the present level of mobility and activity. Nursing interventions then are aimed at accomplishing this goal. If the person's responses/strengths are not used to help meet the goal, it is likely that an alteration in mobility and activity may become a diagnosis of dysfunction.

Human Needs and Wellness Diagnoses for Assessment

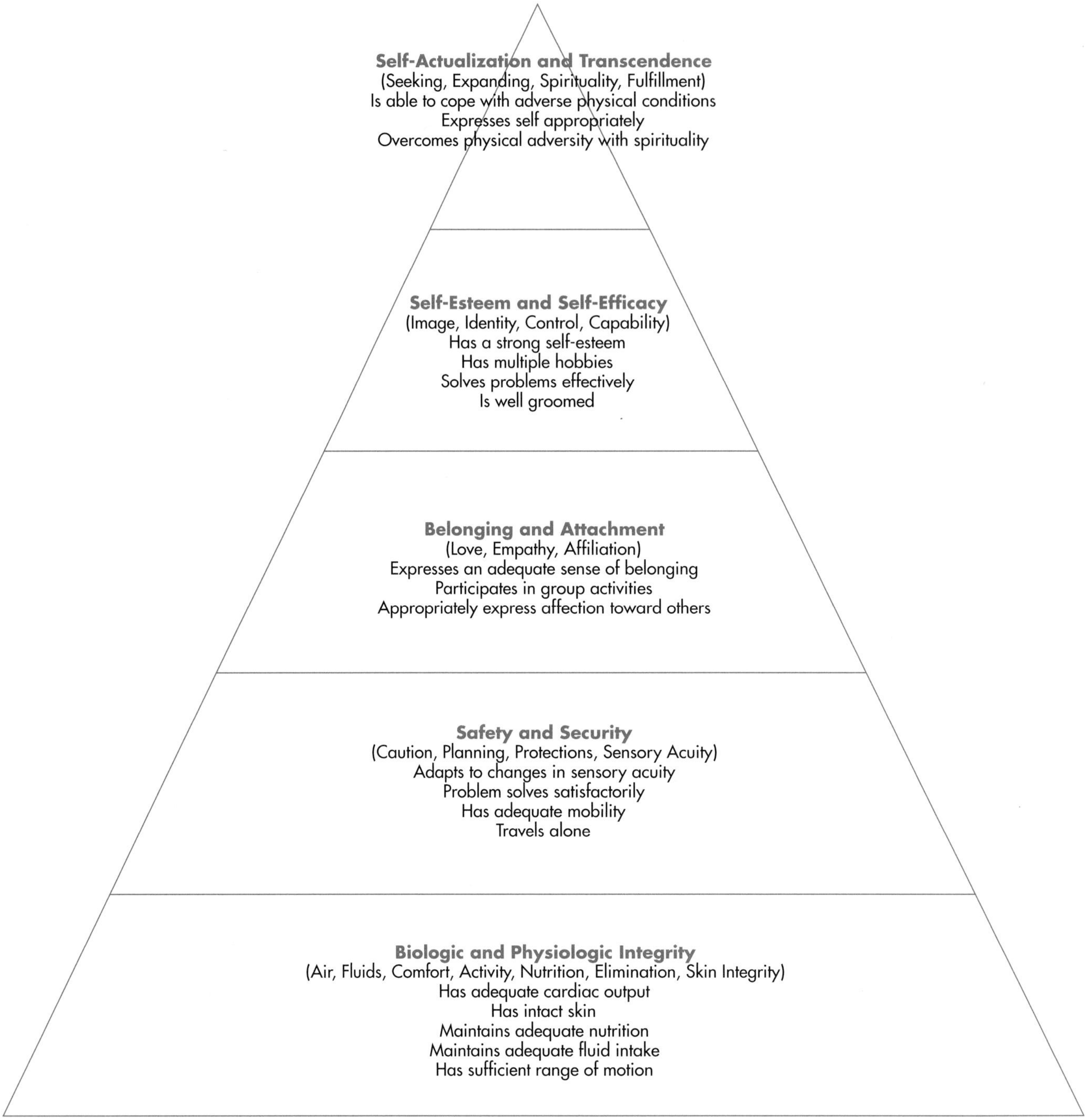

Self-Actualization and Transcendence
(Seeking, Expanding, Spirituality, Fulfillment)
Is able to cope with adverse physical conditions
Expresses self appropriately
Overcomes physical adversity with spirituality

Self-Esteem and Self-Efficacy
(Image, Identity, Control, Capability)
Has a strong self-esteem
Has multiple hobbies
Solves problems effectively
Is well groomed

Belonging and Attachment
(Love, Empathy, Affiliation)
Expresses an adequate sense of belonging
Participates in group activities
Appropriately express affection toward others

Safety and Security
(Caution, Planning, Protections, Sensory Acuity)
Adapts to changes in sensory acuity
Problem solves satisfactorily
Has adequate mobility
Travels alone

Biologic and Physiologic Integrity
(Air, Fluids, Comfort, Activity, Nutrition, Elimination, Skin Integrity)
Has adequate cardiac output
Has intact skin
Maintains adequate nutrition
Maintains adequate fluid intake
Has sufficient range of motion

These are not all the possible wellness diagnoses that may be identified. The above are examples of nursing diagnoses that should be considered when planning care for the older adult.

KEY CONCEPTS

- Age-related changes are the observable, measurable, or felt changes that occur in one's being over time and are chiefly focused on physiologic and biologic changes.
- Physiologic aging is universal, progressive, decremental, intrinsic, and unavoidable.
- There are enormous individual variations in the rate of aging of body systems and functions.
- Individuals normally and gradually lose bone mass, structural integrity of organs, and specificity of bodily processes in the course of aging.
- Physical appearance inevitably changes with a downward shift of skin and tissue integrity brought about by the pressure of gravity over time.
- Lubrication of joints, elasticity, enzymatic processes, and cellular fluids diminish during aging.
- The changes in the cardiovascular system are most likely to progress toward a disease state in late life.
- Hormonal and endocrine changes are significant in the aging process.
- Nervous system acuity and sensory acuity are diminished in aging, and these losses are often compensated for with the use of accoutrements or aids.
- Careful assessment of individual aging changes, lifestyle, and desires is fundamental to good nursing care of the old.

▲ CASE STUDY

Fred was 74 years old and had an active and vital life. He was involved in leather tooling and restoration of classic automobiles. He had developed a cadre of acquaintances, worldwide, of similar interests. His retirement from a lifelong U.S. Air Force commitment was painful, but he had his hobbies and his friends to sustain him. He would chuckle a little when he often said, "Those years in the war were the best years of my life . . . everything since then has been pale by comparison."

Fred is similar to many of the men who were born in the years between 1920 and 1930. When they arrived at their near majority, there were the "war years"; the male youth of the nation took arms. The females, so often left behind, waited and watched for the return of the heroes. The artificial nature of life at that juncture has resulted in a range of problems that are unique to that generation. Separating the age-related problems from the generational and environmental ones can be difficult.

The first difficult problem of growing older that Fred noticed was the diminishment of hearing, especially in situations that were loud and with multiple sources of noise. His nurse friend told him that it was likely related to his years in the war when the unnatural noises of shelling had affected his hearing. Then he gradually became aware that his eyesight was impaired so that he could focus only on distant objects but near objects were fuzzy. But the biggest problem he experienced was in his inability to write notes to his acquaintances with the same fluidity he had previously experienced. Sometimes the words were lurking on the tip of his tongue but simply would not come. Another thing that troubled him was the decreasing strength of his grip. Recently it had become more difficult to repair automobiles because of this decreasing strength. He did not know whether these were normal age-related changes that he must adjust to or whether they were indications of serious pathologic problems that required active medical intervention.

Based on the case study, develop a nursing care plan using the following procedure:

List comments of client that provide subjective data.

List information that provides objective data.

From these data identify and state, using accepted format, two nursing diagnoses you determine are most significant to this client at this time. List two client strengths that you have identified from data.

Determine and state outcome criteria for each diagnosis. These must reflect some alleviation of the problem identified in the nursing diagnosis and must be stated in concrete and measurable terms.

Plan and state one or more interventions for each diagnosed problem. Provide specific documentation of source used to determine appropriate intervention. Plan at least one intervention that incorporates the client's existing strengths.

Evaluate success of intervention. Interventions must correlate directly with the stated outcome criteria in order to measure the outcome success.

STUDY QUESTIONS

Which of the changes Fred experienced are the normal consequences of aging?

Which of Fred's disabilities do you think has created the most distress in his life?

What problem would you address first if Fred asked for your assistance?

What wellness nursing diagnosis (or diagnoses) could you develop for Fred?

How would you assist Fred to adapt to the changes of aging that he cannot avoid?

What resources would you suggest to Fred to enhance his coping?

Discuss the aging changes you would find most difficult to accept.

RESEARCH QUESTIONS

It is most difficult for elders to cope with which age changes?

Which are the inevitable sensory changes of aging?

Where do individuals seek knowledge of the aging process?

Is chronologic age more significant than physiologic age in determining functional efficacy?

When does one become aware of changes in function that are related to aging? Which change is likely to appear first? How much influence does environment have on reduced hearing capacity?

How do age-related changes differ in males and females?

REFERENCES

Altman DF: Changes in gastrointestinal, pancreatic, biliary, and hepatic function with aging, *Gastroenterol Clin North Am* 19(2):227, 1990.

Anderson W: Aging and the lung. In Beers MH, Berkow R, editors: *The Merck manual of geriatrics*, ed 3, Whitehouse Station, NJ, 2000, Merck Research Laboratories.

Anderson WF: *Practical management of the elderly*, ed 3, Oxford, 1976, Blackwell Scientific Publications.

Baltimore Longitudinal Study of Aging, National Institutes of Health no 84-2450, Washington, DC, 1984, US Government Printing Office.

Banaski JL: Cardiac function. In Copstead LEC, editor: *Perspectives on pathophysiology*, Philadelphia, 1995, WB Saunders.

Barthel Index, *Med Care* 19:491, 1981.

Bartz B: Mechanisms of endocrine control and metabolism. In Copstead LEC, editor: *Perspectives on pathophysiology*, Philadelphia, 1995, WB Saunders.

Beare P, Meyers J: *Principles and practices of adult health nursing*, ed 2, St Louis, 1994, Mosby.

Benner P: *From novice to expert*, Menlo Park, CA, 1984, Addison-Wesley.

Boult C: Comprehensive geriatric assessment. In Beers MH, Berkow R, editors: *The Merck manual of geriatrics*, ed 3, Whitehouse Station, NJ, 2000, Merck Research Laboratories.

Campbell EJ, Lefrak SS: How aging affects the structure and function of the respiratory system, *Geriatrics* 33:68, 1978.

Cassmeyer VL, Blevin DB: The patient with biliary and pancreatic problems. In Long BC, Phillips WJ, Cassmeyer VL, editors: *Medical-surgical nursing: a nursing process approach*, ed 3, St Louis, 1993, Mosby.

Chiu N: Aging and the skin. In Beers MH, Berkow R, editors: *The Merck manual of geriatrics*, ed 3, Whitehouse Station, NJ, 2000, Merck Research Laboratories.

Coni N, Davison W, Webster S: *Aging: the facts*, New York, 1984, Oxford University Press.

Cooper LT, Cooke JP, Dzau VJ: The vasculopathy of aging, *J Gerontol Biol Sci* 49(5):B191, 1994.

Cornell RC: Aging and the skin: what is normal aging, *Geriatr Med Today* 5(pt 20):24, 1986.

Costa PT, Andres R: Patterns of age changes. In Rossman I, editor: *Clinical geriatrics*, ed 3, Philadelphia, 1986, JB Lippincott.

Cunningham WR, Brookbank JW: *Gerontology: the psychology, biology, and sociology of aging*, New York, 1988, Harper & Row.

Diettert G: Circulation time in the aged, *JAMA* 183:1037, 1963.

Eliopoulos C: *Gerontological nursing*, ed 4, Philadelphia, 1997, Lippincott.

Frohlich EV: Hypertension. In Abrams WB, Beers MH, Berkow R, editors: *The Merck manual of geriatrics*, ed 2, Whitehouse Station, NJ, 1995, Merck Research Laboratories.

Fujino M, Okada R, Arakawa K: The relationship of aging to histologic changes in the conduction system of the normal heart, *Jpn Heart J* 24:13, 1982.

Furukawa C: Adult health conference: community-oriented health maintenance for the elderly. In Wells T, editor: *Aging and health promotion*, Rockville, MD, 1982, Aspen Systems Corp.

Gallo JJ, Reichel W, Andersen L: *Handbook of geriatric assessment*, ed 2, Rockville, MD, 1995, Aspen Publishers.

Gardin JM et al: Echocardiographic measurements in normal subjects: evaluation of an adult population without apparent heart disease, *J Clin Ultrasound* 7:85, 1979.

Gardner AW, Poehlman ET: Predictors of the age-related increase in blood pressure in men and women, *J Gerontol Med Sci* 50A(1):M1, 1995.

Gawlinski A, Jensen GA: The complications of cardiovascular aging, *Am J Nurs* 9:221, 1991.

Gerstenblith G et al: Echocardiographic assessment of a normal adult population, *Circulation* 56(2):273, 1977.

Gilchrest B: Aging and the skin. In Beers MH, Berkow R, editors: *The Merck manual of geriatrics*, ed 3, Whitehouse Station, NJ, 2000, Merck Research Laboratories.

Goldman R: Decline in organic function with age. In Rossman I, editor: *Clinical geriatrics*, ed 2, Philadelphia, 1979, JB Lippincott.

Gordon M: *Manual of nursing diagnosis 1986-1987*, New York, 1987, McGraw-Hill.

Grove GL, Kingman AM: Age associated changes in human epidermal cell renewal, *J Gerontol* 38:137, 1983.

Gugoz Y, Munro HN: Nutrition and aging. In Finch CE, Schneider EL, editors: *Handbook of the biology of aging*, ed 2, New York, 1985, Van Nostrand Reinhold.

Gulya AJ: Ear disorders. In Abrams WB, Beers MH, Berkow R, editors: *The Merck manual of geriatrics*, ed 2, Whitehouse Station, NJ, 1995, Merck Research Laboratories.

Ham RJ: Assessment. In Ham RJ, Sloane PD: *Primary care geriatrics: a case-based approach*, ed 3, St Louis, 1997, Mosby.

Harvard Medical School Health Letter, Department of Continuing Education, Harvard Medical School 9:5, 1983.

Healthy People 2000, Washington, DC, 1991, US Department of Health and Human Services, Public Health Service, US Government Printing Office.

Hirsh B: Normal changes in host defenses. In Abrams WB, Beers MH, Berkow R, editors: *The Merck manual of geriatrics*, ed 2, Whitehouse Station, NJ, 1995, Merck Research Laboratories.

Hogstel MO: Vital signs are really vital in the old-old, *Geriatr Nurs* 15(5):253, 1994.

Horowitz M: Aging and the gastrointestinal tract. In Beers MH, Berkow R, editors: *Merck manual of geriatrics*, ed 2, Whitehouse Station, NJ, 2000, Merck Research Laboratories.

Houldin AD, Saltstein SW, Ganley KM: *Nursing diagnoses for wellness*, Philadelphia, 1987, Lippincott.

Jacobs R: Physical changes in the aged. In Deveraux MO et al, editors: *Elder care: a guide to clinical geriatrics*, New York, 1981, Grune & Stratton.

Jarvis C: *Physical examination and health assessment*, ed 2, Philadelphia, 1996, WB Saunders.

Johns Hopkins Medical Letter, Health After 50: The next five years: our experts look ahead, 6(1):1, 1994.

Johns Hopkins Medical Letter, Health After 50: Important new advice for treating hypertension, 8(2):7, 1996.

Joynt JR: Aging and the nervous system. In Beers MH, Berkow R, editors: *The Merck manual of geriatrics*, ed 3, Whitehouse Station, NJ, 2000, Merck Research Laboratories.

Katz S et al: Studies of illness in the aged: the index of ADL, *JAMA* 185:914, 1963.

Kee JL, Paulanka BJ: Fluids and their influence on the body. In Kee JL, Paulanka BJ: *Handbook of fluids, electrolytes and acid-base imbalances*, Albany, NY, 2000, Delmar.

Kenney RA: *Physiology of aging: a synopsis*, Chicago, 1982, Mosby.

Krumpe P et al: The aging respiratory system, *Clin Geriatr Med* 1:143, 1985.

Kupfer C: Ophthalmologic disorders. In Abrams WB, Beers MH, Berkow R, editors: *The Merck manual of geriatrics*, ed 2, Whitehouse Station, NJ, 1995, Merck Research Laboratories.

Lakatta E: Cardiovascular regulatory mechanisms in advanced age, *Physiol Rev* 73(2):413, 1993.

Lakatta EG: Normal age changes. In Abrams WB, Beers MH, Berkow R, editors: *The Merck manual of geriatrics*, ed 2, Whitehouse Station, NJ, 1995, Merck Research Laboratories.

Lakatta EG: Aging in the cardiovascular system. In Beers MH, Berkow R, editors: *The Merck manual of geriatrics*, ed 3, Whitehouse Station, NJ, 2000, Merck Research Laboratories.

Lamb KV: Musculoskeletal function. In Leuckenotte AG, editor: *Gerontologic nursing*, St Louis, 1996, Mosby.

Leyden JJ, Grove GL, Ginley JK: Age-related differences in the rate of desquamation of skin surface in the aging process. In Adelman R, Roberts J, Christofalo VJ, editors: *Pharmacological interventions in the aging process*, New York, 1978, Plenum Press.

Lindemann RD: Aging and the kidney. In Beers MH, Berkow R, editors: *The Merck manual of geriatrics*, ed 3, Whitehouse Station, NJ, 2000, Merck Research Laboratories.

Lindsay R: The aging skeleton. In Haug M, Ford A, Sheafor D, editors: *Physical and mental health of aged women*, New York, 1985, Springer.

Malasanos L, Barkauskaus V, Stoltenberg-Allen K: *Health assessment*, ed 4, St Louis, 1989, Mosby.

Manolagas S: Aging musculoskeletal system. In Beers MH, Berkow R, editors: *The Merck manual of geriatrics*, ed 3, Whitehouse Station, NJ, 2000, Merck Research Laboratories.

Meisami E: Aging of the sensory system. In Timiras PS, editor: *Physiological basis of aging and geriatrics*, ed 2, Boca Raton, FL, 1995, CRC Press.

Meisami E, Brown CM, Emerle HF: Sensory systems: normal aging, disorders, and treatments of vision and hearing in humans. In Timoras PS, editor: *Physiological basis of aging and geriatrics*, ed 3, Boca Raton, FL, 2003, CRC Press.

Mendez MF, Ala T, Underwood KL: Development of scoring criteria for the clock drawing task in Alzheimer's disease, *J Am Geriatr Soc* 40:1095, 1992.

Michel J: Aging and the immune system. In Beers MH, Berkow R, editors: *The Merck manual of geriatrics*, ed 3, Whitehouse Station, NJ, 2000, Merck Research Laboratories.

Miller RA: Aging and the immune response. In Schneider EL, Rowe JW, editors: *Handbook of biology of aging*, ed 3, San Diego, 1990, Academic Press.

Moore J et al: A functional dementia scale for assessment, *J Fam Pract* 16:499, 1993.

Morgan S: Effects of age on cardiovascular functioning, *Geriatr Nurs* 14(5):249, 1993.

Nolan KA, Mohs RC: Screening for dementia in family practice. In Richter RW, Blass JP, editors: *Alzheimer's practical management part II*, St Louis, 1994, Mosby.

Nursing diagnoses: definitions and classifications 1995-1996, Philadelphia, 1994, North American Nursing Diagnosis Association.

Pfeiffer E: Physical and mental assessment—OARS. Workshop Intensive, Western Gerontological Society, San Francisco, April 28, 1979.

Pierson DJ: Effects of aging on the respiratory system. In Pierson DJ, Kacmarek RM, editors: *Foundations of respiratory care*, New York, 1992, Churchill Livingstone.

Podsiadlo D, Richardson S: Timed "up and go": a test of basic functional mobility for frail elder persons, *J Am Geriatr Soc* 39:142, 1991.

Pope E: News and trends: 51 top scientists blast anti-aging idea, *AARP Bull* 43(6):3, 2002.

Proust J: Aging and the immune system. In Beers MH and Berkow R, editors: *Merck manual of geriatrics*, ed 3, Whitehouse Station, NJ, 2000, Merck Research Laboratories.

Richard C: Renal function. In Copstead LEC, editor: *Perspectives on pathophysiology*, Philadelphia, 1995, WB Saunders.

Richey MI, Richey HK, Fenske NA: Age-related skin changes: development and clinical meaning, *Geriatrics* 43:49, 1988.

Rossman I, editor: *Clinical geriatrics*, ed 3, Philadelphia, 1986, Lippincott.

Rowe JW: Aging process: renal changes and disorders. In Abrams WB, Beers MH, Berkow R, editors: *The Merck manual of geriatrics*, ed 2, Whitehouse Station, NJ, 1995, Merck Research Laboratories.

Schumann L: Alterations in respiratory function. In Copstead LEC, editor: *Perspectives on pathophysiology*, Philadelphia, 1995, WB Saunders.

Schuster MM: Effects of aging on the GI system. In Abrams WB, Beers MH, Berkow R, editors: *The Merck manual of geriatrics*, ed 2, Whitehouse Station, NJ, 1995, Merck Research Laboratories.

Sheahan SL, Musialowski R: Clinical implications of respiratory system changes in aging, *J Gerontol Nurs* 27(5):26, 2001.

Sloane PD: Normal aging. In Ham RJ, Sloane PD, editors: *Primary care geriatrics: a case-based approach*, ed 3, St Louis, 1992, Mosby.

Solomon DH: Age-related endocrine and metabolic changes: normal and diseased thyroid gland. In Abrams WB, Beers MH, Berkow R, editors: *The Merck manual of geriatrics*, ed 2, Whitehouse Station, NJ, 1995, Merck Research Laboratories.

Special report on aging, NIH pub no 81-2328, Washington, DC, 1981, US Department of Health and Human Services, Public Health Service, National Institute on Aging.

Special report: a review of the sixth report of the Joint National Committee on Prevention, Detection, Evaluation, and Treatment of High Blood Pressure, Washington, DC, 1998, American Pharmaceutical Association.

Stengel GB: Oral temperature in the elderly, *Gerontologist* 23:306, 1983 (special issue).

Stolte KM: Health-oriented nursing diagnoses: development and use. In Carroll-Johnson RM, Paquette M, editors: *Classification of nursing diagnoses: proceedings of the 10th conference North American Nursing Diagnosis Association*, Philadelphia, 1994, Lippincott.

Stolte KM: *Wellness nursing diagnosis for health promotion*, Philadelphia, 1996, Lippincott.

Tappan RM: Development of the refined ADL assessment scale for patients with Alzheimer's and related disorders, *J Gerontol Nurs* 20(6):36, 1994.

Tichy AN, Malasanos LJ: Physiologic parameters of aging, *J Gerontol Nurs* 5:42, Jan/Feb 1979; 5:38, April/May 1979.

Timiras PS: *Physiological basis of aging and geriatrics*, ed 2, Boca Raton, FL, 1994, CRC Press.

Timiras PS: The nervous system: structured and biochemical changes. In Timiras PS, editor: *Physiological basis of aging and geriatrics*, ed 3, Boca Raton, FL, 2003a, CRC Press.

Timiras PS: The thyroid, parathyroid and pineal glands. In Timiras PS, editor: *Physiological basis of aging and geriatrics*, ed 3, Boca Raton, FL, 2003b, CRC Press.

Timiras PS, Leary J: Kidney, lower urinary tract body fluids and the prostate. In Timiras PS, editor: *Physiological basis of aging and geriatrics*, ed 3, Boca Raton, FL, 2003.

Tockman MS: The effects of aging on the lungs: lung cancer. In Abrams WB, Beers MH, Berkow R, editors: *The Merck manual of geriatrics*, ed 2, Whitehouse Station, NJ, 1995, Merck Research Laboratories.

Tockman MS: Aging and the lung. In Beers MH, Berkow R, editors: *The Merck manual of geriatrics*, ed 3, Whitehouse Station, NJ, 2000, Merck Research Laboratories.

Tompkins RG: Surgery: preoperative evaluation and interoperative and postoperative care: surgery of the gastrointestinal tract. In Abrams WB, Beers MH, Berkow R, editors: *The Merck manual of geriatrics*, ed 2, Whitehouse Station, NJ, 1995, Merck Research Laboratories.

Tumosa N: Aging and the eye. In Beers MH, Berkow R, editors: *The Merck manual of geriatrics*, ed 3, Whitehouse Station, NJ, 2000, Merck Research Laboratories.

Tuokko H: The clock test: a sensitive measure to differentiate normal elderly from those with Alzheimer's disease, *J Am Geriatr Soc* 40:579, 1992.

Wardell S: *Acute intervention: nursing process throughout the life span*, Reston, VA, 1979, Reston.

Weber F, Barnard RJ, Ray D: Effects of a high–complex carbohydrate low-fat diet and daily exercise on individuals 70 years of age and older, *J Gerontol* 38:155, 1983.

Wei JY: Cardiovascular system. In Rowe JW, Besdine RW, editors: *Geriatric medicine*, Boston, 1988, Little, Brown.

Welch CE: Surgery: preoperative evaluation and intraoperative and postoperative care: surgery of the gastrointestinal tract. In Abrams WB, Beers MH, Berkow R, editors: *The Merck manual of geriatrics*, ed 2, Whitehouse Station, NJ, 1995, Merck Research Laboratories.

Williams M: Functional assessment, gerontological nursing. Contemporary Forums, San Francisco, May 7-13, 1995.

Williams TF: History and physical examination. In Beers MH, Berkow R, editors: *The Merck manual of geriatrics*, ed 3, Whitehouse Station, NJ, 2000, Merck Research Laboratories.

Wilson WR: Nose and throat disorders. In Abrams WB, Beers MH, Berkow R, editors: *The Merck manual of geriatrics*, ed 2, Whitehouse Station, NJ, 1995, Merck Research Laboratories.

Yehuda AB: Normal change in host defense. In Abrams WB, Beers MH, Berkow R, editors: *The Merck manual of geriatrics*, ed 2, Whitehouse Station, NJ, 1995, Merck Research Laboratories.

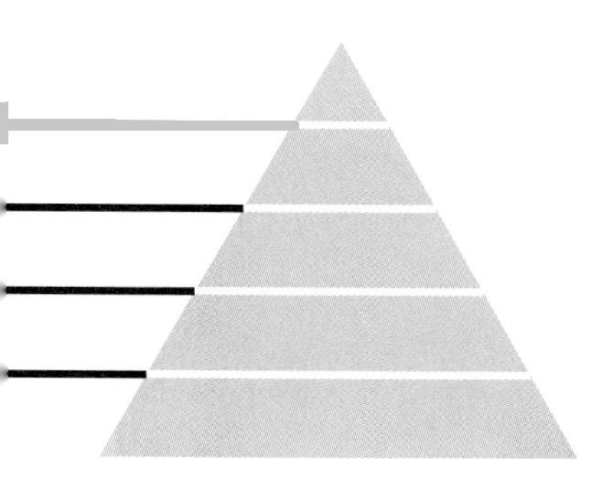

APPENDIX 4-A

Normal Physical Assessment Findings in the Elderly

CARDIOVASCULAR CHANGES

Cardiac output	Heart loses elasticity; therefore decreased heart contractility in response to increased demands
Arterial circulation	Decreased vessel compliance with increased peripheral resistance to blood flow resulting from general or localized arteriosclerosis
Venous circulation	Does not change with age in absence of disease
Blood pressure	Significant increase in systolic (at or above 140 mm Hg) suggestive of hypertension, slight increase in diastolic (at or above 90 mm Hg) suggestive of hypertension, increase in peripheral resistance and pulse pressure
Heart	Dislocation of apex due to kyphoscoliosis; therefore diagnostic significance of location can be lost Increased premature beats, rarely clinically important
Murmurs	Systolic murmurs in over half the aged; the most common heard at base of heart due to sclerotic heart valves
Peripheral pulses	Easily palpated due to increased arterial wall narrowing and loss of connective tissue; feeling of tortuous and rigid vessels Possible that pedal pulses may be weaker as a result of arteriosclerotic changes; colder lower extremities, especially at night; possibility of cold feet and hands with mottled color
Heart rate	No change with age at rest

RESPIRATORY CHANGES

Pulmonary blood flow and diffusion	Decreased blood flow to pulmonary circulation; decreased diffusion
Anatomic structure	Increased anterior-posterior-lateral diameters
Respiratory accessory muscles	Decreased strength; increased rigidity of chest wall, muscle atrophy of pharaynx and larynx muscles
Internal pulmonic structure	Decreased pulmonary elasticity creates senile emphysema; shorter breaths taken without decreased maximum breathing capacity, vital capacity, residual volume, and functional capacity; airway resistance increased; less ventilation at lung bases and more at apices

INTEGUMENTARY CHANGES

Texture	Skin loses elasticity; wrinkles, folding, sagging, rough, dry
Color	Spotty pigmentation in sun-exposed areas; face paler even in the absence of anemia
Temperature	Extremities cooler; decreased ability to perspire
Fat distribution	Less on extremities; more on trunk
Hair color	Dull gray, white, yellow or yellow-green
Hair distribution	Thins on scalp, axilla, pubic area, upper and lower extremities; decreased facial hair in men; development of chin and upper lip hair in women
Nails	Slower growth rate; chipping, flaking, brittle ridging, longitudinal lines, flat or concave; thicken; yellow to gray in color; lunulae poorly defined

GENITOURINARY AND REPRODUCTIVE CHANGES

Renal blood flow	Reduced filtration rate and renal efficiency due to decreased cardiac output; possible subsequent loss of protein from kidney
Micturition	
Men	Increase due to enlarged prostate
Women	Decreased perineal muscle tone— potential for urgency and stress incontinence
	Increased nocturia in both men and women
Incontinence	Increases with age, specifically in those with dementia
Male reproduction	
Testosterone	Decreases
Intercourse	No change in libido and sexual satisfaction; phases of intercourse slower; longer refractory time; decreased frequency of intercourse to once or twice a week
Testes	Decreased size; decreased sperm count; less seminal fluid viscosity
Penis	Smaller; decreased penile sensation
Prostate	Atrophy with hyperplasia
Female reproduction	
Estrogen	Decreased production; menopause
Breasts and nipples	Decreased breast tissue; decreased breast and nipple size
Uterus	Smaller; mucous secretions cease; potential for uterine prolapse from pelvic muscle weakness
Vagina	Narrowing and shortening of canal; epithelial lining atrophies
Vaginal secretions	Increased alkalinity as glycogen content increases

GASTROINTESTINAL CHANGES

Mastication	Impaired by partial loss or total loss of teeth, malocclusive bite, ill-fitting dentures
Swallowing and carbohydrate digestion	Swallowing more difficult; saliva secretions diminish
Esophagus	Decreased peristalsis (presbyesophagus); increased incidence of hiatus hernia with accompanying gasous distention or reflux
Digestive enzymes	Decreased production of hydrochloric acid, pepsin, pancreatic enzymes
Fat absorption	Delayed; affects absorption rate of fat-soluble vitamins A, D, E, K
Intestinal peristalsis	Reduced peristalsis; resultant constipation not uncommon with decreased motility
Sphincters	Weaker anal sphincter tone

MUSCULOSKELETAL CHANGES

Muscle strength and function	Decrease with loss of muscle mass; bony prominences normal in aged with loss of muscle mass; more strength lost in legs than arms (proximal more than distal)
Bone structure	Normal demineralization, more porous; intervertebral space narrowing; shortened trunk
Joints	Tightening and fixation occur with less mobility; range of motion limited; normal posture changes: bent forward, kyphosis; activity may maintain function longer
Anatomic size and height	Decrease in total size as losses of body protein and body water occur in proportion to diminished metabolic rate; increased body fat: more in trunk, less in arms and legs; loss of 2 inches in height from young adulthood

NERVOUS SYSTEM CHANGES

Response to stimuli	All voluntary and autonomic reflexes slower; decrease ability to respond to multiple stimuli; more time needed to learn and perform cognitive process; benign forgetfulness
Sleep patterns	Stage IV sleep reduced from young adulthood; increased frequency of spontaneous awakening; stay in bed longer but less sleep; insomnia should be investigated
Reflexes	Deep tendon: responsive in healthy aged, have decrease or absent knee, ankle jerk, biceps, triceps reflexes
Ambulation	Kinesthetic sense less efficient; may exhibit an extrapyramidal Parkinson-like gait
Gait	Women have narrow walking and standing base and waddle; men have a wide walking and standing base and use small steps
Voice	Decreased range, duration, and intensity; higher pitched and monotonous

SENSORY CHANGES

Vision:	
Peripheral vision	Decreased
Lens accommodation	Decreased; need corrective lenses
Ciliary body	Atrophy, alter accommodation of lens
Iris	Develop arcus senilis
Choroid	Atrophy around disc
Lens	Yellows; decreased discrimination of blue-colored objects; opacity formation (cataracts)
	More light needed to see
Color	Fades or disappears
Macula	Degeneration
Conjunctiva	Thins; looks yellow
Pupil	May be smaller
Cornea	Presence of arcus senilis
Retina	Observable vascular changes; blue, green, red cones decline, color discrimination altered, more difficult seeing contrasts of color
Tearing	Decreases; increased irritation and infection
Stimuli threshold	Increases for light touch and pain; ischemic paresthesias common in extremities
Hearing	Perceive high-frequency tones less, seems to create impaired understanding of conversations; promotes confusion and creates increased rigidity of thought
Gustatory	Decreased taste bud acuity; may increase amount of food seasoning
Temperature	Threshold stimulus, higher temperature; normal usually 96°-97° F; decreased thermal regulation, heat/cold tolerance
Proprioception	Decreased sense of position and balance
Touch	Decreased stereognosis

ENDOCRINE CHANGES

Thyroid	Decreased production or clearance of thyroid hormone
Aldosterone	Inactive to active rennin
Insulin	Increased levels
Glucagon	Increased levels

Data from Ham RJ, Sloane PD, editors: *Primary geriatrics,* ed 3, St Louis, 1997, Mosby, Copstead LEC: *Perspectives on pathophysiology,* Philadelphia, 1995, WB Saunders; Malasanos L et al: *Health assessment,* ed 3, St Louis, 1985, Wardell S, editor: *Acute interventions: nursing process throughout the life span,* Reston, VA, 1979, Reston.

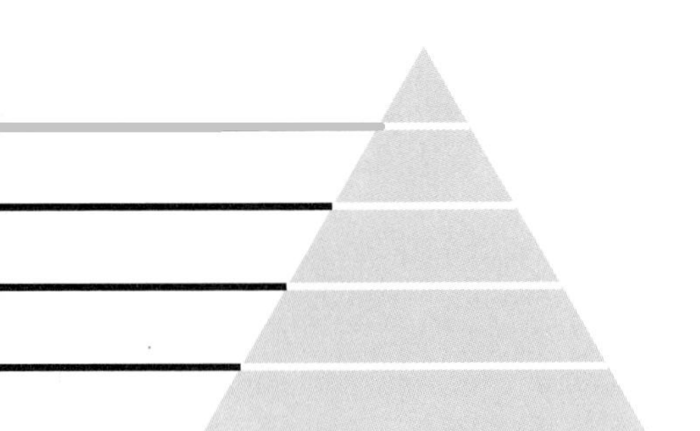

APPENDIX 4-B

Geriatric Assessment Instrument to Be Used in Primary Care

DAILY FUNCTION

Basic and instrumental activities of daily living

ASSISTIVE DEVICES

Use of personal devices (cane, walker, wheelchair, oxygen)

CAREGIVERS

Use of paid caregiver such as nurse, aide
Use of unpaid caregivers such as family members, friends, volunteers

DRUGS

Name of prescription drugs used
Name of over-the-counter (nonprescription) drugs used

NUTRITION

Height
Weight
Stability of weight (loss of 10 lb) in last 6 months without trying

PREVENTIVE MEASURE

Regular blood pressure measurements, guaiac test for occult blood in stool, sigmoidoscopy, immunizations (influenza, pneumococcal, tetanus), thyroid-stimulating hormone assessment, dental care, intake of calcium and vitamin D, regularity of exercise (walking or other forms), use of smoke detectors

COGNITION

Ability to remember three objects after 1 minute

AFFECT

Feeling sad, depressed, or hopeless

ADVANCE DIRECTIVE

Possesses a living will
Has a durable power of attorney for health care

SUBSTANCE ABUSE

Use of alcohol determined by the CAGE questionnaire
Use of cigarettes
Use of other substances, licit or illicit

GAIT, BALANCE

Number of falls in past 6 months
Positive Romberg test (sways while standing, feet together, eyes closed)
Time required to rise from a chair, walk 9-10 feet, turn around, return, and sit down
Extent of maximum forward reach while standing

SENSORY ABILITY

Ability to report three numbers whispered 2 feet behind head
Ability to read Snellen chart at 20/40 or better with corrective lenses, if used

UPPER EXTREMITIES

Able to clasp hands behind head and neck

Modified from Boult C: Comprehensive geriatric assessment. In Beers MH, Berkow R: *The Merck manual of geriatrics,* ed 3, Whitehouse Station, NJ, 2000, Merck Research Laboratories, pp 41-42.

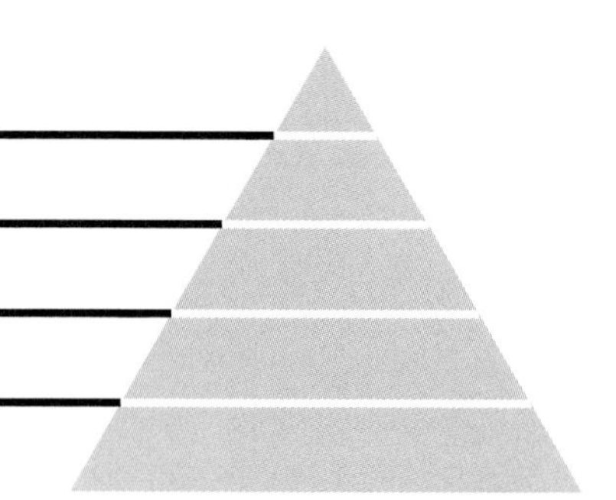

APPENDIX 4-C

Katz Index, Modified Barthel Index, and Functional Performance Tests

Katz Index of Activities of Daily Living

1. Bathing (sponge, shower, or tub):
   - I: Receives no assistance (gets in and out of tub if tub is the usual means of bathing)
   - A: Receives assistance in bathing only one part of the body (such as the back or a leg)
   - D: Receives assistance in bathing more than one part of the body (or not bathed)
2. Dressing:
   - I: Gets clothes and gets completely dressed without assistance
   - A: Gets clothes and gets dressed without assistance except in tying shoes
   - D: Receives assistance in getting clothes or in getting dressed or stays partly or completely undressed
3. Toileting:
   - I: Goes to "toilet room," cleans self, and arranges clothes without assistance (may use object for support such as cane, walker, or wheelchair and may manage night bedpan or commode, emptying it in the morning)
   - A: Receives assistance in going to "toilet room" or in cleansing self or in arranging clothes after elimination or in use of night bedpan or commode
   - D: Doesn't go to room termed "toilet" for the elimination process
4. Transfer:
   - I: Moves in and out of bed as well as in and out of chair without assistance (may be using object for support such as cane or walker)
   - A: Moves in and out of bed or chair with assistance
   - D: Doesn't get out of bed
5. Continence:
   - I: Controls urination and bowel movement completely by self
   - A: Has occasional "accidents"
   - D: Supervision helps keep urine or bowel control; catheter is used, or is incontinent
6. Feeding:
   - I: Feeds self without assistance
   - A: Feeds self except for getting assistance in cutting meat or buttering bread
   - D: Receives assistance in feeding or is fed partly or completely by using tubes or intravenous fluids

Adapted from *JAMA* 185:915, 1963.
I, Independent; *A,* assistance; *D,* dependent.

Modified Barthel Index

	Independent		Dependent	
	Intact	Limited	Helper	Null
Feed from dish	10	5	3	0
Dress upper body	5	5	3	0
Dress lower body	5	5	2	0
Don brace or prosthesis	0	0	−2	0
Grooming	5	5	0	0
Wash or bathe	4	4	0	0
Bladder incontinence	10	10	5	0
Bowel incontinence	10	10	5	0
Care of perineum/clothing at toilet	4	4	2	0
Transfer, chair	15	15	7	0
Transfer, toilet	6	5	3	0
Transfer, tub or shower	1	1	0	0
Walk on level 50 yards or more	15	15	10	0
Up and down stairs for one flight or more	10	10	5	0
Wheelchair 50 yards (only if not walking)	15	5	0	0

Adapted from *Medical Care* 19:491, 1981.

Functional Performance Tests

Standing Balance

Instructions: Semi-tandem stand.* The nurse:

a. First demonstrates the task.
(The heel of one foot is placed to the side of the first toe of the other foot.)
b. Supports one arm of the older adult while he or she positions the feet as demonstrated above. The elder can choose which foot to place forward.
c. Asks if the person is ready, then releases the support and begins timing.
d. Stop timing when the older adult moves the feet or grasps the nurse for support, or when 10 seconds have elapsed.

*Start with the semi-tandem stand. If it cannot be done for 10 seconds, the **side-by-side** test should be done. If the semi-tandem can be accomplished for the requisite 10 seconds, follow the same instructions as above, except the **full tandem** requires placing the heel of one foot directly in front of the toes of the other foot.

Scoring	Full tandem	Semi-tandem	Side-by-side
0	________	<10 seconds or unable	<10 seconds or unable
1	________	<10 seconds or unable	10 seconds
2	<3 seconds or unable	10 seconds	________
3	3 to 9 seconds	10 seconds	________
4	10 seconds	10 seconds	________

Standing Balance Score: ________

Walking Speed

Instructions: The nurse:

a. Sets up an 8-foot walking course with an additional 2 feet at both ends free of any obstacles.
b. Places an 8-foot rigid carpenter's ruler to the side of the course.
c. Instructs the older adults to "walk to the other end of the course at your normal speed, just like walking down the street to go to the store." Assistive devices should be used if needed.
d. Times two walks. **The fastest of the two is used as the score.**

Scoring:	
0	Unable
1	>5.6 seconds
2	4.1 to 5.6 seconds
3	3.2 to 4 seconds
4	<3.2 seconds

Walking Speed Score: ________

Chair Stands

Instructions: The nurse:

a. Places a straight-backed chair next to a well.
b. Asks the older adult to fold the arms across the chest and stand up from the chair one time. If successful:
c. Asks the older adult to stand and sit five times as quickly as possible.
d. Times from the initial sitting position to the final standing position at the end of the fifth stand.

Scores are for the five rise-and-sits only. If the older adult performs less than five repetitions, the score is 0.

Scoring	
0	Unable
1	>16.6 seconds
2	13.7 to 16.5 seconds
3	11.2 to 13.6 seconds
4	<11.2 seconds

Chair Stands Score: ________ **Total of all performance tests (0-12)** ________

Modified from Guralnik JM et al: A short physical performance battery assessment of lower extremity function: association with self-reported disability and prediction of mortality and nursing home admission, *J Gerontol Med Sci* 49(2):M85, 1994; and Bennett JA: Activities of daily living: old-fashioned or still useful? *J Gerontol Nurs* 25(5):22, 1999.

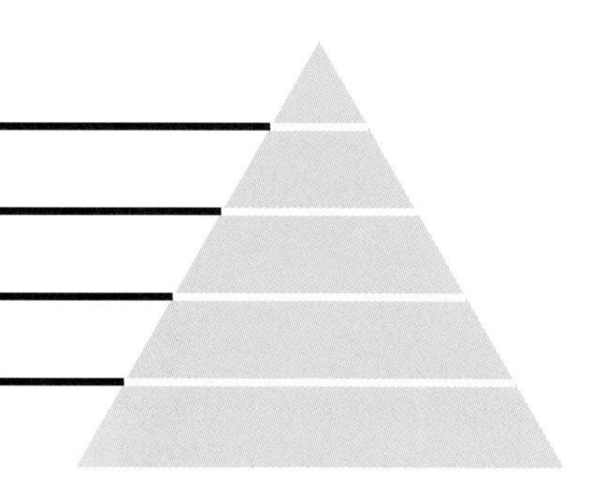

CHAPTER 5

Laboratory Values and Diagnostics

Ann Schmidt Luggen

A student speculates

I believe self-care is important and, sure, I watch my cholesterol intake every day and get it checked annually. I worry about my mother as I'm not sure she takes her diabetic diet seriously. Sometimes she forgets to check her blood sugar.

Leslie, age 37

An elder speaks

You know, in the old days when my grandfather was practicing he would diagnose by sight, feel, smell, and taste. Yes, taste! But, of course, nobody ever heard of a malpractice suit either.

Daisy, age 82

LEARNING OBJECTIVES

On completion of this chapter, the reader will be able to:

1. Identify the laboratory values that increase or decrease with normal aging.
2. Understand the implications and deviations of abnormal laboratory values in the aged.
3. Define cautions the nurse should take when interpreting laboratory values in the aged.
4. Distinguish between clinical findings of hypothyroidism and hyperthyroidism in the elderly.
5. State common causes of hypokalemia and hyperkalemia.
6. Describe symptoms and signs suggestive of diabetes in the elderly.
7. Identify laboratory values in the elderly that frequently fall out of the so-called *normal range.*
8. Discuss laboratory tests necessary for minimally adequate screening of elderly residents in long-term care institutions.

This chapter is intended to give a background of the importance of laboratory diagnostic findings. Some are exceedingly complex and sophisticated, but each nurse needs a basic knowledge because the review and reporting of laboratory values constitute a significant task of nursing. More frequently now they are reported directly to the client by the nurse, and the nurse will need to explain the significance of findings. Additionally, the gerontologic nurse depends on laboratory values because the ill elderly person often has vague clinical signs and symptoms. When reviewing laboratory values seen in older adults, the nurse knows that many values are outside normal ranges for younger adults and whether those values reflect illness or normal aging changes.

Normal laboratory values are determined by a random sample of "healthy" individuals, obtaining the mean, and considering normal a range of two standard deviations on either side of the mean. "Normal" has little meaning because healthy individuals of all age-groups often have asymmetric distribution of test results (Malone et al, 2000). Reference values or reference ranges have mainly been gathered from young college-aged men. Now we are using "reference intervals" of age, sex, and race that can be defined via demographics. As people age, they become *less* like each other. Organ function declines with aging (Beers and Berkow, 2000), but the rate of change varies from person to person and system to system. Geriatric *reference ranges* are those intervals within which 95% of values for persons over 70 years of age will fall.

Reference values, a term recommended by the International Federation of Clinical Chemistry, will be used synonymously with *reference ranges* throughout this chapter. International standards are important because laboratory values for an individual remain relatively stable over time and observed changes may be due to differing laboratory methods. Thus knowledge of reference values, standardized procedures, and individual biologic variations would allow a subject to follow throughout life the evolution of his or her biologic constituents and to detect any deviation suggestive of a pathologic condition. Some of the standardized procedures that should be observed are listed in Table 5-1.

Another issue is the difficulty of defining a healthy elderly population for the development of normal laboratory values. The majority of elders have one or more disease entities and are taking one or more medications, which may affect the laboratory values. In a study of over 5000 participants in a cardiovascular health study, Medicare-eligible, ostensibly healthy individuals residing in the community were used to define a healthy subset of the older population. Blood samples revealed that levels of cholesterol, high-density lipoprotein (HDL) and low-density lipoprotein (LDL) cholesterol, fasting and 2-hour postload glucose and insulin, fibrinogen, factors VII and VIII, potassium, creatinine, albumin, uric acid, white blood cell count, hematocrit, hemoglobin, and platelet count were all significantly different than the generally accepted reference ranges used in clinical laboratories (Robbins et al, 1995). Further, lower hemoglobin and hematocrit values, elevated total cholesterol levels, the presence of antinuclear antibodies and rheumatoid factor, and elevated systolic blood pressure were more frequent in aged women than aged men.

This chapter discusses the laboratory values that significantly change with aging. Tables are provided for general reference values for the aged. Because normal reference ranges vary with institutions, depending on the instrumentation used for performing tests, Table 5-1 should be used as a guideline within institutional laboratory parameters. Also see Table 5-2.

HEMATOLOGY

Age-related hematologic changes occur mainly from changes in the bone marrow; few of these changes are clinically significant (Beers and Berkow, 2000). There is a diminished capacity to make new blood cells quickly in the presence of acute disease; this can be a significant problem for elderly adults and is termed *decreased marrow reserve.* Other elements that may impair the hematologic system, such as inadequate nutrition, sensory deficits, and impaired physical mobility, may reduce circulatory red blood cells, granulocytes, and lymphocytes.

Bone Marrow

The bone marrow space with the hematopoietic tissue diminishes from birth through age 30; then it levels off. At about age 70, it diminishes again in a progressive fashion starting with the long bones, mainly the femur (Beers and Berkow, 2000). The cause of this age-related diminution is not known. The number of stem cells in the marrow decreases with increasing age. There is decreased erythropoiesis, which decreases the absorption of iron into red blood cells (RBCs). Bone marrow iron (and total body iron) increase with age, and folate and vitamin B_{12} in healthy elders remains in the individual's normal range.

Red Blood Cells

There is little evidence of age-related differences in RBCs; the RBC life span, total blood volume, and RBC volume do not change with increasing age (Beers and Berkow, 2000). There may be changes in red cell enzymes that affect the life span of the cell, but the significance is uncertain.

Anemia is a condition indicated by a decrease in the number of RBCs; this may be related to decreased production or increased destruction of RBCs. The hemoglobin level is the screen for anemia (Brown et al, 1999). Signs and symptoms of severe anemia such as apathy, depression, confusion, general fatigue, and pallor may be incorrectly attributed to old age or other concomitant chronic illnesses instead of anemia. A blue tint to the sclerae may be a sign of iron deficiency anemia in older adults. Pale conjunctivae may also be present. Anemia is a common disease state of the elderly person, but it is not a normal aging process. Anemias that may be found in elderly people include vitamin B_{12} deficiency anemia, folate deficiency anemia, iron deficiency anemia, anemia of chronic disease, anemias of malignancy, anemia of liver disease, anemia of acute or chronic blood loss, and anemia of chronic renal insufficiency (Desai and Isa-Pratt, 2002). Evaluation of the etiology of any hemoglobin or hematocrit levels below the individual's normal values is necessary at any age but is more complicated in the aged.

Hemoglobin

Hemoglobin is the main component of the red blood cell. It is a conjugated protein whose main function is to transport oxygen and carbon dioxide. In the elderly person the hemoglobin concentration in both sexes decreases slightly after about 65 years of age. However, there is debate as to whether this is normal aging or a "clue to occult chronic disease" (Desai and Isa-Pratt, 2002). The decrease is more prevalent in men than women and may be related to the reduction in androgen production in men. In healthy young adults, male hemoglobin levels are normally higher than those of females. However, in elderly people the hemoglobin concentrations in both sexes are nearly the same. A decrease in hemoglobin may indicate chronic disease or physiologic changes caused by illness. When a low hemoglobin level is present, there is lowered oxygen content and a delay in wound healing. Therefore older individuals with pressure sores or any slow-healing wounds should have hemoglobin levels monitored.

Hematocrit

Hematocrit is the ratio of the volume of red blood cells to that of whole blood. Studies show that elderly women and men

Text continued on p. 121

Table 5-1 Laboratory Values for the Elderly

Test	Normal aged	Standard reference ranges*	Implications and deviations†
Hematology			
Hemoglobin	Slight decrease	Male: 14.0-18.0 g/dl Female: 12.0-16.0 g/dl	
Hematocrit	Slight decrease	Male: 40%-54% Female: 38%-47%	
White blood cells	Slight decrease	4.3-11.0 × $10^3/mm^3$	
Erythrocyte sedimentation rate (ESR)			
Minivess method	Slight increase	Male: 0-20 mm Female: 0-20 mm	
Differential lymphocytes			
Neutrophils	Unchanged	46%-82%	Increase: Diabetes mellitus Gout Rheumatoid arthritis Stress Bacterial infections Thyroiditis Hemolytic anemia Rheumatic fever Carcinoma Acute hemorrhage Cushing's disease Increased corticosteroids Lead poisoning Pancreatitis Decrease: Vitamin B_{12} deficiency Acute viral infection Folic acid deficiency Bone marrow damage
Lymphocytes	Increased B cells Decreased T cells	11%-45%	
Monocytes	Increased both sexes	2.0%-10.0%	Increase: Tuberculosis Subacute bacterial endocarditis
Eosinophils	Increase or decrease	0%-4.0%	Increase: Parasitosis Allergy Colitis Collagen disease Eosinophilic granulomatosis Eosinophilic leukemia
Basophils	Unchanged	0%-2.0%	Increase: Polycythemia vera Myelofibrosis
Serum chemistry			
Iron‡	Decrease 50%-75% of young adult value at about age 71-80 yr	Male: 49-181 μg/dl Female: 37-170 μg/dl	Increase: Pernicious anemia Hemolytic anemia Hemochromatosis Hepatitis Decrease: Iron deficiency anemia Anaphylactic reaction

Source: Garner B: Guide to changing lab values in the elderly, *Geriatric Nurs* 10(3):144, 1989.
*Standard reference ranges used at St Francis Hospital Laboratory, Beech Grove, IN, 1996.
†The deviations listed are not an all-inclusive list but a helpful guide for many of the frequent deviations seen in the elderly. Modified from Eliopoulos C: *Health assessment of the older adult,* Reading, MA, 1990, Addison-Wesley; and Eliopoulos C: *A guide to the nursing of the aging,* Baltimore, 1987, Williams & Wilkins.
‡Must be differentiated between normal age changes and anemia.

Continued

Table 5-1 Laboratory Values for the Elderly—cont'd

Test	Normal aged	Standard reference ranges*	Implications and deviations†
B_{12}‡	Decrease 60%-80% of young adult value at about age 70+ yr	179-1132 pg/ml	
Folate‡	Unchanged	3.1-12.4 ng/ml	
Thyroid			
T_4	Slight functional decrease	4.5-12.0 μg/dl	
T_3	Male decrease after age 70 yr Female decrease around age 70-80 yr	86-181 mg/dl	
TSH		0.49-4.67 μu/ml	
Blood chemistry			
Urea nitrogen (BUN)	Slight increase	Male: 9-20 mg/dl Female: 7-17 mg/dl	Increase: Dehydration Gastrointestinal hemorrhage Intestinal obstruction Renal disease Acute glomerulonephritis Prostatic hypertrophy Burns High-protein intake Mercury poisoning Protein catabolism Decrease: Cirrhosis Liver disease Low-protein intake Starvation
Creatinine	Slight increase	Male: 0.8-1.5 mg/dl Female: 0.7-1.2 mg/dl	Increase: Renal dysfunction Chronic glomerulonephritis Tetanus Typhoid fever Salmonella infection Decrease: Anemia Muscular atrophy Leukemia Renal failures
Potassium	Age-related increase after sixth decade	3.6-5.0 mEq/L	Increase: Addison's disease Bronchial asthma Renal disease Tissue breakdown Trauma Anuria Decrease: Steroid therapy Vomiting Cirrhosis Diarrhea Diuretic therapy Diabetic acidosis Cushing's disease Intravenous therapy
Glucose	Increases	70-110 mg/dl	Increase: Diabetes mellitus Emotional stress Hyperthyroidism

Table 5-1 Laboratory Values for the Elderly—cont'd

Test	Normal aged	Standard reference ranges*	Implications and deviations†
			Infections Thiazide therapy Increased intracranial pressure Pituitary disorder Decrease: Hyperinsulinism Hypothyroidism Starvation
Fasting blood sugar	Minimal increase		
1 hour postprandial blood sugar	Increases by 10 mg/dl per decade after age 30		
2 hour postprandial blood sugar	Increases up to 100 plus age after age 40		
CPK	May not be elevated	Male: 55-170 U/L Female: 30-135 U/L	
Alkaline phosphatase	Increases	38-126 U/L	
LDH	1-1½ times higher, especially in females	313-618 U/L	
SGPT or ALT	Unchanged	Male: 21-72 IU/L Female: 9-52 IU/L	
SGOT or AST	Unchanged	Male: 17-59 IU/L Female: 14-36 IU/L	
Total protein		6.3-8.2 g/dl	
Serum albumin	Decrease	3.9-5.0 g/dl	
Cholesterol (total)	Gradual increase with age	200 mg/dl	Increase: Chronic renal disease Hypothyroidism Diabetes mellitus Liver disease Pancreatic dysfunction Decrease: Fasting state Tuberculosis Hypermetabolic states Hyperthyroidism Intestinal obstruction Liver disease Malnutrition Pernicious anemia Hemolytic anemia
HDL	Women consistently higher than men, then difference disappears in elders§	>35 mg/dl	
Triglycerides	Increases	35-160 mg/dl	
Calcium	Men decrease Women increase	8.4-10.2 mg/dl	
Phosphorus	Men decrease Women increase	2.5-4.5 mg/dl	
Uric acid	Males increase more than females Females over 44 years	3.5-8.5 mg/dl 2.5-7.5 mg/dl	Increase: Thiazide diuretic therapy Pneumonia Multiple myeloma Leukemia High salicylate intake Gout Fasting Chronic renal failure Chronic lymphocytic granulocytic leukemia Decrease: Allopurinol therapy

Continued

Table 5-1 Laboratory Values for the Elderly—cont'd

Test	Normal aged	Standard reference ranges*	Implications and deviations†
Urinalysis			
Protein	Slight increase	Negative	
Glucose	Unchanged	Negative	
Specific gravity	Decrease	1.005-1.030 o.d. (refractometer)	
Creatinine clearance			
Male	Decrease	85-125 ml/min	Decrease: Renal disease
Female	Decrease	75-115 ml/min	
Arterial blood gases			
Pco_2	Increase or decrease	34-46 mm Hg	Increase: Metabolic alkalosis; Respiratory acidosis. Decrease: Metabolic acidosis; Respiratory alkalosis
Po_2	Decrease	85-95 mm Hg	Increase: Administration of pure O_2. Decrease: Circulatory disorders; Decreased hemoglobin; Decreased O_2 supply; High altitudes; Poor O_2 uptake and utilization; Respiratory exchange problems

Table 5-2 Special Considerations for Laboratory Testing in the Aged

Test	Cautions*
Hemoglobin	Just because hemoglobin declines with age, do not assume a low hemoglobin is normal in an elder. When hemoglobin and hematocrits are low, look for other signs of anemia: pale skin, pale conjunctiva.
Lymphocytes	Protect elders from infection since they have fewer and weaker lymphocytes with which to fight invading organisms. Immune system changes diminish antibody-antigen response. Encourage elders to have pneumococcal, tetanus, and influenza vaccines.
BUN	A slightly elevated BUN causes no problems unless such stressors as infection or surgery are added.
Creatinine	Consider the creatinine and the creatinine clearance levels to prevent toxicity when giving drugs excreted via the urinary system.
Potassium	Avoid salt substitutes, largely composed of potassium. Teach elders to check food labels for potassium and to learn signs of hyperkalemia.
Glucose	Drugs such as alcohol, MAO inhibitors, and beta blockers can contribute to a rapid fall in glucose. A rise in glucose can quickly precipitate nonketotic hyperosmolar acidosis. A drop in glucose triggers confusion as brain cells are deprived of glucose.
Urinalysis protein	Proteinuria is more common in elders than younger adults. 1 + (30 mg/100 ml) may be of no clinical significance, but renal pathology or a urinary tract infection should be ruled out.
Glucose	Glycosuria may not occur until the plasma glucose exceeds 300 mg/100 ml. Urine glucose checks in diabetic elders are highly unreliable.
Serum albumin	Low serum albumin produces edema. If there is no liver dysfunction, teach the elder to increase protein intake by eating fish, meat, nuts, grains, peanut butter, vegetables, eggs, and milk products. Elders need more protein per kilogram of body weight than does a younger person.
Cholesterol	After menopause, women's risk of cardiovascular problems increases to the male level. Diet high in fiber and in fish oils (e.g., from tuna, salmon, sardines, trout) can lower cholesterol. Weight loss and exercise can raise HDL.

*Source: Garner B: Guide to changing lab values in elders, *Geriatr Nurs* 10(3):144, 1989.

may have a slight decrease in their hematocrit levels. Other laboratory tests should always be evaluated along with hemoglobin and hematocrit values in making a diagnosis. The hematocrit test is to be used along with other laboratory tests in evaluating the patient with anemia. Recent data from the Second National Health and Nutrition Examination Study (NHANES II) suggest a complex relationship between a high hematocrit and death from cardiovascular disease (Brown et al, 1999). However, further research is needed to enhance our understanding of this relationship.

Erythrocyte Sedimentation Rate

When well-mixed venous blood is placed in a vertical tube, erythrocytes will tend to fall to the bottom. The distance the red blood cells fall in an interval of time is the erythrocyte sedimentation rate (ESR). The ESR is often increased in the elderly. The changes in plasma constituents in the elderly may possibly increase the ESR; however, it is most likely due to the presence of chronic inflammatory processes such as rheumatic disease or cancer. The elevations in serum proteins are usually due to inflammatory activity. If an elderly person has an unexplained rise in ESR, further testing should be accomplished. The American Geriatric Society offers formulas to determine a normal ESR for older adults (2002). For women, the formula is age plus 10, divided by 2. For men, the formula is age divided by 2.

Monoclonal gammopathy is a diagnosis that the practitioner should have an awareness of because it occurs in about 10% of older adults ages 62 through 95 who appear to be healthy, but in about 35% of those with an elevated ESR (Beers and Berkow, 2000). The C-reactive protein, a measure of inflammation, also increases with age.

White Blood Cells

White blood cells (WBCs), or leukocytes, protect the body by phagocytosis of microorganisms and other foreign debris. They exist in tissues and in the circulatory and lymph systems. The average adult has 5000 to 10,000 WBCs. The elderly person has a diminished response to infection that involves WBCs. We observe clinically that chronic inflammation with fever, elevated WBCs, swelling, pain, and lymph node enlargement may be reduced or absent. Often there is no increase in total leukocyte count but a shift to the left, which is an increase in the number of bands (neutrophils), also called *bandemia* (Desai and Isa-Pratt, 2002). The left shift is a more definitive indication of bacterial (and sometimes viral) infection in the aged. The types of WBCs present and changes of those present must be determined by ordering a differential when ordering a complete blood count, or WBC count.

There are five major types of leukocytes in the blood: neutrophils, lymphocytes, monocytes, eosinophils, and basophils. Each type of WBC plays a different role in fighting infection.

Neutrophils. The largest percentage of white blood cells are neutrophils (55% to 70%), which are produced daily in the bone marrow (Pagana and Pagana, 2001). Neutrophils are granulocytes (as are basophils and eosinophils). They are also all called polymorphonuclear leukocytes (PMNs), or "polys." Neutrophils play an important part in the localization of infections by phagocytizing bacteria. Aging does not appear to change the neutrophil count in older adults. Neutrophilia, or increased neutrophils, may be caused by infections, connective tissue diseases such as rheumatoid arthritis, malignancies, medications such as corticosteroids, trauma, and metabolic conditions such as gout, uremia, thyrotoxicosis, and lactic acidosis (Desai and Isa-Pratt, 2002).

Lymphocytes. Lymphocytes are nongranulocytes, or agranulocytes (as are monocytes), and are divided into two types: T cells and B cells. Lymphocytes are the primary cells in the immune response. Clinically, we observe that the immune response seems to diminish with increasing age. T cells are produced by the thymus and are concerned with cell-mediated immunity; B cells are bone marrow related and produce antibodies, or humoral immunity, while working with T cells in the immune process. The differential does not separate out T cells and B cells, but counts them together. In some disease situations, it is important to separate them, but rarely. Normally, 80% of lymphocytes are T cells and most of the remaining cells are B cells. The effect of age on total lymphocyte counts is not evident, but studies have shown a consistent finding of an increased number of B cells in the elderly population and an age-related decline in T-cell function. Monoclonal gammopathy, common in older adults, is a T cell lymphocyte dysfunction (Beers and Berkow, 2000).

Monocytes. Monocytes and macrophages are large leukocytes that fight viral, bacterial, parasitic, and rickettsial infections through phagocytosis. Monocytes, immature macrophages, later migrate into lymph tissue. They may be present for months or even years before they migrate to an inflammatory site to phagocytose microorganisms, dead RBCs, and foreign debris. Monocytes do not seem to change with increasing age.

Eosinophils and Basophils. Eosinophils are involved in allergic reactions. They ingest antigen-antibody complexes induced by IgE-mediated reactions to attack parasites. High eosinophil counts are found in people with type I allergies such as hay fever or asthma. Eosinophils are involved in the mucosal immune response, which is known to diminish in the aged (Beers and Berkow, 2000). Increased eosinophils in the peripheral blood smear may be caused by infections such as tuberculosis or pulmonary fungal infections, rheumatoid arthritis, ulcerative colitis, regional enteritis, seasonal allergic rhinitis, atopic dermatitis, solid tumor cancers, and various lymphomas and leukemias (Desai and Isa-Pratt, 2002). Basophils transport histamine (all the histamine in the body), a factor in immune and antiinflammatory responses. They are not involved in bacterial or viral infections.

Platelets. There is a decline in baseline platelet count and a higher likelihood of thrombocytopenia after bleeding that has been observed with increasing age (HealthandAge.com and American Geriatric Society, 2000). Platelet function has been reported as normal, decreased, or increased (Beers and Berkow, 2000). Not all elders with thrombocytopenia have petechiae or ecchymoses or bleeding gums. Often the abnormal platelet count is found serendipitously with the complete blood cell count (CBC) (Desai and Isa-Pratt, 2002). Causes include vitamin B_{12} and folate deficiencies (diminished production); leukemias, lymphomas, and solid tumor cancers; medications (estrogen and thiazides); radiation; alcohol; infection; immune disorders, such as systemic lupus and polyarteritis nodosa; and hepatitis. Clotting factors VII and VIII increase with age (Beers and Berkow, 2000; HealthandAge.com and American Geriatric Society, 2000).

SERUM CHEMISTRY

Vitamins, minerals, and hormones circulate throughout the body, and these in combination with cellular processes influence individual function in gross and subtle ways.

Serum Iron

The most common cause of anemia in the aged (and in the world) is deficiency of iron, especially among older individuals with low incomes and chronic disease. It is a microcytic (small red cells) anemia but can be normocytic and the cells are pale. Normally, total body and bone marrow stores increase with age (Beers and Berkow, 2000). This indicates that no iron deficiency anemia is normal in elderly people. Dietary iron deficiency in adults is virtually unknown in the United States (Beers and Berkow, 2000) and occurs only with severe malabsorption or gastrectomy. In the elderly patient, changes in serum iron reflect blood loss from the gastrointestinal or genitourinary tract in most instances. Causes include decreased erythropoiesis, overall reduction of hematopoietic reserve, inflammatory disease, neoplastic disease, or poorly managed use of anticoagulant, antiinflammatory, or nonsteroidal drugs. Diagnosing iron deficiency anemia is more difficult in older persons. The mean corpuscular hemoglobin (Hb) and the mean corpuscular Hb concentration may be normal in elderly people with this anemia (Beers and Berkow, 2000). Further, a ratio often used to diagnose it in younger people, the transferrin saturation ratio of serum iron to total iron-binding capacity (TIBC), is not useful because serum iron and TIBC both decrease with age and in individuals with chronic disease. Serum ferritin usually reflects bone marrow iron; however, in older adults with infection, inflammation, and liver disease, this laboratory value may be falsely elevated. In this instance, a bone marrow aspirate is advised.

Vitamin B_{12}

Vitamin B_{12} deficiency is recognized as an important cause of anemia in the elderly population. This is a macrocytic (large red cells) anemia that accounts for about 9% of anemias in elders (Beers and Berkow, 2000). Vitamin B_{12} decreases with advancing age in many older adults. The most common cause is the inability to split vitamin B_{12} from the proteins in food to which it is bound. This may be due to deficiency in hydrochloric acid or pancreatic enzymes. Mainly in elders, low acidity is the cause. However, in diagnosing this, other causes must be considered. These are pernicious anemia, strict vegetarian diet, alcoholism, cancer, hyperthyroidism, fistulae, diverticulosis, regional ileitis, fish tapeworm, and medications such as colchicine (Desai and Isa-Pratt, 2002); and aminoglycoside antibiotics, aspirin, and anticonvulsants (Pagana and Pagana, 2001).

Undiagnosed pernicious anemia (PA) in the aged is thought to afflict as many as 1% of all people older than 60 years (Beers and Berkow, 2000). It is characterized by antiparietal cell antibodies, which are present in 85% of PA. Formerly, we would identify anti—intrinsic factor antibodies, but the test is only about 50% sensitive and negative results do not exclude the diagnosis of PA (Desai and Isa-Pratt, 2002).

The initial presentation of PA or vitamin B_{12} deficiency may be a dementia. If untreated, anemia of vitamin B_{12} deficiency may ultimately be fatal, so the diagnosis must be foremost in mind when an elder has dementia (Brown et al, 1999). Other clinical manifestations include glossitis, increased lactate dehydrogenase (LDH) levels, paresthesias of feet and hands, and vibratory and proprioception disturbances. Ataxias will occur without treatment. Cerebral manifestations include memory impairment, change in taste and smell, irritability, and somnolence.

Folic Acid

Folic acid deficiency is more commonly dietary in origin than is vitamin B_{12} deficiency. Despite adequate stores of folate, serum folate levels may decline within several days without folic acid intake (Desai and Isa-Pratt, 2002). They will be decreased if the patient has had recent alcohol intake. Folate levels may be increased if the patient in the laboratory has just eaten, confusing the diagnosis. Folate levels may be falsely normal in patients with severe iron deficiency anemia. Folic acid deficiency can be distinguished from vitamin B_{12} deficiency (both megaloblastic anemias) through the use of homocysteine and methylmalonic acid levels. Only the homocysteine level will be elevated with folate deficiency.

Causes of folate deficiency include dietary deficiencies and malnutrition, malabsorption syndromes, cancers, liver disease, some anticonvulsant drugs, alcohol, and methotrexate (usually given with folic acid to manage the antagonist effect). Elevated folic acid levels are caused by vegetarian diets and blood transfusions (Pagana and Pagana, 2001).

Endocrine

The normal aging process causes a number of alterations in hormone production, secretion, and biologic effect. All endocrine glands in older people change. Therefore proper diagnosis and treatment of endocrine problems are especially critical for the aged. In addition, the normal aging changes in the renal, pulmonary, gonadal, gastrointestinal, and hepatic systems complicate endocrine test result interpretation.

Thyroid. The prevalence of hypothyroidism and thyroid nodules increases dramatically in older adults (Beers and Berkow, 2000). Screening for thyroid disease is a component for any primary health provider visit, especially in women older than 50. The thyroid gland normally becomes atrophied with increasing age. The production of T_4 (thyroxine) decreases about 30% at advanced age; however, serum T_4 levels remain unchanged, probably because less T_4 is used by the body. Serum T_3 (triiodothyronine) decreases with age (Cotter and Strumpf, 2002) perhaps as a result of decreased secretion of thyroid-stimulating hormone (TSH) by the pituitary gland.

Hypothyroidism. Hypothyroidism (myxedema) occurs in 10% of women and 2% of men older than 65 (Cotter and Strumpf, 2002). About 15% of those 70 years and older have hypothyroidism. It increases with aging and occurs 10 times more often in women than men. The most common causes are Hashimoto's disease and previous irradiation or surgery of the thyroid gland. In hypothyroidism, the TSH is elevated and the T_3 and T_4 levels are diminished. In subclinical hypothyroidism, which occurs in about 5% to 10% of older adults, the TSH is increased and the T_3 and T_4 levels are normal.

Things that may affect these laboratory values include the following:

- TSH: Severe illness, aspirin, dopamine, heparin, and steroids decrease TSH. Potassium iodide and lithium increase TSH.
- T_3: Anabolic steroids, androgens, phenytoin, propranolol, reserpine, and salicylates decrease T_3. Estrogen and methadone increase T_3.
- T_4: Anabolic steroids, androgens, lithium, phenytoin, and propranolol decrease T_4. Estrogen, methadone, and clofibrate increase T_4.

The classic clinical presentation includes dry skin, brittle hair and alopecia, weight gain and fluid retention, facial puffiness, pallor, cold intolerance, malaise, myalgias, fatigue, lethargy, confusion, decreased concentration, insomnia, constipation, delayed deep tendon reflexes (DTRs), and decreased basal metabolic rate (BMR) (Cotter and Strumpf, 2002). Elderly people may have atypical signs and symptoms. The onset may be insidious and subtle. Dementia may be suspected. Most people older than 70 have fatigue and weakness. Other typical signs and symptoms include heart failure, depression, confusion, anorexia, gastrointestinal (GI) disorders, falls, incontinence, and decreased mobility (Beers and Berkow, 2000). Atrial fibrillation may occur with hypothyroidism, and increased LDLs increase the risk of atherosclerosis. Subclinical hypothyroidism may be a risk factor for cardiac disease (Cotter and Strumpf, 2002).

Hyperthyroidism. Hyperthyroidism, or thyrotoxicosis, occurs more frequently in women and with advancing age (Cotter and Strumpf, 2002). Its prevalence is 0.5% to 6% of older adults. It is usually caused by multinodular and uninodular toxic goiter rather than Graves' disease. A common cause is iodine-induced hyperthyroidism from the use of amiodarone, a cardiac drug (Beers and Berkow, 2000). In elderly people, hyperthyroidism is more difficult to diagnose than hypothyroidism. Elderly patients have fewer signs and symptoms than young patients. In older patients there is a classic triad of tachycardia, weight loss, and fatigue (or lack of energy or weakness). It is uncommon to have ocular signs, which are common in young patients. Constipation is present in about 20% of older patients. One may observe tremor. Symptoms of heart failure or angina may cloud the clinical presentation and prevent the correct diagnosis. The most common complication is atrial fibrillation, present in 27% of elderly hyperthyroid patients. If not converted, heart failure and early death may occur (Beers and Berkow, 2000).

Diagnosis is characterized by increased T_4 or T_3 (Cotter and Strumpf, 2002). Diagnosis of hyperthyroidism is difficult in the elderly for several reasons: (1) The patient exhibits fewer diagnostic clues, (2) other existing diseases may mask symptoms, and (3) symptoms that are present in young people with hyperthyroidism are often absent in older adults. Confirmation of the diagnosis of hyperthyroidism relies heavily on laboratory test results.

BLOOD CHEMISTRY

Blood chemistry studies form a profile of the characteristics and properties of the circulating plasma and elements and particles of the blood: glucose, proteins, amino acids, nutritive materials, excretion products, hormones, enzymes, vitamins, and minerals. Those conveying significant diagnostic information are discussed.

Glucose

Glucose metabolism changes with increasing age. Endocrine changes include a decrease in glucose tolerance and increased levels of insulin and glucagon. Factors that may contribute to decreasing glucose values in the aged are the increase in adiposity and decrease in lean body mass without significant change in total body weight, although obesity is a major risk factor for the development of diabetes mellitus (DM). Physical activity is known to enhance the sensitivity of insulin. Unfortunately, many older people still have a sedentary lifestyle despite recent widespread national interest in exercise. The American Diabetes Association recommends screening all persons at risk for DM; everyone over 45 should be screened every 3 years. Screening consists of a fasting plasma glucose level.

Type 2 diabetes (non–insulin-dependent DM) is the form that occurs most often in elderly people, and its prevalence is increasing dramatically. It is characterized by a fasting plasma glucose level of 126 mg/dl or greater, which must be confirmed on a subsequent day. Fasting means that there is no caloric intake for 8 hours before the test. At the time of diagnosis, a glycosylated hemoglobin (HbA_{1c}) should be drawn, which measures overall blood glucose for the past 60 to 120 days (Desai and Isa-Pratt, 2002). This test is then used to measure management of type 2 DM every 3 months of the year. The goal is an HbA_{1c} less than 7%. It is extremely important to diagnose DM as early as possible because it is believed that the pathology that occurs with diabetes occurs long before the clinical onset of symptoms.

Urine glucose testing is commonly done. However, there is not a good correlation between serum glucose and urine glucose concentrations (Desai and Isa-Pratt, 2002). In some patients, glucose spills into the urine even when plasma glucose is normal. There is great individual variability. It is not advised to use urine glucose levels to manage diabetes, but rather plasma glucose levels. Therapeutic targets for plasma glucose are 80 to 120 mg/dl for premeal glucose and 100 to 140 mg/dl at bedtime.

Creatine Kinase

Data on age-related laboratory values are important tools for nurses who are caring for elderly patients. Creatine kinase (CK) values are especially important in aiding the diagnosis of myocardial infarction (MI), myocardial muscle injury, unstable angina, shock, malignant hyperthermia, myopathies, and myocarditis (Pagana and Pagana, 2001). After an MI, the CK-MB, specific for myocardial cells, rises 3 to 6 hours after infarction occurs. It peaks at 12 to 24 hours (unless the infarction extends) and returns to normal after 12 to 48 hours. Drugs that can cause elevation of CK-MB are anticoagulants, aspirin, clofibrate, dexamethasone, furosemide, captopril, colchicine, alcohol, lovastatin, lidocaine, propranolol, and morphine. Clinical presentation of an MI in elderly people is often atypical, with nausea, weakness, dyspnea, diaphoresis, and palpitations (Cotter and Strumpf, 2002). In a suspected MI, myoglobin level should be determined. Myoglobin is the first protein released when myocardial cells are injured and can be detected 1 to 4 hours after symptoms begin.

Troponin

This is the most specific of the cardiac markers available. Troponin I and troponin T are levels useful in diagnosing myocardial damage. These can be drawn 3 hours after onset of chest pain. Levels peak 24 to 48 hours after the event and remain elevated for 2 weeks after the acute event (Desai and Isa-Pratt, 2002). Troponin I replaces the use of LDH levels.

Alkaline Phosphatase

An important enzyme test for aiding diagnosis and identifying liver and bone disease is the serum alkaline phosphatase (ALP). ALP gradually increases with age in both men and women. The increase is more marked in women (see Table 5-1) but may be abnormally high in 6% of well adults (Fitzgerald, 2000). Increases may be related to extrahepatic sources such as renal insufficiency, bone disorders, malabsorption, statin use, improper specimen handling, intestinal mucosa disturbances, heavy alcohol consumption, systemic infection, pancreatitis, and neoplasms. Food ingestion can cause an increase in ALP and should be drawn fasting. In patients with blood groups B and O, this can last up to 12 hours (Desai and Isa-Pratt, 2002). ALP is higher in African American men (15%) and higher in African American women (10%). It is also higher in smokers (10%). The level of 5′-nucleotidase, which is specific for the hepatobiliary tree, should be determined to differentiate it from other sources. Low ALP levels occur with hypothyroidism, pernicious anemia, hypophosphatemia, and medications such as estrogens, theophylline, clofibrate, and alendronate.

Alanine Aminotransferase/Serum Glutamic Pyruvic Transaminase

Alanine aminotransferase/serum glutamic pyruvic transaminase (ALT; previously serum glutamate pyruvate transaminase [SGPT]) is found mainly in the liver and is a specific and sensitive index of acute hepatocellular injury. ALT is also present in the kidney, heart, and skeletal muscles; the release of this enzyme indicates tissue injury.

Aspartate Aminotransferase

Aspartate aminotransferase (AST; previously serum glutamic-oxaloacetic transaminase [SGOT]) is found primarily in heart and skeletal muscle, liver, kidney, pancreas, and red blood cells. Increased levels indicate cellular damage or myocardial infarction, hepatitis, liver necrosis, and skeletal muscle damage.

Laboratory values for LDH, ALT, and AST may significantly change with normal aging, although additional research is needed in this area. Values of these enzymes are used to determine the functional status of the organs mentioned and the presence of disease. All three of these enzyme levels may need to be appraised to determine the nature of a problem and to rule out hepatic origin of the enzymes.

Serum Albumin

Lower serum albumin occurs in older adults compared with children. It is a measure of liver function, and with liver damage the serum albumin is greatly reduced. Serum albumin and globulin are measures of nutrition (Pagana and Pagana, 2001) and are reduced after surgery, in malnutrition, and in some protein-losing enteropathies. In some instances the albumin is selectively reduced with normal globulins. This occurs in collagen vascular diseases such as lupus erythematosus and also in chronic liver diseases. One must measure the albumin/globulin ratio to know this because total protein may be normal. Serum protein electrophoresis can further specify causation. Estrogens, hepatotoxic drugs, and ammonium ions cause decreased protein levels. Anabolic steroids, corticosteroids, dextran, insulin, phenazopyridine, and progesterone cause increased protein levels.

A low serum albumin level may be an indicator of malnutrition in the elderly. A serum albumin level of less than 3.5 g/dl is a criterion for justifying a diagnosis of malnutrition serious enough to qualify for Medicare or Medicaid reimbursement. However, a normal or increased serum albumin level alone does not ensure the nutritional adequacy of an older adult. Drawing a serum prealbumin is a marker for nutritional status. The half-life is 2 to 3 days and responds to current and recent nutritional imbalance. Prealbumin responds to infection, inflammation, and other stress, but not to malnutrition itself. Lymphocytes may be diminished with malnutrition, but they are decreased in other pathologic processes and are not specific. A thorough nutritional screening, along with laboratory values, is essential for assessing the nutritional status of an elder.

Pressure ulcer development and low serum albumin levels have been positively correlated (Cotter and Strumpf, 2002). A diet deficient in protein places the older adult at risk for pressure ulcers, wound infection, and delayed healing. The elderly who have stage II, III, or IV pressure ulcers should have albumin levels monitored routinely to determine effectiveness of the dietary and nursing care therapeutic regimen.

Cholesterol

Cholesterol levels are increased with age in both men and women (Beers and Berkow, 2000). Women have higher levels of HDL (the so-called good lipids) in all age-groups. With changes in lipid metabolism, cholesterol rises to a maximum at age 65 and then decreases, but never to a level as low as that of young adults. Total cholesterol is a measure of coronary risk, although almost half of the people who suffer myocardial infarcts have a total cholesterol level of 200 mg/dl or less. Fractionation into the dominant fractions HDL, LDL, and very-low-density lipoprotein (VLDL) yield more accurate and sophisticated indices of risk factors that can be monitored and quantitated during therapy. The LDL and HDL fractions, in combination with systolic blood pressure, are significant in predicting coronary disease risk in the elderly. These levels are used as indicators of risk and may be decreased by diet and exercise. The purpose of cholesterol screening (every 5 years in those over 65 years of age) is to identify those at risk for coronary heart disease (Pagana and Pagana, 2001). It is done with lipid profiling, because cholesterol alone is not a very accurate predictor, but with triglycerides and lipoproteins it is a good predictor. If the cholesterol is high, it should be repeated and averaged. Drugs that increase cholesterol include adrenocorticotropic hormone, anabolic steroids, beta-adrenergic blocking agents, corticosteroids, phenytoin, sulfonamides, thiazides, and vitamin D. Drugs that decrease serum cholesterol levels include allopurinol, androgens, bile salt binding agents, captopril, chlorpropamide, clofibrate, colchicine, erythromycin, isoniazid, lovastatin, monoamine oxidase (MAO) inhibitors, neomycin (taken orally), niacin, and nitrates. Low serum cholesterol is indicative of severe liver disease or malnutrition. However, suffering an acute MI can account for a 50% reduction in serum cholesterol. A cholesterol level below 160 mg/dl in a frail elder is a risk factor for increased mortality (Johnson, 2002).

For some time, it has been debated regarding the importance, or even the advisability, of pharmacologic intervention in hypercholesterolemia for individuals over 70 years old. Primary prevention studies have not demonstrated a decrease in mortality rate with interventions (Beers and Berkow, 2000). However, the American Geriatric Society suggests treating older adults with overt atherosclerosis, angina, previous MI, transient ischemic attack, or previous stroke, and considering it for those without overt risk factors (Reuben et al, 2002).

Triglycerides

Triglyceride values gradually increase with age until about middle age, when, for women, estrogen production diminishes. The increase is greater in women than in men after age 50. As men age, values stay elevated or drop slightly. With age, women have significantly higher levels than younger females. Abnormal triglyceride levels may indicate obesity, alcohol abuse, or estrogen use; these should be considered when determining a course of action. Treatment includes weight loss, decreasing alcohol intake, avoiding estrogens, and reducing intake of total fats, saturated fats, and dietary sugars (Beers and Berkow, 2000). Elevated triglyceride levels may lead to premature coronary artery disease and pancreatitis.

Calcium

Calcium levels decline with age. This may be due to decreased daily intake of calcium-containing products, lower serum albumin levels, and decreased intake of vitamin D or activation of vitamin D. This vitamin is known to be frequently deficient in the healthy aged and most particularly in the institutionalized aged. Factors such as reduced exposure to sunlight, decrease in production from liver disease or chronic renal failure, or use of anticonvulsants may contribute to this deficiency. Calcium may be reduced as a result of increased elimination from loop diuretics (Beers and Berkow, 2000) or reduced absorption. Low calcium levels are common in chronically ill elderly patients; however, when serum calcium is corrected using a standard formula, it is normal (9 to 11 mg/dl). The formula is to add 0.8 mg/dl to the total calcium concentration for each 1 g/dl decrease in albumin below its normal concentration of 4 g/dl. When the patient has true hypocalcemia, causes include hypoparathyroidism, hypomagnesemia (common), vitamin D deficiency, acute pancreatitis, or malignancy. Medications that cause hypocalcemia include calcitonin, bisphosphonates, phenobarbital, fluoride, and radiographic contrast dyes (Desai and Isa-Pratt, 2002).

Hypercalcemia can result from dehydration. True hypercalcemia may be caused by hyperparathyroidism, lithium therapy, malignancy, vitamin A or D intoxication, hyperthyroidism, granulomatous diseases, immobilization, and drugs such as thiazides and theophylline (Desai and Isa-Pratt, 2002). Mild hypercalcemia is asymptomatic and easily detected. Related abnormalities include hypertension, muscular weakness, irritability, GI disturbances, renal colic, bone cysts, polyuria, and diminished bone mass (Beers and Berkow, 2000).

Uric Acid

Uric acid levels are known to increase with aging, beginning in middle age (40s to 50s in men and 60s in women). Males, at all ages, have higher uric acid levels than females but have a less dramatic increase as they age. The upper limit of reference values for adults is 7 mg/dl, which is when gout symptoms begin to occur; however, the upper limit may be higher in elderly people. Most people who have elevated uric acid levels never have symptoms, but 30% of those who have an acute attack have normal uric acid levels (Desai and Isa-Pratt, 2002).

Thiazide diuretics are the most common cause of increased uric acid levels in older adults. Obesity, alcohol ingestion, and infections have all been associated with significant elevations in uric acid. Gout is the formation of needle-like monosodium urate crystals in joint synovial fluid. These crystals cause inflammation and discomfort and if not treated will greatly incapacitate the older person. Environmental stressors such as trauma, fatigue, cold, and surgery have been associated with acute attacks of gout. Dietary indulgences in protein foods that contain glutamic acid must also be considered. Gout becomes a chronic and painful condition in the aged.

Prostate-Specific Antigen

Prostate cancer is the most common type of cancer found in men. Rare in men younger than 50, it has a median age of onset of 72 years and is more prevalent in African American men compared with whites (Cotter and Strumpf, 2002).

The primary screening tools are digital rectal examination (DRE) and prostate-specific antigen (PSA). The PSA value increases with increasing age, with a reference range that varies with age and race. Asians have the lowest levels at all ages, then African Americans, and whites have the highest normal levels. Using adjusted levels helps make the test more sensitive. However, controversy continues over the value of this screen because studies do not show a decease in mortality rate when using it (Desai and Isa-Pratt, 2002). The upper limit of normal for PSA is 4 ng/ml; however, 20% to 30% of affected men have normal PSA values. There are a number of causes of increased levels of PSA in addition to prostate cancer, including infection, physical activity, DRE, benign prostatic hyperplasia, and ejaculation within 1 day of the laboratory test.

RENAL TESTS

Kidney function decreases substantially with age (Beers and Berkow, 2000). A decrease in glomerular filtration rates occurs with aging and is the most important functional defect caused by aging; however, about one third of elders do not have this decrease. Blood urea nitrogen (BUN) and creatinine are relatively unchanged with aging, although elderly patients may have a higher BUN (Pagana and Pagana, 2001) and women have a normal lower creatinine (Desai and Isa-Pratt, 2002). BUN and serum creatinine levels are both related to renal function and glomerular filtration rate. Dietary intake of protein, metabolism, and previous physical activity contribute to the increase in these values along with reduction in lean body mass. Because serum creatinine levels can overestimate renal function in the elderly, serum creatinine values must be related to the creatinine clearance values for a true assessment of renal function.

Many factors can interfere with these levels. Protein intake affects BUN, and many drugs increase the levels. Some are allopurinol, aminoglycosides, cephalosporins, furosemide, methotrexate, aspirin, bacitracin, gentamicin, carbamazepine, probenecid, corticosteroids, propranolol, thiazides, and tetracyclines (Pagana and Pagana, 2001).

The Cockcroft-Gault equation was developed to estimate creatinine clearance using the serum creatinine value. This is frequently used by clinicians in estimating doses when prescribing drugs for elders with probable diminished renal function (Desai and Isa-Pratt, 2002). It replaces obtaining a 24-hour urine collection for creatinine clearance, which is difficult to do, especially in frail elders. The formula is

$$\frac{(140 - \text{Age}) \times \text{Weight in kg}}{(72 \times \text{Serum creatinine})}$$

In women, multiply the value obtained by 0.85.

Urine

Urine is the fluid that carries waste products from the body as they are filtered from the blood through the kidneys. There are many changes in the kidneys with aging. By age 80 they have shrunk 20% with major loss (30%) of glomeruli that filter urine. Renal blood flow diminishes. With age, there is a diminished capacity to conserve salts and increased antidiuretic hormone (ADH) but decreased responsiveness to ADH. Renin and aldosterone decrease production (30% to 50%) with age, and there is diminished ability to concentrate and conserve water. With all these changes, "old" kidneys do not respond to stress (such as surgery, fever, or disease) as well as when they were "young." Elders are susceptible to fluid and electrolyte imbalances. Table 5-3 summarizes normal values and their clinical significance.

Urinalysis

Most urinalysis values do not change with advancing age but may reflect the chronic diseases so common in older adults. Urine color and clarity and odor are important to note (Desai and Isa-Pratt, 2002). Colorless urine may be the result of large fluid intake. Dark urine often is the result of poor fluid intake, common in elderly people. A microscopic examination should be done on any turbid urine specimen; turbidity is often due to *phosphaturia,* phosphate crystals in alkaline urine, which is benign and occurs after a high-protein meal. However, another reason for cloudy and turbid urine is *pyuria,* infected urine. The odor is pungent rather than the normal, slightly ammonia smell.

Table 5-3 Urinalysis: A Summary of Normal Values and Their Clinical Significance in the Elderly

Determination	Normal value	Clinical significance
Macroscopic analysis		
Color	Pale yellow to dark amber	Very pale: diabetes insipidus, excess fluid intake, chronic renal disease, nervousness Very amber: dehydration. Note: medications may alter color
Appearance	Clear to slightly hazy	Cloudy, turbid: presence of bacteria, WBCs or RBCs
Odor	Faintly aromatic	Fetid odor: bacterial infection Ammonia: urea breakdown by bacteria
Specific gravity	1.017-1.028	Decreased: overhydration; diabetes insipidus; diet (NA, restriction) Elevated ↓ fluid intake; fever; diabetes mellitus. ◆ Note: lower maximum value in the elderly
pH	4.5-8.0	>8.0: bacterial infection due to *Pseudomonas* or *Proteus,* chronic renal failure <4 metabolic/respiratory acidosis, starvation
Protein	Negative	Increased: renal disease, cardiac failure, febrile states, hematuria, amyloidosis
Glucose	Negative	Positive: uncontrolled diabetes mellitus; pituitary disorders; ↑ intracranial pressure Renal threshold for glucose rises after age 50, ♀ > ♂
Ketones	Negative	Positive: uncontrolled diabetes mellitus; prolonged vomiting; fasting
Blood	Negative	Positive: infection, renal calculus
Bilirubin	Negative	Positive: liver dysfunction
Nitrite	Negative	Positive: bacterial infection
Leukocyte esterase	Negative	Positive: pyuria
Microscopic analysis		
RBSs	Rare per high-power field	Increased: renal genitourinary disorders
WBCs	0-4 per high-power field	Increased: bacterial infection ◆ Not always a reliable indicator of infection in the elderly; if clinically asymptomatic, is not significant
Epithelial cells	0-3	Increased: probable perineal contamination
Casts	Rare per high-power field	Increased: renal disease
Bacteria	<105 colonies/ml	Increased: bacterial infection ◆ Significance is dependent on specimen collectior technique and specific gravity of sample

From Brazier AM, Palmer MH: Collecting clean-catch urine in the nursing home: obtaining the uncontaminated specimen, *Geriatr Nurs* 16(5):217, 1995.

Specific gravity is a simple test that measures the density of urine relative to the density of water. Urine is 95% water. This test is helpful in determining the adequacy of the renal concentrative mechanism; it measure hydration (Desai and Isa-Pratt, 2002). Specific gravity declines to 1.024 by age 80. This decline has been related to the 33% to 50% decline in the number of nephrons, which impairs the ability of the kidney to concentrate urine. Lower maximum values for specific gravity should be evaluated and a low-sodium, protein-restricted diet instituted when necessary, or the use of diuretics may need to be considered. The limitations of specific gravity testing must be considered when using this test as a diagnostic tool.

The pH indicates acid-base balance of the patient. An alkaline pH is caused by bacteria with urinary tract infections, a diet high in citrus fruits and vegetables, or taking sodium bicarbonates. Acidic urine occurs with starvation, dehydration, and diets high in meats and cranberries.

Protein is a sensitive indicator of kidney function. It is normally not present in urine except perhaps in trace amounts in concentrated urine. In dilute urine, it is pathologic and should always be considered with the specific gravity of the urine. Ketones, blood, and glucose should all remain negative at any age. Ascorbic acid and aspirin can cause false-negative results for glucose. Ketones may be positive in high protein diets, "crash" diets, or starvation. Gross blood is never normal in urine; white blood cells are normal (0 to 5 per high-power field), but an increase suggests an inflammatory process (Desai and Isa-Pratt, 2002).

Creatinine Clearance

Creatinine clearance is a urine test used to estimate glomerular filtration rate (GFR) as an indicator of glomerular function. This test is a more reliable measure of renal function than BUN or serum creatinine. Because urine collection can be a problem with the elderly person and a complete and timed collection is essential for accuracy of this test, catheterization often may be necessary. However, it is possible to estimate the creatinine clearance using the Cockcroft-Gault formula. The average creatinine clearance excretion rate declines from about 24 mg/kg per 24 hours in persons 18 to 29 years of age to about 12 mg/kg per 24 hours in those 80 to 90 years of age.

Bacteriuria

Both older men and women are subject to bacteriuria, the presence of bacteria in the urine. Infection increases because of diminished defenses of the body resulting in less phagocytosis of bacteria. Cystitis is common in older men and institutionalized elders (10% to 30% rate of infection) (Malone et al, 2000). Men should be evaluated for prostate enlargement and tenderness. Women should be evaluated for vaginal discharge or erythema. Typical signs and symptoms of urinary tract infection such as incontinence, urgency, frequency, fever, flank pain, or suprapubic pain may not occur in the elderly population. Confusion is often a sign of a urinary tract infection. Urinalysis is an imperative screening test.

Obtaining the clean-catch or midstream urine specimen for culture and sensitivity is often difficult in elderly patients. Contamination is common from hands, vaginal secretions, stool, or clothing (Pagana and Pagana, 2001). Catheterization may be necessary to obtain the specimen; however, this is uncomfortable and may introduce organisms. If the patient has an indwelling catheter, the specimen is obtained by inserting a 25-gauge needle into a distal point from the balloon and aspirating. The specimen should be sent to the laboratory immediately, or it may be refrigerated for up to 2 hours. A specimen with greater than 100,000 bacteria per milliliter of urine is positive and will be cultured; sensitivities are obtained to determine appropriate antibiotics to be administered.

ELECTROLYTES

The elderly are susceptible to electrolyte imbalances because of medications and poor fluid intake. Dehydration is the most common fluid and electrolyte disturbance of older adults. One of the most significant electrolyte disturbances is the potassium level, which decreases with aging so that hypokalemia is common.

Dehydration

Nurses need to help prevent dehydration by monitoring fluid balance in elderly patients (Beers and Berkow, 2000). Dehydration occurs from decreased fluid intake, fever, hot environment, polyuria, diuretic use, vomiting, diarrhea, orthopedic impairment, diabetes, and renal disease. Elders have a diminished thirst response and may be unaware of dehydration.

The percentage of body fluids decreases in elders, from 60% of body weight to 50%. Dehydration is diagnosed clinically and with laboratory data. Mild dehydration is less than 5% loss of body weight; moderate dehydration is 10% loss of body weight; and severe dehydration is greater than 15% loss of body weight. Clinically, there is altered mental status, lethargy, and syncope (Beers and Berkow, 2000). There will be dry mucous membranes, decreased turgor of skin, and tachycardia, although these may occur in elders with normal volumes. Laboratory values affected by volume depletion are the hematocrit, BUN, and creatinine, all of which are increased. The BUN/creatinine ratio may be increased because slow urine flow allows reabsorption of urea, but not creatinine. The urinary sodium level may be increased more than 20 mEq/L with volume depletion.

Potassium

Potassium (K) is the electrolyte in highest concentration within cells and is the chief intracellular cation. Serum potassium levels decrease as lean body mass decreases, because most potassium (75%) is stored in lean body mass (Beers and Berkow, 2000). Serum potassium may not reflect potassium body stores.

Hypokalemia. Hypokalemia is important to recognize in elderly patients because it is associated with cardiac arrhythmias and may cause glucose intolerance and renal tubular dysfunction. Mild hypokalemia is asymptomatic. Severe hypokalemia (less than 2.5 mEq/L) produces muscle weakness, cramping, confusion, fatigue, adynamic ileus, atrial and ventricular ectopy and tachycardia, fibrillation, and sudden death (Beers and Berkow, 2000). The electrocardiogram (ECG) will demonstrate a characteristic response to hypokalemia. Chronic hypokalemia may lead to significant renal tubular dysfunction. Some of the many causes or risk factors for low K levels include low K intake, pernicious anemia therapy, leukemias and lymphomas, parenteral nutrition, increased catecholamine release such as myocardial infarction, head trauma, delirium tremens, hypothermia, and GI losses through vomiting and diarrhea. Excessive exercise in a hot environment may cause hypokalemia, as can diuretic therapy and many renal disturbances associated with hypertension (Desai and Isa-Pratt, 2002). In a susceptible individual with borderline K levels, the blood should be drawn regularly, especially if some of the risk factors are present.

Hyperkalemia. Hyperkalemia (greater than 5 mEq/L) is most commonly exhibited by a shift of potassium (K) from the intracellular to the extracellular compartment, which increases the plasma concentration while body stores may be normal or low (Beers and Berkow, 2000). It may also be caused by decreased renal excretion of K (Desai and Isa-Pratt, 2002). Common causes of hyperkalemia in the elderly patient include the concurrent use of potassium-sparing diuretics with prescribed potassium supplements, excessive K intake in the presence of acute or chronic renal failure, hyperglycemia, nonsteroidal antiinflammatory drugs (NSAIDs), angiotensin-converting enzyme (ACE) inhibitors, and beta-blocking drugs. High K may be asymptomatic until cardiac toxicity occurs (Beers and Berkow, 2000). Characteristic ECG changes indicate the problem. It causes ventricular arrhythmias, vague weakness, paresthesias, flaccid paralysis, ventricular fibrillation, and asystole. For more specific causes and clinical manifestations of hypokalemia and hyperkalemia, see Boxes 5-1 and 5-2.

Sodium/Hyponatremia

Aging is associated with impaired water conservation and sodium balance (Beers and Berkow, 2000). Sodium balance is further influenced by renal filtration and blood flow, cardiac output, blood pressure, and GFR. Serum sodium (Na) concentration is determined mainly by body water balance.

Box 5-1

Causes of Hypokalemia and Hyperkalemia

Hypokalemia	Hyperkalemia
Intake	
Decreased intake Increased secretions	Increased intake or intravenous administration
Gastrointestinal Losses	
Vomiting Diarrhea or repeated enemas Pyloric and other forms of intestinal obstruction Biliary or gastrointestinal fistulas Suction or tube drainage Laxative use	Active gastrointestinal bleeding
Renal Losses	
Increased loss Renal tubular acidosis (proximal & distal) Thiazide diuretic use Loop diuretic use (furosemide, bumetanide, ethacrynic acid) Antibiotic use (gentamycin, penicillins, amphotericin B) Secondary hyperaldosteronism (heart failure, cirrhosis) Cushing's syndrome Exogenous glucocorticoids/mineralocorticoids Hyperreninemic renovascular hypertension Postobstructive diuresis Chronic renal insufficiency	*Decreased excretion* Acute renal disease Dyrenium diuretic therapy (triamterene) Spironolactone therapy Adrenal insufficiency ACE inhibitors β-Adrenergic blockers NSAIDs Tetracycline
Transcellular Shifts	
Alkalosis Insulin administration	Metabolic acidosis Hyponatremia (potassium moves out of cell to replace sodium) Anorexia
Hemotologic Disorders	
Vitamin B_{12} treatment of megaloblastic anemia Acute myeloid leukemia	
Miscellaneous	
Acidosis of any cause Trauma or burns with tissue breakdown Intravenous administration of potassium-free liquid	

Adapted from Collins R: *Fluid and electrolyte disorders*, Philadelphia, 1976, Lippincott; Miller M: Water and electrolyte disorders. In Abrams WB, Beers MH, Berkow R, editors: *The Merck manual of geriatrics*, ed 2, Whitehouse Station, NJ, 1995, Merck Research Laboratories.

Hyponatremia occurs with excessive water retention; hypernatremia occurs with excessive water loss.

There is an age-related decrease in serum sodium concentration, but it produces no apparent symptoms (Beers and Berkow, 2000). The most common cause of hyponatremia in elderly people is dilutional; it is the most severe cause in that it results in the highest morbidity and mortality rates. A common cause is the taking of nutritional supplements such as Ensure, Osmolite, and Isocal, which are all low in sodium. Occasionally, intravenous administration of hypotonic fluids causes low Na. Other causes include hyperglycemia, GI fluid loss via nausea and vomiting, excessive sweating, pancreatitis, bowel obstruction, thiazide diuretic therapy, syndrome of inappropriate antidiuretic hormone (SIADH), hypothyroidism, tea-and-toast diets, congestive failure, cirrhosis, and acute and chronic renal failure (Desai and Isa-Pratt, 2002).

Hyponatremia is one of the most common causes of delirium in older adults. When severe, there will be diminished DTRs; hypothermia; Cheyne-Stokes respirations; pathologic reflexes; and a depressed sensorium, coma, or seizures. A hypertonic sodium solution should be carefully infused in severe cases, or sometimes 0.9% sodium chloride is given

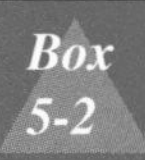

Box 5-2 Clinical Manifestations of Hypokalemia and Hyperkalemia

Hypokalemia	Hyperkalemia
Generalized muscle weakness	Impaired muscle activity
Fatigue	Weakness
Diminished or absent reflexes	Muscle pain/cramps
Decreased GI motility	Increased GI motility
Anorexia	Nausea
Abdominal distention	Diarrhea
Paralytic ileus	Intestinal colic
Vomiting	Oliguria
Hypotension	Dizziness
Dysrhythmias	Bradycardia
Weak pulse	Irritability
Shallow respirations	ECG changes:
Shortness of breath	P wave flattened
Apathy	T wave large, peaked
Drowsiness	QRS broad
Irritability	
Tentany	
Coma	
ECG changes:	
QT interval prolonged	
T wave flattened or depressed	
ST segment depressed	

Modified from Miller M: Water and electrolyte disorders. In Abrams WB, Beers MH, Berkow R, editors: *The Merck manual of geriatrics*, Whitehouse Station, NJ, 1995, Merck Research Laboratories; Clark JM: Endocrine clinical assessment and diagnostic procedures. In Thelan LA, Davie JK, Urden LD, Lough ME: *Critical care nursing diagnosis and management*, ed 2, St Louis, 1994, Mosby.

concomitantly with furosemide for a gentle correction (Beers and Berkow, 2000). In milder hyponatremia, such as that caused by nutritional supplements, an increase in salt intake is suggested.

Hypernatremia

Hypernatremia is an elevation of plasma sodium (greater than 146 mEq/L) that is caused by a deficit of water relative to solute. There is excessive loss of water without concurrent loss of sodium. This is a problem in up to 2% of older adults in hospital and long-term care facilities (Desai and Isa-Pratt, 2002). Low body weight is a risk factor. The mortality rate for this is 40% in hospitalized elders, especially if it occurs quickly. The sodium level will be greater than 160 mEq/L if this occurs. Moderately high Na may cause weakness and lethargy. Signs of water loss such as diminished skin turgor, dry mucous membranes, and orthostatic hypotension will not be present. Severely high Na (greater than 152 mEq/L) may cause hemiparesis, stupor or coma, and seizures. There is a continuing functional decline in elders who survive an episode of hypernatremia (Beers and Berkow, 2000). Laboratory findings include high serum sodium and increased hematocrit, BUN, and creatinine. Serum osmolality may not be increased because of the impaired ability to concentrate urine that occurs with advancing age. Treatment is replacement of water deficits with hypotonic fluid slowly over 48 hours. The "rule of sevens" applies in estimating the deficit: for every 10 mEq/L the serum sodium is elevated, a 7% deficit of total body water exists (Beers and Berkow, 2000).

Acid-Base Metabolism

Normal pH does not increase with age. There are age-related changes that affect the response in maintaining the normal pH (Beers and Berkow, 2000). Where a younger person may hyperventilate when challenged with metabolic acidosis, the elderly person's response may be blunted, allowing the condition to deteriorate. Many common problems that occur in older age contribute to acid-base disturbances. Some are heart failure, anemia, diabetes, pulmonary disease, renal disease, and sepsis. Many drugs also contribute, such as salicylates, diuretics, and laxatives. This combination makes acid-base problems common in older adults.

LONG-TERM CARE

Admission laboratory tests and regular screening tests are commonly employed when caring for a nursing home resident. Laboratory tests are often viewed positively by both nurses and physicians in long-term care because they are a fast and accurate way to assess the older person's physical status. Older adults and their families view the tests as factual presentations of their conditions. Protocols for establishing routine laboratory testing procedures for long-term care vary widely from one institution to the next. Nurses advocate good resident care by ordering laboratory tests or by encouraging physicians to order and develop protocols to comply with recommended minimal standards for screening and monitoring laboratory tests for elderly residents in long-term care institutions.

The American Geriatric Society has a list of primary prevention and secondary prevention screens (Reuben et al, 2002). The following should be done at least annually: blood pressure, diabetes screen, influenza immunization, obesity, height and weight, hearing impairment screen, skin examination, mammography, vision screen, cognitive impairment screen, PSA and DRE, and TSH. Smoking cessation should be discussed at every visit, breast self-examination should be performed monthly, and pneumonia immunization should be given once at age 65 with consideration of repeating every 6 to 7 years. Bone densitometry and other osteoporosis testing should be done often enough to prevent deterioration. Tetanus immunization should be done every 10 years.

Dementia is a widespread problem in long-term care. Laboratory investigation can reveal the cause of reversible dementia. Recommended laboratory tests for screening elders with dementia include urinary assay, CBC, electrolytes, tests for liver and kidney function, BUN, syphilis serology, thyroid function tests, chest x-ray, calcium and phosphorous, serum B_{12}, and folate. Additional tests should be considered when conditions warrant.

Poor dietary intake continues to be a significant problem in long-term care institutions. Protein-calorie malnutrition is a major medical problem for long-term care residents and hospitalized elders. Because vitamin deficiency testing is expensive, multivitamins should probably be given to any elder suspected of having poor nutrition. Other tests described earlier in the chapter will help elucidate nutrition problems. Albumin and globulin levels, albumin/globulin ratios, prealbumin, vitamin B_{12}, and folate levels are examples of some tests to order.

Older adults in long-term care institutions may be seen by a nurse practitioner or physician infrequently but are monitored daily by nursing staff. It is therefore imperative that the bedside nurse be knowledgeable about the importance of routine and specific laboratory tests when vague and atypical signs and symptoms of disease arise.

SPECIMEN COLLECTION

Nurses in long-term care, home care, and hospitals are responsible for obtaining many laboratory specimens. The importance of meticulous specimen collection cannot be overemphasized if accurate laboratory results are to be derived.

The most important step in specimen collection is identification. Institutionalized elders should be identified by full name, and identification bands should be matched to requisition orders. Even if the nurse is familiar with the elder, the verification process must not be skipped. Obtaining a specimen from the wrong person can have serious and even fatal results. Standard precautions must be observed throughout the specimen collection process.

Phlebotomy

The main purpose of phlebotomy is to collect blood for diagnostic testing to assist physicians in establishing the cause and nature of illness. Many nurses perform phlebotomy procedures, especially in home care, acute care hospitals, health maintenance organization (HMO) clinics, and physicians' offices. This cost-containment strategy is particularly helpful to the elder in the home with limited mobility and lack of transportation to outpatient laboratory facilities.

Venipuncture involves collecting blood by penetrating a vein with a needle and syringe or an adapter with attached needle and vacuum tube. Most elders tolerate the phlebotomy process with little or no difficulty. Some people become faint at the thought of having blood drawn. There is no way to predict how someone will react to a venipuncture except to ask how the patient has responded in past procedures. Always have the individual sitting or lying down before performing the procedure. There may be complications associated with the phlebotomy procedure. Some complications, such as bruising and hematoma, may be unavoidable. Most complications can be minimized by proper collection technique and knowledge. The nurse performing the phlebotomy procedure should be aware of the seven precautions listed in Box 5-3.

Box 5-3 Phlebotomy Collection Guidelines

Never draw above an intravenous (IV) or indwelling line. There is no exception to this rule. If this is not observed, the specimens will be contaminated with IV fluid, causing erroneous results.

Do not try to obtain a specimen from a damaged or sclerosed vein. These veins are hard, and no specimen can be obtained.

Hematomas are caused by leaking from the vein underneath the skin. If this occurs, release the tourniquet and needle and apply pressure to the site. Never restick the hematoma area.

Edema is caused by abnormal accumulation of fluid in the intracellular spaces, which may be localized or diffused over a large area. Do not stick this area because specimens may be contaminated with tissue fluid.

Do not attempt a venipuncture in an area of a burn or scar. Burns are sensitive and susceptible to infections.

If the patient exhibits petechiae, which are small red spots on the skin, this should alert the nurse that this person has the potential for bleeding problems and special attention should be given to the puncture site.

Reflex sympathetic dystrophy (RSD) is a complication that can occur as a result of injury to a peripheral nerve during the venipuncture/arterial puncture procedure. The patient experiences severe pain, swelling, vasomotor instability, and sweating. This is a severe complication, and a physician should be notified immediately.

Some venipuncture specimens need to be placed on ice after collection; others need to be kept warm. There may also be a time requirement for delivery to the laboratory. Current policies, procedures, ongoing inservice training, and skills verification are necessary for nurses to be competent in obtaining laboratory specimens. The nurse should be familiar with the specimen requirements before performing the procedure.

Clean-Catch Urine Specimens

Obtaining uncontaminated urine specimens from frail, often incontinent, elders in nursing homes is a difficult task. Their ability to move about and their ability to control urine flow are often impaired. Some instructions for obtaining urine specimens in these situations is detailed in Tables 5-4 and 5-5.

In summary, nurses are in a primary position to note and interpret laboratory values. The aged person's changing laboratory values reflect normal aging, as well as disease states. This presents a challenge for the nurse to make valid interpretations of the changing status of the older individual. The importance of laboratory testing cannot be overemphasized. Laboratory testing can be the major factor in supporting or disproving diagnoses. Many of the age-related laboratory changes are fractional. However, the clinical impact cannot be minimized.

Reference values for the aged are imperative before laboratory test results can guide treatment in the elderly person. The variance of values at both ends of the laboratory range could be misinterpreted as abnormal or questionable when they are within normal range for that sex and age-group. The "normal ranges" in the population over 65 years are often different from those of the younger population, and these differences should be and are slowly being established so that we have standards to indicate real pathologic age-related differences (Boxes 5-4 and 5-5). We must not compare those patients over 65 years with those between 20 and 50 years,

Table 5-4 Technique for Obtaining Clean-Catch Midstream Voided Specimen

A clean-catch midstream specimen is the best clinically effective method of securing a voided specimen for urinalysis. It is not a simple procedure and requires patient education and active assistance of the female patient.

Equipment

- Antiseptic solution or liquid soap solution
- Sterile water
- 4 × 4–inch sponges
- Disposable gloves for nurse assisting female patient
- Sterile specimen container

Procedure

Nursing action	Rationale/amplification
Male patient	
1. Instruct the patient to expose glans and cleanse area around the meatus. Wash area with mild antiseptic solution or liquid soap. Rinse thoroughly.	1. The urethral orifice is colonized by bacteria. Urine readily becomes contaminated during voiding. Rinse thoroughly because these agents can inhibit bacterial growth in a urine culture.
2. Allow the initial urinary flow to escape.	2. The first portion of urine washes out the urethra and contains debris.
3. Collect the midstream urine specimen in a sterile container.	3. The midstream sample reflects the status of the bladder.
4. Avoid collecting the last few drops of urine.	4. Prostatic secretions may be introduced into urine at the end of the urinary stream.
5. Send specimen to laboratory immediately.	5. A culture should be performed as soon as possible to avoid multiplication of urinary bacteria and lysis of cells.
Female patient	
1. Ask the patient to separate her labia to expose the urethral orifice. If no one is available to assist the patient, she may sit backward on the toilet seat facing the water tank or sit on (straddle) the wide part of the bedpan.	1. Keeping the labia separated prevents labial or vaginal contamination of the urine specimen. By straddling the toilet seat/bedpan, the patient's labia are spread apart for cleansing.
2. Cleanse the area around the urinary meatus with sponges soaked with antiseptic/soap solution. Rinse thoroughly. a. Wipe the perineum from the front to the back. b. Do not use sponges more than once.	2. The urethral orifice is colonized by bacteria. Urine is readily contaminated during voiding.
3. While the patient keeps the labia separated, instruct her to void forcibly.	3. This helps wash away urethral contaminants.
4. Allow initial urinary flow to drain into bedpan (toilet) and then catch the midstream specimen in a sterile container, make sure that the container does not come in contact with the genitalia.	4. The first portion of urine washes out the urethra. Have patient remove the container from the stream while she is still voiding.
5. Send the specimen to the laboratory immediately.	5. Too long an interval between collection and analysis causes contaminants to multiply in the urine and cells to lyse.

From Suddarth D, editor: *The Lippincott manual of nursing practice,* ed 5, Philadelphia, 1991, Lippincott; Brazier AM, Palmer MH: Collecting clean-catch urine in the nursing home: obtaining the uncontaminated specimen, *Geriatr Nurs* 16(5):217, 1995.

Table 5-5 Adaptations to the Standard Guidelines for Obtaining Clean-Catch Urine Specimen in Frail Elders

Tip	Advantage (rationale)
1. Know the patient's voiding habits by using a bladder log or by consulting the nursing assistant caring for the patient.	1. Decreases time spent in specimen collection.
2. Collect the specimen in the early morning (morning specimens are more concentrated).	2. Ensures accuracy of results.
3. Avoid collection after giving diuretics.	3. Ensures accuracy of results (alters concentration).
4. Perform perineal care on bedridden or incontinent patients before collection.	4. Decreases risk of contamination.
5. When possible, have patients void in the bathroom, sitting upright.	5. Decreases risk of contamination.
6. Use an assistant when the patient is physically impaired.	6. Decreases collection time and increases risks of contamination.
7. Hold the patient's labia apart throughout the procedure.	7. Decreases risk of contamination.
8. Use distractionary tactics with the confused or embarrassed patient (speak in calm voice, singing, involve patient in conversation, use assistance of a caregiver more familiar with the patient).	8. May decrease time spent in specimen collection. Facilitates patient cooperation.
9. Ensure good lighting in bathroom with a 75-watt bulb.	9. Increases visibility. Decreases risk of contamination.
10. Prompt resident to increase fluid intake.	10. Decreases time spent in specimen collection.
11. Use physical prompts (running water, spirit of wintergreen).	11. Decreases time spent in specimen collection.
12. Utilize a portable bladder scanner to determine bladder volume prior to specimen collection.	12. Decreases time spent in specimen collection.

From Brazier AM, Palmer MH: Collecting clean-catch urine in the nursing home: obtaining the uncontaminated specimen, *Geriatr Nurs* 16(5):217, 1995.

just as we should not compare infants with children or young adults. Each age-group must have its own established norms.

Laboratory values are helpful tools in understanding clinical signs and symptoms, although clinical decisions based on laboratory values alone are not enough for treatment of the elderly person. The nurse should perform a comprehensive baseline assessment of the older adult, obtaining information about clinical signs and symptoms, patient history, and psychosocial and physical assessments. The nurse synthesizes this information along with the interpretation of laboratory values to establish appropriate nursing care for the aged. This "building-block" approach to obtaining and synthesizing information about the older adult helps nurses and other health care professionals to provide quality care for the aged.

Box 5-4 Summary of Laboratory Values Unchanged with Age

Serum bilirubin
AST
ALT
Gamma-glutamyl transpeptidase (GGTP)
Prothrombin time (PT)
Partial thromboplastin time (PTT)
Serum electrolytes
Total protein
Calcium
Phosphorus
Serum folate
pH
$Paco_2$
Serum creatinine
T_4
RBC indices
Platelets

Modified from Cavalieri T, Chopra A, Bryman P: When outside the norm is normal: interpreting lab data in the aged, *Geriatrics* 47(5):66, 1992.

Box 5-5 Summary of Laboratory Values that Change with Age

Alkaline phosphatase (increase)
Serum albumin (decrease)
Uric acid (increase)
Total cholesterol (increase):
- HDL:
  - Male (increase)
  - Female (decrease)
- Triglycerides (increase)

Serum B_{12} (decrease)
Serum magnesium (decrease)
$Paco_2$ (decrease)
Creatinine clearance (decrease)
T_3 (decrease)
T_4 (increase)
Fasting blood sugar (increase)
1-Hour postprandial blood sugar (increase)
2-Hour postprandial blood sugar (increase)
WBC count (decrease)

Modified from Cavalieri T, Chopra A, Bryman P: When outside the norm is normal: interpreting lab data in the aged, *Geriatrics* 47(5):66, 1992.

KEY CONCEPTS

- The range of laboratory values that are considered normal and appear on laboratory reports usually does not make allowance for age differentials.
- The subtle changes in laboratory values that accompany subsets of aging, such as gender, young-old versus old-old, and ethnicity, have not been thoroughly studied.
- The tolerable variance in serum, enzyme, and cellular processes and changes that can occur without causing negative consequences becomes narrower the older one becomes.
- Medications and chronic disorders complicate the measurement of laboratory values in elders because most elders are taking several medications at any given time that may interact to alter the reliability of laboratory measurements.
- Some measurable deficiencies in elders may be due to consistently poor dietary patterns. These deficiencies, when serious, may produce dementia and confusion, mistakenly assumed to be irreversible.
- Thyroid disorders are so common in elders that thyroid screening of all elders is recommended, especially for women older than 50.
- The definitive diagnosis of diabetes in the aged cannot be accurately made based on decreased glucose tolerance.
- Creatinine kinase values are especially important in aiding the diagnosis of myocardial infarction in the aged.
- Cholesterol levels and their significance in those over 70 are being studied because it is not clear that reducing high cholesterol lowers mortality rates.
- Specific protocols and a panel of routine requirements for laboratory tests on admission to nursing homes have not been developed. It is urged that nurses become active in advocating for these.

▲ CASE STUDY

For several months following an episode of pneumonia, Helen had been experiencing disturbing symptoms such as mental clouding, anorexia, periodic episodes of weakness and unsteadiness of gait, general lethargy, hypertension, sensitivity to cold, and constipation. She was resigned to the inevitability of such problems because she remembered her mother had experienced similar problems in her later years. Helen said, "Oh, this is just part of getting old. Mother had these problems, too." Helen's daughters insisted that she be given a complete medical and laboratory workup, though her physician tended to agree with Helen and appeased her with platitudes about adjusting to aging. However, he recognized the daughters' concern and ordered a serum electrolyte and metabolic panel, T_4, CBC, and urinalysis. Helen was careful to follow directions regarding obtaining the laboratory specimens; even though she did not believe they were needed, she would agree that there was a problem if it was revealed through the laboratory tests. All were within normal limits as ordinarily expected for adults, with the exception of a slightly low serum thyroid hormone concentration (T_4) and an elevated TSH. The physician ordered 0.125 mg of L-thyroxine daily for Helen.

Based on the case study, develop a nursing care plan using the following procedure:

List comments of client that provide subjective data.

List information that provides objective data.

From these data identify and state, using accepted format, two nursing diagnoses you determine are most significant to this client at this time. List two client strengths that you have identified from the data.

Determine and state outcome criteria for each diagnosis. These must reflect some alleviation of the problem identified in the nursing diagnosis and must be stated in concrete and measurable terms.

Plan and state one or more interventions for each diagnosed problem.

Provide specific documentation of the source used to determine the appropriate intervention. Plan at least one intervention that incorporates the client's existing strengths.

Evaluate success of intervention. Interventions must correlate directly with the stated outcome criteria in order to measure the outcome success.

STUDY QUESTIONS/ACTIVITIES

Do you believe the physician was justified in ordering replacement thyroid hormone, or is the normal thyroid function reduced during aging?

Are there other laboratory tests that would further clarify Helen's condition, and do you believe they should have been done before prescribing L-thyroxine?

Did Helen's symptoms relate in any way to her recent bout with pneumonia?

Refer to a physiology book and list all the symptoms of hypothyroidism; determine which might be considered part of normal aging.

Discuss the meanings and the thoughts triggered by the student's and elder's viewpoints expressed at the beginning of the chapter. How do these vary from your own experience?

Discuss whether you believe mandatory human immunodeficiency virus (HIV) testing should be required for any elder living in a congregate setting.

Discuss how you would proceed with a phlebotomy in an elder's home.

RESEARCH QUESTIONS

What endocrine functions are normally altered as a consequence of aging?

What endocrine functions are altered in response to specific nonendocrine disease states?

What particular laboratory tests are indicative of endocrinopathy?

What differences in laboratory values are characteristic of aged men, and do these differ from those of women of the same age?

What percentage of health professionals are cognizant of the parameters of normal laboratory values for older adults and the variances from those of the young and middle-aged adult?

What is the number of specimens obtained in the client's home that are obtained without proper instruction or precautions?

REFERENCES

Beers MH, Berkow R: *Merck manual of geriatrics,* ed 3, Whitehouse Station, NJ, 2000, Merck Research Laboratories.

Brown JB, Bedford NK, White SJ: *Gerontological protocols for nurse practitioners,* Philadelphia, 1999, Lippincott.

Cotter V, Strumpf NE: *Advanced practice nursing with older adults,* New York, 2002, McGraw-Hill.

Desai SP, Isa-Pratt S: *Clinician's guide to laboratory medicine,* ed 2, Cleveland, 2002, Lexi-Comp.

Fitzgerald M: What are the reasons for an elevated alkaline phosphatase? Available at *www.medscape.com/Medscape/Nurses/AskExperts/2000/04/NP-ae15.html*

HealthandAge.com, American Geriatric Society: Laboratory values, 2000. Available at *www.healthandage.com/syllabus/aging/aging2/labor.htm*

Johnson LE: Nutrition. In Ham RS, Sloane P, Warshaw G, editors: *Primary care geriatrics*, ed 4, St Louis, 2002, Mosby.

Malone LK, Fletcher KR, Plank LM: *Management guidelines for gerontological nurse practitioners,* Philadelphia, 2000, FA Davis.

Pagana KD, Pagana TJ. *Mosby's diagnostic and laboratory test reference,* ed 5, St Louis, 2001, Mosby.

Reuben D et al: *Geriatrics at your fingertips,* Malden, MA, 2002, Blackwell Science.

Robbins J et al: Hematological and biochemical laboratory values in older cardiovascular health study participants, *J Am Geriatr Soc* 43(8):855, 1995.

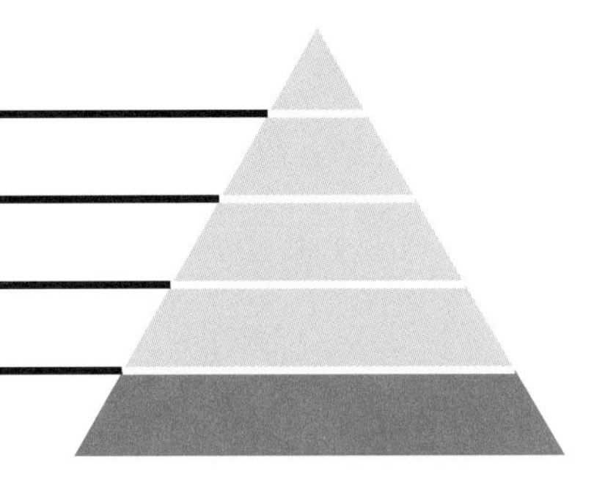

CHAPTER 6

Managing Basic Physiologic Needs

Ann Schmidt Luggen

An elder speaks

I began thinking how my own sleep patterns have changed. As an active young woman I needed a great deal of sleep. My husband marveled at my ability to sleep 9 and 10 hours a night. Sleep was never a problem unless my mind got locked in high gear over regrets or anticipated disagreeable projects. The mind whirled around getting nowhere like a squirrel in a cage. Instead of sheep I counted lists of people or tried to recall the sequence of events on a trip or in a novel. Still sleepless at 1 or 2 o'clock in the morning, I resorted to warm milk or hot cocoa with Tylenol or cheese and crackers with a slug of brandy.

The years have changed the sleep patterns. Bedtime rituals take longer. Nature wakens me two or three times a night for trips to the bathroom. Sleep returns at once unless my mind turns on and it gets launched on a needless project. The earlier remedies are called on to slow down the activities or the next day is a disaster. My 90-year-old aunt, who slept very little and lightly and lay awake many nights, said she went to the bathroom several times just for something to do instead of just lying there.

Ricarda, 90 years old

LEARNING OBJECTIVES

On completion of this chapter, the reader will be able to:

1. Identify age-related changes that affect the basic biologic support needs.
2. List the types of outcomes that occur because of age-related changes in the basic biologic support needs.
3. Describe the nursing assessment relevant to basic biologic support needs.
4. Explain nursing interventions useful in the promotion of the individual's basic biologic support needs.
5. Discuss individualizing nursing care plans for each of the basic biologic support needs.

Life support or survival requirements are no different for the aged than for other human beings. Fluctuations in homeostatic balance of these needs, however, make each of these needs more precarious. Assessing and monitoring survival functions are basic to ensuring the aged person's opportunity to reach his or her highest level of health and wellness.

This chapter addresses these crucial needs in the context of the biologic needs of Maslow's hierarchy. Unless the biologic needs are fulfilled adequately, the individual cannot be expected to ascend to the higher levels of coping and health. Attention has been devoted to nutrition, elimination, rest, and activity because these are areas of function in which the nurse can make a significant difference in health and wellness. Elimination is discussed here with regard to normal function in the section on chronic problems, as it pertains to urinary and fecal incontinence. The nurse's role in the maintenance of neurologic, renal, and cardiopulmonary function in the aged is indirect. Nurses cannot directly change the existing physiologic or pathologic conditions of heart, lungs, nervous system, or kidneys, but they can promote and maintain rest, exercise, and nutrition, which affect the function of these systems.

Two important questions should be considered in assessing the life support needs of the aged: What is bothering the client, and what threatens his or her life or health? Keeping these two questions in mind will assist the nurse in providing the most appropriate and realistic approaches to the survival needs of the aged.

NUTRITIONAL NEEDS

Well-being is influenced by the triad of aging, nutrition, and health. Proper nutrition means that all the essential nutrients—carbohydrates, fat, protein, vitamins, minerals, and water—are adequately supplied and used to maintain optimum health and well-being. Detailed discussion of each of these nutrients can be found in textbooks devoted to nutrition.

Proper nutrition provides the energy and building blocks necessary to maintain body structure and function. The variances in nutritional requirements throughout the life span are not well established for the aged. Increased amounts of calcium and vitamins A and C are needed in late life but tend to be deficient in the average diet of the aged or are affected by alterations in storage, use, and absorption. Total caloric intake should decline in response to corresponding changes in metabolic rate and a general decrease in physical activity. Serious nutritional deficits may also be induced by drugs. Nutritional needs of the aged and food sources of required nutrients are provided in condensed form in Table 6-1.

Several approaches in the past few decades were applied to the education and evaluation of the nutritional status of individuals and of nations. Four commonly used approaches are the Food Guide Pyramid, the Recommended Dietary Allowances (RDA), the Dietary Guidelines for Americans (developed by the U.S. Department of Agriculture [USDA] and U.S. Department of Health and Human Services), and the Nutrition Screening Initiative.

Food Guide Pyramid

The Modified Food Guide Pyramid for adults older than age 70 has been adapted from the USDA's Food Guide Pyramid. Adults older than 70 need fewer calories because they are less physically active, in general, than younger adults. Older adults are susceptible to nutrient deficiencies, and the Modified Food Guide Pyramid adds vitamin and mineral supplements that should be included in the daily diet. The Modified Food Guide Pyramid provides the types and amounts of food that should be eaten to optimize nutrient intake. Figure 6-1 illustrates the Modified Food Guide Pyramid. This food pyramid emphasizes a higher ratio of nutrients to calories. Fluid is emphasized in the pyramid because elderly individuals' thirst mechanisms are less responsive than a younger person's. With proper instruction the Modified Food Guide Pyramid is an easy and systematic way for a person to evaluate his or her own nutritional intake and independently make corrective adjustments. Pictures can be used to transcend cultural and speech barriers and educational limitations. Box 6-1 translates guidelines into daily food choices useful in clinical practice.

Box 6-1 Tips for Following the Dietary Guidelines

1. *Eat a variety of foods.*
   Provide more servings of fruits and vegetables.
   Frequently include dark green vegetables, dried bean dishes, and starchy vegetables.
   Use more grain products.
2. *Maintain ideal weight.*
   Reduce fats, sugars, and alcohol in diet.
   Cut back on size of serving.
   Increase physical activity.
3. *Avoid too much fat, saturated fat, and cholesterol.*
   Select lean hamburger and lean roasts, chops, and steak; trim visible fat.
   Drain meat drippings.
   Limit the amount of margarine or other fat used on bread and vegetables.
   Emphasize low-fat and skim milk and reduce the amount of fat in other foods when whole milk and cheese are used.
   Reduce the amount of fat used in recipes, added to food in cooking, or added at the table.
   Limit the number of fried foods, especially breaded or batter-fried foods.
   Use moderate amounts of organ meats and egg yolk.
   Use fewer creamed foods and rich desserts.
   Limit the amount of salad dressing used.
4. *Eat foods with adequate amounts of starch and fiber.*
   Provide more vegetables and fruits.
   Eat potatoes, sweet potatoes, yams, corn, peas, and dried beans more often.
   Increase consumption of whole-grain cereal products such as brown rice, oatmeal, and whole wheat cereals and breads.
5. *Avoid too much sugar.*
   Avoid or cut down on very sweet foods.
   Reduce the amount of sugar in recipes for baked goods.
   Rely more on fresh fruit and canned fruits packed in juice or light syrup.
   Limit the amounts of sugar, jams, jellies, and syrups.
6. *Avoid too much sodium and salt.*
   Use fewer salty, processed foods.
   Use little or no salt and assume that none is added at the table.
   Make only sparing use of commercially prepared sauces and condiments; these include such foods as catsup, Worcestershire or soy sauce, mustard, relishes and pickles, bouillon cubes, meat tenderizer, monosodium glutamate (MSG), gravy mixes, and canned soups.
   Use more fresh and frozen vegetables than canned or seasoned frozen vegetables, which have added salt.
   Limit the use of salty snack foods such as chips, pretzels, and crackers.
7. *If you drink alcohol, do so in moderation.*
   Provide more fruit and vegetable juice.
   Measure your drink.
   Eat something before drinking.
   Offer nonalcoholic beverages at parties.

Table 6-1 Special Nutritional Considerations for the Older Adult

Nutrient	Comments	Major food sources
Essential nutrients		
Fiber	Intakes are often inadequate. Increasing fiber in the diet may aid in preventing constipation.	Whole-grain breads (such as whole wheat, rye, Roman Meal, and pumpernickel); Wheatena, Ry-Krisp, and whole wheat crackers; cereals (such as shredded wheat, oatmeal, four-grain, and seven-grain); whole wheat pastas, and brown rice Fresh fruits and vegetables
Protein	The recommended level for older adults is as high as 1 g/kg body weight. Intakes are usually adequate. (Aged individuals may need to be shown portion sizes that would provide the necessary protein.)	Dried peas, dried or canned beans, lentils (especially in combination with whole grains such as brown rice and whole wheat bread), or peanut butter Cheese, milk, and nonfat dry milk Eggs Canned clams, salmon, sardines, and tuna
Calcium	Intakes are often inadequate. Older women may need generous amounts, 1 to 2 g daily, to protect against demineralization of the bones, leading to osteoporosis.	For those who are lactose intolerant: Tofu (soybean curd) All cheeses except cottage cheese Corn tortillas treated in lime All greens such as turnip, mustard, and collard (except spinach) Sardines Milk in small quantities (may be tolerated by some individuals) For those who are not lactose intolerant: All foods listed above Whole, low-fat, skim, evaporated, or dried milk Yogurt, buttermilk, and cottage cheese
Iron	Intakes are often inadequate.	Dried or canned beans Cereals, whole wheat pastas, whole-grain breads, and brown rice Liver Canned oysters
Zinc	Widespread deficiency is found in aged men and women.	Legumes Whole grains Meat
Folic acid	Folic acid deficiency may be linked to dementia.	Leafy green vegetables (such as spinach, collard, mustard, turnip, and kale greens) Dried beans and peas, lentils, and nuts Whole-grain breads, pastas, and cereals Liver
Vitamin A	Intakes are often inadequate.	Green vegetables (such as spinach, turnip, mustard, and collard greens, and broccoli) Carrots, winter squash, and sweet potato Watermelon and cantaloupe Liver
Vitamin B_6 (pyridoxine)	Intakes are sometimes inadequate. Age per se has been shown to influence blood levels, which decrease markedly with age.	Liver Vegetables Nuts and seeds, dried beans and peas Bran and whole grains Bananas, raisins, and cantaloupe
Vitamin C (ascorbic acid)	Intakes are sometimes inadequate, even in nursing home diets. Age per se influences blood levels, which decrease markedly with age. Vitamin C aids in the absorption of iron from vegetable sources.	Oranges, lemons, tomatoes, grapefruit, cantaloupe or other melon, strawberries Broccoli, cabbage, green peppers, fresh chili peppers, and dark, leafy greens Baked potatoes
Vitamin E (tocopherol)	Several researchers have demonstrated that 3-4 months of treatment with vitamin E (300-400 IU—about 30 times the recommended dietary allowance) relieves intermittent claudication (severe cramps in calf muscles during walking).	Fats of vegetable origin Some nuts and seeds Cereal products, especially whole grains Some vegetables

Compiled from *Recommended Daily Allowance*, ed 10, Washington, DC, 1989, National Academy Press; Linder MC: *Nutritional biochemistry and metabolism with clinical application*, New York, 1991, Elsevier; Roe D: *Geriatric nutrition*, ed 3, Englewood Cliffs, NJ, 1992, Prentice Hall.

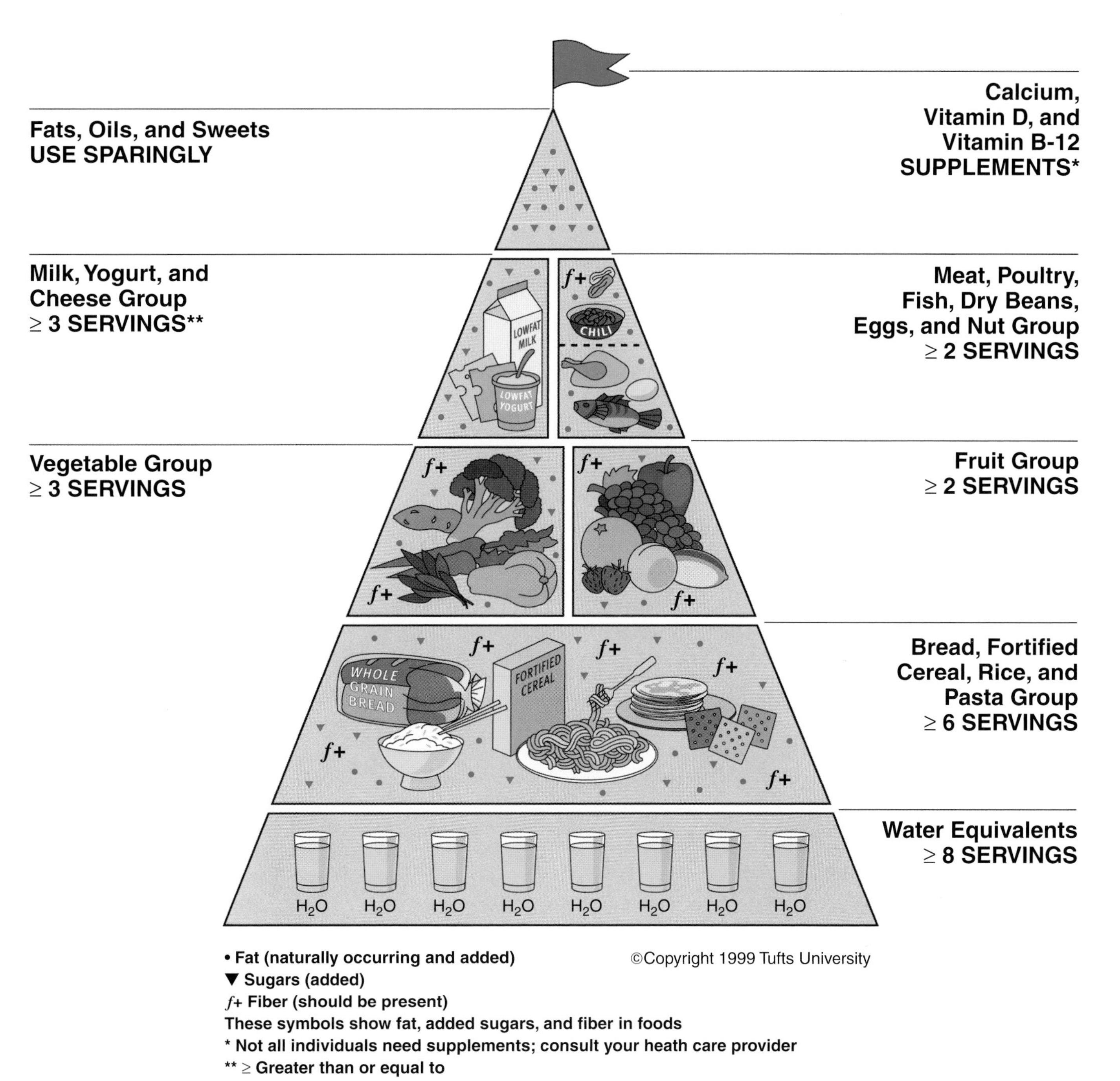

Figure 6-1. Modified Food Guide Pyramid for Mature (70+) Adults. (Copyright 1999 Tufts University, Medford, MA.)

Recommended Dietary Allowance

Another approach to evaluating nutritional status of individuals is the use of the RDA, established by the National Academy of Science Research Council. The RDA is a guideline for assessing the intake of energy and specific nutrients up to age 50. It establishes the daily minimum amount of vitamins and minerals needed by young and middle-aged healthy individuals based on body size. Some adjustment is required for many individuals. The RDA does not consider requirements for additional nutrients as a result of infection, metabolic disorders, and chronic illness, nor does the RDA address requirements of those older than 65 (*Recommended Dietary Allowances,* 1989). This is due, in part, to disagreement about the elderly's need for increased amounts of nutrients. However, recently the RDA for folate has increased in older adults, from 200 to 400 µg per day for men and from 180 to 400 µg per day for women; the RDA for vitamin A has decreased to 900 µg per day (3000 IU) for men and 700 μg per day (2300 IU) for women, 100 μg per day lower than the previous RDAs established in 1989 (National Policy and Resource Center on Nutrition and Aging, 2002). This applies to the retinol form but not the carotene form of vitamin A. The safest way to obtain vitamin A is not with supplements, even beta-carotene, but with increased intake of tomatoes for lycopene and dark green leafy vegetables for lutein—think "deep color."

Dietary reference intakes (DRIs) and dietary guidelines (DGs) have been developed for Older Americans Act (OAA) nutrition programs, Title III and Title VI. The programs provide congregate and home-delivered meals to about 3 million older adults each year (National Policy and Resource Center on Nutrition and Aging, 2002). These programs and all federal programs must comply with DGs and DRIs, which are revised every 5 years.

Factors Affecting Fulfillment of Nutritional Needs

Fulfillment of the aged person's nutritional needs is affected by numerous factors, including lifelong eating habits, socialization, income, transportation, housing, and food knowledge.

Lifelong Eating Habits. The nutritional state of a person reflects an individual's dietary history, as well as present food practices. Lifelong eating habits are developed out of tradition, ethnicity, and religion, all of which collectively can be termed *culture*. Food habits established in childhood may influence the intake of older adults.

Eating habits do not always coincide with fulfillment of nutritional needs. Rigidity of food habits increases with age as familiar food patterns are sought. Ethnicity determines if traditional foods are preserved, whereas religion affects choice of foods possible. Throughout life, then, preferences for particular foods bring deep satisfaction and possess emotional significance. Such foods are called "soul food" or comfort foods. Preferences for soul food influence food choices and affect nutrient intake. Foods prepared or served in a special way provide "soul." Rice with every meal or homemade chicken soup given to the individual when ill are examples of what some people consider their soul food. Foods of this nature are not unique to any one group but rather are found all over the world. Table 6-2 lists cultural food patterns for various ethnic groups and the dietary excesses or omissions associated with the pattern.

Lifelong habits of dieting or eating fad foods echo through the later years. The aged, in particular, are taken in by food fads that profess to partially or completely cure various ailments or to make one look younger or feel more vital. Skipping meals is another practice that one finds with the aged. The quantity of food eaten diminishes and the adequacy of nutrition becomes questionable. It is difficult to reach an adequate nutritional intake if the total calories are fewer than 1200 per day. Individuals who are on self-imposed diets of 1000 calories or less per day are inviting malnutrition.

Socialization. Food and eating are behavioral and social symbols. Many aged are forced to remain isolated from the

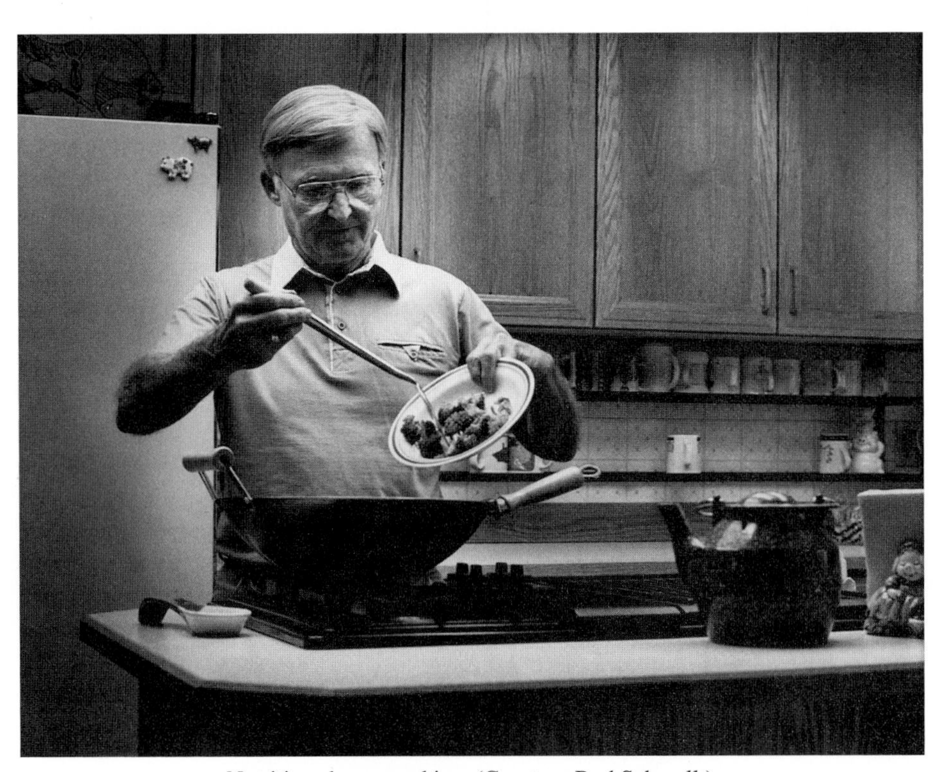

Nutritious home cooking. (Courtesy Rod Schmall.)

Table 6-2 Ethnic Food Patterns

Ethnic group	Cultural food patterns	Dietary excesses or omissions
Mexican (native)	Basic sources of protein—dry beans, flan, cheese, many meats, fish, eggs. Chili peppers and many deep-green and yellow vegetables. Fruits include: zapote, guava, papaya, mango, citrus. Tortillas (corn, flour); sweet bread; fideo; tacos, burritos, enchiladas.	*Limited* meats, milk, and milk products. Some are using flour tortillas more than the more nutritious corn tortillas. *Excessive* use of lard (manteca), sugar. Tendency to boil vegetables for long periods of time.
Filipino (Spanish-Chinese influence)	Most meats, eggs, nuts, legumes. Many different kinds of vegetables. Large amounts of rice and cereals.	May *limit* meat, milk, and milk products (the latter may be due to lactose intolerance). Tend to prewash rice. Tend to fry many foods.
Chinese (mostly Cantonese)	Cheese, soybean curd (tofu), many meats, chicken and pigeon eggs; nuts; legumes. Many different vegetables, leaves, bamboo sprouts. Rice and rice-flour products; wheat, corn, millet seed; green tea. Mixtures of fish, pork, and chicken with vegetables—bamboo shoots, broccoli, cabbage, onions, mushrooms, pea pods.	Tendency among some immigrants to use *excess* grease in cooking. May be *low* in protein, milk, and milk products (the latter may be due to lactose intolerance). Often wash rice before cooking. Large amounts of soy and oyster sauces, both of which are *high in salt.*
Puerto Rican	Milk with coffee. Pork, poultry, eggs, dried fish; beans (habichuelas). Viandas (starchy vegetables; starchy ripe fruits). Avocados, okra, eggplant, sweet yams. Rice, cornmeal.	Use *large* amounts of lard for cooking. *Limited* use of milk and milk products. *Limited* amounts of pork and poultry.
Black American	Milk with coffee. Pork, poultry, eggs, dried fish; beans (habichuelas). Viandas (starchy vegetables; starchy ripe fruits). Avocados, okra, eggplant, sweet yams. Rice, cornmeal. Cereals (including grits, hominy, hot breads). Molasses (dark molasses is especially good source of calcium, iron, vitamins B_1 and B_2, and niacin).	*Limited* use of milk group (lactose intolerance). Extensive use of frying, "something," simmering for cooking. *Large* amounts of fat: salt pork, bacon drippings, lard, gravies. May have *limited* use of citrus and enriched breads.
Middle Eastern (Greek, Syrian, Armenian)	Yogurt. Predominantly lamb, nuts, dried peas, beans, lentils. Deep-green leaves and vegetables; dried fruits. Dark breads and cracked wheat.	Tend to use *excessive* sweeteners, lamb fat, olive oil. Tend to fry meats and vegetables. *Insufficient* milk and milk products (almost no butter—use olive oil, which has no nutritive value except for calories); deficiency in fresh fruits.
Middle European (Polish)	Many milk products. Pork, chicken. Root vegetables (potatoes); cabbage; fruits. Wheat products. Sausages, smoked and cured meats; noodles, dumplings; bread; cream with coffee.	Tend to use *excessive* sweets and to overcook vegetables. *Limited* amounts of fruits (citrus), raw vegetables, and meats.
Native American (American Indian—much variation)	If "Americanized," use milk and milk products. Variety of meats: game, fowl, fish; nuts, seeds, legumes. Variety of vegetables, some wild; variety of fruits, some wild, rose hips; roots. Variety of breads, including tortillas, cornmeal, rice.	*Limited* quantities of high-protein foods depending on availability (flocks) and economic situation. *Excessive* use of sugar.
Italian	Staples are pasta with sauces; bread; eggs; cheese; tomatoes and vegetables such as artichokes, eggplant, greens, and zucchini. Only small amount of meat is used.	*Limited* use of whole grains; *insufficient* servings from milk group; tendency to overcook vegetables; enjoy sweets.

From Swanson J: *Community health nursing*, Philadelphia, 1993, WB Saunders.

mainstream of life because of impinging factors. When one eats alone, the outcome is often either overindulgence or disinterest in food.

Some aged spend much of their time in neighborhood bars, a center for social interaction. In seeking this type of fleeting social support, they spend money on alcohol that is needed for adequate nutrition. The perception that drinking is a sanctioned way to maintain social contact, which is preferable to not drinking and becoming isolated, is a powerful consideration, particularly for men who are single-room occupants. Drinking alcohol depletes the body of necessary nutrients and often replaces meals, thus making an individual susceptible to malnutrition.

There are more constructive means of maintaining social contact and nutritional status. Title VII of the OAA provides funding for strategically located outreach centers or nutrition sites whose purposes are to provide at least one nutritionally sound meal daily and to facilitate congregate dining to foster social contact and relationships. No one age 60 or over (all spouses are also included) can be denied participation in the nutrition program because of his or her economic situation. Those who are able to pay for their meal do so according to their ability.

Meals-on-wheels is another community program that encourages both the attainment of good nutrition and human contact for those who are unable to prepare meals or go out to obtain them. Most cities and rural areas throughout the United States have such programs. Delivery in the rural areas may be limited. Other congregate or group feeding programs exist through church and other community auspices such as food cooperatives, home grocery delivery services, and chore services for shopping and meal preparation. The federal government awards grants to the Congregate Housing Services Project to provide meals to elderly residents who need them to remain independent.

The social essence ascribed to eating is sharing a meal, which provides a sense of belonging. We use food as a means of giving and receiving love, friendship, or belonging.

Informational Needs. With the rising cost of health care, most of us are turning to the Internet or other information sources to help us understand our health needs, as well as our disease processes. Physicians, geriatric nurse practitioners, and other primary care health providers have less and less time for the provision of education. The Nutrition Screening Initiative (NSI) surveyed 600 Americans older than age 60 and found that although 80% knew that nutrition played an important role in their health management, only one third reported that their physician emphasized nutrition. The vast majority said they would use nutrition strategies in their self-care if they received information from their health care provider (Nutrition Screening Initiative, 2002). Effective January 1, 2002, Medicare began covering nutrition therapy for select diseases, such as diabetes or kidney disease, which creates unprecedented opportunities for older Americans to access information (Pear, 2001).

National Goals. One objective for *Healthy People 2000* has been to increase to at least 80% the receipt of home food services by people ages 65 and older who have difficulty in preparing their own meals or are otherwise in need of home-delivered meals. *Healthy People 2010* further addresses nutrition and considers it a leading health indicator to be used over the next 10 years to measure the health of the nation (U.S. Department of Health and Human Services, 2002).

There are federal regulations in place in the form of the Omnibus Budget Reconciliation Act of 1987 (OBRA) that ensure nutritional standards in long-term care facilities. These standards include assessment of nutritional status; assurance of the maintenance of nutritional status unless the clinical state renders this impossible; and a therapeutic diet for nutritional problems. The Joint Commission on Accreditation of Healthcare Organizations (JCAHO) has also set standards for nutrition (Box 6-2).

Income. There is a strong relationship between poor nutrition and low income (Wakefield, 2001). The United States has a stringently defined poverty rate. Poverty rates in those older than 65 dropped to 10.2%, or 3.36 million people, in 2000 (Butler, 2001). Although it is encouraging that the rate is declining, it does not reflect the economically fragile situation of many of America's older people. Older adults with low incomes need to choose among needs such as food, heat, telephone bills, medications, and health care visits. Some aged eat only once a day in an attempt to make their income last through the month. Aged individuals accustomed to eating meat, fish, and poultry as their main sources of protein have watched the cost climb to heights beyond their purchasing power. Inexpensive alternative protein sources such as tofu (soybean curd) are foreign to the diets of many aged in Western society today but have slowly been making their way into acceptance. At present the development of a taste for alternative protein sources and an understanding of what foods to mix to obtain complete dietary protein requires some knowledge and practice to ensure adequate protein intake and to prevent monotony. If at all possible, the aged should be encouraged to use vegetable protein sources to meet daily needs. This is a more economical form of protein that may help the aged conserve their income for other necessities, medications, unexpected bills, or special treats. Combinations such as milk or cheese with bread or pasta; cereal with milk; rice and cheese or rice and bean casseroles; wheat soy or corn soy bread; wheat bread with baked beans, beans, or pea curry; tortillas and beans; and legume soup with bread are sources of protein.

More older adults live in poverty than younger adults, according to the 2000 census (U.S. Bureau of the Census, 2001). Median household income for those older than 65 is $22,812 compared with $40,816 for all householders. Programs such as the food stamp program have the potential for increasing the purchasing power of the aged who qualify, but these are vulnerable to federal budget cutting. Transportation may be limited and the distance too far for the older adult to travel to grocery stores or to acquire food stamps, which are sold only at designated locations in cities.

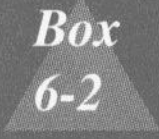

Joint Commission on Accreditation of Healthcare Organizations (JCAHO) Nutrition Standards

- Screen for nutritional risk
- Provide nutritional intervention and counseling
- Plan for nutritional care
- Prescribe nutrition products
- Prepare, distribute, and administer food and nutrition products
- Monitor response to nutritional care plan

Free food programs, such as donated commodities, are also available at distribution centers (food banks, churches, senior centers) for those with limited incomes. Although this is another valuable option for the aged, use of it is not always feasible. One takes a chance on the types of food available any particular day or week; quantities distributed are frequently too large for the single aged person or the aged couple to use or even carry from the distribution site; the site may be too far away or difficult to reach; and the time of distribution of the food may be inconvenient.

Cafeterias and restaurants that provided special meal prices for the aged have had to increase their prices as food costs have risen; thus the previous advantages of eating out have diminished. Yet many single elders rely on them for most meals.

Though rapidly disappearing, "mom-and-pop" stores in the neighborhoods where many elderly live do not have a rapid turnover of fresh products, and this may cause the aged to spend money on partially spoiled items. Those who purchase semispoiled food and discover the spoilage when they return home rarely return the items.

Transportation. Availability of transportation may be limited for the aged. Many small, long-standing neighborhood food stores have been closed in the wake of larger supermarkets, which are located in areas that serve a greater segment of the population. It may become difficult to walk to the market, to reach it by public transportation, or to carry a bag of groceries while using a cane. Fear is apparent in the elderly's consideration of transportation. They fear walking in the street and being mugged, not being able to cross the street in the time it takes the traffic light to change, or being knocked down or falling as they walk in crowded streets. Despite reduced senior citizen bus fares, many elders are fearful of attack when using public transportation. Transportation by taxicab for an individual on a limited income is unrealistic, but sharing a taxicab with others who also need to shop may enable the aged to go where food prices are cheaper and to take advantage of sale items. For the aged, convenience foods, devoid of many essential nutrients, are lighter to carry or pull along in a cart than fresh fruits and vegetables. Today, many markets can be accessed on the Internet or by telephone and will make home deliveries.

Senior citizen organizations have been helpful in providing the elderly with van service to shopping areas. In housing complexes it may be possible to schedule trips to the supermarket. Most communities have multiple sources of transportation available, but the aged may be unaware of them. Local departments of aging and senior centers are a good source of information.

Housing. Poor and near-poor aged are likely to reside in substandard housing. Some live in single rooms that lack storage space for food, a means of refrigeration, and a stove for cooking. At certain times of the year some of the single-room dwellers use the window ledges and fire escapes to keep perishables cool for several days' use. Box 6-3 lists items suitable for the single-room occupant's pantry and items that can be purchased to be eaten the same day. Of foremost concern to the nurse is tailoring an acceptable diet. Additional factors affecting dietary intake include living arrangements, number of meals eaten daily, who cooks and shops, presence of physical impediments affecting cooking and shopping, problems with chewing, use of dentures, alcohol use, and medication use.

Problems in Nutrition

Hydration, adequate fiber, lactose intolerance, weight loss, vitamin and mineral deficiencies, osteoporosis, sarcopenia, malnutrition, and obesity are factors that affect or are affected by the nutritional status of elders. Figure 6-2 shows a Nutrition Screening Initiative checklist to determine nutritional health.

Dehydration. The aged are vulnerable to fluid and accompanying electrolyte imbalance. In children, 80% of their body composition is water. In elderly people, 43% to 51% is water (Bennett, 2000). Even small decreases in fluid intake can cause more dehydration in an elder than in a child. The concentrating ability of old kidneys decreases, so urine flow is not diminished with dehydration until late. Thirst decreases in advancing age, resulting in the loss of an important defense against dehydration.

Box 6-3 Nonperishable Foods Suitable for Single-Room Occupant

Milk Products
- Box of dry skim or whole milk
- Small can of evaporated milk
- Instant cocoa
- Instant pudding to use with dry milk
- Small pieces of cheese (if wrapped airtight and kept in cool place)

Meat Products
- Small can of tuna fish, sardines, salmon
- Canned potted meat
- Peanut butter
- Cottage cheese
- Hard-cooked eggs

Fruits and Vegetables
- Small cans of any fruits and vegetables
- Dried fruit (raisins, apricots, dates)
- Fresh apples, oranges, seasonal fruits

Miscellaneous Foods
- Instant coffee
- Tea
- Sugar
- Condiments of choice

Read the statements below. Circle the number in the Yes column for those that apply to you or someone you know. For each "yes" answer, score the number listed. Total your nutritional score.	YES
I have an illness or condition that made me change the kind or amount of food I eat.	2
I eat fewer than two meals per day.	3
I eat few fruits, vegetables or milk products.	2
I have three or more drinks of beer, liquor, or wine almost every day.	2
I have tooth or mouth problems that make it hard for me to eat.	2
I don't always have enough money to buy the food I need.	4
I eat alone most of the time.	1
I take three or more different prescriptions or over-the-counter drugs each day.	1
Without wanting to, I have lost or gained 10 pounds in the past 6 months.	2
I am not always physically able to shop, cook, and/or feed myself.	2
Total Nutritional Score	______

0-2 indicates good nutrition
3-5 moderate risk
6+ high nutritional risk

Figure 6-2. Nutrition Screening Initiative checklist to determine nutritional health. (From The Nutrition Screening Initiative, 1010 Wisconsin Avenue NW, Suite 800, Washington, DC 20007. The Nutrition Screening Initiative is funded in part by a grant from Ross Products Division of Abbott Laboratories, Inc.)

Dehydration can cause confusion as a result of electrolyte imbalance. Adequate amounts of fluid not only prevent confusion associated with dehydration but also are essential for individuals who are receiving specific medications. Constipation, a common problem among elderly people, can be minimized with adequate fluid intake. Other consequences of dehydration include thromboembolism, pressure ulcers, periodontal sepsis, orthostasis, falls, and kidney stones (Morely, 2000). Use of diuretics requires that fluid intake be maintained unless specifically ordered to the contrary. Coffee has a diuretic effect that requires fluid intake to compensate for fluid loss through diuresis. In hot weather increased perspiration and evaporation deplete the individual of needed body fluid. Fever and upper respiratory infections also cause dehydration in the aged. Older adults often have a diminished thirst sensation. Adequate fluid intake is as important to total nutrition as food. Daily fluid needs fluctuate widely in older adults and depend on general health status, medications, and activity level. To maintain water balance, eight servings of water, or about 2 liters, is recommended each day (Wakefield, 2000).

Standard indicators for dehydration among the aged are not always reliable. In general, in *mild dehydration* the nurse will find diminished skin turgor best evaluated on the forehead or sternum, dry mucous membranes, and orthostatic hypotension (Beers and Berkow, 2000). There may be tachycardia. *Moderate dehydration* causes the same symptoms plus oliguria or anuria, confusion, and a resting hypotension. The older adult with *severe dehydration* will be in shock or near shock. The difficulty of a definitive diagnosis is that many of the symptoms may be present in the older adult without volume problems. Weighing on a regular basis can be useful in assessing volume loss. However, weighing may be impracticable in the nursing home setting for some patients. Dry mucous membranes may be misleading because many elderly are mouth breathers. Intake and output charts are all too often unreliable.

Laboratory Assessment. Urine specific gravity is not well correlated with serum biochemical parameters of hydration status. However, urinary sodium concentration is usually less than 20 mEq/L when sodium intake is reduced or the patient has vomiting or diarrhea. A urinary sodium concentration greater than 20 mEq/L can occur with volume depletion. Hematocrit, blood urea nitrogen (BUN), and creatinine will be elevated. BUN/creatinine ratios are also increased (Beers and Berkow, 2000). Laboratory parameters can be used, but other conditions that can occur in elderly people can alter these laboratory findings.

Prevention of dehydration is essential. Nursing staff in long-term care facilities can identify dehydration based on poor oral intake and the occurrence of vomiting or diarrhea. Staff education to increase awareness of the need for fluids and the symptoms of dehydration is encouraged. Box 6-4 is a Hydration Assessment Checklist from the Hartford Institute for Geriatric Nursing (Zembruski, 2000).

Dehydration Management. When dehydration occurs, treatment is based on the type of dehydration experienced and the amount of dehydration (Box 6-5). Oral hydration is the

Box 6-4 Hydration Assessment Checklist

1. Symptoms of hydration requiring immediate interventions—fever, thirst, dry and warm skin, furrowed tongue, decreased urinary output
2. Associated factors: older than 85, immobility, cognitive impairment, fluid intake less than 1500 ml, lack of awareness of thirst
3. Increasing vulnerability—osteoporosis, congestive failure, dementia
4. Dietary restrictions of fluids, salt, potassium, protein
5. Medications—diuretics, tricyclic antidepressants, laxatives
6. History of dehydration, infections, difficulty swallowing
7. Return from a 24-hour hospitalization, dental or eye surgery, procedures that require fasting
8. Laboratory reports with increasing sodium, blood urea nitrogen, creatinine, hematocrit, urine specific gravity

Adapted from Zembruski C: *Hydration checklist,* New York, 2000, Hartford Institute for Geriatric Nursing.

Box 6-5 Estimates of Dehydration

Mild dehydration: Less than 5% loss of body weight
Moderate dehydration: 10% loss of body weight
Severe dehydration: 15% loss of body weight

Adapted from Beers MH, Berkow R: *Merck manual of geriatrics*, ed 3, Whitehouse Station, NJ, 2000, Merck Research Laboratories.

first treatment approach if the patient is able to ingest fluids. Two to three liters of water or clear fluids may be necessary (Beers and Berkow, 2000). If there is impaired mental status or larger fluid deficits, intravenous therapy is required, usually with 0.9% sodium chloride. A general rule is to replace 50% of the loss within the first 12 hours (or 1 L/day in afebrile elders) or sufficient quantity to relieve tachycardia and hypotension. Further fluid replacement can be administered more slowly over a longer period of time. Inadequate rehydration in a reasonable time can result in complications such as renal failure, myocardial infarction, stroke, or rhabdomyolysis (Beers and Berkow, 2000). Box 6-6 lists measures to help prevent dehydration of institutionalized elders.

Hyponatremia. *Hyponatremia* is defined as a decrease in sodium plasma concentration less than 136 mEq/L and is caused by an excess of water relative to solute. It is one of the most common causes of delirium in elderly patients. There is, in general, an age-related decrease in serum sodium without any clinical symptomatology. Dilutional hyponatremia is associated with the highest mortality rate and may be caused by nutritional supplements such as Ensure, Isocal, or Osmolite, all of which are low in sodium. Hyponatremia caused by vomiting or diarrhea, suctioning of the gastrointestinal (GI) tract, and diuretics stimulate antidiuretic hormone (ADH) production, which causes retention of water but not sodium. This is usually mild, but the nurse may want to consider irrigation of gastric tubes with normal saline or administer saline intravenous fluids. Hyponatremia can also occur in chronic diseases such as congestive heart failure, cirrhosis, and nephrosis (Beers and Berkow, 2000). In this instance, patients often have edema and there is impaired renal ability to dilute urine.

Hypernatremia. *Hypernatremia* is defined as an elevated plasma sodium concentration greater than 145 mEq/L that is caused by a deficit of water relative to sodium (Desai and Isa-Pratt, 2002). Common causes include decreased water intake, increased sodium intake, and increased water loss from the GI tract and loop diuretics. Low body weight is a risk factor for hypernatremia. The mortality rate for hypernatremia is approximately 40% in older hospitalized patients, especially if it is of rapid onset, and also if the sodium is higher than 160 mEq/L (Beers and Berkow, 2000). Weakness and lethargy are common symptoms, although they are not specific. If the sodium level is greater than 152 mEq/L, seizures, stupor, and coma may occur. Body water deficits require hypotonic fluid replacement using 0.45% sodium chloride solution or 5% dextrose in water.

Adequate Fiber. Fiber is an important dietary component that some aged persons do not consume in sufficient quantities. Fiber, the undigestible material that gives plants their structure, is abundant in raw fruits and vegetables and unrefined grains and cereals.

Fiber facilitates the absorption of water, increases bulk, and improves intestinal motility. It helps prevent constipation, hemorrhoids, and diverticulosis. Various types of fiber exist, but all possess the common characteristic of indigestibility. Individuals who can chew foods well could benefit from eating increased amounts of fresh fruits and vegetables daily or combining unsweetened bran with other types of food. Those who have difficulty chewing could sprinkle oat bran on cereals or in soups, meat loaf, or casseroles. The quantity of bran used depends on the individual, but generally 1 to 2

Box 6-6 Measures to Help Prevent Dehydration of Institutionalized Elderly

- Ensure a 24-hour intake of at least 1500 ml of oral fluid. (Food intake and metabolic oxidation should provide additional fluid for hydration.)
- Offer fluids hourly during the day. Include fluids with an evening snack.
- Ask the physician to order intravenous fluids if the elder is not able to take oral fluids.
- Accurately record intake and output for all elders. (The 24-hour urine volume should be 1000 to 1500 ml.)
- Note the urine color and specific gravity.
- Listen to bowel sounds. Note any change in activity. (Extra soft or loose stool means losing water, and hard stool means dehydration.)
- Be familiar with tests or examinations that the patient may have had. If they involved enemas or laxatives before the tests, there will be a fluid loss.
- Replace fluids when there has been nothing consumed orally or fluids have been lost from test preparation.
- Obtain a drug history.
- Provide cups, glasses, and pitchers that are not too big or heavy for the aged to handle. (Help those who cannot help themselves to fluids.)
- Offer other fluids in addition to water. Find out the types of beverages liked and fluid temperature preferred.
- Remember that coffee acts as a diuretic. Fluid loss by coffee should be supplemented to compensate for the fluid loss.
- Note skin turgor and mucous membranes.
- Note increases in pulse and respiration rates and decrease in blood pressure (suggestive of dehydration).
- Check laboratory values for changes: sodium, blood urea nitrogen, hematocrit, hemoglobin, urine and serum osmolarity, and creatinine. Also check for signs of acidosis.
- Weigh the patient daily at the same time and on the same scale.

From Reedy DF: Fluid intake: how can you prevent dehydration? *Geriatr Nurs* 9:224, 1988.

tablespoons daily is sufficient to facilitate intestinal motility. Individuals who have not used bran should begin with 1 teaspoon and progressively increase the quantity until the fiber intake is enough to accomplish its purpose. If used in larger amounts to start, bloating, gas, diarrhea, and other colon discomforts will initially occur and discourage further use of this important dietary ingredient.

Cooked dried beans are a good source of fiber. Pinto beans, split peas, red beans, and peanuts can be served in casseroles, soups, and dips. These are all relatively inexpensive and nutritious in addition to having high fiber content. See Box 6-7 for fiber choices and amounts of fiber in each (Moore, 2001). The discussion of elimination in this chapter presents recipes for promoting bowel elimination. Each of these recipes has fiber agents.

Milk/Lactose Intolerance. The use of milk and other dairy products is a major and efficient source of protein and calcium for the aged. For some persons, lactose intolerance is a problem that must be considered in nutritional counseling. Lactose intolerance is thought to be a genetic characteristic occurring in blacks, Asians, American Indians, Eskimos, and other ethnic groups for whom animal milk is not a traditional food. Whites of northern European descent retain the lactase enzyme in adulthood, and other whites begin to experience some degree of intolerance at about age 45. Even low levels of ingested lactose cause such symptoms as gas, bloating, cramping, and diarrhea.

Lactose intolerance resembles milk intolerance. The symptoms displayed are similar and occur when more than 8 ounces of milk is consumed. Intolerance does not always occur when other products such as hard cheese yogurt, acidophilus milk, and buttermilk are consumed. It is difficult to know exactly if the milk intolerance is a direct reflection of lactose intolerance. Lactase enzyme can be added to milk to hydrolyze the lactose in order to obtain the benefit of milk. Also, foods high in calcium, such as greens and dried beans, also can provide essential calcium for those who are lactose intolerant and do not like milk. It may be necessary to supplement the diet with calcium carbonate or calcium lactate, sodium fluoride, and B-complex vitamins to maintain skeletal integrity.

Box 6-8 provides osteoporosis nutrition interventions, and Box 6-9 lists causes of calcium malabsorption. Table 6-3 lists leading sources of calcium.

Malnutrition. Malnutrition encompasses both overnutrition and undernutrition. It may result from inadequate intake, malabsorption, digestive disorders, or excessive intake of food (Moore, 2001). These can be detected in physical examinations, biochemical studies, and physiologic tests. Included in malnutrition are specific nutrient deficiencies, nutritional imbalances, and obesity. Figure 6-3 provides the malnutrition trajectory. See Box 6-10 for factors potentiating malnutrition.

Undernutrition. *Undernutrition* may be defined as "imbalanced nutrition: less than body requirements." About 16% of elderly people in the community eat less than 1000 kcal/day, which is insufficient for adequate nutrition (Beers and

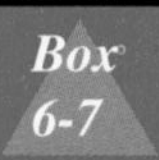

Foods High in Dietary Fiber

Highest
All wheat bran types
Figs
Dried peaches
Prunes (dried or cooked)

Moderate
Oat bran
Apple with skin
Dried apricots
Whole grain or bran English muffin
Bran muffin
Ry-Krisps
Mueslix
Beans (kidney, lima, red, northern)
Brussels sprouts
Corn
Peas
Avocados
Blackberries
Dates
Oranges
Pears

Low
Cracked wheat bread
Brown rice
Cornbread
Corn flakes
Cheerios
Applesauce
Grapes
Green beans
Onions
Peppers
Potatoes
Pears (canned)
French toast
Raisins
Strawberries
Pineapple
Granola
Pancakes
Grape Nuts
Cantaloupe
Blueberries
Nonbran muffins
Kiwifruit
Carrots
Cauliflower
Broccoli
Cherries
Mushrooms

Adapted from Moore MC: *Pocket guide to nutritional care,* ed 4, St Louis, 2001, Mosby.

Box 6-8

Osteoporosis Nutrition Interventions

- Assess height and weight yearly (body mass index less than 22 is a risk factor).
- Assess bone density with DEXA scan.
- Assess dietary intake of calcium and vitamin D and sun exposure.
- Screen for medications causing calcium or bone loss.
- Increase calcium intake to 1200 mg/day and vitamin D intake to 200-400 IU/day.
- Reduce or eliminate alcohol intake.
- Encourage sun exposure 10-30 min/day.
- Consider calcium and vitamin D supplements.
- Weight-bearing exercises daily if able.
- Provide analgesia to reduce pain of osteoporosis and fracture.

Box 6-9

Causes of Calcium Malabsorption

- Inadequate vitamin D
- Lactose intolerance (causing lack of milk in the diet)
- Excessive intake of phosphorus (competes with calcium for absorption; present in meat and carbonated drinks)
- High-sodium diet (interferes with calcium absorption)
- High-protein diets
- Diets high in oxalates (spinach and very deep green vegetables)
- Diets high in phytates (bran and whole grains or fiber)
- Achlorhydria (calcium absorption requires acid rather than alkaline environment)
- Corticosteroids and anticonvulsants
- Smoking, moderate to high alcohol intake, and excess caffeine intake (all of which promote bone loss)

Adapted from Moore MC: *Pocket guide to nutritional care,* ed 4, St Louis, 2001, Mosby.

Table 6-3 Leading Calcium Sources

Food	Amount	Milligrams of calcium
Dairy products		
Low-fat milk, 1% to 2%	1 cup	310
Skim milk	1 cup	300
Whole milk	1 cup	290
Buttermilk	1 cup	290
Nonfat dry milk	2 tablespoons	105
Eggnog	1 cup	330
Ice cream	1 cup	208
Plain yogurt (whole milk)	1 cup	300
Plain yogurt (low fat)	1 cup	400
Mozzarella cheese	1 ounce	210
Parmesan cheese	1 ounce	340
Swiss cheese	1 ounce	270
Cottage cheese, 2% fat	1 cup	160
Vegetables		
Collard greens	1 cup	360
Turnip greens	1 cup	250
Kale	1 cup	200
Bok choy	1 cup	250
Broccoli	1 cup	150
Fish		
Canned sardines (with bones)	4 ounces	500
Canned red salmon	4 ounces	290
Canned mackerel	4 ounces	300
Nuts		
Brazil nuts and hazelnuts	½ cup	125
Almonds	½ cup	160
Miscellaneous		
Tofu	3½ ounces	128
Chocolate fudge	3½ ounces	100
Light molasses	5 tablespoons	165
Black strap molasses	5 tablespoons	579
Seaweed, kelp, agar	3½ ounces	1093

Compiled from *Reader's Digest*: The hidden health risk most women face, 1985; *Family Circle NBC Special Section:* For women only: your body, your health, 1985; *Kaiser Permanente Fact Sheet*, 1983. Women and calcium; Sardana R: Nutritional management of osteoporosis, *Geriatr Nurs* 13(6):317, 1992.

Berkow, 2000). Undernutrition affects 17% to 65% of elders in hospitals and many of the elders in long-term care facilities. In one study by the University of Oklahoma (Rahman, 2001), 26% of ambulatory geriatric patients were identified as malnourished, with a body mass index (BMI) less than 22, unintentional weight loss greater than 10% in 6 months, serum albumin less than 3.5 mg/dl, and cholesterol less than 160 mg/dl. Another 45% who had no objective signs of malnutrition were found to be at risk based on the NSI nutrition assessment score of greater than 2.

A study by Thomas and associates (2000) shows that malnutrition in elders is predictive of poor clinical outcomes and risk for increased mortality. The triad of depression, impaired immune function, and unexplained weight loss of 5% or more is predictive of death within 6 months. Many medical conditions common to elders increase metabolism, thus exacerbating undernutrition. These individuals are also likely to suffer from dehydration and poor fluid intake. Persons with severe malnutrition are at higher risk for chronic medical conditions that could be prevented by early correction of reversible nutritional deficits.

The "skeleton in the nursing home closet" is the problem of malnutrition in long-term care facilities (Nutrition Screening Initiative, 2001). A clinical guideline to manage involuntary weight loss and malnutrition in residents focuses on a number of factors, including reporting of medical conditions, declines in ability to perform activities of daily living, and cognizance of delirium, depression, and mood disorders.

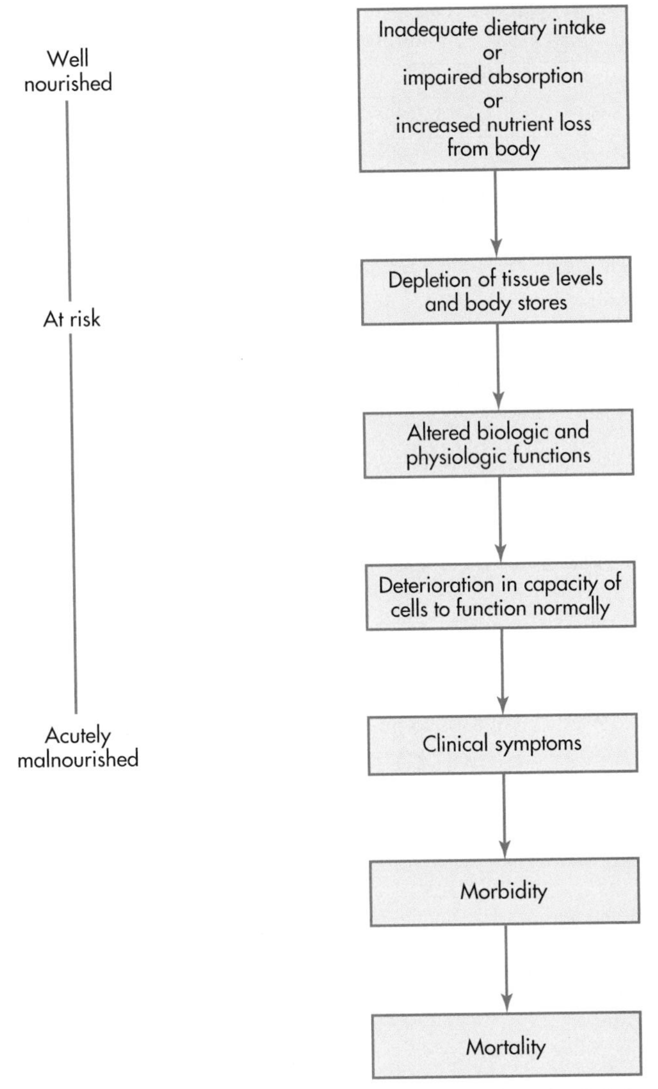

Figure 6-3. A trajectory for malnutrition. (Modified from Prodrabsky M: In Mahan LK, Arlin MT, editors: *Krause's food nutrition and diet therapy,* ed 8, Philadelphia, 1992, WB Saunders.)

Box 6-10 Factors Potentiating Malnutrition in the Aged

Social Factors
Poverty
Lack of help with food shopping and preparation
No socialization at meals

Psychologic Factors
Bereavement
Confusion
Depression

Physical Factors
Immobility
Inability to feed self
Bad oral hygiene
Poor dentition or ill-fitting dentures

Physiologic Factors
Decreased metabolic rate
Decreased enjoyment (diminished taste, smell, vision)
Decreased feeding drive (neurotransmitters, nutritional factors)
Increased satiety (peptide hormones, stomach emptying)
Disease

Psychosocial Risk Factors
Limited income
Abuse of alcohol and other central nervous system depressants
Bereavement, loneliness, or living alone
Removal from usual cultural patterns
Confusion, forgetfulness, or disorientation
Working toward intentional or subintentional death

Mechanical Risk Factors
Decreased or limited strength and mobility
Neurologic deficits, arthritis, handicap, impairment of hand-arm coordination, loss of tongue strength, and dysphagia
Decreased or diminished vision or blindness
Inability to feed self
Decubitus ulcers
Loss of teeth, poor-fitting dentures, or chewing problems
Difficult breathing
Polypharmacy
Surgery, nothing by mouth (NPO) for extended periods of time, or intravenous therapy only

Depression is a major cause of weight loss in long-term care residents and perhaps accounts for 36% of the residents who lose weight. The guideline recommends consultation with pharmacy on medications that may cause anorexia and medications that may stimulate appetite and reverse malnutrition. In an effort to deal with the malnutrition in long-term care facilities, the Council for Nutritional Strategies in Long-Term Care was established (Morely, 1999). The interdisciplinary council developed an evidence-based recommendation on nutrition management for health disciplines. The one developed for nurses is seen in Figure 6-4.

Obesity. Body fat increases until about age 50 in women and age 40 in men, remains steady, and then decreases after age 70 (Beers and Berkow, 2000). Those who weigh 120% to 130% of their ideal weight are considered moderately obese; those who weigh more than 130% of their ideal weight are morbidly obese. At this time, however, the ideal body mass for elderly people has not been established.

Obesity results from decreased physical activity that frequently occurs in elderly individuals. The loss of estrogen and growth hormone (GH) contributes to obesity in women; loss of GH contributes to obesity in men. Other causes of obesity in the aged include hypothyroidism, hypothalamic tumors, glucocorticoid therapy, monoamine oxidase inhibitors, and moderate dosages of phenothiazines (Beers and Berkow, 2000).

It has long been known that obese adults have more medical problems compared with thin and normal-weight adults, including diabetes, hypertension, colon cancer, and increased death rates. A recent study by Grabowski and Ellis (2001) supported by the Agency for Healthcare Research and Quality suggests that extra weight may be protective for elderly people. Fat is a storage "organ" for excess calories and provides protection during times of acute illness (Beers and Berkow, 2000). It protects the vital organs from injury in falls, and it helps maintain the body's core temperature. Excess fat, however, causes medical complications (Box 6-11) (Beers and Berkow, 2000).

The prevalence of obesity is rising in the United States. Certain groups have classified obesity as an epidemic, including the World Health Organization and the National Heart, Lung, and Blood Institute of the National Institutes of Health (National Institutes of Health, 2001). More than 20% of Americans are obese. These obese people have a BMI greater than 30 (National Institutes of Health Consensus Statement, 2000).

Screening for obesity is usually done by calculating the BMI normalized for height. The National Center for Health Statistics uses the 85th percentile sex-specific values for persons ages 20 through 29 (27.8 kg/m^2 or greater for men and 27.3 kg/m^2 or greater for women). This was derived from the U.S. National Health and Nutrition Examination Survey (NHANES II) (National Center for Health Statistics, 2000). Risk of mortality is increased for severely obese people, although the thinnest people also have this risk. An elevated waist/hip circumference ratio (WHR), which indicates central adiposity (fat), correlates with BMI and may be a better predictor of complications of obesity. Waist circumferences greater than 40 inches (102 cm) in men and greater than 35 inches (88 cm) in women indicate high risk. Although we can identify obese individuals from physical examination, precise methods should be used to evaluate mild to moderate obesity. The easiest and most common clinical method is the evaluation of body weight and height based on a table of "desirable" weights. The tables reflect the weight at which risk of mortality is minimized. An alternative is the calculation of BMI. *Overweight* is defined as a BMI of 27.8 or greater for men and 27.3 or greater for women. The formula is weight (kg) divided by height (m^2) or, using pounds instead of kilograms, weight (lb) times 703 and then divided by height (in^2).

Obesity management risk/benefit ratios should be evaluated before intervention. Excessive weight loss may be a cause of higher mortality rates (Beers and Berkow, 2000). A walking program such as mall walking may help with gradual loss of weight and can also be a social occasion. Weight-loss drugs are not recommended for older persons because the side effects may outweigh the positive effect. Orlistat (Xenocal), which inhibits fat absorption, may be used in elderly obese patients, especially those with diabetes and hypertension. Orlistat can produce weight loss of 8% to 10%. It can cause soft stools and decreased absorption of fat-soluble vitamins (National Institutes of Health, 2001). Stomach surgery would be considered only in those with sleep apnea and BMI greater than 40 or BMI greater than 35 with comorbid conditions.

Box 6-11 Complications of Obesity

Moderate Obesity
Coronary artery disease
Hypertension
Osteoarthritis
Gallbladder disease
Diabetes mellitus
Colon and prostate cancer (in men)
Breast and ovarian cancer (in women)

Morbid Obesity
Immobility
Intertrigo
Drug problems
Increased mortality rate
Increased surgical risk
All complications of moderate obesity

Ethics of Nutrition

Fads, megavitamins, feeding, and intentional starvation are ethical issues to be addressed in nutrition of the older adult.

Food Fads. Aged individuals are not immune to food faddism and may fall prey to advertisements that claim specific foods maintain youth and vitality or rid one of chronic conditions. Fad foods are often more costly than a balanced diet and can sometimes be obtained only in health food stores or by mail order. Even if the food is easily obtained in a supermarket, which is becoming common, such large quantities may be called for that some nutrients are obtained in excess, whereas others are excluded.

Megavitamin therapy, the ingestion of large amounts of a specific vitamin or many different vitamins, can also be considered a fad. Unless the individual is severely depleted of vitamins, which can usually be obtained in an adequate diet, megavitamin therapy is nonessential and dangerous. Risks exist in megavitamin therapy: Bone meal, a source of calcium, may contain lead and thus cause lead poisoning; high doses of zinc cause zinc toxicity; and kelp, with its high iodine content, can cause goiter in those with preexisting thyroid enlargement. High intake of niacin is discouraged because of a high incidence of cardiac arrhythmias, abnormal biochemical findings, and gastrointestinal problems. Excess vitamin A has two detrimental effects in elderly individuals: liver disease and bone demineralization. The RDA has recently been decreased for the desired amount of vitamin A (the retinol form, not the carotene form) by 100 μg per day. The money spent on food fads and unneeded vitamins by the aged could buy more economical foods that benefit the individual's health. Megavitamin therapy has a role in maintaining nutrition when illness, malnutrition, or excessive demands are placed on body function. Table 6-4 compares and contrasts fad diets (Russell et al, 2002).

Many of our older adults are lowering the cholesterol in their diets. A soy-containing diet, fatty fish (salmon, herring, mackerel, and anchovies) in the diet at least four times a week, and other low-fat diets have been found to decrease total cholesterol and low-density lipoprotein (LDL) measurements. Following the Food Guide Pyramid for adults older than 70 is the best idea for an ideal diet, with changes based on particular problems such as hypercholesterolemia and following the primary health care provider's recommendations.

Fast foods and snack foods also constitute a substantial component of the American diet. Cross and colleagues (1995) evaluated snacking behavior among 335 community-based older adults. They found that the majority of seniors snacked at least once daily, with only 2.1% reporting that they never snack. Evening was the most common time for snacking, with the most often reported foods being salty/crunchy foods. When selecting snacks, taste outranked nutrition as a selection criteria.

Feeding the Impaired Aged. It is not uncommon in long-term care facilities to hear over the public address system at mealtime, "Feeder trays are ready." This reference to the need to feed those unable to feed themselves is, in itself, degrading and erases any trace of dignity the aged person is trying to maintain in a controlled environment. It is not malicious intent by nurses or other caregivers but rather a habit of convenience. Feeding the aged who do not respond intelligibly becomes mechanical and devoid of conversation and feeling. The feeding process becomes rapid, and if it bogs down and becomes too slow, the meal may be ended abruptly, depending on the time the caregiver has allotted for feeding the patient. Any pleasure is destroyed that could be derived through socialization and eating, as is any dignity that could be maintained while dependent on others for food.

Food should be given with variety throughout the meal; that is, serve a bite of one item, then another, or follow the pattern of eating that the person had before he or she lost the ability to feed himself or herself (if that is known). When an elder needs encouragement to eat, small, frequent servings of foods that he or she likes are better tolerated. Touch and verbal cueing during a meal are thought to help increase nutritional intake.

Lack of eating competence may result in a lessened intake of food. Older adults accustomed to certain table manners may feel ashamed at their inability to behave in what they feel is an appropriate manner.

A qualitative study of eating behaviors in long-term care facilities concluded that the quality of feeding interactions with demented residents was poor. It was attributed to the inadequate number of trained staff (Pierson, 1999), a problem that continues to exist. Residents were fed too fast, with excessive amounts of food for each bite, putting them at risk for aspiration. Adequate nutrition for the helpless aged depends on the conscientiousness of the individual doing the feeding. It is the nurse's responsibility to ensure that all patients unable to feed themselves not only receive a tray but also are actually fed the food that has been brought to them. Any time a patient has refused three consecutive meals, it is essential that a nutritional assessment be done to prevent malnutrition and its complications.

Table 6-4 Fad Diets

Diet	Claim	Composition	Claimed mechanism
Zone	Increased energy Decreased hunger	40% carbohydrate, 30% protein, 30% fat Restricted calories Three meals and two snacks a day Less than 400 kcal per meal	Lower insulin and eicosanoid levels are a master switch for decreasing hunger
Atkins	Carbohydrates cause obesity High protein and high fat cause decreased hunger	36% protein, 8% carbohydrate, 53% fat; then 24% protein 40% fat, 31% carbohydrate No calorie restriction	Ketogenic diet does not oxidize fatty acids in the liver
Pritikin	Low fat Increases energy	8%-12% fat, 12%-15% protein, 80% carbohydrate Less than 100 mg of cholesterol per day	Reduces cholesterol (especially low-density lipoproteins) Low-fat dies carries more oxygen to the cells
Ornish	Low-fat diet lowers cholesterol Diet reverses heart disease	Less than 10% fat, 15%-20% protein, 70%-75% carbohydrate	Reduces cholesterol (especially low-density lipoproteins) Causes documented atherosclerosis regression

Adapted from Russell RM, Saltzman E, Rasmussen H: *Comparison of diet claims*. Available at *www.cyberounds.com/conferences/nutrition.*

In the acute care hospital setting it is equally important to give consideration, care, and attention to the feeding of the dependent aged patient. Sufficient time should be provided to accommodate the aged person who has a slow eating pace.

Dysphagia. Difficulty swallowing is a common problem of older adults. Malnutrition may occur rapidly after onset of the problem, especially in instances such as stroke or Parkinson's disease (Mosqueda and Brummel-Smith, 2002). Although a feeding tube may facilitate better nutrition, about one half of elderly patients will aspirate with a nasogastric or gastric tube. The speech therapist will be able to assess the elder to determine the best type of food and food consistency for the swallowing problem.

Those with late-stage dementia will also have problems of malnutrition because of dysphagia. With poor attention and concentration, the elder also forgets to swallow (Ham, 2002). In this instance, it may be that inserting a feeding tube constitutes "extraordinary treatment." Maintaining oral and spoon feeding of the elder should continue as long as possible. The risk of aspiration is present with or without the feeding tube. The oral gratification one derives from eating, as well as pleasure it gives a family member, should be weighed against the risk of aspiration in the demented patient with a poor prognosis.

Tube feeding. Some of the reasons that tube feeding is considered are mechanical problems with eating, psychologic disorders, unconsciousness, esophageal stricture or obstruction, anorexia of chronic illness, and neurologic disorders (Moore, 2001). Most commercial products are lactose free because of intolerance in many older adults and those with malabsorption syndromes. Formulas for feedings should vary based on certain diseases such as glucose intolerance, which would entail finding a formula with low carbohydrate content, high fiber to reduce glucose response, and high monounsaturated fatty acids to reduce risk of heart disease. Tube feedings may be given in the esophagus, stomach, or small intestine. Nasogastric, nasoduodenal, and nasojejunal tubes are used for short-term feedings, often a good idea after a hip fracture when the serum albumin is low. For long-term feedings for very debilitated elders, percutaneous endoscopic gastrostomies are popular because they can be inserted without general anesthesia. Other types for long-term feeding include esophagostomy, gastrostomy, and jejunostomy. Most of the formulas given through tube feedings are concentrated, and the hydration status of the patient must be closely monitored.

Intentional starvation. Refusal of food can be an acceptable means of suicide for the aged person. Some elders truly have given up and wish to die. Not eating is one last bastion of control over life and dignity. It is essential for the nurse to differentiate between the individual who is refusing food because it is unpalatable and the person who is depressed and really wishes to die. Intentional starvation is easier and more successful when one is not institutionalized. The institutionalized person is often denied this right and is robbed of the option by forced feeding via a nasogastric tube. The American Nurses' Association (1992) developed a position statement on forgoing artificial nutrition and hydration. The position states: "The decision to withhold artificial nutrition and hydration should be made by the patient or surrogate with the health care team. The nurse continues to provide expert care to patients who are no longer receiving artificial nutrition and hydration."

Watching someone starve is difficult for the nurse, but if intentional starvation is the patient's desire, the nurse should continue to order the tray, take it to the person, and acknowledge that the individual has the right to eat or not eat. It is important to leave the tray so that the person can exercise the option to change his or her mind. If the person is unable to feed himself or herself, check shortly after the first offering of food has been refused to see if the person does wish to eat. An empathetic and nonjudgmental approach by the nurse to the aged person who demonstrates starvation behavior will convey that the individual is still in control, and if for some reason the individual decides to exercise the option to eat again, this too is all right. Either way, the caregiver has provided support and respect for that individual. Professional team conferences are needed to deal with the client's mental status and ethical issues involved in referral and the right to die. Superficial judgments are not adequate to encompass these profound issues.

Assessment

A nutritional assessment that provides the most conclusive data about a person's actual nutritional state consists of four steps: interview, physical examination, anthropometric measurements, and biochemical analysis. The collective results can provide the nurse with data needed to identify the immediate and potential nutrition problems of the client. The nurse can then begin to establish plans for supervision, assistance, and education in the attainment of adequate nutrition for the aged person. The Nutrition Screening Initiative presents an algorithm for nutritional assessment and approaches (see Figure 6-4).

Interview. The interview provides background information and clues to the nutritional state and actual and potential problems of the elderly person. Questions about the individual's state of health, social activities, normal patterns, and changes that have occurred should be asked. The nurse must explore the individual's needs, the manner in which food is obtained, and the client's ability to prepare food. Information concerning the relationship of food to daily events will provide clues to the meaning and significance of food to that person. The aged who eat alone are considered candidates for malnutrition. Information about daily activities will suggest the degree of energy expenditure and caloric intake most correct for the overall activity. One's economic state will have a direct bearing on nutrition. It is therefore important to explore the client's financial resources to establish the income available for food. Knowledge of medications taken should be included in the nutrition history. Additional medical information

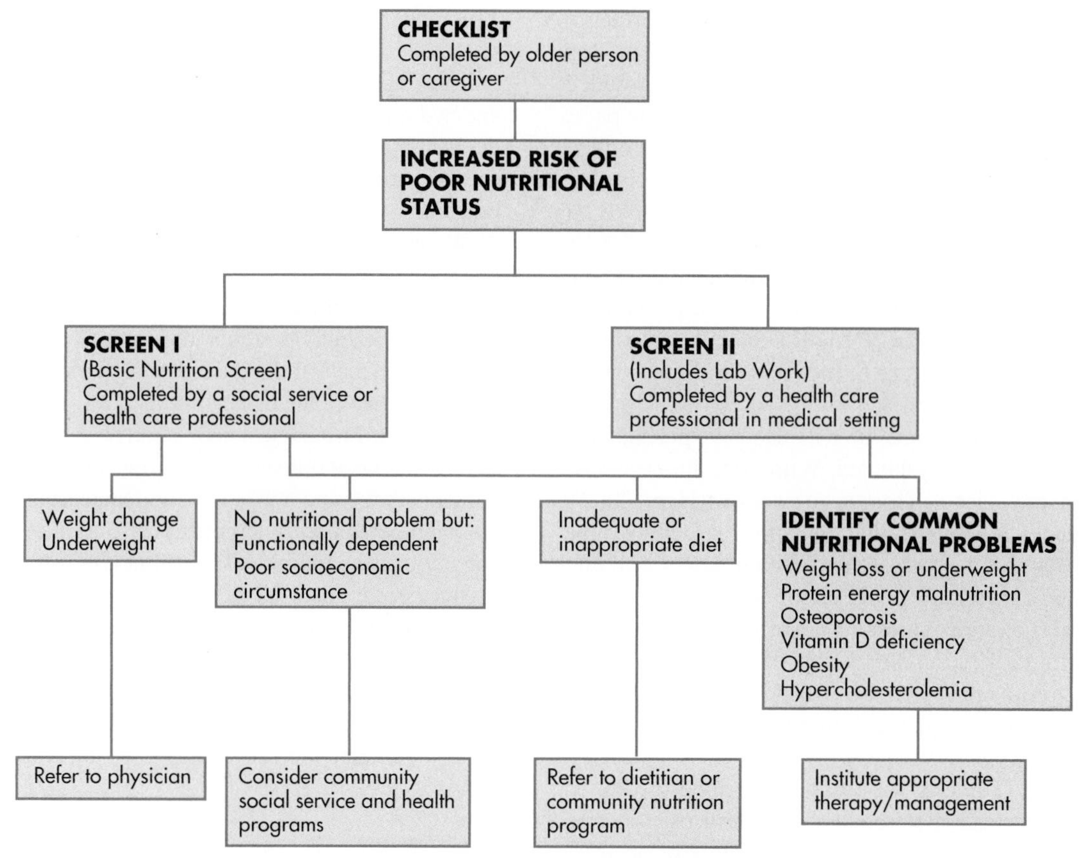

Figure 6-4. Nutritional assessment and approaches. (Courtesy The Nutrition Screening Initiative, Washington, DC.)

should be included in the interview. The presence or absence of mouth pain or discomfort, visual difficulty, bowel and bladder function, and food intake patterns should be explored. Frequently a 24-hour diet recall compared with the Food Guide Pyramid can present an estimate of nutritional adequacy. When the aged person cannot provide all the information requested, it may be possible to obtain data from a family member or another source. There will be times, however, when information will not be as complete as one would like, or the aged person, too proud to admit that he or she is not eating, will furnish erroneous information. The nurse will still be able to obtain additional data from the other three areas of the nutritional assessment.

Keeping a dietary record for 3 days is another assessment tool. Careful recording of when one ate, what was eaten, and amounts eaten must be made. This approach should be attempted only with dependable, cooperative elders. Computer analysis of the dietary records provides information on energy and vitamin and mineral intake. Printouts can provide the elderly and the health care provider with a visual graph of their intake.

Physical Examination. The second step of the nutritional assessment, the physical examination, furnishes clinically observable evidence of the existing state of nutrition. Data such as height and weight; vital signs; condition of the tongue, lips, and gums; and skin turgor, texture, and color are assessed, and the general overall appearance is scrutinized for evidence of wasting.

Debate continues in the quest to determine the appropriate weight charts for the aged. Weight, however, is not the only issue; fat distribution must be considered.

Anthropometric Measurements. Anthropometric measurements are the third part of the nutritional assessment and should include height, weight, midarm circumference, and triceps skinfold thickness. These include simple body measurement procedures, which take less than 5 minutes to perform. These measurements obtain information about the status of the aged person's muscle mass and body fat in relation to height and weight. In some instances an individual is bedridden or confined to a chair, or the individual has a spinal curvature preventing accurate height measurement. Unlike stature, knee height changes little with age. It should be noted that blacks have proportionally longer lower extremities and Chinese have shorter extremities than whites (Moore, 2001). An estimation of stature can be made using knee height and a sliding broad-blade calipers, similar to the apparatus used to measure the length of an infant. This device consists of an adjustable blade attached to each end at a 90-degree angle.

Muscle mass measurements are obtained by measuring the arm circumference of the nondominant upper arm. The arm hangs freely at the side, and a measuring tape is placed around the midpoint of the upper arm, between the acromion of the scapula and the olecranon of the ulna. The centimeter circumference is recorded and compared with standard values (see Table 6-4).

Body fat and lean body mass are assessed by measuring specific skinfolds with Lange or Harpenden calipers. Two areas are accessible for measurement. One area is the midpoint of the upper arm, the triceps area, which is also used to obtain arm circumference. The nondominant arm is again used. The nurse lifts the skin with the thumb and forefinger so that it parallels the humerus. The calipers are placed around the skinfold, 1 cm below where the fingers are grasping the skin. Two readings are averaged to the nearest half centimeter. Results should be compared with standard values such as those cited in Moore (2001). If there is a neuropathologic condition or hemiplegia following a stroke, the unaffected arm should be used for obtaining measurements.

There are more sophisticated methods of assessing body composition. Magnetic resonance imaging (MRI), computed tomography (CT), ultrasound, DEXA scans, and densitometry are a few. They are becoming available in most communities but are expensive.

The BMI, or body mass index, discussed earlier, is a simple tool for evaluation of the appropriateness of weight to height. It does not, however, assess lean body mass or fat, but does correlate well with many of the other measures of body fat content and does correlate with the risk of morbidity. It has the additional virtue of ease of assessment if accurate measures of height and weight are available (Moore, 2001).

Biochemical Examination. The final step in a nutritional assessment is the biochemical examination. A decreased albumin may indicate protein deficiency, but albumin is slow to change during malnutrition (Moore, 2001). Serum albumin less than 4 is desired. Prealbumin levels are a better indicator of protein loss because it changes rapidly in malnutrition. It also decreases in inflammatory diseases and injury situations. Transferrin, an iron transport protein, is diminished in protein malnutrition; like prealbumin, it responds quickly (diminishes) with undernutrition. However, it increases in iron deficiency anemia, which is common in older adults and those with protein calorie malnutrition, so it is not a sensitive indicator of protein calorie malnutrition. A normocytic red blood cell (RBC) anemia with low hemoglobin and hematocrit indicates protein deficiency, and a microcytic (small RBC) anemia indicates iron or copper deficiency. A macrocytic (large RBC) anemia is caused by vitamin B_{12} or folate deficiency.

Intervention

Interventions are formulated around the identified nutritional problem or problems. Perhaps the most significant intervention for the community-dwelling elder is nutrition education and problem solving with the elder in how to best resolve the potential or actual nutritional deficit.

Education in the area of reading nutritional information on labels is needed. Since 1994, the U.S. Food and Drug Administration (FDA) has required producers of processed foods to list nutrition information based on daily values. Daily values represent the maximum amounts of nutrients and fiber that are desirable in daily diets of 2000 to 2500 calories. The nutrients were chosen based on evidence suggesting that eating too much or too little of these substances has the greatest impact on one's health. FDA defines a "good source" as a food that contains 10% to 19% of the daily value per serving. The daily totals for fat, cholesterol, and sodium should be less than 100%. Balance should be emphasized as the key to a healthful diet.

Practical suggestions for increasing intake when an older person is experiencing a poor appetite or is known to have protein calorie undernutrition are as follows:

- Determine food preferences, including ethnic preferences.
- Ensure that the resident has adequate time to eat.
- Provide snacks between meals and at night.
- Do not interrupt meals with medications.
- Encourage family members to share the mealtimes for a heightened social situation.
- If calorie supplements are given, offer between meals or with the "medication pass."
- Encourage eating in the dining room with others for a more enjoyable social atmosphere.
- Recommend an exercise program, which often increases appetite.
- A small amount of wine or alcohol before meals may stimulate the appetite.
- For those with dysphagia (difficulty swallowing), discourage talking during meals and remind to swallow.
- Encourage denture use.
- Wear glasses with meals.
- Conduct calorie counts, because they serve as a useful indicator that progress is being made and show foods that are tolerated.

It is important for those elders who are institutionalized to receive appropriate supervision at mealtime so that they are able to eat their food, have their food cut for them (if necessary), and have any other requirements met that will enable them to meet their nutritional intake needs.

ELIMINATION

The body must remove waste products of metabolism to sustain healthy function, but bladder and bowel activity are fraught with social implications. Bladder and bowel function of the aged, although normally only slightly altered by physiologic changes of age, can develop problems severe enough to interfere with the ability to continue independent living and seriously threaten the body's capacity to function and to survive. The effects of uncontrolled bladder and bowel action are a threat to the person's independence and well-being.

Elimination is a private matter not publicized socially. However, the media places emphasis on specific procedures of eliminating and disposing of waste and advertises laxatives to maintain evacuation of fecal matter. Bowel preoccupation costs millions of dollars in laxative expenditures, mainly to the older patient. As children, correct behavior in dealing with our own body waste is taught early. Deviations from this are socially unacceptable and can lead to chastisement, ostracism, and social withdrawal.

Bowel Function

Attention to bowel function occurs when there is a deviation from what is perceived as normal elimination. The aged are known for their concern with their bowel function and frequently complain to physicians and other health care personnel about problems, particularly constipation. Whatever the complaint, one needs to know exactly what the individual means when he or she says there is a problem. Bowel function problems that the nurse will encounter among aged clients are constipation, fecal impaction, irritable bowel syndrome, and fecal or bowel incontinence.

Constipation. Constipation has different meanings to different people. Some individuals consider constipation infrequent bowel action; others perceive it as difficulty in passing feces. In one study, half the elders who complained of constipation moved their bowels at least once a day (Edwards, 2002). To the health professional, constipation occurs when there are less than three bowel movements a week or there is a decrease in usual stool frequency. It is the most common GI complaint to the health care provider, with about 60% of community-based elders reporting laxative use (Beers and Berkow, 2000). About 74% of older adults in long-term care use laxatives daily.

Normal elimination should be an easy passage of feces, without undue straining or a feeling of incomplete evacuation or defecation. The urge to defecate occurs when the distended walls of the sigmoid and rectum, which are filled with feces, stimulate pressure receptors to relax the sphincters for the expulsion of stool through the anus. Evacuation of feces is accomplished by relaxation of the sphincters and contraction of the diaphragm and abdominal muscles, which raises intraabdominal pressure.

Constipation appears to be a problem of the elder because of age-related physiologic changes (Beers and Berkow, 2000). There is impaired rectal sensation so that larger volumes are required to elicit the sensation to defecate. There is also reduced resting anal sphincter pressure and diminished maximum sphincter pressure, predisposing to fecal incontinence. It is perhaps more correct to consider the extensive use of laxatives by the aged as a cultural habit. During their formative years, weekly doses of rhubarb, cascara, castor oil, and other types of laxatives were consumed to promote health. This belief that cleaning out the colon was paramount to maintaining good health still persists with many elderly persons.

Constipation is a symptom. It is a reflection of poor habits, postponed passage of stool, and many chronic illnesses—both physical and psychologic. Numerous precipitating factors or conditions can cause or worsen constipation (Beers and Berkow, 2000). Table 6-5 lists these factors. Diet plays a significant role in problems with intestinal motility and constipation.

Assessment. The precipitants and causes of constipation must be included in the assessment of the patient. A review of these factors will also determine if a patient is at risk for altered bowel function. It is recognized that elderly people at high risk for constipation and subsequent impaction are those who are immobilized and debilitated or who have central nervous system lesions. It is also important to know that confusion, increased agitation, incontinence, or unexplainable falls may be the only clinical symptoms of constipation in the elderly person.

Table 6-5 Precipitating Factors for Constipation

Physiologic	Psychologic
Dehydration	Avoidance of urge to defecate
Insufficient fiber intake	Confusion
Poor dietary habits	Depression
	Emotional stress
Functional	**Systemic**
Decreased physical activity	Diabetes mellitus
Inadequate toileting	Hypercalcemia
Irregular defecation habits	Hyperparathyroidism
Irritable bowel disease	Hypothyroidism
Weakness	Hypokalemia
	Pheochromocytoma
	Porphyria
	Uremia
Mechanical	**Pharmacologic**
Abscess or ulcer	Aluminum-containing antacids
Cerebrovascular disease	Anticholinergics
Defective electrolyte transfer	Anticonvulsants
Fissures	Antidepressants
Hemorrhoids	Bismuth salts
Hirschsprung's disease	Calcium carbonate
Neurological disease	Calcium channel blockers
Parkinson's disease	Diuretics
Postsurgical obstruction	Laxative overuse
Prostate enlargement	Iron salts
Rectal prolapse	Nonsteroidal antiinflammatories
Rectocele	Opiates
Spinal cord injury	Phenothiazines
Strictures	Sedatives
Tumors	Sympathomimetics
Other	
Lack of abdominal muscle tone	Obesity
Recent environmental changes	Poor dentition

From Allison OC, Porter ME, Briggs GG: Chronic constipation: assessment and management in the elderly, *J Am Acad Nurse Pract* 6(7):311, 1994.

A physical examination is needed to rule out systemic causes of constipation. A neurologic examination is important because constipation is a common problem of many neurologic illnesses (Edwards, 2002). The assessment will also focus on the GI system and an assessment for signs of dehydration. The abdomen is examined for bowel sounds, pain, localized masses (retained stool), distention, and evidence of prior surgery (Edwards, 2002).

A rectal examination is important to reveal painful anal disorders such as hemorrhoids or fissures that will impede the evacuation of stool and to evaluate sphincter tone, rectal prolapse, stool presence in the vault, strictures, masses, anal reflex, and enlarged prostate (Edwards, 2002).

Biochemical tests should include a complete blood count, fasting glucose, chemistry panel, and thyroid studies. These will rule out a number of causes of constipation such as anemia, diabetes, electrolyte imbalances, and hypothyroidism. If the constipation is of recent or sudden onset, or is accompanied by bleeding, a colonoscopy or other GI examination may be warranted to rule out obstruction or tumor. If there is stool seepage and impaction is suspected with an empty vault, abdominal x-ray films will reveal a high impaction, intussusception, or other obstruction (Edwards, 2002).

Many tests are available for intractable constipation. Colonic transit and anorectal function can be evaluated (Beers and Berkow, 2000). These tests include radiopaque markers, defecating proctography, and anorectal manometry.

Intervention. The first intervention is to examine the medications the patient is taking and eliminate those that are constipation producing or change to medications that are not constipation producing. Edwards (2002) states that it is better to start a bowel regimen with an empty colon, which may require removal of impaction manually or the use of enemas. Any regimen should be started slowly and with the patient's preferences included in order to improve compliance. This will also avoid bloating and cramping gas pains that occur with a faster implementation time.

Nonpharmacologic interventions for constipation that have been implemented and evaluated can be grouped into four areas: (1) fluid/fiber, (2) exercise, (3) environmental manipulation, and (4) a combination of these. Fluids should be mainly water, because many beverages cause diuresis. Adequate hydration is the cornerstone of constipation therapy (Beers and Berkow, 2000). The use of bran fiber and fruit and vegetable fiber and nuts is recommended. Bran fiber results in a functioning colon with higher fecal bulking action. See Box 6-7 for foods high in dietary fiber. This may minimize or obviate the need for supplemental fibers such as psyllium and methylcellulose. Decreasing the fat in the diet is useful because fat slows down the transit time of digestion (Edwards, 2002). If megacolon or colonic dilation from bowel obstruction is suspected, fiber supplements are not advised. Indeed, most of these patients are on a fiber-restricted diet.

Laxatives. One consideration besides fiber is senna tea. Senna is an effective laxative that is safe for elderly patients and is nontoxic. Senna tea is slightly absorbed systemically, is effective in small doses, and has a local action that increases colon peristalsis. Another laxative often prescribed is cascara. They can both be taken orally or rectally. They can cause abdominal cramping and fluid and electrolyte disturbances, especially if impaction is present (Beers and Berkow, 2000). These stimulant laxatives should be used short term because they can cause dependency. Hyperosmolar laxatives such as polyethylene glycol (GoLYTELY) are used for bowel preparations for procedures and are safe. Lactulose and sorbitol increase fluid in the colon and promote soft stools. They work slowly but are effective in frail elderly (Edwards, 2002). Emollient laxatives include mineral oil and docusate sodium. Mineral oil should not be used because of the risk of oil aspiration and vitamin depletion if used too often. Saline laxatives work by drawing water into the small bowel and stimulating peristalsis; the bowel empties within hours. They should not be used in those elders with poor renal function if they contain magnesium, phosphate, or sulfate salts (Edwards, 2002). See Box 6-12 for a natural laxative recipe.

Stool softeners. These medications help soften hard stools but do not actually affect constipation. Docusate sodium is the most common stool softener prescribed. They may be a useful adjunct to other methods, especially in bedridden patients.

Enemas. Soapsuds and phosphate enemas irritate the rectal mucosa and should not be used (Edwards, 2002). Enemas of any type should be reserved for situations where other methods produce no response or when it is known that there is an impaction. Normal saline or tap water enema at a temperature of about 105° F is the best choice. Perforation is a possibility, and the enema should be administered with care. The amount of water should be about 500 to 1000 ml (Beers and Berkow, 2000).

Position. The squatting position facilitates bowel function if the patient is able to squat. A similar position may be obtained by leaning forward and applying firm pressure to the lower abdomen or placing the feet on a stool. Massaging the abdomen may help stimulate the bowel.

Exercise. Exercise is important as an intervention to stimulate colon motility and bowel evacuation. Daily walking for 20 to 30 minutes is helpful, especially after a meal. Pelvic tilt

Box 6-12 Natural Laxative Recipe That Really Works

Power Pudding

Standard recipe:

- 1 cup wheat bran
- 1 cup applesauce
- 1 cup prune juice

Mix and store in refrigerator. Start with administration of 1 tbsp/day. Increase *slowly* until desired effect is achieved and no disagreeable symptoms occur.

exercises and range-of-motion (passive or active) exercises are beneficial for those who are less mobile or even bedbound.

Regularity. Establishing a routine for toileting promotes or normalizes bowel function. The gastrocolic reflex occurs after breakfast or supper and may be enhanced by a warm drink (Edwards, 2002). Given privacy and ample time (a minimum of 10 minutes) many will have a daily bowel movement. However, any urge to defecate should be followed by a response toward the bathroom.

A program to prevent as well as treat constipation that incorporates a high-fiber diet, liberal fluid intake, daily exercise, and environmental modifications that promote a regular pattern of bowel elimination needs to be developed for each client. The interventions for clients in any setting are based on a thorough assessment.

Fecal impaction. This situation is a major complication of constipation. It is especially common in incapacitated and institutionalized elderly people. Symptoms of fecal impaction include malaise, urinary retention, incontinence of bladder or bowel, confusion, fissures, hemorrhoids, and intestinal obstruction. The causes are similar to those of constipation. Unrecognized, unattended, or neglected constipation eventually leads to fecal impaction and incontinence or paradoxic diarrhea, which results from a ball-valve effect that allows liquid stool to seep around the obstructing fecal mass during normal colon contractions. Removal of a fecal impaction is at times worse than the misery of the condition. Continued obstruction by the fecal mass may eventually impair sensation, leading to the need for larger stool volume to stimulate the urge to defecate, which contributes to megacolon (Edwards, 2002). Valsalva maneuvers done during straining at stool defecation can cause transient ischemic attacks and syncope, especially in frail elderly.

Management of fecal impactions requires the digital removal of the hard, compacted stool from the rectum with use of lubrication containing lidocaine jelly. Generally this is preceded by multiple enemas or an oil-retention enema to soften the feces in preparation for manual removal. Use of suppositories is not effective, because their action is blocked by the amount and the size of the stool in the rectum as compared with the capacity of the sphincter to dilate. Suppositories do not facilitate the removal of stool in the sigmoid, which may continue to ooze once the rectum is emptied.

Several sessions or days may be required to totally cleanse the sigmoid colon and rectum of impacted feces. Once this is achieved, attention should be directed to planning a regimen that includes adequate fluid intake, increased dietary fiber, administration of stool softeners if needed, and many of the suggestions presented for prevention of constipation.

REST AND SLEEP

The human organism needs rest and sleep to conserve energy, prevent fatigue, provide organ respite, and relieve tension. Sleep is an extension of rest, and both are physiologic and mental necessities for survival. Rest depends on the degree of physical and mental relaxation. It is often assumed that lying in bed constitutes rest, but worries and other related stressors cause muscles throughout the body to continue to contract with tension even though physical activity has ceased. Attainment of rest depends on this interrelationship of psyche and soma. Body functions possess refractory times and rest periods in the continuous cycle of activity (biorhythms). Drastically or continually altered sleep and rest cycles disrupt homeostatic balance and create physical or mental aberrations.

Sleep is a basic need. Rest occurs with sleep in sustained unbroken periods. Sleep is restorative and recuperative and is necessary for the preservation of life.

Biorhythm and Sleep

Our lives are a series of rhythms that influence and regulate physiologic function, chemical concentrations, performance, behavioral responses, moods, and the ability to adapt. The most obvious rhythm is the day-night cycle known as the diurnal or circadian rhythm. The most important and obvious biorhythm is the circadian sleep/wake rhythm. Abnormalities of this cycle, termed *circadian dysrhythmia,* are common among elderly people (Beers and Berkow, 2000). They take a longer time to resolve than in younger adults.

Several different types of dysrhythmia can occur. *Jet lag* is a transient shift in sleep/wake patterns caused by travel across time zones. *Shift work dysrhythmia* occurs when one switches from a day work pattern to a night work pattern. *Delayed sleep phase syndrome* is when one falls asleep later and wakes later than usual or desired. *Advanced sleep phase syndrome* is falling asleep earlier and waking earlier than desired. *Non–24-hour syndrome* is a sleep/wake pattern reflecting a circadian cycle longer or shorter than 24 hours. *Irregular sleep/wake patterns* are when one falls asleep and wakes at irregular times (Beers and Berkow, 2000).

Institutions that provide care for the aged adhere to specific time schedules, which may not correspond to the biorhythm of the aged person and which may place the individual out of synchronization with his or her body functions. Attention to biorhythms can help establish the normal sleep/wake pattern of the aged person and identify the best times to introduce activities, periods of rest, and therapeutic measures.

Bright light therapy has been found to be effective, especially for jet lag and for those with advanced sleep phase syndrome in which the elder falls asleep early. It is helpful for readjusting sleeping schedules (Rosto, 2001). The author suggests exposure to bright outdoor light or the use of a light box later in the afternoon to reset the circadian rhythm. Melatonin is another therapy used for jet lag. The use of hypnotics such as zolpidem tartrate (Ambien) or zaleplon (Sonata) appears to cause little residual sleepiness and may be helpful in reestablishing a regular sleep pattern (Hill-O'Neill and Shaughnessy, 2002). The nonbenzodiazepine hypnotics should be used only short term, for 7 to 10 days, and then reevaluated.

Normal Sleep Pattern

Sleep structure is the term for the stages and cycles of sleep. It is characterized by non–rapid eye movement (NREM) sleep and rapid eye movement (REM) sleep. Sleep structure is shown in Box 6-13.

About 50% of elderly people complain of sleep problems, most often the problem of falling asleep and staying asleep (Beers and Berkow, 2000). Age-related changes in sleep include the timing and amount of sleep. Elderly people tend to fall asleep earlier and wake earlier and are less tolerant of changes in the sleep/wake cycle. Daytime naps may compensate for poor nocturnal sleep, or poor nocturnal sleep may be due to daytime naps. One study of more than 400 community-based elders found that 19% were troubled by poor sleep, 21% felt that they got too little sleep, 24% reported difficulty falling asleep at least once each week, and 39% reported excessive daytime sleepiness (Schoenfelder and Culp, 2001).

Insomnia. *Insomnia* is defined as difficulty falling asleep or staying asleep. Insomnia can be classified by duration. Transient insomnia occurs in times of acute stress, which may be due to bereavement, hospitalization, or even retirement. Short-term insomnia occurs with prolonged stress, new medications or stopping a medication, or a psychologic disorder. Chronic insomnia lasts longer than 3 weeks and is what usually occurs with aging, but it may occur with chronic stress such as nursing home placement, continued bereavement, a forced retirement, medications, or a psychiatric disorder (Beers and Berkow, 2000). Insomnia is more common in women and can be a serious problem to the older person and family. Its effects include mood changes, memory deficits, difficulty with concentration, poor judgment, impaired performance, and changes in the immune system (Fielo, 2001).

There is a Diagnostic and Statistical Manual of Mental Disorders (DSM-IV-TR) classification and an International Classification of Diseases (ICD) classification for insomnia. Most primary health providers use the ICD classification; psychiatrists use the DSM criteria. Depression is a common cause of insomnia in older adults. The prevalence of insomnia is difficult to document, but the use of hypnotics is more common in older adults than in younger people. A number of drugs may cause sleep disturbances (Box 6-14). In addition to medications, depression, and daytime naps, other causes of insomnia include worry and anxiety, hospitalization, new environments, pain, heat or cold, dementia, Parkinson's disease, allergies, changes in routine, alcohol use or abuse, inadequate exercise, and periodic limb movement of sleep (PLMS; also called nocturnal myoclonus) (Schoenfelder and Culp, 2001). In addition, melatonin, which is naturally secreted during evening hours and promotes sleep, is decreased in older adults.

Narcolepsy. Narcolepsy is a disorder of unknown etiology and is underdiagnosed (McCullough, 2001). Symptoms include excessive sleepiness and sleep "attacks";

Box 6-13 Sleep Structure

Four Stages of Non–Rapid Eye Movement (NREM) Sleep

Stage 1

Lightest level
Easy to awaken
5% of sleep in young

Stage 2

Decreases with age
Low-voltage activity on electroencephalogram (EEG)
May cease in old age

Stage 3

Decreases with age
High-voltage activity on EEG
May cease in old age

Stage 4

Decreases with age
High-voltage activity on EEG
15% of sleep in elders

Rapid Eye Movement (REM) Sleep

Alternates with NREM sleep throughout the night
Rapid eye movements the key feature
Breathing increases in rate and depth
Muscle tone relaxed
85% of dreaming occurs

Adapted from Beers MH, Berkow R: *Merck manual of geriatrics,* ed 3, Whitehouse Station, NJ, 2000, Merck Research Laboratories.

Box 6-14 Drugs That Cause Sleep Disturbances

Caffeine (prolongs sleep latency and interferes with sleep maintenance)
Bronchodilators and sympathomimetics (stimulate central nervous system [CNS])
Diuretics (if used late in the day, produce nocturia, waking the person)
Decongestants, ephedrine, β-agonists, and methylxanthines (if used at night, prolong sleep initiation)
Antihypertensives, α-agonists, and central-acting (CNS effects alter sleep physiology)
β-Blockers (cause nightmares; CNS effects cause changes in sleep physiology)
Carbidopa and levodopa (cause nightmares)
Benzodiazepines (cause rebound insomnia with discontinuation; tolerance with prolonged use)

Adapted from Beers MH, Berkow R: *Merck manual of geriatrics,* ed 3, Whitehouse Station, NJ, 2000, Merck Research Laboratories.

hallucinations or dreamlike perceptions at sleep onset; a sleep paralysis, in which the person does not move at sleep onset and sometimes on awakening; and disturbed nighttime sleep. REM sleep occurs at sleep onset, which is premature, usually occurring later in the sleep cycle. Modafinil (Provigil), a newer drug, promotes daytime alertness and is technically a stimulant (Gorman, 2001). Provigil has side effects of headache, nausea, and anxiety. This drug is not recommended in patients with a history of cardiac ischemia, arrhythmia, myocardial infarction, or left ventricular hypertrophy.

Sleep Apnea. Sleep apnea syndrome is a disorder characterized by repetitive cessation of respiration during sleep. Obstructive sleep apnea affects about 10% of those older than 65 and is the most common type of sleep apnea in elderly people (Drazen, 2002) and occurs twice as often in men as women (McCullough, 2001). Although we usually associate it with obesity, and it is common in obese elders, this is not a risk factor for sleep apnea. Box 6-15 lists sleep apnea risk factors. Normal ventilation does not occur in those with sleep apnea, and there is cessation of airflow for greater than 10 seconds. When breathing is inadequate, a "fire alarm" goes off and the person is aroused from slumber, normal ventilation then occurs, and the person tries to go back to sleep. Sleep is then very fragmented and not restoring. After months or years of living with this problem, severe psychologic and physiologic consequences occur, including right-sided heart failure, hypertension, cardiac arrhythmias, and death (Drazen, 2002). Other consequences include an increased number of automobile accidents, more work-related accidents, poor performance, depression, and decreased quality of life (McCullough, 2001).

Assessment includes information from the sleeping partner and consideration of a sleep study because assessment of patients during sleep is important. The sleeping partner's sleep is often disturbed by this treatment, and the sleeping partner may move to another room to sleep. Therapy will depend on the severity of the sleep apnea. Some of the clinical features of sleep apnea include gasping and choking on awakenings; uncertainty of reason for awakenings; restless sleep; nonrestoring sleep; poor memory and intellectual functioning; irritability and personality change; and morning headache or confusion (McCullough, 2001). The family will reveal that the person has daytime sleepiness, which is often unrecognized by the patient. If questioned about automobile accidents, the assessor will find that there have been some or some near misses. The patient will sleep in inappropriate settings such as in social situations or at work.

Physical assessment often reveals that the individual is obese, although this is not a specific risk factor. The neck is often short and thick. The uvula is large and the soft palate hangs low. Tonsils may be enlarged; adenoids are enlarged. There may be micrognathia or retrognathia, that is, small chin or receded chin. Look for upper airway tumors or cysts (McCullough, 2001).

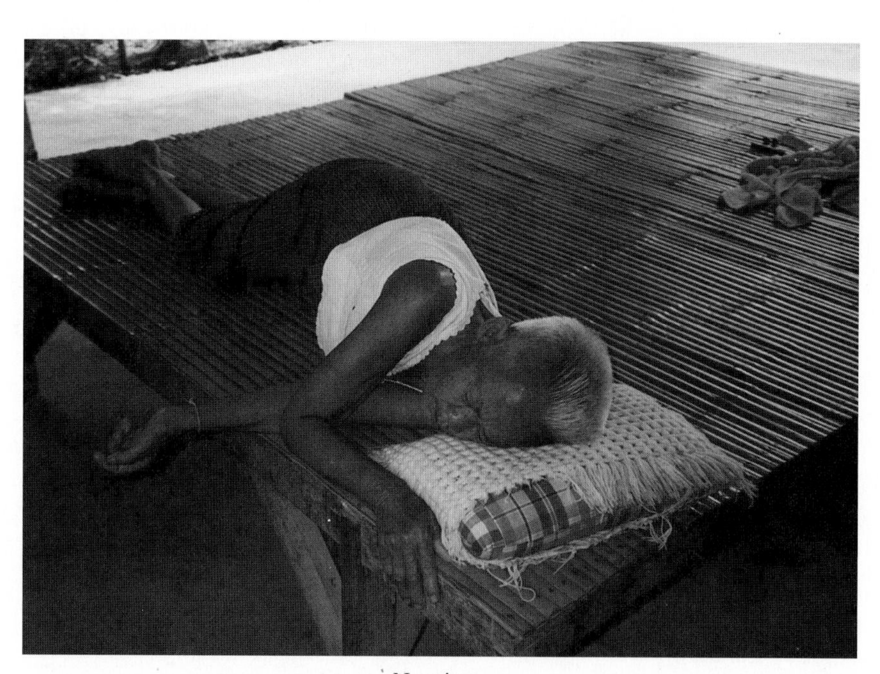

Napping.

Box 6-15 Sleep Apnea Risk Factors

- Increasing age
- Male gender
- Anatomic abnormalities of the upper airway
- Family history
- Alcohol or sedative use
- Smoking
- Associated conditions

Adapted from McCullough P: *How well do you sleep?* Presentation at the Kentucky Council of Nurse Practitioners and Midwives, Lexington, KY, April 2001.

Specific treatment of sleep apnea has the goals of reducing morbidity and mortality and increasing quality of life. There should be risk counseling about impaired judgment from sleeplessness and possibility of accidents if driving. The patient should be encouraged to lose weight, avoid alcohol and sedatives, stop smoking, avoid supine sleep positions by using pillows or sleeping in a chair, and avoid situations where there would be sleep deprivation (McCullough, 2001). Medical interventions include nasal mask continuous positive airway pressure (CPAP), which presents the difficulty of compliance. Oxygen may be used because it can reduce arrhythmias; humidifiers, oral appliances, decongestants, nasal steroids, antihistamines, selective serotonin reuptake inhibitor (SSRI) antidepressants, and tricyclic antidepressants may also be used. Surgery to reconstruct the upper airway can be considered; this involves tonsillectomy, uvula surgery, and a number of other procedures. In severe cases, tracheostomy is used to bypass the upper airway. Interestingly, because sleep apnea causes arrhythmias in older adults, pacemakers have been inserted. A significant finding with the pacemaker is that patients have fewer and less severe episodes of apnea if the pacemaker is set to achieve atrial overdrive (15 beats per minute faster than usual night heart rate without the pacer) (Drazen, 2002).

Nocturnal Myoclonus. The syndrome of periodic limb jerks or movements in sleep (PLMS) is nocturnal myoclonus. The incidence of PLMS increases with age and may occur in up to 45% of community-based elders (Beers and Berkow, 2000). It may occur in up to 80% of those with restless leg syndrome (RLS) (McCullough, 2001). The etiology is unknown, although it has been suggested that the cause may be an age-related decrease in dopamine receptors because carbidopa-levodopa can be used to manage the myoclonus. PLMS occurs only during sleep. Often, the patient is unaware of the occurrence; however, it is very disruptive to the sleep partner.

Diagnosis is difficult to make, but usually there are periodic movements with an interval of 20 to 40 seconds with a duration of 2 to 4 seconds; movements occur only during sleep. It typically manifests as flexion of the big toe, rapid ankle flexion, and some flexion of the knee and hip (Beers and Berkow, 2000). The upper extremities also may move. Carbidopa-levodopa is a preferred treatment and is effective in low doses. If this treatment is ineffective, clonazepam (a benzodiazepine) or bromocriptine may be tried. Use of opioids is another option if symptoms are severe and other treatments are ineffective.

Restless Leg Syndrome. Restless leg syndrome (RLS) is characterized by the need to move the legs. Other symptoms include paresthesias, creeping sensations, crawling sensations, tingling, cramping, burning sensations, pain, or even indescribable sensations (McCullough, 2001). It is worse at rest and at night, and is relieved by activity. It is a motor restlessness that in daytime is characterized as leg rubbing, stretching, flexing, body rocking, marching in place, and floor pacing. This can occur at any age but most severely affects those in middle to old age. It is often progressive but may have remissions. About 30% of cases report family history of RLS, but it can occur as a side effect of some pharmaceuticals.

Assessment focuses on the neurologic examination, which is usually normal. There may be a peripheral neuropathy or radiculopathy. In secondary RLS, patients usually have one of the following: polyneuropathies, lumbosacral radiculopathy, amyotrophic lateral sclerosis (ALS), Parkinson's disease, multiple sclerosis, or poliomyelitis. It has also occurred after gastrectomy and with anemia (especially iron or folate deficiency), diabetes, cancers, chronic obstructive pulmonary disease (COPD), rheumatoid arthritis, hypothyroidism, renal failure, and amyloidosis (McCullough, 2001). It can be caused or precipitated by drugs and medications such as SSRIs. Implicated are caffeine, neuroleptics, lithium, calcium channel blockers, and withdrawal of sedatives or narcotics.

Diagnosis and management can be long and cumbersome. A number of laboratory tests can be performed to rule out certain conditions, such as anemia and diabetes. If a neuroleptic is implicated, changing medications may stop the symptoms entirely. Walking, stretching, and rubbing the legs usually help. Carbidopa-levodopa or bromocriptine may relieve chronic symptoms (Beers and Berkow, 2000). Opioids or benzodiazepines may also be effective, but these are used only for patients with severe symptoms that do not respond to other drugs.

Sleep Disorders of Dementia. Patients with Alzheimer's disease have more arousals and awakenings and spend more time in stage 1 sleep and less time in stage 3 and 4 NREM sleep than do elders without dementia (Beers and Berkow, 2000). This becomes more pronounced with disease progression. Patients with Alzheimer's disease and multiinfarct dementia may also have a higher incidence of sleep apnea than do nondemented elders. Suggestions for management include reviewing medications for those causing sleep disruption, providing only short daytime naps, relieving daytime boredom, and providing adequate daylight or light exposure.

Sleep and Drugs. Drug tolerance, physical dependence, daytime delirium, drowsiness, and depression of mental alertness occur with chronic use of bedtime hypnotic agents. Some major tranquilizers and sedatives are responsible for loss of equilibrium and falls. Hypnotic drugs often induce night terrors, hallucinations, and such paradoxic responses as agitation instead of relaxation, hangover, depression, and changes in memory, balance, and gait. If hypnotic drugs are necessary, those that are the least disruptive to the sleep cycle should be employed, particularly the nonbenzodiazepine hypnotics.

Assessment

Nurses are in an excellent position to assess sleep, to improve the quality of the aged person's sleep, and to study sleep or assist in sleep research by being available at customary sleep times. Sleep history interviews are important and should be obtained from all elderly clients. The nurse should learn how well the person sleeps at home, how many times the aged person is awakened at night, what time the person retires, and what rituals occur at bedtime. Rituals include bedtime snacks, watching television, listening to music, or reading, which, unless carried out, interfere with the individual's ability to fall asleep. Other assessment data should include the amount and type of daily exercise, favorite position when in bed, room environment, temperature, ventilation, illumination, activities engaged in several hours before bedtime, and sleep medications, as well as other medications taken routinely. Information about involvement in hobbies, life satisfaction, and perception of health status is also important to establish possible depression. The history should be cross-checked with the caregiver or family members. Some of the numerous medical conditions, the related reasons for sleep alterations in the elderly, and possible interventions are listed in Table 6-6.

Subjective and objective measures of sleep assessment available to nurses include visual analogue scales, subjective rating scales (e.g., 0 to 10 or 0 to 100), questionnaires that determine if one's sleep is disturbed, interviews, and daily sleep charts. Objective measures include polysomnography conducted in sleep laboratories, including electroencephalograms (EEGs), electromyograms (EMGs), and direct observation (Schoenfelder and Culp, 2001).

A nursing standard-of-practice protocol for sleep disturbances in elderly patients was developed as part of the Nurses Improving Care of the Hospitalized Elderly (NICHE) Project supported by a grant from the Hartford Foundation. Assessment standards are presented in Table 6-7. The assessment is to elicit information relative to indicators or defining characteristics of sleep disturbance. The sleep diary or log is noted as an important part of assessment. This information will provide an accurate account of the person's sleep problem and identify the sleep disturbance. Usually a family member or the caregiver, if the aged person is unable, records specific behaviors on a flow sheet. Two to four weeks is required to obtain a clear picture of the sleep problem. Important items to record are the following:

1. The number of times a call for assistance to the bathroom, pain medication, or subjective symptoms of inability to sleep, such as anxiety, occur
2. If the person is out of bed
3. Whether the person appears to be asleep or awake on rounds or when checked
4. Episodes of confusion or disorientation
5. If sleep medication was given and if repeated
6. Time the person awakens in the morning (approximation)
7. Where the person falls asleep in the evening
8. Daytime nap

Intervention

Interventions begin after a thorough sleep history has been recorded. Management is directed at identifiable causes. Transient sleep disorders or short-term sleep problems do not require treatment with medications. For chronic sleep problems, use the lowest dose of the mildest drug first—for example, a hypnotic such as zolpidem (Ambien) or zaleplon (Sonata); trazodone (Desyrel) may be used if there is depression, because this antidepressant has good sleep profile. Although pharmacologic treatment is clearly beneficial, the benefits may not persist over time (Griffith, 2002).

Nonpharmacologic interventions are of benefit either alone or in combination with drug therapy as demonstrated from one research study (Griffith, 2002) looking at three treatment methods, one being placebo. The drug treatment in this study was beneficial for about 3 months, but subjects were less well maintained in the subsequent 21 months without the drug than those subjects with behavioral treatments. This is not surprising, because behavioral changes have a longer-lasting effect. Interestingly, the combined treatment of behavioral therapy plus drug therapy was less effective than behavioral therapy alone. The behavior treatment consisted of the following: associate bed with sleep or sex; do not go to bed unless sleepy; if unable to sleep in 15 minutes, go to another room and repeat as necessary; arise at the same time every morning; naps are permitted until 3 PM; education about sleep requirements; and corrections about mistaken concepts on how to promote sleep. The researcher states that the optimal management regimen may be to begin with a hypnotic, followed by behavioral therapy after discontinuing the

Box 6-16 Stimulus Control for Insomnia

- Go to sleep only with the intention of sleep and when sleepy.
- Use the bed only for sleep and sexual activity.
- If you cannot fall asleep, get up and go to another room. Stay up as long as needed to feel sleepy. Return to bed when sleepy. If unable to sleep again after 10 minutes, repeat and get up as long as needed.
- Set the alarm clock and get up at the same time every morning, regardless of how long you slept.
- Do not nap during the day.

Adapted from Kirkwood C: *Treatment of insomnia,* New York, 2001, Power-Pak, CE Publishers. Available at *www.powerpak.com.*

Table 6-6 Causes, Reasons, and Potential Interventions for Sleep Alterations in the Aged

Causes	Reasons	Potential interventions
Arthritis	Pain builds; joints stiffen during periods of activity; pain relief medicine may wear off	Provide comfortable pillows; offer pain medication before pain becomes too intense
Angina pectoris	Pain likely to occur during REM sleep	Keep nitroglycerine at bedside
Chronic obstructive pulmonary disease	Abnormal increases in alveolar tension; decrease in oxygen saturation; prone position causes dyspnea and stasis of mucus	Patient education regarding self-care Toilet before bedtime; use bronchial dilators; prevent fatigue; rest during day; no diuretics in late afternoon; caution to avoid cola, coffee, tea, chocolate; use sedatives and OTC medication with caution
Heart failure	Nocturnal dyspnea Nocturia	Appropriate cardiotonic regimen; extra pillows; do not take diuretics late in day or in the evening
Diabetes	Inadequate regulation of blood sugar may lead to glycosuria and nocturia; overly tight control of blood sugar	Control by diet, insulin, or oral medication Adjust diabetic regimen
	Hypoglycemic attacks (can mimic anxiety attacks)	Teach regular, adequate caloric intake; bedtime snack
Disturbed sensory perception	Poor environmental lighting; visual difficulties; nocturnal hallucinations; alterations in REM-NREM cycle	Modify environment; check hearing aid; put glasses nearby; reduce noise at home or in hospital; reassure frequently
Alzheimer's disease (AD)	AD patients' sleep shows reduction in stages III and IV sleep early in disease; late in AD these stages disappear; daytime sleepiness increases as disease progresses	Assist staff and family with wandering behavior and sundowning syndrome; major tranquilizers may be needed; be sure person has comfortable chair in which to rest; strict scheduling of nighttime bed hours, day naps, and activity periods and needs; for wanderers and behavior problems, stop all drug treatment to see if normal sleep rhythm returns
Depression	Disturbed sleep pattern: problem falling asleep, early morning awakening, decreased total sleep time; barbiturate use can cause fragmented sleep and nightmares	Assess sleep; check for recent discontinued drugs; frequent reassurance; have same caregiver relate to client; tricyclic antidepressants if depression diagnosed
Congestive heart failure	Fluid buildup produces symptoms	Restrict fluids at bedtime; prop up on pillows
Peptic ulcers	Gastric juices and stomach acid increases during REM sleep	Provide nightly ulcer medicine
Alcoholism	Abnormal EEG pattern results; as effects wear off, sleeper may awaken with withdrawal symptoms and a hangover	No alcoholic beverages; explain that reformed alcoholics may experience insomnia for a year or so after withdrawal of alcohol
Parkinsonism	Total wake time increases, decreased REM	L-Dopa at bedtime may help decrease rigidity that occurs during the night
Surgical procedures	Premature arousal related to blood drawn at 5 AM or 6 AM; anxiety and worry about outcome; pain	Analyze rituals and routines in place. Can they be changed? Keep pain free; monitor vital signs frequently, and promote rest
Cardiac	Discomfort due to environment (noise, temperature, lights); postoperative psychosis (usually follows 24-day lucid interval)	Modify environment Establish therapeutic rapport early; instruct patient preoperatively; orient frequently when postoperative; elicit family support
Situational insomnia	On admission to institution; after visit by relative; after move to new residence; after recent loss or death	Establish one-to-one relationship; provide short-term use of hypnotic

Data from Wagner D: On sleep and Alzheimer's disease, *Alzheimer's Disease and Related Disorders Newsletter* 5(1), 1985; Pacini C, Fitzpatrick J: Sleep patterns of hospitalized and nonhospitalized aged individuals, *J Gerontol Nurs* 8(6):327, 1982; de Brun S: Insomnia: the common sense approach, *Occupational Health Nursing* 29:36, 1981; Hemenway J: Sleep and the cardiac patient, *Heart Lung* 9(3):453, 1980; Raskind M, Eisdorfer C: When elderly patients can't sleep, *Drug Therapy* 7(8):44, 1977.

hypnotic. This study was based on "stimulus control" or "sleep restriction therapy." Guidelines for stimulus control are listed in Box 6-16. A meta-analysis of treatment protocols revealed that 70% to 80% of patients will improve with behavioral therapy (Kirkwood, 2001). The patient who is self-directed may benefit from these behavioral routines or other rules of sleep hygiene (Box 6-17). Other behavioral techniques include progressive muscle relaxation, meditation, hypnosis, and biofeedback. Often there needs to be referral to a specialist for education of these techniques.

Bright light therapy, as discussed in the section on biorhythms, helps reset the patient's biologic clock. It is also used to treat depression. Bright light therapy is given 30 minutes to 2 hours each day. Duration depends on the brightness of the

Table 6-7 Nursing Protocol: Sleep Disturbance in Elderly Patients

Assessment	Health promotion and maintenance intervention	Evaluation
Sleep-wake patterns Inquire about usual times for retiring and rising, time for falling asleep, frequency and duration of nighttime awakenings; frequency and duration of daytime naps; daytime physical and social activity Have person provide a subjective evaluation of the quality of sleep Have person complete sleep log for 2 wk	**Maintain normal sleep pattern** Maintain usual bedtime/wake time Avoid staying in bed beyond waking hours Encourage to get up at regular time even if did not sleep well Schedule nightime activities to provide uninterrupted periods of sleep of at least 2-3 hr Balance daytime activity and rest Encourage keeping daytime naps to a minimum Promote social interaction Encourage exercise before evening	**Objective evidence** Time required to fall asleep; should fall asleep within 30-45 min Time for awakening, at usual reported time Behavior, alertness, attention, ability to concentrate, reaction time Observe duration of sleep: patient should remain asleep for at least 4-hour intervals
Bedtime routines/rituals Inquire about activities performed by the individual before bedtime (e.g., personal hygiene, prayer, reading, watching TV, listening to music, snacks)	**Support bedtime routines/rituals** Offer a bedtime snack or beverage Enable bedtime reading or listening to music Assist with aspects of personal hygiene at bedtime (e.g., bath) Encourage prayer or meditation Assist to establish a relaxing bedtime routine	**Subjective evidence** Verbalizations about the quality and quantity of sleep (e.g., statements of difficulty falling asleep or frequent awakenings; having slept well; feeling well rested/refreshed; an increased sense of well-being)
Medications Obtain information relative to all prescribed and self-selected over-the-counter medications used by person, especially, sleep aids, diuretics, laxatives Determine types of medications and length of time used by person	**Avoid/minimize drugs that negatively influence sleep** Pharmacologic treatment of sleep disturbances is treatment of last resort Discontinue or adjust the dose or dosing schedule of any/all offending medications Consider drug-drug potentiation Administer meds to promote sleep (i.e., give diuretics at least 4 hours before bedtime)	
Diet effects Obtain information about the consumption of caffeinated and alcoholic beverages	**Minimize/avoid foods that negatively influence sleep** Discourage use of beverages containing stimulants (e.g., coffee, tea, sodas) in afternoon and evening Encourage use of food naturally containing L-tryptophan Provide snacks according to patient preference Generally discourage use of alcoholic beverages Decrease fluid intake 2-4 hours before bedtime Encourage to have lighter meal in evening	
Environmental factors Evaluate noise, light, temperature, ventilation, bedding Inquire about distance of bathroom from bedroom Inquire about use of night-lights	**Create optimal environment for sleep** Keep noise to an absolute minimum Set room temperature according to preference Provide blankets as requested Use night light as desired Provide soft music or white noise to mask noise Encourage bed and bedroom for sleep and not other activities Use light exposure during day and evening to maintain wakefulness	
Physiologic factors Evaluate breathing pattern with sleep, with attention to pauses Observe for periodic movement or jerking during sleep Inquire about sleeping position Note diagnoses of sleep disorder Note diagnoses of specific health problems that adversely affect sleep (e.g., CHF, COPD)	**Promote physiologic stability** Elevate head of bed as required Provide extra pillows per preference Administer bronchodilators, if prescribed, before bedtime Use medical therapeutics (e.g., continuous positive airway pressure machine) as prescribed	

Modified from Forman MD, Wykle M: Nursing standard-of-practice protocol: sleep disturbances in elderly patients, *Geriatr Nurs* 16(5):238, 1995.

Table 6-7 Nursing Protocol: Sleep Disturbance in Elderly Patients—cont'd

Assessment	Health promotion and maintenance intervention	Evaluation
Illness factors	**Promote comfort**	
Inquire about pain, affective disturbances (e.g., depression, anxiety, worry, fatigue, and discomfort)	Provide analgesia as needed 30 min before bedtime (Note that some over-the-counter analgesics may have caffeine) Massage, back or foot, to help relax Warm and cool compresses to painful areas as indicated Use relaxation methods—deep breathing, progressive relaxation, mental imagery Encourage to urinate before going to bed Keep path to bathroom clear/provide bedside commode	

light (Beers and Berkow, 2000). Outdoor light or a commercially made light box can be used. Room light is inadequate.

Melatonin, which is classified as a dietary supplement, has been the topic of talk shows and numerous popular magazines over the past several years. It has been cited not only as a sleep aid, but also as an age-reversing, disease-fighting hormone. It is an over-the-counter drug and its use is controversial. There are no studies known to have been conducted in older adults. The preparations that are available lack control and are unregulated, and quality is unknown.

Drugs should be a last resort and are not intended for long-term treatment. Rebound insomnia and episodes of confusion and nightmares are common when sleep medications are withdrawn. The key to selection of a hypnotic is to consider the half-life and the adverse effects of the agent. Long-acting benzodiazepines should not be used in elderly patients. They are twice as likely to fracture a hip compared with elders using short-acting or intermediate-acting benzodiazepines. Table 6-8 presents the characteristics of selected medications used as hypnotics in treatment of elderly patients.

Evaluation

The nursing standard-of-practice protocol presented in Table 6-7 includes an evaluation component. Observation of the person when awake and asleep is necessary. Physiologic changes observable for each stage of sleep reviewed previously can be evaluated to give clues to the phases of sleep cycle experienced. It is essential to obtain subjective evidence of the quality and quantity of sleep.

ACTIVITY

Activity is a direct use of energy in voluntary and involuntary physical and mental ways that alter the microenvironment and macroenvironment of the individual. The focus of this section is on physical activity. The Administration on Aging (AOA) at the National Institute on Aging (2002) gives the facts:

- Exercise helps older people feel better and enjoy life more, even if they think they are too old or too out of shape.
- Most older adults (more than two thirds) do not get enough physical activity.
- The combination of lack of physical activity and poor diet is the second highest underlying cause of death in the United States (smoking is the leading cause).
- Regular exercise improves existing diseases and disabilities in older people. It improves mood and relieves depression.
- Staying physically active on a regular, permanent basis helps prevent certain diseases such as cancers, heart disease, diabetes, and disabilities as we grow older.

Box 6-17 Sleep Hygiene Rules

1. Have a regular bed time and wakeup time even on weekends.
2. Avoid naps. If you must nap, sleep no longer than 30 minutes in early afternoon.
3. Exercise at least 3 hours before bedtime.
4. Wind down during the evening; have a bedtime routine, such as brush teeth, set alarm clock, and read.
5. Limit caffeine (tea, cola, coffee, chocolate), nicotine, and diuretics, especially late in the day.
6. Do not use alcohol to sleep. It maintains a light sleep, not a restful deep sleep.
7. If you have reflux, eat the evening meal at least 3 to 4 hours before bedtime; have a light snack if needed before bedtime.
8. Give attention to the bed environment (comfortable bed, pillows between the knees, quiet, darkness, warm temperature).
9. Do not watch the clock, which increases anxiety and pressure to sleep; if anxious, take a warm bath.

Adapted from Sleep Clinic of San Francisco: *Rules for good sleep hygiene,* press release, Aug 30, 2001; Beers MH, Berkow R: *Merck manual of geriatrics,* ed 3, Whitehouse Station, NJ, 2000, Merck Research Laboratories.

Table 6-8 Characteristics of Selected Medications Used as Hypnotics in Treatment of Elderly Patients

Medication	Class	Hypnotic efficacy	Risk of hangover	Risk of tolerance or dependence	Other complications
Diphenhydramine	Antihistamine	Unpredictable	High	Low	Anticholinergic
Amitriptyline	Tricyclic	Unpredictable	High	Low	Anticholinergic
Trazodone	Triazolopyridine	High	High	Low	Priapism
Flurazepam	Benzodiazepine	Very high	High	High	Falls, worsens obstruction sleep apnea
Temazepam	Benzodiazepine	Very high	Low	High	Falls, worsens obstruction sleep apnea
Triazolam	Benzodiazepine	Very high	Low	High	Memory disturbance
Zolpidem	Imidazopyridine	Very high	Low	Low	Unknown

From McCall WV: Management of primary sleep disorders among elderly persons, *Psych Services* 46(1)51, 1995.

Public perceptions of the aged and how they spend their time continue to reflect the belief that retirement ushers in the pursuit of sedentary, private, isolated activity and the assumption of a passive role in society. Physical activity is often the barometer by which an individual's health and wellness are judged. The inability to exercise, perform physical work, and complete activities of daily living are among the first indicators of decline. Research in gerontologic exercise physiology is relatively young, but results indicate that maintenance of a physically active lifestyle arrests, delays, or significantly improves age changes associated with cardiovascular, respiratory, and musculoskeletal function.

Physical inactivity is a risk factor for many conditions experienced by the elderly, including obesity, diabetes, and cardiovascular, respiratory, and musculoskeletal diseases. Regular exercise reduces mortality rates even for smokers and obese elders (Beers and Berkow, 2000). Indirect benefits of regular exercise include increased social interaction, increased sense of well-being, and improved quality of sleep.

The National Institute on Aging has a guide in Spanish in order to make health information about exercise available to Hispanic elders (National Institute on Aging, 2002). The guide has been extensively tested in Hispanic senior centers, ensuring cultural appropriateness. "It's never too late to start" is an accompanying "fotonovela" with a case study of an older woman who convinces her friends to join her exercise group.

Direct benefits of exercise include preservation of muscle strength, increased aerobic capacity, greater bone density, and greater mobility and independence (Beers and Berkow, 2000). Regular exercise is known to increase insulin sensitivity and glucose tolerance and therefore is part of the management plan of anyone with diabetes. Exercise, if done on a regular basis, reduces systolic and diastolic blood pressures and can lessen the need for drug therapy. Exercise increases high-density lipoproteins (HDLs, or the so-called "good" lipoproteins) and lowers triglycerides. It is of benefit in mood disorders such as depression, so common in older adults. Karani and colleagues (2001) describe a study of 32 elderly people in a 10-week exercise program who improved in social functioning and depressive symptoms during the program. Other physical benefits include improved cardiac muscle tone, decreased percentage of body fat, improved ability to breathe deeply and effectively, reduced tension, favorable bowel control, and appetite control.

Regular exercise can help prevent falls and injury by improving strength, balance, neuromuscular coordination, joint function, and endurance (Beers and Berkow, 2000). To avoid falls during active exercise, balance training should be part of the exercise program. Benefits in both physical and psychosocial aspects of function have been found for community-living and institutionalized elderly. All elders, whether frail or healthy, can benefit from various forms of exercise programs.

Assessment

An assessment should be initiated before allowing an older adult to participate in an exercise program. The assessment must include a medical history; knowledge of the individual's physical activity level and any physical limitations; current medication regimen; and emotional, psychologic, and social needs.

In addition to the medical history, a physical examination with emphasis on cardiovascular, pulmonary, musculoskeletal, and neurologic systems should be done. The examination should focus on those aspects that may have an impact on functional status and that may give clues to potential risk. Attention should be focused on joint range of motion, flexibility, and strength. Previous injuries and the presence of active inflammation must be assessed. Conditions that must be stabilized before starting an exercise program include unstable angina, thrombophlebitis, cardiomyopathy, uncontrolled arrhythmias, uncompensated heart failure, and high systolic (greater than 200 mm Hg) and diastolic (greater than 110 mm Hg) blood pressures (Beers and Berkow, 2000).

Fitness Testing. Fitness testing may be warranted in some elders with chronic illnesses. Performance on a 6-minute walk test can help determine the intensity level to start fitness training (Beers and Berkow, 2000). It also provides feedback to the person as he or she improves in performance over time. The American College of Sports Medicine recommends exercise tolerance testing (ETT) for the elderly before recommending a moderately intense or vigorous exercise program. This test provides information regarding metabolic equivalents and target heart rate of the older person. ETT for frail elderly is not recommended. A frail elder's functional impairments may hinder the ability to perform an adequate test. The strength required for ETT may exceed the aerobic capacity of a frail elder. ETT is not essential for the elder who desires to start a simple walking program or perform a moderate level of exercise as a means to improve mobility and performance of activities of daily living.

Exercise Supervision. Some patients should be supervised during exercise testing and the exercise program. This may be done in a rehabilitation center. These patients include those with acquired valvular heart disease, congenital heart disease, angina, ventricular arrhythmias, severe coronary artery disease of three vessels or the main vessel, two previous myocardial infarctions, an ejection fraction of less than 30%, heart disease symptoms at rest or in very low intensity activity, and those who have a drop in systolic blood pressure with exercise (Beers and Berkow, 2000).

The risk of cardiac events in sedentary older women is greater than in younger individuals. Elderly women exercise less than elderly men and are at higher risk for deconditioning. However, a review of randomized, controlled exercise trials confirms a low rate of myocardial infarction and cardiovascular complications (George and Goldberg, 2001). A concern is the increase in blood pressure during resistance exercise. Large changes in blood pressure during exercise can be avoided if older women are educated about avoiding the Valsalva maneuver and maintaining normal breathing patterns.

Laboratory. Laboratory analysis should include a hematocrit ratio and a hemoglobin level. A low hematocrit ratio and hemoglobin level will increase the workload on the heart to maintain an adequate oxygen supply. In addition, analysis of electrolyte and fluid balance is necessary to evaluate conductivity and contractility of the cardiac muscle and its ability to function adequately. Lipid levels may be obtained to evaluate positive change, and thyroid studies may be obtained if this is a possible reason for inactivity.

Exercise Prescription. Four types of exercise may be prescribed that will be therapeutic for different patients: endurance exercises, muscle strengthening, balance training, and flexibility exercises. The patients' levels of fitness and medical problems will be considered before prescribing. Those who are markedly deconditioned will need to start very slowly. For example, a patient with severe COPD can begin treadmill exercises at a slow rate (Beers and Berkow, 2000). Patients with difficulty standing can perform seated exercise programs using cuff weights for strength training. Patients with arthritis benefit from water exercises. The prescription is most effective if the nurse finds one that consists of activities the patient most enjoys, or activities chosen by the patient.

The Centers for Disease Control and Prevention (CDC) recommends that all adults participate in at least 30 minutes of exercise over a 24-hour period. Three 10-minute activities meet the goal and may work best for elders who cannot do 30 minutes at one time. The ability to talk while exercising suggests how well or how long one can exercise; if one can talk easily while exercising, the exercise intensity level is low or moderate for that person. If talking is difficult, the intensity may be high. The elder may be able to integrate activity into daily life rather than doing a specific exercise. Examples are walking to the store instead of driving, golfing, swimming, hiking, raking leaves, and gardening. When there is a need for especially low intensity exercise, the person can work for 2 to 3 minutes, rest for 2 to 3 minutes, and continue the pattern for 15 to 20 minutes. Patients who are extremely deconditioned will improve markedly with this program.

Low-intensity exercise includes walking, cycling on level terrain, light stretching exercises, swimming on a float, and light housework. Moderate-intensity exercise includes walking fast, cycling fast, golfing with a cart or walking, light calisthenics, treading water, and heavy housework or yard work (Beers and Berkow, 2000). High-intensity exercises for the very fit include walking or jogging at 5 mph, cycling at 11 to 12 mph, swimming 0.5 mile in 30 minutes, playing tennis (not competitively), and hiking.

Walking is the most common exercise of older adults in the United States; about 50% walk for exercise (Beers and Berkow, 2000). Mortality rate is reduced 50% in those elders who walk at least 2 miles per day. Walking reduces the risk of new heart disease and falls.

Patients may want to learn to monitor their heart rates during exercise. An exercise stress test will determine the maximum heart rate and target heart rate range. A conservative formula for estimating maximum heart rate is 220 minus age (Beers and Berkow, 2000). Moderate-intensity exercise is defined as that which produces 60% to 79% of maximum heart rate. If the patient has a maximum heart rate of 160, the target rate will be 96 to 128 beats per minute. The exercise stress test is the best way to calculate maximum heart rate.

A rating of perceived exertion can be used to assess tolerance to exercise. The Borg scale has been used successfully to measure perceived exertion among elderly individuals (Table 6-9). It is recommended that a rating of perceived exertion be used rather than a pulse rate for monitoring exertion during exercise.

The respiratory system indicates intolerance to activity when dyspnea is evident or when a decrease in respiratory rate occurs during the activity. The cheeks, lips, and nailbeds become red (flushed), pallid, or cyanotic with intolerance, and exercise should cease immediately. Fatigue, tiredness, and the need to sit down are additional signs of inability to tolerate the activity. Obviously, tightness and heaviness in the chest and tightness in the legs are indicative of activity that has gone too far.

Table 6-9 Borg Scale of Perceived Exertion

Rating	Perceived intensity
6, 7, 8	Very, very light
9, 10	Very light
11, 12	Fairly light
13, 14	Somewhat hard
15, 16	Hard
17, 18	Very hard
19, 20	Very, very hard

From Barry HC, Eathorne SW: Exercise and aging issues for the practitioner, *Med Clin North Am* 78(2):357, 1994.

If nothing occurs within the expected tolerance level, but the nurse notices that the aged person is slowing down, shows signs of decreased dexterity or coordination, and needs frequent rests, that aged person is not able to tolerate that level of activity.

A sustained brisk walk is one of the most popular and accessible forms of activity for the aged. Those who have done little walking are encouraged to start slowly by first walking to the corner of the block and eventually being able to develop the capacity for distance walking of several miles. Those limited to institutional facilities should also be encouraged to increase the amount of walking. First it may be only from the bed to the bathroom, then with time down the hall, and eventually around the total facility. If the person can go outside, walking around the block might be a long-term goal.

Exercise Programs

Participation in exercise programs is influenced by a number of factors. Among a group of mall walkers, those told to exercise by their physician perceived significantly greater susceptibility and severity of health problems if they did not walk than those not told by their physician to walk. Motivating the elderly to change their behavior is not always easy, but usually, if the exercise or activity is one that the elder chooses, compliance will be greater.

The following variables reflect critical characteristics of exercise programs that improve long-term compliance:

1. Low to moderate intensity, duration, and frequency of exercise
2. Group participation and social pleasure
3. Emphasis on variety and pleasure, including use of games as exercise
4. Setting of personal goals or develop contracts
5. Evaluation of response to training and demonstration of improvement
6. Involvement of friends, family, or spouse
7. Use of music
8. Positive feedback
9. Enthusiastic leadership and role models

Enjoyment and individualization of the program to meet individual goals and needs are key factors in improving long-term participation. Another consideration for many older adults is the expense associated with the exercise program. Many elderly have limited financial reserves for recreational purposes.

It is also important that the individuals who conduct aerobic exercise programs and classes consider differences between the abilities of young and old. Classes are generally taught by young and fit persons who may become so involved in what they are doing that they are unaware that the elderly may not be able to do the number of repetitions they consider necessary for toning muscles. These programs can damage the muscles, tendons, ligaments, and joints of the older adult. Training older fit women or men to lead aerobic exercise programs is helpful; participants can identify and bond with the leaders, which increases compliance. A variety of exercise programs exist for the elderly. The existing programs need to be evaluated on an individual basis to determine if they are appropriate. Sample programs for endurance, muscle strengthening, balance training, and flexibility are seen in Figure 6-5.

Senior Games

Senior centers throughout the United States have instituted physical fitness programs, which include Ping-Pong, boccie, golf, horseshoes, and many other activities enjoyed by the aged. These activities incorporate rhythmic action and stretching and provide improvement in or maintenance of cardiopulmonary function, muscle tone, and mental stimulation.

Nearly all of the states of the United States promote "Senior Games" in collaboration with public service and private corporations. These are Olympic-style competitions for men and women 55 years of age and older. Some companies have established par courses or 1-mile exercise fitness trails for the older adult.

Dancing. For those accustomed to it, ballroom, folk, or square dancing should be encouraged. This form of activity done properly can have as much aerobic benefit as workouts to music videotapes. Dancing is kind to the joints and can burn as many calories as swimming, biking, or walking. However, it should not be done as the only form of activity because it does not develop upper body strength. To enhance cardiovascular and respiratory fitness, one would have to engage in 20 to 30 minutes of sustained dancing. Dancing provides another means of obtaining pleasant, sociable, vigorous exercise, which tones the body and benefits cardiopulmonary and mental health.

Swimming. Swimming, one of America's most popular sports, or water exercise facilitates muscle tone and improves circulation, muscle strength, endurance, flexibility, and weight control; it can also be relaxing and a mood elevator. The benefits of aquatic activity or exercise therapy are that arm and leg movements against water are less painful and do not seem to require as much effort because of the buoyancy of the water. Some aged maintain a swimming program begun earlier in life; others enjoy this as a relaxing new way to get activity and socialize. Those who are nonswimmers or who do not swim well might benefit from water exercise classes such as "water walking" held in the shallow end of the pool. The

LYING DOWN

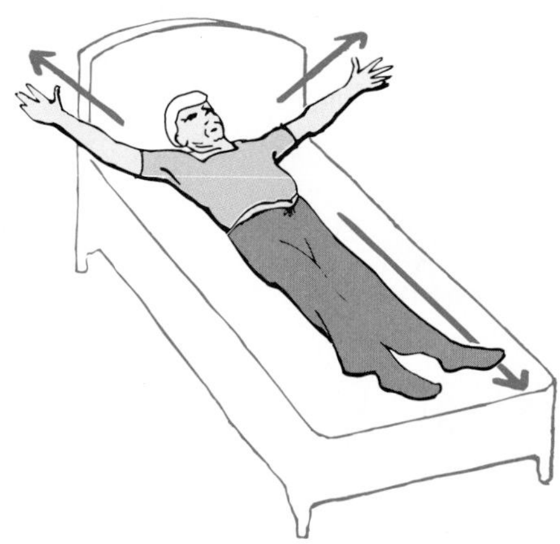

Stretch your arms and legs; take a deep breath.

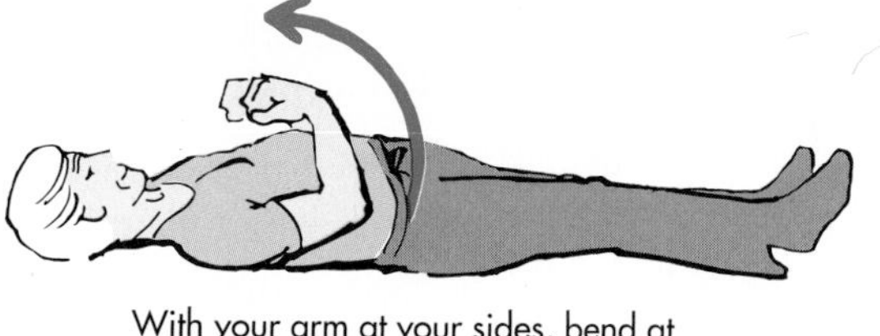

With your arm at your sides, bend at the elbow and curl your arms as if "making a muscle."

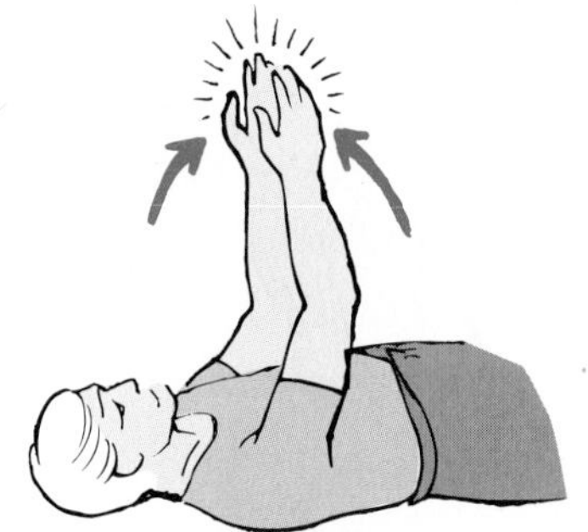

Clap your hands directly above your head.

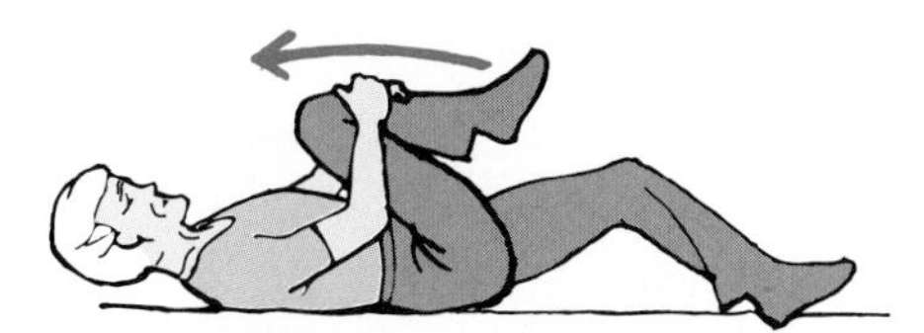

Grab each leg with both hands below the knee and pull toward your chest slowly.

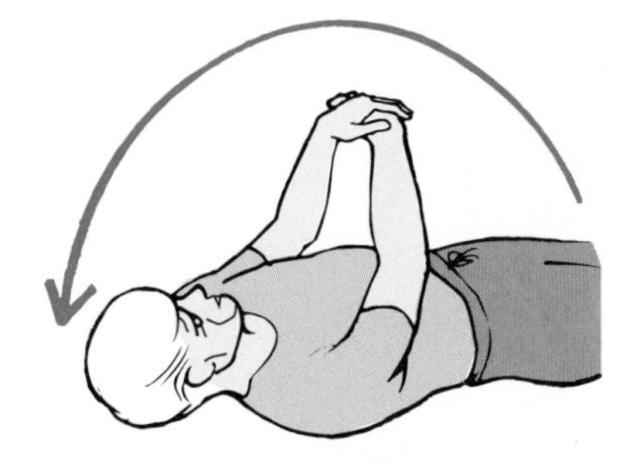

Fold your hands on your stomach; raise your arms over your head toward the headboard.

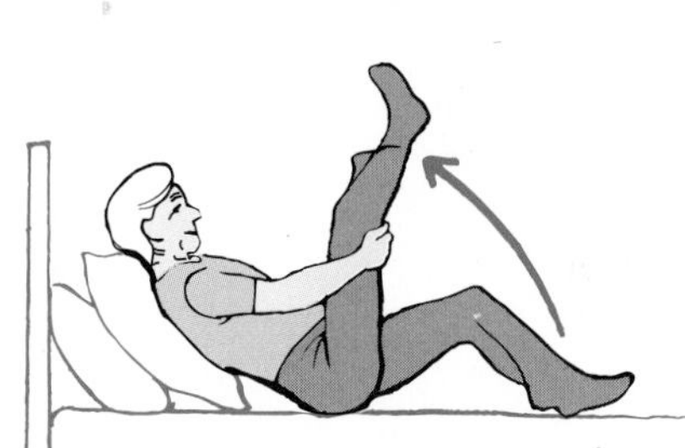

Lift each leg off the bed, but try not to bend your knee. Use an arm to help.

SITTING

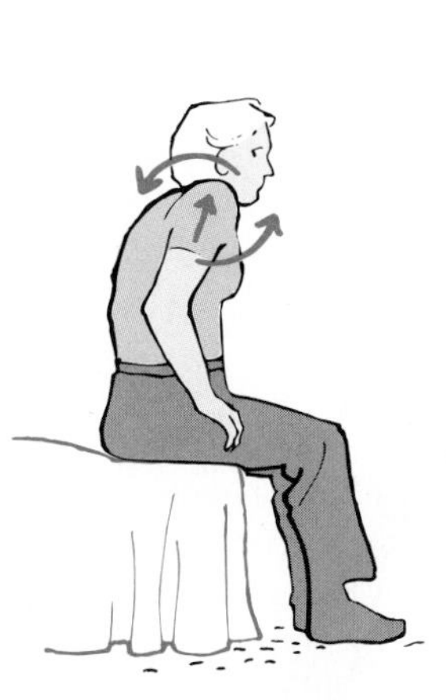

Shrug your shoulders forward, then move them in a circle, raising them high enough to reach your ears.

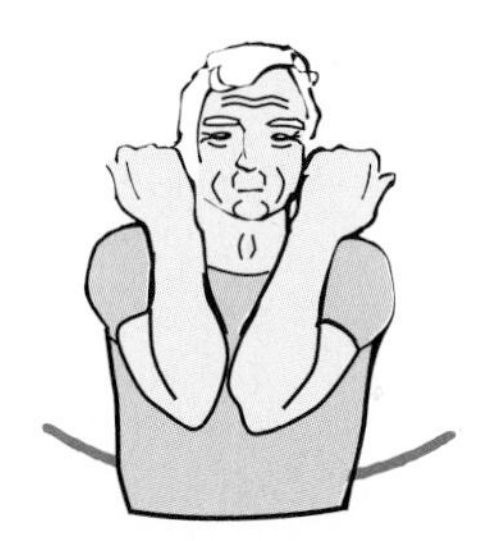

Touch your elbows together in front of you.

Twist your whole upper body from side to side with your hands on your hips.

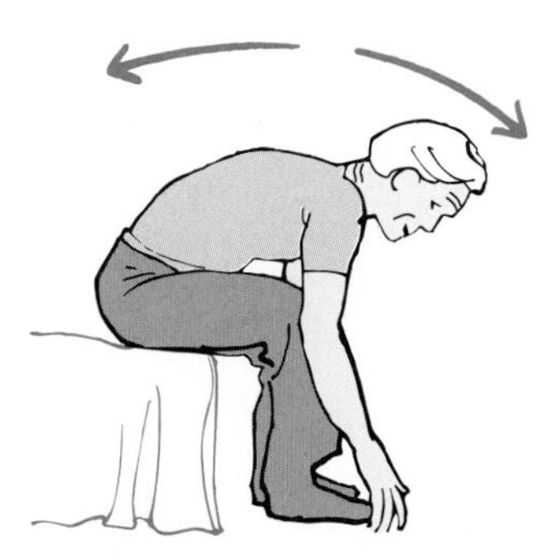

Bend forward and let your arms dangle; try to touch the floor with your hands.

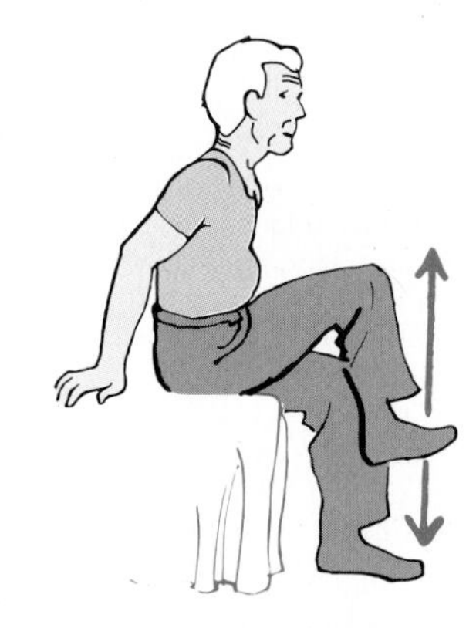

While still sitting, move each of your knees up and down as if you are walking; each time your right foot hits the ground, count it as one. Lift your knee high.

Figure 6-5. Exercises: lying down, sitting, standing up, and walking places. (From Johnson-Paulson JE, Kosher R: *Geriatr Nurs,* pp 322-325, 1985.)

Continued

STANDING UP

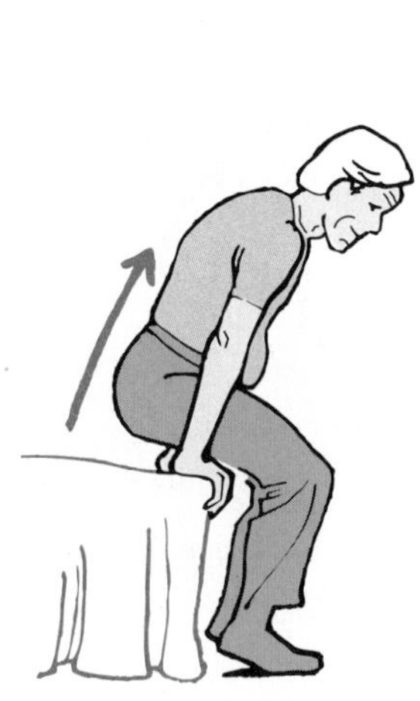

Using your arms, push off from the bed and stand up; if you get dizzy, sit down and try again.

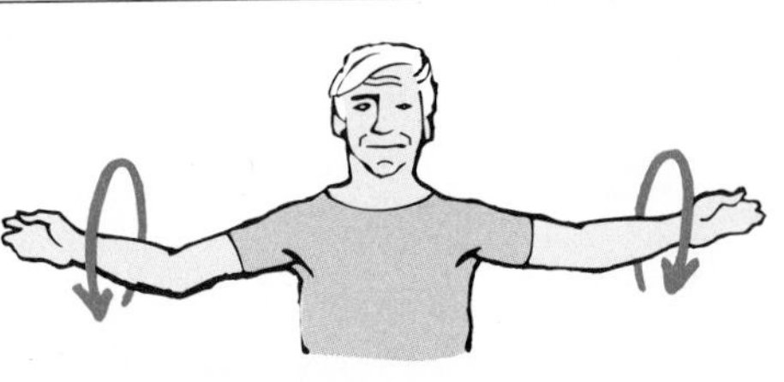

Hold your arms out and turn them in big circles.

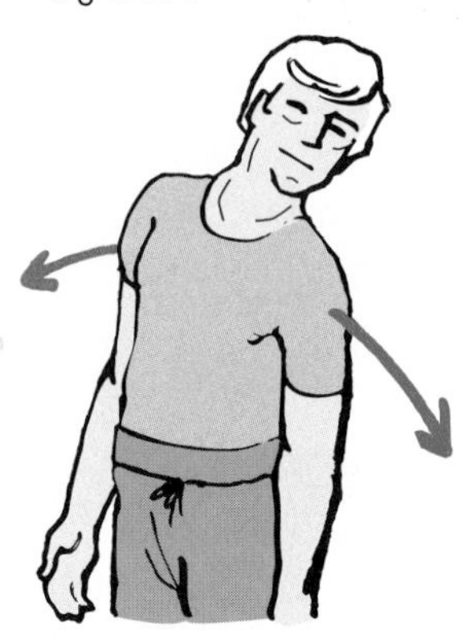

With hands at your side bend at the waist as far as you can to the right side, then to the left.

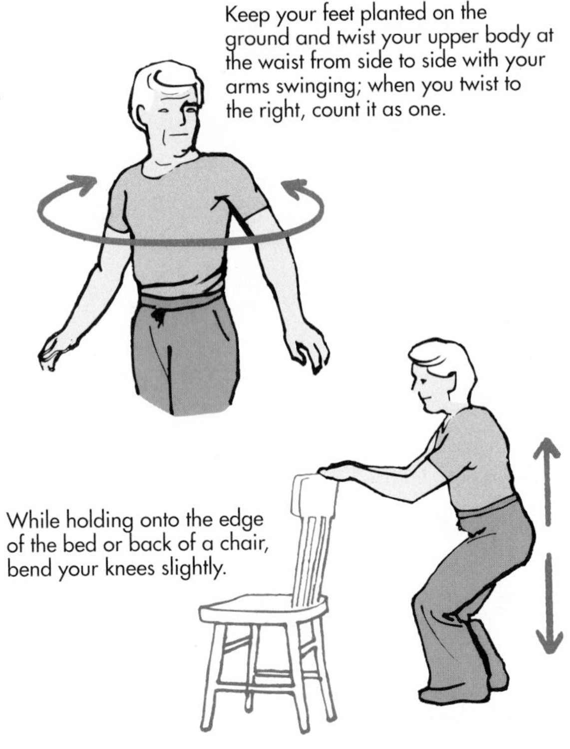

Keep your feet planted on the ground and twist your upper body at the waist from side to side with your arms swinging; when you twist to the right, count it as one.

While holding onto the edge of the bed or back of a chair, bend your knees slightly.

WALKING PLACES

Walking is good exercise. It helps in toning muscles, maintaining flexibility of joints, and also is good exercise for the heart and circulatory system. Walking briskly for 20 minutes a day, 3 times a week can be as effective a heart conditioner as jogging, but it does take a longer time to achieve the same effect as jogging. For those who cannot walk rapidly for long periods, walking to the point of muscular fatigue also helps maintain good muscle tone.

There are signs your body may give you to indicate you are overdoing exercise. Stop, rest, and if necessary call your physician if you experience any of these symptoms:

- SEVERE SHORTNESS OF BREATH
- CHEST PAIN
- SEVERE JOINT PAIN
- DIZZINESS OR FAINT FEELING
- HEART FLUTTERS

In all walking exercises, go only as fast as you are able to walk and still carry on a conversation. If you cannot, slow down.

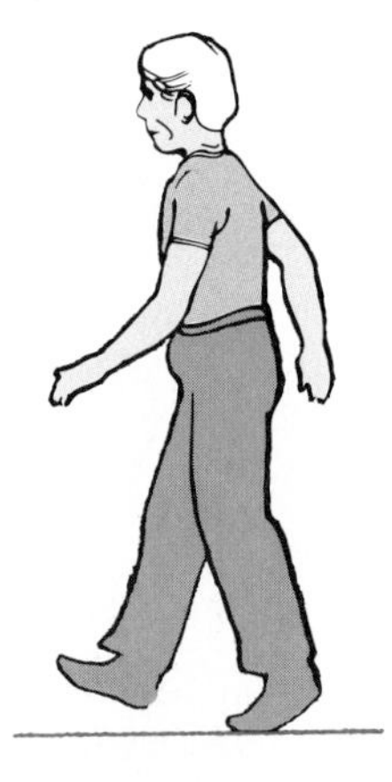

INSIDE

It is important to maintain walking ability. Determine how far you can walk and each day walk to 3/4 of that distance, building endurance. Wear supportive shoes and use whatever aids are necessary.

OUTSIDE

Wear soft-soled shoes with good support, i.e., jogging shoes. When walking, push off *from* your toes and land on your heels. Swing arms loosely at your sides. Begin with 10-minute walks and build to 20 to 30 minutes.

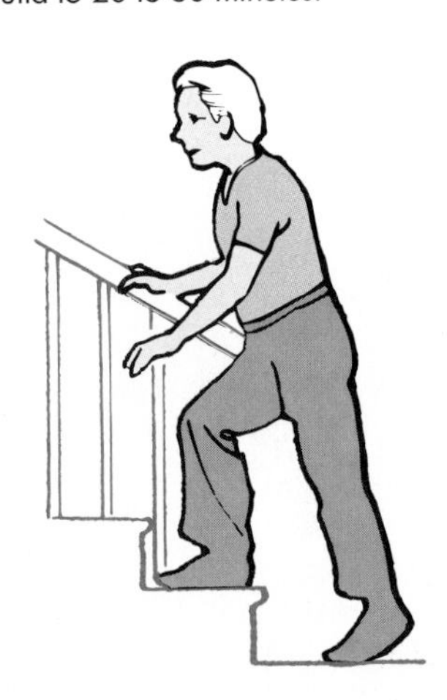

Walking upstairs requires effort. Place one foot flat on a step, push off with the other and shift your weight. Use a railing for balance if necessary.

Figure 6-5. Cont'd.

YMCA, the YWCA, and the American Red Cross offer classes in these types of activities. The Arthritis Foundation sponsors water exercise programs, "senior splash" aerobic swim classes, or arthritic aquatic programs, which conform to guidelines. Elders with mobility problems move at ease in water.

Different Forms of Exercises

Yoga is another form of exercise that can be practiced regardless of one's condition. It can foster mental alacrity, independence, and good health in the aged through simple exercise, relaxation, meditation, and nutritional education.

Isotonic exercises train the cardiovascular and skeletal muscles. Isometrics mainly work with the cardiovascular system. Persons who are confined to a bed or chair or who are ambulatory can do these rhythmic tasks or calisthenics. Tai Chi is popular with older adults at this time, but research on its benefits is conflicting. Exercise should be aerobic in nature, easily attained, and not produce an oxygen debt. Numerous programs have been developed in which simplicity and flexibility of the program make it easily adaptable to a variety of settings. Guidelines include the following:

- Teach to avoid sudden twisting movements, rapid movements, and rapid transitions from one movement to the next.
- Avoid sustained isometric contractions of greater than 10 seconds.
- Assess ability to tolerate low-level activity without signs and symptoms of muscle fatigue, shortness of breath, angina, arrhythmias, abnormal blood pressure, or intermittent claudication.
- Stop exercising if arrhythmias, angina, or excessive breathlessness occur.
- Avoid exercise during acute viral infections.
- Increase activity slowly by intensity, duration, and frequency.
- Monitor exercise intensity by perceived exertion and exercise heart rate.
- Perform a gradual, extended exercise warm-up (at least 15 minutes) to maximize flexibility and decrease muscle injury.
- Perform cooldown until heart rate returns to resting level.
- Modify exercise program up or down based on individual responses.

Special Needs of Elderly People

It is also important to address the special needs of elderly people when initiating an exercise program. The elderly are less able to adapt to the environment during exercise. They should dress in layers to adjust to different environmental temperatures. Well-fitting footwear and stockings are essential to prevent injury because of impaired foot sensation. Blisters and friction injuries may occur without the elderly person knowing it if there is impaired perception, such as in diabetes. Maintaining hydration is essential. Consumption of fluid before exercising and regularly while exercising is recommended. Environments with poor air quality should be avoided for exercise, including areas near roadways.

Often when beginning a physical exercise program muscles will be sore. Warm, not hot, baths or soaks are excellent. Another way to minimize muscle soreness is a 5- to 10-minute cooldown period of slow walking or stretching to keep the primary muscle groups active, to decrease venous pooling and increase venous return to the heart and to prevent vagal responses.

Nurses should capitalize, more than they do, on activities of daily living, such as providing the aged with bath brushes to wash their own backs in the shower or bathtub and encouraging the aged to dry body parts or rub the back dry with a towel. Reaching for objects while cleaning house can be included in an activity program, as can washing dishes in warm water to provide finger exercises. Warm water aids in the relief of stiffness and enables the fingers to move more easily without discomfort. Various exercises for bed, chair, and standing are presented in Figure 6-5. This does not cover the numerous maneuvers that exist but rather gives a sampling of possible movements.

Housekeeping activities can be utilized for strength and flexibility. Community-dwelling elders can be taught simple approaches in utilizing household chores for activity. The elderly in long-term care who respond to the work ethic can be encouraged to push wheelchairs, clean tables, and run errands.

Other activities that can be done while watching television or whenever there are a few spare minutes during the day are rolling a pencil between the hand and a hard surface, exaggerating the chewing motion of the jaw, holding the stomach in, tightening the buttocks, flexing the fingers, and rotating the head and the ankles.

Activity, in general, should be paced and occur regularly every day. Activities that will help eliminate stiffness should be planned for the morning, when stiffness is most prevalent. Relaxation exercises should be considered before bedtime to help induce sleep. With any activity in which the aged are involved, sufficient intermittent rest periods should be provided. An example of a small-group exercise program is presented in Box 6-18.

Safety Considerations

Those who are frail should not engage in strenuous activity, nor should their joints be forced past the point of resistance or discomfort. If the frail have regularly participated in activity that the nurse deems too stressful to their skeletal systems, it is important to keep in mind that an activity done for many years is not as difficult as if it were just introduced. When the activity is new, serious consideration should be given to levels of stress produced.

Many aged are fearful of falling because of altered balance or the inability to reach or bend. Some fear that if they get down on the floor they will not be able to get up again. Sometimes all that is necessary to alleviate this fear is to ensure that the aged person has his or her glasses or other appliances that provide security, stability, and mobility. Activity should not be thought of as something to keep the aged busy but should be purposeful to enhance their physical and mental well-being.

In summary, this chapter has looked at the life support needs individually. It is apparent that each area influences the function of others. The aged would not continue to survive if these needs could not be met independently or with assistance of others. The quality and the overall perception of life can be augmented when the nurse monitors these specific functions and provides support or assistance according to identified problems.

Human Needs and Wellness Diagnoses

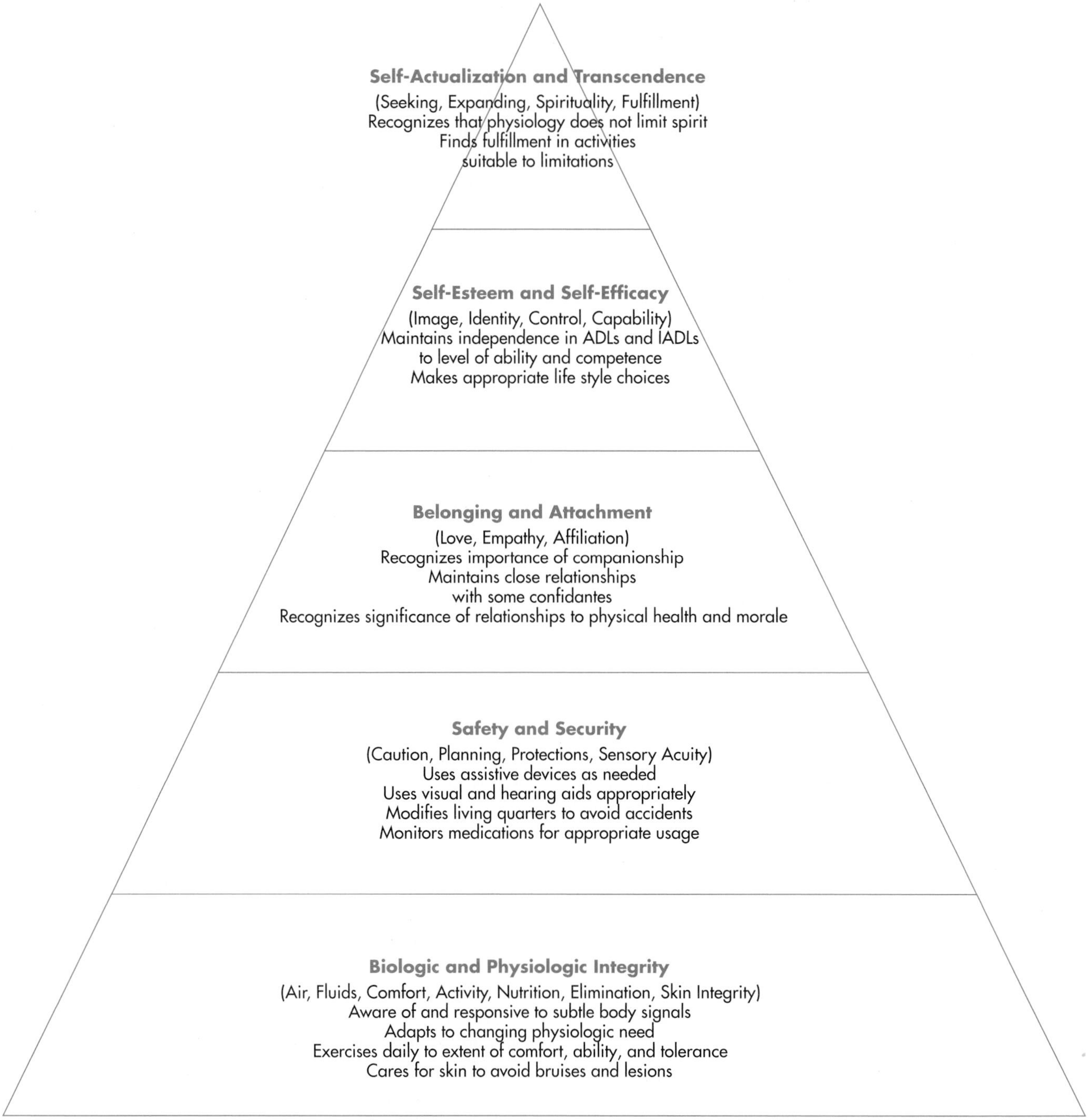

Self-Actualization and Transcendence
(Seeking, Expanding, Spirituality, Fulfillment)
Recognizes that physiology does not limit spirit
Finds fulfillment in activities
suitable to limitations

Self-Esteem and Self-Efficacy
(Image, Identity, Control, Capability)
Maintains independence in ADLs and IADLs
to level of ability and competence
Makes appropriate life style choices

Belonging and Attachment
(Love, Empathy, Affiliation)
Recognizes importance of companionship
Maintains close relationships
with some confidantes
Recognizes significance of relationships to physical health and morale

Safety and Security
(Caution, Planning, Protections, Sensory Acuity)
Uses assistive devices as needed
Uses visual and hearing aids appropriately
Modifies living quarters to avoid accidents
Monitors medications for appropriate usage

Biologic and Physiologic Integrity
(Air, Fluids, Comfort, Activity, Nutrition, Elimination, Skin Integrity)
Aware of and responsive to subtle body signals
Adapts to changing physiologic need
Exercises daily to extent of comfort, ability, and tolerance
Cares for skin to avoid bruises and lesions

These are not all the possible wellness diagnoses that may be identified. The above are examples of nursing diagnoses that should be considered when planning care for the older adult.

Box 6-18 Movements for Geriatric Patients

The progression should be from smaller, more personal movements to larger ones that may involve communication with the rest of the group. Movements should begin slowly and later develop speed. The amount of balance required should be minimal at first and more later when the patients feel more secure and uninhibited. A sample class might be as follows:

1. Scratch the small of your back against the chair. Now, try your upper back, too.
2. Begin by pretending to wash your face, then your arms and shoulders and neck.
3. Stretch up as high as you can; now sink down as low as you can. Now try to reach as far forward as possible, now out to each side.
4. Can you nod your head up and down as if to say "Yes?" Now try "No." Now an even stronger *"No!"*
5. Let's try marching in place to the music. You may use one or both feet.
6. Let's try making circles with different parts of our body. Start with one shoulder. Try both shoulders. Try one hand, now the other hand. Can you reverse directions?
7. How about kicking one leg at a time up in the air as the music gets louder?
8. Let's have one half of the group kick while the other half stomps. Now let's reverse.
9. Can you now reach out as if you're trying to shake hands with the person across the circle from you?
10. Now try actually shaking hands with the person next to you. How about the person on the other side?
11. Now, let's all take a huge deep breath and stretch as tall and as long as possible. Now let the air out slowly and let your head, back, and arms deflate slowly as a balloon. Try it again, take in even more air. Now deflate even more slowly.

The above is a simple example of what can be done with a small group of 6 to 10 patients. It is advisable, if possible, to have one aide present to help encourage patients and monitor safety.

The goals that may be achieved are many and varied. They include increased range of motion and strength, increased balance and coordination, and increased cardiovascular function if the class takes place for at least 20 minutes on a regular basis. Non-physical goals may be greater social interaction, communication with others who are limited in function or disabled in the same or different ways, and greater self-awareness.

From Fond D: Group movement class model for geriatric patients, *Coordinator* 2:30, Mar 1983.

KEY CONCEPTS

- Interruptions in the basic requirements for nutrition, fluids, elimination, activity, and rest may trigger exacerbations of subclinical and chronic disorders.
- When basic needs are out of balance, it is common for the very old to demonstrate the deficiency by becoming confused.
- Recommended dietary patterns for the aged are similar to those of younger persons, with some reduction in caloric intake based on decreased metabolic requirements.
- Adequacy of nutrition is affected by lifelong eating habits and patterns, accessibility of food, mood disorders, capacity for food preparation, and income.
- Medications may interfere with adequate food intake, absorption, digestion, and elimination. A common nutritional deficiency is a lack of sufficient calcium, especially for women.
- Making mealtimes pleasant and attractive for the aged who are unable to eat unassisted is entirely a nursing challenge; mealtimes must be made enjoyable.
- Elimination is often a preoccupation of the aged, signifying sluggishness of involuntary responses or a loss of control. Nursing attention to these functions is critical for client satisfaction and comfort.
- Deep, stage 4 sleep is not attained by the aged. They tend to be easily aroused. The nursing focus is to help them understand the changes and their sleep pattern and that their individual needs to obtain sufficient rest will vary.
- Sleep apnea is an interruption in breathing during sleep that has been linked to excess pharyngeal tissue, cardiac problems, cerebral infarction, and hypertension. It is often demonstrated by long periods without inspiring and loud snoring on expiration. The long periods of anoxia may have effects, over time, on cerebration.
- Physical activity (and the ease with which it is performed) is often the barometer by which an individual's health and wellness are judged.

▲ CASE STUDY

Nutrition

Carlotta, 73 years old, had dieted all her life—or so it seemed. She often chided herself about it. "After all, at my age who cares if I'm too fat? I do. It depresses me when I gain weight and then I gain even more when I'm depressed." At 5 ft 5 in tall and 140 lb, her weight was ideal for her height and age, but Carlotta, as so many women of her generation, had incorporated Donna Reed's weight of 105 lb as ideal. She had achieved that weight for only a few weeks three or four times in her adult life. She had tried high-protein diets, celery and cottage cheese diets, fasting, commercially prepared diet foods, and numerous fad diets. She always discontinued the diets when she perceived any negative effects. She was invested in maintaining her general good health. Her most recent attempt at losing 30 lb on an all-liquid diet had been unsuccessful and left her feeling constipated, weak, irritable, mildly nauseated, and experiencing heart palpitations. This really frightened her. Her physician upbraided her regarding the liquid diet but seemed rather amused while reinforcing that her weight was "just perfect" for her age. In the discussion the doctor pointed out how fortunate she was that she was able to drive to the market, had sufficient money for food, and was able to eat anything with no dietary restrictions. Carlotta left his office feeling silly. She was an independent, intelligent woman; she had been a successful manager of a large financial office. Before her retirement 2 years ago her work had consumed most of her energies. There had been no time for family, romance, or hobbies. Lately, she had immersed herself in reading the Harvard Classics as she had promised herself she would when she retired. Unfortunately, now that she had the time to read them she was losing interest. She knew that she must begin to "pull herself together" and "be grateful for her blessings" just as the doctor had said.

Based on the case study, develop a nursing care plan using the following procedure:*

List comments of client that provide subjective data.

List information that provides objective data.

From these data identify and state, using accepted format, two nursing diagnoses you determine are most significant to this client at this time. List two client strengths that you have identified from data.

Determine and state outcome criteria for each diagnosis. These must reflect some alleviation of the problem identified in the nursing diagnosis and must be stated in concrete and measurable terms.

Plan and state one or more interventions for each diagnosed problem. Provide specific documentation of source used to determine appropriate intervention. Plan at least one intervention that incorporates the client's existing strengths.

Evaluate success of intervention. Interventions must correlate directly with the stated outcome criteria in order to measure the outcome success.

STUDY QUESTIONS/ACTIVITIES

What factors may be involved in Carlotta's preoccupation with her weight?

What are some of the reasons that fad diets are dangerous?

Discuss how you would counsel Carlotta regarding her weight.

If Carlotta insists on dieting, what diet would you recommend, considering her age and activity level?

What lifestyle changes should Carlotta make?

*Students are advised to refer to their nursing diagnosis text and identify possible or potential problems.

What lifestyle changes would you suggest to Carlotta?

What are the specific health concerns that require attention in Carlotta's case?

RESEARCH QUESTIONS

What are the ideal weights for older men and women?

What are the dietary patterns of older career women living alone?

What percentage of women over 60 are satisfied with their weight? Men?

What eating disorders are most common among aged men? Women?

What is the compliance rate in regard to major dietary changes suggested for elders by dietitians or physicians?

What percentage of men and women over 80 years old are overweight? Obese?

▲ CASE STUDY

Elimination

Flora, at 82 years old, could truthfully say she had never had problems with her bowel movements. They had been regular—each morning about 30 minutes after breakfast. In fact, she hardly thought of them at all because they had been so consistent. Following a hospitalization for a fractured hip last year she had never regained her reliable pattern of bowel function. She was greatly distressed by this because bowel function was a symbol to her of good health. Admittedly, she did not move about as much now and used a walker when she did. And she had heard that pain medications sometimes made one constipated, but she tried to use them very sparingly. She had even reestablished her pattern of attempting a bowel movement every morning after breakfast. She began to worry considerably about her constipation and to use laxatives almost routinely. She said, "This constipation really upsets me. I just don't feel like myself if I don't have a bowel movement every day."

Based on the case study, develop a nursing care plan using the following procedure:*

List comments of client that provide subjective data.

List information that provides objective data.

From these data identify and state, using accepted format, two nursing diagnoses you determine are most significant to this client at this time. List two client strengths that you have identified from data.

Determine and state outcome criteria for each diagnosis. These must reflect some alleviation of the problem identified in the nursing diagnosis and must be stated in concrete and measurable terms.

*Students are advised to refer to their nursing diagnosis text and identify possible or potential problems.

Plan and state one or more interventions for each diagnosed problem. Provide specific documentation of source used to determine appropriate intervention. Plan at least one intervention that incorporates the client's existing strengths.

Evaluate success of intervention. Interventions must correlate directly with the stated outcome criteria in order to measure the outcome success.

STUDY QUESTIONS/ACTIVITIES

What information will you need to obtain from Flora to help her isolate the causes of her constipation?

What advice will you give her regarding the use of laxatives?

What dietary changes will you suggest, and how will you do this in order to cultivate compliance?

What information regarding the relationship of medications to constipation will be useful to Flora?

When you are constipated, how do you feel?

Do you know any elders who focus a lot of their conversation on elimination? How do you handle that?

RESEARCH QUESTIONS

What are the specific concerns elders harbor related to constipation?

Is concern with constipation a sociocultural artifact?

Do childhood training experiences affect one's eliminatory functions in late life?

What are the remedies for constipation most often deemed effective as perceived by elders?

Does fecal impaction affect urinary incontinence?

▲ CASE STUDY

Rest and Sleep

Daniel had a sleep disorder and consequently was torpid during the day and lonely at night. His wife of 35 years had recently insisted on moving into the guest room because she could no longer cope with his loud snoring and periods of interrupted breathing. Daniel suffered from obstructive sleep apnea. In recent years, he often wakened abruptly with a feeling of drowning and gasping for air. However, he simply tolerated it because he thought nothing could be done about it. Now that it had become a threat to his marriage he became more motivated to investigate possible solutions. Daniel said, "This doesn't amount to anything, but it bugs my wife." Though he did not admit it, he was also worried because he was beginning to feel rather sleepy during the day. On consulting the clinic nurse he found that there were some very practical means of dealing with sleep apnea, and if these were not effective there were additional medical interventions that could be helpful.

Based on the case study, develop a nursing care plan using the following procedure:*

List comments of client that provide subjective data.

List information that provides objective data.

From these data identify and state, using accepted format, two nursing diagnoses you determine are most significant to this client at this time. List two client strengths that you have identified from data.

Determine and state outcome criteria for each diagnosis. These must reflect some alleviation of the problem identified in the nursing diagnosis and must be stated in concrete and measurable terms.

Plan and state one or more interventions for each diagnosed problem. Provide specific documentation of source used to determine appropriate intervention. Plan at least one intervention that incorporates the client's existing strengths.

Evaluate success of intervention. Interventions must correlate directly with the stated outcome criteria in order to measure the outcome success.

STUDY QUESTIONS/ACTIVITIES

What lifestyle factors may be increasing Daniel's episodes of sleep apnea?

In what circumstances is sleep apnea particularly dangerous to health?

Compose a list of 10 questions you would ask Daniel to obtain a clear picture of factors contributing to his sleep apnea. Discuss the rationale behind each.

Look up and discuss the terms *hypnagogic* and *hypnopompic* and relate any episodes you may have experienced and how these affected you.

RESEARCH QUESTIONS

How do sleep patterns correlate with various disease states?

How do sleep patterns change with each decade after age 60?

How are hypnagogic and hypnopompic states related to sleep patterns of the aged?

What is the average time of the total sleep cycle as experienced by a healthy individual over 70 years of age?

REFERENCES

American Nurses' Association: *Position statement on forgoing artificial nutrition and hydration,* Washington, DC, 1992, The Association.

Beers MH, Berkow R: *Merck manual of geriatrics,* ed 3, Whitehouse Station, NJ, 2000, Merck Research Laboratories.

Bennett JA: Dehydration: hazards and benefits, *Geriatr Nurs* 21(2):84, 2000.

*Students are advised to refer to their nursing diagnosis text and identify possible or potential problems.

Butler R: *Old and poor in America,* issue brief, New York, 2001, International Longevity Center—USA.

Cross AT, Babicz D, Cushman LF: Snacking habits of senior Americans, *J Nutr Elderly* 14(2/3):27, 1995.

Desai SP, Isa-Pratt S: *Clinical guide to laboratory medicine,* ed 2, Cleveland, 2002, Lexi-Comp.

Drazen JM: Perspective, sleep apnea syndrome, *N Engl J Med* 346(6):390, 2002.

Edwards WF: Gastrointestinal problems. In Cotter VT, Strumpf NE, editors: *Advanced practice nursing with older adults,* New York, 2002, McGraw-Hill.

Fielo S: The mystery of sleep: how nurses can help the elderly, *Nursing Spectrum,* p 30, Oct 2001.

George B, Goldberg N: The benefits of exercise in geriatric women, *Am J Geriatr Cardiol* 10(5):260, 2001.

Gorman C: Sleeplessness in America, *Time,* p 43, Dec 17, 2001.

Grabowski D, Ellis: *Extra weight is protective for elderly people,* 2001, Agency for Healthcare Research and Quality.

Griffith R: *Treating insomnia in the elderly,* 2002. Available at *www.healthandage.com*

Ham RJ: Dementia (and delirium). In Ham RJ, Sloane PD, Warshaw GA, editors: *Primary care geriatrics,* ed 4, St Louis, 2002, Mosby.

Hill-O'Neill KA, Shaughnessy M: Dizziness and stroke. In Cotter VT, Strumpf N, editors: *Advanced practice nursing with older adults,* New York, 2002, McGraw-Hill.

Karani T et al: Exercise in the healthy older adult, *Am J Geriatr Cardiol* 10(5):269, 2001.

Kirkwood C: *Treatment of insomnia,* New York, 2001, Power-Pak, CE Publishers. Available at *www.powerpak.com*

McCullough P: How well do you sleep? Presentation at the Kentucky Council of Nurse Practitioners and Midwives, Lexington, KY, April 2001.

Moore MC: *Pocket guide to nutritional care,* ed 4, St Louis, 2001, Mosby.

Morely JE: Dehydration. Available at *www.cyberounds.com/conferences/geriatrics*

Mosqueda L, Brummel-Smith K: Rehabilitation. In Ham RJ, Sloane PD, Warshaw GA, editors: *Primary care geriatrics,* ed 4, St Louis, 2002, Mosby.

National Center for Health Statistics: *NHANES II.* Available at *http://text/nlm.nih.gov/tempfiles/is/tempBrPg43432.html*

National Institute on Aging: *It's never too late to start* (exercise pamphlet, Spanish). Available at *www.nia.nih.gov/news/pr/2002*

National Institutes of Health Consensus Statement: *Osteoporosis prevention, diagnosis and therapy,* 17(2):1, Mar 2000. NIH Consensus Programs, Information Service, Kensington, MD.

National Institutes of Health: National Heart, Lung, and Blood Institute. Available at *www.medscape.com/endocrinology/clinicalmanagement*

National Policy and Resource Center on Nutrition and Aging, Issue Panel: *Dietary reference intakes and dietary guidelines in Older Americans Act (OAA) nutrition programs,* press release, Jan 31, 2002.

Nutrition Screening Initiative: *Older Americans want more information on nutrition to manage chronic disease—but many don't receive it from their doctors,* press release, Jan 15, 2002.

Nutrition Screening Initiative: Skeleton in the nursing home closet, *Geriatr Nurs* 22(1):46, 2001.

Pear R: Nutritional therapy to fall under Medicare umbrella, *New York Times,* Dec 31, 2001.

Pierson CA: Ethnomethodologic analysis of accounts of feeding demented residents in LTC, *Image* 31(2):127, 1999.

Rahman S: Impaired nutritional status in the geriatric population, *Geriatric Medicine Focus* 2(2):1, Spring 2001.

Recommended dietary allowances, ed 10, Washington, DC, 1989, National Academy Press. Available at *www.cyberounds.com/conferences/nutrition*

Rosto L: Sleep and the elderly, *Advance for Providers of Post-Acute Care* 4(6):27, 2001.

Russell RM, Saltzman E, Rasmussen H: Comparison of diet claims. Available at *www.cyberounds.com/conferences/nutrition*

Schoenfelder DP, Culp KR: Sleep pattern disturbance. In Maas ML et al, editors: *Nursing care of older adults: diagnoses, outcomes, and interventions,* St Louis, 2001, Mosby.

Thomas DR, Ashmen W, Morley JE, Evans WJ: Nutritional mangement in long-term care: development of a clinical guideline, *J Gerontol* 55A(12):M725, 2000.

U.S. Bureau of the Census: *Statistical abstract of the United States, 2000,* Washington, DC, 2001. Available at *www.census.gov/press-release*

U.S. Department of Health and Human Services: *Healthy people 2010,* Hyattsville, MD, 2002, Public Health Service.

U.S. Department of Health and Human Services, Public Health Service, Centers for Disease Control: *Healthy people 2000: review 1994,* DHHS pub no (PHS) 95-1256-1, Hyattsville, MD, 1995.

Wakefield B: A food pyramid for the elderly, *Women's Health in Primary Care* 3(1):36, 2000.

Wakefield B: Altered nutrition: less than body requirements. In Maas ML et al, editors: *Nursing care of older adults: diagnoses, outcomes, and interventions,* St Louis, 2001, Mosby.

Zembruski C: *Hydration checklist,* New York, 2000, Hartford Institute for Geriatric Nursing.

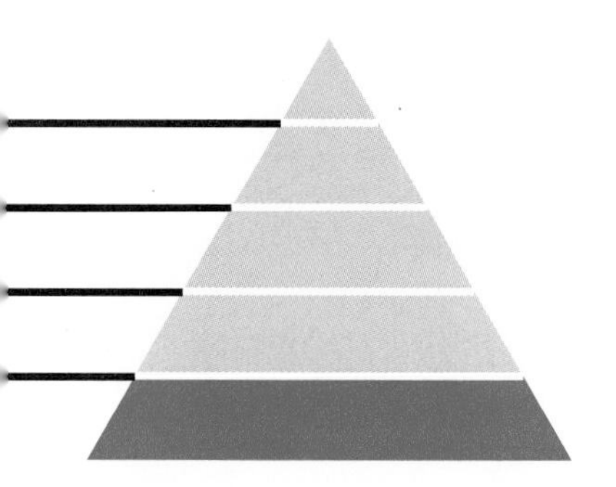

CHAPTER 7

Biologic Maintenance Needs

Ann Schmidt Luggen

An elder speaks ***If I'd known I was going to live so long, I would have taken better care of myself!***

George Burns, nearing his 100th birthday

LEARNING OBJECTIVES On completion of this chapter, the reader will be able to:

1. Describe health promotion components of maintenance needs.
2. Identify normal age changes of the buccal cavity, feet, and skin.
3. Identify common dental, foot, and skin problems of the elderly.
4. Use standard assessment tools to assess buccal cavity, feet, and skin.
5. Identify preventive, maintenance, and restorative measures for dental, foot, and skin health.
6. Establish selected nursing diagnoses on the basis of assessment for dental, foot, and skin health and care.
7. Make a plan of care for prevention and maintenance of dental, foot, and skin health.

Maintenance needs are adjuncts to life support needs. The maintenance needs discussed in this chapter also have direct and indirect effects on the psychosocial well-being of the aged. For some unexplainable reason, patients are well cared for from neck to ankles, instead of from head to toe. Under normal circumstances, teeth and feet receive cursory or minimum attention in the overall care of the client. When care is rushed because of a "busy day" or a "heavy assignment," the care of the teeth and feet is most frequently omitted. Skin care fares better. Much attention is directed to alleviating pressure, but other important integumentary influences such as friction, shearing force, moisture, and nutrition are not addressed as carefully.

DENTAL HEALTH

Dental health of the aged is a basic need that is increasingly neglected with advanced age, debilitation, and limited mobility. One reason for this neglect may be the general assumption that most older people are edentulous. The aged, themselves, believe that losing their teeth is a natural consequence of growing old. The problem with this attitude is that it fosters neglect of an essential body part: the mouth. Orodental status can affect well-being in a variety of ways. Gum or dental problems can put the older person at risk for systemic disease. The mouth is an important zone for communication between people through speech, but much of socialization and pleasure is derived from food and drink. Orodental health is integral to general health. Poor oral function, poor hygiene, and chronic oral problems can raise concern with self-presentation and fear of embarrassment that affects socialization and self-esteem.

The percentage of elders without teeth is greater than 50%, primarily as a result of periodontitis, which occurs in about 95% of those older than age 65. More than one third have moderate to severe periodontal disease (National Institutes of Health, 2000; Vargas et al, 2001). This should improve in coming generations as knowledge increases and more people use fluorides, improve nutrition, use new oral hygiene practices, and use improved dental health care. However, the caregiver should realize that whether with natural teeth or full or partial dentures, the teeth need care. In the existing health care system dental care is a low priority, reflected by the inadequacy of third-party reimbursement for the type of dental care needed by the aged. Dental insurance generally terminates at 65 years of age or is too expensive for the aged to continue the premium payments, and the older adult population is less likely to go to the dentist when compared with any other age group (Centers for Disease Control and Prevention [CDC], 2001). Average out-of-pocket dental expenses are higher for the retired aged than the working population because national programs such as Medicare and Medicaid do not provide adequate reimbursement for tooth and dental repair. Although some states include certain dental services under Medicaid, those elderly in nursing homes who are eligible for dental treatment often do not receive it. Elders are finding that even with insurance their past employers and health maintenance organizations (HMOs) are paying less of the premiums and the policy holder is paying more. Dental services should be more readily available if the aged are to use them. A recent report from the CDC indicates that both male and female elders have fewer dentist visits than any other age-group (*HealthandAge.com*, 2002). Black elders have the fewest dentist visits of any ethnic or racial group. The poor elderly have about one half the number of dentist visits of other poor age-groups. Nurses could render a valuable service to older persons by referring them to a specific dentist who will develop an ongoing relationship with the older patient.

Primary and secondary prevention strategies are effective in older adults with potential or actual dental problems (Rubenstein and Nahas, 1998). This approach will ensure good health in the successive levels of Maslow's hierarchy of needs.

Lack of teeth alters articulation of speech, jaw alignment, and general appearance. Persons without teeth rarely smile; they feel embarrassed and cover their mouths or withdraw from social contacts. The type and consistency of food chosen to eat becomes limited and monotonous. Frequently, food eaten by those who are edentulous is inadequate and deficient in nutritive value. Further, oral pain is common and prevents eating normally. At least 7% of elders report having tooth pain twice during the past 6 months (CDC, 2001). Older adults in racial/ethnic minorities with low levels of education are more likely to report dental pain, which usually signifies advanced dental problems. Difficulty eating can be caused by lack of teeth, dental pain, ill-fitting dentures, infections, or temporomandibular joint (TMJ) problems. Trouble chewing is also related to educational level: 23% of those with 0 to 8 years of education have trouble chewing, whereas 10% of those with at least 13 years of education have problems (Centers for Disease Control and Prevention, 2001; Vargas et al, 2001).

Changes in the Buccal Cavity during the Aging Process

Aging teeth become worn, become darker in color, and tend to develop longitudinal cracks. The dentin, or layer beneath the enamel, becomes brittle, and the inner layer, the pulp, atrophies with age. The most common change is in tooth loss (Reese, 2001). With tooth loss, the alveolar bone beneath shrinks (Box 7-1).

Box 7-1 Age Changes of the Buccal Cavity

- Decrease in the cellular compartment
- Loss of submucosal elastin in oral mucosa
- Loss of connective tissue (collagen)
- Increase in thickness of collagen fibers
- Decrease in function of minor salivary glands
- Decrease in number and quality of blood vessels and nerves
- Attrition on occlusive contact surfaces
- Enamel less permeable and teeth more brittle
- Tooth color change
- Excessive secondary dentin formation
- Decrease in rate of cementin deposition
- Decrease in size of pulp chamber and root canals
- Decrease in size and volume of the tooth pulp
- Increase in pulp stones and dystrophic mineralization

Dental caries is the major reason for tooth loss. It is usually thought that periodontal disease, a group of diseases affecting the teeth and gums, is the major reason, but caries (either on the crown or enamel or beneath the surface of the gum in the root or cementum surface) is thought to be the major factor in loss. Severe periodontitis is uncommon in elders because most have lost their diseased teeth (Valdez and Berkey, 2002). Loss is similar in men and women. Elders in poverty are twice as likely to be edentulous as those above the poverty line (Vargas et al, 2001). About 52% of nursing home residents are edentulous. Further, 92% of elders have both upper and lower dentures. In this group, 24% of black elders and 19% of Hispanic elders do not use their dentures. In long-term care, 80% of those who lost all their teeth had both dentures, but they were not worn by nearly 20% (Vargas et al, 2001).

Susceptibility to caries may be related to insufficient fluoride applied preventively and from toothpastes. Salivary hypofunction may also contribute. Saliva provides lubrication and protection from dehydration and infection (Reese, 2001). It contains antimicrobials that interfere with caries development. Saliva is stimulated by cholinergic innervation, and anticholinergics interfere with its release. Xerostomia (dry mouth) is related to saliva underproduction in nearly 25% of cases. Xerostomia is common in older adults but probably is more related to medical problems and medications than to the aging process.

Gum recession occurs because of periodontal disease and lack of good oral hygiene. Periodontal changes should be minimal in the healthy aged, but the attention given to oral care by health care professionals and by the aged themselves is inadequate. Inattention to periodontal conditions results in layers of plaque composed of food particles, bacteria, and saliva. Plaque should be removed every day. When it is not, inflammation, swelling, pain, and bleeding occur, and there may be discomfort from odors and an unpleasant taste in the mouth. Tartar, or calculus, forms over plaque; if not removed regularly, gum recession and periodontal disease will occur. Periodontal disease does not appear to be a specific disease of the elderly but the result of chronic periodontitis from young and middle-aged adulthood. The prevalence of periodontal disease is about 6% in adults ages 25 through 34 and 41% in those age 65 and older (Vargas et al, 2001).

Periodontitis can be a significant infection. It has been linked to diabetes complications, heart disease, and respiratory diseases, as well as tooth loss (Centers for Disease Control and Prevention, 2000). It warrants more attention and care than we have given it to this point. According to the CDC, although water fluoridation has drastically improved the incidence of tooth decay and has a minimal cost, and is a method of primary prevention, more than 100 million Americans have no access to it (Box 7-2).

Taste. Many older adults do not enjoy taste as they once did. The number of taste receptors, however, remains consistent. The problem may be in other parts of the sensory system—olfactory, thermal, tactile, or textural sensors (Reese, 2001). Drugs, diseases, and tobacco use reduce or alter taste sensation. Common among postmenopausal women is the burning mouth syndrome (Beers and Berkow, 2000). Proposed causes are poor-fitting dentures; deficiencies of vitamins B_1, B_2, B_6, and B_{12}; and deficiency of folic acid. Other possible causes are local trauma such as abrasive teeth, gastrointestinal (GI) disorders, allergies, salivary dysfunction, and diabetes.

Box 7-2 Contributing Factors in Periodontal Problems in the Aged

Anatomic
Tooth malalignment
Thinning gingival mucosa

Bacterial
Plaque accumulation
Invasion of organisms at or below gumline
Food impaction

Drugs and Metallic Poisons
Allergic responses
Phenytoin
Cytotoxins
Heavy metals (lead, arsenic, mercury)

Emotional and Psychomotor
Bruxism (grinding of teeth)
Cerebrovascular accident
Mental impairment

Intrinsic (Systemic)
Endocrine
Metabolic
Altered immune system

Mechanical
Calculus
Retention of impacted food
Moveable and spreading teeth
Ragged-edged fillings and crown overhangs
Poorly designed or poorly fitting dentures

Data compiled from Zach L, Trieger N: In Rossman I: *Clinical geriatrics,* ed 3, Philadelphia, 1986, Lippincott; Odslehage JC, Magilvey K: *Geriatr Nurs* 7:238, 1986; and Papas AS, Niessen LC, Chauncey HH: *Geriatric dentistry, aging and oral health,* St Louis, 1991, Mosby.

Common Dental Problems

Xerostomia. Dry mouth is a condition often found in the elderly as a result of salivary gland dysfunction, although salivary gland output remains stable in healthy persons but is brought on by diseases and medical treatments (Administration on Aging, 2000). Dry mouth makes eating, swallowing, tasting, and speaking difficult. Some of the causes of hyposalivation are radiation therapy to the head and neck, chemotherapy, and at least 400 common medications. Medications that interfere with saliva production include hydrochlorothiazide, a common therapy of older adults (Reese, 2001). Other drugs include sedatives, antidepressants, antihistamines, and antipsychotics. There is some evidence that estrogen replacement in postmenopausal women reduces tooth loss (Hammond, 2001). Other causes include dehydration, tumors, duct obstruction, sarcoidosis, diabetes, Alzheimer's disease, acquired immunodeficiency syndrome (AIDS), and Sjögren's syndrome (a connective tissue disorder that includes decreased lacrimal and salivary gland function). The primary form of Sjögren's syndrome affects salivary and lacrimal glands; the secondary form includes a connective tissue disease, usually rheumatoid arthritis, scleroderma, or thyroiditis (Beers and Berkow, 2000). Treatment includes discontinuing the offending drug; drinking more water; and avoiding sugary snacks, beverages with caffeine, tobacco, and alcohol, all of which increase mouth dryness. With some remaining secretion, stimulation occurs with sugarless candies, mints, and chewing gum. Pilocarpine, a cholinergic drug, can be prescribed but is to be avoided in those with Parkinson's disease, peptic ulcer, asthma, heart failure, urinary tract infection, and glaucoma.

Root Caries. Root caries can occur on any tooth surface. Most root caries are found on the proximal and buccal surfaces of the teeth, appearing initially as small, round, shallow, pigmented defects at the root surface. As these caries advance, they usually spread laterally and may undermine the tooth crown. With the new preventive measures available for tooth decay, the incidence has diminished. However, for the most economically disadvantaged elderly people, the decline has not occurred. The percentage of older black persons and poor persons with untreated caries has increased since 1974; poor whites went from 33% in 1974 to 39% in 1994, and blacks went from 42% in 1974 to 47% in 1994 (Vargas et al, 2001).

Gingivitis and Periodontitis. Gingivitis and periodontitis are major causes of tooth loss and are caused by accumulation of bacterial plaque on the teeth (Box 7-3). The bacteria invade periodontal tissues, causing an inflammatory response and destruction of connective tissues that support the tooth (Figure 7-1). Resulting problems cause loss of tooth anchorage and eventually the loss of teeth from bacterial sources. A number of drugs and medications aggravate periodontal disease. Phenytoin, calcium channel blockers, and cyclosporine cause gingival hyperplasia that bleeds easily. Antihypertensives, anticholinergics, and antipsychotics reduce the saliva, which contains antimicrobials. If allowed to continue, the tooth loses stability, and deep pockets around the tooth appear. Although the disease progresses and remits, it eventually leads to tooth loss if not stopped.

Stomatitis. Burning mouth syndrome, or stomatopyrosis, is common in postmenopausal women. It is called glossopyrosis when it occurs on the tongue. It occurs frequently with candidal infection and is painful. Proposed causes include vitamin deficiencies and poor oral hygiene with infrequent cleaning of dentures (Ettinger, 2001). It occurs in about 20% of elders who wear dentures. The burning pain increases and remits during the course of a day; nothing seems to alleviate the pain. If lesions are present, the diagnosis is incorrect and is probably candidiasis, which also causes a burning sensation. Prevention is the best management. Consultation with a dietitian may clarify the need for vitamin supplements.

Box 7-3

Signs of Periodontal Disease*

- Gums bleeding when teeth are brushed (even a little bleeding is not normal; if you have a "pink" toothbrush, see your dentist)
- Red, swollen, or tender gums
- Detachment of the gums from the teeth
- Pus that appears from the gum line when the gums are pressed
- Teeth that have become loose or change position
- Any change in the way your teeth fit together when you bite
- Any change in the fit of partial dentures
- Chronic bad breath or bad taste

*Not limited to elders alone.

Candidiasis. Candidiasis is a common infection in elderly persons. It resembles leukoplakia in that in some types, it cannot be scraped away, and that they both cause white patches in the oral cavity. They are often painful especially when beneath the dentures. Diagnosis is easily made by a smear and Gram stain. The cause is usually an immunocompromising situation such as diabetes, antibiotics, corticosteroids, or antineoplastics (Beers and Berkow, 2000). Treatment is a topical or systemic antifungal agent such as nystatin or clotrimazole. The dentures should be soaked in benzoic acid, chlorhexidine, or sodium hypochlorite and rinsed thoroughly and worn infrequently during treatment.

Leukoplakia. Leukoplakia is a precancerous lesion that manifests as a slightly raised, slightly circumscribed patch that cannot be scraped away. It is generally found on the lips, tongue, gums, or buccal mucosa. It should be evaluated by a dentist or an oral surgeon and a biopsy taken. One should look for lymphadenopathy, which might indicate a cancerous lesion that has (hematogenously) spread.

Oral Cancers. Oral cancers are more frequent in the aged. Adults age 65 and older are seven times more likely to be diagnosed with oral cancer than people younger than age 65 (Vargas et al, 2001). Oral cancers represent about 3% to 5% of all cancers; one half occur in adults older than age 65. Although white elders have more oral cancers, black men have a much higher mortality rate from oral cancers (Vargas et al, 2001). The 5-year survival rate for oral cancers is about 50% (Beers and Berkow, 2000). The male/female ratio is 2:1, down considerably from previous years. The major factors for risk of oral cancer are tobacco use and alcohol use. Pipe, cigar, and cigarette smoking are all implicated. Chewing tobacco is associated with an uncommon type of squamous cell carcinoma. The other risk factors are age, leukoplakia of long

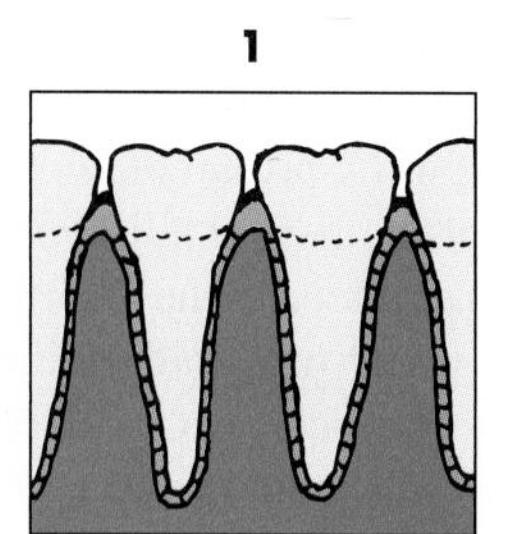

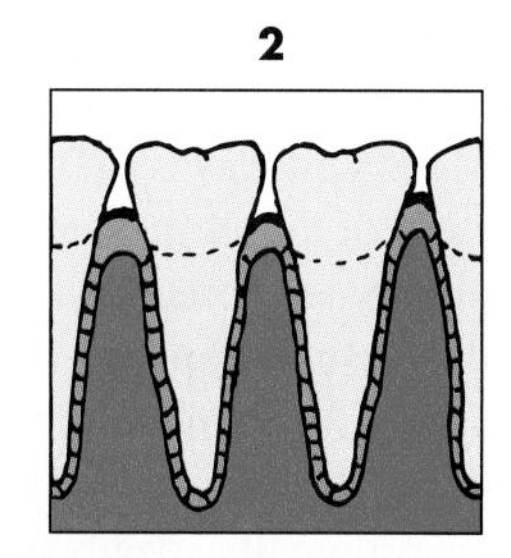

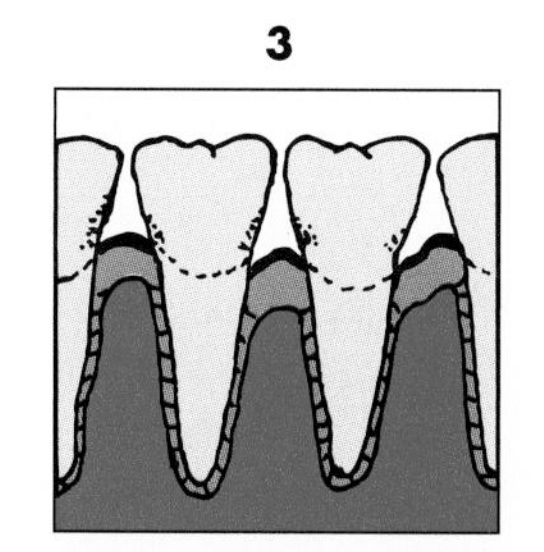

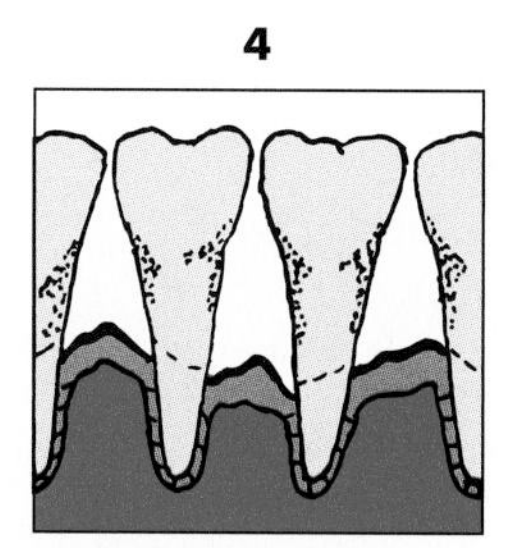

Figure 7-1. Progression of periodontal disease. *1,* Normal, healthy gingivae (gums). Healthy gums and bone anchor teeth firmly in place. *2,* Gingivitis. Plaque and its by-products irritate the gums, making them tender, inflamed, and likely to bleed. *3,* Periodontitis. Unremoved, plaque hardens into calculus (tartar). As plaque and calculus continue to build up, the gums begin to recede (pull away) from the teeth, and pockets form between the teeth and gums. *4,* Advanced periodontitis. The gums recede farther, destroying more bone and the periodontal ligament. Teeth—even healthy teeth—may become loose and need to be extracted. (Courtesy Karen L. Merrill, Wellesley, MA.)

standing or longer than 3 weeks, erythroplakia (flat red mucosal patches) of similar duration, ulcerations, dysplasias, and human papillomavirus infection. Having an oral cancer predisposes one to a second primary cancer by up to 33%.

Oral cancers are difficult to diagnose without biopsy because they are varied. Many lesions are benign. Malignant tumors usually occur between ages 50 and 70 in older people. The 50% survival rate has not improved over the years (Valdez and Berkey, 2002). Screening has the potential to improve this prognosis. Most cancers are on the lip or tongue; however, the floor of the mouth and oropharynx are also common. Benign tumors occur most often on the gingivae and occur between ages 30 and 60. Squamous cell carcinoma is the most common malignancy of the oral cavity, and most cases occur in older individuals. Mortality rate is lowest in lip cancer and highest in cancer of the tongue (Reese, 2001). Treatment is surgery with or without radiation therapy. Chemotherapy is used for advanced or unresectable tumors.

Assessment

Assessment of the oral cavity should be a regular part of nursing assessment (Box 7-4). It is much better preventive care to periodically inspect the aged person's mouth than to wait until there is a problem. All aged persons with or without dentures should have their gums, tongue, teeth (natural or dentures), and mucous membranes inspected on a regular basis. Federal regulations mandate an annual examination for institutionalized elderly people. The American Cancer Society recommends an annual oral examination. This is easily performed during a dental examination, but nurses can also perform them capably (Figure 7-2).

Box 7-4 Important Points of Oral Assessment

- Salivation
- Tongue:
  - Texture
  - Moisture
  - Coloring
- Palates
- Gingival tissues (gums)
- Teeth
- Dentures/bridgework
- Soft tooth debris
- Lips:
  - Texture
  - Moisture
  - Coloring
- Voice
- Swallowing ability

Modified from Danielson KH: Oral care and adults, *J Gerontol Nurs* 14(11):6, 1988.

Gums should be inspected for color and palpated for lesions and swelling. Ill-fitting dentures are responsible for ulcerations, which resemble cancerous lesions. Generalized inflammation, or sore mouth, is demonstrated by a reddened mucosa and a granular-looking outline of the denture bases along the gingival borders. Papillary hyperplasia is a warty papular type of condition of the palate created by the suction of the upper denture. Skinfolds at the mouth corners can overlap, causing lesions that resemble lesions seen in vitamin deficiencies such as riboflavin or an infectious process such as candidiasis. It is important not to overlook this possibility.

Teeth, if present, should be checked for jagged edges, fractures, lost fillings, caries, the number of teeth, and adequate occlusion. Dentures, if partial or full, should be removed and inspected for excessive wear, breakage, and rough spots. It is also necessary to learn when dentures were last checked by a dentist for relining, rebasing, and replacement, which is necessary whenever denture fit is too loose or causing pressure sores on the gums. This is frequently difficult for the aged person to understand or to accept. Equally difficult to accept is that no dentures will ever fit or feel exactly like one's own teeth because the mouth is always changing, especially when there is weight loss or weight gain.

The tongue should be inspected for color, swelling, and lesions and palpated on all surfaces for tenderness and lesions. The mucous membranes, in general, should be observed for color, moistness, smoothness, and the appearance of lesions. Assessment should also consider and utilize the strengths of the older adult when developing nursing diagnoses and interventions for oral care. These strengths may include maintenance of dignity, increased socialization, the desire to be well groomed and well dressed, and taking an active role in maintenance of one's own health.

It cannot be emphasized too strongly how vital dental care is to the well-being of the aged individual. For too long, health care providers have been too naive, unconcerned, or remiss in the maintenance of this important need, which influences so many other equally and more important physiologic, psychologic, and social needs. It is heartening to note that dental schools include dental care of geriatric patients in their curricula, and students receive practice by going into the community with mobile dental vans to senior centers and to visit homebound and institutionalized elders.

Interventions

Care of the Teeth. Generally, the aged are seen by the dentist when it is too late to salvage the teeth. It is therefore imperative to conscientiously include appropriate dental care to maintain and preserve the existing teeth of the aged person. Dental care begins at home and should be reinforced by the caregiver when the aged person requires assistance in meeting this activity of daily living. Prescribed oral hygiene for the individual with some or all teeth is to brush, floss, and use a fluoride dentifrice and mouth rinse daily. It is best if individuals can brush their teeth after each meal. Elders with

KAYSER-JONES BRIEF ORAL HEALTH STATUS EXAMINATION

Resident's Name ______________ Date ______________

Examiner's Name ______________ TOTAL SCORE ______________

CATEGORY	MEASUREMENT	0	1	2
LYMPH NODES	Observe and feel nodes	No enlargement	Enlarged, not tender	_Enlarged and tender_*
LIPS	Observe, feel tissue, and ask resident, family or staff (e.g., primary caregiver)	Smooth, pink, moist	Dry, chapped, or _red at corners_*	_White or red patch, bleeding or ulcer for 2 weeks_*
TONGUE	Observe, feel tissue, and ask resident, family or staff (e.g., primary caregiver)	Normal roughness, pink and moist	Coated, smooth, patchy, severely fissured or some redness	_Red, smooth, white or red patch; ulcer for 2 weeks_*
TISSUE INSIDE CHEEK, FLOOR, AND ROOF OF MOUTH	Observe, feel tissue, and ask resident, family or staff (e.g., primary caregiver)	Pink and moist	_Dry, shiny, rough red, or swollen_*	_White or red patch, bleeding, hardness; ulcer for 2 weeks_*
GUMS BETWEEN TEETH AND/OR UNDER ARTIFICIAL TEETH	Gently press gums with tip of tongue blade	Pink, small indentations; firm, smooth and pink under artificial teeth	_Redness at border around 1-6 teeth; one red area or sore spot under artificial teeth_*	_Swollen or bleeding gums, redness at border around 7 or more teeth, loose teeth; generalized redness or sores under artificial teeth_*
SALIVA (EFFECT ON TISSUE)	Touch tongue blade to center of tongue and floor of mouth	Tissues moist, saliva free flowing and watery	Tissues dry and sticky	_Tissues parched and red, no saliva_*
CONDITION OF NATURAL TEETH	Observe and count number of decayed or broken teeth	No decayed or broken teeth/roots	_1-3 decayed or broken teeth/roots_*	_4 or more decayed or broken teeth/roots; fewer than 4 teeth in either jaw_*
CONDITION OF ARTIFICIAL TEETH	Observe and ask patient, family or staff (e.g., primary caregiver)	Unbroken teeth, worn most of the time	1 broken/missing tooth, or worn for eating or cosmetics only	_More than 1 broken or missing tooth, or either denture missing or never worn_*
PAIRS OF TEETH IN CHEWING POSITION (NATURAL OR ARTIFICIAL)	Observe and count pairs of teeth in chewing position	12 or more pairs of teeth in chewing position	8-11 pairs of teeth in chewing position	_0-7 pairs of teeth in chewing position_*
ORAL CLEANLINESS	Observe appearance of teeth or dentures	Clean, no food particles/ tartar in the mouth or on artificial teeth	Food particles/tartar in one or two places in the mouth or on artificial teeth	Food particles/tartar in most places in the mouth or on artificial teeth

Upper dentures labeled: Yes ____ No ____ None ____ Lower dentures labeled: Yes ____ No ____ None ____ _Italic_*—refer to dentist immediately

Is your mouth comfortable? Yes ____ No ____ If no, explain: ______________

Additional comments: ______________

Figure 7-2. Kayser-Jones Brief Oral Health Status Examination. (With permission of Jeanie Kayser-Jones, RN, PhD, School of Nursing, University of California, San Francisco.)

cognitive problems or problems with dexterity require regular assistance and dental prophylaxis more often than every 6 months (Beers and Berkow, 2000), especially if caries are present.

Mechanical Plaque Removal. A soft, round-bristled toothbrush minimizes the chance of causing trauma to the gums yet stimulates the gums to retain firmness and adequate circulation. Dental experts recommend inclining the soft toothbrush at a 45-degree angle to the gum line and using a gentle scrubbing motion of short back-and-forth strokes over one or two teeth at a time. All surfaces—inner, outer, and chewing—should be brushed accordingly. It may be easier for the elder to use a child's toothbrush rather than an adult brush. A brush of this size and type is generally made of soft bristles and is a third smaller than the adult brush. It is easier to brush individual teeth and into the back angles of the mouth. Disclosure tablets or drops will stain the plaque that collects at the gum line and tooth appositions red or deep pink. It can help the person see the areas of plaque accumulation that otherwise are not visible on inspection. Brushing teeth routinely for approximately 2 minutes each time should adequately remove debris and stimulate the gums.

Interproximal Plaque Removal. Dental flossing is an integral part of the cleaning process; once a day is sufficient if done properly. The person should use about a 46-cm length of lightly waxed or unwaxed floss; a seesaw motion places the floss between the tooth surfaces; removal of plaque requires up-and-down movement under the gum line and side surfaces of teeth. Many people floss just between the teeth but forget to include under the gum line and the single surface of the last molar. Use of a commercial floss handle may provide the leverage and ease necessary for the aged person to continue flossing. If the floss handle is too delicate to grasp, the section on adaptive aids suggests modifications. Persons with sensitive or ulcerated gums might find a Water Pik device appropriate. The forced water device cleans teeth and provides a gentle massage to the gums.

Rinses. There are a variety of rinses that individuals use; most are cosmetic or therapeutic. Cosmetic rinses primarily function to refresh the mouth, but there are major disadvantages. Depending on the brand, cosmetic rinses contain 6% to 29% alcohol by volume, which can be an oral tissue irritant and can exacerbate or create xerostomia. Second, alcoholism is a problem of elderly people, so caution is advised in the use of alcohol-containing rinses. A third disadvantage of cosmetic rinses is that the effect of the mouth-flushing rinse is transient and may mask underlying causes of oral disease such as halitosis.

Therapeutic rinses contain an agent that is beneficial to the surface of the teeth and the oral environment. Some therapeutic rinses require a prescription such as Peridex (chlorhexidine), which contains alcohol but is also a broad-spectrum antimicrobial agent that helps control plaque. Listerine, which is in this same category, is an over-the-counter product that carries the American Dental Association approval, but it should not be used by persons on Antabuse or who have severe oral mucositis. Listerine also contains a high quantity by volume of alcohol (26.9%). Fluoride rinses such as the over-the-counter ACT and Fluorigard act to prevent caries development by incorporating fluoride into developing enamel, by enhancing or increasing remineralization of enamel, and by antibacterial action. Remineralizing rinses are used to replace calcium and phosphate lost from enamel or cementum during the caries process.

Nurses often use hydrogen peroxide or sodium bicarbonate (Coleman, 2002). There is no good evidence that these are particularly useful. In fact, there is evidence that peroxide damages the oral mucosa. The taste is not preferred by most patients. Bicarbonate is also unpleasant to taste, changes the mouth pH, and may cause mucosal burns if not diluted properly. Rinsing the mouth with plain water is also not sufficient because bacterial plaque will continue to form.

Electronic devices. Plaque control toothbrushes may be useful for the aged person because they have large handles for easier grasp, require little or no arm or wrist movement, provide a consistent motion, and are relatively lightweight. Some plaque removal devices stop when too much pressure is applied. (My own dentist has prescribed one for me, and I actually enjoy it!)

Adaptive aids for oral care. The handle of a toothbrush or floss holder can be easily customized for elders with a grasp weakened by arthritis, stroke, or other conditions. Enlisting the elder's assistance and creativity in designing the home care device is important because he or she is the best judge of what works well. Box 7-5 and Figure 7-3 provide possible adaptations.

Assisting Dependent Elders

It is essential to provide oral care daily regardless of whether the elder is severely disabled, physically handicapped, comatose, or mentally incapable of carrying out his or her own oral hygiene. Debilitated elders are at a greater risk of developing oral disease. They take more medications; they have decreased saliva production; they lack resistance to bacterial toxins that cause periodontal disease; and they eat softer

Box 7-5 Toothbrush and Floss Holder Adaptations

Wrap Handle with:
- Washcloth
- Aluminum foil
- Thin foam sheets

Insert Handle into:
- Sponge ball
- Sponge hair roller
- Plastic bicycle handle grip

Secure to Handle:
- Velcro or elastic strap to handle to slip over hand
- Attach handle to curved handle of nail brush with bristles removed, slip over fingers

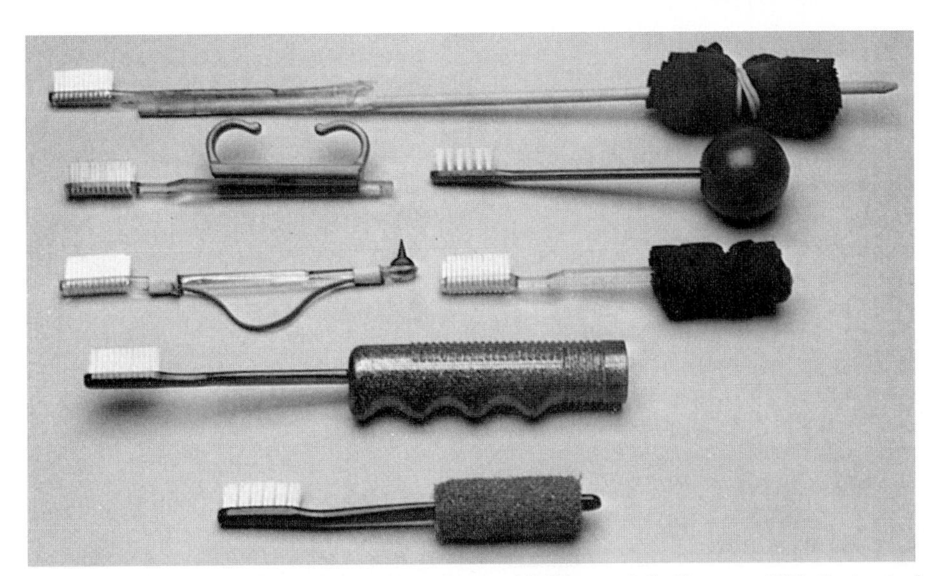

Figure 7-3. Adaptive aids for brushing. (From Papas AS, Niessen LC, Chauncey HH: *Geriatric dentistry, aging and oral health,* St Louis, 1991, Mosby.)

foods, more liquids, and foods higher in sugar, which tend to remain in their mouths longer.

Homebound

Daily oral home care should be a part of general hygiene care. Having the proper equipment and using the appropriate techniques can greatly simplify the task and ensure better results. Caregivers should be shown and provided with written instructions to reinforce the verbal instructions and demonstration. Box 7-6 provides directions for caregivers.

To make oral hygiene complete, the tongue should be brushed. With age a white coating is formed on the tongue by mouth organisms, and this coating must be brushed or scraped off. This can most easily be done at the time of brushing teeth. It is preferable to brush the tongue or wipe it with a gauze when brushing the teeth after each meal. Cleaning the tongue may be difficult for some people because it elicits the gag reflex if brushed too far back on the tongue.

The type of dentifrice is not as important as the mechanical action employed in the teeth-cleaning process, although it should contain fluoride. With the effects of fluoride in reducing gum line and root caries and preventing bacterial invasion of teeth, the use of a commercial fluoride toothpaste is beneficial.

When the aged person with natural teeth is unable to carry out his or her own dental regimen, it is the responsibility of the caregiver to do so. In the institutional setting it may not be possible to brush a person's teeth three or four times each day, but if the teeth are thoroughly brushed for 2 minutes and flossed at least once in 24 hours, the integrity of the mouth can be maintained; however, after each meal is preferred. It is common to see nurses using foam swabs with or without lemon glycerine. These swabs are ineffective for cleaning teeth and controlling plaque and should not be used (Coleman, 2002).

A curved-bristle toothbrush for those in nursing homes who need assistance allows greater access to harder-to-reach dental surfaces. These are readily available commercially. They remove more plaque than straight-bristle brushes. The benefit to the caregiver is reduction in time and degree of difficulty in giving oral care. Use of disclosure liquid or chewing tablets would help the caregiver identify whether proper brushing and flossing was actually accomplished.

To ensure that the aged person receives thorough oral hygiene, it might be necessary to write it as a routine part of the nursing care plan, which can be evaluated daily.

Box 7-6 Dental Care: Instructions for Caregiver

1. If the patient is in bed, elevate his or her head by raising the bed or propping it with pillows and have the patient turn his or her head to face you. Place a clean towel across the chest and under the chin, and place a basin under his or her chin.
2. If the patient is sitting in a stationary chair or wheelchair, stand behind the patient and stabilize his or her head by placing one hand under the patient's chin and resting his or her head against your body. Place a towel across his or her chest and over the shoulders. (It may be helpful to secure it with a safety pin.) The basin can be kept handy in the patient's lap or on a table placed in front of or at the side of the patient. A wheelchair may be positioned in front of the sink.
3. If the patient's lips are dry or cracked, apply a light coating of petroleum jelly.
4. Brush and floss the patient's teeth as you have been instructed (sulcular brushing, if possible). It may be helpful to retract the patient's lips and cheek with a tongue blade or fingers in order to see the area that is being cleaned. Use a mouth prop as needed if the patient cannot hold his or her mouth open. If manual flossing is too difficult, use a floss holder or an interproximal brush to clean the proximal surfaces between the teeth. Use a dentifrice containing fluoride.
5. Provide the conscious patient with fluoride rinses or other rinses as indicated by the dentist or hygienist.

From Papas AS, Niessen LC, Chauncey HH: *Geriatric dentistry, aging and oral health,* St Louis, 1991, Mosby.

Care of the Dentures

A significant number of elders are edentulous and wear complete dentures. Dentures help maintain adequate nutrition and psychologically aid to preserve appearance, social contacts, and relationships that a person has cultivated. Many elders believe that once they have dentures there is no longer a need for oral care. Older adults with dentures should be taught the proper home care of their dentures and oral tissue. This prevents odor, stain, and plaque buildup, and removes debris under dentures that causes pressure and shrinkage of the underlying support structures. Dentures and other dental appliances such as bridges should be cleaned after each meal and anytime they are removed (Box 7-7).

Dentures must be worn constantly during the day. They should be removed at bedtime and replaced in the mouth in the morning to allow relief of the compression on the gums. If the elder prefers to sleep with dentures in place, he or she should be encouraged to remove them for at least 4 hours during the day and relinquish them for daily cleaning. See Box 7-8 for tips on proper care of dentures. If cleaning must be done by the caregiver, brushing with a denture brush or a medium-firm toothbrush should be done on all surfaces of the dentures. If there are removable bridges or other wires (or prong-type attachments), these should be thoroughly cleaned to remove any debris and food. When cleaning dentures, fill the sink over which the washing will be done one third or half full of water; hold the dentures close to the water so that if the dentures do slip, the water will break the fall and no damage will result.

Some immersion (soaking) cleaners assist in cleaning dentures. These products should be nonabrasive to the denture

Box 7-7

Instructions for Denture Cleaning

1. Rinse your denture or dentures after each meal to remove soft debris.
2. Once a day, preferably before retiring, brush your denture according to the method described below. Then place it in a denture-cleaning solution and allow it to soak overnight or for at least a few hours. (Acrylic denture material must be kept wet at all times to prevent cracking or warping.)
3. Remove your denture from the cleaning solution and brush it thoroughly.
   a. Although an ordinary soft toothbrush is adequate, a specially designed denture brush may clean more effectively. (CAUTION: Acrylic denture material is softer than natural teeth and may be damaged by being brushed with very firm bristles.)
   b. Brush your denture over a sink lined with a washcloth and half-filled with water. This will prevent breakage if the denture is dropped.
   c. Hold the denture securely in one hand, but do not squeeze. Hold the brush in the other hand. It is not essential to use a denture paste, particularly if dentures are soaked before being brushed to soften debris. Never use a commercial tooth powder because it is abrasive and may damage the denture materials. Plain water, mild soap, or sodium bicarbonate may be used.
   d. When cleaning a removable partial denture, great care must be taken to remove plaque from the curved metal clasps that hook around the teeth. This can be done with a regular toothbrush or with a specially designed clasp brush.
4. After brushing, rinse your denture thoroughly and insert it into your mouth.

From Papas AS, Niessen LC, Chauncey HH: *Geriatric dentistry, aging and oral health,* St Louis, 1991, Mosby.

material, require little handling of the dentures, and reach all parts of the dentures. If used daily in conjunction with brushing, this should be sufficient to keep dentures clean. The elder or caregiver should always brush and rinse the dentures before and after the immersion soak. The gums, tongue, and palate should be cleansed by using a soft-bristled brush or by wiping the soft tissue with a gauze-wrapped finger. It does little for tissue integrity to clean the dentures and leave a residual film of debris on the gums. Gums, too, should be cleansed with a gloved finger wrapped in gauze or with a soft toothbrush to remove the film and residual food particles caught under dentures. This is an opportune time to massage the gums to increase circulation and inspect them for irritations.

Dentures are very personal and expensive possessions. In communal living situations of nursing homes, hospitals, and other care centers, dentures have often been misplaced or mixed up with others. Dentures should be marked; in fact, it should be a mandatory procedure for all persons who wear dentures to have their name, initials, or an identification number, such as their social security number, imprinted on the denture plates. Dentists, laboratory technicians, and dental hygienists are now marking dentures. Some states require all newly made dentures to contain the client's identification. If dentures have not been marked, the caregiver can write the name, initial, or appropriate identification number on the dentures either on the buccal flange or on the palate. This is a temporary measure that must be repeated after a short time. This is not ideal, but it is better than not having dentures marked at all. A commercial denture marking system called Identure, produced by 3M Company, provides a simple, efficient, and permanent means of marking dentures. It contains a special marking pen to mark the denture base and a permanent transparent film to cover the marking.

Broken or damaged dentures are a common problem for the aged. This generally happens when dentures are accidentally dropped during cleaning because of poor neuromuscular coordination or because they are slippery to handle. Do-it-yourself fix-it kits are not advisable.

Dentures should be correctly repaired by a dentist. Relining of dentures is usually a temporary measure; rebasing dentures is more successful. A new impression is made of the remaining dental ridge. The teeth are removed from the original pink denture and used in the new better-fitting denture base that has been adjusted to the changes in the dental ridges. This is less costly than a new denture because the original teeth are used. Prosthetic failure generally results from tissue changes in the mouth. These alterations can develop from the

Box 7-8

Take Care of Your Dentures

1. When your denture is out of your mouth, it should be stored in a water-filled container. This will prevent the denture material from drying out.
2. Place the container in a secure location where it will not be knocked onto the floor or disturbed by pets or children.
3. Never place your denture in hot water—use only cool or lukewarm water.
4. Never soak dentures with metal parts in bleach.
5. Never try to adjust or repair your denture. Let an expert do it.
6. Never use abrasive powders or a hard toothbrush to clean your denture.
7. Never soak your denture in a product that contains alcohol, such as mouthwash, or clean it with regular toothpaste.
8. *ALWAYS rinse your denture thoroughly* under running water before inserting it into the mouth.

From Papas AS, Niessen LC, Chauncey HH: *Geriatric dentistry, aging and oral health,* St Louis, 1991, Mosby.

prostheses themselves, from the physical and emotional status of the aged person, or from significant weight fluctuations.

Dentures should be checked once a year. The average time a denture base will be able to support the denture is 10 to 20 years. Many elders lose as much as 50% of supporting bone in as few as 5 to 10 years. Rapid bone loss occurs with ill-fitting dentures (loose dentures). Denture adhesive helps only temporarily.

Dental Implants

During recent years several new approaches to dealing with missing teeth have been devised, such as dental implants. There are diverse reasons for the cause and inability of elders to wear dentures. Current research indicates that providing a stable prosthetic may be the single most important determinant in fulfilling client aesthetic expectations. Osseointegrated dental implants have become reliable and safely provide long-term prosthetic stability for edentulous clients of all ages. Dental implants are not an appropriate treatment for all persons. The basic objective of dental implantation is to provide an attachment mechanism for teeth or dentures. Dental implants can anchor lower or upper dentures, usually with a metal screw surgically placed into the jaw bones (National Institutes of Health, 2000). They provide a method to replace partial or full dentures with fixed bridgework, provide a method of replacing a single tooth, improve chewing function and restore the feeling of natural tooth function, and improve the quality of life by removing the frustration associated with using dentures or removable bridgework.

The procedure is done in several steps, which cover approximately 3 to 5 months from start to completion. Elderly candidates for dental implantations must be fit enough to undergo minor oral surgery and have a jaw that can accommodate the implant system. A major problem for implants is the lack of jaw bone that occurs in 10% of prospective patients. In addition, the candidate for implants can have no history of drug abuse (potential for misuse of pain management drugs) and must possess realistic expectations of the outcome. Cost of implants varies widely from area to area, but implants are costly and are not covered by insurance. Figure 7-4 demonstrates several types of implant supports.

FEET

The feet undergo a great deal of use, trauma, misuse, and neglect as a part of everyday living. Most aged accept foot problems as an inescapable accompaniment of aging. Nurses and people in general have a fairly strong negative reaction to having

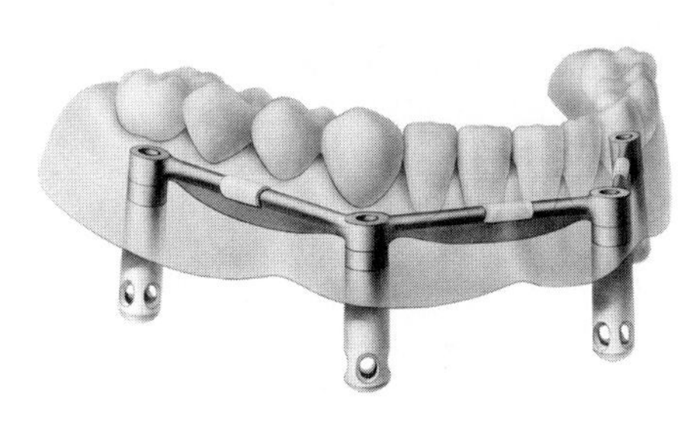
Bar-supported lower denture

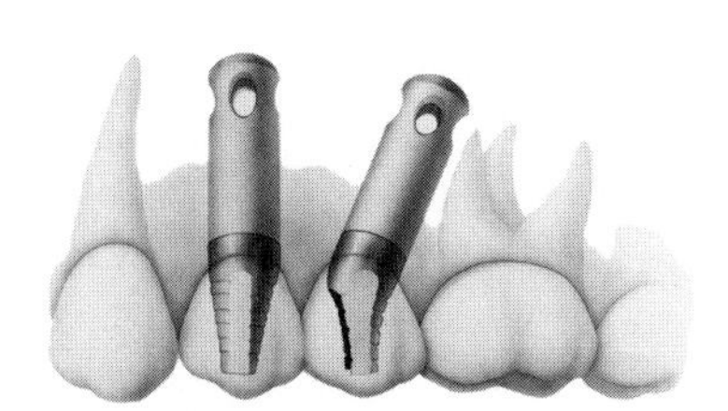
Implant-supported crowns

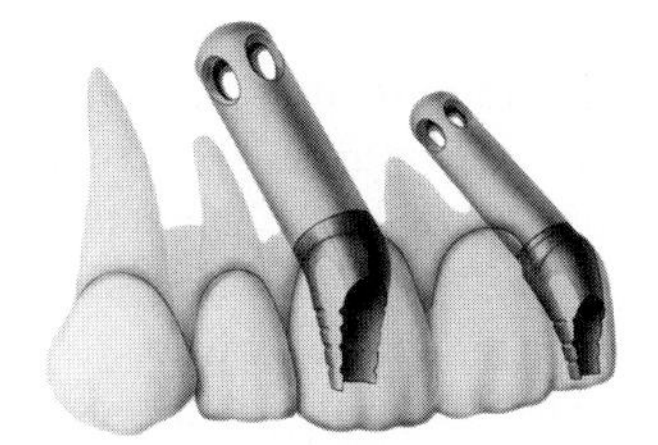
Implant-supported upper bridge

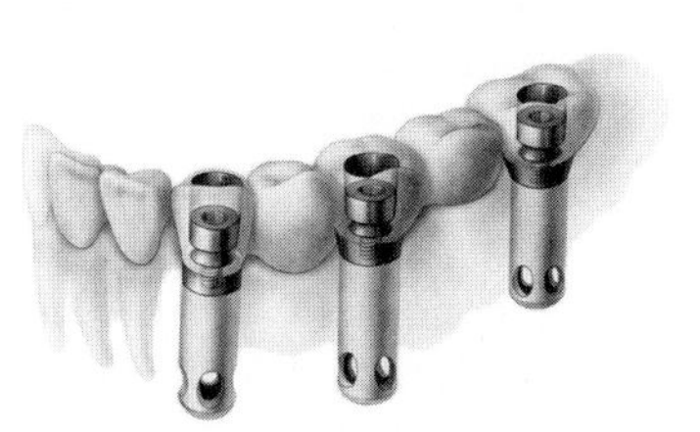
Implant-supported lower bridge

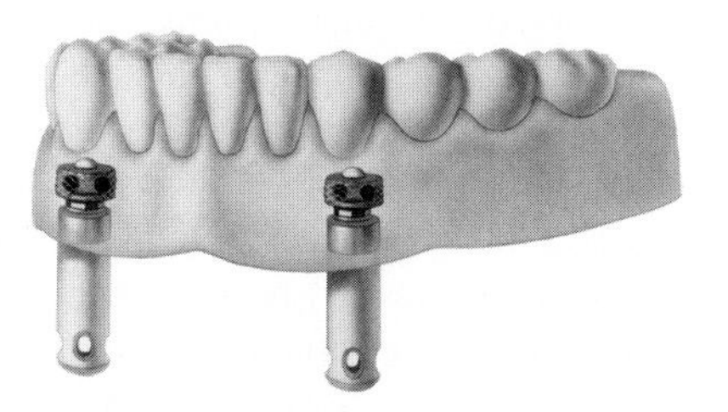
Ball-supported lower denture

Figure 7-4. Type of dental implant supports. (Courtesy Sulzer Calcitek, Inc., Carlsbad, CA.)

contact with the feet. It is aesthetically unpleasant to us. Yet adequate care of the feet can alleviate disability, pain, and the propensity for falling. It is for these reasons that the importance of feet to the well-being of the aged is emphasized more extensively in this chapter than in most texts.

Feet influence the physical, psychologic, and social well-being of the individual. Feet carry one's body weight, hold the body erect in an upright and stationary position, coordinate and maintain balance in walking, and must be rigid yet loose and adaptable enough to conform to the surfaces underfoot (all the while holding the legs and body in an upright position). Little attention is given to these valuable appendages until the feet interfere with ambulation and the ability to maintain independence.

Feet have been symbolically significant from biblical times, when respect and concern were shown by washing the feet, particularly of religious leaders and those held in esteem. The expressions "cold feet" (when we are reluctant to do something) and "he has both feet on the ground" (indicating someone with a good deal of common sense) are examples of the metaphors we use to symbolize the meaningfulness we attribute to feet. We contend that the symbolic significance of the feet is present today, and attending to the feet is a gesture of response to the total individual.

Feet often reflect systemic disease conditions or give clues to physical ailments before their actual appearance. Sudden or gradual changes in nail or skin condition of the feet or appearance of recurring infections may be the precursors of more serious health problems. Feet have a significant effect on one's productivity, amiability, and mobility. The effect is comparable to the influence that the automobile has had in our society. Like the automobile, if there is something wrong, it is difficult to get around and the routine of the day is upset. Feet, like the automobile, are taken for granted and accorded little attention as long as they work. Unlike the automobile, though, the feet do not have easily replaceable parts. Neglect of the feet throughout one's active years can result in painful conditions later. Uncomfortable and painful feet may force the elderly person to become sedentary and deprived of social contacts. Foot discomfort can cause irritability, fatigue, and chronic complaints. Socrates is thought to have said, "To him whose feet hurt, everything hurts."

The aged person's feet are subjected to functional and physical neglect and traumatic stresses over the years. The residual effect from these varied stresses, compounded by a decreased ability of the aged to clearly see their feet (because of visual impairment) and to bend to give their feet routine care, often results in conditions that need not exist or at least could be controlled (Box 7-9).

Mobility for the aged may mean the difference between an independent, active community life, self-respect, motivation, and responsibility for one's health versus institutionalization. Even in an institution, foot problems may mean the difference between confinement to bed or wheelchair and the ability to ambulate in the protective setting.

Box 7-9 Age-Related Foot Changes

- Skin becomes drier, less elastic, and cooler.
- Subcutaneous tissue on dorsum and sides of foot thins.
- Plantar fat pad shrinks and degenerates.
- Toenails become brittle, thicken, and are less resistant to fungal infections.
- Degenerative joint disease decreases range of motion.

Foot Problems in Old Age

Foot disorders begin early in life and may be affected by heredity, gait patterns, and level of activity, as well as foot care. Shoe styles affect the foot and can even affect the hip or leg. See Box 7-9 for age-related foot changes. At least 50% of people have foot problems. The number and severity of the problems increase with age. Almost 80% of persons over age 50 have at least one significant foot problem. Three of every four persons age 65 years and over complain of foot pain. Most individuals over 55 years of age (88% of women and 83% of men) demonstrate arthritic changes in the foot on x-ray. Of these older adults, 25% have symptoms of foot problems. Major abnormalities occur gradually with discomfort, not with pain. Without proper care and treatment these conditions become disabling and a threat to the person's independence. Consult the podiatrist for common problems of the feet in the aged.

Arthritis. Osteoarthritis, a disease occurring in virtually all elders, can cause pain and deformity in the feet and make difficulty in fitting shoes. It is the most common cause of foot pain (Beers and Berkow, 2000). It usually involves the ankle and first metatarsophalangeal joint of the hallux. Palpation reveals stiffness, pain, and limited range of motion (ROM). There is narrowing of the joint space, loss of cartilage, and osteophyte formation. Treatment is usually with nonsteroidal antiinflammatory drugs (NSAIDs) and Cox-2 inhibitors or corticosteroid injections. Exercising the joint and traction of the toe will help increase ROM. Orthotics may help with pain when walking.

Rheumatoid arthritis causes progressive stiffening of joints, which leads to deformity and ankylosis. Periods of rest from weight bearing are essential. Specially made shoes should be obtained to accommodate painful plantar areas. Local injections of corticosteroids are helpful for joint pain, and NSAIDs are useful on a regular basis.

Gout usually starts in the metatarsophalangeal joint of the big toe. It is painful, swollen, red, and hot (Meiner, 2002). Prevention of further attacks includes losing weight, reducing alcohol intake, increasing fluid intake, and management with colchicine (at the beginning of an attack) and allopurinol (after the acute attack has subsided). Pain medications are given for acute attacks, as well as corticosteroid injections at the painful site.

Corns. Corns, conical-shaped layers of compacted skin usually on the dorsal surface of the proximal interphalangeal joint of smaller toes, occur as a result of friction and pressure on the skin rubbing against bony, protuberant areas of the toes when shoes are worn. Once the small, hard, white corn is established, continued pressure elicits pain. Unless the cause of the corn is removed, it will continue to enlarge and cause increasing pain. Soft corns (heloma molle) form in the same manner but occur between opposing surfaces of the toes. Both corns and calluses interfere with the ability to walk comfortably and wear shoes. If not managed, corns can lead to inflammation and infection. Many elders usually follow what they or their parents have done for years to correct their foot discomfort. *Over-the-counter preparations for corns, in particular, damage normal tissue as well as remove the corn; they do not treat the cause.* Chemical burns and ulcerations can result in the loss of toes or a leg for the aged person with diabetes, neurologic impairment, or poor circulatory function to the lower extremities. Some elderly use razor blades and scissors to remove corns and calluses; this is a dangerous solution. Moleskin or lamb's wool can be used, with a hole cut in the center for the corn. This can be placed around the corn, protecting it from pressure without restricting circulation to healthy tissue. Soft corns between the toes can be eased by loosely wrapping small amounts of lamb's wool around the involved toe (Figure 7-5).

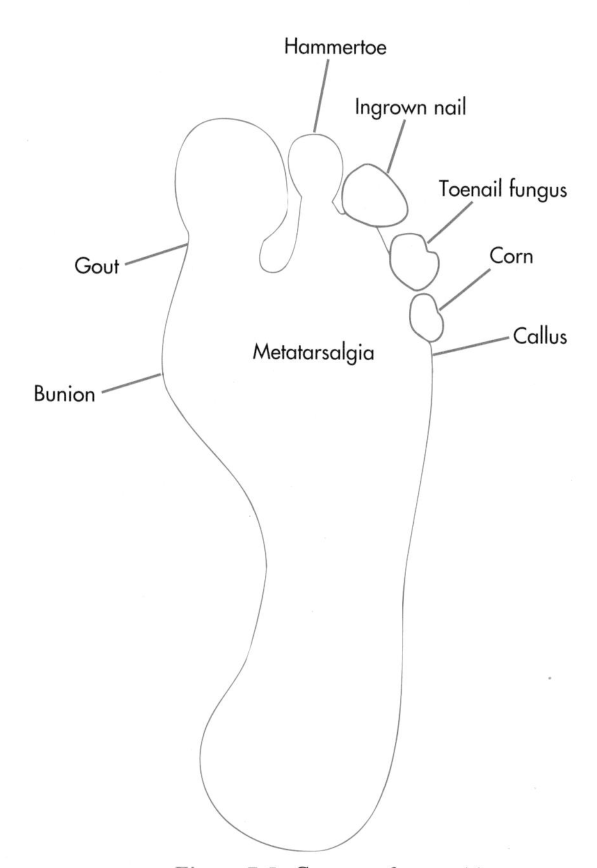

Figure 7-5. Common foot problems.

Calluses. Calluses are also layers of compacted skin that usually occur on the soles and heels of the feet because of chronic irritation and friction from shoes. Calluses can be eased with moleskin or lamb's wool applied to those areas that receive undue friction. Moleskin adheres for several days or longer but should be removed when it becomes wet or excessively soiled. Removing moleskin from the feet of the elderly should be done slowly to prevent tearing of skin. An emollient cream with a urea base, used routinely, will also be helpful in reducing keratosis and increasing hydration.

Bunions. Bunions (hallux valgus) are deviations of the first metatarsal head (the joint of the great toe) causing it to protrude medially. Bunions are long-standing residual effects from occupational activity and the influence of shoe styles. They are most common in women. Women's shoes, which draw the toes together, and the improper weight transmission and restrictive hose all contribute to the problem. Bunions are also thought to have a hereditary predisposition. Walking can be markedly compromised. Bunions may be treated with corticosteroid injections or the use of antiinflammatory pain medications. A custom-made shoe should be considered. Surgery is available.

The nurse should educate the person on the need to obtain shoes that properly support, protect, and provide comfort for the foot and encourage the client to wear them. Shoes that provide enough forefoot space laterally and dorsally, such as running shoes, generally have a wide toe box and fit well. Depth inlay shoes made by the Alden Shoe Company (Middleborough, MA 02346) have been cited as providing significant relief. Extra depth in shoes for women is offered by Miller Shoes, now owned by Drew Shoe Company (252 Quarry Road, Lancaster, OH 43130).

Hammer Toe. Hammer toe is malalignment of the toe in a contracted position of the proximal interphalangeal joint with hyperextension of the distal interphalangeal joint. It results from years of wearing improper shoes. Over time, the toe, usually the second toe, is pushed against the great toe, slanting toward and under it. Balance and comfort are affected. Treatments include use of professional orthotics; use of properly fitting, nonconstricting shoes; and surgical intervention, such as débriding the lesion or other surgery.

Metatarsalgia. Metatarsalgia is pain in the ball of the foot caused by atrophy of the fat pad on the plantar surface of the foot (Beers and Berkow, 2000). Other causes include a narrow, high-arched foot, which focuses stress on the ball of the foot; legs that are unequal in length, thus adding stress to the metatarsal joints of the shorter leg; rheumatoid arthritis; stress fractures; fluid accumulation; muscle fatigue; flat feet; and excessive pressure from obesity. Without care, bursitis or arthritis of the involved joints may occur. Bunions or tender calluses under the metatarsophalangeal joint or a Morton's neuroma may also be responsible for this foot problem. Relief is obtained with redistribution of the pressure away from the metatarsal head. Orthotics and the use of NSAIDs are helpful for symptomatic relief. Orthotics can be a reasonably priced alternative (rather than custom-made shoes) for the elder with foot problems.

Morton's Neuroma. Morton's neuroma is a painful, disabling deformity caused by entrapment of nerves of the foot. The affected nerves lie between the metatarsal heads, and the diagnosis is made by applying direct pressure on the plantar surface of the foot. Massage provides symptomatic relief of pain. Corticosteroid injections also provide temporary relief. For permanent correction, surgery must be done.

Heel Pain. Heel spurs caused by abnormal pronation of the foot are the most common cause of heel pain. This may be from a long history of wearing high heels. Atrophy of the fat pad beneath the calcaneus is a common cause in elderly persons. Rheumatoid arthritis and gout are other causes of heel pain. Plantar fasciitis (pain in the longitudinal arch with associated heel pain) is another possible diagnosis. It is not uncommon to see a "pump bump," or Haglund's deformity (Beers and Berkow, 2000), on the posterior aspect of the heel; Haglund's deformity is a calcaneus exostosis. It may lead to bursitis because it creates pressure on the heel. Treatment is similar to other foot problems with corticosteroid injections, NSAIDs, and Cox-2 inhibitors. In addition, physical therapy with hydrotherapy, heel cups, and plantar paddings will reduce heel pain. Slippers should be worn when pain is acute.

Fungal Infections. Fungal infections are common in the aged foot. Nail fungus, onychomycosis, is characterized by degeneration of the nail plate and brittleness and hypertrophy of the nail. It is often caused by a *Trichophyton* species and some *Candida* species (Figure 7-6). Laboratory testing for dermatophytes makes the definitive diagnosis. Diminished blood supply to the feet in elderly people often decreases the treatment options. Itraconazole or terbinafine, antifungals for toenails, and clotrimazole are therapies for *Candida.* Griseofulvin has many systemic side effects and is usually not given to older adults. Nails should be under the care of a podiatrist on a regular basis. This is imperative if there is vascular impairment or diabetes. Hands should be washed each time the feet of a patient with a fungus infection are handled. Feet, especially between the toes, should be dry and exposed to sun and air. Topical application of antifungal drugs may prevent complications such as fissures with subsequent opportunistic infection.

Peripheral Vascular Disease and Diabetes. Peripheral vascular disease (PVD) affects the legs and feet. The skin becomes discolored, cold, burning, and numb. There is loss of hair on the legs and feet, and they are often edematous. Ulcers are not uncommon. Onychomycosis is common with advancing disease. Infection is difficult to combat because of poor circulation. Diabetes causes symptoms similar to those of PVD. There may be color and temperature changes, dry scaly skin, and edema. Weakness, paresthesias, numbness, burning, and cramping may occur (Beers and Berkow, 2000). Management of risk factors for elders with diabetes is extremely important, because morbidity due to foot ulcers and amputation is significant (American Diabetes Association, 2002). Box 7-10 provides information for risk identification for people with diabetes.

Care of the Feet

Foot care is a prime factor in determining mobility and quality of life in retaining independence. Elders with painful foot problems and resultant activity limitations are usually forced to remain within the boundaries of their homes. Nursing care of the aged foot should be directed toward maintaining comfort and function, removing possible mechanical irritants, decreasing the likelihood of infection, and helping to enhance and preserve maximum function. These goals are consistent with podiatric goals. The nurse has the important function of assessing the feet of the aged person for clues to well-being and functional ability, not just bathing and applying lotion to the

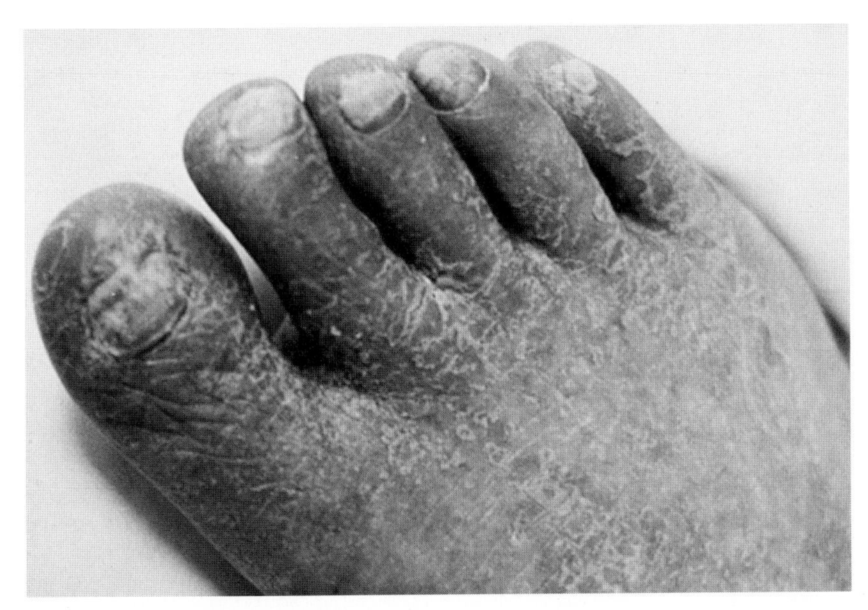

Figure 7-6. Dry scaly foot with toenail fungus. (Courtesy Stewart H. Bloom.)

Box 7-10 Risk Identification for People with Diabetes

Diabetes for longer than 10 years
Male
Poor glucose control
Cardiovascular, retinal, or renal complications
Increased risk for amputation with the following:
- Peripheral neuropathy with loss of sensation
- Evidence of increased pressure (redness, bony deformity)
- Peripheral vascular disease (diminished or absent pedal pulses)
- History of ulcers
- History of amputation
- Severe nail pathology

Source: American Diabetes Association: Position statement on preventive foot care in people with diabetes, *Diabetes Care* 25:S69, 2002.

feet. Nurses can identify potential and actual problems and refer or seek podiatric assistance for the foot problems of the patient.

Assessment

Nursing care of the feet should include a thorough assessment. Figure 7-7 illustrates some of the important aspects to look for and evaluate, and it includes simple explanations of specific items to ensure uniform evaluation regardless of who performs the assessment. A foot assessment includes careful inspection of gait, postural deformities, physical limitations, and position of the foot with the heel strike. Inspect feet for irritation, abrasions, and other lesions; check for hazards to the maintenance of adequate circulation to the lower extremities and the existing circulatory status; and observe the individual's general mobility. A variety of tools are available, which speaks to the need for individualization to the client population with whom one is working and to the expertise of the individual who is doing the assessment and giving the care (Figure 7-8).

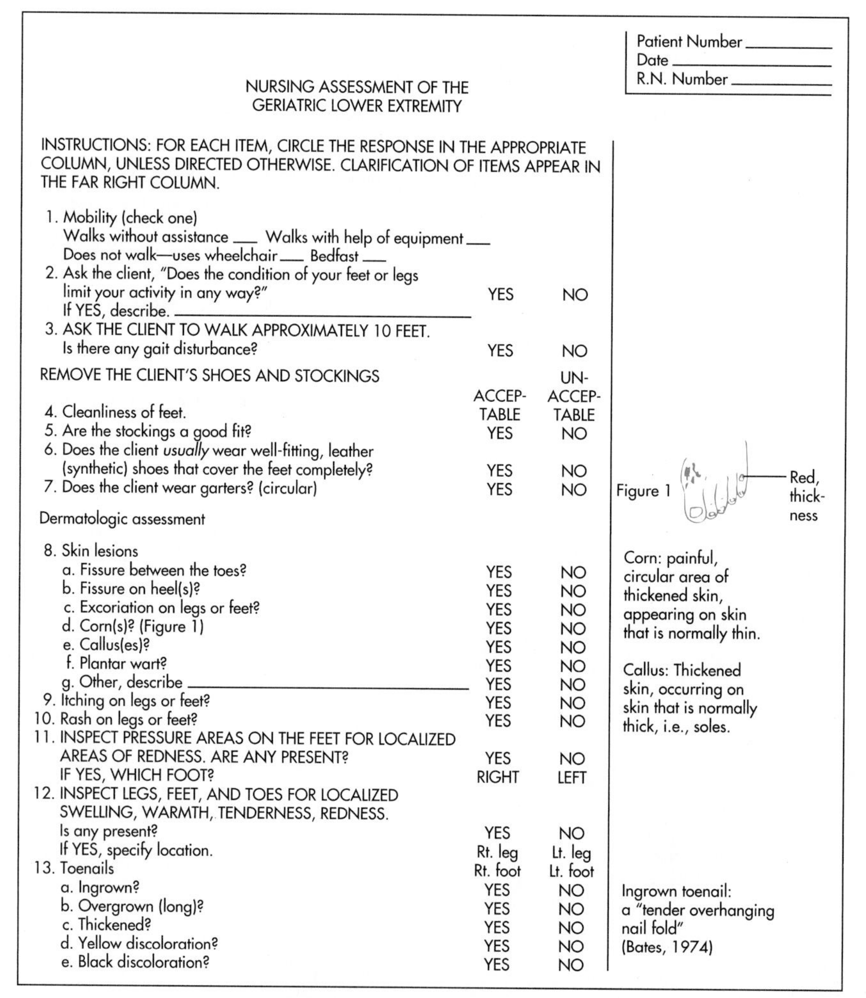
Patient Number ______
Date ______
R.N. Number ______

NURSING ASSESSMENT OF THE
GERIATRIC LOWER EXTREMITY

INSTRUCTIONS: FOR EACH ITEM, CIRCLE THE RESPONSE IN THE APPROPRIATE COLUMN, UNLESS DIRECTED OTHERWISE. CLARIFICATION OF ITEMS APPEAR IN THE FAR RIGHT COLUMN.

Item			Clarification
1. Mobility (check one) Walks without assistance ___ Walks with help of equipment ___ Does not walk—uses wheelchair ___ Bedfast ___			
2. Ask the client, "Does the condition of your feet or legs limit your activity in any way?" If YES, describe. ______	YES	NO	
3. ASK THE CLIENT TO WALK APPROXIMATELY 10 FEET. Is there any gait disturbance?	YES	NO	
REMOVE THE CLIENT'S SHOES AND STOCKINGS	ACCEPTABLE	UNACCEPTABLE	
4. Cleanliness of feet.			
5. Are the stockings a good fit?	YES	NO	
6. Does the client *usually* wear well-fitting, leather (synthetic) shoes that cover the feet completely?	YES	NO	
7. Does the client wear garters? (circular)	YES	NO	Figure 1 — Red, thickness
Dermatologic assessment			
8. Skin lesions			
a. Fissure between the toes?	YES	NO	Corn: painful, circular area of thickened skin, appearing on skin that is normally thin.
b. Fissure on heel(s)?	YES	NO	
c. Excoriation on legs or feet?	YES	NO	
d. Corn(s)? (Figure 1)	YES	NO	
e. Callus(es)?	YES	NO	Callus: Thickened skin, occurring on skin that is normally thick, i.e., soles.
f. Plantar wart?	YES	NO	
g. Other, describe ______	YES	NO	
9. Itching on legs or feet?	YES	NO	
10. Rash on legs or feet?	YES	NO	
11. INSPECT PRESSURE AREAS ON THE FEET FOR LOCALIZED AREAS OF REDNESS. ARE ANY PRESENT?	YES	NO	
IF YES, WHICH FOOT?	RIGHT	LEFT	
12. INSPECT LEGS, FEET, AND TOES FOR LOCALIZED SWELLING, WARMTH, TENDERNESS, REDNESS. Is any present?	YES	NO	
If YES, specify location.	Rt. leg	Lt. leg	
13. Toenails	Rt. foot	Lt. foot	
a. Ingrown?	YES	NO	Ingrown toenail: a "tender overhanging nail fold" (Bates, 1974)
b. Overgrown (long)?	YES	NO	
c. Thickened?	YES	NO	
d. Yellow discoloration?	YES	NO	
e. Black discoloration?	YES	NO	

Figure 7-7. Nursing assessment of the geriatric lower extremities. (From King PA: *J Gerontol Nurs* 4:47, Nov/Dec 1978.)

Continued

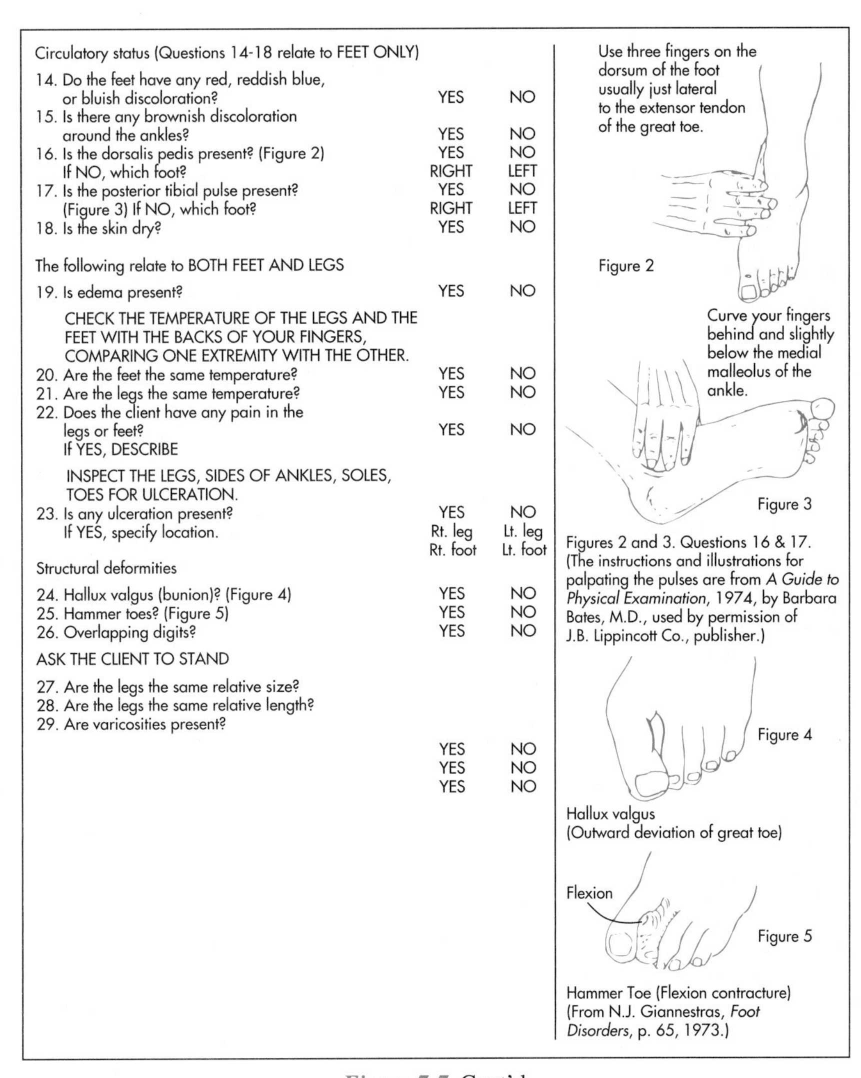

Circulatory status (Questions 14-18 relate to FEET ONLY)		
14. Do the feet have any red, reddish blue, or bluish discoloration?	YES	NO
15. Is there any brownish discoloration around the ankles?	YES	NO
16. Is the dorsalis pedis present? (Figure 2)	YES	NO
If NO, which foot?	RIGHT	LEFT
17. Is the posterior tibial pulse present?	YES	NO
(Figure 3) If NO, which foot?	RIGHT	LEFT
18. Is the skin dry?	YES	NO
The following relate to BOTH FEET AND LEGS		
19. Is edema present?	YES	NO
CHECK THE TEMPERATURE OF THE LEGS AND THE FEET WITH THE BACKS OF YOUR FINGERS, COMPARING ONE EXTREMITY WITH THE OTHER.		
20. Are the feet the same temperature?	YES	NO
21. Are the legs the same temperature?	YES	NO
22. Does the client have any pain in the legs or feet?	YES	NO
If YES, DESCRIBE		
INSPECT THE LEGS, SIDES OF ANKLES, SOLES, TOES FOR ULCERATION.		
23. Is any ulceration present?	YES	NO
If YES, specify location.	Rt. leg Rt. foot	Lt. leg Lt. foot
Structural deformities		
24. Hallux valgus (bunion)? (Figure 4)	YES	NO
25. Hammer toes? (Figure 5)	YES	NO
26. Overlapping digits?	YES	NO
ASK THE CLIENT TO STAND		
27. Are the legs the same relative size?	YES	NO
28. Are the legs the same relative length?	YES	NO
29. Are varicosities present?	YES	NO

Use three fingers on the dorsum of the foot usually just lateral to the extensor tendon of the great toe.

Figure 2

Curve your fingers behind and slightly below the medial malleolus of the ankle.

Figure 3

Figures 2 and 3. Questions 16 & 17. (The instructions and illustrations for palpating the pulses are from *A Guide to Physical Examination*, 1974, by Barbara Bates, M.D., used by permission of J.B. Lippincott Co., publisher.)

Figure 4

Hallux valgus (Outward deviation of great toe)

Figure 5

Hammer Toe (Flexion contracture) (From N.J. Giannestras, *Foot Disorders*, p. 65, 1973.)

Figure 7-7. Cont'd.

Assessment is the key to maintenance of the aged person's highest level of function and mobility (Box 7-11). Elderly persons with diabetes mellitus, cardiac conditions, PVD, thyroid conditions, or renal conditions are prone to foot problems. Those individuals with residual foot and leg impairment from strokes may develop foot ulcers from pressure exerted by their shoes or braces and from pressure and persistent friction and irritation caused by altered walking patterns.

Interventions

Care of Toenails. The inability of the aged to care for their toenails is influenced by poor vision, hand tremors, the inability to bend, obesity, or increased nail thickness. Nails that are neglected or do not receive treatment may become unusually long and curved. This type of nail is known as ram's horn because of its appearance. Hard, thickened nails indicate inadequate nutrition to the nail matrix from trauma or poor circulation. Once the nail becomes thickened, it will remain so. These conditions should be brought to the attention of the podiatrist. Any attempt by the nurse or other caregiver to cut these nails may result in further damage to the matrix or precipitate an infection. This problem can be crippling if neglected.

Normal nails that become too long or begin to interfere with stockings, hose, or shoes should be cut straight across and even with the top of the toe (Figure 7-9). Nails that are hard can easily split, causing trauma to the matrix, pain, and possibly infection. Feet should be soaked in warm water to soften the nails before they are clipped. Ideally, toenails should be trimmed after the bath or shower, but if this is not appropriate, soaking the feet for 20 to 30 minutes will facilitate the procedure. Box 7-12 provides suggestions for a variety of foot soaks for specific aspects of foot care. Foot soaks are not recommended for elders with diabetes.

Shoes. Shoes should be worn that cover, protect, and provide stability for the foot, maximize toe space, and minimize the chance of falls. In essence, shoes should be functional. Slip-on shoes are helpful for those aged who are unable to bend or lace shoes. Velcro closures are also useful to those

ASSESSMENT

Medical history

____________ Arthritis
____________ Diabetes
____________ Peripheral vascular disease
____________ Smoking
____________ Vision problems
____________ Falls in past year

Does client do a daily foot inspection? _____ yes _____ no, comments:

Footwear

Does client ever go barefoot? _____ yes _____ no, comments:
____________ Canvas or leather shoes
____________ Shoes fitted properly
____________ Socks
____________ Restrictive leg wear
____________ More than one pair of shoes
Appearance of footwear: ____________________

Type of footwear most often worn: ____________________

Ambulation _____ with _____ without assistance.
Type of device used if assisted: ____________________
Color and temperature of extremity: ____________________
Presence of pedal pulses: Right _____ Left _____

Structure

Presence of:

		Location/remarks
_____ Bunions	_____ Spurs	__________
_____ Corns	_____ Ulcerations	__________
_____ Callus	_____ Cracks	__________
_____ Edema	_____ Dry skin	__________
_____ Hammertoes	_____ Blisters	__________

Description of toenails: ____________________

Skills performed: Foot soak
Nail trim

Follow-up date:

Figure 7-8. Foot assessment tool. (From Ruscin C, Cunningham G, Blaylock A: Foot care protocol for the older client, *Geriatr Nurs* 14(4):211, 1993.)

who have limited finger dexterity. Low-heeled shoes with a wide toe box and a ridged sole minimize falls, place less stress on the legs and back, and are ideal for comfort. The proverbial "thumb's width" is the correct space between the big toe and toe of the shoe.

Fitting shoes appropriately is useful in preventing foot ailments (National Institute on Aging, 2000). Our feet change size as we grow older, and foot size increases as the day grows longer. Usually, one foot is larger than another. Shoes should be fitted to the largest foot. Select a shoe that is shaped like your foot. There should be about one-half inch of space from the longest toe to the end of the inside of the shoe while standing. Shoes are not likely to "stretch" and become more comfortable. Make sure the shoe does not slip and ride up and down on the heel during walking. Take new shoes home and walk on the carpet to make sure they "work" right.

Dependent Edema. Circulatory efficiency in the lower extremities, especially the feet, is sluggish. Edema of the ankles and feet is evident after periods of prolonged sitting and standing. It is helpful if the elder does not wear constricting circular garters, socks with snug bands, or support hose, which constrict the feet. Sitting with the feet elevated on a footstool or hassock is helpful in reducing edema and facilitating better venous circulation. Foot exercises are a means of reducing edema by encouraging more efficient venous return. Exercises can be done at any time. It may be helpful to develop the habit of doing foot exercises after rising and before going to bed. Other times would be during television commercials.

The exercises are simple, and in addition to helping reduce edema, they facilitate foot flexibility. Toe bends, or curling and relaxing the toes, should be done at least five times on each foot. These can be done one foot at a time or both feet together followed by rotating the feet at the ankles clockwise and then counterclockwise 5 to 10 times, and finally, bringing the knees to the chest 5 to 10 times. These exercises can be done consecutively or with short rest periods in between, depending on the stamina of the individual.

Foot Massage. Foot massage is another useful means of reducing edema, stimulating circulation, and improving pedal flexibility. Not only does massage aid in accomplishing these

Box 7-11 Essential Data of Foot Assessment

Observation of Mobility
Gait
Ambulation
Foot hygiene
Footwear

Past Medical History
Systemic diseases
Musculoskeletal problems
Vascular disease, ulcerations, or peripheral vascular disease
Vision problems
Falls
Trauma
Smoking history
Pain

Bilateral Assessment
Color
Circulation
Pulses
Structures (hammer toe, bunion, overlapping digits)
Temperature
Dermatologic aspects:
- Skin lesions (fissures, corns, calluses, warts, excoriation)
- Edema
- Itching
- Rash

Toenails:
- Long, thick
- Discoloration

things, but it also relaxes the feet and stimulates relaxation of the rest of the body. However, not all elderly are candidates for foot massage. Individuals with foot lesions or vascular problems of the lower extremities should be seen by their physician for a definitive decision before massage is considered. Foot massage requires little lubrication and can use the lotion or oil applied after the bath or shower, if done at that time.

Box 7-12 Foot Soaks

Cleansing
Add several drops of mild liquid soap or detergent to warm water.

Callus Softening
Add ½ cup vinegar or ¼ cup baking soda to 1 qt of warm water.

Dry Skin
Use warm water only.

Wound or Mild Infection
Add 2 tbsp of Epsom salts or 1 tsp of table salt to 1 qt of warm water.

Modified from Kaiser Permanente patient information sheet.

To give a foot massage, the nurse should be positioned so that the client's feet are easily accessible; sit at the foot of the bed, if the client is reclining, or opposite the client, if seated, with the foot to be massaged cradled between the nurse's knees or resting on something comfortable for support.

Steady the foot to be massaged with one hand, and with the knuckles of the other hand make small, firm circles over the entire sole of the foot, including the heel (Figure 7-10, *A* and *B*). Light touch tends to tickle, whereas firmness does not; however, the feet of the aged may be more sensitive to pressure than those of the young, so the nurse must modulate the firmness of the massage accordingly. There is an overpowering urge when about to touch someone's feet to say, "I hope you aren't ticklish"—stifle that urge! The power of suggestion is tremendous. Use firm smooth movements, and you should have satisfying results. You may also find that the person seems to spontaneously come forth with conversation. Continue to massage the foot; support the foot with the fingers of both hands while the thumbs repeat the small circles over the entire sole of the foot. As you move your thumbs from the toes you may find that the fingertips are less awkward when you massage around the ankle and the heel (Figure 7-10, *C*

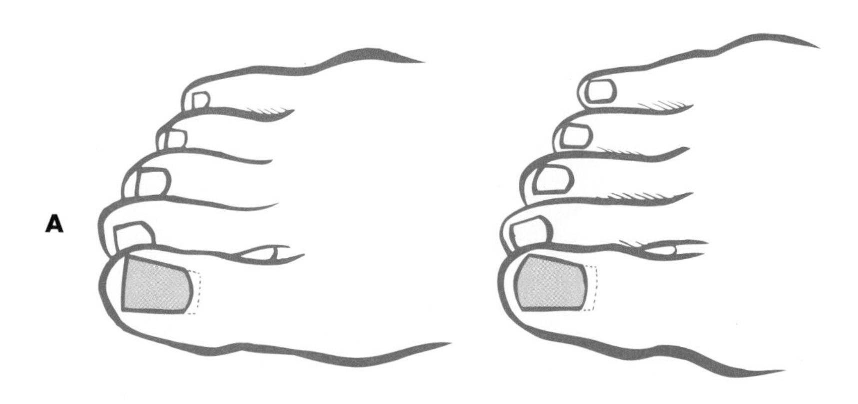

Figure 7-9. Cutting of toenails. **A,** Correct method. **B,** Incorrect method.

and *D*). When your fingers reach the heel, take one hand and gently lift the foot under the ankle, and with the other hand use the fingertips and thumb to firmly make circles on the heel. More pressure will be required here because of the thicker horny layer of skin (see Figure 7-10, *D*).

On the top of the foot, starting at the ankle, look at the long tendons that run from the base of the ankle to each toe. Support the heel of the foot with one hand, and with the tip of the thumb on your other hand firmly but gently run your thumb between each tendon groove and off between the toes (Figure 7-10, *E*). (This can be uncomfortable, so adjust your pressure.) Next grasp the foot between both hands; fingers should be touching on the sole of the foot, heels of the hands touching on the top of the foot (Figure 7-10, *F*). Press the heels of your hands firmly downward on the foot and push up on the sole of the foot with your fingers (like breaking a cracker in half). At the same time slide your hands toward the edges of the foot. Repeat this motion three times. With one hand, steady the foot, and with the thumb and forefinger of the other hand grasp the base of the big toe. Gently stretch and rotate it from side to side, using a corkscrew motion, until your fingers slide off the tip of the toe. Do this to each toe in sequence (Figure 7-10, *G*). To finish the massage, place the foot between your hands; hold the foot gently for several seconds (Figure 7-10, *H*); replace it next to the other foot; gently pick up the other foot; and repeat the massage sequence. The nurse will find that foot massage can be easily modified to incorporate ROM exercises for the toes and ankles. In addition to foot massage, lukewarm oil (baby oil or mineral oil) applied to the feet followed by wrapping in warm moist towels and elevation for 10 to 15 minutes not only facilitates a few minutes of relaxation but aids in improving integrity of the skin of the feet. Feet are then washed in sudsy warm water, dried thoroughly, and dusted with powder, or excess oil can be simply removed with a soft towel.

Diabetic foot care is similar to that suggested for good foot care but is critical. A summary of good foot care and diabetic foot care, identifying the similarities and differences, is presented in Table 7-1. If an individual follows the recommendations for diabetic foot care, feet can usually be maintained in comfort.

INTEGUMENT

The skin is looked on as having aesthetic and cosmetic appeal. Artists have portrayed its delicate, flawless qualities, and poets have extolled its virtues through descriptive phrases. Today art, poetry, and conversation still include similar depictions.

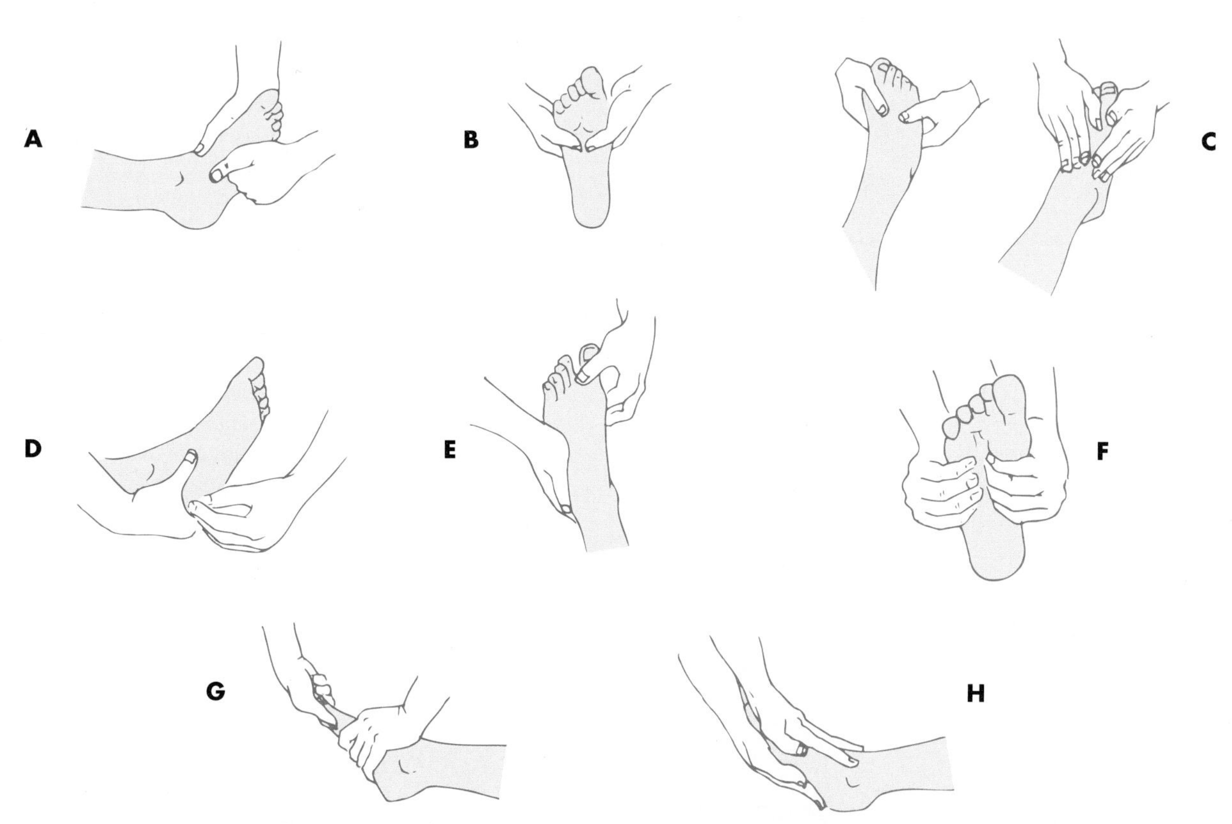

Figure 7-10. Foot massage. **A,** With knuckles make small circles over sole of foot. **B** and **C,** With thumbs and fingers make circles over entire foot. **D,** With tips of fingers make circles on heel. **E,** Gently run thumb between tendon grooves from ankle to toes. **F,** As if breaking a cracker, move the foot back and forth. **G,** Gently stretch and rotate each toe. **H,** End by placing foot between hands.

Table 7-1 Essentials of Good Foot Care: Standard and Diabetic

Standard foot care	Applicable to both	Diabetic foot care
	Inspect feet daily for cuts, blisters, reddened areas, and scratches. Use a magnifying glass or mirror to inspect the feet or have someone else do it for you if you can't reach or see well.	
Wash feet daily (if unable to do by self, ask someone else).		Wash feet daily but DO NOT soak feet daily (causes excessive dryness).
	Blot dry rather than rub dry to avoid injury to sensitive skin. Pay particular attention to between toes. Use emollients, cocoa butter, lanolin lotion, mineral oil, or vegetable oil to soften dry skin to help retain moisture and prevent cracking. DO NOT put between toes; it may contribute to fungal infections.	
		Dust lightly with a nonscented powder between toes (can prevent excessive perspiration).
	Soak toenails 10-15 minutes in warm water only on day you trim your toe nails. Cut toenails straight across using a toenail clipper. Never cut down the corners.	
Seek help if unable to trim toenails alone.		Have a podiatrist cut toenails if they are too thick to cut yourself, or if you are unable to cut your toenails alone. DO NOT cut corns or calluses. Have a podiatrist treat them. DO NOT apply harsh chemical corn and wart removing products to the toes and feet. These can remove tissue as well as the corn or wart. DO NOT apply heating pads, chemical or battery operated, to feet.
	Wear clean socks, hose, stockings daily. Cotton socks absorb perspiration for feet that sweat. Keep feet warm with thick fleecy insoles inside slippers to protect from cold or wear cotton socks with comfortable slippers.	
		DO NOT walk barefooted at any time. Sandals for the beach protect the feet from hot sand, sharp objects, etc. At home wear shoes or slippers.
	Wear comfortable well-fitting shoes with broad toe space and low heels.	
Avoid shoes that do not feel comfortable or need to be "broken in."		Good quality athletic shoes, while expensive, outlast regular shoes and are less expensive in the long run. Shake out shoes before putting them on to remove foreign objects that might cause injury. Carefully break in new shoes. Begin by wearing shoes an hour a day, gradually increase the time worn.
	DO NOT pop blisters. Infections can occur.	
If blister breaks, wash area, apply antiseptic, keep covered during the day, uncovered at night.		See physician immediately.
	Avoid wearing tight-fitting hose, tight stockings, stocking, or garters; DO NOT sit with crossed legs. All of these constrict blood flow to the lower extremities. Review the condition of your orthotics regularly. Mark a date with a laundry marker as a reminder for the podiatrist to reevaluate the effectiveness of the device. Stop smoking. Smoking constricts blood vessels, reducing blood flow to the lower extremities. Report foot injuries promptly to the physician.	
		Call physician for any problems such as tenderness, redness, warmth, drainage, ingrown toenail, athlete's foot, pain in the feet or calves.

Modified from Jarvik L, Small G: *Parent care*, New York, 1988, Crown; Helfand AE, issue editor: *The aging foot: focus on geriatric care and rehabilitation*, 2(10):1, 1989; Dellasega C, Yonushonis MEH: Diabetes mellitus in the elderly. In Stanley M, Beare PG: *Geronological nursing*, Philadelphia, 1995, Davis.

As the largest, most visible organ of the body, the skin serves as a "window" on the person (Kagan et al, 2002). The effects of time and exposure are visible; the skin wrinkles, epidermis thins, dermal blood vessels recede, dermal-epidermal ridges flatten, and the skin appears thin and fragile and pale. Sensation is lost, as is tissue resistance to pressure. Skin becomes dry, rough, and lax, and there is an increase in benign and malignant neoplasms. Thermoregulation is diminished, barrier functions are lessened, and wound healing is delayed and diminished. Although there are intrinsic changes with aging, most obvious skin changes are due to *photoaging,* chronic exposure to ultraviolet (UV) radiation superimposed on intrinsic aging (Beers and Berkow, 2000).

There is decreased skin capacity for vitamin D (cholecalciferol) synthesis with increasing age (Moore, 2001). Also, there is often impaired ability for vitamin D to stimulate calcium absorption. A response to calcium absorption is hyperparathyroidism, common in older adults. Other reasons for insufficient vitamin D include lack of sun exposure in many elderly people, especially those who are institutionalized; paradoxically, we know that avoidance of sun exposure is a cornerstone to prevention of skin cancer. It is suggested that small amounts of sun exposure, exposing hands, face, and arms for 5 to 15 minutes per day, three times per week, may be sufficient to ensure adequate levels of vitamin D (Fuller and Casparian, 2001). Poor intake of dairy products is another reason for insufficient vitamin D. The recommended amount of vitamin D has recently been increased for adults older than age 50, and some researchers are urging even higher doses for the entire population, to prevent osteoporotic fractures (Fuller and Casparian, 2001).

Skin is important in both health and illness. It provides clues to hereditary, racial, dietary, physical, and emotional conditions. It is also an important means of communication. The integument provides at least seven physiologic functions. It protects underlying structures, serves as a heat-regulating mechanism, serves as a sense organ, is involved in the metabolism of salt and water, and stores fat. The skin facilitates two-way gaseous exchange and converts sunshine into vitamin D. When the integument malfunctions or is overwhelmed by outside trauma, discomfort, or disfigurement, morbidity increases. Healthy skin, despite exposure to heat, cold, water trauma, friction, and pressure, maintains a homeostatic environment. Healthy skin is durable, pliable, and strong enough to protect the body by absorbing, reflecting, cushioning, and restricting various substances and forces that might enter and alter its function. It is sensitive enough to relay messages to the brain.

The epidermis, dermis, and subcutaneous layers of the skin have specific functions that affect nursing assessment and intervention. Figure 7-11 outlines the layers of the integument, their structures and functions, and the conditions that frequently

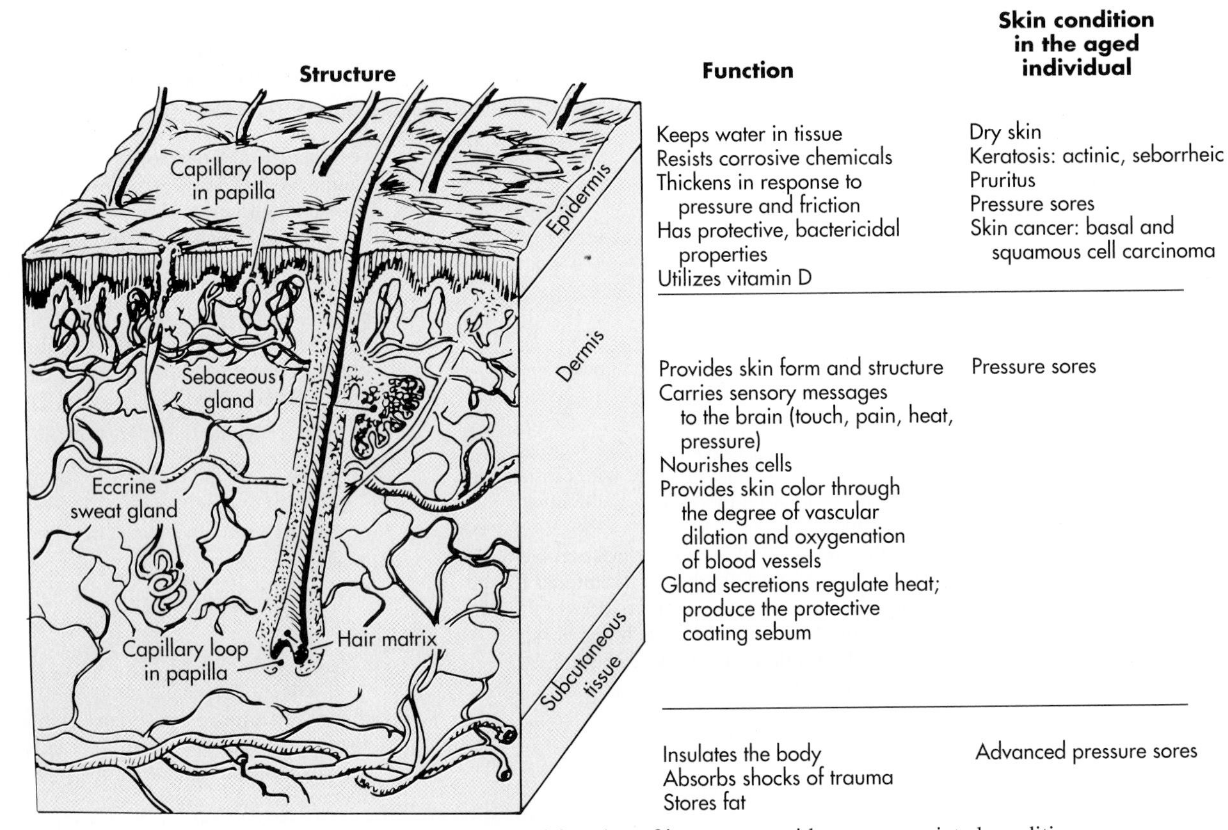

Figure 7-11. Correlation of structure and function of integument with some associated conditions.

occur in the aged. The aged epidermis produces varying cell shapes and sizes. The dermis, lying beneath the epidermis, is a supportive layer of connective tissue composed of a matrix of elastic fibers that provide stretch and recoil, fibrous collagen fibers that provide tensile strength, and an absorbent gel between the two fibers. The dermis also supports hair follicles, sweat and sebaceous glands, nerve fibers, muscle cells, and blood vessels. With age the dermis elasticity and suppleness is lost because of cross-link changes of the elastin and collagen components. Blood flow diminishes to the hair bulbs and to the eccrine, apocrine, and sebaceous glands, thereby contributing to their senescence. Epidermal cells are replaced about 30% to 50% more slowly between age 30 and age 80 (Beers and Berkow, 2000), and sensory receptors do not transmit sensations as rapidly, although pain is probably not affected (Box 7-13).

Circulatory disorders affect skin. Skin loses color, and blood vessels become fragile. Although the aged may appear less attractive physically to many people, like younger people, elders take pride in their appearance.

Box 7-13 Structural and Functional Changes of the Aging Skin

Compared with a healthy younger person, age-related changes are as follows:

- Epidermis (outer layer) thins gradually
- Loss of integrity between epidermis and dermis increases susceptibility to trauma and shearing forces
- Dermis becomes thin and less flexible
- Dermis has fewer fibroblasts, resulting in decreased production of elastin (reduced skin elasticity) and collagen (decreased skin strength, increased wrinkling)
- Dryness, xerosis
- Damaged skin is replaced slowly
- Fewer Langerhans cells (immune surveillance cells)
- Keratoses appear, especially on the back of the hands
- Loss of melanocyte function, less tanning of skin, and less protection from sun, increasing likelihood of cancers
- Pigmentation areas of melanin clumps form telangiectasias on the face
- Senile purpura on hands and arms due to vulnerable blood vessels

Photoaging effects seen in elderly people include the following:

- Increased elastin so that epidermis thickens and atrophies
- Wrinkles
- Increased loss of Langerhans cells
- Increased loss of collagen
- Increased predisposition to skin cancers

Adapted from *Skin*. Available at *www.healthandage.com/html/res/primer/skin.htm*.

Pigmentation Changes

Pigmented moles and nevi are benign melanocytic neoplasms. These lesions are common in younger people, peaking between 20 and 40 years of age, and are rare in elders older than age 70 years (Beers and Berkow, 2000). Presence of lesions signals the loss of melanin and DNA repair capacity, increasing the risk of photocarcinogenesis. Lentigines, called "age spots" or "liver spots," are similar to freckles. They can occur at any age. In those under 40 or 50 years of age, there does not seem to be a correlation with sun exposure. However, from the sixth decade on, they are thought to be sun related. The development of lentigines is also thought to be caused by uneven melanin production; melanin decreases in later years. Lentigines are dramatically seen on the back of the hands and wrists of light-skinned persons.

Nerves

About one third of our cutaneous sensory end organs decrease between ages 10 and 90 (Beers and Berkow, 2000). This results in age-related loss of sensation of touch, vibration, two-point discrimination, spatial acuity, and corneal sensitivity. The skin's pain threshold increases (perceives less pain) by about 20%.

Glands

The sweat glands, or eccrine glands, respond to thermostimulation and neurostimulation. They decrease by about 15% during adulthood (Beers and Berkow, 2000). The usual body response to heat is to produce moisture or sweat from these glands and thus cool the skin by evaporation. Because sweating is diminished in the aged (up to 70% in one study), overheating and heat intolerance are important problems. The aged should avoid spending long periods in the heat, both indoors and outdoors. The summer, in particular, poses a major threat in areas in which there is persistent high humidity and heat. In these areas the death rate among the aged from heat is high because these changes are compounded by diminished vascularity of the skin. The aged should be encouraged to wear a hat when in the sun, to wear light, cool clothing, and to drink sufficient amounts of fluid.

Apocrine glands are also diminished with aging. There does not seem to be much of an effect in terms of health. There is a decline in body odor. Secretions are odorless until bacteria begin to act on the moisture to produce odors. Deodorants and antiperspirants are often used to suppress odors from the apocrine glands in younger adults. Dusting powder with baking soda is a natural, inexpensive substance that can keep the axilla dry and free from odor in elders, if needed at all.

Sebaceous glands, which secrete sebum, depend on hormonal stimulation and do not appear to decrease with age. However, because of a decrease in androgen levels and blood supply to sebaceous glands, sebum production decreases with age, about 23% per decade beginning after puberty (Beers and Berkow, 2000). Sebum protects the skin by preventing the evaporation of water from the keratin, or horny, layer of the epidermis; it possesses bactericidal properties.

Hair

As part of the integument, hair has biologic, psychologic, and cosmetic value for both men and women. A hair is tightly fused horny cells that arise from the dermal layer and obtain coloration from melanocytes. Hair coloration usually correlates with skin coloration; however, there are exceptions. With age, melanin is reduced, causing graying of hair, or is lost, causing white hair. The age at which hair falls out is mainly genetically determined; women, as well as men, lose their hair with age (*HealthandAge.com*, 2002). If the hair does not grey with age, the person may be hypothyroid. Hair becomes more brittle, turning from "terminal" to "vellus" hair, and grows more slowly. The opposite trend occurs on the chin and above the upper lip on many women, with a conversion from vellus hair to terminal hair. Older men have an increase in ear, nostril, and eyebrow hair (*HealthandAge.com*, 2002).

The hormone testosterone influences hair distribution in men (androgenetic alopecia). Hair loss begins in the twenties, and by their sixties, 80% of men are substantially bald (Beers and Berkow, 2000). After menopause, the same pattern of hair loss occurs in women, but is less pronounced. Diffuse alopecia occurs in both sexes with aging. It can also occur because of iron deficiency, hypothyroidism, anabolic steroids, chronic renal failure, hypoproteinemia, or inflammatory skin diseases. Granulomatous disorders such as sarcoidosis and inflammatory disorders such as discoid lupus or lichen planus can cause hair loss due to scarring.

Axillary and pubic hair tends to diminish with age in women and in some instances disappears. Older women may develop chin and facial hair because of the estrogen/androgen balance in hormonally sensitive hair follicles (Beers and Berkow, 2000).

The various races have definite hair characteristics, which should be kept in mind when caring for or assessing the aged. Almost all Asians have sparse facial and body hair that is dark, straight, and silky. Blacks have slightly more head and body hair than Asians; however, the hair texture varies widely. It can range from long and straight to short, spiraled, thick, and kinky. Whites have the most head and body hair, with an intermediate texture and form ranging from straight to curly and fine to thick and coarse.

Nails

The aged often complain about the splitting and breaking of their nails. The aged nail becomes harder and thicker, more brittle, dull, and opaque and grows more slowly. Nails change shape, becoming at times flat or concave instead of convex. Vertical ridges appear because of decreasing water, calcium, and lipid content. Longitudinal pigment bands are common among blacks, seen in 96% in one study (Beers and Berkow, 2000). The blood supply decreases, as does the rate of nail growth. The half moon (lunula unguis) of the fingernail may entirely disappear, and the nails become gray or yellow. With onychogryphosis, the nails become thick and distorted. If the nails separate from the nail bed (onycholysis), the patient probably has a fungal infection (onychomycosis). There is no effective treatment for age-related nail changes. Wearing gloves during housework will protect brittle nails. Discourage use of nail polish remover, because it significantly dries the nails. A nightly massage with oils and wearing white cotton gloves to bed is helpful.

Photoaging

Solar elastosis, or photoaging, is the result of environmental damage to the skin by UV sun rays. Many of the changes associated with photoaging are preventable. Ideally, preventive measures should begin in childhood, but clinical evidence has shown that some improvement can be achieved by avoidance of sun exposure and regular use of sunscreens, even after actinic damage has occurred. Elders with sun damage appear older than those who have been protected. Skin cancers occur almost exclusively in sun-damaged skin.

Sunscreens offer protection from harmful ultraviolet A and B rays. Effectiveness of sunscreens is measured in terms of the sun protection factor (SPF). The following formula provides the length of time, in minutes, that an individual can be in the sun without burning: minimal erythema dose (the amount of time it takes to cause the skin to become red) times the SPF. Older persons may not have had sunscreens available in their youth.

Sun-induced damage varies with skin type. Individuals who always burn, never tan, or minimally tan, or who burn moderately and tan to a light brown, should be considered to have sensitive to very sensitive skin, which requires an SPF greater than 15, preferably much higher. Individuals who minimally burn and always tan to a moderate brown should use a sunscreen with an SPF of 6 to 10. The use of sunscreens should not be limited to summer use or sunny days. Damaging UV rays penetrate clouds and overcast skies. It must be remembered that the normal skin changes, such as fragility and diminished melanocyte activity, that occur in older adults may not coincide with the level of SPF protection that was adequate when they were younger. The aged individual may require a higher SPF sunscreen preparation. Box 7-14 offers sun protection recommendations.

Skin Problems

Consensus in the literature is that the common skin problems of the aged are dry skin, pruritus, seborrheic keratosis and actinic keratosis, skin cancer, and pressure sores.

Dry Skin. Dry skin (xerosis) is perhaps the most common problem of the aged and is poorly understood. Xerosis is probably a reflection of alteration in lipid composition of the stratum corneum and other changes in the epidermis. The use of statins (HMG-CoA reductase inhibitors), commonly used in management of lipid disorders, may produce acquired ichthyosis and severe xerosis.

Box 7-14

Sun Protection Recommendations

Avoid getting sunburned. Persons of all skin types and races can sunburn, but fair-skinned persons burn more easily.
Do not consider tanning healthy. Do not try to get a suntan, and avoid tanning booths.
Avoid the midday sun (10 AM to 3 PM) when the ultraviolet radiation is most intense.
Wear protective clothing such as a broad-brimmed hat, long sleeves, long pants; however, be aware that clothing alone does not provide complete protection.
Use sunscreen daily (if going outside), even on a cloudy day because clouds do not block ultraviolet radiation.
Select and use a sunscreen with a sun protection factor (SPF) greater than 15 that is appropriate for your skin type. Apply to sun-exposed areas 45 minutes before going outside and reapply periodically after perspiring heavily or swimming. If using cosmetics on face, apply sunscreen first.
Use a lip balm that contains a sunscreen.
Be aware of reflection from sand, snow, and water, which will intensify the radiation.
Avoid sun if using photosensitizing drugs.
Avoid para-aminobenzoic acid (PABA) sunscreens if allergic to procaine, sulfonamides, or hair dyes because of cross sensitization.

Adapted from Hogstel MO: *Clinical manual of gerontological nursing*, St Louis, 1992, Mosby.

Xerosis is a problem for 59% to 85% of elderly people (Hardy, 2001). It occurs primarily in the extremities, especially the legs, but can affect the face and trunk as well. Experts vary on theories of causation. Skin that is aged becomes less efficient at holding moisture. It may be that dry skin results from a lack of water, not a lack of skin oils; this theory continues to be debated. The thinner epidermis allows more moisture to escape from the skin. Inadequate fluid intake has a systemic effect; it pulls moisture from the skin to assist in overall hydration of the body.

Exposure to environmental elements, decreased humidity, use of harsh soaps, frequent hot baths, nutritional deficiencies, and smoking contribute to skin dryness and dehydration of the stratum corneum. Hospital care promotes dry skin through routine bathing, use of soap, prolonged bed rest, and the action of bed linen on the patient's skin. Repeated wetting and drying of the skin layer causes subsequent tissue drying. Chapping, drying, and major skin changes occur more slowly and later in those individuals who routinely use emollient skin care products that afford good skin protection. These skin care items are more apt to contain moisturizers and sun-screening agents. Based on the number of commercial skin preparations on the market today, it is obvious that dry skin and protection from UV rays are recognized problems.

Treatment of dry skin in the aged is focused on the relief of symptoms; the underlying problem cannot be cured. The nurse should be alert to signs of rough, scaly, flaking skin on the legs and feet, face, hands, forearms, sides of the lower trunk, and the exterior and lateral aspects of the thighs. Itching (pruritus) frequently accompanies dryness and may be evident as skin irritation or scratch marks in those areas. Dry skin may be just dry skin, but it may also be a symptom of a more serious systemic disease, such as diabetes mellitus, hypothyroidism, or renal disease. Dry skin is more common in winter months because of lower humidity of air indoors and outdoors. A complication of xerosis that occurs during these months is xerotic eczema, also called eczema craquelé or asteatotic eczema. This disorder causes fissures and excoriations that allow the environment's irritants to penetrate skin and cause inflammation and infection (Beers and Berkow, 2000).

The management of dry, itchy skin is to rehydrate the epidermis, especially the keratin, or horny layer. Bathing should occur only once each day or less often, and the person should not use strong soaps, rubbing alcohol, and other drying agents. Use only soft material next to the skin (not rough woolens). The skin's only moisturizer is water. Substances may be used to enhance water's ability to stay on the skin. Use an emollient liberally after bathing, when the skin is moist. This is accomplished with binders (bind water to the skin) and humectants (attract moisture from the air to the skin), but other products such as oils, Vaseline (petrolatum), and zinc oxide serve to keep moisture that is already in the skin from evaporating and are effective and inexpensive. Oils and ointments also are designed to coat the skin and replace the skin's natural oil barrier (sebum). Use of superfatted soaps without hexachlorophene is most effective in helping to restore the protective lipid film to the skin surface. Dove, Tone, and Caress are the most common of the superfatted soaps used, but scented soaps and emollients should be avoided because they may irritate dry skin.

Incorporation of bath oils and other hydrophobic preparations into the bathing routine temporarily helps hold moisture and retards its escape from the skin. However, bath oil poured into the bathtub creates the potential for falls. It is safer and more effective to have the aged person bathe or shower, lightly towel dry, and apply the substance directly onto the moist skin; mild, water-laden emulsions are best. Light mineral oil or petrolatum as a bath aid is as effective as commercial brands and is less costly.

Prescription lotions with urea or α-hydroxy acid (lactic acid) help remove scales, hydrate skin, and prevent itching. Also, a topical corticosteroid ointment containing 1% to 2% hydrocortisone will cool inflamed skin. Apply after bathing and at bedtime. Corticosteroid ointments should not be used for a long period of time because there is some systemic absorption.

Maintaining an environment with 60% humidity, alleviating mechanical irritation caused by clothing, encouraging baths and showers with water temperatures at 90° to 105° F, and applying mineral oil after bathing helps control dry skin (Hardy, 2001). The need for "squeaky clean" skin is an American cultural oddity. Boxes 7-15 and 7-16 offer tips for healthy skin and care of dry skin. Use of humidifiers in the house or bedroom is helpful.

Pruritus. Pruritus (itching), an unpleasant cutaneous sensation, is a symptom, not a diagnosis or a disease, and is an additional threat to skin intactness. Pruritus is a common complaint of the elderly and often is caused by xerosis. It is aggravated by heat, sudden temperature changes, sweating, contact with articles of clothing, fatigue, and emotional upheavals. Pruritus accompanies systemic disorders such as chronic renal failure, biliary or hepatic disease, lymphomas, iron deficiency anemia, leukemias, parasitosis, human immunodeficiency virus (HIV) infection, and drugs (e.g., opioids). Box 7-17 lists the various causes of pruritus in the elderly.

The urge to scratch is an ineffective response to the urge to remove the irritant itch from the skin. When one scratches, a counterstimulus is introduced, which is stronger than the original itch stimulus. The nerve messages become confused or eliminate the itching sensation by the intensity of the scratch stimulus. Itching is akin to pain. The nerve endings that produce cutaneous pain also respond to itching. When rehydration of the stratum corneum is not sufficient to control itching, cool compresses of saline solution or oatmeal or Epsom salt baths may be indicated. Use of a lotion such as Lubriderm or Nutraderm is helpful. Vigorous towel drying intensifies

Box 7-15 Tips for Healthy Skin

Pay attention to any break in the skin.
Use a humidifier if necessary to keep room humidity above 40%.
Bathing every 2 to 3 days is sufficient.
Use a nondeodorant mild soap with lanolin or other creams in its base.
Add bath oil to water—there is a risk of slipping.
Use a moisturizer that applies easily, leaves no greasy film, and does not stain clothing.
Apply moisturizers as often as necessary to maintain continuous coverage.
Choose clothing made of soft cotton or other nonabrasive materials.
Drink several glasses of pure water every day.
In cold and windy weather, wear a warm hat, gloves, and scarf to protect extremities.
Wear a wide-brimmed hat to shade from the sun.
Use a sunscreen lotion with the appropriate sun protection factor (SPF) (usually SPF 15 or higher) on all exposed areas.
Avoid direct sunlight for extended periods.

Box 7-16 Care of Dry Skin

To soften dry skin and keep it soft, do as little as possible to break the skin's natural protective oils; do as much as possible to maintain and replenish them.

- Take fewer and faster soaking baths. In winter, one tub or shower per week is plenty. None is OK too, for the person with dry skin. Sponge bathe armpits, groin, and perianal areas and any other parts of the body that need daily (or more frequent) care.
- Use warm water rather than hot to bathe, whether in the tub or shower. The hotter the water, the more natural oils are washed away.
- Limit the use of soap. One lathering is enough to cleanse most of the normally moist body areas; a damp cloth without any soap is sufficient to clean extremities and body areas that stay dry. Consider using superfatted soap; it need not be expensive—Dove, Tone, and others are superfatted and relatively inexpensive. A soap made of cocoa butter or olive or coconut oil (castile soaps) may be preferred.
- If skin is both dry and itchy, apply an oil freely and often. Do not use rubbing alcohol or rubs containing alcohol, because these destroy natural oils on the skin and make it dry out faster.
- Use hand or body oils that work on all of the dry areas and be sure to apply immediately after bathing, while the skin is moist.
- Avoid long periods in the sun. When going out in the sun or when staying in the sun is unavoidable, use a sun barrier oil. Be sure to reapply after swimming.
- Use an oil that is easily affordable. The most expensive is not necessarily the best. Hydrogenated shortening (Crisco or Spry) or the least expensive mineral oil will do a good moisturizing job.
- If dry skin is a problem only in winter, consider installing an efficient, whole-house humidifier in the home heating system. Not only will it help the skin hold its natural moisture (less evaporation into dry air), but it will help lower heat costs. Moist air feels warmer than dry; the same degree of comfort at lower temperatures will be experienced.
- If living or working in air-conditioned areas, try to keep the temperature high enough for the air to stay moist. Most air-conditioning systems reduce humidity as well as temperature, and air cooled much below 21° C (about 75° F) is likely to be too dry for dry skin.
- Take tepid baths using bath oil so as not to further dehydrate skin.
- Apply soothing creams or emollients several times daily, especially on hands, feet, and face.
- Wear soft, absorbent clothing such as cotton.
- Use the following with caution: topical steroid creams (unpredictable absorption); low-dose systemic steroids (likely to result in complications).
- Persons over age 75 should not use antihistamines (may experience sudden, severe side effects).

Box 7-17 Causes of Pruritus in the Elderly

Dermatitis
Eczema
Contact
Seborrhea
Lichen simplex chronicus (neurodermatitis)
Xerosis (dry skin)
Microvascular (stasis dermatitis, erythema)

Papular Scaling Disorders
Psoriasis, Lichen planus

Drug Reactions
Drug withdrawal (delirium tremens)
Erythema multiforme:
- Antidepressants, opiates
- Acetylsalicylic acid, idiosyncratic responses

Metabolic Responses
Liver and biliary disorders
Renal failure (uremia)
Diabetes mellitus
Hypothyroidism

Neoplastic Disorders
Benign (seborrheic keratosis)
Malignant (central nervous system tumors)

Hematopoietic Responses
Iron deficiency anemia
Leukemia, lymphoma

Psychogenic Etiologies
Involutional psychoses
Hallucinatory aberrations (dementias)

Infections and Infestations
Bacterial (impetigo, chlamydia)
Viral (herpes zoster)
Yeast infections (candidiasis, monilial intertrigo)
Parasitic (scabies, pediculosis)

pruritus by overstimulation of the skin and by removing the needed water from the stratum corneum. Hot bath water should be avoided.

For relief of itching, ammonium lactate moisturizer is suggested (Webster, 2001), as well as antipruritic creams without steroids. The addition of 10% coal tar, 0.25% phenol, or 0.25% menthol to a moisturizing lotion is useful. Ultraviolet phototherapy has also been used, is a great antipruritic, and may be tried if other measures are not successful. It is especially useful for liver disease and renal disease itches.

Keratoses

Seborrheic keratosis. Seborrheic keratosis is a benign growth that appears mainly on the trunk, face, and scalp as single or multiple lesions. One or more benign lesions are present on nearly all adults over age 65. Most elderly individuals have dozens of benign lesions. The keratosis is a waxy, raised, verrucous lesion, flesh-colored or pigmented in varying sizes. They have the appearance of being "stuck on the skin." Sebaceous keratotic lesions can at times be picked off with a fingernail, but the lesion soon returns. Generally, this neoplasm is removed by a dermatologist, by curettage and light cautery or by freezing with liquid nitrogen for 15 to 20 seconds. There is a variant seen in blacks mostly on the face with numerous small, dark, possibly pedunculated papules (Beers and Berkow, 2000).

Actinic keratosis. Actinic or solar keratosis, unlike the benign seborrheic keratosis, is a precancerous lesion, or even perhaps carcinoma in situ (Webster, 2001). It is the result of years of overexposure to the sun or UV light, which induces mutations. Risk factors are older age, fair complexion, blue eyes, and history of freckles in childhood. It is found on sun-exposed areas such as bald head, hands, face, ears, nose, upper trunk, and arms. Actinic keratosis is characterized by scaly sandpaper-like patches, with varied coloration from pink to reddish-brown to yellow-black. Lesions may be single or multiple; they may be painless or mildly tender. Actinic keratosis has a long latency, but it may develop into squamous cell carcinoma. Early recognition, treatment, and removal of this lesion are important to prevent serious problems later. Persons with actinic keratoses should use a protective sunscreen with a minimum SPF of 15. They should be seen by a dermatologist every 6 to 12 months for evaluation. Topical 5-fluorouracil (5-FU) may be used and applied once or twice a day. Resistant lesions may be treated with the addition of tretinoin cream. Cryotherapy with liquid nitrogen or curettage and light cautery are also often used to treat the lesions.

Rosacea. This disorder begins in late middle age, forties to sixties, and is characterized by erythema and telangiectasia, possibly with papules and pustules in the central areas of the face (Beers and Berkow, 2000). The etiology is not known, but it is thought to be related to hereditary predisposition, hormonal influences, and psychologic factors. It may be triggered by sunlight, alcohol, hot drinks, and heat. Skin may be sensitive to cosmetics. Eye involvement is common, including soreness, grittiness, burning, and tearing. More severe eye problems can also occur, such as iritis, episcleritis, scarring, and even corneal perforation. End-stage disease in men includes rhinophyma, a bulbous hypertrophy of the nose. Treatments include antibiotics such as topical metronidazole gel or ketoconazole, erythromycin, clindamycin, or sulfacetamide/sulfur. Patients should avoid known triggers and use sun protection. With eye involvement, an oral antibiotic is warranted with tetracycline, doxycycline, or micocycline for 1 month. Telangiectasias respond to pulsed dye laser therapy, an outpatient procedure.

Stasis Dermatitis. Stasis dermatitis is an inflammation of the lower legs associated with venous hypertension. The cause is unknown, but it may be exacerbated by edema, scratching, or contact dermatitis. It is a risk factor for venous ulcers. Edema fluid is inflammatory (Webster, 2001) and, if not drained by lymphatic or venous systems, causes persistent swelling, redness (hemosiderin deposition), a woody induration, and itchy eruptions. Chronic edema impairs healing, and even very small wounds may become large, chronic ulcerations. Control of edema is paramount in avoiding or resolving the problem. Diuretics are of little use. Compressive dressings are paramount and should begin with elastic bandages. They should be applied immediately on arising, and rewrapped several times during the day to maintain the pressure. The legs should be elevated to at least heart level to facilitate venous return. After most of the fluid is gone, use prescription stockings (requiring fitting) to maintain the new unedematous state. Not all elderly patients are able to put on the stockings, and they may prefer to keep using the bandages. The pressure dressings or stockings should continue long after the swelling appears to be gone. Aggressive compression can cause ischemia in patients with arterial insufficiency, particularly in elders with diabetes. If arterial insufficiency is a possibility, ankle-brachial indexes and vascular studies should be performed before initiating compression therapy. Topical steroids may help calm a swollen, itching stasis dermatitis; however, use should be minimized. Avoid topical contact allergens such as fragrances, bacitracin, and neomycin.

Venous ulceration is the result of untreated edema. Ulcers will not resolve because of the edema. The chronic inflammation retards reepithelialization. With edema control, hydrocolloid dressings will greatly benefit the ulceration (Webster, 2001). The ulcers are serious and compromise mobility. They are expensive to treat. Débridement may be necessary if fibrinous debris persists. It should be recognized that squamous cell carcinoma (SCC) can occur in leg ulcers and metastasize.

Skin Cancers. Nearly 1 million cases of skin cancer are diagnosed each year (National Institutes of Health, 2000). More than 95% of these are basal cell carcinoma (BCC) or SCC, which are the nonmelanomatous skin cancers (NMSCs). They are highly treatable and rarely metastasize. However, local invasion can cause disfigurement and functional impairment if not detected and treated early. Risk factors are listed in Box 7-18.

Box 7-18 Risk Factors for Nonmelanomatous Skin Cancers

- History of nonmelanomatous skin cancer
- Older age
- Light eyes
- Light skin
- Light hair
- Poor ability to tan
- Substantive cumulative lifetime sun exposure

Adapted from National Institutes of Health: Screening for skin cancer including counseling to prevent skin cancer. Available at *http://text.nlm.nih.gov/temppfiles/is/tempBRPg43432.html.*

Basal cell cancer begins to appear in about the fifth decade and is the most common malignant lesion of epithelial tissue. It is precipitated by extensive sun exposure, chronic irritation, and chronic ulceration of the skin. It is more prevalent in light-skinned races. This is a slow-growing neoplasm, which appears as a pearly papule with prominent telangiectasias (blood vessels) or as a scarlike area where no history of trauma has occurred. Basal cell carcinoma is also known to ulcerate. Early detection and treatment are advisable, even though metastasis is rare; however, it can occur and be quite disfiguring.

Squamous cell carcinoma is the second most common skin cancer and predominantly affects older adults. Sun exposure is the major cause, and it is more prevalent in fair-skinned, elderly men who live in sunny climates. Bowen's disease, or SCC in situ, is a premalignant lesion that often gives rise to SCC. Other causes that may lead to the development of this type of skin cancer include chemical carcinogens, such as exposure to arsenic, and human papillomavirus (HPV). It is a persistent, erythematous, scaly plaque (Beers and Berkow, 2000), with well-defined margins.

Squamous cell carcinoma is more aggressive than basal cell carcinoma; it has a higher incidence of metastasis and cannot be ignored. It arises from Bowen's disease or actinic keratoses. Although many occur in sun-exposed areas, about 25% occur in sites of chronic inflammation or persistent ulceration such as chronic venous ulcers, a burn scar, radiodermatitis, or lupus vulgaris of long standing. Those in areas of chronic inflammation or irritation have the greatest incidence of metastasis. Early signs are erythema and induration. The epidermis may be scaly or hyperkeratotic. Later, ulceration occurs with crusting. About 2% to 5% metastasize. Those on the lip, the ear pinna, and the genitals are most likely to metastasize. They are treated with excision, radiotherapy, and cryotherapy.

Melanoma. Melanoma is a highly malignant skin cancer that metastasizes readily. The malignancy is associated with intermittent, high-intensity sun exposure (Fuller and Casparian, 2001). The incidence has risen dramatically—in 1981 an American's lifetime risk was 1 in 250; today the risk is 1 in 87. In older adults, the superficial spreading melanoma is most common, accounting for about 60% of all melanomas (Beers and Berkow, 2000). It increases through the eighth decade. Nodular melanoma accounts for 15% of all melanomas and also occurs mostly in elderly people. Lentigo melanoma accounts for 5% to 10% of melanomas and occurs mainly in elderly patients. Mean age at diagnosis is 67 years of age.

The common superficial spreading melanoma is a plaque, variably pigmented, with irregular borders. Colors may be red, white, black, or brown. It is asymptomatic. Pruritus and bleeding occur with advanced lesions.

Nodular melanoma is a papule with dark pigmentation, blue to brown to black, that enlarges rapidly. Lesions contain little pigment.

Lentigo melanoma is nodular, changes color, and ulcerates when long standing.

Any suspicious lesion should be referred to a dermatologist. A biopsy will be performed. The rate of progression differs among the subtypes, and prognosis relates to tumor thickness at the time of biopsy. Morbidity is high among men, probably because of delays in referral and diagnosis. Metastatic melanoma is fatal, and cure depends on early diagnosis and excision.

Treatment depends on the risk category based on the size of the lesion. Enlarged lymph nodes will be removed. Wide local excision of the lesion often requires a skin flap or graft. Mohs' surgery is the most successful type and conserves tissue. Long-term follow-up is done at 6-month intervals. Advanced melanoma is incurable and treated palliatively. Radiation with corticosteroids may prolong comfort. Opioids and other end-of-life measures will be necessary, and advance directives should be in place.

Total body skin examinations should be part of the yearly assessment. The nurse should ask about skin cancer prevention, teach about risk, and ask about history of sun exposure (Agency for Healthcare Research and Quality, 2001). Training in basic skin cancer triage can improve primary care providers' practice of skin cancer control measures. Suspicious lesions should be referred for expert consultation by dermatologists, because research shows that primary care providers (physicians, in this case) make significantly fewer correct diagnoses of skin lesions, including malignant melanoma and BCC (National Institutes of Health, 2000). The ABCDs of melanoma assessment are listed in Box 7-19.

The ABCD Rules of Melanoma

Asymmetry: One half does not match the other half.
Border irregularity: The edges are ragged, notched, or blurred.
Color: The pigment is not uniform in color, having shades of tan, brown, or black, or a mottled appearance with red, white, or blue areas.
Diameter: The diameter is greater than the size of a pencil eraser or is increased, increasing in size.

Herpes Zoster. Herpes zoster (HZ), or shingles, is frequently seen in older adults. The peak incidence occurs between ages 50 and 70. Immunosuppressed elders are at greatest risk; however, HZ can also occur in healthy people. The onset may be preceded by a prodrome of chills, fever, GI disturbance, malaise, and pain or paresthesia along the affected dermatome. Soon it develops clusters of papulovesicles in the dermatomal distribution. Most HZ occurs in the thoracic area (50% to 60%), 10% to 20% are trigeminal, 10% to 20% are cervical, 5% to 10% are lumbar, and less than 5% are sacral. HZ may be very painful. As many as 20% of elderly patients may have pain (postherpetic neuralgia) lasting weeks or months after resolution of the acute infection (Webster, 2001). HZ is infectious until dry crusts appear (Beers and Berkow, 2000). Early treatment of the infection with oral antiviral drugs (acyclovir or famciclovir) substantially reduces the incidence of postherpetic neuralgia, which is common with increasing age (40% in those over age 60) and increases in severity more than incidence with increasing age. Analgesics are usually needed (acetaminophen, NSAIDs, or opioids, depending on the patient's pain). Post-HZ scarring and discoloration is common in elderly patients. Topical drugs are not effective, nor are steroids effective in management. Oral antidepressants may be helpful. Burow's solution (aluminum acetate 5%) diluted 1:20 or greater helps remove crusts and soothes the skin. Gauze dressings can be applied after soaking in the solution, but they must be changed every 2 to 3 hours. If impetigo develops, antibiotics must be given (Beers and Berkow, 2000). HZ recurs in about 6% of patients.

Complications of HZ depend on the dermatome involved. Eye involvement requires immediate consultation with an ophthalmologist. Encephalitis may occur, as well as motor neuropathies such as Guillain-Barré syndrome and urinary retention. With severe HZ or HZ affecting more than one dermatome, intravenous therapy of antivirals should be given. Postherpetic neuralgias are difficult to treat. The pain can be described as lancinating and intermittent, constant deep aching or burning, or dysesthetic pain that is provoked by trivial stimuli (Beers and Berkow, 2000). Treatment may range from simple analgesics to capsaicin cream or EMLA patches to opioids, although opioids are not very useful for neuropathic pain. Gabapentin or nerve blocks and tricyclic antidepressants may work best.

Diagnosis is made by a biopsy of a vesicle or a Tzanck smear. HZ is distinguished from herpes simplex by fluid culture or direct fluorescent antibody analysis.

Human Needs and Wellness Diagnoses

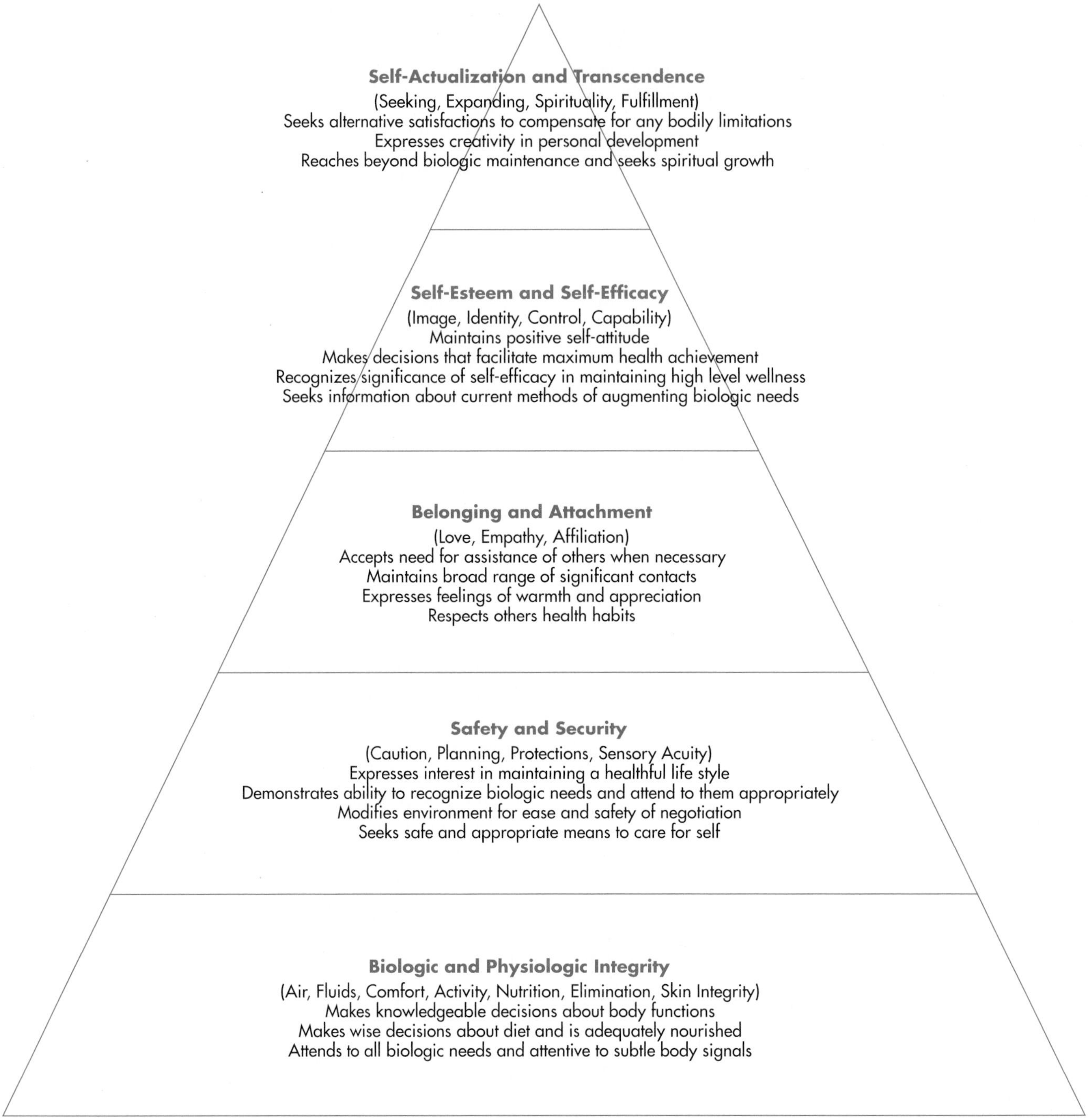

Self-Actualization and Transcendence
(Seeking, Expanding, Spirituality, Fulfillment)
Seeks alternative satisfactions to compensate for any bodily limitations
Expresses creativity in personal development
Reaches beyond biologic maintenance and seeks spiritual growth

Self-Esteem and Self-Efficacy
(Image, Identity, Control, Capability)
Maintains positive self-attitude
Makes decisions that facilitate maximum health achievement
Recognizes significance of self-efficacy in maintaining high level wellness
Seeks information about current methods of augmenting biologic needs

Belonging and Attachment
(Love, Empathy, Affiliation)
Accepts need for assistance of others when necessary
Maintains broad range of significant contacts
Expresses feelings of warmth and appreciation
Respects others health habits

Safety and Security
(Caution, Planning, Protections, Sensory Acuity)
Expresses interest in maintaining a healthful life style
Demonstrates ability to recognize biologic needs and attend to them appropriately
Modifies environment for ease and safety of negotiation
Seeks safe and appropriate means to care for self

Biologic and Physiologic Integrity
(Air, Fluids, Comfort, Activity, Nutrition, Elimination, Skin Integrity)
Makes knowledgeable decisions about body functions
Makes wise decisions about diet and is adequately nourished
Attends to all biologic needs and attentive to subtle body signals

These are not all the possible wellness diagnoses that may be identified. The above are examples of nursing diagnoses that should be considered when planning care for the older adult.

KEY CONCEPTS

- Physical adaptation is immeasurably enhanced by good dentition, well cared for and comfortably shod feet, and soft, lubricated skin.
- The appearance, alignment, and anchoring of teeth are subject to negative effects during aging.
- Routine dental care, foods requiring vigorous chewing, and thorough brushing and flossing after meals are helpful in preventing periodontal disease.
- The enjoyment of food and pride in personal appearance are enhanced by care of the teeth and mouth.
- Caring for the feet and toenails is important to maintain mobility, and mobility is fundamental to independence. Foot care should not be neglected.
- Feet often reflect systemic disease or give clues to physical ailments before their actual appearance.
- Foot massage with a good lubricating lotion reduces edema, stimulates circulation, improves pedal flexibility, and tends to relax the entire body.
- Individuals with foot lesions or vascular problems of the extremities should have a qualified podiatrist care for their feet routinely. Massage only with the doctor's approval.
- The skin is the largest and most visible organ of the body; it is the direct mediator with the environment.
- Showering is best for elders (but not more than two or three times weekly), followed by the use of moisturizing lotion. Avoid prolonged direct exposure to sunlight.

▲ CASE STUDY

For two reasons Philip's teeth, like many others of those 70 years old or older, had loosened and deteriorated: He had ignored regular care, and he smoked a pipe. His teeth were stained and detracted markedly from his appearance, and, because they were loosening, his ability to chew was affected. He stubbornly ignored them even though he was fastidious about his appearance and his health in every other respect. Why did he neglect his teeth? Philip grew up in a time when the dentist had a most amazing array of torture tools and knew exactly how to use them to produce the strongest reaction. Dentists were to be feared. Second, it seemed to be in God's plan that all folk lose their teeth around age 70; his parents had, his relatives had, and several of his friends had. He was, in fact, fortunate to still have his teeth and with only one bridge. He had not been to a dentist in more than a decade. He said, "Well, I'm waiting until I get these eyeglasses fitted and the hearing aids taken care of; then I'll go to the dentist." When his two lower front teeth loosened to the point that he feared swallowing them, he went to the dentist armed with the idea that dental implants would remedy the problem. After thorough discussion of the procedures and alternatives, he opted for having all his teeth removed. It seemed to him the best solution, because all his teeth and gums were ravaged by periodontal disease. There was little problem extracting the teeth. Dentures had been made before the extractions and were immediately placed in his mouth. The swelling subsided, 2 or 3 weeks elapsed, and the dentures were physically more comfortable—but then the psychosocial aspects of the situation began to predominate. Philip was adamant that he could not adapt to these horrible devices for eating. They would not stay in place, and food strayed beneath them and felt uncomfortable. He couldn't taste his food or enjoy the texture and feel of chewing. He lost interest in food and lost 15 pounds. His socialization had often centered around dining, especially going to lovely restaurants. Now he was ashamed to eat in public and thought everyone was aware of how difficult it was for him to chew. He insisted that the removal of his teeth was the most devastating thing that had ever happened to him. He did not think it amusing when one of his insensitive friends suggested that he was much better off than George Washington had been with his wooden teeth. He returned to the dentist, insisting on implants. The dentist assured him that they would consider the possibility if he was unable to adapt to the dentures within a few months. His speech was affected, and articulation was slurred. Sometimes he sounded as if he had imbibed a bit too much. He called friends who had dentures and sought their advice and support. They assured him that he would, in time, become unaware of the dentures, and they would feel very natural. They seemed not to understand that the loss of teeth was the first and most undeniable evidence that his body parts were wearing out. He was confronted many times a day with his loss of youth. Factors to consider: Eating was an important social aspect of Philip's life; Philip had been remarkably free from health problems, and this was his first confrontation with loss of bodily capacity; Philip's friends were unable to provide empathetic support; Philip felt guilty and angry that he had not taken care of his teeth; and Philip took great pride in his appearance.

Based on the case study, develop a nursing care plan using the following procedure:*

List comments of client that provide subjective data.

List information that provides objective data.

From these data identify and state, using accepted format, two nursing diagnoses you determine are most significant to this client at this time. List two client strengths that you have identified from data.

Determine and state outcome criteria for each diagnosis. These must reflect some alleviation of the problem identified in the nursing diagnosis and must be stated in concrete and measurable terms.

Plan and state one or more interventions for each diagnosed problem. Provide specific documentation of source used to determine appropriate intervention. Plan at least one intervention that incorporates the client's existing strengths.

---

*Students are advised to refer to their nursing diagnosis text and identify possible or potential problems.

Evaluate success of intervention. Interventions must correlate directly with the stated outcome criteria in order to measure the outcome success.

STUDY QUESTIONS/ACTIVITIES

How do you think this physical change has affected Philip's self-view and his self-esteem?

How can you assist Philip to identify and determine previous coping capacities that can assist him to get through this present identity crisis?

Discuss ways you can assist Philip to avoid a disturbance in nutritional intake.

Develop a teaching plan that you would like to initiate with individuals before getting dentures.

What anticipatory guidance might have reduced the stress in this situation?

What preventive strategies can you suggest to avoid loss of teeth and consequent need for dentures?

RESEARCH QUESTIONS

How frequently do older clients see their dentist?

How many old people have access to a specialist in geriatric dentistry, and how many would use these services?

Do most elders believe that dentures are an inevitable outcome of aging?

What are the common podiatric problems for which elders seek attention?

How many elders regularly have pedicures?

What percentage of elders have mobility problems related to correctable podiatric problems?

What do elders know about precancerous skin lesions?

Which ingredients in skin-cleansing agents (lotions, creams, soaps) facilitate the retention of moisture in the skin and eliminate dry skin and pruritus?

REFERENCES

Administration on Aging: Age page: taking care of your teeth and mouth. Available at *www.aoa.gov/aoa/pages/agepages/teethmou.html*

Agency for Healthcare Research and Quality: Training in basic skin cancer triage can improve primary care providers' practice of skin cancer control measures, *AHRQ Research Activities* 252:4, Aug 2001.

American Diabetes Association: Position statement on preventive foot care in people with diabetes, *Diabetes Care* 25:S69, 2002.

Beers MH, Berkow R: *Merck manual of geriatrics,* ed 3, Whitehouse Station, NJ, 2000, Merck Research Laboratories.

Centers for Disease Control and Prevention: *CDC fact book 2000/2001,* Washington, DC, Sept 2000, Department of Health and Human Services, Centers for Disease Control and Prevention.

Centers for Disease Control and Prevention: *Health U.S. 2001,* Washington, DC, 2001, Department of Health and Human Services, Centers for Disease Control and Prevention.

Coleman P: Improving oral health care for frail elderly, *Geriatr Nurs* 234:189, 2002.

Ettinger RL: Oral health. In Swanson EA, Tripp-Reimer T, Buckwalter K, editors: *Health promotion and disease prevention in the older adult,* New York, 2001, Springer.

Fuller KE, Casparian JM: Vitamin D: balancing cutaneous and systemic considerations, *Southern Med J.* Available at *http://rheumatology.medscape.com/SMA/SMJ*

Hammond R: Confronting aging and disease: the role of HRT. Available at *www.medscape.com/womenshe.ment/update*

Hardy M: Impaired skin integrity: dry skin. In Maas ML et al, editors: *Nursing care of older adults: diagnoses, outcomes, and interventions,* St Louis, 2001, Mosby.

HealthandAge.com: Treating insomnia in the elderly. Available at *www.healthandage.com/Phome/gid2=272.*

Kagan S et al: Pressure injury and ulceration: a holistic context for advanced practice nurses. In Cotter V, Strumpf N, editors: *Advanced practice nursing with older adults,* New York, 2002, McGraw-Hill.

Meiner S: Gout. In Luggen AS, Meiner S, editors: *Care of the older adult with arthritis,* New York, 2002, Springer.

Moore MC: *Nutrition care,* ed 4, St Louis, 2001, Mosby.

National Institute on Aging: Age page: footcare 2000. Available at *www.aoa.gov/aoa/pages/agepages/footcare.html.*

National Institutes of Health: Counseling to prevent dental and periodontal disease. Available at *http://nlm.nih.gov/tempfiles/is/tempBrPg4342*

National Institutes of Health: Screening for skin cancer including counseling to prevent skin cancer. Available at *http://text.nlm.nih.gov/temppfiles/is/tempBRPg43432.html*

Reese JL: Altered oral mucous membrane. In Maas ML et al, editors: *Nursing care of older adults: diagnoses, outcomes, and interventions,* St Louis, 2001, Mosby.

Rubenstein LZ, Nahas R: Primary and secondary prevention strategies in the older adult, *Geriatr Nurs* 19(1):11, 1998.

Valdez IH, Berkey DB: Mouth and teeth. In Ham RJ, Sloane PD, Warshaw GA, editors: *Primary care geriatrics,* St Louis, 2002, Mosby.

Vargas et al: The oral health of older Americans, *Aging Trends,* p 1, Mar 2001.

Webster GF: Common skin disorders in the elderly, *Clin Cornerstone* 4(1):39, 2001.

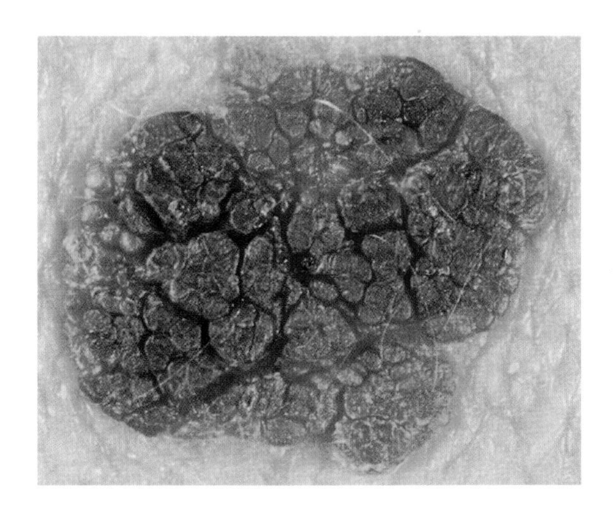

Figure 1. Seborrheic keratosis in an older adult. (From Habif TP: *Clinical dermatology: a color guide to diagnosis and therapy,* ed 3, St Louis, 1996, Mosby.)

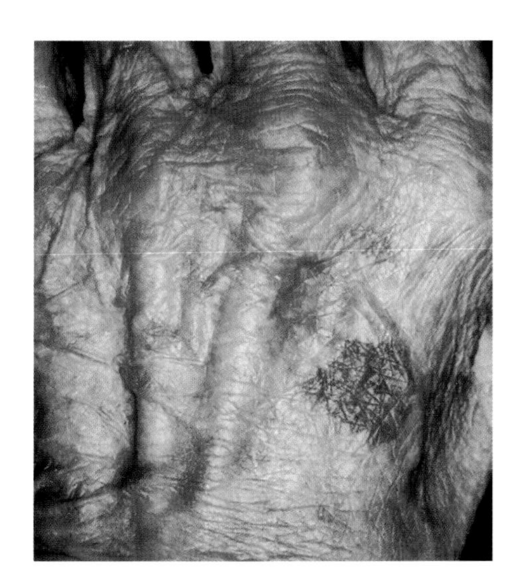

Figure 2. Lentigo, a brown macule that appears in chronically sun-exposed areas. (From Habif TP: *Clinical dermatology: a color guide to diagnosis and therapy,* ed 3, St Louis, 1996, Mosby.)

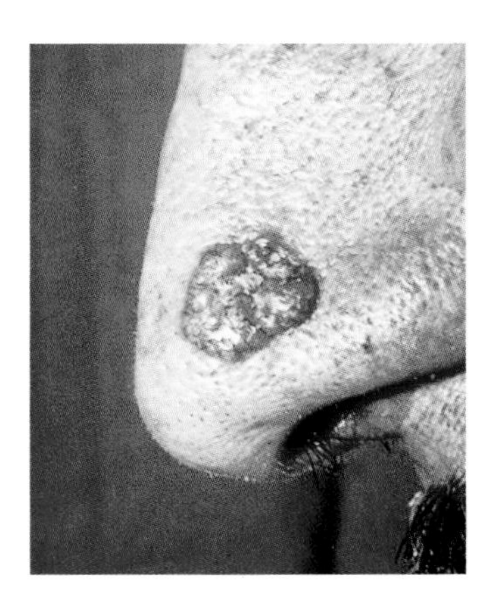

Figure 3. Basal cell carcinoma, the most commonly occurring skin cancer. (Courtesy Gary Monheit, MD, University of Alabama at Birmingham School of Medicine.)

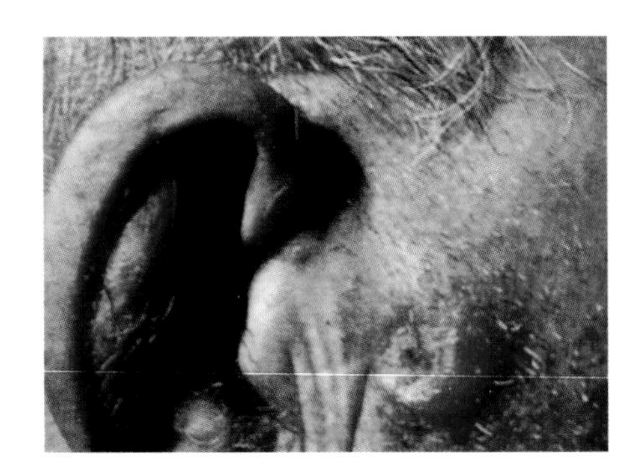

Figure 4. Squamous cell carcinoma. (Courtesy Gary Monheit, MD, University of Alabama at Birmingham School of Medicine.)

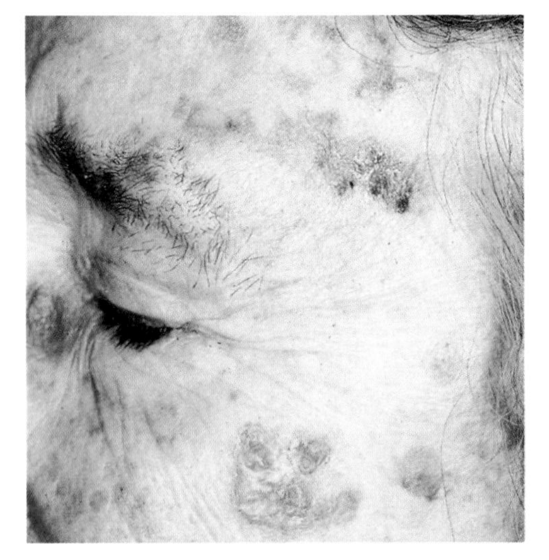

Figure 5. Actinic keratosis in an older adult in an area of sun exposure. (From Habif TP: *Clinical dermatology: a color guide to diagnosis and therapy,* ed 3, St Louis, 1996, Mosby.)

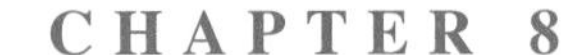
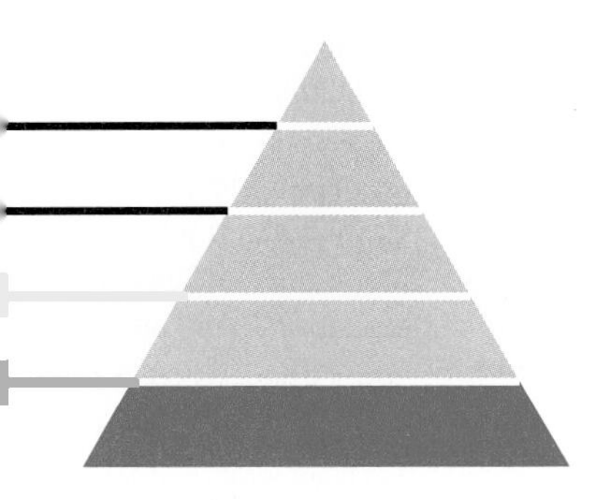

CHAPTER 8

Common Chronic Problems

Catherine Hill
Ann Schmidt Luggen

An elder speaks ***If I'd known I was going to live this long, I'd have taken better care of myself.***

Eubie Blake, on his 100th birthday

LEARNING OBJECTIVES

On completion of this chapter, the reader will be able to:

1. Identify the most common chronic disorders of the aged and their sequelae.
2. Relate strategies that have been used successfully to maintain maximum function and comfort in the client with a chronic disorder.
3. Complete a nursing care plan appropriate to the care of an individual with a chronic disorder.
4. Explain lifestyle factors that frequently exacerbate chronic disorders.
5. Discuss activities of daily living (ADLs) and instrumental activities of daily living (IADLs) in relation to chronicity.
6. Describe some of the effects on self-concept of chronic disorders.
7. Explain the trajectory concept and its relationship to chronicity.

As a result of scientific advances, it is likely that you will grow old more slowly than your parents. Some experts are forecasting an increase in your "health span" along with your life span, as health is defined by functional standards (Peterson, 1999). The family you are a part of will gradually become adult dominated and transgenerational as a result of the lower birth rate. Once a rarity, four-generation families will become more commonplace. We are headed into a "senior boom," as the leading edge of the baby boomer generation approaches 65 (Dychtwald and Flower, 1990). These population trends are significant in chronic illness as they relate to the number of family "caregivers" available for elders, the prevalence of prolonged health problems, and our approach as nurses interested in promoting self-care.

CHRONICITY

Lubkin (1995) provides the most cogent, inclusive, and appropriate definition for chronic illness that we have found: "Chronic illness is the irreversible presence, accumulation, or latency of disease states or impairments that involve the total human environment for supportive care and self-care, maintenance of function and prevention of further disability" (p. 8). Though we particularly ascribe to Lubkin's definition, in 1956 Mayo provided a good definition as well: "All impairments or deviations from normal which have one or more of the following characteristics: are permanent, leave residual disability, are caused by non-reversible pathological alteration, require special training of the patient for rehabilitation, and may be expected to require a long period of supervision, observation or care." Those disorders that truly fit Lubkin's and Mayo's definitions are ongoing, poorly recognized, and largely ignored by everyone except those directly affected by them.

Healthy People 2000: National Health Promotion and Disease Prevention Objectives is a historic document developed in 1991 by the U.S. Department of Health and Human Services (1991) for the express purpose of moving forward into a preventive, wellness attitude toward health and to decrease the "wait and see what develops and then diagnose and treat" approach to health care. For the elderly this is a significant change in perspective because most of the disorders of aging are chronic ones that must be treated within a framework of lifestyle changes, living situation adaptations, and attention to the whole person coping with a disorder. *Healthy People 2000: Midcourse Review and 1995 Objectives* (U.S. Department of Health and Human Services, 1995) measures progress toward specific target goals for older adults that were defined as desirable. Some of these were specific to the reduction of the incidence and degree of chronic impairment.

Currently, *Healthy People 2010* guides our comprehensive, national disease prevention and health promotion efforts (U.S. Department of Health and Human Services, 2000). Building on the initiatives of the previous 20 years, it provides a 10-year plan for continued improvement in the health of all Americans and can be accessed on the World Wide Web at *www.health.gov/healthypeople/*. Age data in *Healthy People 2010* are not included in the minimum population table (provided on the website) to reduce the complexity of information management; however, age-specific subobjectives are included based on the current understanding of relevance. As a collaborative effort among scientists, the government, and the public, *Healthy People 2010* is designed to address citizen health concerns. It is important for nurses to contribute to the evaluation of the plan as it relates to aging and chronic illness. Your comments by fax, Internet, or letter and in person to the U.S. Department of Health and Human Services on the utility and comprehensiveness of *Healthy People 2010* are encouraged.

The present concern we have is that those who are now coping with chronic illness be provided sufficient support, assistance, accoutrements, and comforts to enjoy the extended life span that is more and more possible for an aging population. Current projections identify a life expectancy of approximately 65 years for men and 71 years for women born in 1950; children born in 2000 will enjoy 73 years and 80 years, respectively (U.S. Department of Health and Human Services, 2000). A longer and healthier life, therefore, requires effective management, if not cure, of chronic illnesses and their attendant disability risk. This text and particularly this chapter are devoted to those ends.

We recommend that nurses or students unfamiliar with the specific illnesses and medical management of their clients review the excellent *Merck Manual of Geriatrics*, third edition (Beers and Berkow, 2000). The *Merck Manual* is the most widely used medical text in the world. Now in its sixteenth edition, it has been the bible of diagnosis and therapy since the first edition was published in 1899. In 1990, in response to the massive increases in the aged population, Merck issued the first edition of the *Merck Manual of Geriatrics*. The necessity of nursing input was soon realized, and that perspective is included in the third edition of the *Merck Manual of Geriatrics* (Beers and Berkow, 2000).

Why do we recommend a medical text in addition to the healthy aging text we are presenting? We believe it is essential that nurses be extremely well grounded and that one nursing text cannot give sufficient guidance in illness and wellness, both of which are important to elders. Given the degree of knowledge necessary today and the level of nursing responsibility for patient management, it is imperative that the nurse be thoroughly prepared for each case. The nurse is often the primary care manager and must lay the foundation for all other services. Chronic illnesses create limitations, and when we consider the physiology of the disorder as it affects the quality of life, we implicitly accept the reality of illness.

Chronic disorders and acute illness cannot truly be separated, because so many conditions are intricately intertwined; acute disorders have chronic sequelae, and many of the commonly identified disorders tend to intermittently flare up and then go into remission. Many elders have several chronic disorders simultaneously and have great difficulty managing the complexity of these overlapping and often contradictory demands. The management of chronic illness largely relies on the patient and caregiver. Health care coverage is usually limited and available only when a particular improved outcome is expected.

Physical disabilities are often multiple and serious but need not kill the spirit nor define the person. Psychologic functioning may be more affected than physical or social functioning. The diagnosis, duration of the disease, and economic status are factors influential in psychologic adjustment. The challenge to the aged individual with multiple disabilities and chronic problems may simply become overwhelming. Women with severe arthritis may be as psychologically distressed as those with breast cancer, and strong social networks will have more positive effect on both conditions than other factors. Additionally, social functioning may mediate psychologic adjustment, but that is largely dependent on education and occupation, as well as age, sex, marital status, and economic status.

One of the earliest geriatric nurse pioneers, Eldonna Shields, once said, "Old age is a losing game when focused on function" (Shields, 1990). Our culture values independence, and winning is among our most revered goals. We, as nurses, are challenged to authenticate necessary dependency and to respect those who have the courage to let go of function when necessary. The things nurses "do" and the order in which they are done is probably far less important in chronic disease management than how they are done and with what attitude.

Carrie (a home health nurse) knelt on the carpet while applying dressings to open, nonhealing leg wounds that were a result of impaired circulation in an elder. She laughed and chatted, sharing some of her own interests and concerns as she worked. She had brought a book of hummingbird photographs for the patient to enjoy. She said, "I practice down on my knees." This, from our perspective, was nursing in its highest sense. It is symbolic of much of our practice with elders: conducted "down on our knees," pleading to powers beyond our understanding to restore health and function.

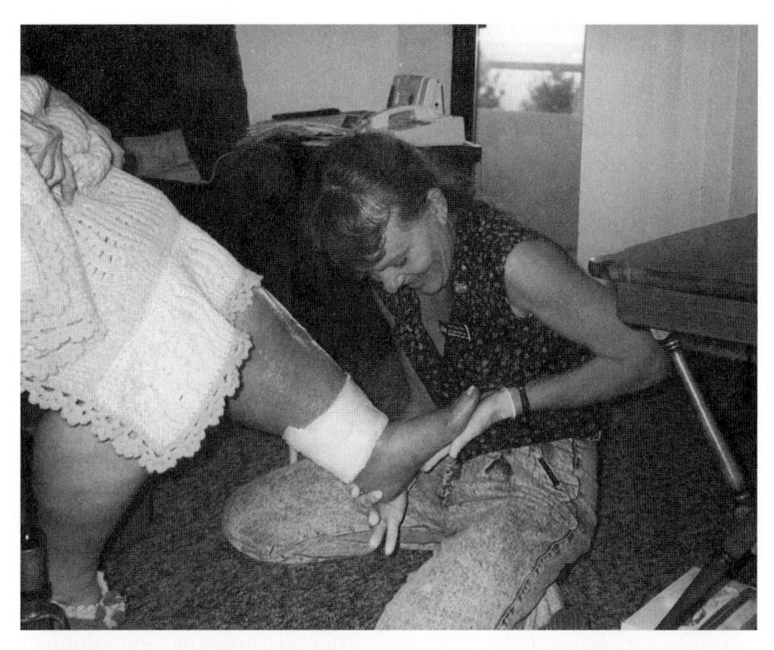

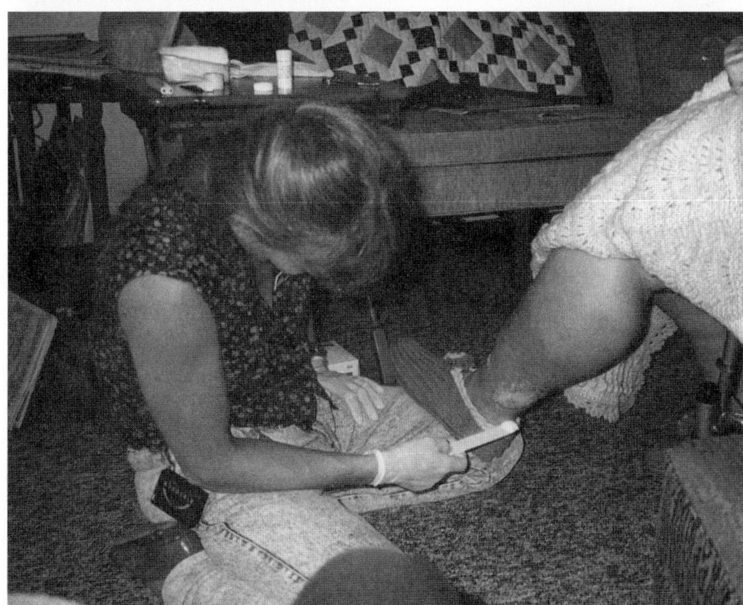

Care of venous stasis ulcer. (Courtesy Priscilla Ebersole.)

The nurse's greatest challenge in working with the chronically ill is to assist them to maintain hope, to sustain interest in their own welfare, and to develop the capacity to view the restrictions imposed by the disorder as having the potential for personal enrichment. Work with the neurologically disabled provides insight into a humanistic and expansive manner of dealing with functional deficits. Nurses must "educate" the client about his or her illness with care. The giving of information by one who has not experienced the particular condition and knows not the outcome or the subjective resources of the individual is presumptuous at best and often insulting. The good and helpful intentions must be in the direction of supplementing, and enhancing when possible, the individual's knowledge of resources, both objective and subjective. Knowledge of the client and caring about the client are crucial, and in the case of chronic disorders the patient must educate the nurse before a plan of care can be developed.

WELLNESS IN CHRONIC ILLNESS

The aged with one or more chronic conditions can be supported toward the achievement of wellness and maximization of life satisfaction by caregivers who ascribe to a holistic philosophy that incorporates efforts directed toward the maintenance of the elderly person's self-care and self-esteem. Figure 8-1 shows how the wellness continuum and Maslow's

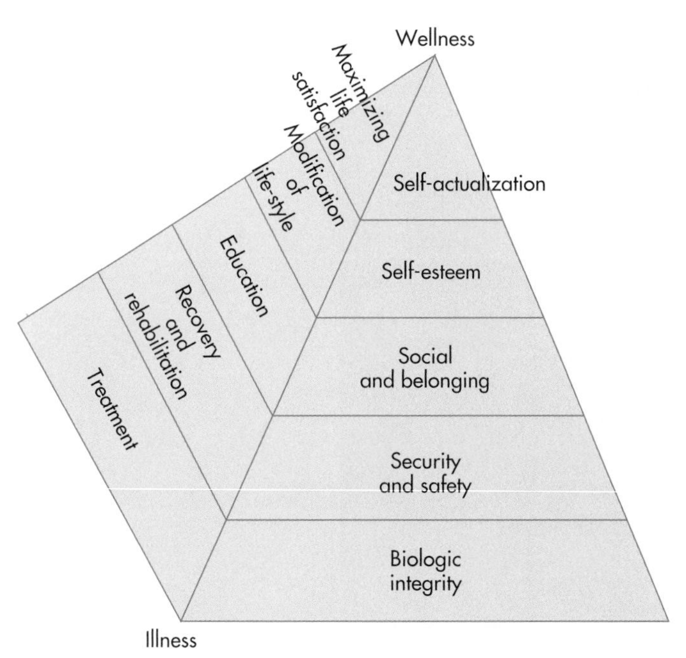

Figure 8-1. Correlation between illness-wellness continuum and Maslow's hierarchy of needs. (Developed by Patricia Hess.)

hierarchy of needs can complement each other in the attainment of wellness and self-actualization. A reorganization of thinking is needed by many aged persons and those associated with them: kin, friends, and caregivers. Physical manifestations of chronic illness should not be the sole determinative factor in the establishment of the elder's state of health or wellness. The greatest factor in establishing wellness is adaptation. The illness-wellness continuum illustrates this well. To achieve maximization of life satisfaction, adaptation of lifestyle is necessary.

What is wellness in the face of chronic illness? This produced a lively discussion from the contentious voices of an assertive group of elders. Comments included "Let's get real!" and "I'm like the old one-hoss shay* . . . losing a little something every day. Someday, I'll wake up and find that nothing works."

CHRONIC ILLNESS AND AGING

Chronic illness is the accrual of life's earnings, sometimes self-generated, often inherent or as a result of imposed lifestyles and environmental hazards. Often treating an acute disorder yields a chronic residual disability. The thought has been, "It's a small price to pay for staying alive." For years, individuals with strokes or intractable pain of arthritis were simply told, "You must just learn to live with it." But, finally, chronic disorders are being taken seriously as we confront the individual, social, and economic costs of chronic impairment.

*A "one-hoss shay" was a cart drawn by a horse, popular around 1910.

The development of geriatric nursing has been largely based on caring for those with persistent disorders that kill slowly but erode joy and function.

In this chapter we consider ways in which nurses may assist their clients toward an enriched capacity for living in the shadow of chronic disabilities, so many of which are common to the aged. Arthritis is almost universal but more troublesome for some than others; often there is some mild to severe cardiovascular problem; breathing becomes more difficult; digestive disorders and nutritional problems go hand in hand, often including elimination problems; and diabetes is common and sometimes out of control, creating many other problems. Several of these disorders may intermingle to put a damper on the vitality of all but the most mentally robust. However, a state of wellness may be achieved and maintained consistently if the individual feels capable of managing and is motivated to manage the problems, with or without assistance.

Scope of the Problem

There is a growing recognition that chronic illness is the major area of health concern and that health care professionals and the lay public have inadequate knowledge of chronic illness, its management, and the priorities and economics that have dictated inadequate policies and services. The prevalence of chronic diseases continues to rise with the lengthening of frail aged life span and highly technical medical care.

In 1995 the direct medical cost for treating chronic conditions was $470 billion; it is expected to be as high as $864 billion by 2040 (Holden, 2001). It is estimated that 90 million people in the United States are afflicted by chronic disease and comorbidities. The National Chronic Care Consortium based in Bloomington, Minnesota, notes that these conditions plunder the personal bank accounts of elders. The average Medicare enrollee spends well over $3000 annually in out-of-pocket expenses on these disorders. In the past the predominance of short-term, cure-oriented conditions consumed most health resources. This balance is shifting, although we still do not have a full grasp of the problems of chronic disorders. Medicare stringently limits home care support for chronic disorders. Verbrugge and Patrick (1995) analyzed seven chronic conditions, three nonfatal (arthritis, visual impairment, and hearing impairment) and four fatal (ischemic heart disease, chronic obstructive pulmonary disease, diabetes mellitus, and malignant neoplasms), for impact on activity levels and use of medical services. The nonfatal conditions limited functioning considerably more than the fatal conditions but received far fewer health services.

Chronic illnesses tend to be composed of multiple diseases; are long term, unpredictable, and expensive; intrude into life course and self-concept; and require extensive palliative care. The incidence of chronic illness triples after 45 years of age but is thought to decrease markedly in relation to higher socioeconomic status.

Certain terms describing the accompaniments of chronic disease, such as *handicap*, *impairment*, and *physical limita-*

tion, are used rather indiscriminately. The term *decreased function without incapacitation* also needs to be stated consistently. Because these and other terms are often used interchangeably, available statistics may be easily misinterpreted if one does not use caution. The most prevalent chronic conditions in individuals over 75 years in rank order are arthritis, hypertension, hearing impairments, heart disease, and cataracts (Holden, 2001). Interestingly, individuals between 65 and 74 years old have a higher incidence of dermatitis, sinusitis, ulcers, and asthma than those over 75.

At some point, even in the face of devoted family caretakers, it is highly likely that a very old woman, and about 10% as many very old men, will require care in a nursing home as a result of numerous, ongoing chronic problems that have become devastatingly disabling. It is also likely that resources of family and individual will by then have become exhausted. Elders and others with disabilities make up 27% of Medicaid beneficiaries but account for 59% of the total Medicaid spending, most of it on long-term care. Recent figures show that annual spending of Medicaid dollars per capita for elders averages $9,293. This leaves many recipients extremely vulnerable to legislation that is rapidly shifting responsibility entirely to states. Numerous governors of poorer states may need to make very difficult choices. Long-term health care, chiefly represented by the American Health Care Association (AHCA) and Association of American Homes and Services for the Aged (AAHSA), are mounting extensive and expensive campaigns to prevent this shift for fiscal reasons. Ideally, long-term care would be a fundamental service, a benefit of citizenry, that could be relied on at minimal cost when needed by individuals and their families in late life. However, at present it is not a social service but an enormous profit-making endeavor that will remain so in the foreseeable future. Numerous abuses and federal regulations remain. However, the progress in quality of nursing home care is visible. Primarily nurses, and some other health care providers, have managed in the face of almost insurmountable challenges, through sheer courage and tenacity, to bring the quality of care in nursing homes ever higher. This will continue, with or without federal regulations, because of the commitment of numerous nurses and others.

Chronic Illness Trajectory

In considering an appropriate conceptual framework for the study of chronic illness we have tried to blend Corbin and Strauss with Maslow. The trajectory model of chronic illness, originally conceptualized by Anselm Strauss (Strauss and Glaser, 1975), has aided health care providers to better understand the realities of chronic illness. Later, Corbin and Strauss (1988) presented a view of chronic illness as a trajectory that traces a course of illness through eight phases, which may be upward, downward, or at a plateau. In its entirety, a chronic illness may include a preventive phase, a definitive phase, a crisis phase, an acute phase, a comeback, a stable phase, an unstable phase, deterioration, and death. Key points of the model are based on the theoretic assumptions listed in Box 8-1.

Box 8-1 Theoretic Assumptions Regarding Chronic Illness Trajectory

- The prevalent form of disease at this time is chronic illness.
- These presumably incurable illnesses may appear at any time in the life span but are most frequent in late life.
- Chronic illnesses are lifelong and entail lifetime adaptations.
- Those with chronic illnesses are likely to experience the trajectory phases identified by Strauss and Corbin (1988).
- The acute phase of illness management is designed to stabilize physiologic processes and promote a comeback from the acute phase.
- Other phases of management, except the severely deteriorating, are primarily designed to maximize and extend the period of stability in the home with the help of family and augmented by visits to physicians or clinics.
- Maintaining stable phases is central in the work of managing chronic illness.
- Chronic illness and its management often profoundly affect the lives and identities of the afflicted and the family members.
- The management in the home by the family, self, or significant other is central to care and is not peripheral to medical management (Strauss and Corbin, 1988).
- Recommended actions require appropriate timing and patience of the family and the practitioner.
- A primary care nurse able to coordinate multiple resources may be needed.
- Finally, creativity and ability to use what is available are essential to successful management.

Maslow's concept of five major levels of need that affect function and self-perception fits nicely with the Corbin-Strauss model (see Figure 8-1). The patient's perceptions of needs met and basic biologic functional limitations are paramount to predicting movement within the illness trajectory (Woog, 1992). In this respect, our wellness approach largely hinges on assisting the elder to meet as many of the Maslow-defined needs as possible at any given time. These efforts enhance the individual's potential for remaining on a plateau or gaining ground in any of the trajectory phases (Table 8-1).

Strauss and Corbin (1988) emphasized the changing nature of health care needed for an aging population in which chronic disorders are by far the most prevalent forms of illness. The incidence of chronic disease is increasing in proportion to lifesaving technologies. Until the late 1930s, illness was primarily caused by bacterial or parasitic infection. With the advent of antibiotics and immunizations these diseases decreased markedly in the industrialized nations. Instead,

Table 8-1 Definitions of Phases and Goals

Phase	Definition
1. Pretrajectory	Before the illness course begins, the preventive phase, no signs or symptoms present
2. Trajectory onset	Signs and symptoms are present, includes diagnostic period
3. Crisis	Life-threatening situation
4. Acute	Active illness or complications that require hospitalization for management
5. Stable	Illness course/symptoms controlled by regimen
6. Unstable	Illness course/symptoms not controlled by regimen but not requiring hospitalization
7. Downward	Progressive deterioration in physical/mental status characterized by increasing disability/symptoms
8. Dying	Immediate weeks, days, hours preceding death

Examples of goals that nurses might establish include the following:

1. To assist a client in overcoming a plateau during a comeback phase by increasing adherence to a regimen so that he or she might reach the highest level of functional ability possible within limits of the disability.
2. To assist a client in making the attitudinal and life-style changes that are needed to promote health and prevent disease.
3. To assist a client who is in a downward trajectory make the adjustments and readjustments in biography and everyday life activities that are necessary to adapt to increasing physical deterioration.
4. To assist the client who is in an unstable phase to gain greater control over symptoms that are interfering with his or her ability to carry out everyday activities.
5. To assist a client in maintaining illness stability by finding a way to blend illness management activities with biographical and everyday life activities.

Goals can be broken down into specific client-oriented objectives. Built into the objectives are the criteria that will be used to evaluate the effectiveness of each intervention. What is important here is to look at what takes place in the process (the steps) of working toward a goal, as well as the end to be reached, and to be realistic about what can be achieved in what time period, taking into consideration the desires, wants, and abilities of the client and family.

From Woog P: *The chronic illness trajectory framework: the Corbin and Strauss nursing model*, New York, 1992, Springer Publishing Company, Inc. Used by permission.

cancers, arthritis, and cardiovascular conditions have become the most common health problems. Recently, cancers and cardiovascular conditions have decreased somewhat, and infectious diseases are returning with a vengeance.

Since the last edition of this text was published, we have seen enormous restructuring of the health care system in ways that are beginning to more realistically serve the large numbers of chronically ill. In many ways the acquired immunodeficiency syndrome (AIDS) epidemic has been the catalyst for change. As the society becomes unhealthy in terms of environment, diet, infectious agents, and stress inducers, more attention is being paid to seeking a healthy lifestyle. Anselm Strauss, a pioneer in conceptualizing chronic illness, died in September of 1996. We believe he accomplished much toward achieving some of the goals of understanding chronic illness that we are advancing toward at present.

Special Considerations

Regardless of the nature of chronic problems, there are special considerations that almost universally need attention and must be addressed actively by nurses. It is not sufficient to wait until the client brings up the topic.

Gender and Chronic Illness. Because women typically live longer than men and more frequently live alone, the issues of management of chronic disorders have a large gender component. The Rand Corporation found from a large study of elders (sample of 11,242) hospitalized with congestive heart failure (CHF), heart attack, pneumonia, and stroke that elderly men receive more care and more expensive, highly technical services than do women (Shoben, 1992).

With the growing concern and scientific interest in women's health, in April of 1991, Dr. Bernadine Healy, then Director of the National Institutes of Health (NIH), launched the Women's Health Initiative (WHI) to address the most common causes of death, disability, and impaired quality of life in postmenopausal women. Sponsored by the NIH and the National Heart, Lung, and Blood Insititute (NHLBI), the WHI addresses cardiovascular disease, cancer, and osteoporosis. The research from this project, to be completed in 2006, has already raised serious questions about the approriate use of hormone replacement therapy (HRT) *(www.nhlbi.nih.gov/whi/index/html)*. The major components of WHI include a randomized controlled clinical trial of promising but unproven approaches to prevention, an observational study to identify predictors of disease, and a study of community approaches to developing healthful behaviors. Dr. Claude Lenfant, Director, and Dr. Vivian Pinn, Associate Director, are presently guiding the research endeavors.

Fatigue from Living with Chronic Disorders. Fatigue from living with chronic disorders is seldom considered in its full significance. It is a variable and unpredictable condition that is often ignored or relegated to an insignificant and incidental aspect of growing old. It may occur in the presence or absence of any other disorder but cannot be ignored. The lassitude that one experiences is often evidence of depression as well as chronic illness. Zest for life is gone, and every action seems to involve an inordinate amount of energy, hardly worth the effort. Nurses confronted by this attitude tend to become either impatient or caught up in the feeling of futility. The most important intervention is undoubtedly to validate the reality and debilitating effects of the disorder. Discussing patterns of fatigue and identifying the precipitants are important. If the elder can be engaged in keeping a log of the low points of energy, it may prove useful. It is also helpful to emphasize the wisdom of the body and the assumption that it is presently necessary for the individual to move in "low gear." Permission to rest periodically and engage in brief periods of mild activity may reassure elders that they can indeed cope with this overwhelming inertia.

Energy to enjoy life's activities becomes more precious with advancing age. Chronic problems tax this existing energy level. Direct assistance by caregivers or families may be necessary to aid the aged person in exploring lifestyle adaptations that decrease energy expenditure and permit continued involvement in valued interests. Throughout the process, the aged disabled person must remain involved in decision making on every level of need. The aged often have different priorities than the caregiver. Elderly clients may relegate their health needs to a lower priority to fulfill other needs or life demands. One must understand and respect the priorities established by the elder.

When caregivers work with the aged who have disabling chronic conditions, the concept of time is important. More time is required. A slower pace of activity and large segments of time for direct care are needed. The slower movements of the aged and the response to physiologic stress require more time for care activities with rest periods in between.

Pain and Chronic Illness. Chronic health problems of the elderly person usually involve not only certain painful physical impairments, but frequently depressed moods that exacerbate pain perception. There is great variance in cohorts in the relationship between pain and depression. The older one becomes, the more likely is the correlation between pain and depression. It is common for individuals to be told, "You must learn to live with it."

Often an antidepressant is needed in combination with analgesics. However, our attachment to the belief that only Western medicine really works and all else is adjunctive has limited our thinking about pain management. "Alternative" strategies can be extremely effective, especially when sought and managed by the individual. We do not suggest that they are always effective, but in many cases therapeutic benefits are obtained from a combination of scientifically undefined qualities, personal idiosyncrasies, placebo effects, and individual control. However, chronic conditions often do produce excruciating pain. Most adjunctive therapies are just that and not adequate for management of extreme pain without medication as well. In fact, one elder got very angry when asked to visualize to relieve his pain. It seemed to him a superficial dismissal of him and his very real problem. Chronicity and pain often go hand in hand, and one of the major management issues is the control of pain.

Box 8-2 **PLISST**

Permission to masturbate, fantasize, and claim feelings
Limited **I**nformation related to problem being experienced
Specific **S**uggestions—Only when the nurse is clear about the problem
Intensive **T**herapy—Referral to professional with advanced training if necessary

Sexuality and Chronic Illness. Sexual problems and misinformation are pervasive in society in spite of generally high levels of exposure to knowledge about sex and near-toxic exposure to sexuality in media, schools, and politics. In spite of this, little attention is paid to those who are living daily with chronic disorders that interfere with sexual intercourse and the fundamental feelings of sexual attractiveness. Individuals with chronic disorders also experience the sexual problems that beset most individuals. Various disorders may produce mechanical problems, erectile problems, decreased libido, and decreased lubrication. Certain disorders involving ostomies and incontinence may produce revulsion in the partner and sexual anxiety in the afflicted. Discussing and assessing medication regimens, the expected dysfunctions that accompany particular diseases, and the individual's expectations are all important. A sexual history may provide important clues regarding the individual's needs and desires. The nurse's responsibility is toward an open, accepting discussion of the patient's sexuality and the provision of information and resources appropriate to the client's situation. PLISST is an acronym that is helpful in reminding us of a useful format for discussing sexuality (Box 8-2). Additional discussion of sexuality is in Chapter 17.

ASSESSMENT

Assessment of the elderly involves selection of appropriate tools, repeated testing, careful observation, periodic monitoring, alert watchfulness, and, most important, discussion and corroboration with elders of their perceptions and the meaning their illness has for them. In the case of chronic illness and the great variability in presentation and impact on individual lifestyle, adequate assessment is critical. Functional assessments strive to identify the quantity and quality of disability in chronic illness. These measures, although sometimes not specific to the medical treatment regimen, are often a good measure of the patient's response and adaptation to chronic health problems. Subjective age and objective age can vary widely. Disability assessment helps identify the gap between the existing patient self-care abilities and needed self-care resources. The difference between these two, existing abilities and needed resources, identifies areas of nursing care. In this approach to assessment we are embracing the idea of an illness as chronic; patients can achieve various degrees of adaptation, and as nurses we can help maximize their function and therefore their quality of life. Consider most assessment tools and measurement instruments as possible methods of ongoing assessment in chronic illness. Incorporate validated assessment tools and Nursing Outcomes Classifications whenever possible, but avoid depending on them exclusively because none of our health care assessment research tools is all-inclusive (Nursing Outcomes Classification, 2002).

Activities of Daily Living and Instrumental Activities of Daily Living: ADLs and IADLs

It is difficult if not impossible to estimate the number of individuals with functional disabilities. Estimates vary enormously from one study to another and from one agency to another (Figure 8-2). Many of the needs for assistance are going unmet. Fundamental to adaptation and life satisfaction are the activities of daily living (ADLs) and those that go beyond basic bodily tasks necessary to daily life, the instrumental activities of daily living (IADLs). ADLs include eating, bathing, dressing, toileting, walking, and transferring. IADLs include shopping, using the telephone, paying bills, obtaining medical and dental attention, preparing meals, and light housework. ADLs and IADLs are the major thrust of any type of chronic care. The goal is to sustain or improve all functions as much and as long as possible with a minimum of discomfort. Chronic disorders become problems only when they involve pain or self-care deficits in ADLs.

Assessment of capacity for self-care in both ADLs and IADLs can be accomplished through the use of the Barthel Index (Appendix 8-A) and the ADLs/IADLs charts (see Appendix 8-C).

Chronic disorders and the qualification for home care are defined by the degree of impairment in ADLs. The more complex and higher-level functions are categorized as IADLs. It is apparent that ADLs are largely mechanical, and IADLs are largely cognitive. To qualify for Medicare coverage of home care one must be homebound, be expected to improve with treatment, have a signed order from a physician, and require the services of a professional. Impairment in ADLs is not sufficient to receive Medicare reimbursement. However, it is useful to assess the level of ability of an individual for self-care. There are many tools designed to accomplish this. One of the simplest and most used is the previously mentioned Barthel Index. This scale, which measures ADLs and IADLs with values weighted toward difficulty or complexity, is a useful assessment of a person's capacity to manage with or without assistance.

According to the U.S. Bureau of the Census (2001), assistance needs of elders receiving home health care were as follows: bathing (52%), dressing (46%), transferring (35.9%), taking medications (20.7%), light housework (36.4%), toileting (27.8%), and meal preparation (21.8%). Medicare and Medicaid paid for 81.3% of this care.

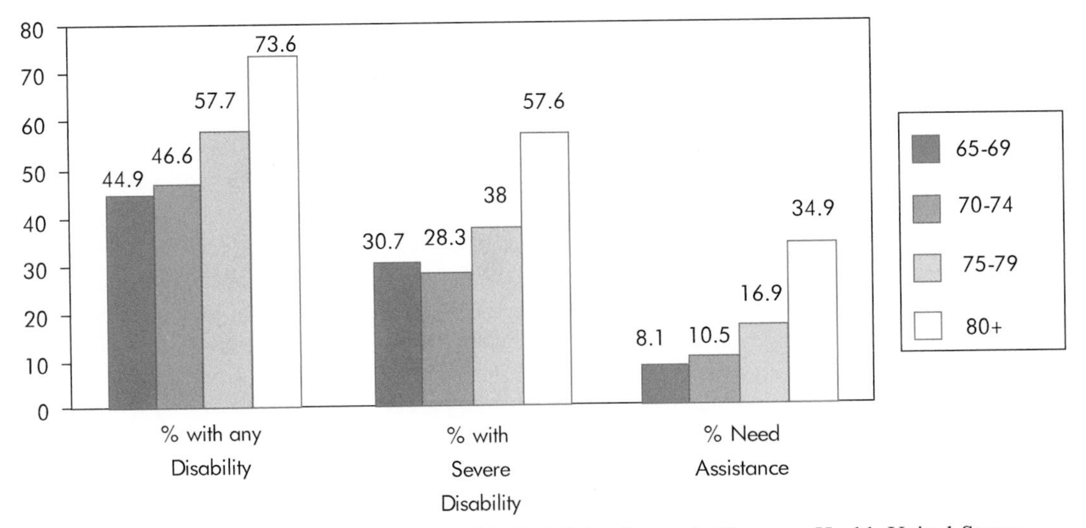

Figure 8-2. Percentage of older adults with disabilities (by age). (Sources: Health United States: 2002; *Americans with Disabilities, 1997,* pp 70-73, February 2001 and related Internet data; Internet releases of the U.S. Census Bureau, National Center on Health Statistics, and the U.S. Bureau of Labor Statistics.)

INTERVENTIONS

Caring

Caring, continuity, commitment, competence—a litany of *C*s have historically formed the foundation of nursing care. Today, in the face of information overload, pandemics, media irresponsibility, ethical confusion, and the ever-growing capability to technologically accomplish things that are humanely questionable, caring may be fundamental to the continuance of civilization. Caring and compassion form the difference between civilization and corruption. Compassion has been seen as a distinguishing aspect of being human.

Numerous definitions of caring in nursing have been presented in the past. One commonly accepted definition is Watson's: "The moral idea of nursing consists of transpersonal human-to-human attempts to protect, enhance, and preserve humanity" (Watson, 1988, p. 54). It is helpful to understand the roots of the word *care* in order to find its place in nursing. We have often heard that care is the nurse's domain and cure belongs to the physician. Of course, these delineations have weakened considerably in the overlapping roles, managed care, and advanced practice nursing models. However, it is enlightening to look into the origins of the words. Care is derived from the Old English word of the commoners, *carian*, meaning to trouble oneself for another, whereas cure is of high Latin derivation, meaning priest. Dunlop (1994) believes this class difference has influenced medicine and nursing, in that the lower orders cared while the higher orders cured. Although this digression is not a central point in caring, it is significant to nursing in general. In our present system "caring time" is a rare commodity. Milne and McWilliam (1996) surveyed doctors, nurses, and nurse managers and found that they understood caring primarily as "spending time with," "being with," and "doing for." They concluded that there was insufficient time and they must take leadership roles in achieving promotion and allocation of "caring time" within each of their agencies.

Nursing Interventions Classification (NIC) is a language developed to describe nursing care in all settings. It is linked to North American Nursing Diagnosis Association (NANDA), addresses the Nursing Minimum Data Set, and is useful in planning and documenting nursing care in chronic illness (Nursing Interventions Classification, 2001). Compatible with resident assessment protocols (RAPs) and OASIS outcome measures, NICs are research based, reflect current practice, and have been embraced by the American Nurses' Association. Organized into 7 domains, 30 classes, and 486 interventions, NIC provides a helpful, concise body of information to supplement your intervention development for individual patients. As we discuss common chronic problems, NICs will be suggested. As discussed in the assessment section, NICs provide an important resource but should not be considered all-inclusive at this time.

Self-Care. In chronic care, self-care is of the greatest importance and must be cultivated beyond all else. The very nature of chronicity demands it. It is important in understanding the self-care movement to know its origins. As it became more apparent that the present system was incapable of providing ongoing care for most of the conditions of elders, self-care as an idea grew in popularity. The self-care movement is rooted not only in the economic imperative of self-care but also in the primacy of the biomedical ethical principle of respect for autonomy and self-governance. This has been a radical change in perspective. Less than 20 years ago the prevailing ethical principle was that of beneficence, conferring good on others—sometimes against their desires. Orem's self-care movement in nursing has grown popular based partially on the increasing awareness of the individual's direct impact on disease and the impotence of nursing and medicine to effect positive change in a depressed, declining individual who no longer cares (Orem, 1980).

According to Carpenito (2002), a self-care deficit is experienced when an individual is unable to carry out basic functions without assistance. These deficits are primarily the result of pathophysiologic disorders that impinge on neuromuscular, musculoskeletal, or sensory integrity. The interruption in function may also stem from situational conditions or treatment sequelae. Thus, when all three situations coalesce, it may require more adaptive capacity than an individual has at the time. The appropriate approach is highly individual and may involve changing the situation, modifying the treatment, or retraining the individual to compensate for the pathophysiologic changes. The impact of chronic illness is also highly individual and may include identity erosion, expectation of death, dependency conflicts, and feelings of failure and fatalism. Interestingly, many of the largest health maintenance organization (HMO) providers now offer reimbursement for alternative medicine therapies such as therapeutic massage, touch therapy, acupuncture, chiropractic, biofeedback, homeopathy, and naturopathy. This trend arises from studies showing that alternative medicine is less expensive, demands fewer hospitalizations, and tends to be used by individuals who are more concerned about managing their own health in a holistic manner. Now it is possible for individuals to direct their own care, order their own special supplies without physician approval, and, in many cases, purchase their medications over the counter. Although this is an important trend, it places even greater responsibility on the client for making wise decisions, sometimes with insufficient information or education. Nursing will be more often called on to assist clients in obtaining background information and sorting out options in health management.

Maintaining a Health Diary. The health diary has multiple purposes in the assessment and management of chronic disorders (see earlier section on assessment). Its most important function is probably to serve as a mechanism by which an elder may develop self-awareness regarding perception and management of a chronic disorder. It has no recommended form or structure and is thus designed according to individual preference. The entries may be lengthy, with much embellishment, or brief, precise descriptions of daily activities and body responses. Some persons make daily entries, whereas others do so only occasionally. Kept over time, the health diary reveals progression or remission of the condition and provides concrete longitudinal assessment data that may long since have been forgotten by the diarist. It also reveals something of the individual's personality style in the way perceptions are recorded, and, most important, it serves as a coping mechanism. A diarist is able to convey, at will, any thoughts or feelings and have full freedom of expression. The act of expressing brings control and solace. The intended, or unintended, recipient of the information becomes incidental to the process when it is considered as a therapeutic mode of self-care, personal integration, and release. Gerontic nurses might encourage clients with prolonged disorders to keep a health diary. It is extremely useful in many ways, the most important being the acute awareness in the nurse of the true meaning of "wellness" and courage.

Another method used to assist elders to become aware of the body and its signals was developed in Idaho. Elders in a senior center wrote about their bodies, aches, and pains in both poetic and prose forms. They were able in doing so to get a new perspective on an ailing heart, an aching shoulder, and feet that had lost their spring. The collective effort and publication of their small book gave substance to their efforts and built a feeling of community that helped objectify their distress and develop a new appreciation for the body.

Small-Group Approaches to Chronic Illness

Group meetings are among the most effective and economic ways of assisting clients to meet informational and psychosocial needs. They can also be designed to provide family support and counseling. Self-help groups can be seen as support systems, consumer participant systems, expressive-social influence groups, or homogeneously identified therapeutic groups. Facilitating adjustment to new roles and activities and redefinition of self and meanings constitute a large part of working with the physically challenged in groups.

The first meeting should set the tone and expectations for the group and also make clear any necessary ground rules. It is important to involve the group in identifying topics and issues they wish to focus on during the groups. These ideally should be planned sufficiently in advance to allow the group facilitator to gather information, brochures, and other resources that may be valuable to the group members. In addition to information there are many psychologic issues to be addressed, such as the following:

1. Fears about incapacitation, pain, abandonment, isolation, and death
2. Expressions of low self-esteem and loss of confidence
3. Feelings of helplessness and uselessness; a desire to be whole and well again
4. A desire to fit into the family system once again
5. Willingness to redefine role relationships with significant others
6. A desire to face and handle public situations without fear or embarrassment

Group Support by Telephone

Organized telephone group therapy may counteract feelings of isolation and loneliness experienced by persons housebound by various degrees of immobility or functional impairment. This mode of intervention has not been thoroughly explored in relation to effectiveness, but telephone support is readily available and conceivably could be very useful.

As common as telephone contact is with community-based elders, formal adoption and integration of this mode for nursing intervention has been slow to develop. Sporadic, specialized applications in chronic disease populations contrasts with widely used, structured telephone interviews for research purposes. Congestive heart failure, diabetes mellitus, post–coronary artery bypass graft, pacemaker, stroke, and smoking cessation follow-up are the most frequently found application areas in the literature. Limited research, contradictory findings, time constraints, litigation risk, and lack of reimbursement are often cited as barriers to its use. Castro and King (2001) studied telephone versus mail interventions in 140 patients and found improved maintenance in prescribed exercise adherence with mailed reinforcement materials. Mental health nursing, however, is aggressively pursuing telephone interventions to intervene in community-based patients with psychologic distress (Hemingway, 2002). Telephonic social problem solving has enjoyed popularity and success in the United Kingdom since the mid-1990s (Grant et al, 2001). Although elderly patients routinely receive a phone call as an appointment reminder, routine telephonic nursing is not utilized.

Adaptive Devices

About 71% of all assistive devices are used by individuals over 65 years of age. The most common devices used by the aged are (in rank order) handrails (65%), canes (49%), hearing aids (38%), raised toilets (30%), hospital beds (24%), and walkers (24%). Overall, 63% of the payment for these items is out-of-pocket. Many varieties of adaptive feeding and homemaking devices are available to compensate for deficits in function. Gerontology experts have identified many useful products that can help people deal with problems caused by arthritis, stroke, reduced hearing or vision, diminished strength, and other impairments (Figure 8-3).

An occupational therapist should be contacted for assistance solving individual adaptive needs. At present this is a highly specialized field. High technology has been used to provide assistive devices, computerized training programs, programmed pillboxes, patient distance monitoring, and robotic aids for the handicapped. Voice-activated computer programs are now highly developed and can assist elders who are completely disabled to accomplish many things.

As computer applications affect the delivery of care for the elderly, new difficulties are created. Computer-assisted

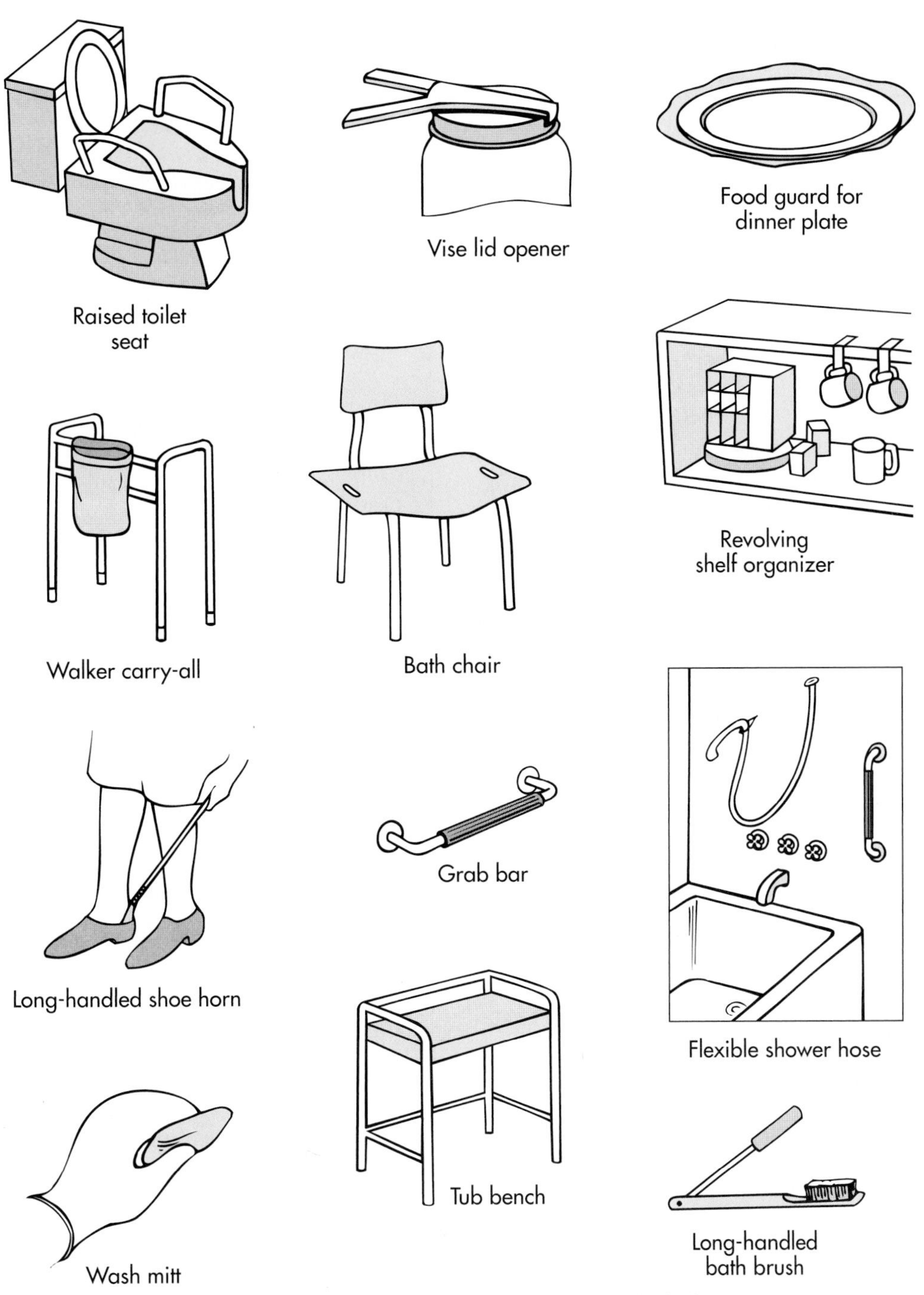

Figure 8-3. Adaptive equipment commonly used in the home.

retraining can be applied to stroke rehabilitation, aphasia, and cognitively impaired clients. Speech synthesis and telecommunication devices are available for the verbally and orally handicapped. Electronic monitoring of status, activity, and location of hospital and nursing home clients is increasingly feasible. Pocket-sized computer notebooks may be useful for the mildly memory impaired. Electronic monitors can locate the wandering individual. The many potential applications of computer technology must be surveyed and correctly applied for maximum benefit. Given the possibilities, it is imperative that health care providers become educated regarding potentials and serve as advocates for the elderly who could benefit from assistive devices.

Each year more training is required for families and professionals simply to use the equipment; in addition, as these become more sophisticated they often become too expensive for most elders. The challenge of the future is to use computer advances to enhance the quality of life for the elderly

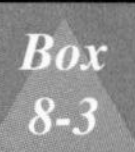

Box 8-3 Common Iatrogenic Disorders of the Old Due to Hospitalization

Loss of mobility due to insufficient ambulation
Temporary incontinence due to inattention when needed; sometimes becoming a permanent problem
Confusion due to medications, treatments, anesthesia, and translocation
Pressure sores due to infrequent changes of position
Dehydration due to limited access to fluids
Fluid overload due to improper use of intravenous fluids
Nosocomial infections due to infectious agents in surroundings
Urinary tract infections due to improper perineal care and catheter usage
Upper respiratory tract infections due to immobility and shallow breathing; pneumonia
Fluid and electrolyte imbalances due to medications and treatments
Falls due to unfamiliar environment and instability
Impaired sleep due to treatments and environment
Malnutrition due to anorexia and insufficient assistance in eating

while lowering the ultimate cost. At this time, the challenge is to provide some of the many assistive devices that should be made generally available.

Substitute Activities

Mrs. L bemoaned the fact that with her advanced arthritis she could no longer knead bread. Because she had built a reputation as an excellent bread baker, she not only lost an enjoyable activity but some of her personal recognition. The home health nurse suggested to the family that they purchase a bread-making machine and a book on how to make bread. This is only one substitute activity that could be suggested for an individual with special skills or interests.

PREVENTION OF IATROGENIC DISTURBANCES

In this era of rapid patient turnaround and numerous treatments compressed into a few days, nurses are well aware of the deleterious iatrogenic effects of hospitalization superimposed on the acute illness that required treatment (Box 8-3). Hospitalized individuals with some functional disabilities often rapidly regress into a helpless state. Simple interventions, noted time and again, have proved helpful in retaining functional status during episodic illness. A geriatric clinical specialist facilitated the following interventions that were found most helpful: staff education regarding special needs of the hospitalized elder, daily orientation cues for the patient and reassurance regarding the probability of transient delirium, getting the patient up and out of the room at least once daily, using physical and occupational therapy daily for particular therapeutic exercises, environmental modifications, personalization of environment, minimal use of medications, and interdisciplinary discharge planning with frequent revisions. (Box 8-4 includes specifics.)

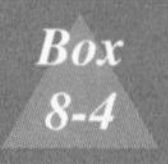

Box 8-4 Minimizing the Effects of Hospitalization on Functional Capacity

Staff Education

Mental and functional status assessment
Management of sensoriperceptual function
Mobility
Environmental modifications

Orientation and Communication

Use of cues and repetition
Discussion of condition
Providing anticipatory guidance regarding procedures
Reassurance regarding likelihood of delirium

Mobilization

Getting patients up, out of bed, and out of room
Involving physical and occupational therapy in exercise

Environmental Modifications

Glasses and hearing aids available and working well
Calendars
Favorite programs on radio and TV available
Increased lighting, night-lights from dusk until dawn

Caregiver Education and Consultation

Families asked to bring in significant items; photos

Medication Management

Daily medication review; discouraged use if not clearly necessary; particularly discouraged neuroleptics and anticholinergics, which tend to exacerbate delirium

Discharge Planning

Weekly, or more frequent, case conferences with primary nurse, social worker, physical and occupational therapist, nutritionist, and discharge planner

Telephone Follow-up after Discharge

Recent emphasis on cost savings and what often seem to be precipitous discharges of individuals from acute care hospitals has revived interest in telephone follow-up after treatment. Although it is geared to individuals rather than groups and those in the hospital for acute care, it has shown that individuals have numerous questions when contacted, although they rarely initiated contact themselves even though encouraged to do so. Their most common concerns were not directly related to the disorder or illness for which they were treated but rather dealt with comfort and daily living.

For those individuals with frequent exacerbations of chronic disorders, a consistent and frequent telephone follow-up by the nurse and primary provider is helpful for general

Box 8-5 Telephone Communication Tips

1. Cultivate the skill of active listening for spoken and unspoken messages.
2. Use clear, slow speech at low pitch.
3. Speak clearly and directly into the telephone.
4. Eliminate or reduce background noises such as music or talking.
5. Maintain focus.
6. Remain open to cues.
7. Engage in complete assessment and avoid premature diagnosis.
8. Verify the elder's understanding of information.
9. Demonstrate sensitivity to and respect for racial-ethnic and cultural differences.
10. Provide telephone care with discretion and competence.
11. Terminate the call in a pleasant, cordial manner.
12. Document care.

From Guy DH: Telephone care for elders: physical, psychosocial, and legal aspects, *J Gerontol Nurs* 21(12):27, 1995.

discussion and problem solving. Anderson and colleagues (2000) studied and confirmed its positive impact on and effectiveness in integrating the continuum of care for rural elderly. They found that attentiveness to possible sensory impairments and interpersonal, cultural, and educational factors are important. They also caution that proper written documentation is a significant aspect of telephone care and counseling. Box 8-5 lists suggestions for increasing telephone follow-up effectiveness.

REHABILITATION AND RESTORATIVE CARE

Restorative care is rehabilitative care within a humanistic framework provided under the guiding assumption that the care and services are thoughtfully designed to capitalize on the individual client's needs and strengths in a manner that will help him or her achieve the "highest practicable level of function" (Klusch, 1995). We prefer the term *restorative* because it implies the capability of individual renewal, whereas the term *rehabilitative* seems to focus on restoration of function. This is actually a moot point that we bring out only because of our personal interpretation of meanings and because we always lean toward the elusive and away from the mechanical aspects of aging.

Considerations in Planning Rehabilitation Care

Rehabilitation is long term. During acute hospitalizations rehabilitative plans should begin. The following issues are important to consider:

1. The client is in a crisis when admitted to the hospital, and personal strengths are not always visible or easily assessed.
2. Client anxiety impairs learning during hospitalizations, yet clients are more motivated toward change when physical status is threatened.
3. Early discharge to home or a nursing home may impede continuation of rehabilitative efforts.
4. Multidisciplinary discharge planning must begin on admission, and a nurse or case manager should be assigned to each client who will need rehabilitation.
5. Twenty-four–hour rehabilitative focus is necessary; it is insufficient to consider physical therapy two or three times per day as "rehabilitation."

Medicare requirements influence inpatient hospital stays for rehabilitative care. A client's medical or surgical needs alone may not warrant inpatient hospital care, but hospitalization may nevertheless be necessary because of the client's need for rehabilitative services. A hospital level of care is required by a client needing rehabilitative services if that client needs a relatively intense program that requires a multidisciplinary, coordinated team approach to upgrade ability to function. Two basic requirements must be met for inpatient hospital stays for rehabilitation care to be covered by Medicare:

1. The services must be reasonable and necessary (in terms of efficacy, duration, frequency, and amount) for the client's condition.
2. It must be reasonable and necessary to furnish the care on an inpatient hospital basis, rather than in a less intensive facility such as a skilled nursing facility or on an outpatient basis.

Comprehensive nursing assessment is critical. Nursing assessment includes a comprehensive biopsychosocial history and a client care plan with long- and short-term goals. Weekly interdisciplinary team conferences are held to evaluate client progress and revision of goals. Discharge goals and family conferences are a part of these weekly conferences. The following services should be available to patients in acute rehabilitation programs:

1. Rehabilitation nursing
2. Physical therapy
3. Occupational therapy
4. Speech therapy
5. Social service
6. Discharge planning
7. Psychologists
8. Prosthetist and orthotist services
9. Audiology
10. Physician
11. Consultation with vocational rehabilitation specialists

When assessing individual needs it is important to focus on loss of function rather than the specific disease because therapeutic treatments will be designed to improve function (Box 8-6).

Legislation. The landmark Rehabilitation Act of 1973 was originally intended to provide rehabilitation services

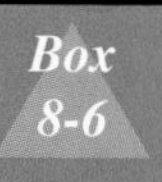

Box 8-6 Common Conditions and Diagnoses Appropriate for Home Health Rehabilitation Referrals

1. Patients who have sustained fractures of dislocations
2. Patients who have undergone orthopedic surgeries, including joint replacements or reconstructive surgeries
3. Patients suffering from degenerative joint or disk disease
4. Patients suffering from rheumatoid arthritis
5. Patients who have undergone amputations or require prosthetic training
6. Patients who have sustained burns with joint involvement or have physical impairment with an associated decrease in function
7. Patients who have suffered cerebral vascular accidents
8. Patients who have suffered head injuries or spinal cord injuries
9. Patients with multiple sclerosis
10. Patients with amyotrophic lateral sclerosis
11. Patients with Parkinson's disease
12. Patients with a decrease in function as a result of neuropathies and/or myopathies
13. Patients with chronic obstructive pulmonary disease who require postular drainage and teaching
14. Patients with cardiac impairment requiring cardiac rehabilitation
15. Patients with severe immobility as a result of any disease process requiring instruction to the caregiver in hoyer life transfers or any assistive device
16. Patients suffering from newly diagnosed blindness
17. Patients with head/neck cancer resulting in partial or total laryngectomies or glossectomies
18. Patients whose underlying disease process, illness, or injury has resulted in dysphagia
19. Patients suffering from a hearing loss

Source: Health Care Financing Administration: *Health insurance manual,* No. 11-T273, Washington, DC, rev 3/95, U.S. Department of Health and Human Services.

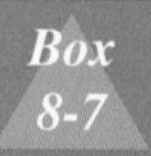

Box 8-7 Comparison of Disability Issues of Young and Old

Youth	Aged
Loss of attractiveness	Loss of role/status
Anxiety regarding future	Anxiety regarding dependency
Interference with social life	Fear of institutionalization
Loss of friendships	Loss of mobility
Rapid recuperation	Prolonged recuperation
Traumatic disabilities	Secondary incapacitation
High energy reserves	Diminished endurance
Resistance to infection	Compromised resistance
Lack of health care coverage	Fragmented benefits

Summarized from Frengley MB, Murray P, Wykle ML: Policy and philosophic issues. In *Practicing rehabilitation with geriatric clients*, New York, 1990, Springer.

regardless of whether or not the disabled recipient could be expected to return to gainful employment. The legislation also required alterations to provide access for the disabled to all institutions receiving any federal funding. Amendments in 1985 gave the National Council on the Handicapped independent status, which in effect gave it more strength and influence. The American Disabilities Act of 1990 went beyond that of 1973 to require physical and vocational access to private as well as federally funded businesses and vocational and educational institutions.

Three subgroups of disabled elderly are increasingly using rehabilitative medicine. The first two are those who are developmentally disabled and those who were traumatically disabled in childhood, who, because of medical advances, are for the first time in history remaining alive into old age. The third group, and by far the largest, is composed of individuals who suffer stroke or injury in later life and have been left with residual impairment following treatment or lack of treatment. The aged with long-standing physical disabilities to which they have adapted well may find that the adaptation sustained earlier may be more difficult in late life because of generally decreased functional ability and coping energy. The normal changes of aging must be incorporated into life patterns. It is important to recognize that the issues of the disabled elderly are distinct from those of the young (Box 8-7).

There is a fourth group, sometimes difficult to identify as such: those who have iatrogenically induced disabilities. These may be the result of aggressive, passive, or neglectful treatment patterns. Recent observations emphasize the need for intense and immediate rehabilitation efforts during acute illnesses to avoid prolongation, iatrogenic responses, and chronic sequelae. No longer is it appropriate to withhold rehabilitation procedures until the client is medically stable, particularly considering that Diagnosis Related Group (DRG)–incited early discharge patterns may then preclude rehabilitation in some settings. Thus professionals treating the early phases of an individual's disorder must be able to provide both necessary medical support and rehabilitation services to achieve maximum wellness potential (Melvin, 1988).

Rehabilitation Services. It is estimated that there are 5 million severely disabled persons over 65 years old in the United States today. Many could live independently with rehabilitative and supportive services, but because a return to employability is one driving force in rehabilitation, there may be little assistance available when there is no expectation of improvement. In fact, there is great variation among Medicare, Medicaid, HMOs, and private insurance regarding coverage for various services. Rehabilitation facilities are reimbursed through Medicare under the Tax Equity and Fiscal Responsibility Act (TEFRA) of 1982 at a flat rate regardless of diagnosis, length of stay, or other variables. Over half of those units are losing money. Given managed care and subacute developments, as well as numerous Health Care Financing Administration (HCFA) state waivers, it appears that the excellent rehabilitation units financed through TEFRA that flourished in the 1980s may be destined for abandonment.

The best of the geriatric rehabilitation units being developed now under various funding mechanisms are specially designed to foster function and teach individuals how to influence their environment to adapt to whatever their disability may be. These are also the units where health care providers become most acutely aware of the need for interdisciplinary teamwork and planning. Resnick and Fleishell (2002) report in the *American Journal of Nursing* on a "restorative care unit," developed by the Department of Medicine at the University of Maryland, that is designed to bridge the gap between acute care and home care. In the 6 years of the unit's existence, orthopedic procedures have been the major reason for admission to the unit. Individuals with joint replacements, fractures, stroke, amputations, and arthritis make up most of the unit's clientele. More than 86% of the individuals are discharged to home, and 80% of those are able to remain there for 2 years or longer. We expect many more restorative care units to emerge along the lines of this model. The National Council on the Handicapped recognizes the increasing problems of secondary and iatrogenically induced disabilities such as pressure sores, contractures, and cognitive impairment as important issues that must be considered in any future rehabilitation models.

Problems in Rehabilitation. Staff members who have worked intensively with the aged in rehabilitation settings have noted the following problems:

- The aged are reluctant to engage in activities that employ objects that are childish or seemingly irrelevant to daily tasks.
- Individuals suffering traumatic injury early in life are now living until old age; however, the problems they experience are exacerbated by the normal aging changes, such as bowel and bladder atony.
- Individuals who have taken care of others for much of their lives and are then stricken with a chronic disorder seem prone to develop excess disability reactions and lose motivation to participate in their own care. It seems as if they feel they have earned the right to be taken care of.
- Frustration, agitation, and irritation are often the overt expressions of the functionally impaired. Rather than focusing entirely on the visible symptoms, it may be more productive to establish groups to teach ways to enhance function. Memory training groups, sensorimotor skill training, and physical therapy are some of the methods of restoring the maximum potential of impaired persons. Remodeling of the environment for ease of adaptation and function should also be considered (Lapp, 1987).

Rehabilitation and the Future. Lack of education in rehabilitation among health care professionals in acute care settings results in inadequate care and even further disabilities. Most health care professionals poorly understand the potential of rehabilitative care. Better education, appropriate policies and protocols, and definitions of roles in rehabilitative care for allied health professionals are needed to bring rehabilitative care into the mainstream of the health care system. Services to Medicare beneficiaries with chronic diseases provide more than half the revenues of rehabilitation units and hospitals. Other sources of revenue are from the Disability Insurance Program (Supplemental Security Income [SSI]), Medicaid, workers' compensation programs, and private disability insurance plans. These need to be more extensive and inclusive.

Rehabilitative care providers often have difficulty demonstrating precise outcomes, because services are provided through multiple disciplines: medicine, physical and occupational therapy, speech therapy, nursing, and psychology. Consequently, outcome measures are extremely difficult to develop.

In the future, we expect wider acceptance of rehabilitation by all professionals and increased integration of its principles into all medical and social activities. Greater accountability will be expected of all professionals and institutions. This accountability will seek a balance between the resources expended and the practical outcomes achieved. Effective rehabilitation for aged disabled persons is consistent with the philosophy that all persons should have the opportunity for optimum personal development and function. The penalty for lack of accessibility to appropriate rehabilitation is increased dependence on family, nursing homes, or other care providers at an even greater cost to society. The agenda for rehabilitation in the twenty-first century includes increased numbers of rehabilitation hospitals, reimbursement, and rehabilitation educational programs.

Nurses advocating for the needs of the aged and disabled, armed with clinical examples, anecdotal evidence, and empirical research findings, have the power to affect the character of legislation proposed in the U.S. House of Representatives and Senate, as has been shown by the responsiveness of Congress to the lobbying power of nurses in Washington, DC. Cost-effectiveness is the strongest argument in today's political climate. The increased number of disabled elders who will be alive because of technologic advances but will require decades of rehabilitative services is an extremely important issue. How will their care be financed, and will services generally be available? What will happen to Medicare after 2010, and will exorbitant home care costs be sustainable? Numerous questions need answers very soon.

COMMON CHRONIC DISORDERS

Numerous textbooks on geriatric diseases and chronic illness are available as references. Although we may begin our patient encounter with the medical diagnosis given to the patient by the physician, we look beyond the diagnosis to the broader implications of chronic illness to the aged and their families, and thus to nurses. Given support, many elders with chronic disabilities can transcend the physical and emotional adversity of chronicity to maintain feelings of self-esteem and self-fulfillment. Expecting and reckoning with episodes of depression in all involved parties, claiming discouragement at times, and grieving for the lost capacities are all legitimate responses that should be expected in the search for meaning. Many persons have found meaning in suffering and have transcended physical limitations to discover values that those of us without physical disabilities cannot understand.

Certain disorders are encountered frequently enough among the old to merit special attention. Diabetes mellitus, stroke, pressure ulcers, incontinence, diverticulitis, coronary artery disease, congestive heart failure, vascular insufficiency, pernicious anemia, chronic obstructive pulmonary disease (COPD), asthma, tuberculosis, and polymyalgia rheumatica are among the most common chronic disorders. Osteoporosis, osteoarthritis, rheumatoid arthritis, and related disorders are dealt with in Chapter 13, rather than in this chapter, because they so often impair mobility. Parkinson's disease primarily produces problems with mentation and movement, so these are dealt with in Chapters 13 and 23. We do not intend to include comprehensive medical management of these disorders, but they will be addressed individually to focus on the holistic needs and nursing responses.

For medical management refresher and review we refer the reader to the excellent, detailed, and comprehensive *Merck Manual of Geriatrics*, third edition (Beers and Berkow, 2000). We also refer readers to the Agency for Health Care Policy and Research series of practice guidelines, now available at www.ahrq.gov. These provide algorithmic decision-making protocols for incontinence, heart failure, unstable angina, urinary incontinence, pressure ulcers, acute low back pain, and several other common conditions. They have been developed by panels of experts, including nurses, and can be obtained free of charge.

Diabetes Mellitus

As many as 20% of elders (8 million people) 65 years and older have diabetes (Daly, 2001). The Centers for Disease Control and Prevention (CDC) reports that in the past 10 years the incidence of diabetes mellitus (DM) rose 70% among those ages 30 to 39, by 40% in those ages 40 to 49, and by 31% in those ages 50 to 59. In the next decades, the incidence will be much higher than 20% of elders. At this time, over 50% of DM occurs in people older than 65 (Reed and Mooradian, 2002). About 90% of elders with DM have type 2 DM.

Definition. Diabetes is a number of complex disorders of metabolism that involve glucose intolerance (Piano and Huether, 2002). Diabetes mellitus is characterized by chronic hyperglycemia and disturbances of carbohydrate, fat, and protein metabolism. There are two major types of DM: type 1 DM, characterized by absolute lack of insulin due to autoimmune destruction of the insulin-producing pancreatic beta cells; and type 2 DM, characterized by diminished insulin secretion from beta cells and by insulin resistance, which results from impaired ability of insulin to decrease glucose production in the liver and to stimulate glucose uptake by skeletal muscle (Whitehead, 2002). Two other categories of DM are (in addition to gestational diabetes) impaired glucose tolerance (IGT) and impaired fasting glucose (IFG).

Risk Factors. The risk of developing type 2 DM increases with age, obesity, and lack of physical activity (American Diabetes Association, 2000). In some groups, it is considered an epidemic (Baldridge, 2001). The Pima Indians in southern Arizona have the highest known DM rates in the world; more than 80% of the tribe's elders are afflicted. The major risk factors for type 2 DM are as follows:

- Family history of diabetes
- Obesity—especially abdominal, the most powerful risk factor (more than 20% over desired body weight or body mass index [BMI] greater than 27 kg/m^2)
- Race/ethnicity—African Americans, Native Americans, Hispanic Americans, Asian Americans, Pacific Islanders
- Age greater than 45 years
- Polycystic ovary syndrome—increases risk sevenfold
- Inactivity
- High-carbohydrate, high-fat, low-fiber diet
- Syndrome X—a cluster of disorders such as hypertension, insulin resistance, high lipids, hyperinsulinism
- High-density lipoproteins (HDLs) less than 35 mg/dl or triglycerides greater than 250 mg/dl (or both)
- Chronic pancreatitis, especially in alcoholics

Clinical Signs and Symptoms. In elderly people, DM often has an atypical presentation (Reed and Mooradian, 2002). Because of this, older adults are often not diagnosed and are left untreated. Whereas polydipsia occurs in young patients, the presentation in elders is dehydration, confusion, delirium, obtundation, and decreased visual acuity. Glycosuria often causes incontinence. The catabolic state caused by lack of insulin causes polyphagia in younger persons but causes weight loss and anorexia in elders. It may also manifest as nonketotic hyperglycemic-hyperosmolar coma (NKHHC) (Beers and Berkow, 2000). Other vague signs and symptoms include fatigue, nausea, recurrent infections, delayed wound healing, and paresthesias (Piano and Huether, 2002). The presentation of DM in black patients is atypical (McCulloch, 2002). Ketosis occurs in obese blacks with type 2 DM. It is often mistakenly thought that ketosis occurs only in type 1 DM.

Recently, syndrome X (also called *metabolic syndrome*, *dysmetabolic syndrome*, or *insulin resistance syndrome*) has been described (Roseman, 2002). It is a network of atherogenic factors that, if not treated, ensure coronary artery disease and heart failure. The factors in the atherogenic network are described in Box 8-8. According to Brashears (2002), glucose intolerance, hyperinsulinemia, dyslipidemia, and obesity probably share a genetic etiology. There is a role of insulin resistance in atherogenesis and coronary artery disease,

Box 8-8 Syndrome X (Dysmetabolic Syndrome or Insulin Resistance Syndrome)

- Insulin resistance (or acanthosis nigricans)
- Central obesity (apple-shaped, not pear-shaped, body type)
- High-density lipoprotein less than 45 mg/dl in women, less than 35 mg/dl in men
- Triglyceride level greater than 150 mg/dl
- Hypertension
- Impaired fasting glucose or type 2 diabetes
- Hyperuricemia

Adapted from Boyle P: *Diabetes, part B*, presentation, Primary Care Updates, Oct 4-5, 2002, Cincinnati, OH.

although it is not clear what the role is other than that it is an important risk factor for heart disease. With syndrome X, multiple therapeutic interventions are prescribed to lower the risk of atherosclerotic heart disease, even when the client has no clinical evidence of diabetes. The diagnosis of syndrome X is described in Box 8-8 (Roseman, 2002). Interestingly, though about 18 million people have diabetes and another 22 million have IGT, it is estimated that about 36 million people have syndrome X (Robertson, 2001). The syndrome accelerates with age and with obesity.

Diabetes often hampers sexual function in men, and this presents a great psychologic problem for some. Fifty percent of men with diabetes develop erectile impotence because of reduction in vascular flow, peripheral neuropathy (PN), and uncontrolled plasma glucose. Orgasmic and ejaculatory capacity remain unchanged. The patient may need counseling regarding sexual activity modifications to provide satisfaction by alternative methods. Women seem to retain their sexual responsiveness and orgasmic capacity when diabetic.

Acute Complications. Hypoglycemia can occur by many causes, such as from exercise or alcohol intake. It occurs when blood glucose is less than 60 mg/dl (Piano and Huether, 2002). If the decrease is rapid, some elders will have signs and symptoms with blood glucose greater than 60 mg/dl. It occurs mainly in those taking insulin. The assessment may reveal tachycardia, palpitations, diaphoresis, tremors, pallor, and anxiety. Later symptoms may include headache, dizziness, fatigue, irritability, confusion, hunger, visual changes, seizures, and coma. Immediate care involves giving the patient glucose to avoid the late signs.

NKHHC manifests with very high plasma glucose levels. It may occur in the elder whose diabetes has not been diagnosed. Large amounts of fluid are then lost, causing volume depletion and dehydration. Physical findings include neurologic changes such as stupor, which correlates with the degree of hyperosmolarity (Piano and Huether, 2002).

Progressive Signs and Symptoms. Diabetes progresses via large vessel and small vessel disease (Reed and Mooradian, 2002). Large vessel complications include myocardial infarction, stroke, and peripheral vascular disease due to accelerated atherosclerosis. Small vessel complications include retinopathy, neuropathy, and nephropathy. Other common complications are foot ulcers, gastroparesis, impotence, glaucoma, cataracts, myopathy, and cognitive deficits.

Assessment. Physical examination of the newly diagnosed diabetic elder should be directed toward the associated acute and chronic complications. Assess for risk factors that can be modified. Hyperglycemia enhances the risk for macrovascular complications fivefold (Beers and Berkow, 2000). Hypertension and smoking increase the risk 10 to 20 times. Assess lipid levels because diabetics often have high low-density lipoprotein (LDL) levels.

Laboratory assessment. The laboratory assessment is used to diagnose and manage diabetes. Maintaining blood glucose at optimal levels is a major goal of diabetic management, and glycemic control is particularly important in the elderly person with diabetes. Many of the effects of diabetes occur before diagnosis. Even mildly elevated glucose levels cause retinopathy, neuropathy, and nephropathy. Obtain a microalbumin urinalysis to screen for the presence of nephropathy. Glycosylated hemoglobin (HbA_{1c}) should be monitored because it reflects the average blood-glucose level over time. The glucose tolerance test is not necessary in elderly patients (Reed and Mooradian, 2002). Other tests to order include urinalysis, blood urea nitrogen, creatinine, electrocardiogram (ECG), chest x-ray, and possibly a stress test (Mayhew et al, 2001).

Financial assessment. Another area of assessment should be financial. Many elders live on fixed incomes and cope with a number of chronic problems with high costs for medications and care. However, researchers in Scotland found that only one third of patients with type 2 DM have their prescriptions filled often enough to take at least 90% of the desired amount of medication (American Diabetes Association, 2002). In Scotland, prescription medications are purchased by the National Health Service, so compliance is not financially related.

Management of Diabetes. Good glucose control is primary. Maintaining the HbA_{1c} level at less than 7 is considered successful management (Cook et al, 2001). We know that the risk of complications is high even with mild hyperglycemia. The goal is a fasting blood glucose level below 120 mg/dl in healthy elders (Mayhew et al, 2001). Through management of diet, weight reduction, exercise, and drug therapies, blood glucose levels can usually be kept near normal levels. Experiential teaching, encouragement, and reinforcement of mastery are important factors that promote successful self-management.

Laboratory. Maintaining blood glucose at optimal levels is a major goal of diabetes management. In older individuals the determination of acceptable levels is not generally agreed on. Most adults maintain blood sugar between 60 and 130 mg/dl. For elders the norms are higher because the pancreas does not produce as much insulin, even in those without diabetes. The goal is to maintain levels that do not harm the

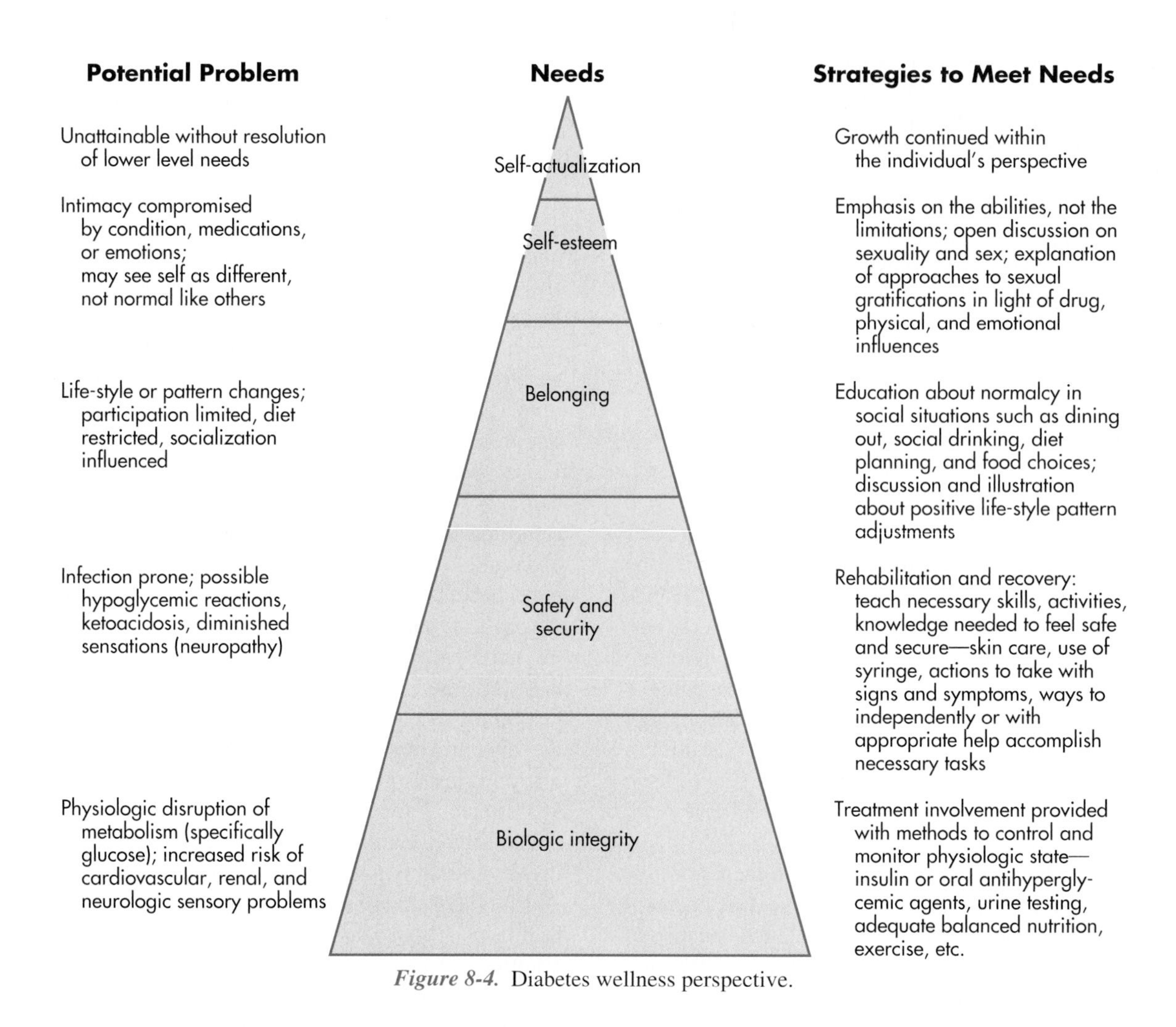

Figure 8-4. Diabetes wellness perspective.

blood vessels. Rather than become overly concerned about occasional blood glucose surges, it is recommended that glycosylated hemoglobin be monitored because it reflects the average blood glucose level over a 1- to 4-month period (Kee, 2001). Focusing on maintaining normal ranges of weight, blood pressure, and lipids is also important. Elders need to know that during times of illness or stress they may temporarily need insulin even though they usually manage well through nutritional control or oral medication. Figure 8-4 shows the management of diabetes mellitus from a wellness perspective.

Diet. The new American Diabetes Association guidelines focus on controlling glucose without restricting foods (American Diabetes Association, 2002). A healthful diet is a good diabetes diet. Again, the goal is keeping the glucose level under control through regular exercise; losing weight (if obese); limiting saturated fats in the diet; eating carbohydrates that are whole grains, fruits and vegetables, and low-fat milk—a healthful diet. Foods high in monounsaturated fats are thought to be good for patients with diabetes. The American Diabetes Association (2002) reports a study from the University of Texas in the mid-1990s that found that patients with diabetes "thrived" on this diet. Foods high in monounsaturated fats include nuts, avocados, and olive, canola, and peanut oils.

Self-care. A "Diabetes To-Do List" has been developed that may be useful to elders (Box 8-9). For good self-care, the elder must learn what affects the blood sugar level. Eating and drinking increase blood sugar. Therefore testing should occur before meals or 2 hours after meals and at bedtime. Exercise decreases blood sugar; the elder should test before and after exercise. Skipping a meal decreases blood sugar. Testing should occur if the elder feels clammy or cold, sweaty, shaky, or confused because these are signs of low blood sugar. Hypoglycemia is the most common problem for elderly diabetics. The elder should have a list of warning signs for high and low blood sugar levels. High blood sugar levels result in the following:

- Frequent urination
- Increased appetite
- Increased thirst, parched lips
- Fatigue, tiredness, or weakness
- Dry and itchy skin
- Flulike achiness
- Tachycardia

Box 8-9 Diabetes To-Do List

Every 3 Months
1. Visit health care provider
2. Have glycosylated hemoglobin checked (HbA_{1c})
3. Discuss prevention of high and low glucose levels and signs and symptoms of each
4. Discuss management of high and low glucose levels
5. Have health care provider check feet
6. Discuss any problems with diabetes management; discuss glucose goals
7. Visit podiatrist for foot care

Every Year
1. Visit dentist
2. Visit eye doctor to look for signs of diabetic eye disease
3. Have urine albumin/protein checked for signs of diabetic kidney disease
4. Have cholesterol and triglycerides checked
5. Ask health care provider how to manage any of the diseases that have developed, such as eye disease, kidney disease, or neuropathy of the feet, due to diabetes

The elder should have a good exercise plan for good self-care. Awareness of the need for good shoes that fit well is essential, as is self-examination of the feet on a regular basis. An identification bracelet is a consideration because confusion may be a manifestation of low blood sugar. Nutrition counseling should be made available on diagnosis, and a weight loss program should be undertaken if the elder is obese.

Medications. The mainstay of treatment of type 2 DM in elders is oral medication (Whitehead, 2002). Sulfonylureas and meglitinides increase insulin secretion. Insulin action is improved with biguanides or thiazolidinediones. One can delay or reduce the intestinal absorption of carbohydrates with alpha-glucosidase inhibitors and reduce absorption of fats with lipase inhibitors (e.g., orlistat). The last and rarely used treatment option is exogenous insulin. The preferred oral agents for elderly diabetics are glimepiride (the standard, given once per day), glipizide, glipizide XL, and tolbutamide (Tangalos, 2002). According to the Tangalos group, acetohexamide and chlorpropamide should not be used in elders. All patients with type 2 DM should be on an angiotensin-converting enzyme (ACE) inhibitor, according to the Joslin Diabetes Center (2001).

Herbal approaches to diabetes management were in place before the discovery of insulin in 1921. Approximately 400 different plants affect blood glucose, and many are still in use. Stevia is a sweet herb that is used as a sugar substitute. Fenugreek as a tea can induce a hypoglycemic response. Licorice and rosemary raise blood sugar but have the risk of overdose. Goldenseal, bilberry, and Spanish nettle lower blood sugar; the nettle has been used in Hawaii to treat type 2 DM, but it can be toxic. At least 30% of people (probably more) use herbals or alternative therapies. As health professionals, we need to know about the herbs and we need to ask our patients about usage. Further discussion is in Chapter 11.

Long-term effects. The long-term incidence of lower extremity amputation in the elder diabetic is over 7% and is higher in those who have a history of leg ulcers, higher diastolic pressure, high HbA_{1c}, proteinuria, and a 10-year history of diabetes (Moss, Klein, and Klein, 1996). In one study of over 300 people, 43% of elders with diabetes had PN, which impairs sensation and may result in foot injury and subsequent loss (Abrams, 2000). Further, prevalence increases with the duration of diabetes; an average of 49% of elders have PN more than 19 years after diagnosis. Nurses are well aware of the need for routine examination and care of the feet of diabetics. Evaluation of the foot should be done at a minimum of annually using a quantitative somatosensory threshold test, that is, the Semmes-Weinstein 5.07 (10 g) monofilament. Also, check peripheral pulses to assess vascular status. Some nurses are reluctant to provide foot care regardless of the patient's condition. However, when PN and ulceration are detected, the client should see a foot specialist.

In addition to PN and subsequent foot problems, many older diabetics die of myocardial infarction or stroke (O'Conner, 2001). Further, severe eye problems (leading to blindness) and kidney problems are long-term effects of poorly managed diabetes. In addition to maintaining a lowered glucose level, attention must be given toward preventing these problems by lowering lipid levels, stopping smoking, lowering blood pressure, starting exercise programs, and adding drugs that help prevent the problems. These may be ACE inhibitors, statins, minidose aspirin, and blood thinners if indicated.

Standards of Care for Patients with Diabetes Mellitus. The three most important evaluations recommended by the American Diabetes Association (2000) are regular medical visits (at least two office visits per year), annual lipid profiles, and a thorough annual ophthalmology examination. Nurses must advocate for elders and encourage them to demand quality care to prevent the devastating end results of poor management. The following evaluation is recommended:

- History should include dietary habits, weight patterns, previous treatment programs, current treatment regimen, exercise and activity levels, infections, illnesses, and complications of diabetes.
- Physical examination should include blood pressure; eye ground examination; thyroid palpation; auscultation of pulses; foot, periodontal, and skin examination; and neurologic examination.
- Laboratory tests should include fasting plasma glucose; glycosylated hemoglobin; fasting lipid profile; serum creatinine if proteinuria is present; urinalysis, including microalbuminuria, urine culture, and thyroid function (T_4 or thyroid-stimulating hormone [TSH]); and ECG.

Screening and Prevention. About one half of those with diabetes are undiagnosed (National Institutes of Health, 2001). A recent study that included more than 3000 prediabetic subjects, the Diabetes Prevention Program, gave lifestyle advice plus metformin to one group; gave advice plus placebo to another group; and gave intensive lifestyle advice, including encouragement to lose weight and get more exercise, to a third group (Health and Age, 2002). Nearly 3 years later, group 1 had a 58% lower incidence of diabetes compared with placebo (group 2); in group 3, the intensive lifestyle advice had a 31% lower risk for developing diabetes. This demonstrates that preventive medication and lifestyle changes both play an important role in lowering the risk of diabetes.

Stroke and its Consequences

Epidemiology. Stroke is the leading cause of long-term disability among adults in the United States. It is the third leading cause of death in the United States, behind heart disease and cancer (Sica, 2002). In the United States each year, about 750,000 people have a stroke, 150,000 of whom die (Beers and Berkow, 2000). Morbidity and mortality rates increase with age and increase greatly after age 65. Stroke occurs more frequently in men and in black persons. The complications of stroke are devastating. There may be impairment of walking, seeing, feeling, clotting, remembering, speaking, and thinking.

Strokes are cerebrovascular accidents that affect cerebral circulation through occlusive thrombi and emboli or, less often, hemorrhagic incidents occurring in the intracerebral or subarachnoid space. These variations account for differences in severity and symptoms. Hemorrhagic strokes are more life threatening but much less frequent than thrombotic strokes. Thrombotic strokes are most frequently a consequence of atrial fibrillation, which predisposes one to systemic emboli.

Risk Factors. Hypertension, hyperlipidemia, obesity, diabetes, and cardiac disease such as atrial fibrillation, valvular diseases, acute myocardial infarction, and having had a coronary artery bypass graft are the primary risk factors for stroke (Kistler et al, 2002). The risk of stroke with high blood pressure is very high. Other risk factors are smoking, use of amphetamines and hard drugs, overeating and undereating, severe fatigue, anemia, and bleeding problems (Beers and Berkow, 2000). A stroke risk worksheet is available from the National Institutes of Health, National Institute of Neurological Disorders and Stroke, via the Internet.

Prevention. The best approach to stroke, despite new therapies and medications, is prevention. Identifying high-risk or stroke-prone elders is something nurses can do in their own homes or at the health facilities where they work. Reducing the blood pressure 5 mm Hg in a hypertensive person reduces risk of stroke 34%; with reduction of 10 mm Hg, it is reduced 56% (Sica, 2002). The target blood pressure in elders is 130/85 mm Hg; however, any reduction should be done very slowly because the risk of stroke increases with rapid reduction.

When a patient has had a stroke, there is a high likelihood of another stroke. Therefore much attention needs to be given to preventing that next stroke (Sica, 2002). ACE inhibitors reduce risk of a second stroke by 28%. Other medications used to prevent further strokes include diuretics, beta-blockers, calcium channel blockers, and aspirin. However, it is known that women who take more than 15 aspirin tablets per week are twice as likely to have a hemorrhagic stroke, especially if they also have high blood pressure (American Stroke Association, 2002).

We have all seen someone turn "purple" with rage or distress and thought, "He's going to have a stroke if he doesn't calm down." A recent study has determined that abrupt changes in body position can trigger a stroke; sharing this information with clients and their family members may prevent such an incident (Koton, 2002). Emotional stress, anger, sudden physical effort, sudden change in temperature, sudden change in body position, and sudden movement, such as jumping when the doorbell rings, can all trigger a stroke in a susceptible person. The highest-risk trigger was sudden change in body position or posture, followed by negative anger or stress.

One study revealed that moderate alcohol consumption is protective for ischemic stroke (Sacco et al, 1999). Moderate alcohol consumption (up to two drinks per day) had a protective effect in the study's nearly 700 subjects (an elderly, multiethnic, urban population). Heavy alcohol consumption, however, has deleterious effects, and increases the risk of hemorrhagic stroke.

Transient Ischemic Attacks. *Transient cerebral ischemia* is defined as the sudden onset of a focal neurologic symptom or sign that lasts less than 24 hours; 75% last less than 5 minutes. The cause may be interrupted blood flow or vasospasm of brain arteries. The flow is usually restored in time to avoid a brain infarction. However, when the symptoms last for more than 1 hour, there has been some infarction. Transient ischemic attacks (TIAs) may herald a stroke (Beers and Berkow, 2000); however, most strokes are not preceded by TIAs (American Stroke Association, 2002). Symptoms and signs of TIA and stroke include the following:

- Sudden weakness or numbness on one side of the body (face, arm, or leg)
- Dimness or loss of vision in one eye
- Slurred speech, loss of speech, difficulty comprehending speech
- Dizziness, difficulty walking, loss of coordination, balance, a fall
- Sudden severe headache
- Difficulty swallowing
- Sudden confusion
- Nausea and vomiting

To prevent a stroke from occurring, endarterectomy or stent placement should be considered in those with greater than 70% carotid stenosis. Warfarin therapy should be used in those with atrial fibrillation. Aspirin, 30 to 325 mg/day, is the mainstay of therapy for elders with TIAs because it reduces the incidence 15% to 25% (Kistler et al, 2002). However, for those who are aspirin sensitive, clopidogrel or ticlopidine may be used (Reuben et al, 2002).

Management. An acute stroke can be diagnosed with a computed tomography (CT) scan. Thrombolytic therapy (tissue plasminogen activator or eptifibatide) may be started immediately by paramedics in some areas of the United States. If there is delay in administration of more than 3 hours, there is often "little brain to salvage" because most damage (90%) occurs in the first 3 hours (Flanagan, 2001; Saver, 2002). Newer drugs for management (experimental) include citicoline, which is neuroprotective and neuroreparative; magnesium; and erythropoietin, which is antiinflammatory and neuroprotective.

Recovery. Stroke is one of the most traumatic medical events one can face (Flanagan, 2001). Recovery from stroke is affected by the location and extent of the cerebrovascular accident. Difficulties and handicaps following stroke often involve neurologic and functional aspects. A common complication of acute stroke is deep vein thrombosis (DVT) in a flaccid lower limb (Young and Hoffberg, 2001). Aspiration pneumonia occurs and is often "silent." A speech therapy evaluation early in the recovery period will uncover this problem. Spasticity is also a common occurrence after stroke. Low-dose baclofen is commonly used in rehabilitation centers to treat this. Dantrolene sodium is also used. Spasticity can lead to contractures if it is not managed.

About 90% of neurologic recovery occurs within 3 months of the stroke; 10% occurs more slowly, especially in those with hemorrhagic stroke (Beers and Berkow, 2000). At 18 months following the stroke there tends to be a small decline. The inverse relationship between functional improvement and advanced age, social isolation, and emotional distress is clear. Up to one third of stroke victims become profoundly depressed in the year following stroke. Improvements in functional performance tend to be seen mainly in severely and moderately disabled patients. Some of the methods of measuring characteristic functional disorders of the poststroke patient are listed in Box 8-10.

Curly, a 72-year-old African American, is admitted with a stroke and has a right hemiparesis. Nell, the nurse, says "Good morning," but Curly raises his eyebrows and with his left hand points toward the bathroom; with frustration, he mutters some fragmented speech. He reaches out with his left hand and slaps at the siderail. He has become very agitated and unable to say any word intelligibly.

Nurses are becoming aware of the devastation a stroke produces because they have experienced it and have written about it from a personal perspective. Curly has a number of problems, including aphasia and weakness on his right side, due to a left frontal lobe stroke, often from obstruction of the middle cerebral artery. The anxiety and depression that will probably result cause further problems in his rehabilitation.

Assessment of Needs. Nowhere in the care of elders is the multidisciplinary team more essential than in the evaluation of the needs of an elder following stroke. We know now that this must be done as soon as the individual is physiologically stabilized in order to maximize the benefits of interventions. See Box 8-10 for some of the disabilities that follow stroke and how to test for them. The assessment of needs following stroke is extremely complex; it requires evaluation by a team that is often coordinated by nursing: a neurologist; a physiatrist; speech, occupational, and physical therapists; an ophthalmologist; a rehabilitation specialist; a psychologist; and an environmental planner. Caretakers of the patient must be included at every stage of planning, as well as the elder to every extent possible. An important role for nursing is documenting clearly and in detail the functional capacities that are retained and those that are impaired. The assessment must be redone routinely to carefully evaluate and document areas of progress and areas of need.

Nurses must be active in preventing skin breakdown, preventing falls, identifying confusion, monitoring the lungs for

Box 8-10 Tests of Specific Disabilities That Commonly Follow Stroke

Hemianopia (Loss of Part of Visual Field)

Sitting opposite patient, hold up simultaneously two pens of different colors 30 cm in front of patient and 30 cm apart; patients with hemianopia will be unable to see one of the pens or may turn head toward hemianopic side in an effort to see.

Proprioception (Awareness of Body in Space)

The wrist of the affected arm is held between the thumb and forefinger of the examiner; patient's hand is raised and lowered and patient, with closed eyes, is asked the position of the hand; this exercise can also be done with fingers to determine even more specific loss of proprioception.

Sensation (Feeling Generated by Sensory Receptors)

With patient's eyes closed the examiner strokes the back of the unaffected hand and then the affected hand and in both cases asks the patient to describe the sensation. The affected side may have varying degrees of loss of sensation or total loss of feeling.

Balance (Bodily Poise)

Patient asked to sit on side of bed with feet off floor and maintain balance and sit unaided for 1 minute; it is usually readily apparent if individual has a problem maintaining balance.

Arm Function (Range of Motion and Control)

Patient asked to lift affected arm to shoulder height and press against examiner's upheld hand:

- Complete paralysis = inability to move arm
- Severe weakness = can move arm but not lift up or push
- Moderate weakness = able to lift arm but unable to push
- Slight weakness = able to do task requested but cannot push as hard as with unaffected arm
- No weakness = no difference in abilities of either arm

Data summarized from Anderson R: *The aftermath of stroke: the experience of patients and their families,* Cambridge, 1992, Cambridge University Press.

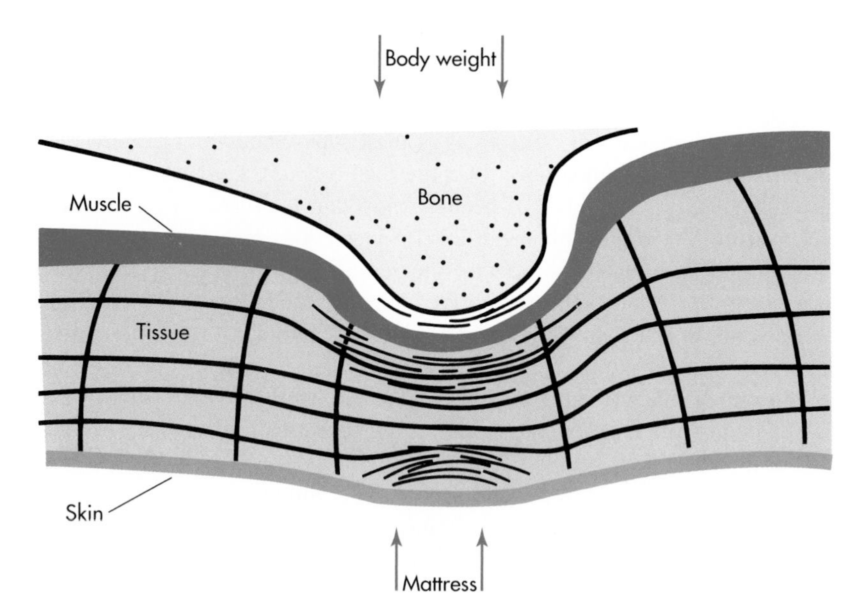

Figure 8-5. Tissue under pressure.

pneumonia, helping with ambulation, dealing with eating and feeding problems, maintaining fluids, managing incontinence, and identifying sleep problems (Beers and Berkow, 2000). The Barthel Index is a useful tool for assessing activity of the elder and is readily available on the Internet. Assess for depression, which is common after a stroke. The discharge plan is complex and should be started at the time of diagnosis. The elder is included in this plan because he or she needs to be willing to have a caretaker such as a nursing assistant in the home. There will be medications to take, food to be prepared, appointments to arrange to get to, and continuing passive and active therapy at home.

Stroke Support. Group support for victims of stroke can provide an environment for problem solving and feedback, acceptance, and encouragement from others with similar limitations and struggles to relearn. When members have great difficulty verbalizing, it may be useful and relieve some tension to have part of each group meeting time designed toward nonverbal expressions such as art, music, or psychomotor activities. It would be useful to have a nurse with neurosurgical, gerontologic, and rehabilitation expertise. When such specialized nurses are not available, it may be best to have cofacilitators whose combined skills most closely align with members' biopsychosocial needs.

New support services on the horizon are primary stroke centers. The major elements of a stroke center are patient care areas, acute stroke teams, written care protocols, emergency medical services, stroke unit, neurologic service, support services, a stroke center director with support from the medical organization, neuroimaging services, laboratory services, outcome and quality improvement activities, and continuing education (Brain Attack Coalition, 2001).

Pressure Sores (Pressure Ulcers)

Definition. Pressure sores, or pressure ulcers as they are also called, tend to be a chronic problem of debilitated elders who are mainly bed or chair bound or unable to reposition themselves. The pressure ulcer is a localized area of tissue necrosis that develops when soft tissue is compressed against a bony prominence and an external surface for a long period of time. Pressure ulcers are the consequence of skin breakdown, pressure, friction, shearing, and maceration. They can develop anywhere on the body but most frequently occur from the waist down. See Figure 8-5 for how pressure ulcers develop.

Epidemiology. The prevalence is 1.8 million elders, 10% to 23% of nursing home patients in long-term care settings (Nutrition Screening Initiative, 2001) and 10% to 29% of patients in acute care settings. The prevalence is 41% of critical care patients and about 13% of home care patients (Beers and Berkow, 2000; Cobb and Durfee, 2002). Seventy percent of pressure sores occur in elders older than 70 (Tangalos, 2002). The cost of pressure ulcers is estimated to be nearly $1.5 billion per year.

Risk Factors. Risk for the development of pressure ulcers is associated with severity of illness, involuntary weight loss with decreasing immune status, dehydration, incontinence and catheter use, history of pressure ulcers, diabetes, male sex, and dependency in more than seven ADLs (Nutrition Screening Initiative, 2001). The first two factors account for 74% and 42%, respectively, increased risk. Other factors identified include immobility, old age with decreased hormone levels, dementia, and extended hospitalization or nursing home stay (Cobb and Durfee, 2002). With involuntary weight loss the risk increases by 74%. Other authors contribute more risk factors: decreased level of consciousness, smoking, corticosteroid use, anemia, infections, peripheral vascular disease, edema, stroke, alcoholism, fractures, and malignancies (Beers and Berkow, 2000).

Staging, Assessment, and Management. Pressure sores are staged in four categories (Figure 8-6). Stage I can heal rapidly with avoidance of pressure and modification of risk factors (Ferrell, 2002). Stage II can resolve quickly with

Stage I

Erythema not resolving within thirty (30) minutes of pressure relief. Epidermis remains intact. REVERSIBLE WITH INTERVENTION.

Epidermis
Grade I
Dermis
Subcutaneous fat
Muscle

Stage II

Partial-thickness skin loss involving epidermis. May penetrate the dermis superficially. Presents as bulla or blister with erythema and/or induration. Wound base moist, pink, and painful.

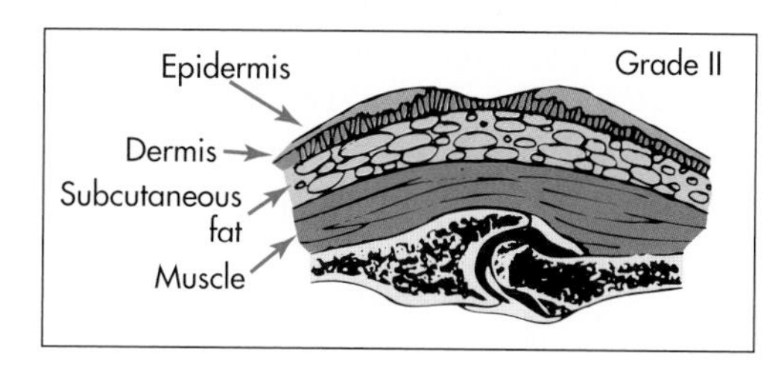

Stage III

Full-thickness tissue loss extending through dermis to involve subcutaneous tissue. Presents as shallow crater unless covered by eschar. May include necrotic tissue, undermining, sinus tract formation, exudate, and/or infection. Wound base is usually not painful.

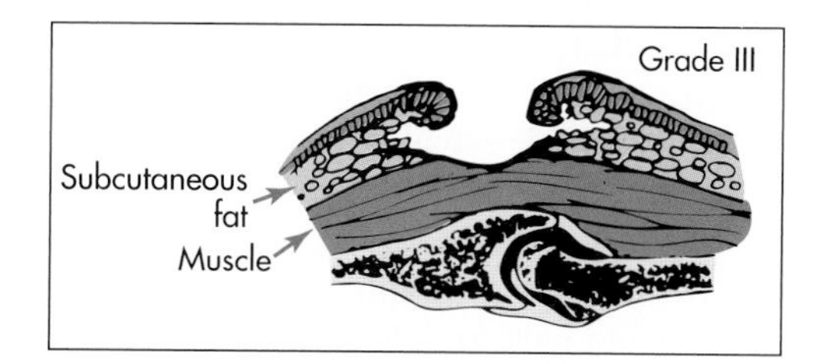

Stage IV

Deep tissue destruction extending through subcutaneous tissue to fascia and may involve muscle layers, joint and/or bone. Presents as a deep crater. May include necrotic tissue, undermining, sinus tract formation, exudate and/or infection. Wound base is usually not painful.

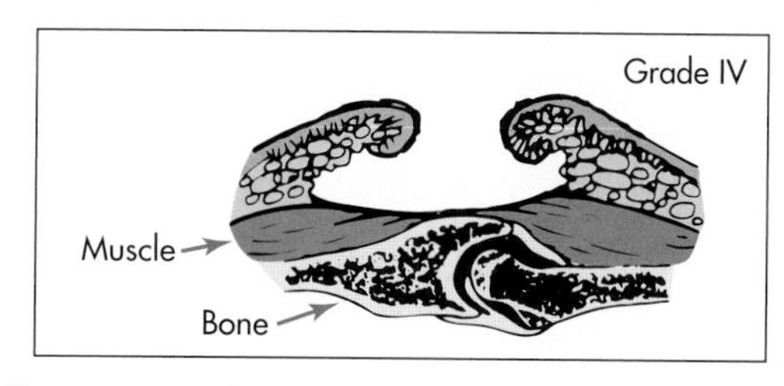

Figure 8-6. Pressure sore development.

avoidance of pressure, modification of risk factors, and treatment with a moist, flat, nonocclusive dressing. Stage III manifests as a deep crater and requires topical antiinfective agents such as bacitracin-polymyxin ointment (preferred) if the ulcer does not heal in 2 to 3 weeks or if it appears infected (Tangalos, 2002). Before treatment, obtain a culture and sensitivity. The pressure sore may require enzymatic debridement; however, this is not done on heel ulcers. Coverage against gram-negative, gram-positive, and anaerobic organisms should be administered, avoiding topical antiseptics. Stage IV ulcers are large and deep and often require surgical debridement of necrotic tissue, opening pockets for drainage and irrigation of the site, and possibly skin grafting (Huether, 2002). However, chemical debriding may be tried using proteolytic enzymes, especially if the elder is not a good candidate for surgery. The preferred enzyme is collagenase or papain-urea applied once per day. Collagenase is better tolerated, but papain-urea with or without chlorophyll has better action (Tangalos, 2002). Stage IV ulcers may result in extensive tissue destruction and osteomyelitis.

Primary areas of breakdown in the posterior aspects include the occiput, spine, sacrum, ischium, and heels (Ferrell, 2002). Lateral areas of breakdown include the trochanter, lateral condyles of the knee, and ankle. The pinna of the ears is another common lateral aspect for breakdown, as are the elbows and scapulae. If one is lying prone, the knees, shins, and pelvis sustain undue pressure. It is particularly important to consider the underside of the scrotum and inspect it for pressure and excoriation. This area is subject to the friction and shearing forces of the sheets without the benefit of a pull sheet. The warm, moist tissue is particularly susceptible to bacterial action from sustained moisture and soil.

The Braden Scale (Bergstrom, Allman, and Alvarez, 1994), the Norton Risk Assessment Scale (Norton et al, 1962), and Gosnell's Scale, which is a refinement of the Norton Scale, are risk assessment tools used frequently in the clinical setting in predicting individuals at risk for pressure sores. Because development of pressure sores is a dynamic process, it requires constant vigilance and reassessment. The use of either the Braden Scale or others provides the means for a systematic evaluation and periodic reevaluation of a person's risk for pressure sores. See the Braden Scale in Appendix 8-B.

Nurses play a vital role in the prevention of pressure sores, and prevention is much better than treatment. They must be able to identify early signs and initiate appropriate interventions to prevent further skin breakdown and to promote healing. Failure to do this jeopardizes the health and life of the elderly person. Pressure sores are costly to treat and may require extended separation from friends and loved ones. For many it can prolong recovery and extend rehabilitation. The acquisition of iatrogenic complications such as pressure ulcers and complications from them such as the need for grafting or amputation, sepsis, and even death may lead to legal action by the individual or his or her representative against the caregiver.

Visual and tactile inspection is essential to establish a normal skin characteristic baseline for a particular patient. We highly recommend photographic recording along the trajectory of development and healing (Box 8-11). Photographic documentation and inspection should include actual and potential areas for breakdown, with special attention directed to specific areas when an individual uses orthotic devices such as corsets, braces, prostheses, postural supports, splints, slings, and casts. Visual inspection should look for hyperemia; if it is present, the area should be rechecked in an hour. Even though it is more difficult to see hyperemia in dark-skinned people, a red tone can be detected no matter how dark the skin may be (Giger and Davidhizar, 1991).

A nutrition assessment and serum albumin should be obtained. A serum albumin below 3.5 g/dl, total lymphocyte count below $1800/mm^3$, or body weight loss of greater than 15% is considered malnutrition (Bates-Jensen, 1998). Malnutrition diminishes the immune response, and nutritional supplementation should be considered. Adequate nutritional intake should be monitored, as well as the serum albumin level, hematocrit, and hemoglobin. Diets high in protein, carbohydrates, and vitamins are necessary to maintain and promote tissue growth. Supplements of vitamin B help in the metabolism of carbohydrates, and pyridoxine and vitamin C assist in protein use. Bergstrom and colleagues (1994) have developed a clinical practice guideline for the treatment of pressure ulcers. A goal of nurses is to help maintain skin integrity against the various environmental, mechanical, and chemical assaults that are potentials for skin breakdown. For those elders who are independent, mobile, and active, an appropriate nursing diagnosis would be health maintenance of skin integrity. For those in dependent-care situations not only is the nursing diagnosis of actual impaired skin integrity pertinent, but a nursing diagnosis of potential for impaired skin integrity is also germane.

Interventions. Nursing interventions should focus on prevention: actions that eliminate friction and irritation to the skin by lifting, turning, placing, and rolling (using two or more persons) the patient; reducing moisture; and displacement of body weight from prominent areas to facilitate circulation to the skin. Turning every 2 hours is not sufficient.

Interventions for prevention and early skin care treatment are presented in Box 8-12. Mechanical and surface support apparatus are discussed in Table 8-2. Common types of topical agents and dressings used in the treatment of pressure sores are presented in Table 8-3. It should be remembered that solutions such as alcohol, certain soaps, iodine, and hydrogen peroxide are damaging to newly formed, fragile skin. It should also be noted that wounds heal best in their own natural environment (clean, moist, normal pH). Never occlude an infected wound.

Consultation with a wound care specialist is advisable for wounds that do not follow the pattern of healing. These consultants are experienced nurses or nurse practitioners who often work with surgeons and may consult in nursing homes, offices, or clinics.

Box 8-11 General Skin Assessment Guidelines

- General inspection:
  - Exposed body parts
    - Color: generalized with regard to light- and dark-skinned individuals; variations
  - Unexposed parts (if individual is inactive, confined to bed or chair)
- General palpation:
  - Texture, temperature, moisture, turgor, edema
  - Inspection and palpation of lesions
    - Size, location, mobility, consistency, pattern, type (primary/secondary)
  - Hair: inspection and palpation
    - Color, amount, distribution, texture, parasites
  - Scalp: inspection and palpation
    - Texture, lesions
  - Nails: inspection and palpation
    - Color, shape, texture, condition of nail bed

Polymyalgia Rheumatica and Giant Cell Arteritis

Epidemiology. The average age of onset of polymyalgia rheumatica (PMR) is 65 to 70 years (Woolley, 2002), and the incidence increases with age. Both PMR and giant cell arteritis (GCA) are common in elders. GCA may be seen in more than one third of elders with PMR at some time in the course of the disorder. About one half of those with GCA will develop PMR. PMR occurs more often in older women than men (2:1) and is seen more in whites in the United States and Europe; it is uncommon in blacks.

Definition. PMR is a chronic inflammatory disease characterized by an insidious onset of stiffness and moderate to severe aching pain of the neck, shoulders, and hips that lasts longer than 30 minutes in the morning. It may be so severe that the elder cannot get out of bed. GCA is a granulomatous inflammation of the aorta and its branches

Box 8-12 Interventions by Risk Factor

Bed or Chair Confinement
Inspect skin at least once daily.
Bathe when needed for comfort or cleanliness.
Prevent dry skin.

Bed confinement
Change position at least every 2 hours.
Use a special mattress that contains foam, air, gel, or water.
Raise head of bed as little and for as short a time as possible.

Inability to Move
Bed confinement
Place pillow under legs from midcalf to ankles to keep heels off bed.

Loss of Bowel and Bladder Control
Clean skin as soon as soiled.
Assesss and treat urine leaks.
If moisture cannot be controlled:
- Use absorbant pads and/or briefs with a quick-drying surface.
- Protect skin with a cream or ointment.

Poor Nutrition
Eat a balanced diet.
If a normal diet is not possible, talk to health care provider about nutritional supplements.

Lowered Mental Awareness
Choose preventive action that applies to person with lowered mental awareness. For example: if person chair-bound, refer to specific prevention action as outlined in the above risk factors.

Chair confinement
Change position every hour.
Use foam, gel, air, cushion to relieve pressure.
Reduce friction by:
- Lifting rather than dragging when repositioning.
- Using corn starch on skin.

Avoid use of donut-shaped cushions.
Participate in a rehabilitation program.

Chair confinement
Reposition every hour *if unable* to do by self.
Shift weight and position at least every 15 minutes *if able* to do by self.
Use pillows or wedges to keep knees or ankles from touching each other.

From *Clinical practice guidelines, preventing pressure ulcers, a patient's guide*, Rockville, MD, 1992, U.S. Department of Health and Human Services, Public Health Service, Agency for Health Care Policy and Research.

and the cranial arteries. It is often called *temporal arteritis* or *cranial arteritis* because these arteries are often involved. Both disorders are immunologic and systemic. The serum from each contains circulating immune complexes when the diseases are active. There is a strong relationship between the two diseases.

Clinical Signs and Symptoms. The systemic manifestations of both disorders include low-grade fever, weight loss, malaise, fatigue, depression, myalgias, and arthralgias. They begin and progress slowly over time in most cases, but may develop rapidly in some elders. Symptoms in PMR may be unilateral at onset, but eventually they become bilateral. There may be limited range of motion. Early symptoms of GCA are similar to those of flu but may include headache, pain in the temples, double vision or blurred vision, ptosis, and transient or permanent blindness; blindness may occur early or late in the disease process. Jaw and tongue pain occurs in about one half of patients. GCA can also occur in large arteries such as the subclavian or the aorta.

Diagnosis. An elevated erythrocyte sedimentation rate (ESR) or C-reactive protein is the most typical manifestation of both disorders; however, the ESR can be elevated in any inflammatory state such as arthritis. With PMR, the health care provider must suspect the disorder because the diagnosis is made clinically from symptoms in addition to a positive ESR and ruling out other diseases such as rheumatoid arthritis. If an elder is diagnosed with PMR, GCA should be suspected immediately because of the possibility of blindness occurring without treatment. If it is suspected because of a tender or red temporal artery or other signs, a biopsy of the temporal artery should be taken. It should be suspected in an elder with new-onset headache, because headaches are not common in elderly people. Those elders with GCA of the larger vessels may have a negative temporal artery biopsy, making diagnosis difficult. Diagnostic criteria exist for GCA and PMR; those for GCA are highly sensitive and specific (Box 8-13).

Management. The laboratory data may be followed periodically to determine quiescence or relapse. The mainstay therapy for both problems is glucocorticoids. Therapy for PMR may continue for 1 to 2 years, although the patient feels better almost immediately after treatment begins. In some cases of PMR, methotrexate will need to be added. The side effects of steroid therapy can be problematic, especially osteoporosis, increased susceptibility to infection, and increased glucose levels. Efforts should be made to lower the dose to the optimum level that suppresses symptoms. Relapse is common if therapy is lowered too quickly (Hunder, 2002). Elders with GCA also need steroid therapy, and at higher doses than those used for PMR.

Bisphosphonates should be given to prevent bone loss and fractures, which are not uncommon in elders treated for PMR and GCA. Calcium and vitamin D are also important. Follow blood glucose levels for onset of diabetes. If the elder has diabetes already, there will need to be a change in therapy.

Table 8-2 Mechanical Loading and Support Apparatus

Apparatus	Indications	Advantages	Disadvantages
Convoluted foam pad (high density, solid, 3 to 4 in foam pad)	Those patients whose activity limitation is short lived (postoperative; those in OR undergoing lengthy procedures)	Inexpensive, lightweight, comfortable	Minimum pressure relief, may cause retention of body heat (increasing moisture; possible maceration); fire hazard—many emit lethal fumes if ignited
Vinyl air-filled mattress (inflates and deflates air cells at regular intervals by electric pump)	Those at high risk for skin breakdown; those with stage I or II pressure sores	Mechanically alters the points of pressure against body; provides a moderate degree of protection against pressure; decreases maceration if mattress has air vents; lightweight; easily cleaned if wet or soiled	Minimizes but does not prevent pressure; uncomfortable because feels lumpy; costly because of electric pump operation
Water mattress (heavy vinyl, water-filled mattress placed on top of bed mattress)	Those at high risk for stage I, II, or III pressure sores; those who already have stage I, II, or III pressure sores	Distributes patient's weight evenly; provides moderate protection against pressure; comfortable; easy to maintain; easy to clean if wet or soiled	Minimizes but does not prevent pressure; heavy when filled (130-150 lb) costs approximately the same as an air mattress
Air-fluidized bed (Clinitron, Fluid Air, Mediscus Heavy Duty System)	Those patients with any stage of pressure sore, especially stage III or IV; those undergoing graft or flap surgery	Supports patient at subcapillary closing pressure (<15 to 33 mm Hg); maximum protection against pressure, shearing, friction, maceration; comfortable	Has fixed height; immovable head; patient transfer from bed difficult; unable to maintain a semi-Fowler's position to eat or if there are pulmonary problems; equipment heavy (1800 lb); circulating warm air may dehydrate patient and wound; turning of patient difficult (bed moves and molds) claim is that less turning is necessary; however, it creates risks of immobility; respiratory, mobility, and renal problems, and flexion contractures if not turned or range-of-motion exercises done frequently; rental equipment—expensive fee/day; difficult to adapt to home care Expensive rental fee
Alternating air mattress (some have vents that allow air between mattress and client)	High risk for stage I and II pressure ulcers	Moderate protection against pressure and shearing; decreased maceration; lightweight; easy to clean	Expensive; does not prevent pressure; uncomfortable
Low-air loss bed (Flexicair, Mediscus Air Support System) (air-filled cushions arranged in segmented configuration that fit into hospital bed)	Same as above	Exerts lowest pressure for patient's weight, height, and body type; uniformly supported over a maximum area with little pressure on bony prominences; bed may be raised or lowered; easy patient transfer in and out of bed; provides low pressure; decreases friction and shearing; prevents moisture buildup; reduces dehydration; patient can sit in semi-Fowler's position	
Adjunctive devices			
Sheepskin	Those who may be predisposed to skin breakdown from friction (e.g., under heels)		
Heel and elbow protectors (pads of sheepskin)	Those needing protection from friction		
Trapeze	Those who have upper arm strength and the ability to grasp	Allows patient to move or shift weight independently or assist with moving	

Compiled from Bergstrom N, Allman RM, Alvarez OM: *Treatment of pressure ulcers, clinical practice guidelines*, no 15, pub no 95-0652, Rockville, MD, 1994, U.S. Department of Health and Human Services, Public Health Service, Agency for Health Care Policy and Research; Pajk M: Pressure sores. In Abrams WB, Beers MH, Berkow R. editors: *The Merck manual of geriatrics*, ed 3, Whitehouse Station, NJ, 2000, Merck Research Laboratories.

Table 8-3 Dressings and Topical Agents in the Treatment of Pressure Sores

Type	Description	Action	Guidelines	Advantages	Disadvantages
Liquid barriers (e.g., United Skin Prep, Tegaderm)	Contains plasticizing agents and alcohol applied as spray, wipe, or roll-on	Protective waterproof coating over affected areas; reduces maceration and shearing	Gently clean, rinse, and dry skin; apply and allow to dry for 1 minute (will momentarily sting excoriated skin)	Does not irritate, unaffected by urine, perspiration, or digestive acids; dissolvable by soap solution	High alcohol content causes stinging; fragile skin may be inadvertently pulled
Film dressings (e.g., Biooclusive, Tegaderm, Op-Site)	Polymer based; permeable to gases and vapors but not to fluids	Healing occurs more quickly in a moist environment; maintains wound exudate against the wound surface, promoting epithelial cell migration across wound	Wound and surrounding tissue cleansed and dried to enable dressing to adhere; needs a 1-inch margin around the wound; do not stretch dressing tightly over wound, this creates shearing against tissue	Oxygen can get to tissue but contaminated fluid cannot; can be left on wound for 5-7 days if wound is not infected	Excessive exudate may collect under dressing; aspirate it out via small-bore needle through dressing
Hydrocolloid dressings (e.g., DuoDerm, Tegasorb, Restore)	Inert hydroponic polymers containing fluid-absorbing hydrocolloid particles, occlusive	When hydrocolloid particles contact wound exudate, they swell and form moist gel; optimal wound healing occurs in a closed, moist environment	Cleanse and dry wound and surrounding skin; dressing to extend 1.5 inches beyond the wound	Promotes cell migration, cleaning, debridement, and granulation; dressing may be left in place 7 days unless leakage occurs	Not usable if infection is present; may initially enlarge the wound because of debridement properties
Debriding enzymes (e.g., Comfeel Powder, Panafil, Accuzyme, Collagenase, Santyl)	Protolytic and fibrinolytic agents	Acts against devitalized tissue	Enzymes must be in contact with wound substrate; some enzyme preparations must be reconstituted every 24 hours (Elase powder) for each use; povidone-iodine, hexachlorophene, silver nitrate, and hydrogen peroxide inhibit action of Travase	Chemical debridement; useful as an adjunct to mechanical or surgical debridement	Must remove hardened or dry eschar; antibacterial and antiseptic inhibit enzyme
Absorption dressings (e.g., Comfeel Powder, Chronicure, Bard Absorption Dressing, HydraGran)	Hydrophilic beads, grains, flakes	Absorbs excess exudate	Reconstituted per directions; packed into wound; covered with dry dressing	Absorbs excess exudate and necrotic debris; deodorizes wound; keeps wound moist	Need to change once or twice a day; not effective on dry eschar
Hydrogels (e.g., Curafil, Carrington gel, Geliperm, Nu-gel)	Polymers	Absorbs exudate to form water-soluble gelatinous substance	Cleanse and dry wound; hydrogel may be refrigerated for patient comfort; dressing should extend 1.5 inches beyond wound	Dressing may be left on 1-3 days if remains intact; provides a moist environment for wound healing; use with Urgosorb results in better healing	Occasionally causes maceration of surrounding tissue
Calcium alginate dressings (e.g., Sorbsan, Kaltostate, Calcicure, Urgosorb)	Natural polysaccharides from brown seaweed dye; high-quality textile fiber pad; provides a moist environment	Absorbs 20 times its weight in exudate	Wound irrigated with normal saline; dry dressing	As wound heals can be left on longer, for up to several days; on contact with wound exudate forms a soft gas-permeable gel	Alginate as forms gel emits seaweed odor (a charcoal pad can be placed over outer gauze dressing to absorb odor)

Box 8-13 Criteria for Diagnosis of Giant Cell Arthritis and Polymyalgia Rheumatica

Giant Cell Arthritis

Age of onset older than 50
New headache or pain in head
Temporal artery abnormality (tender or diminished pulsation)
Increased erythrocyte sedimentation rate (ESR) of more than 50 to 100
Abnormal artery biopsy

Polymyalgia Rheumatica

Age of onset older than 50; peaks at 60 to 80 years
Increased ESR of more than 50 to 100
Normochromic/normocytic anemia
Malaise and severe fatigue
Fever
Stiffness and soreness in neck, shoulders, and pelvic girdle
Rapid improvement with low-dose steroids

Source: American College of Rheumatology (ACR): 1990 criteria for GCA; Paget S: Polymyalgia rheumatica. In ACR: *Clinical care in the rheumatic diseases*, ed 2, Atlanta, 2001, ACR.

Box 8-14 Risk Factors for Incontinent Older Adults

Immobility of chronic degenerative diseases
Diminished cognitive status, dementia
Delirium
Medications including diuretics
Smoking
Fecal impaction
Low fluid intake
Environmental barriers
High-impact physical exercise
Diabetes
Stroke
Estrogen dificiency
Pelvic muscle weakness

From Fantl JA et al: Managing acute and chronic urinary incontinence. In *Clinical practice guideline: quick reference guide for clinicians*, no 2, pub no 96-0686, 1996 update, Rockville, MD, 1996, U.S. Department of Health and Human Services, Public Health Service, Agency for Health Care Policy and Research.

Because the symptoms of PMR are similar to those of arthritis and other musculoskeletal problems that occur with increasing age, it is difficult to diagnose. Depression is common in PMR and GCA and will require management. The elder may become dependent, lose strength, and become discouraged because of stiffness and pain. Pitting edema may occur and cause additional discomfort. Assistance or a short stay in an assisted living facility may be required until the disease is well managed. Education is important so that the elder and family understand the course of the disease. Attention to the routine of therapy is important, as are the laboratory tests needed during the course of treatment. Pain management is important, especially early in the course until steroid therapy has been given for several days. COX-2 inhibitors may alleviate some pain but are usually not sufficient.

Complications. In addition to the possibility of temporary or permanent blindness with GCA, elders may also develop tenosynovitis and carpal tunnel syndrome (Hunder, 2002). Another serious complication is thoracic aortic aneurysm, which may occur late in the disease.

Incontinence

Incontinence, or the loss of ability to control the elimination of urine or feces on an occasional or a consistent basis, has caused considerable embarrassment and astronomic costs both socially and economically. The economic costs are $11.2 billion annually in the community and nearly $5.3 billion in long-term care settings (Fourcroy, 2001). Estimates of costs and numbers of individuals enduring incontinence vary widely because many people isolate themselves and keep silent about the problem unless institutionalized, when it may become apparent, or episodes of incontinence may be present only during a hospitalization, lifestyle change, or physiologic disruption. One study reported that in women older than 60, 34% had urinary incontinence (UI) at least once, and 12% report daily UI (Thom, 1998). Frenchman (2001) reports that 50% of institutionalized elders may suffer UI. Elders in rural settings and small towns are more likely than those in metropolitan areas to be institutionalized when afflicted with incontinence (Coward et al, 1995). See Box 8-14 for risk factors for incontinent older adults. Continence must be routinely addressed in the initial assessment of every aged person in the nurse's care. Initial and periodic assessments are necessary to maintain an individualized nursing care plan.

Bladder Function in Old Age. Normal bladder function requires an intact brain and spinal cord, a competent bladder, and active sphincters that will sustain maximum urethral pressure against rising bladder pressure. A full bladder increases pressure and signals the spinal cord and the brainstem center the desire to micturate. Social training then dictates whether micturition should be attended to or should be postponed until there is an appropriate opportunity to seek out toilet facilities. However, when the bladder contents reach 500 ml or more, the pressure is such that it becomes more difficult to control the urge to void. As volume increases, emptying the bladder becomes an uncontrollable act. The bladder of the aged retains its tonus, but the volume that it can hold decreases. If cerebrovascular disease is present, dementia being the most severe form, the changes are exaggerated and bladder control becomes diminished.

Many healthy aged are annoyed by frequency and some degree of urgency. The warning period between the desire to void and actual micturition is shortened or lost. Severe illness, difficulty in walking or handling the bedpan or urinal, problems manipulating clothing, and emotional disturbances (such as those that occur during a change in living situation or resentment, anger, or bereavement) may be responsible for some incontinence. In some instances micturition is uncontrolled as a deliberate means to gain attention or demonstrate hostility. Drugs that increase urinary output and medications that produce drowsiness or confusion facilitate incontinence by dulling the transmission of the desire to micturate.

Urinary Incontinence. Urinary incontinence is one of the most prevalent symptoms encountered in the care of the aged. Many families cannot cope with incontinent relatives. It is therefore not surprising that incontinence is a leading cause of institutionalization of the aged person.

Incontinence is defined as involuntary loss of urine that is sufficient to be a problem (Cefalu, 2002). Incontinence is not a result of advancing age, nor is it a disease. It is a symptom of existing environmental, psychologic, drug, or physical disturbances and can become a catastrophic event when it interferes with mobility, sociability, and the ability to remain in one's home. Risk factors common to women are parity, severe lacerations during birth, maternal age, baby birth weights, and hysterectomy. Caesarean section is protective (Fourcroy, 2001). Box 8-14 enumerates some of the many risk factors associated with UI.

Incontinence ushers in dependence, shame, guilt, fear, and depression. The aged who are aware of a problem of continence are mortified by their state. If it is assumed that all aged eventually become incontinent, a resolution of the problem will not be sought, and it will become a self-fulfilling prophecy. Health care personnel must begin to change their thinking about incontinence and acknowledge that incontinence can be cured. If it cannot be cured, it can be treated to minimize its detrimental effects. The nurse who cares for the incontinent person needs sensitivity, insight, patience, and understanding. Reassurance rather than guilt should be promoted. The Agency for Health Care Policy and Research increased awareness of and knowledge about incontinence through its clinical practice guideline, *Urinary Incontinence in Adults* (U.S. Department of Health and Human Services, 1992, 1996). This information attempts to improve reporting, diagnosis, and treatment of the ambulatory and nonambulatory individual and to educate health care professionals and consumers about urinary incontinence.

Urinary Problems. The most common types of UI in older adults are stress incontinence, urge incontinence, and overflow incontinence (U.S. Department of Health and Human Services, 1992). Overactive bladder, iatrogenic, functional, and mixed incontinence are also commonly cited in the literature.

Stress incontinence occurs more often in elderly women and occurs when intraabdominal pressure exceeds urethral resistance. Muscles around the urethra become weak so that even a small amount of urine may pass. It occurs frequently in obese individuals, especially apple-shaped (rather than pear-shaped) individuals (Fourcroy, 2001). It occurs more commonly in white women than in African American women. UI may occur during everyday activities, when the elderly individual sneezes, coughs, bends over, or lifts a heavy object. The amount of urine leakage is small, and the volume is low when postresidual urine is obtained.

Urge incontinence, or overactive bladder, more common in younger women, may be caused by central nervous system lesions such as stroke, diabetes, demyelinating diseases, or local irritating factors such as bladder tumors or (perhaps most often) urinary tract infections. Individuals sense the urge to void but cannot inhibit urination long enough to reach a toilet. The volume of urine lost is small or moderate, and episodes occur every few hours. Postresidual urine reveals a low volume.

Overflow incontinence is a result of neurologic abnormalities of the spinal cord that affect the contractility of the detrusor muscle of the bladder. Any factor disrupting detrusor stability such as drugs, tumors, strictures, and prostatic hypertrophy will cause the bladder to become overdistended, leading to frequent or constant loss of urine.

Functional incontinence refers to a situation in which the lower urinary tract is intact but the individual is limited by musculoskeletal disability or severe cognitive impairment. Urine is lost because the individual is unaware of the need to void or is unable to reach a toilet because of arthritis, Parkinson's disease, or, for hospitalized patients, their condition or raised bed rails. Environmental conditions and prescribed drug use are additional examples of factors that can create functional incontinence.

Iatrogenic incontinence is associated with medication side effects. This can be managed by decreasing the dosage of medication to maintain the primary drug effect but eliminate the secondary effects. It may be necessary to change a drug to another class of medication that is not associated with incontinence. Other iatrogenic causes of incontinence include expanded extracellular fluid compartmentalization with the development of nocturia and polyuria, as occurs in CHF, chronic venous insufficiency, and metabolic states such as polyuria with increased glycosuria or increased calcemia.

More than one urinary incontinence problem may exist in the same individual, which is called *mixed incontinence.* These conditions can be caused by anatomic, physiologic, or pathologic factors (internal factors) or by external factors such as mobility, dexterity, motivation, and environment. Box 8-15 summarizes the types of urinary incontinence and associated causal factors.

Assessment. Nurses are often the ones to identify urinary incontinence, but neither nurses nor doctors have been particularly aggressive in management. Assessment is multidimensional. It includes a health history, physical examination, and urinalysis. More extensive examinations are considered after the initial findings are assessed. A thorough health history should focus on the medical, neurologic, and genitourinary history; a medication review of both prescribed and over-the-

Box 8-15 Types of Incontinence and Associated Causal Factors

Type	Causal Factors
Stress	Obesity
	Estrogen deficiency
	Pelvic floor muscle weakness
	Radiation or prostate surgery
	Urethral sphincter weakness
	Drugs
Urge	Stroke
	Dementia
	Parkinsonism
	Urinary tract infection
	Detrusor overactivity or instability
	Drugs
Overflow	Fecal impaction
	Enlarged prostate
	Diabetic neuropathy
	Severe pelvic prolapse
	Drugs
Functional	Mobility limitations
	Cognitive impairment
	Depression
	Bipolar/schizophrenic disorders
	External factors:
	Restraints
	Caregiver inattention
	Drugs
	Environmental barriers
Iatrogenic	Extracellular fluid compartment
	Congestive heart failure
	Chronic venous insufficiency
	Metabolic states:
	Glycosuria
	Calcemia
	Drugs

Adapted from Resnick NM: Urinary incontinence. In Abrams WB, Beers MH, Berkow R, editors: *Merck manual of geriatrics,* ed 2, Whitehouse Station, NJ, 1995, Merck Research Laboratories; Staab AS, Hodges LC: *Essentials of gerontological nursing,* Philadelphia, 1996, JB Lippincott; Palmer MH: *Urinary incontinence,* Gaithersberg, MD, 1996, Aspen; Miller CA: *Nursing care of older adults,* ed 2, Philadelphia, 1995, JB Lippincott; Fantl JA et al: Managing acute and chronic urinary incontinence. In *Clinical practice guideline: quick reference guide for clinicians,* no 2, pub no 96-0686, 1996 update, Rockville, MD 1996, U.S. Department of Health and Human Services, Public Health Service, Agency for Health Care Policy and Research.

counter drugs; and a detailed exploration of the symptoms of the urinary incontinence and associated symptoms and other factors, which can assist the physician or advanced practice nurse in accurate diagnosis and treatment. Data should include the duration, frequency, and volume of the incontinence.

The type of incontinence should be validated and described with a voiding diary (Figure 8-7). Accurate notations should be made of significant burning, itching, or pressure. The character of the urine (odor, color, sedimentary, or clear) and difficulty starting and stopping the urinary stream should be recorded. Activities of daily living such as ability to reach a toilet and use it and finger dexterity for clothing manipulation should be documented.

Use of problematic medications such as sedatives, hypnotics, anticholinergics, and antidepressants should be assessed. Diuretics, narcotics, calcium channel blockers, alpha-adrenergic agonists, minor tranquilizers, antispasmodics, and major tranquilizers are among the drugs commonly prescribed. In addition, the nurse should not forget to ask about caffeine and alcohol. Assess for vaginal discharge or constipation or investigate fecal impaction, which occurs more often in institutional settings and in bed-bound elders in the home. The nurse may do the physical examination, which includes evaluation of mental status; mobility; dexterity; and a neurologic, abdominal, rectal, and pelvic examination.

Laboratory tests should include urinalysis; serum creatinine or blood urea nitrogen; postvoid residual, which can be done by abdominal palpation, percussion, bimanual examination, catheterization, or bladder ultrasound; and urine culture, blood sugar, and urine cytology, as necessary. Based on these findings, a decision can be made on how to treat the incontinence or the need for additional tests and consultation with a urologist for urodynamic testing (cystometrogram, electrophysiologic sphincter testing, ultrasound of kidney and bladder, cystourethroscopy, or uroflowmetry).

In summary, assessment of urinary incontinence can identify incontinence as either transient—the result of temporary conditions that are amenable to medication, surgery, or other interventions—or established, the result of neurologic damage to the urinary system. Transient incontinence is curable; established incontinence is treatable or controllable but not usually curable.

Interventions. When there is sufficient understanding of the problem, various therapeutic modalities and concomitant nursing interventions can be initiated. Selection of a modality and interventions will depend on the type of incontinence and its underlying cause and whether the outcome is to cure or to minimize the extent of the incontinence. Box 8-16 lists the numerous modalities available for the treatment of incontinence. Colposuspension and slings are most effective for stress incontinence. Pessaries are useful for elderly women and those with prolapse, especially if they are poor candidates for surgery. Collagen injections can help support the urethra, especially in those with diabetes, poor surgical risk, or multiple sclerosis. It is an office procedure. Medical therapies include the use of estrogen vaginal creams, alpha-blockers for prostate problems, oxybutynin, and tolterodine. The latter may cause cognitive changes in the frail elder. Nursing interventions focus primarily on the therapeutic modality of supportive measures and may also be involved in designing restorative therapeutic modalities.

"URO-Log" (Voiding Diary)

To be completed before your doctor's appointments.

Name ______________________ Date ______________________

Time of day	Type and amount of fluid intake	Type and amount of food eaten	Amount voided (in ounces)	Amount of leakage (small, medium, large)	Activity engaged in when leakage occurred	Was urge present?

Figure 8-7. Example of voiding diary. (From HIP, Union, SC.)

Box 8-16 Therapeutic Modalities in the Treatment of Incontinence

Support Measures

Appropriate attitude
Accessible toilet substitutes (bedpan, urinal, commode)
Avoidance of iatrogenic complications (urinary tract infections, excessive sedation, inaccessible toilets, drugs adversely affecting the bladder or urethral function)
Protective undergarments
Absorbent bed pads
Behavioral techniques (bladder training, toilet scheduling, conditioning, biofeedback, Kegel exercises)
Good skin care

Drugs

Bladder relaxants
Bladder outlet stimulants

Surgery

Suspension of bladder neck
Prostatectomy
Prosthetic sphincter implants
Urethral sling
Bladder augmentation

Mechanical and Electric Devices

Catheters

External (condom or "Texas" catheter)
Intermittent
Suprapubic
Indwelling

Attitude. An appropriate attitude is most important when providing nursing care to an incontinent individual. Caregivers are often unaware of the many causes of incontinence and passively accept a client's urinary incontinence and feel that it is an inevitable part of aging, only adding to the elder's feelings of low self-worth, dependence, and social isolation. Caregivers who regard incontinence as an unpleasant and demanding hygienic problem emphasize only keeping the patient clean and dry with little consideration of what causes the problem. The fact that incontinence is curable if the patient has the will and resolve to work on it, and that the nurse and other health care providers will work with the elder to resolve the incontinence, is an important idea to foster in the elder who is not cognitively impaired. The role of the nurse in the community is to give the older adult information and tools that will allow the individual to maintain body control.

Toilet Accessibility. Accessibility to the toilet is an intervention that is often not considered in providing assistance for the incontinent patient. Environmental circumstances can contribute to incontinence. If the distance the aged person must either walk or travel by wheelchair to reach the toilet is longer than the time between the onset of the desire to micturate and actual micturition, incontinence is certain to occur. Toilet substitutes for the infirm and ill have been around for hundreds of years. Four types are used: commodes for the bedside, overtoilet chairs for transport, bedpans for beds or commodes, and urinals for both men and women that can be used in bed, chair, or a standing position. The criteria for use of a commode are that the toilet is too far for the elder's mobility or it requires too much energy for the elderly person to get to the toilet. A bedside commode can also substitute for an inadequate number of available toilets. Overtoilet chair criteria are similar to those for a commode. However, it cannot be used as a substitute for available toilets. Urinals are generally used by men; however, bottle-shaped urinals have been designed for women and are used on occasion. They can be obtained from a surgical supply store or various mail order catalogs.

Protective Undergarments and Padding. A variety of protective undergarments or adult briefs are available for the incontinent older adult (Box 8-17). Disposable types come in several sizes determined by hip and waist measurement; rarely does one size fit all. The lining of these disposable pants may be fiber filled or made with an absorbent polymer or gel substance. Polymer and gel substances are more absorbent and tend to keep a protective layer between the skin and wet material. Washable garments with inserts also do a reasonable job of containing urine. However, they tend to be made of plastic or rubber and therefore are hot and cause skin discomfort. If pants are going to leak, they will do so at the groin. It is important to fit them firmly but comfortably around the leg (Figure 8-8).

A variation of the standard drawsheet is a protective washable pad used along with a plastic sheet. The Australian Kylie pad is a sophisticated version of the drawsheet that is successful in keeping both the bed and the incontinent person dry. It is composed of two layers, with a water-repellent layer next to the individual. Urine is absorbed by the liner. Disposable protective pads are available in the United States, but it is important to know the amount and type of fill in the pads. A polymer gel is more economical. It is unwise to purchase pads because they are inexpensive if it means using several more per day than if more expensive and more absorbent pads were bought (Figure 8-9).

Behavioral Techniques. Behavioral techniques such as scheduled toileting, habit training, bladder training, biofeedback, and conditioning focus on improving the person's awareness of his or her lower urinary tract (Box 8-18). These techniques are usually effective in urge and stress incontinence. In some instances the goal is not to regain a normal voiding pattern but to decrease the number of wetting episodes, to decrease laundry costs and use of absorbent protection, and to improve the quality of life and social activity. The methods are free of side effects and do not limit future options. However, they do require time, effort, practice, and an individual who is cognitively intact and highly motivated.

Scheduled toileting consists of a fixed toileting schedule, such as every 2 hours, with techniques to trigger voiding and emptying the bladder completely (National Institutes of Health Panel, 1989; Newman, 1992; Palmer, 1996). Habit training uses frequent checks (every 1 to 2 hours) for dryness. The client is reminded to void and praised frequently when successful. The objective of habit training is to allow the person to regain a normal voiding pattern and continence. It involves cognitive function, mobility, dexterity, and motivation (Newman, 1992; Rousseau and Fuentevilla-Clifton, 1992; Palmer, 1996). Bladder retraining uses an interplay of methods. It teaches the individual to void at regular intervals and attempts to lengthen these intervals between voidings. Bladder training has been effective in reducing the frequency of urge and stress incontinence (Agency for Health Care Policy and Research [AHCPR], 1996; Newman, 1992; Palmer, 1996).

Conditioning of the pelvic muscles employs use of the Kegel exercise. Conditioning also refers to improving mobility. Pelvic floor exercises strengthen the periurethral and pelvic floor muscles. The contractions exert a closing force on the urethra. Kegel exercises are one approach to the problem of stress incontinence. They can be either slow or rapid. The muscle contraction is held for 3 seconds then relaxed. This is repeated 10 times working up to 20 times. The exercise is repeated five times a day. Quick Kegel exercises begin with tightening and relaxing the pubococcygeal muscle without a pause between. These are done as quickly as possible beginning with a count of 15 seconds and working up to 2 minutes. Initially it is difficult to identify, tighten, and relax this muscle, but with repeated work the exercise becomes easier. Mandelstam and Robinson (1977) first described the following exercise useful in improving perineal and sphincter muscle control:

Box 8-17 Factors to Consider for Use of Absorbent Products

Functional disability of person
Type and severity of incontinence
Gender
Availability of caregivers
Failure with previous treatment program
Client preference
Comorbidity

Box 8-18 Forms of Behavioral Modification

- Diet modification
- Bowel retraining
- Behavioral interventions
  - Habit training
  - Prompted voiding
  - Bladder training
  - Pelvic floor exercises (Kegel exercises)
- Used in conjunction with behavioral interventions
  - Vaginal cones
  - Biofeedback
  - Electrical stimulation

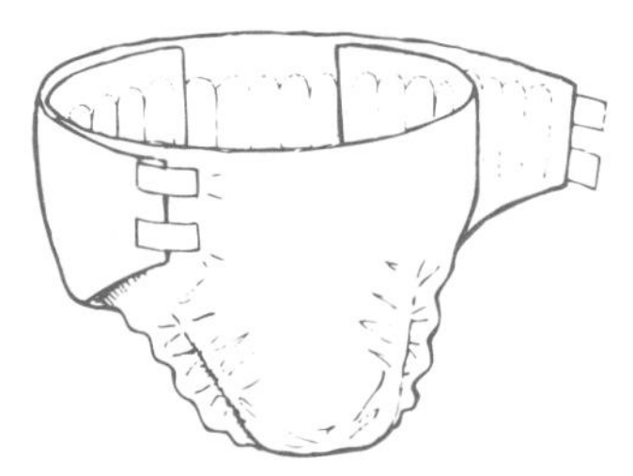

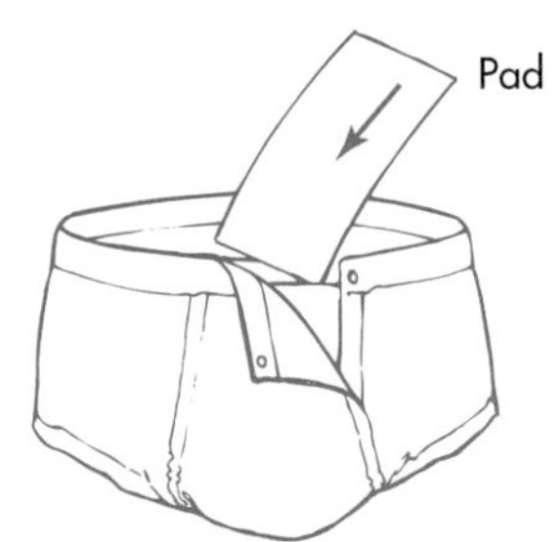

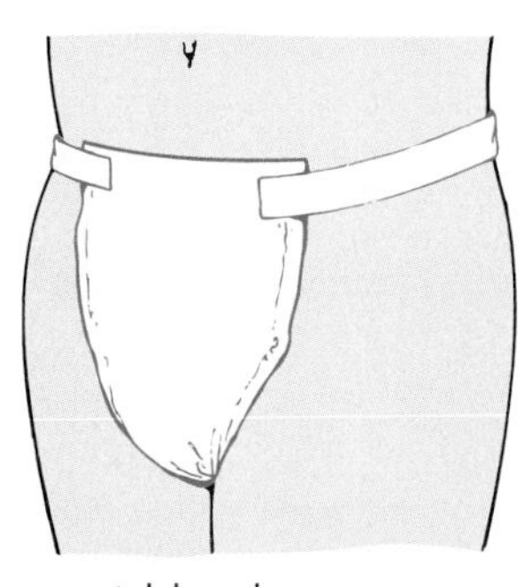

Figure 8-8. Disposable and reusable incontinence garment for men and women. (From Gray M: *Genitourinary disorders,* St Louis, 1992, Mosby.)

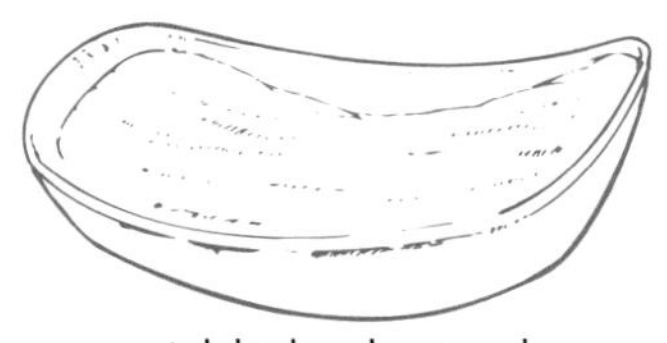

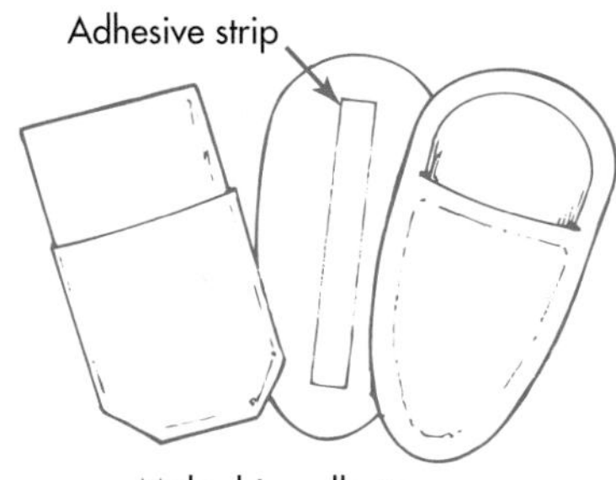

Figure 8-9. Disposable incontinence pads. (From Gray M: *Genitourinary disorders,* St Louis, 1992, Mosby.)

standing, sitting, or lying, tighten the anal sphincter (as if to control the passage of flatus or feces) and then the urethra/vaginal muscles (as if to stop the flow of urine). This should be done at least four times each hour and can be done in any position or any place.

Biofeedback employs visual or auditory instruments to give the individual immediate feedback on how well he or she is controlling the sphincter, the detrusor muscle, and abdominal muscles. Those who are successful learn to contract the sphincter and relax the detrusor and abdominal muscles automatically. Complete continence can occur in 20% to 25% of individuals and improvement in an additional 30%. Biofeedback requires sophisticated equipment. Table 8-4 provides a summary of behavioral modalities, the type of incontinence, outcomes, and appropriate populations for these approaches.

Skin Care. Skin care maintains the first line of defense against infection. Skin that is in contact with urine should be washed with mild soap and warm water, then dried thoroughly. Application of a skin lubricant or an ointment such as A&D provides a thin protective layer to skin repeatedly exposed to urine. It is tempting to neglect an individual who wears protective pants, but it is important that the person be checked every few hours for wetness in order to maintain skin intactness. To minimize the episodes of incontinence, it is prudent to establish the incontinence pattern and place the individual on a toilet or commode before voiding.

Medications. Drugs to eliminate or improve incontinence include bladder relaxants and bladder stimulants. Bladder relaxants include anticholinergic agents that delay, decrease, or inhibit detrusor muscle contractions, especially the involuntary contractions, and may increase bladder capacity. The most commonly used drug is probably oxybutynin, an antispasmodic that reduces the urge to void and reduces contractions of the detrusor muscle. Dry mouth, dry eyes, constipation, and palpitations may occur. Other drugs exert mild anticholinergic side effects. Calcium channel blockers, also used for cardiovascular problems, have a depressant effect on the bladder. More study is needed to determine if there is a significant benefit for their use in urge incontinence. Imipramine (Tofranil), a tricyclic antidepressant, exerts both anticholinergic and direct relaxant effects on the detrusor muscle, as well as a contractile effect on the bladder outlet, enhancing continence. Two important side effects to be aware of in the elderly client are hypotension and sedation. Bladder outlet stimulants include alpha-adrenergic agonist agents and estrogen replacement preparations. Alpha-adrenergic agonists, pseudoephedrine and ephedrine, cause contractions of smooth muscle at the bladder outlet and improve stress incontinence. Estrogen replacement therapy, although not definitively used for stress incontinence, has been effective in improving postmenopausal urgency, frequency, and urge incontinence. Use of medications must be thoughtfully considered for possible undesirable side effects.

Surgery. Surgical intervention is appropriate for some conditions of incontinence. Surgical suspension of the bladder

Table 8-4 Behavioral Intervention Options for Incontinence

Type of incontinence	Intended population	Behavioral intervention	Purpose of intervention	Expected outcome
Urge, stress, mixed	Cognitively intact; able to discern urge sensation; able to understand or learn how to inhibit urge; able to toilet themselves with or without assistance	Bladder training	Restore normal pattern of voiding and normal bladder function Inhibit involuntary destrusor contractions	↓ Number of wet episodes ↓ Amount of urine lost ↓ Number of voidings ↑ Bladder capacity ↑ Quality of life
Urge, functional	Cognitively impaired; functionally disabled; incomplete bladder emptying; caregiver dependent	Scheduled toileting	Timed with individuals voiding habits Decrease wet episodes; no attempt to regain normal voiding pattern	↓ Number of wet episodes ↓ Laundry costs and/or use of absorbent devices ↑ Life quality ↑ Social activity
Functional, urge, mixed	Same as above	Habit training	Develop a pattern for voiding	↓ Frequency of incontinent episodes ↑ Comfort ↑ Quality of life
Urge, functional	Functionally able to use toilet or toileting device; able to feel urge sensation; able to request toileting assistance; caregiver is available	Prompted voiding	Heighten individual awareness of need to void	↑ Interaction between caregiver and individual ↓ Wet episodes
Stress, urge, mixed	Able to identify and contract pelvic muscles; able and willing to follow instructions and committed to actively participate	Pelvic floor training	Strengthen pubococcygeus muscle efficient urethral closure during sudden increases in intravesical pressure	↑ Strength and size of pubococcygeus ↑ Duration of muscle contraction with increased urethral pressure ↓ Urine loss ↑ Ability to stop urine flow once initiated Self-report of ↓ urine loss ↑ Self-esteem; enhance quality of life ↓ Reliance on pads, pantyliners, or absorbent products
Stress, urge, mixed	Cognitively intact Compliant with instructions Able to stand Sufficient muscle strength to contract muscle and retain the lightest weight No pelvic organ prolapse	Vaginal weight training	Same as above	Same as above
Stress, mixed	Ability to understand analog or digital signals using auditory or visual display Motivated, able to learn voluntary control through observation of biofeedback A health care provider who can appropriately assess the incontinence problem and provide behavior interventions	Biofeedback	Same as above	Same as above
Stress, urge, mixed	Ability to discern stimulation	Electrical stimulation	Reeducation of pelvic muscle; inhibit bladder instability and improve striated sphincter and levator anti contractility and efficiency	↑ Resistance of the pelvic floor; block uninhibited bladder contractions

Adapted and compiled from Fantl JA. et al: Managing acute and chronic urinary incontinence. In *Clinical practice guideline: quick reference guide for clinicians*, no 2, pub no 96-0686, 1996 update, Rockville, MD, 1996, U.S. Department of Health and Human Services, Agency for Health Care Policy and Research; Staab AS, Hodges LC: *Essentials of gerontological nursing*, Philadelphia, 1996, JB Lippincott; Palmer MH: *Urinary incontinence*, Gaithersburg, MD, 1996, Aspen, Anderson MA, Braun JV: *Caring for the elderly client*, Philadelphia, 1995, FA Davis.

neck in women has proved effective in 80% to 95% of persons electing to have this surgical corrective procedure. Outflow obstruction incontinence due to prostatic hypertrophy is generally corrected by prostatectomy. Sphincter dysfunction due to nerve damage following surgical trauma or radical perineal procedures is 70% to 90% repairable through sphincter implantation. Complications related to this type of surgery are greater than 20% and may require an additional surgery. A urethral sling of fascia increases urethral elevation and compression. Continence is restored in approximately 80% of clients who have this surgery. Currently periurethral bulking has been added to the number of surgical procedures that address urinary incontinence. Collagen or polytetrafluoroethylene (PTFE) is injected into the periurethral area to increase pressure on the urethra. This adds bulk to the internal sphincter and closes the gap that allowed leakage to occur.

Nonsurgical Devices. The Food and Drug Administration (FDA) has approved two devices, available through prescription, to manage stress incontinence. The Miniguard is about the size of a postage stamp and fits over the urethral opening. It is contoured with an adhesive-foam backing. The other device, the Reliance Urinary Control Insert, is designed for moderate to severe incontinence in women. The device is a balloon-tipped plug, about one fifth the diameter of a tampon, which is inserted by applicator. The force of the insertion inflates the balloon, so that the neck of the bladder is then obstructed. The device must be removed by pulling a string before urination or intercourse. Trials of both of these devices have been on a limited number of women at present. Women using the devices gained complete or limited continence but also experienced urinary tract infections (UTIs), particularly with the Reliance Control Insert. However, it was thought that as the women gained skill in use of the devices, the UTIs and urethral irritation would decline (Harvard Medical School Health Publications, 1996).

Catheters. As a last resort, appliances may need to be used. Too frequently, abuse of appliances occurs because they are convenient for the caregivers. Foley and condom catheters, diapers, and rubber pants carry with them inherent hazards of iatrogenic infection and skin irritation and breakdown. Psychologically the aged person feels and is treated differently, no longer as an adult but rather as a dependent and, perhaps, childlike individual. The aged person who has an indwelling catheter soon loses awareness of the sensations of bladder pressure and the habit of toileting. Persons with catheters often lose the micturition function completely. Women have fewer appliance options than men. In addition to the Foley catheter, men can use condom and sheath catheters, which are soft and pliable.

Catheter care is important regardless of the type of catheter used. The condom catheter should be removed daily to allow the penis to be scrupulously cleansed, dried, and aired to prevent irritation, maceration, and the development of pressure areas and skin breakdown. Foley catheter care should be performed at least twice a day. Cleansing of the external urethral meatus with a gentle cleanser, maintaining a closed system with unobstructed flow, maintaining an acid urine (Box 8-19), and meticulous care of equipment are essential in acute care or long-term care facilities, as well as at home, if a Foley catheter is used. Regular Foley catheter care ensures cleansing and removal of secretions and fecal matter, which can become the media for bacterial growth in the perineal area. See Box 8-20 for other helpful interventions to control or eliminate incontinence.

Diverticulosis

Epidemiology. The prevalence of diverticulosis in Americans 65 years and older is greater than the 28% found in younger adults, although broad population-based studies in the elderly are limited (Camilleri et al, 2000). Considered a functional bowel disease of developed countries, the incidence of diverticulosis increases as a country's population enlarges their dietary intake percentage of processed foods (Melange and Vanheuverzwyn, 1990). Age appears to contribute to the preponderance of the disorder in those above 40 years old, consuming less than 25 g of fiber daily, and living in an industrialized country (Halphen and Blain, 1995).

Constipation. Associated with the development of diverticulosis and a common complaint in the elderly, constipation has been identified as contributing to the herniation of the mucosa through a weakened colon wall (Nadel, 2001). Although liquid barium studies in healthy humans have not demonstrated an age-related change in transit times, and jejunal manometry research indicates that the movement patterns during the fasting period are the same in younger (mean age 25) and older (mean age 72) adults (Nådel, 2001), chronic constipation's causative effect on the aging colon continues. Constipation-related increases in intraluminal pressures and colonic segmentation, combined with physiologic aging–induced inhibited neuromuscular function and collagen deposition in the wall of the colon (Camilleri et al, 2000), produce diverticula most commonly found in the sigmoid colon. The inhibition of neurohormonal control on fecal transit times is the product of animal model studies, and the clinical significance continues to be in question (Nadel, 2001).

Culture. Cultural variations in diverticular disease prevalence are impressive, with the United States, Europe, and Australia yielding a higher percentage of affected adults than in Asia and Africa, where the population eats a high-fiber, vegetable-based diet (Yap and Hoe, 1991). Culturally competent nursing care for patients with diverticular disease is therefore important (Estes, 2002). The social influences and implications related to food selection and preparation can be multicultural and significant to diverticular disease development. Holidays, religious beliefs, racial group, and regional considerations all affect dietary consumption or restriction and have yet to be definitively studied in diverticular disease; however, the meaning individuals of different cultures attach to health and illness has been discussed (Giger and Davidhizar, 1999).

Box 8-19 Foods That Do and Do Not Acidify Urine

Do	Do Not
Juices	
Prunce Plum Cranberry	Citrus: Orange Lemon Lime Tomato
Dairy products	
No more than 8 oz milk 3 oz cheese: Cottage Cream Cheddar Swiss Gruyère	Avoid excesses of milk as in milk-shakes, malts, etc.
Vegetables	
Small servings (3) Corn Lentils White beans	Potatoes Lima beans Soybeans Beet greens Parsnips Spinach Dried vegetables
Fruits	
2 or more servings except those listed to the right—prunes, plums, cranberries eat freely	Cantaloupe Raisins Dates Dried fruits (except prunes) Citrus fruits
Beverages	
Coffee Tea	Flavored sodas Fruit ades
Soups	
Bouillon Meat broths Soup with allowed foods	
Concentrated sweets	
White sugar Corn syrup Cranberry sauce Plum jelly Candy	Molasses Almonds Chestnuts Coconut
Cereal, breads, potato substitutes	
2 or more servings white/brown rice Noodles/macaroni/spaghetti Barley 1 or more servings dry or cooked cereal (whole grain/enriched preferred) 4 or more slices whole grain/enriched bread	

Adapted from Newman DK: The treatment of urinary incontinence in adults, *Nurse Pract* 14(6):32, 1989.

Box 8-20 Helpful Interventions for Noninstitutionalized Elders to Control or Eliminate Incontinence

Empty bladder completely before and after meals and at bedtime.
Urinate whenever the urge arises, never ignore it.
A schedule of urinating every 2 hours during the day and every 4 hours at night is often helpful in retraining the bladder. An alarm clock may be necessary.
Drink $1\frac{1}{2}$ to 2 quarts of fluid day before 8 PM. This helps the kidneys to function properly. Limit fluids after supper to $\frac{1}{2}$ to 1 cup (except in very hot weather).
Drink cranberry juice or take vitamin C to help acidify the urine and lower the chances of bladder infection.
Eliminate or reduce the use of coffee, tea, brown cola, and alcohol since they have a diuretic effect.
Take prescription diuretics in the morning upon rising.
Limit the use of sleeping pills, sedatives, and alcohol because they decrease sensation to urinate and can increase incontinence, especially at night.
If overweight, lose weight.
Exercises to strengthen pelvic muscles that help support the bladder are often helpful for women.
Make sure the toilet is nearby with a clear path and good lighting, especially at night. Grab bars or a raised toilet seat may be needed.
Dress protectively with cotton underwear, sanitary pads for women, and protective pants or incontinent pads if necessary.

Disease as an imbalance between "hot" and "cold" factors is a commonly held health belief among many Eastern and Hispanic cultures. Diverticular disease is primarily a "hot" illness, and self-care practices to aid in health promotion and maintenance may include the use of folk remedies. Common culturally influenced dietary beliefs held by many Hispanic, Arabic, and Asian ethnic groups on the "hot" and "cold" nature of diverticular symptoms and routinely consumed foods may affect treatment approaches (Giger and Davidhizar, 1999).

Definition. Diverticulosis is characterized by small pouches, called *diverticula*, that bulge outward through weak areas in the colon wall (Nadel, 2001). Although they may be found along the entire length of the colon, they are most common in the sigmoid colon. Noninflamed sacklike protuberances, usually less than 1 cm, diverticula have thin, compressible walls if empty or firm walls if full of fecal matter (Nadel, 2001). Occasionally the fecal matter in one of these pouches (diverticula) will become quite desiccated, even calcified. Usually there is a tract, or lumen, which leads from the colon into the diverticula. The serosal surface of these saccular formations is typically the same color as the surrounding mucosa, free of erythema and exudates. Often confused with diverticulosis, diverticulitis is an acute inflammatory complication of diverticulosis.

Risk Factors. Low dietary intake of fiber, use of medications that slow fecal transit time, overuse of laxatives, family history, gallbladder disease, and obesity are common risk factors in the development of diverticulosis in the elderly (Cotran et al, 1994).

Sign and Symptoms. Although the prevalence of diverticulosis is high in the elderly, greater than 28% (Camilleri et al, 2000), 80% of those affected are free of symptoms (Nadel, 2001). Of the 20% who do experience symptoms, most will have some intermittent mild lower gastrointestinal blood loss (Nadel, 2001), but only 3% to 5% will ever experience severe acute blood loss.

Acute Complications. The most common complication is an acute inflammatory process called diverticulitis (Nadel, 2001). Often unknown in etiology, a relatively sudden onset (hours or days versus weeks) of abdominal pain is the hallmark of an "attack" of diverticulitis (Sleisenger and Fordtran, 1993). The serosal surface, usually of a limited number of diverticula, becomes erythematous, exudates are produced, abscesses may form, and the surrounding area becomes indurated (Nadel, 2001). Necrotic tissue may develop, although surrounding colonic mucosa can remain normal (Cotran et al, 1994). When severe, fever, nausea, vomiting, chills, cramping, and constipation may occur as well (Sleisenger and Fordtran, 1993).

Lower gastrointestinal hemorrhage, related to diverticular disease, although rare (1%), is the most common cause of massive bleeding from the colon (Nadel, 2001). It is postulated that vessels lining the diverticulum weaken and burst to produce copious bright red bleeding from the rectum (Sleisenger and Fordtran, 1993). Different from the minor blood loss that commonly occurs in chronic diverticular disease, surgery may be necessary (Nadel, 2001). In all cases, physician or nurse practitioner evaluation of bright red blood from the rectum should determine the etiology, medical follow-up, and treatment parameters.

Abscess, perforation, and peritonitis are possible complications if the initial acute diverticulitis does not improve with antibiotics and rest of the colon (Nadel, 2001). An abscess is an infected area of diverticula that has localized swelling and pus accumulation (Sleisenger and Fordtran, 1993). On occasion, physicians drain recalcitrant abscesses. Sometimes the abscess can damage mucosal tissue sufficiently to perforate the colon wall (Cotran et al, 1994). A small hole in the saccular protuberance may allow the infection to leak into the peritoneum, causing peritonitis (Nadel, 2001).

Fistula formation can occur after diverticular perforation (Sleisenger and Fordtran, 1993). A fistula is an abnormal tissue formation that connects two organs or an organ with the skin. Damaged tissue may come in contact with each other after infection or perforation and heal to form a lumen. Most commonly the bladder, small intestine, and skin are involved. The most common fistula affects men more than women and occurs between the bladder and the colon. Surgery is generally required to avoid a severe, long-term infection (Nadel, 2001).

Partial or total intestinal obstruction may follow multiple episodes of diverticulitis, infection, and scarring in the large intestine. Partial obstruction may allow some time for planning surgery; total obstruction, however, is an emergency (Sleisenger and Fordtran, 1993).

Progressive Signs and Symptoms. A chronic disorder, the progression of diverticulosis is judged by the frequency of acute complications and the severity of functional bowel impairment. The serial utilization of Nursing Outcomes Classification (NOC) can serve to quantify the frequency and severity of signs and symptoms while facilitating communication with other nursing disciplines and facilitating the development of nursing knowledge (Nursing Outcomes Classification, 2002). Scales of measurement used with NOC are Likert type, from 1 to 5, describing extremely compromised to not compromised or never demonstrated to consistently demonstrated, respectively. These gradations can be useful in the sequential monitoring of an elder's experience of diverticular disease.

Assessment. Although the physician diagnoses diverticular disease through medical history, physical examination, and one or more diagnostic tests, nursing assessment of the patient with diverticular disease is distinctly more wholistic. Data collection involves the patient, the patient's family, and other health care providers. Although self-report of the older adult is the most common source of the information in a geriatric assessment, the patient may have poor recall or may deliberately minimize symptoms in order to "please" the health care professional. Older adults, particularly the frail elderly, may have multiple and chronic complaints. Rather than having specific, well-defined symptoms and signs of disease, older adults may have vague complaints or report deterioration in their ability to do everyday tasks. Numerous North American Nursing Diagnosis Association (NANDA) nursing diagnoses are relevant in cases of diverticulosis.

Systematic and ongoing nursing assessment in diverticular disease should include standardized assessment tools whenever possible to supplement our traditional "history and physical" approach. Standardized instruments enhance the professional's ability to recognize problems, evaluate them, and monitor progress in solving them. Selective use of the Folstein Mini-Mental Status examination (see Chapter 21) (Folstein et al, 1975), Geriatric Depression Scale (see Chapter 23), Barthel Index (see Appendix 8-A), ADLs/IADLs charts (see Appendix 8-C), and Minimum Data Set (MDS) (see Appendix 8-D) in addition to a theory-based assessment tool should be the gold standard in herontic nursing. The Orem Self-Care Deficit Nursing Theory (SCDNT)–based assessment for the senior patient with diverticulosis may be useful (Orem, 1995).

Management. Avoidance of constipation through the use of fiber intake, fluid intake, and daily exercise is fundamental to patient management and nursing intervention in diverticular disease. Often, though, it is nursing's attention to psychosocial, developmental, financial, and environmental aspects that provides crucial support and helps make the patient successful over the long run. Nursing Interventions Classification (NIC) offers a standardized language describing nursing interventions for patients with diverticulosis. These interventions are suitable for all care settings and address the health promotion, physiologic, psychosocial, and illness treatments for patients and their families (McCloskey and Bulechek, 2002). NIC interventions are linked to NOCs, NANDA nursing diagnoses, long-term care resident assessment protocols (RAPS), and OASIS outcome measures to improve the continuity of care. Diverticulosis care is complex and demanding.

Fiber. Gradually increasing the amount of fiber in the diet may reduce symptoms of diverticulosis and prevent complications such as diverticulitis. Fiber keeps stool soft and lowers pressure inside the colon so that bowel contents can move through easily. The American Dietetic Association recommends 20 to 35 g of fiber each day. Oat bran, psyllium, and wheat bran are commonly available in retail stores. The addition of 4 to 6 g of fiber to the daily diet every 2 weeks is a reasonable pace. Appreciable amounts of fiber can be added to one's diet with little effort. Planning, procuring, storing, preparing, and recording are important steps toward healthful eating. The nurse may also recommend drinking a fiber product such as Citrucel or Metamucil once a day. These products are mixed with water and provide about 4 to 6 g of fiber in an 8-ounce glass. Alternative medicine providers routinely recommend that fiber supplements be taken separately from other medicines (Balch and Balch, 2000).

Fluid. Drinking eight glasses of water per day is recommended to soften the stool and facilitate easy passage through the colon and rectum. Water intake, like fiber, should be gradually increased. The patient can be taught intake and output measurement methods until optimum intake is achieved. Often the use of a diet diary will include tracking of fluid intake.

Diet. Until recently, many doctors suggested avoiding foods with small seeds such as tomatoes or strawberries because they believed that particles could lodge in the diverticula and cause inflammation. However, this is now a controversial point and no evidence supports this recommendation. During episodes of diverticulitis, a clear liquid diet is helpful to rest the colon.

Pain Management. If cramps, bloating, and constipation are a problem, a physician may prescribe a short course of pain medication. However, many medications affect emptying of the colon, an undesirable side effect for people with diverticulosis. Massage, hot or cold packs, stretching exercises, and relaxation or meditation techniques offer reasonable relief in most cases without the adverse side effects of medication.

Education. It may be difficult to alter the health behaviors of older adults. Use these strategies to enhance the likelihood of effecting change in those behaviors:

1. Develop a therapeutic provider-patient partnership.
2. Make a concerted effort to respond to the educational needs of all patients. Quieter patients are often those who require more education.
3. Do not assume that patients understand the association between certain behaviors and health.
4. Help patients identify obstacles to changing behaviors.
5. Ask patients to commit to change. By doing so they indicate their agreement that their behaviors may be related to their health outcomes.
6. Let the patient choose which risk factor to change. Success in one area may stimulate a patient to attempt to modify behaviors in other areas.
7. Use multiple educational strategies, including counseling classes, written materials, audiovisual aids, and community resources. Individualized, personalized, and prioritized interventions are most effective.
8. Design an action plan that points out what patients should do, rather than what they should know.
9. Monitor progress through close follow-up, either through a follow-up appointment or telephone call.
10. Finally, view your own health-promoting behavior as a role model for your patients. It is difficult to help patients exercise or change diet if you have not made these changes in your own behavior. Nurses who both practice and preach health behaviors are better able to foster a healthy lifestyle for themselves and their patients.

Collaboration. Patients with diverticulosis generally benefit from collaborative care, especially if acute complications occur. Nutritional and physical therapy consultations can reduce the nursing care intensity and provide a significant patient motivation to initiate and maintain changes in eating habits and physical activity. Problems are identified in frequent collaborative sessions.

Prevention and Screening. High fiber generally refers to an intake greater than 25 to 30 g per day and is cited in American, European, and Asian studies as protective against diverticulosis (Rubio, 2002). Trowell and Burkitt developed the "fiber theory" 30 years ago by contending that there was a link between a diet rich in fiber and the avoidance of "first world diseases" such as constipation and diverticulosis (Rubio, 2002). Since that time many studies have analyzed the relationship between diet and health. Despite the evidence for fiber consumption as healthy, no consensus exists on the type or amount of fiber that should be consumed (Rubio, 2002).

Routine screening for diverticulosis is not currently recommended. Most people do not have symptoms, and diverticulosis is often discovered incidentally by a physician (Hazzard et al, 1990). Screening for risk factors and some of the symptoms of diverticulosis, however, is included in the current preventive care guidelines adapted from the U.S. Preventive Service Task Force Report. These may be useful.

Coronary Disease

Epidemiology. Coronary problems are the major cause of morbidity, disability, and mortality of the aged. Cardiovascular disease is the most prevalent of the disorders of the aged. However, the concept of the "golden years" as a time of inactivity and confinement is no longer valid, with 85% of elders 65 and older reporting their health as good, very good, or excellent; 80% of seniors also reported no difficulty with any ADLs. Exercise, leisure physical activities, and competitive sports are an important part of the life of many retired elders. Although chronic conditions, such as arthritis (47.7% of seniors) and heart disease (59.8% of seniors), frequently occur in this age-group, they are not contraindications to regular activity, especially the continuation of modified forms of prior exercise.

Cardiovascular changes do occur with aging; however, some cardiovascular functions do not decline as a result of age alone. According to Hill (2001), exercise cardiac output is maintained with advancing age in healthy human subjects. The mechanism of increased cardiac output is achieved by cardiac dilation and increased stroke volume, which compensate for a diminished heart rate in the elderly. The variability of senescence and the range of physical activity levels seen in elder athletes make aging physiology important in their assessment and treatment. Cardiopulmonary and musculoskeletal systems have intrinsic changes related to aging, some of which are slowed by fitness activities, others of which may increase or affect speed of recovery from injury. The interplay of these systems often is measured by maximum oxygen consumption to quantify cardiopulmonary endurance as a marker of fitness. As people age past the thirties, their maximum work capacity declines at a rate of about $^1/_{37}$ per year (Williams, 1999). A person's highest level of conditioning influences his or her final level of decline. Therefore athletes and untrained or sedentary seniors will have very different functional abilities. Unfortunately, the inactive senior will decline twice as fast as his or her physically active counterpart.

Coronary Artery Disease. The beating heart, like other muscles, needs oxygen and other nutrients to provide energy for its work. The coronary arteries are the vessels that bring the blood to the heart muscle. Despite all of the blood that passes through the heart, it cannot use the nutrients from the blood that passes through its chambers. The heart muscle, like all other muscles, receives its oxygen from arteries. Blockage in these arteries is the cause of most of the heart disease in the United States. Cholesterol is widely discussed and blamed for the development of coronary artery disease, but current research suggests that this may not be accurate. Several systems in the body are involved in the atherosclerotic process (Farmer and Gotto, 1997), which narrows the cardiac arteries:

- Inflammatory system (system that responds to infection and injuries)
- Blood-clotting system
- Inner lining of the coronary arteries
- Cholesterol-handling system
- Body's wound-healing system

Narrowed arterial lumens probably result from a complicated interaction of these systems, a process that begins before birth. Researchers have established that atherosclerosis, the process that produces narrow, hard vessels, can begin in the first year of life. Common in most diseases, coronary artery disease develops from an interaction of genetic and environmental influences. Over 250 genes have been proposed to be involved in coronary artery disease (Higgins, 2000). There is continuing research regarding these. It is probably a matter of nature and nurture, not nature versus nurture. It makes sense that genes and environment both play a role in coronary artery disease. Since Nightingale's time, nursing has embraced the importance of the patient and his or her environment. A narrowing starts forming after an injury to the inner lining of the coronary artery. The inflammatory system responds to this injury, but overreacts, spurred on by elements of the blood-clotting system. The injury to the inner lining of the artery does not heal properly. If the cap ever comes loose or breaks off (rather like a scab), the underlying gelatin core will trigger the formation of a blood clot. If the blood clot is small, the person may never know it happened.

Definition. Coronary artery disease (CAD) is blockage of the vessels that supply the heart with blood. This disease process is termed *arteriosclerosis,* commonly called "hardening of the arteries." In this process, cholesterol and other fats are deposited in the layers of the arteries, narrowing the channel for blood to flow.

Risk Factors. Today, the controllable risk factors for CAD are generally well known among the public. Understanding these contributions to CAD was one of the great scientific achievements of the twentieth century. The changes in nursing, medicine, and culture that came from this understanding have dramatically reduced the death rate from coronary disease in the United States. Risk for CAD is higher if a relative developed coronary disease at an early age. "Early age" is before age 55 in men and before age 65 in women. This follows a general rule in genetics: The earlier in life a disease occurs, the greater is the influence of genes.

Signs and Symptoms. Angina is a recurring pain or discomfort in the chest that happens when some part of the heart does not receive enough blood. It is a common symptom of coronary heart disease (CHD), which occurs when vessels that carry blood to the heart become narrowed and blocked due to atherosclerosis. Angina feels like a pressing or squeezing pain, usually in the chest under the breastbone, but sometimes in the shoulders, arms, neck, jaws, or back. Angina is usually precipitated by exertion. Unfortunately, many elderly patients with heart attacks do not have this classic presentation. Their discomfort may be relatively mild and may be localized to the back, abdomen, shoulders, or either or both arms. Nausea and vomiting, or merely a feeling of heartburn, may be the only symptom. These less classic symptoms may not make patients think of a heart problem and may keep them from seeking medical help. In fact, up to 30% of heart attacks are diagnosed by taking a routine ECG long after the fact. This is why seniors with one or more risk factors for CAD need to pay close attention to any unusual symptoms involving the upper half of the body.

Acute Complications. Myocardial infarction (MI) is the death of heart muscle caused by a blockage in one of the coronary arteries. A heart attack occurs when a blood clot forms at the site of an atherosclerotic plaque in a coronary artery. The clot blocks the artery, and blood flow stops. The heart muscle being supplied by that artery immediately becomes starved for oxygen (i.e., the muscle becomes ischemic), and if blood flow is not restored within a few hours, the heart muscle dies.

Heart attacks, heart failure, angina, and sudden death all can occur from the blockages that occur in these vessels (strokes occur with blockages in the vessels to the brain). Typically, there is one artery on the right side and one on the left, with the left one generally being the larger. The left main coronary artery divides into two sizable branches, the left anterior descending (supplying the front of the heart) and the left circumflex (wrapping around the left side and back of the heart). The right coronary artery supplies the back of the heart. Coronary artery disease generally refers to the buildup of cholesterol in the inside layers of the arteries. This gradually narrows the flow of blood through the vessel, and the muscle it supplies eventually will not get enough blood. The plaque weakens the wall. When the vessel is narrowed 90%, there is the potential for lack of blood supply at rest. When the vessel becomes 100% closed, a myocardial infarction ("heart attack") generally occurs. If the vessel closes gradually enough, the muscle may obtain flow from other vessels.

The patient's reluctance to get medical help is the most common reason for critical delays in therapy for heart attacks. The first 3 to 6 hours after the onset of the heart attack are critically important. Most of the lethal arrhythmias seen with acute heart attacks occur during the first few hours. If these arrhythmias occur while the victim is under medical attention, they can virtually always be stopped in time to prevent a catastrophe. If the artery can be opened within the first few hours after the blockage occurs, much of the dying heart muscle can be saved, much of the permanent heart damage can be avoided, and the patient's risk of death or permanent disability can be greatly diminished. But if treatment is delayed beyond 6 hours, the amount of heart muscle that can still be saved drops off significantly.

Progressive Signs and Symptoms. If the amount of heart damage is only mild or moderate, heart failure does not occur—at least, not right away. However, in the effort to heal itself, the heart goes through a period of "remodeling," in which the heart enlarges and changes shape. This remodeling eventually leads to a decrease in cardiac pumping efficiency, and it can lead to a more gradual onset of heart failure months or years after the heart attack. As coronary artery damage progresses, systemic signs may affect function.

Assessment. Because older adults often overestimate their ability to perform ADLs unimpaired by angina or shortness of breath, testing their performance will provide a much more accurate assessment of their abilities. Try to watch the older adult perform ADLs. Increased cardiac output in the elderly is accomplished primarily by increasing stroke volume rather than by increasing heart rate. Most healthy elderly can effectively use this compensatory mechanism to maintain or increase cardiac output during stress or exercise. Elders with artherosclerotic or valvular disease, however, may have difficulty finding reserve cardiac output capacity in the face of a significant stress. Slowing of the electrical activity of the intrinsic cardiac pacemakers of the heart with age has also been shown. This phenomenon has been said to make the older person more susceptible to arrhythmias and extrasystoles. Keep this in mind when assessing the older adult. Question the senior regarding major symptoms for each major body system. Emphasize symptoms common to aging clients. Ask regarding pain, pressure, or discomfort in every system. Box 8-21 suggests important assessment aspects in CHF.

Management. Coronary problems can produce a "cardiac cripple" when an individual believes that any exertion burdens the overtaxed heart and may potentiate heart attack and death. In reality, few elders develop activity-induced ischemia. They are much more likely to trigger an attack by complicating illnesses that increase myocardial oxygen demand, such as infections and bleeding episodes. Cardiac exercise rehabilitation programs must be encouraged for the physical and mental health of the individual. It has been found that exercise training of elderly coronary patients increases work capacity and

Box 8-21 Assessment for Clients with CHF

Brief history of onset and course of condition
Vital signs
Cardiac and respiratory inspection and auscultation of heart and breath sounds
Mental status check
Activity capabilities
Lifestyle
Genitourinary (nocturia, oliguria)
Weight change
Client's perception of condition, reaction to diagnosis, and treatment
General laboratory values (electrolytes, hemoglobin, hematocrit, coagulation)

Compiled from Saunders SA: Atherosclerotic heart disease: heart failure. In Rogers-Seidl FF, editor: *Geriatric nursing care plans,* St Louis, 1991, Mosby; Havens LL, Weaver JW: Cardiovascular system. In Hogstel MO: *Clinical manual of gerontological nursing,* St Louis, 1992, Mosby.

vagal tone and decreases resting heart rate, body weight, and percentage of body fat (Wenger, 1990). Typical programs begin with light activity and progress to moderate activity under the supervision of a nurse or physical therapist. Seniors generally possess significant time to act on behalf of their health. Their commitment to exercise patterns can be easily reinforced because of the rapid benefits, such as enhanced functional independence and self-esteem (Hill, 2001).

The level of activity may be expressed in metabolic equivalents (METs). For example, light to moderate housework is equivalent to 2 to 4 METs; heavy housework or yard work is equal to 5 to 6 METs. A person would be tested for a baseline ability of between 4 and 5 METs. Results of the testing can guide a prescriptive physical activity program at home or in a structured rehabilitation program.

Appropriately designed exercise programs take into account the need for building in longer periods for the exercise heart rate to return to its resting level and low-level activity between components of exercise training. Postexercise orthostatic hypotension is more likely to occur in the aged because of decreased baroreceptor responsiveness. Thermoregulation is impaired, and therefore exercise intensity must be reduced in hot, humid climates. These factors must be considered. A recommended training heart rate ranges from 50% to 70% of maximal heart rate achieved at exercise testing and does not result in discomfort during exercise. Perseverance and consistency are the keys to success and benefits.

Cardiac rehabilitation programs for the elderly person should emphasize activities that build endurance and self-reliance to facilitate self-care and quality of life. For the more impaired clients it is necessary to help them identify energy conservation measures applicable to their daily tasks. Risk reduction programs should be instituted with a clear understanding of the difficulties these present when attempting to alter harmful lifestyles, such as smoking, overeating, habitual anger or irritation, and sedentary lifestyle with sporadic bouts of excessive activity. These are often deeply embedded in the personality structure and are not easily eradicated by "education." Begin by discussing this with the individual—nonjudgmentally. The nursing role is to provide acceptance, encouragement, resources, knowledge, and affirmation of the individual and his or her right to choose. Group programs focused on these issues have shown that some members' motivation and perceived health status improve (Wenger, 1990).

Gender is a factor in the outcome of cardiac rehabilitation. In a study of men and women participating in a structured or home cardiac rehabilitation program, Schuster, Wright, and Tomich (1995) found that men in the structured programs knew more about heart disease and supportive treatment than women. The women failed to increase their understanding of their cardiac disease whether they were in a structured or home cardiac rehabilitation program. Women also demonstrated the poorest exercise adherence. With the increasing number of postmenopausal women, it is important for the nurse to consider this type of finding. It seems from the conclusions of Schuster that women need the reassurance that they already have some knowledge and that they can build on this knowledge to ensure better cardiac health. Because patients with cardiac disorders ordinarily take several medications to control heart rate, strength of beat, hypertension, and angina, these must be carefully and routinely monitored. Many of these drugs have serious toxic side effects, and when an individual decompensates, a medication assessment is the first order of the day.

One of the major ways that cardiac care differs from that for other chronic problems is that most exacerbations require acute hospitalization and intensive treatment, whereas many of the other chronic disorders are essentially managed at home the majority of the time. Onset of illness or exacerbation of chronic disorders may be quite different in older clients. For those with cardiac and other problems, the following events should always trigger investigation:

- Light-headedness or dizziness
- Disturbances in gait and balance
- Loss of appetite or unexplained loss of weight
- Inability to concentrate or shortened attention span
- Changes in personality
- Changes in grooming habits
- Unusual patterns in urination or defecation
- Vague discomfort, frequent bouts of anxiety
- Excessive fatigue, vague pain
- Withdrawal from usual sources of pleasure

There is no one test that should be done before a senior with CAD embarks on a rehabilitation program. A thorough physical, mental, and functional assessment should be done to determine the extent and severity and to rule out other possible causes of the symptoms of CHD.

What specific recommendations about exercise should you make for a hypothetical 69-year-old who has not exercised for years and is overweight?

- Starting slowly
- Using stretching exercises
- Using flexibility exercises
- Walking at a leisurely pace three times per week
- Increasing pace of walking three times per week
- Advancing to aerobic exercise three times per week (perhaps on a stationary bicycle)

The ultimate goal is regular exercise three times per week at 70% of maximum heart rate (220 minus age in years). Exercise is a very important item in the cardiac rehabilitation of seniors (Wenger, 1990; Carpenito, 2002).

Prevention and Screening. Studies have demonstrated that lowering cholesterol levels results in a reduction of subsequent cardiac morbidity and mortality rates, but not the overall death rate. This failure to lower the overall death rate may be due to adverse drug side effects or the failure to lower cholesterol levels sufficiently to cause regression of atherosclerosis. Few data are currently available about primary prevention of CAD in the elderly. However, a large, multicenter primary prevention trial in the elderly is currently in progress.

Many secondary prevention trials have been completed, with results similar to those of the primary prevention trials: a reduction in cardiac morbidity and mortality rates, but not in the overall death rate. In other studies, sequential coronary angiograms were performed to examine the effects of aggressive intervention on the progression of coronary lesions. In general, intensive intervention has slowed the progression or even caused regression of atherosclerosis. No secondary prevention trials geared specifically to the elderly have yet been carried out.

In low-risk individuals with "desirable" total cholesterol and LDL-C levels, cholesterol levels should be measured every 5 years. More frequent measurements should be made in individuals with other CAD risk factors or in those who might have secondary causes of hyperlipidemia, such as diabetes.

A large percentage of the elderly have evidence of hyperlipidemia; however, treatment of hyperlipidemia in the elderly remains controversial. Most of the available data comes from studies performed in middle-aged men. Therefore extrapolation to the elderly, particularly elderly women, is in question. Two large-scale intervention trials are currently in progress to ascertain whether treatment of hyperlipidemia decreases mortality and morbidity rates from CAD in the elderly, and these results should be valuable in formulating treatment guidelines. Many geriatricians currently advocate aggressive screening and intervention in the "vigorous elderly," particularly those with known heart disease or multiple CAD risk factors.

The resting ECG has a low positive predictive value for CAD. When done on asymptomatic persons with a low probability of CAD, a large proportion of false-positive findings are produced. There is no evidence that treating asymptomatic silent ischemia will reduce the incidence of symptomatic cardiac events later. Therefore obtaining a resting ECG is not currently recommended. However, some clinicians advocate obtaining an ECG in men above age 40 if they have two or more risk factors for CAD. Similarly, the exercise stress test has a low positive predictive value. Only 30% of patients with a positive stress test are found on cardiac catheterization to have more than 50% narrowing of the coronary arteries. As a result, there is no consensus on whether to recommend an exercise stress test.

The American College of Sports Medicine advocates exercise treadmill testing before initiating a vigorous exercise program in individuals above age 45 years. The American Heart Association and American College of Cardiologists advocate exercise treadmill testing in men above age 40, particularly in those with multiple CAD risk factors and in whom a cardiac event would endanger public safety.

A trial of 22,000 asymptomatic male physicians taking 325 mg of aspirin daily versus placebo was conducted in the United States to determine whether low-dose aspirin protected against CAD. After 4 years, the study was discontinued because of a 47% reduced incidence of fatal and nonfatal myocardial infarctions among the group taking the aspirin. However, a study in the United Kingdom of 5139 doctors taking 500 mg per day found no reduction in myocardial infarctions and an increased incidence of side effects with aspirin. Therefore consider low-does aspirin therapy (325 mg daily) for men over 40 with these risk factors for myocardial infarction:

- Hypercholesterolemia
- Smoking
- Diabetes mellitus
- Family history of early CAD
- HDL-C less than 35 mg/dl
- LDL-C greater than 130 mg/dl
- Hypertension
- Obesity
- Previous myocardial infarction
- Transient ischemic attacks
- Post–coronary artery bypass graft (post-CABG)
- Postthrombolysis

Screening and risk assessment can be invasive or noninvasive. The invasive approach, cardiac catheterization and coronary angiography, is the most accurate; however, the inherent risks in the elderly can be substantial. The advantage of the invasive approach is that any guesswork about the overall status of a patient's coronary arteries is removed. The noninvasive approach involves exercise stress testing. If signs of ischemia are seen, the patient is referred for cardiac catheterization to define the precise anatomy involved. If signs of ischemia are not seen during exercise, the odds of having critical coronary artery disease (or an early recurrent heart attack) are statistically low. Deciding whether the invasive or noninvasive approach ought to be used is controversial. Most cardiologists prefer the invasive approach because it removes the guesswork. Often the nurse finds herself or himself in the middle of this controversy when the patient asks for decision-making guidance. A reasonable compromise is to use the noninvasive approach in patients who are judged on clinical grounds to fall into a low-risk category for recurrent coronary events. Low-risk patients are under 60, have had no angina or signs of heart failure, have few if any risk factors, have had a heart attack involving the right coronary artery, do not have diabetes, and have normal blood pressure (Chan and Johnson, 2002).

Coronary artery calcium scanning is a relatively new procedure. Performed by ultrafast CT, often without a physician's order, it holds promise for noninvasive detection of underlying coronary artery disease and an estimate of its extent and severity.

Congestive Heart Failure

Epidemiology. Because heart failure usually develops slowly, the symptoms may not appear until the condition has progressed significantly. During this phase of "silent" disease development, the underlying normal aging of the cardiac muscle potentiates any overlying pathology. The heart adjusts, or compensates, in three ways to cope with the effects of heart failure:

- Enlargement (dilation), which allows more blood into the heart
- Thickening (hypertrophy) of muscle fibers to strengthen the heart muscle, which allows the heart to contract more forcefully and pump more blood
- More frequent contraction, which increases circulation

Although compensating for aging and diseases such as CAD and MI delays the eventual loss in pumping capacity, it does not prevent it. Eventually, the heart cannot offset the lost ability to pump blood, and the signs of heart failure appear. Because cardiomyopathy itself usually does not cause any symptoms until heart damage is severe enough to produce heart failure, the symptoms of cardiomyopathy are those of heart failure.

There are three major types of cardiomyopathy: dilated cardiomyopathy, hypertrophic cardiomyopathy, and restrictive cardiomyopathy. Hypertrophic cardiomyopathy is also known as idiopathic hypertrophic subaortic stenosis (IHSS) or asymmetric septal hypertrophy (ASH). Hypertrophic cardiomyopathy is a genetic disorder that causes a chaotic growth of heart muscle cells within the ventricles (most prominent in the left ventricle), which causes an abnormal thickening of the heart muscle. The disordered, thickened (or hypertrophic) heart muscle can lead to problems pumping sufficient blood to the body's organs and can cause potentially fatal cardiac arrhythmias. Restrictive cardiomyopathy is a rare condition in which the heart muscle is infiltrated by abnormal cells, protein, or scar tissue. Common in the elderly is dilated cardiomyopathy (congestive heart failure), in which a previously normal heart muscle becomes damaged, leading to a generalized weakening of the walls of the cardiac chambers. The weakening and the dilation of the heart muscle eventually lead to heart failure.

Definition. Congestive heart failure is a disease of the heart muscle. In most cases, cardiomyopathy decreases heart muscle function. When the heart can no longer pump enough blood to meet the needs of the body, heart failure is said to be present. Diagnosing dilated cardiomyopathy depends on demonstrating enlargement of the cardiac chambers, especially the ventricular chambers. Such enlargement can be seen on chest x-ray, but it can be more accurately measured using an echocardiogram or a multiple gated acquisition (MUGA) scan.

Risk Factors. Patients who suffer large heart attacks have a high risk of developing heart failure, and its onset can be acute—often within the first few hours or days. But even patients with only a moderate amount of muscle damage can eventually experience heart failure. For these patients, appropriate drug therapy can often delay or prevent the onset of heart failure. For patients with only moderate muscle damage, whether heart failure ensues depends to a large extent on how the remaining normal heart muscle behaves. The behavior of the normal heart muscle in response to damage to another portion of heart muscle is termed *remodeling*. After a heart attack, the normal heart muscle stretches in an attempt to pick up the slack for the muscle that has been damaged. The stretching increases the force of contraction in normal muscle and allows it to do more work. In this way, unfortunately, the heart muscle behaves something like a rubber band—the more it stretches, the more it "snaps back."

Signs and Symptoms. Common signs and symptoms in the elderly include fatigue or shortness of breath with exertion, inability to lie flat without getting short of breath (orthopnea), waking up at night gasping for air (paroxysmal nocturnal dyspnea), weight gain, and swelling in the lower extremities. Clinical heart failure is usually further categorized as left-sided, right-sided, or biventricular heart failure, which correspond to signs and symptoms. There are common symptom clusters for right- and left-sided failure. Left-sided heart failure is the most common form and in turn is responsible for eventual right-sided heart failure (Braunwald and Grossman, 1992). However, the rapidity of disease progression dictates management.

Acute Complications. There is an increased incidence of life-threatening arrhythmias, namely ventricular tachycardia and ventricular fibrillation. In these patients, an episode of syncope should be regarded as a harbinger of sudden death.

Progressive Signs and Symptoms. Heart failure is one of the most serious symptoms of heart disease. Until recently, only 50% of patients with cardiomyopathy survived for 5 years and only 25% survived for 10 or more years after diagnosis of the condition. However, new therapies such as the use of beta-blockers and ACE inhibitors promise to significantly improve those survival figures. It is likely that patients being diagnosed today will have survival figures that are substantially better.

As the disease progresses so do the symptoms. Classically, the clinical pattern of a patient with dilated cardiomyopathy is characterized by episodes of severe heart failure (extreme shortness of breath, extreme fatigue, leg swelling) that lead to hospitalization for stabilization, followed by relatively long periods of "baseline" symptomatology. During this baseline period, patients often have symptoms only with exertion. As time goes by, the episodes of severe heart failure become more and more frequent. A gradually worsened level of cardiac function characterizes the "baseline" periods of CHF. In the year or so before death, frequent hospitalizations are common, and it is usually apparent to both patient and doctor that a steady, unrelenting deterioration is under way.

Fluid balance in the progressively cardiomyopathic patient who is over 65 years poses a considerable nursing challenge. If the lung tissue becomes waterlogged, as it does in uncompensated heart failure, less oxygen can be transferred to the blood. In time a persistent cough will develop, especially coughing that regularly produces mucus or pink, blood-tinged sputum. Some people develop raspy breathing or wheezing. Often patients will have to prop themselves up with extra pillows to sleep. The number of pillows used may indicate the extent or progression of CHF. Nighttime awakenings because of shortness of breath are an important symptom of progression.

Box 8-22 Classification of CHF

Class I	***Basically asymptomatic*** Cardiac disease without resulting limitations of physical activity
Class II	***Mild heart failure*** Slight limitation of physical activity Comfortable at rest An increase in activity may cause fatigue, palpitations, dyspnea, or anginal pain
Class III	***Moderate heart failure*** Marked limitation in physical activity Comfortable at rest Ordinary walking or climbing of stairs can quickly bring on symptoms of fatigue, palpitations, dyspnea, or anginal pain Substantial periods of bed rest required
Class IV	***Severe heart failure*** Almost permanently confined to bed Inability to carry on any physical activity without discomfort or severe symptoms Some symptoms occur at rest Chronic shortness of breath is common

Fluid overload of the CHF patient is complicated by an age-related decrease in kidney function. A fall in creatinine clearance correlates with a decrease in the glomerular filtration rate (GFR) of approximately 50% as one ages from 30 to 90 years. The GFR, because it affects the ability of the elderly to concentrate urine, remove body fluid, and excrete many medications, is an important aspect of managing progressive heart failure. Seniors are less able to respond to stresses that affect acid excretion and sodium transport. Although acid-base parameters may be normal under basal conditions, the ability of the older adult to respond to an acid or sodium load is impaired. Likewise, during periods of sodium deprivation, the elderly are thought to be less able to conserve sodium, and thus stand a greater chance of developing sodium depletion and hyponatremia. Although total serum renin concentration remains stable with age, there is an age-related decline in active renin concentration. This causes a blunted renin response to postural changes, and it is one of the mechanisms postulated for the frequency of postural hypotension in the elderly. Because of the decreased GFR, blunted renin-aldosterone axis, and decreased tubular mass, the elderly may have less ability to protect against hyperkalemia in the face of increased potassium loads.

Chronically stretching normal heart muscle causes it to progressively weaken, and heart failure ensues. Therefore avoidance of ventricular remodeling is the key to halting the progression of heart failure. A formal classification of CHF has been established by the New York Heart Association, which identifies characteristics of disease progression (Braunwald and Grossman, 1992) (Box 8-22 lists the classifications).

A good index of the amount of heart muscle damage that has occurred after a heart attack is to measure the left ventricular ejection fraction (LVEF), which is the percentage of blood ejected by the left ventricle with each heartbeat. If the LVEF is less than 40%, significant damage has occurred. The amount of stretching that has occurred can be assessed by measuring the dimensions of the left ventricle—stretching of the heart muscle produces dilation of the ventricle, so greater-than-normal left ventricular dimensions indicate that significant ventricular remodeling is occurring. The greater the dilation of the ventricle, the poorer the patient's prognosis.

Assessment. Assessment using the aspects listed in Boxes 8-21 and 8-22 will facilitate your interaction and collaboration with physicians; however, the disease focus omits several hallmarks of holistic nursing. Nursing data collection involves the patient, family, and other health care providers. Older adults, particularly the frail elderly, may have multiple and chronic complaints over the course of many years of living with CHF. Rather than having specific, well-defined symptoms and signs of disease, older adults often have vague complaints or report deterioration in their ability to do everyday tasks. Include standardized assessment tools whenever possible to supplement the traditional "history and physical" approach. Standardized instruments enhance the professional's ability to recognize problems, evaluate them, and monitor progress in solving them. Selective use of the Folstein Mini-Mental Status examination (see Chapter 21) (Folstein et al, 1975), Geriatric Depression Scale (see Chapter 23), Barthel Index (see Appendix 8-A), Nursing Outcomes Classification (NOC) (Johnson and Maas, 2000), and Minimum Data Set (MDS) (see Appendix 8-D) in addition to a theory-based assessment tool should be the gold standard in gerontic nursing.

The variability in senescence of the cardiopulmonary systems and the range of physical activity levels currently seen in elders make careful assessment important in the CHF patient (Hill, 2001). Americans are remaining physically active into their seventies, eighties, and nineties. Healthy elderly fitness data may be inappropriately used.

Often it is in discussing an elder's ADLs and IADLs that the nurse obtains the best picture of the patient's response to CHF and its medication regimen. The rate of symptom onset, relationship to activities, exercise tolerance, and nighttime symptoms are easily quantified by the patient when discussed in relationship to his or her usual activities. Orthopnea, dyspnea, palpitations, weakness, chest pressure, and edema, while clearly different symptoms to the nurse, may be more difficult concepts for the elderly. Certainly most are unfamiliar with the medical definitions and logic of symptom cause. The influences of stress, alcohol use, eating, and smoking are less clear to the senior and are often overlooked by the physician. Historically, the American College of Sports Medicine has recommended a rating of perceived exertion (RPE) approach to measuring subjective sensations during exercise on a scale of 0 to 10. Resting and active RPEs solicited by the nurse, for the symptoms of CHF, from the senior is a reasonable approach. Whenever possible, postactivity recovery of vital signs should also be assessed related to each symptom and activity.

Although it is ideal to know the patient's baseline pulse before disease development, the "silent" nature of cardiomyopathic progression would call into question what is truly "normal" or baseline for the patient. In the absence of other quantitative measures of the patient's cardiac function, keeping the patient's target heart rate for exercise in mind can help put the patient's resting and active pulse in some perspective. Calculation of the target heart rate involves subtracting the patient's age in years from 220, then identifying 80% of that value (Estes, 2002). This age-adjusted approach may be more useful in seniors than the generic pulse range.

Accurate assessment of the elderly patient's heart sounds, pulses, and jugular venous distention is of the utmost importance to identifying progressive heart failure or sudden decompensation because the elderly often have nonspecific complaints. The appearance of an S_3 heart sound, heard best during inspiration and occurring just after S_2 (the heart rhythm sounds like "Kentucky"), may be one of the earliest clinical findings of worsening cardiac dysfunction (Estes, 2002). Some hyperkinesis of the pulse in seniors is expected as a result of aging arteries and may blunt the hypokinesis expected in stages of CHF. Assessment of CHF patients using respiratory assistive devices is an additional consideration.

Interventions and Management. Medical interventions for patients with CHF are centered on medications to stabilize the underlying cause of the cardiomyopathy, minimize the symptoms of heart failure, and optimize the efficiency of the failing heart. Common medications include ACE inhibitors, beta-blockers, digitalis, and diuretics. Reduction of dosage of most renally excreted medications is therefore recommended in the elderly, with significant care being taken when prescribing medications that may be renal toxic.

Use of the implantable defibrillator is limited by the FDA, and appropriate indications for using this lifesaving device in patients with heart failure are changing frequently. Newer forms of therapy are being actively evaluated for patients with dilated cardiomyopathy. Biventricular pacing is an investigational form of cardiac pacing that stimulates both ventricles (right and left) simultaneously. Recoordinating ventricular contractions improves the efficiency of the heart and increases the amount of blood pumped with each heartbeat. Preliminary studies with biventricular pacing suggest that a substantial proportion of patients with dilated cardiomyopathy can achieve significant improvement in both cardiac function and symptoms. Meanwhile, work on an artificial heart is quietly and gradually making progress.

Nursing interventions generally address pathophysiologic, treatment-related, environmental, developmental, and collaborative problems. Interventions vary with the degree of congestive failure. They range from teaching the client about lifestyle changes in diet, activity, and rest to acute measures such as administration of oxygen if congestive failure is acute (Box 8-23). Common nursing interventions include the following:

1. Activity tolerance
2. Prescribed exercise program

Box 8-23 Topics for Patient, Family, and Caregiver Education and Counseling on Heart Failure

General Counseling

Explanation of heart failure and reasons for symptoms
Cause or probable cause of heart failure
Expected symptoms
Symptoms of worsening heart failure
What to do if symptoms worsen
Self-monitoring with daily weights
Explanation of treatment/care plan
Clarification of patient's responsibilities
Importance of cessation of tobacco use
Role of family members or other caregivers in the treatment/care plan
Availability and value of qualified local support group
Importance of obtaining vaccinations against influenza and pneumococcal disease

Prognosis

Life expectancy
Advance directives
Advice for family members in the event of sudden death

Activity Recommendations

Recreation, leisure, and work activity
Exercise
Sex, sex difficulties, and coping strategies

Dietary Recommendations

Sodium restriction
Avoidance of excessive fluid intake
Fluid restriction (if required)
Alcohol restriction

Medications

Effect of medications on quality of life and survival
Likely side effects and what to do if they occur
Coping mechanisms for complicated medical regimens
Availability of lower cost medications or financial assistance

Importance of Adherence with the Treatment/Case Plan

Modified from Konstam MA et al: *Heart failure: evaluation and care of patients with left-ventricular systolic of dysfunction,* Clinical practice guideline no 11, pub no 94-0612, Rockville, MD, 1994, U.S. Department of Health and Human Services, Public Health Service Agency for Health Care and Policy Research.

3. Medication administration and the evaluation of medication effects
4. Monitoring for signs and symptoms of CHF
5. Monitoring intake and output
6. Monitoring client's weight
7. Checking for jugular distention
8. Auscultating heart and breath sounds
9. Noting laboratory values
10. Client education: low-sodium diet; medication regimen; signs and symptoms to report to the physician, such as weight gain of 2 to 3 lb in a few days, increased nocturia, increase in shortness of breath, a persistent cough, and ankle and leg swelling

Early clinical trials on the therapeutic potential of a vitamin supplement, coenzyme Q10, focused on congestive heart failure. Dr. Per Langsjoen pioneered research that was subsequently confirmed to produce improved patient outcomes with adjunctive coenzyme Q10 supplementation in those with New York Heart Association (NYHA) class I or II CHF, present for less than 1 year (Langsjoen et al, 1997).

Collaborative problems and continuity of care are facilitated by the utilization of NANDA-linked Nursing Interventions Classification (NIC) labels (available at *www.nursing.uiowa.edu/nic*) and Nursing Outcomes Classification (NOC) indicators (available at *www.nursing.uiowa.edu/noc*). These are recommended.

Screening and Prevention. Among people greater than 70 years old, approximately 8 out of 1000 are diagnosed with congestive heart failure each year. Because almost anything that damages cardiac muscle can lead to dilated cardiomyopathy, there are many causes of, and therefore many ways to prevent, CHF. The most common cause of cardiomyopathy in the United States is coronary artery disease. Heart attacks cause death of heart muscle by obstruction of a coronary artery. Although the damage is localized to the region of muscle supplied by that artery, within a few months the entire left ventricle dilates (or remodels) to compensate for the damage. With a small heart attack, the amount of ventricular dilation is minimal. But with a large heart attack or a series of smaller heart attacks, dilated cardiomyopathy becomes extensive, and heart failure ensues.

CHF is also associated with uncontrolled hypertension, alcohol abuse, cocaine or amphetamine abuse, and chronic hyperthyroidism. Another common cause of dilated cardiomyopathy is inflammation of the heart muscle, a condition termed *myocarditis*. Myocarditis is most often caused by viral infections, but it can also be caused by bacterial infections and by noninfectious causes such as lupus and other inflammatory diseases. Valvular heart disease, especially aortic regurgitation and mitral regurgitation, causes dilated cardiomyopathy. Indeed, the gradual enlargement of the cardiac chambers is an important sign that the time may be right for valve replacement or repair.

In conclusion, cardiac "overwork" is generally the cause of dilated cardiomyopathy. Any condition that causes the heart muscle to work at high loads for prolonged periods of time (weeks or months) can eventually cause cardiac dilation and weakening of the heart muscle. Avoiding or controlling the causes is crucial to avoiding CHF.

Vascular Insufficiency

Epidemiology. Affecting 7 to 12 million Americans (Lawrence, 2000), vascular insufficiency occurs more frequently in those over 70 years of age. Medical diagnoses that are included in this category are (1) peripheral artery disease, (2) arterial insufficiency, (3) vascular claudication, (4) Leriche syndrome, (5) femoropopliteal occlusive disease, (6) peripheral vascular disease, (7) claudication, (8) aortoiliac occlusive disease, and (9) iliofemoral occlusive disease.

The peak incidence of superficial venous insufficiency, which tends to develop from deep venous insufficiency, is the fifth decade in women and the eighth decade in men (Novartis Foundation for Gerontology, 2002).

Definition. Vascular insufficiency includes both arterial and venous systems. Arterial insufficiency occurs when arterial stenoses or occlusions cause severe impairment of blood flow to the point where basal requirements for tissue oxygenation cannot be met (McGee and Boyko, 1998).

Chronic venous insufficiency (CVI) of the lower extremities is a condition caused by abnormalities of the vein walls and valves, leading to obstruction or reflux of blood flow in the veins. Venous insufficiency affects the deep or superficial veins, permitting reverse flow and resulting in raised pressure in the veins during ambulation.

Risk Factors. Risk factors for insufficiency include advanced age. Modifiable causes include tobacco use (risk persists for more than 5 years after cessation), uncontrolled diabetes, uncontrolled systolic hypertension, hypercholesterolemia, and obesity. Current research indicates that claudication remains stable in 80% of patients with a risk of limb loss (amputation) of 4% to 7% at 5 years and 12% at 10 years (Lawrence, 2000).

Signs and Symptoms. Arterial insufficiency symptoms include resting pain that is classically described as an ache, pain, numbness, or squeezing sensation, often in the arch of the foot and toes, that occurs more often when the leg is elevated. Claudication symptom characteristics in arterial insufficiency are as follows:

1. Calf, thigh, or buttock pain
2. Pain worse with exertion
3. Pain relieved with several minutes of rest
4. Pain relieved with dependent position

The most uncomfortable time for the patient with arterial insufficiency is during the evening, while resting. Patients with ischemic rest pain frequently awaken from sleep. Some relief of rest pain occurs when the leg is placed in a dependent position. Patients often experience temporary relief of ischemic pain when they begin walking as a result of improved arteriolar flow related to gravitational effects. Ischemic ulcers may develop with significant disease, and they have a characteristic appearance. Generally, they appear distally, at the ends of the toes and over bony prominences. Arterial insufficiency ulcers are dry, necrotic, without signs of vascularity, and pale at the base. There may be a dense fibrinous exudate over the ulcer. Intense pain is a hallmark of ischemic ulcers.

Venous insufficiency is characterized by a dark bluish-purple discoloration. Over time, long-standing stasis of blood leads to the deposition of hemosiderin, giving the skin a dark, speckled appearance. If the leg is placed in a dependent position, the bluish-purple discoloration may darken dramatically, further suggestive of venous insufficiency. This occurs as a result of gravity working against an already ineffective blood return system. Varicosities of the superficial veins may result if the volume of reverse flow is large enough. Traditionally thought to cause many different symptoms, recent studies document only itching, heaviness, and aching as significant correlates with presence of varicosities. Dependent edema (2 to 5 mm macules of skin depigmentation within areas of hyperpigmentation), dermatitis, and firm induration at the medial ankle are common signs in chronic venous insufficiency.

Acute Complications. A delay in medical diagnosis of arterial insufficiency may increase the risk of limb loss and lack of functional mobility. Patients with diabetes mellitus should have an annual assessment for the presence of claudication symptoms or progressive limitation in pain-free walking distance, along with palpation of leg pulses. If these symptoms are present or if pulses are absent, prompt referral to a physician or vascular center should be performed.

Venous insufficiency ulcers are more common in women and are commonly chronic or recurrent in nature (Lawrence, 2001). Deep vein thrombosis with subsequent postphlebitic syndrome may accompany chronic edema and trophic skin changes.

A secondary infection may develop; the ulcer can become "wet" and develop a malodorous, purulent drainage, along with increased erythema and pain. This often requires prompt hospitalization and aggressive treatment, including intravenous antimicrobial therapy, debridement of necrotic tissue, and eventual evaluation for revascularization surgery.

Progressive Signs and Symptoms. A common test, which can be performed at the bedside of patients and done serially to monitor progression, is the ankle-brachial index (ABI). A resting ABI less than 0.4 strongly suggests the likelihood of arterial insufficiency (greater than 0.9 is normal). A toe systolic blood pressure or segmental pressures are sometimes suggested to help predict the likelihood of wound healing. Loss of viable tissue or gangrene is the end stage of arterial insufficiency. This often appears as a gray or black ulcer base, which is dry and painful.

Venous insufficiency leg ulcers are a major clinical problem among the elderly. Only 50% of leg ulcers heal within 4 months, 20% remain open at 2 years, and 8% remain open at 5 years (The Alexander House Group, 1992). Venous ulcerations tend to occur on the medial ankle; may be single or multiple and tend to last for months to years; are typically tender and shallow, with irregular borders and a red base that may be exudative; can spread to be circumferential; are slightly more common in women; and are much more common in the elderly.

Assessment. It is critical to identify the presence of arterial insufficiency because of the significant difference in the management of arterial versus venous insufficiency. Thoroughly review all patient records and carefully question the patient on arterial and venous symptoms. The aging skin will have decreased moisture and elasticity, loss of subcutaneous fat, grayer and thinning hair, and increased nail brittleness, none of which is diagnostic of vascular insufficiency. Table 8-5 compares assessment findings between arterial and venous insufficiency. Assess claudication symptoms by determining the initial distance the patient can walk before the first onset of exertional pain and the furthest distance the patient is able to walk. Palpation of peripheral pulses is important in the assessment of patients with suspected or established arterial insufficiency. It is unusual to palpate the dorsalis pedis or posterior tibial pulses in patients with severe limb ischemia. In patients with complaints of intermittent claudication, however, pedal pulses may be palpable at rest if disease is only moderate aortoiliac occlusive disease. The bedside assessment of greatest value to suggest advanced arterial insufficiency is elevation followed by dependency (dangling) of the affected limbs. An ischemic limb on testing will become pale distally with elevation and develop a red or purple color with dependency.

Interventions and Management. In arterial insufficiency expect to pace activities based on claudication symptoms, promote range-of-motion exercises, teach optimal positioning for circulation, and reinforce nutritional support, in addition to prescribed circulatory-perfusion medications. Daily skin inspection and protection against the effects of pressure, friction, shear, and maceration are essential because of impaired circulation and associated slow wound healing. Daily application of an alcohol-free protective skin barrier should be encouraged. Instruct the patient to avoid compression stockings. Encourage tobacco cessation, maximize hyperlipidemia interventions (LDL less than 100 mg/dl), maximize hypertension control (less than 130/90 mm Hg), maximize diabetes mellitus management (HbA_{1c} less than 7%), encourage walking exercise three times a week for 30 minutes to improve claudication distance, and advise the patient to rest only when near maximal claudication distance and to continue the program for at least 6 months. Shoe fit is important; remind elders (1) that their feet continued to grow as adults, (2) that both feet should be measured for shoes and the larger size selected, (3) to have feet measured at the end of the day when feet are larger, (4) to stand during the fitting process and verify that there is one-half inch of space for the longest toe at the end of each shoe, (5) to make sure the ball of the foot fits comfortably into the widest part of the shoe, and (6) that the heel should fit comfortably with a minimum of slippage.

Venous Insufficiency. Although medical management may include short-term diuretics for severe edema and pentoxifylline for venous leg ulcers, the use of compression bandaging and hosiery will remain the main treatment for patients with chronic venous insufficiency. Boxes 8-24 and 8-25 iden-

Table 8-5 Comparison of Arterial and Venous Insufficiency of the Lower Extremities

Characteristics	Arterial	Venous
Pain	Sudden onset with acute; gradual onset with chronic Exceedingly painful Claudication relieved by rest Rest pain relieved by dependency (with total occlusion, no position will give complete relief)	Deep muscle pain with acute deep vein thrombosis Relieved by elevation
Pulses	Absent or weak	Normal (unless there is also arterial disease)
Associated changes in leg and foot	Thin, shiny, dry skin Thickened toenails Absence of hair growth Temperature variations (cooler if there is no cellulitis) Elevational pallor Dependent rubor Atrophy or no change in limb size	Firm ("brawny") edema Reddish brown discoloration with postphlebitic syndrome Evidence of healed ulcers Dilated and tortuous superficial veins Swollen limb Increased warmth and erythema with acute deep vein thrombosis
Ulcer location	Between toes or at tips of toes Over phalangeal heads On heels Over lateral malleolus or pretibial area (for diabetic patients) over metatarsal heads, on side or sole of foot	"Garter area" around ankles (rich in perforator veins), especially the medial malleolus
Ulcer characteristics	Well-defined edges Black or necrotic tissue Deep, pale base Nonbleeding	Uneven edges Ruddy granulation tissue Superficial Bleeding

tify guidelines for patient interventions related to venous insufficiency and ulcers, respectively. Compression facilitates wound healing, reduces venous dermatitis, improves sclerotic changes, and counteracts venous hypertension. A number of methods can be used to apply compression: elastic bandages; Unna boots; compression bandages or stockings, which provide gradient pressure; compression pumps; and orthotic devices. Stockings, bandages, and other similar systems provide static compression rather than the intermittent compression provided by pneumatic compression devices. Static compression is thought to help reduce the pressure in the veins by aiding venous return. Arterial insufficiency and uncompensated CHF are relative contraindications to compression therapy.

Elevation of the legs above the heart for 30 minutes, three to four times a day, can reduce edema and improve skin microcirculation. Topical or systemic antibiotics are generally avoided in uncomplicated venous ulcers, and topical antiseptics, if not carefully chosen, can impair wound epithelialization. Enzyme debriding agents (for the removal of fibrin and necrotic tissue) are best selected and ordered by a certified wound care specialist. Growth factors (platelet-derived growth factor, epidermal growth factor, fibroblast growth factor, etc.) are currently undergoing clinical trials. Hyperbaric oxygen for recalcitrant venous ulcers may prove useful. Vein stripping, the previous mainstay of surgical treatment for severe varicose veins, has fallen out of favor with the advent of newer, less invasive sclerotherapy and ligation procedures.

Treatment and resolution of venous stasis ulcers is not the only role for the nurse. Education of the aged person is essential as a means of preventing further episodes or minimizing the severity should ulceration recur. Box 8-25 provides education guidelines and a resource to develop an information sheet that elders can refer to when they need reminders of what to do.

Screening and Prevention. Suspect arterial insufficiency in patients with coronary artery disease, carotid stenosis, stroke, or dystrophic toenail disease.

Pernicious Anemia

Epidemiology. Anemia is a common finding among the elderly. This is often erroneously referred to as anemia of old age. The Framingham study and others, however, have shown that healthy elders do not demonstrate a change in hematocrit with aging. Furthermore, there is no evidence that the stem cell responsible for red cell production is deranged or damaged, nor is the ability of the bone marrow to respond to erythropoietin under basal conditions. Therefore anemia in the elderly is almost always due to a pathologic condition or represents a response to a pathologic condition. Common causes of anemia in the elderly include anemia of chronic disease (30% to 45%), iron deficiency (15% to 30%), hemorrhage (5% to 10%), vitamin B_{12} deficiency (5% to 10%), cancer (5% to 10%), and idiopathic (15% to 25%) (Joosten et al, 1992). One study revealed that undiagnosed pernicious anemia was present in nearly 2% of otherwise healthy individuals age 60 years or older (Carmel, 1996).

Definition. According to World Health Organization criteria for anemia (hemoglobin of less than 12 g/dl [120 g/L] in women and less than 13 g/dl [130 g/L] in men), the prevalence of anemia in the elderly has been found to range from 8% to

Box 8-24 Guidelines for Patients with Venous Insufficiency

Give Legs a Rest

Elevate the feet above heart level while sleeping and several times a day. If necessary, elevate the foot of the bed or mattress.

Change Positions Frequently

Avoid activities that require standing or sitting with feet on the ground for long periods of time.

Give Legs Support

Wear professionally made compression stockings that apply even pressure from ankles to knees.
Learn how to put them on correctly.
Have at least two pairs of the compression hose available so they can be changed daily. After laundering, hang up to dry. DO NOT PUT IN DRYER.
Buy new compression hose every 6 months; after that period of time the elastic is stretched.
Put hose on early in the morning; wear all day; remove at bedtime.
Avoid elastic bandages (e.g., Acc). They are difficult to wrap and exert even pressure.
If a compression pump has been prescribed by the physician, follow the instructions.

Take Care of the Skin

Wash lower legs and feet regularly with mild soap and water to avoid buildup of lotion.
Use moisturizing cream and emollients after washing.
Do NOT use lanolin- or petroleum-based creams when wearing support hose made with latex.
Avoid activities that can injure the legs or feet.
Pay attention to skin changes:
- Swelling—stays when lying down
- Discoloration—especially around ankles and lower legs
- Dryness and/or itching—around ankles and lower legs
- Any bruises or wounds that do not go away in one week

Apply Dressings

Follow ulcer care directions as prescribed.

Modified from San Francisco Wound Care Center, Seton Medical Center, Daly City, CA, 1995; Staab AS, Hodges LC: *Essentials of gerontological nursing*, Philadelphia, 1996, JB Lippincott.

44%, with the highest prevalence in men age 85 years and older (Smith, 2000). The elderly have different signs and symptoms from those of younger adults because the classic changes in erythrocyte size do not often accompany anemia in those over 65 years old. In most elderly patients with anemia, red cell indices disclose normocytic, normochromic anemia, instead of macrocytic, hypochromic anemia.

Risk Factors. The amount of vitamin B_{12} recommended daily for adults is minute, only 2.0 μg, and it can take 1 to 2 years for a deficiency to develop. Vitamin B_{12} deficiency rarely is the result of inadequate intake, except in persons who are strict vegetarians. Malnutrition is defined as poor nourishment from (1) insufficient, unbalanced, or improper diet or (2) impaired absorption, assimilation, or use of foods.

A common cause is reduced intestinal absorption of vitamin B_{12}. Pernicious anemia is a classic example of a disorder that causes this. A person must have sufficient intrinsic factor in order to absorb vitamin B_{12}. In the elderly, the intrinsic factor may be present, but vitamin B_{12} may not be readily absorbed from food because hydrochloric acid, the strong natural acid made by the stomach, is needed to free vitamin B_{12} from its association with animal proteins. As many older adults age, they secrete less stomach acid, and pepsin, the protein-digestive enzyme, declines. The elderly may also take antacids with their meals, such as calcium carbonate as in Tums (regular), as a calcium supplement. Such calcium intake could further lower available stomach acid.

Other risk factors include (1) poverty, (2) social isolation, (3) dependency or disability, (4) acute or chronic diseases or conditions, (5) chronic medication use, and (6) advanced age (age 80 and older).

Signs and Symptoms. Vitamin B_{12} deficiency is difficult to detect in the elderly. Often the signs and symptoms of vitamin B_{12} deficiency are not reliably present in those over 65 years old. Unfortunately, permanent nerve damage can occur before any telltale pernicious anemia symptoms appear, with their abnormal red blood cell size, shape, and number and low serum levels of cobalamin. Only about 60% of patients with vitamin B_{12} deficiency are anemic by traditional laboratory testing. In addition, the neurologic symptoms of vitamin B_{12} deficiency can develop before the patient becomes anemic. Finally, serum vitamin B_{12} levels do not reflect tissue vitamin B_{12} deficiency. Up to 30% of geriatric patients with low-normal serum vitamin B_{12} levels have anemia and neurologic disease (Stabler, 1998). This observation has prompted a search for more reliable ways of detecting vitamin B_{12} deficiency.

Common symptoms are weakness in legs, difficulty in walking and balancing, tingling and numbness in hands and feet, and nerves becoming highly responsive to any mild stimulation. Vitamin B_{12} deficiency can also lead to mental confusion, apathy, and irritability and may progress from mild depression and confusion to obvious dementia. Patients may also suffer loss of appetite and weight, indigestion, and periodic diarrhea. All of this can happen before anyone diagnoses a vitamin B_{12} deficiency. In its early stages, these symptoms can be reversed, but if the deficiency is not caught within a few months, the damage can be permanent. Even mild anemia can reduce oxygen transport in the blood, causing fatigue and a diminished physical capacity.

Acute Complications. Acute presentation in the elderly is typically associated with an insidious onset and development. Typically, urgent or emergent medical evaluation of the symptoms will "rule out" other common causes of anemia or neurologic disease (Kahsai and Roekens, 2001) before considering the possibility of pernicious anemia. Avoiding delay in accurate diagnosis of apparently acute symptoms maximizes the avoidance of permanent neurologic deficits.

Box 8-25 Treatments for Venous Stasis Ulcers

Conservative	
Dressings	
Wet	To absorb weeping fluid Prevent tissue drying out
Change daily initially	Decreases risk of infection Keeps clean and protected from bacteria
(If not infected, an adhesive film or absorbant gel or foam is possible)	
Application of fibrinolytic agents	
Cleaning	Mild soap and water Mechanically removes loose tissue without additional trauma Removes creams/lotions/medications applied
Compression wrap	Increases venous flow Should continue to wear even after lesion is healed
Elevation of legs	Decreases swelling Improves venous return
Ambulation	Improves venous return
Treatment for Severe Ulcers	
Mechanical pump compression	Provides intermittent compression for several hours daily
Elastic stockings or wrap	
Surgery	
Skin graft	For large ulcers
Vein stripping	
Chronic Recurring Stasis Ulcers	
Growth factor from human blood platelets applied to ulcer in combination with other treatment	Stimulates new skin formation over ulcer, enhances healing
Cultured skin grown in laboratory (under FDA review)	To cover ulcer and enhance healing

Assessment. Five stages of vitamin B_{12} deficiency have been identified (Cravens, 1998):

Stage 1: Normal vitamin B_{12} levels (no deficiency).

Stage 2: Negative vitamin B_{12} balance.

Stage 3: Vitamin B_{12} depletion with possible clinical signs and symptoms; reversible neuropsychiatric symptoms may occur.

Stage 4: Vitamin B_{12}–deficient erythropoiesis with possible clinical signs and symptoms; potentially reversible neuropsychiatric symptoms may occur.

Stage 5: Vitamin B_{12} deficiency anemia with probable clinical signs and symptoms; irreversible lateral and posterior column involvement may occur.

Holistic nursing assessment should include the following historical items: Geriatric Depression Scale, ADL and IADL screening, number of falls within the last 12 months, family genogram, weight changes, appetite patterns, consumption patterns, food preparation, means of obtaining food (shopping, etc.), history of digestive symptoms, difficulties with chewing or swallowing, adequacy of balanced diet, sleeping patterns (nighttime and naps), presence of hot and cold running water, adequacy of cooking facilities, presence of chronic diseases, alcohol intake (amount and type), prescription and nonprescription medications taken, evidence of more than 1 day's dirty dishes in sink, accumulation of trash or garbage in and around the senior's home, spoiled food stock, poor vision, and dexterity issues in the equipping of the elder's kitchen.

A comprehensive physical examination should include level of consciousness, Folstein Mini-Mental Status examination, physical appearance, dress and grooming, facial expression, affect, communication, cranial nerves, sensation, motor function, cerebellar function, and reflexes.

Interventions and Management. Medical treatment of pernicious anemia includes vitamin B_{12} supplementation, parenterally or orally. The intramuscular dose is 1000 μg, often given daily for 1 week to build up stores, then weekly for 1 month, and then monthly thereafter. Oral therapy with 1000 to 2000 μg of vitamin B_{12} daily has been shown to be as effective as intramuscular injections and in some ways may be superior (Kuzminski et al, 1998). Laboratory indications of treatment response often occur within a week of the initiation of vitamin B_{12} therapy.

Nursing interventions addressing multifactorial influences on nutrition should include eliminating or reducing the following long-term barriers: (1) access to food, (2) shopping for food, (3) storing food, (4) preparing meals, (5) eating alone, (6) taste and temperature preferences, and (7) poor dentition. Oral supplementation is the best option if the patient can ingest food without aspiration or regurgitation. The use of a high-calorie drink supplement is generally well tolerated. Nasally placed feed tubing can be considered for short-term refeeding, but oral intake should be encouraged if at all possible, in addition to enteral supplementation.

Screening and Prevention. Screening for vitamin B_{12} deficiency should be considered for any senior receiving long-term administration of vitamin-depleting medications. A daily supplement of vitamin B_{12}, in addition to dietary animal protein such as meat, fish, poultry, eggs, and milk products, as well as fortified cereals, is probably all that is necessary to guarantee the prevention of pernicious anemia in the elderly. Folate (another B vitamin) deficiency often accompanies lowered vitamin B_{12} levels, but taking only folate supplements can mask the nerve symptoms and metabolic disturbances associated with vitamin B_{12} deficiency. Therefore folate (also labeled folacin or folic acid) supplements should not be taken as a single supplement. A multiple vitamin supplement of 100% of the recommended daily allowance (RDA) is best (Allen and Casterline, 1994).

Chronic Obstructive Pulmonary Disease

Epidemiology. Chronic obstructive pulmonary disease (COPD) is the only major cause of death whose mortality rate is rising among adults, and it is now the fourth leading cause of death in adults. The increase is largely driven by the increase in smoking prevalence, with a lag of 20 to 30 years (Stoller, 2002). From the National Health Interview Survey, it was estimated a decade ago that 12.6 million Americans have COPD, and 2 million have emphysema. Worldwide, between 1990 and 2020, it is estimated that COPD will rise from the twelfth to the fifth leading cause of disability-adjusted life years lost, a variable that combines premature mortality and disability.

Definition. COPD is a major concern in old age. As a category it includes bronchitis and emphysema because of their overlapping clinical features, risk factors, and symptoms. Research advances in COPD have differentiated bronchitis and emphysema from asthma by the type of inflammatory cells involved (McCrory et al, 2001).

Chronic bronchitis is diagnosed clinically, by a productive cough for 3 consecutive months for 2 consecutive years. The chronic bronchitis of COPD is an inflammatory disease. It starts in small airways and involves increased mucous production, increased neutrophils, and increased macrophages.

Emphysema is a pathologic diagnosis of permanent enlargement of the distal airspaces with destruction of their walls. The development of emphysema is triggered by the exposure of a susceptible individual to noxious particles and gases. In contrast to the eosinophilic inflammation seen in asthma, the predominant inflammatory cell is the neutrophil.

Spirometry is indispensable in establishing the diagnosis of COPD because it is a standardized and reproducible test that objectively confirms the presence of airflow obstruction. Characteristically, spirometry shows a decreased forced expiratory volume in 1 second (FEV_1) and FEV_1/forced vital capacity (FVC) ratio. Measurement of the diffusing capacity for carbon monoxide may help differentiate between emphysema and chronic bronchitis.

Risk Factors. According to Dr. Chatila, Assistant Professor of Medicine in the Division of Pulmonary and Critical Care Medicine at Temple University, the common risk factors medical students are taught to consider include (1) smoking, (2) α_1-antitrypsin deficiency, (3) exposure to environmental air pollution, and (4) a history of childhood respiratory infections.

The FEV_1 value normally declines with age in sedentary adults, less so in those who are physically active. Measurement of the maximal ability of the body to deliver oxygen to the tissues during exercise is known as maximum oxygen consumption (VO_2max). VO_2max is the product of adequate pulmonary ventilation, blood circulation, and muscle tissue extraction of oxygen. In general, the reduced VO_2max seen in elderly individuals with mild to moderate airway obstruction is due to cardiovascular deconditioning associated with lowered levels of habitual physical activity. The sedentary aged have a greater decrease in elastic recoil of lung tissue, flattening of the diaphragm, loss of alveoli, pulmonary wall thickening, and decreased medullary sensitivity to carbon dioxide and oxygen levels (Estes, 2002). However, seniors who remain physically active during their lives have improved functional respiratory capacity, greater endurance, superior functional status, less dyspnea, and improved quality of life (Short and Leon, 1990). Therefore caution is warranted in attributing functional decline or symptoms to deconditioning, age-related decline, or disease. The normal rate of decline is approximately 20 to 30 ml of expired volume per year (McCrory et al, 2001). Among smokers, the rate of decline varies widely, reflecting individual genetic variability, smoking history, smoking technique, or exposure to environmental cofactors. Smokers with rapid loss of lung function, about 100 ml or more per year, are thought to be at greater risk for development of symptomatic COPD. Nevertheless, the normal lung has a great deal of excess capacity relative to the respiratory burdens of a sedentary life.

Signs and Symptoms. COPD has a long presymptomatic stage, and usually about 50% of lung function has been irretrievably lost before patients notice dyspnea (Stoller, 2002). Chronic cough is much more common, affecting the majority of smokers. However, this is frequently present without measurable airflow obstruction and is often dismissed by smokers as insignificant. The most common symptoms of COPD are cough, dyspnea on exertion, and increased phlegm production (Estes, 2002). Common signs include wheezing, prolonged expiration with pursed-lip breathing, barrel chest, air trapping, hyperresonance, pale lips or nail beds, fingernail clubbing, and use of accessory breathing muscles (McCrory et al, 2001). In advanced cases, cyanosis, evidence of right-sided heart failure, and peripheral edema are present. A chest radiograph usually shows hyperinflation of the lungs and flattening of the diaphragm.

Acute Complications. Acute exacerbation of COPD represents an acute worsening of the baseline symptoms and signs of COPD, generally characterized by significantly worsened dyspnea and increased volume and purulence of sputum (McCrory et al, 2001). Additionally, pulsus paradoxus, marked by a decrease of 10 mm Hg or more during inspiration compared with expiration, may occur (Estes, 2002). Spirometry of less than 150 ml, worsening orthopnea, paroxysmal nocturnal dyspnea, and respirations greater than 30 per minute signal an emergent exacerbation of COPD. Exacerbations have numerous inciting factors, including viral or bacterial infections, air pollution or other environmental exposures, or changes in the weather.

Exacerbations are typical features of COPD in its moderate to severe stages, especially in patients with predominantly chronic bronchitis symptoms. They frequently precipitate the need for increased medications, hospitalizations, or respiratory support. Mechanical ventilation, either noninvasively applied through a face mask or by endotracheal intubation, may be needed in patients with respiratory acidosis that progresses despite therapy or with impaired consciousness. The routine use of antibiotics is controversial, because the causal role of bacterial infection is often difficult to document. Antibiotics are generally indicated in patients with new pulmonary infiltrates on chest x-ray, fever, or purulent sputum. Although the acute phase of an exacerbation is usually over in 10 days to 2 weeks, lung function may take 4 to 6 weeks to return to baseline.

Progressive Signs and Symptoms. Several factors influence the natural history and affect survival in patients with COPD. These factors include age, smoking status, resting heart rate, airway responsiveness, hypoxemia, and, most important, the level of FEV_1, which remains the single best predictor of prognosis (Anthonisen et al, 1994). The use of long-term oxygen therapy in hypoxemic patients has been shown to improve survival, and smoking cessation slows the rate of FEV_1 decline. Box 8-26 identifies the objective measures currently accepted for staging COPD.

Currently it is believed identification of "rapid decliners" with COPD will facilitate more aggressive smoking cessation efforts. If a sensitivity marker to tobacco smoke can be identified, it will provide a strong incentive to smoking prevention or cessation. There is some controversy to this approach, however, because patients with little risk of COPD are still at risk for coronary and cerebrovascular disease, cancer, and myriad other smoking-related illnesses.

Assessment. COPD is divided into three stages. There is a rough correspondence between symptoms and stage. Stage 0 refers to patients with chronic cough and sputum, but without spirometry abnormality. Stage I patients have airflow obstruction, defined as an FEV_1/FVC ratio of less than 0.7, but an FEV_1 that is still in the normal range. Stage II patients have an FEV_1 of 30% to 80% of that predicted and begin to experience dyspnea on exertion and worsening cough. Stage III patients have an FEV_1 of less than 30% of that predicted; hypercarbia; or right-sided heart failure. Typically, stage III patients are severely disabled, are dyspneic during simple daily activities, and often experience acute exacerbations requiring hospitalization. The course of COPD disease can be followed by measurement of the FEV_1 regardless of the amount of bronchitis or emphysema present because both cause airflow reduction.

Nursing assessment of the functional impact of COPD symptoms should include the quality of breathlessness, onset, frequency, severity, and triggers and activities that provoke dyspnea. A useful assessment scale to determine the functional impact of dyspnea on a senior's life is the chronic respiratory disease questionnaire (CRQ) (Mahler and Horner, 1990). The patient identifies the five most difficult activities to perform, from a list of 26, due to dyspnea on exertion. The severity of dyspnea on the CRQ is indicated by a total of the five numbers, subjectively ranked on a scale from 1 to 7, corresponding to "not short of breath" to "extremely short of breath," respectively. A total score ranging from 5 to 35 is calculated and then trended over time.

Interventions and Management. Box 8-27 details current management recommendations for COPD.

Box 8-26 COPD Assessment

History
Respiratory distress
Smoking history
Symptoms

Physical Examination
Inspection*
- Posture
- Chest symmetry, shape expansion
- Respirations
- Skin color
- Capillary fill
- Sputum (color, amount, consistency)

Palpation
- Tenderness

Percussion
- Areas of hyperinflation, consolidation

Auscultation*
- Breath sounds

Functional Activity Mobility
Levels of activity before dyspneic
Interferences from sensory impairments

Knowledge
Educational attainment
Understanding of disease processes in COPD

*Most important of the four assessment techniques.

Box 8-27 Interventions for COPD

Nutrition

Eat small, frequent, nutrient-intense meals.
Eat foods with high protein and calories.
Serve meals on small plates (servings will not look overwhelming).
Select foods that do not require a lot of chewing.
Have food cut in bite-size pieces to conserve energy.
Establish a plan for fluid intake; drink 2-3 L of fluid daily (pineapple juice helps cut secretions; keep a liter of water in the refrigerator or on the kitchen counter to be consumed each day in addition to other fluids).
Weigh at least twice a week.

Exercise

(Based on an established plan suggested by physician or rehabilitation team).
Walk daily all year round (in good weather, outdoors; in bad weather, go to the mall and walk indoors).
Walk up and down stairs in home (if present).
Use a stationary bicycle.
When buying shoes for activity and everyday wear, avoid shoes that require bending over to tie; instead get slip-on type and use a long-handled shoe horn to assist the heel into shoe.

Activity Pacing

Avoid high levels of exertion in early morning.
Arrange rest periods throughout day.
Allow plenty of time to complete activities; don't hurry.
Schedule activities in advance to reduce pressure and anxiety.
Obtain and follow prescribed exercise program for maintenance of heart/lung capacity.

ADLs

Allow ample time for bathing and dressing. Have a chair in bathroom for bathing.
Arrange toiletries in easy reach.
Wear shoes that slip on or have Velcro closures, not ties.
Select clothing with elasticized waistbands; avoid constrictive clothing; use suspenders rather than belts.
Select and wear clothing that is easy to put on and remove.

Safety

Attempt to keep a dust-free environment.
Minimize or eliminate use of aerosol sprays, fumes, contaminants, dander.
Place plastic covers over mattresses, use hypoallergenic pillows and blankets.
Avoid carpet and rug floor coverings.

Emotional Support

Accept/encourage expression of emotions.
Be an active listener.
Be cognizant of conversational dyspnea; do not interrupt or cut off conversations.

Education

Teach breathing techniques:
Pursed-lip breathing
Diaphragmatic breathing
Cascade coughing (series)
Teach postural drainage.
Teach about *medications:* what, why, frequency, amount, side effects, and what to do if side effects occur
Teach use and care of inhalers.
Teach signs and symptoms of respiratory infection.
Teach about *sexual activity:*
Sexual function improves with rest.
Schedule sex around best-breathing time of day.
Use prescribed bronchidilators 20 to 30 minutes before sex.
Stay away from the use of alcohol or eating large quantities of food.
Use a position that does not require pressure on the chest or support of the arms.

General Instructions

Listen to weather reports.
Avoid going out in inclement weather.
Wear scarf over nose and mouth in cold and windy weather; wear a hat.
Avoid going out when air pollution is high.
Use air conditioner to filter air and make it drier.
Avoid situations where you may encounter individuals with influenza or upper respiratory infections.
Obtain an annual flu shot if not allergic.
Obtain one-time multivalent pneumococcal immunization.
Notify physician of any temperature above 99° F.
Examine sputum; recognize and report changes to physician.
Do not use over-the-counter drugs unless physician approves.

Screening and Prevention. Health fairs often include spirometry screening with peak expiratory flow measurements that identify height-, age-, and sex-adjusted norms. A spirometer is a machine that measures exhaled airflow and is a good indicator of lung functioning. Findings of less than 80% warrant physician follow-up. Prevention approaches include smoking prevention or cessation, avoiding environmental pollution exposure, and prevention of childhood respiratory infections.

Asthma

Epidemiology. We know little about the epidemiology and natural history of asthma in elderly subjects; available data and clinical observations suggest that it is not rare and may appear as late as the eighth or ninth decades of life (Burrows et al, 1991). The natural history of asthma appears to vary widely. Some elderly patients had childhood asthma that continues into later life, although many aged asthmatics deny any symptoms until late in life. Seniors who have mild asthma symptoms and slight chronic airflow obstruction may remain undiagnosed unless their asthma exacerbates. Additionally, there have been a number of misclassifications of asthma as chronic bronchitis in older patients, leading to inappropriate therapy (Banerjee et al, 1987). It is reported that 15 million people in the United States, including more than 1.5 million Americans over 65 years of age, suffer from asthma (National Center for Health Statistics, 2003). A 1999 report by the American College of Chest Physicians identified asthma as underdiagnosed in the elderly. This population-based research project was designed to assess the epidemiologic risks associated with cardiovascular disease in the elderly. Two thousand, five hundred and twenty-seven seniors were studied with spirometry, standardized questions regarding asthma symptoms, and possible aggravating factors of asthma. The report stated: "Our results suggest that not only is asthma underdiagnosed in elderly persons in the United States and associated with considerable morbidity. But most of those who have had an asthma diagnosis and manifest current symptoms are not being treated properly" (Enright, 1999, p. 603).

Definition. Asthma, in all ages, is a lung disease characterized by airway obstruction, inflammation, and hyperresponsiveness to a variety of stimuli. The specialists' view of asthma has changed from the view of a primary acute disease of the airways recurring in an intermittent fashion to that of a chronic, perhaps lifelong inflammatory disorder. Research and treatment is focusing on cells and mediators playing key roles in the emergence and worsening of asthma symptoms, and away from the aspect of smooth muscle hyperresponsiveness. However, incomplete reversibility of smooth muscle constriction is increasingly common among elderly patients, especially when asthma results from smooth muscle hypertrophy and fibrosis. Available data and clinical observations suggest that asthma occurs frequently among the elderly, interacts with age-related pathophysiologic events, and is more likely to produce irreversible airflow obstruction if the disease is severe and long standing (National Heart, Lung and Blood Institute, 2000).

Risk Factors. Mast cell mediators of inflammation, mucous production, and smooth muscle hyperresponsiveness in the development of asthma are probably influenced by genetics, environment, and lifestyle factors. A positive family history of asthma and personal history of allergies have been implicated in a higher risk for asthma. Whereas males have increased risk in childhood, women seem to experience increased risk with older age. After a patient experiences exposure to antigen, a cascade of reactions are produced that have both immediate and (more important) late and recurrent effects. These reactions not only have direct effects on airway smooth muscle and mucous secretion, but also recruit the participation of the many more monocytes, lymphocytes, neutrophils, and eosinophils. So in considering risk factors, avoidance of repeated exposure to sensitizing agents is fundamental. Repeated exposure may potentiate the patient's inflammatory response or desensitize the patient to the antigen. Interestingly, in this setting we can contemplate some age-related decline of immune system function being helpful in asthma. How does one determine which agents might provoke an inflammatory response in a patient? Usually by the patient's history of response. Common external risk factors include exposure to tobacco smoke, air pollution, viral respiratory infections, and allergens such as pet dander, fumes, and dust. Morbidity and mortality risk factors in existing asthma increase with age.

Signs and Symptoms. The presentation of asthma in the elderly is similar to that of younger adults. Wheezing, nonproductive cough, or mild airflow obstruction is associated with a subsequent diagnosis of asthma (Burrows et al, 1991). Symptoms such as chest tightness, cough, wheeze, or dyspnea provide a reliable measure of an aged patient's need for and response to therapy, although differences among individual patients are highly varied in regard to which symptoms are salient, how symptoms are tolerated, and how they relate to physiologic alterations of lung function as measured by peak expiratory flow (PEF). From 65% to 100% of predicted PEF can be encountered in many symptomatic asthma patients.

Acute Complications. When wheezing occurs throughout inhalation and exhalation, cough occurs more than four times a minute, there is dyspnea on exertion, or nighttime awakenings occur more than two to three times a night, the symptom is considered severe. PEF rates of 65% or less accompanied by severe symptoms signal impending crisis and should prompt the patient to seek medical care as soon as possible.

Symptoms of acute asthma such as wheezing, cough, shortness of breath, or chest tightness may be due to other conditions common among the elderly, such as myocardial ischemia or pulmonary embolism. The assessment of episodic or acute chest symptoms in the elderly must include the possibility of cardiovascular disease because it becomes more prevalent with age.

As a rule, continued treatment of acute asthma in the urgent care or emergency department setting should not be extended beyond 4 hours. If the elderly patient has not achieved sufficient improvement by that time, admission to the hospital is warranted. Alternatively, extended treatment in a holding area, clinical decision unit, or overnight unit with sufficient monitoring and nursing care may be considered.

Discharge medications usually include a short course of oral corticosteroids. Follow-up within 3 days of discharge from an urgent care or emergency department setting is recommended. A health care professional should consider telephone contact after discharge to encourage patient follow-up. Medications should be carefully discussed with the patient, and use of a spacer or peak flow meter, if prescribed, should be reviewed. A written calendar of medication dosing, peak flow diary, and follow-up appointment date, time, and location is helpful. Explore transportation issues to the follow-up appointment in advance with the patient and significant others. Be sure to give patients verbal and written instructions on when and how to communicate with their health care provider.

Progressive Signs and Symptoms. Mild, intermittent asthma exists when the patient experiences symptoms or exacerbations less than two times a week, experiences nocturnal symptoms less than two times a month, and is asymptomatic between exacerbations.

Asthma becomes moderate when the patient experiences exacerbations more than two times a week and the exacerbations affect sleep and activity; the patient has nighttime awakenings because of asthma more than two times a month; the patient has chronic asthma symptoms that require use of a short-acting inhaled β_2-agonist daily or every other day; and the patient's pretreatment baseline PEF or FEV_1 is 60% to 80% of predicted.

Severe asthma exists when the patient has almost continuous symptoms, frequent exacerbations, frequent nighttime awakenings because of asthma, limited activities, and PEF or FEV_1 baseline less than 60% of predicted.

Asthma tends to become more persistent and show increasing chronic airflow obstruction as the patient ages, although the rate of pulmonary function decline in elderly patients with asthma has been contradictory in the research literature. For example, airflow obstruction in diagnosed asthma patients showed little worsening over time in one study (Burrows et al, 1991), but it worsened at an excessive rate with increasing age in another study (Peat et al, 1987). Because elderly patients with asthma can have chronic, persistent airflow obstruction with poor bronchodilator responsiveness, progression of signs and symptoms over time is important to identify.

Assessment. Medical evaluation includes laboratory studies in the differential diagnosis of new-onset asthma in addition to pulmonary function tests, chest x-rays, and electrocardiography. Spirometry standards that are age, height, and gender adjusted are available, but in the older patient these demanding standards can be difficult to meet (Enright et al, 1993). Poor technique because of arthritis, dexterity, or dementia, as well as weakness, dizziness, severe airflow obstruction with air trapping, and bronchoconstriction induced by the forced expiratory effort, can interfere with the test results of aged patients. A consistently decreasing pattern of FEV_1 test results during the evaluation is suggestive of asthma.

Research and clinical experience with the elderly indicate that many patients have a persistent degree of airflow obstruction even when treated optimally (Burrows et al, 1991). Obstruction reversibility following bronchodilator therapy, although diagnostic in the young, does not hold true in geriatric asthma. Long-term therapy, often with corticosteroids, is more frequently necessary to achieve significant improvement in the elderly patient with asthma. FEV_1 improvement of 200 ml or greater is expected in the aged to justify the risk inherent in corticosteroid therapy. Nursing assessment of elders with asthma requires collaborative efforts.

Interventions and Management. The treatment goals of optimizing pulmonary function, controlling cough and nocturnal symptoms, preventing exacerbations, promoting prompt recognition and treatment of exacerbations, reducing the need for emergency department visits, avoidance of aggravating other medical conditions, and minimizing medication adverse effects may be more difficult to achieve in the elderly. The nurse should make sure the elder understands the following: how to monitor and identify symptoms; that there is an increased need for inhaled β_2-agonist to relieve symptoms; the possibility of a diminished response to rescue medications; and the importance of changes in PEF rates that indicate the elder's asthma is worsening. Each patient needs a written management plan that includes clear information on what to do.

In 1991 the National Heart, Lung and Blood Institute's expert panel concluded that no new guidelines for asthma management in the elderly were necessary. However, the panel did offer more details on diagnosis, pharmacologic therapy, and patient/family/caregiver education as they relate to the elderly population. The report was reinforced by two additional publications (National Heart, Lung and Blood Institute, 1992, 1995). Management of seniors with asthma is often complicated by the presence of other chronic disorders.

Screening and Prevention. Although two of the top five killers of seniors are lung diseases, age-specific, population-based screening of pulmonary function is not recommended at this time (Masterson, 1998).

Tuberculosis

Epidemiology. This highly infectious disease continues to affect the elderly (Rajagopalan, 2001), and recent studies in developed countries suggest that its incidence is increasing (Packham, 2001). In the early 1900s infectious diseases, such as tuberculosis (TB), accounted for 25% of all deaths (Guyer et al, 2000). It is estimated that one third of the world's population is infected with *Mycobacterium tuberculosis* (Rajagopalan and Yoshikawa, 2000). With increased longevity, the current population of 70- and 80-year-olds was alive when TB was prevalent in many communities. In one sense, all ethnic and gender groups of today's senior population serve as a large reservoir of tubercle infection (Rajagopalan and Yoshikawa, 2000).

Definition. Several tubercle (knot)–producing organisms can produce classic tuberculosis: *Mycobacterium tuberculosis, Mycobacterium bovis,* and *Mycobacterium africanum.* The weakened strain of *M. bovis,* bacille Calmette-Guérin (BCG), is used for vaccines against TB in some countries, but its efficacy is debatable. The term *tuberculosis infection* refers to a positive TB skin test with no evidence of active disease. *Tuberculosis disease* refers to cases that have positive acid-fast smear or culture for *M. tuberculosis* or radiographic and clinical presentation of TB.

Risk Factors. Commonly recognized risk factors include the following: (1) contacts of person known to be infected; (2) patients with abnormal chest film; (3) human immunodeficiency virus (HIV)–positive patients; (4) organ transplant recipients; (5) immunosuppressed patients; (6) recent immigrants (i.e., less than 5 years) from countries with high incidences of TB; (7) residents of prisons, nursing homes, and institutions; (8) injection drug users; (9) health care workers; (10) children younger than 4 years old or adolescents exposed to high-risk adults; (11) persons with chronic illness; and (12) locally identified high-risk groups (American Thoracic Society, 2000). In the elderly, cancer has been commonly associated with the identification of tuberculosis infection (Kaltenbach et al, 2001).

Signs and Symptoms. Age-specific research has recently compared the clinical, biochemical, and radiologic features for a group of 83 elderly as compared with adults (Kaltenbach et al, 2001). Symptoms of weight loss, fever, and cough were the same in both groups. Laboratory results, however, revealed a significant trend in the elderly to experience an increased sedimentation rate and lymphocytopenia. These findings stand in opposition to a recent United Kingdom study, which postulates that geriatric symptoms are nonspecific and less pronounced (Packham, 2001). If findings from the study by Kaltenback and colleagues (2001) can be extrapolated to American seniors, pleuritic chest pain and fever are less frequent in the elderly person (Rocha et al, 1997). Hemoptysis and night sweats were not mentioned in recent age-specific research.

Assessment. Traditionally, the diagnosis of TB has been made on the basis of clinical findings and chest x-ray and confirmed by sputum or tissue smears that show TB bacilli. These methods remain the "gold standard" for diagnosis. The recent development of DNA probes, polymerase chain reaction (PCR) assays, and liquid media now allow more sensitive and rapid diagnosis.

The most accurate tuberculin skin test is the Mantoux test, in which 5 U of tuberculin purified protein derivative (PPD) are injected intradermally to detect delayed hypersensitivity to TB. The amount of induration is assessed after 48 to 72 hours, and the extent of induration (not erythema) should be measured across two diameters at right angles and the two measurements then averaged.

The Mantoux skin test for tuberculosis infections should be performed on all elderly persons at increased risk for developing TB, including those in nursing homes, recent immigrants, and refugees from countries in which TB is common (e.g., countries in Asia, Africa, Central and South America, the Pacific Islands, and the Caribbean), and persons with certain underlying conditions, such as HIV infection (10% of cases are older than 50) (Wooten-Bielski, 1999). Those with a positive PPD test should receive a chest x-ray and clinical evaluation for TB. In certain geographic areas, cross-reactivity with atypical mycobacteria, as well as previous BCG vaccination, can produce intermediate-sized reactions.

Although repeated exposure to tuberculin itself will not sensitize an uninfected person, it may sensitize patients who were infected previously and have experienced waning immunity. An important consideration in the elderly patient, this "booster effect" can occur with a second skin test even up to a year after the first test. This makes it difficult to assess whether the reaction represents new conversion or boosting of an old infection. One recommendation is to repeat the skin test 1 week after an initial negative test. If the second test is positive, boosting of former infection is likely.

Those with a positive PPD test should receive a chest x-ray and clinical evaluation for TB. Contrary to the skin testing logic in young adults, a positive PPD test in the elderly does not necessarily mandate prophylaxis with isoniazid (INH) because of the treatment risks discussed in the following paragraphs.

Interventions and Management. Successful completion of TB treatment regimens in the elderly patient is complicated by a high mortality rate of 22% during the first 3 months (Kaltenbach et al, 2001). Although a major concern with young adults is the use of directly observed therapy to ensure compliance, in the elderly biweekly liver function monitoring is of equal importance because of the frequency of drug-induced hepatitis (Janssens and Zellweger, 1999). Nursing's role in monitoring laboratory values, assessing for adverse drug reactions, and monitoring drug compliance is crucial to treatment effectiveness and the patient's well-being. Patients generally undergo pretreatment measurement of liver function, serum urea nitrogen, platelets, bilirubin, creatinine, and uric acid levels. Laboratory values should be monitored monthly during treatment and whenever symptoms suggesting adverse effects occur.

Elderly people are extremely intolerant to rifampin (Wada, 1998), possibly due to aging of the liver, poor nutritional status, or polypharmacy. Clinically significant interactions have been reported between rifampin and oral contraceptives, corticosteroids, cyclosporine (Neoral, Sandimmune, SangCya), erythromycin, phenytoin, imidazole antifungals, several antiretroviral agents, warfarin sodium (Coumadin), propranolol (Betachron E-R, Inderal), and opioids. Because it interferes with dihydropyridine calcium channel blockers, rifampin also poses a significant hazard to many seniors with hypertension (Yoshimoto et al, 1996). Ocular toxicity with ethambutol and peripheral neuritis with isoniazid, ethambutol, and ethionamide make the management of drug treatment in the elderly highly complicated (Wada, 1998). Vitamin B_6 supplementation is crucial to avoiding peripheral neuritis.

In reality, the hepatotoxicity risk for the elderly with each of the anti-TB medications, isoniazid, rifampin, pyrazinamide, and ethionamide, is compounded by the frequent use of combination therapy. The high incidence of adverse drug effects often dictates a change in dose, frequency, or drugs. The patient may be changed to drugs that are better tolerated but possibly less effective and therefore have to be taken for a longer time (Davies, 1996).

Sputum culture conversion among TB patients is the most important indicator of successful drug treatment in all patients. However, the elderly and non-Hispanic whites were the most unlikely to yield negative sputum culture results in a recent study (Liu et al, 1999). A positive finding on acid-fast smear or culture of the sputum after 5 months of treatment is considered a treatment failure. Failure can result from prescription of an inappropriate dosage or inadequate number of drugs, patient noncompliance, and malabsorption or organism resistance.

Screening and Prevention. Screening of institutionalized patients, those with chronic medical conditions, TB contacts, low-income patients, recent immigrants, alcoholics, Native Americans, Alaskan Natives, travelers to high-risk countries, and street drug users is recommended by serial Mantoux testing to capture the booster effect (Masterson, 1998; Mikami and Kawasaki, 2000).

Some interesting research on vitamin D's role in reducing risk of TB infection has been published (Chan, 2000). Citing the tendency of TB to occur more frequently in the winter months when skin synthesis of vitamin D is lower and the finding of lower vitamin D levels in disease sufferers, the study suggests that elderly, uremic patients and Asian immigrants may benefit from supplementation. A recent Italian study (Corsini et al, 2002) suggests dehydroepiandrosterone (DHEA) replacement therapy to counteract the age-related decrease in macrophage function as a way of decreasing the elderly's risk of pneumonia, influenza, and TB.

HEALTH BELIEFS AND ADHERENCE IN CHRONIC ILLNESS

Nonadherence to recommended therapeutic regimens is considered a major problem for persons with chronic disorders. Origins and concepts of health from the clients' and professionals' perspectives are important factors to consider. It also may be worth noting that the lack of "recovery" from the disorder may precipitate client-blaming strategies such as, "Well, if they would follow the recommendations, they would surely get better." Individuals who adapt lifestyle to health deviations are often motivated by fear of death, disability, pain, and social consequences such as effects on work, activities, and family. Adherence is influenced by numerous factors such as complexity of the regimen, duration, amount of change imposed, inconvenience of obtaining necessary care, dissatisfaction with the system, and health beliefs. The health belief model investigated by Redeker (1988) was developed to explain response to preventive health behaviors. The major belief factors are the value to the individual of a particular outcome and the individual's estimate of the likelihood of a particular outcome associated with compliance or noncompliance. Belief in the efficacy of an action implies belief that that action will reduce the threat to health. The requirements of compliance must not outweigh the benefits, or the client will rarely feel it is worth the effort. Careful assessment of the client's belief in outcomes and energy needed to comply with the regimen is essential. Questions that need to be addressed are as follows:

- Do health beliefs remain stable over time?
- Is there a difference between the responses of individuals recently diagnosed and those of clients with a long history of chronic disorders?
- How important is symptom severity in compliance?
- What relationship exists between social support and maintenance of health benefits?

Emphasis on the importance of the client's perception of health is consistent with Orem's concept that education, experience, attitudes, and knowledge all color one's response to health requirements (Orem, 1980).

Compliance

Compliance has been defined as the extent to which a person's behavior coincides with medical or health advice. If this is viewed traditionally, it essentially means the client becomes a passive respondent to the authoritarian demands of the health care providers. Compliance is one of the dilemmas of the chronically ill. Noncompliance is a nonspecific symptom that may be caused by numerous factors. Given this assumption, we must not expect any one method of intervention to be particularly successful. Physicians treating elderly persons with chronic diseases are often unaware that their compliance rate can vary from 83% (Bungard et al, 2000) to 10% (Colom, 2000).

Often, the demands of long-term illness conflict with values and needs developed over a lifetime. Nurses must appreciate the interpersonal, cultural, situational, and other factors that underlie what may appear to be simple resistance and negativity. Noncompliance is a complex, multidetermined phenomenon that may involve indirect self-destructive tendencies, quality-of-life issues, family deterrents, or the quality of the client-physician relationship. In many cases society itself contributes to noncompliance by imposing regulations, policies, insurance restrictions, and medical constraints that reward noncompliance. For example, in recent years individuals who were receiving Supplemental Security Income (SSI) for disability were often dropped from the rolls if they demonstrated any increasing capacity for self-care.

Chronic illness is increasing because of endemic risk factors, deeply ingrained cultural values, and medical advances that keep people alive longer. *The task of living with these chronic illnesses for years by following increasingly restrictive regimens has not been given enough consideration.* Knowledge of a medical condition does not significantly affect compliance; however, knowledge of the regimen, a therapeutic alliance with the physician, and higher levels of education all seem to significantly relate to greater levels of compliance. The longer a condition exists, the less one is able or willing to continue complex regimens. Positive coping with chronic illness is contingent on the accomplishment of the following tasks:

1. Ability to neutralize harmful environmental conditions
2. Adjustment to negative events consequent to the illness
3. Maintenance of self-image and self-sufficiency
4. Maintenance of social relationships
5. Coping with emotional reactions of anxiety and depression

Compliance is often directly related to the degree of hope one has for recovery—or maintenance. When this is lost, the individual who has little hope may have a cavalier attitude toward any medical or nursing interventions that may be suggested. Researchers are becoming more interested in the impact of self-rated health on compliance and the expectation of recovery. To some extent it appears that an individual's self-ratings before illnesses become predictive of outcomes and changes in functional abilities (Eisen et al, 1999). If this is a common phenomenon, we might expect individuals with negative self-appraisals of their health to become apathetic or fatalistic.

Some types of noncompliance are healthy, in that they may demonstrate an individual's acceptance of responsibility and taking charge, even though in some cases not in the best possible manner. Therefore noncompliance must be carefully evaluated before we conclude that it is helpful or harmful.

Compliance is considered to be the extent to which an individual adheres to medical and health advice. Sustaining compliance is a dilemma of the chronically ill. As the aged become increasingly vulnerable to illness and in spite of their best efforts may actually lose ground physically, they often lose motivation to continue a regimen that does not produce anticipated results. That, in addition to misunderstandings and lack of sufficient information regarding medications and treatments, results in a low rate of compliance among the aged as a group. Estimates of noncompliance vary considerably, depending on the disorder and treatment being reported. Low motivation and feelings of defeat are often compounded by physical and environmental hindrances to compliance.

For some, an element of self-destruction or subliminal suicidal intent may be present. The biomedicalization of our society has often resulted in medical interference in matters that should be in the domain of the individual. The nurse needs to assess the knowledge base of the client related to the regimen prescribed and keep an awareness that resistance to direction may be a form of autonomy and personality strength.

CHRONIC PROBLEMS AND LONG-TERM CARE

Problems that impair one's ability to maintain basic ADLs with intermittent support and assistive devices will most often require institutionalization. Though family caregivers, particularly aging spouses, bear the brunt of this care, there comes a time when the burden simply cannot be borne by the family member. This is discussed thoroughly in Chapter 18. In this chapter it is important to focus on the kind and quality of support one may see and find in long-term care institutions. Today the traditional nursing home seldom exists. Most provide several levels of care and have moved steadily toward the hospital model of care, particularly with the numerous subacute units that provide sophisticated medical treatments. It is important for the individual needing assistance for chronic impairments to seek a setting that provides the level of independence and the home atmosphere that is most supportive of comfort, satisfaction, appropriate levels of independence, and dignity. Although in the past it was difficult to locate such accommodations, it can be done with appropriate planning.

First, one must consider the eventual need for this sort of support and make plans before the need. The prospective client's name must be on the list for potential admission before need, sometimes a year or more in advance. Individuals rarely want to take this step, but it should be reinforced that top-rated facilities simply are not available on an immediate basis. When the name reaches the top of the list, it will move down again until the client is ready for admission. At this writing, a 3-day hospital stay is still required before nursing home admission. The long-term care providers throughout the nation are promoting legislative changes that will delete this requirement. It is no longer necessary in terms of client assessment because thorough and adequate assessment, in a holistic manner quite different from that in a hospital, is now ensured when the Minimum Data Set (MDS 2.0) is completed. This is required by the federal government within 14 days of admission. See Appendix 8-D for a model of the MDS 2.0 and special strategies for implementing it (Klusch, 1995; MDS, 2002).

CHRONIC FUNCTIONAL DISABILITY AND HOME CARE

The elderly population with chronic functional disabilities primarily reside in their homes. Schnack (1995) notes that nurse-owned community health care agencies are proliferating and assuming an ever-larger share of this $31 billion industry. Interest in integrated home care for the elderly has increased (Landi et al, 2001), significant gender trends have been identified (Katz et al, 2000), and the continuum of care from hospital to home health has been surveyed (Anderson et al, 2000). Initially, a 1990 study by Stone and Murtaugh found that nearly half a million elders need assistance in ADLs and only one tenth of these individuals, potentially eligible for home care benefits, could meet the very restrictive disability criteria. Since that time the field has changed considerably, and it is now estimated that more than 7 million persons annually receive medical care in the home. Unfortunately, the reviews are mixed related to nursing's performance in geriatric discharge planning from an inpatient hospital stay (Anderson et al, 2000) or an emergency department visit (Castro et al, 1998).

More than a million elders indicate that they need and receive active assistance with bathing. Those unable to carry out ADLs most frequently needed active assistance with bathing, dressing, and toileting. For those able to manage basic ADLs, most needed active and standby assistance with grocery shopping, money management, and laundry. Short and Leon (1990) reported that those who use home and community services are most frequently over age 85, female, living alone, and having difficulty with several activities, or covered by Medicaid. These trends continue to be clarified and confirmed (Katz et al, 2000), with large gender disparities in the receipt of home care and a glaring absence of psychosocial or nursing care home health referral information in rural areas of the United States.

Kemper (1992) found that on average disabled persons with a spouse or adult child receive 23 hours more care per week than those with neither. However, Katz and colleagues (2000) explored the gender disparity of this finding in a study of 7444 community-based seniors. Informal (generally unpaid) and formal (generally paid) home care findings revealed that women received much less informal care even within married households. This raises the question of how public home care benefits should be distributed. Strauss and Corbin (1988) suggest that assisting individuals and their support persons to view chronic disorders as having a "trajectory" may help them cope with the ups and downs and the acute exacerbations that may require hospitalization. If they are able to better understand the phases of a disorder, they are likely to weather the difficult periods without undue discouragement. Often it must be seen as a lifetime situation that passes through stages in which resources must be tailored accordingly. In summary, they suggest the following points that practitioners must consider:

1. Chronic illness must be seen through the eyes of the persons experiencing it.
2. The illness is often a lifelong course that passes through many phases.
3. Biographic, medical, spiritual, and everyday needs must be considered.
4. Collaborative rather than purely professional relationships may be most effective.
5. Lifelong support may be necessary, although the type, amount, and intensity of such support will vary.

Effects of Chronic Illness on the Family

Often the ill individual feels like a burden to the family and engages in numerous compensatory behaviors to reduce this feeling of guilt. Home care is inconsistently provided and financed, and caregiver burdens are enormous. These have been explored and described extensively (see Chapter 18 for additional discussion). Most often, families are found to extend themselves far beyond their own limits in attempting to deal with a member with a chronic disorder.

Effects of Chronic Illness on the Individual

In summary, management of chronic problems of the aged becomes an issue of the individual and the family. Nurses are resource persons, advisors, teachers, and at times assistants, but the individual is in control of his or her adaptation. Nurses will assist by performing the following functions:

- Identifying and stating strengths the individual demonstrates
- Discussing healthy lifestyle modifications
- Encouraging the reduction of risk factors in the environment
- Assisting the individual to devise methods of improving function, halting disabilities, and adapting lifestyle to reasonable expectations of self
- Providing access to resources when possible
- Referring appropriately and when needed
- Organizing interdisciplinary case conferences
- Informing the individual of insights gained in management of disorders

The goal of care of the chronically ill may be to slow decline, relieve discomfort, and support preferred lifestyle with as few restrictions as possible (Strauss and Glaser, 1975) (Box 8-28). The ability of the aged individual and the family to manage and cope with the problems encountered determines the need. It is necessary for those who care for the aged with chronic conditions to be reoriented and resocialized to care norms and to recognize a different system of rewards. The basics of the care process emphasize improving function, managing the existing illness, preventing secondary complications,

Box 8-28 Goals in Management of Chronic Problems

Stabilize the primary problem
Prevent and manage medical crises
Control symptoms
Encourage compliance with regimen
Prevent secondary disabilities
Prevent social isolation
Treat functional deficits
Promote adaptation
  Person to disability
  Environment to person
  Family to person
Adjust to changes in progress of problems
Normalize interactions

Compiled from Brummel-Smith K: Geriatric rehabilitation, *Generations* 16(1):27, 1992; Corbin JM, Strauss A: *Unending work and care: managing chronic illness at home,* San Francisco, 1988, Jossey-Bass.

delaying deterioration and disability, and facilitating death with peace, comfort, and dignity (Wells and Brink, 1980). Progress is not measured in attempts to achieve cure but rather in maintenance of a steady state or regression of the condition while remembering that the condition does not define the person. This thinking is essential if realistic expectations for the caregiver and the aged are to be achieved. Beyond that, the individual will in some manner seek to understand the meaning of the intrusive non-self of ongoing impairment and struggle to incorporate it in some manner into the perceived total self. The nurse's involvement in this process is to ask about the meanings of the illness and to listen and learn.

Human Needs and Wellness Diagnoses

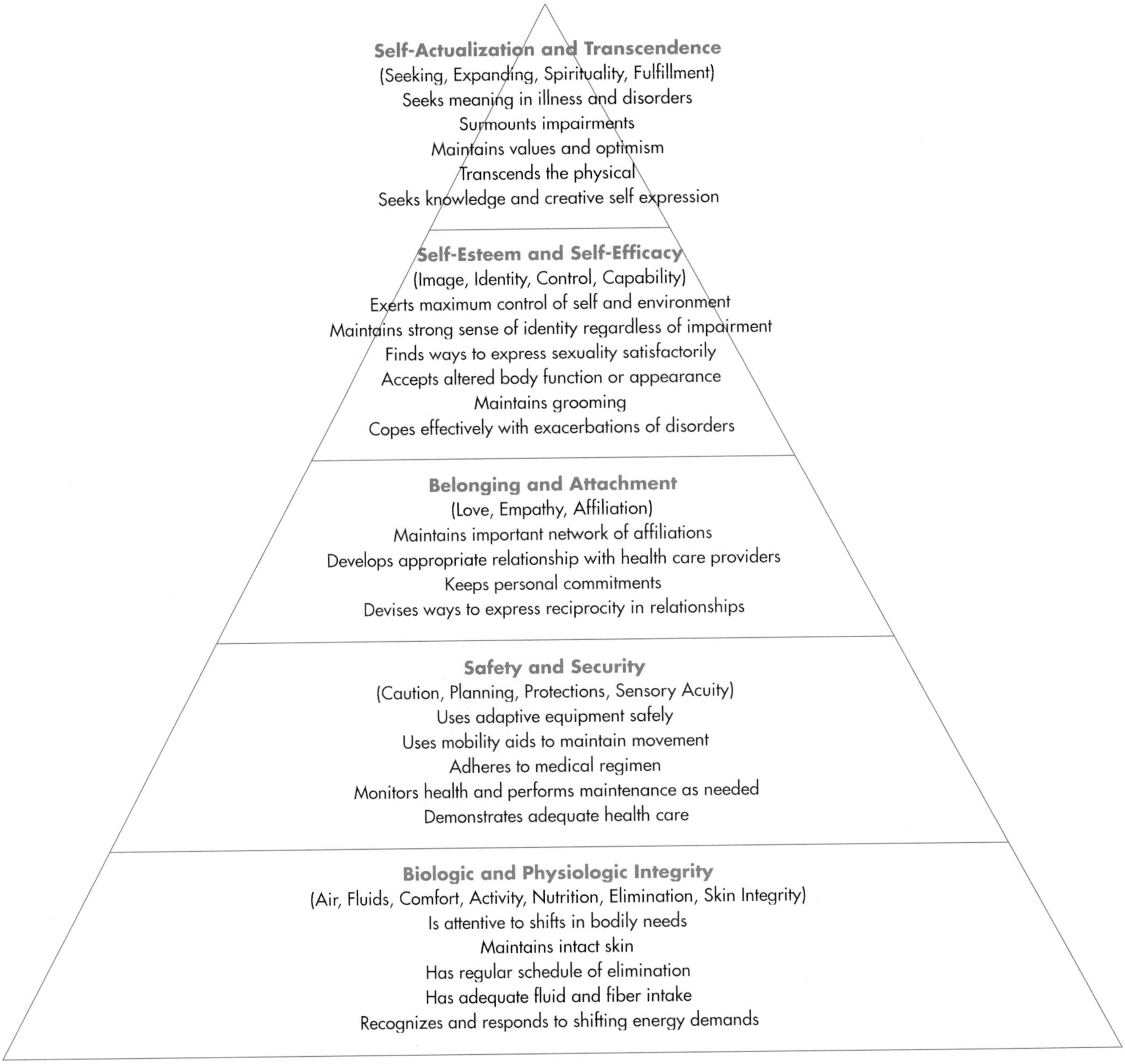

Self-Actualization and Transcendence
(Seeking, Expanding, Spirituality, Fulfillment)
Seeks meaning in illness and disorders
Surmounts impairments
Maintains values and optimism
Transcends the physical
Seeks knowledge and creative self expression

Self-Esteem and Self-Efficacy
(Image, Identity, Control, Capability)
Exerts maximum control of self and environment
Maintains strong sense of identity regardless of impairment
Finds ways to express sexuality satisfactorily
Accepts altered body function or appearance
Maintains grooming
Copes effectively with exacerbations of disorders

Belonging and Attachment
(Love, Empathy, Affiliation)
Maintains important network of affiliations
Develops appropriate relationship with health care providers
Keeps personal commitments
Devises ways to express reciprocity in relationships

Safety and Security
(Caution, Planning, Protections, Sensory Acuity)
Uses adaptive equipment safely
Uses mobility aids to maintain movement
Adheres to medical regimen
Monitors health and performs maintenance as needed
Demonstrates adequate health care

Biologic and Physiologic Integrity
(Air, Fluids, Comfort, Activity, Nutrition, Elimination, Skin Integrity)
Is attentive to shifts in bodily needs
Maintains intact skin
Has regular schedule of elimination
Has adequate fluid and fiber intake
Recognizes and responds to shifting energy demands

These are not all the possible wellness diagnoses that may be identified. The above are examples of nursing diagnoses that should be considered when planning care for the older adult.

KEY CONCEPTS

- Lubkin (1995) states: "Chronic illness is the irreversible presence, accumulation or latency of disease states or impairments that involve the total human environment for supportive care and self care, maintenance of function and prevention of further disability."
- Declines in mortality rates, increasing medical expertise, and sophisticated technologic developments have resulted in a great increase in the survival of the very old with multiple chronic disorders.
- Statistics regarding chronic disease are suspect because they often reflect only those who have sought medical care. In addition, decreased function without incapacitation is rarely reported.
- Women live longer than men and for that and other unknown reasons tend to have a higher incidence of chronic disease.
- One of the most difficult aspects of chronic disease is the unpredictability of the trajectory.
- The management in the home by the family, self, or significant other is central to care and is not peripheral to medical management.
- Adaptations and assistance with ADLs and IADLs are the crux of chronic disease management.
- The most prevalent chronic problems of the aged are arthritis, hearing impairment, heart conditions, and hypertension.
- The most frequent assistance needed by those with chronic disorders is with bathing, dressing, and ambulation.
- The goals of rehabilitation for the aged are to ensure opportunity for optimum personal development and function. Though rehabilitation legislation is chiefly designed to return individuals to productive employment, this is not at this time a goal for most of the aged.

▲ CASE STUDY

Diabetes

Ms. P, an 82-year-old single woman, lives in a life-care community in her own apartment but has the reassurance of knowing her medical and functional needs will be taken care of regardless of the extent of these needs. This is the primary reason she chose to sell her home and live in the tiny apartment in the life-care complex. She is at present independent though she is diabetic (managed with diet, exercise, and oral medications), suffers from CHF, and is having serious problems with her vision. She has also noticed that her toes are cold and somewhat numb. The great toe on her left foot seems to be discolored. Because of the lack of feeling, she often walks around her apartment barefoot because it seems to increase the sensation in her feet. She has also been gaining weight steadily since she moved into the life-care community and attributes that to the fact that she eats much better now that she joins others in the congregate dining room for meals. It is hard for her at times to ignore the delicious desserts that the chef so wonderfully prepares. Overall, she feels quite good and is grateful that she has no severe pains—some mild arthritis but nothing serious. She has not needed to use the health care center and goes to the clinic only to pick up her medication. She sees no reason to bother them with anything else. Her niece stopped by last week to borrow money for her car payment. Ms. P seemed a little confused and lethargic. Her niece asked if she had been sleeping well, and Ms. P responded that, indeed, she slept too well and too much. The niece encouraged her to go to the clinic for a checkup, but Ms. P declined. This week when Ms. P. went to the clinic for her medication and they checked her blood sugar, it was 280 mg/dl. She said, "Oh, I don't think it is anything to worry about. I ran out of medication and didn't take it for 2 days and I ate two pieces of fudge after lunch."

Based on the case study, develop a nursing care plan using the following procedure:*

List comments of client that provide subjective data.

List information that provides objective data.

From these data identify and state, using accepted format, two nursing diagnoses you determine are most significant to this client at this time. List two client strengths that you have identified from data.

Determine and state outcome criteria for each diagnosis. These must reflect some alleviation of the problem identified in the nursing diagnosis and must be stated in concrete and measurable terms.

Plan and state one or more interventions for each diagnosed problem. Provide specific documentation of source used to determine appropriate intervention. Plan at least one intervention that incorporates the client's existing strengths.

Evaluate success of intervention. Interventions must correlate directly with the stated outcome criteria in order to measure the outcome success.

▲ CASE STUDY

Incontinence

Mrs. J, at 82 years old, was hospitalized for an abdominal hysterectomy to remove large benign fibroid tumors. When she awoke from anesthesia, she was quite disoriented and had the illusion that something was crawling into her vagina. She tried repeatedly to pull it away, mildly disoriented and highly agitated because of the presence of a Foley catheter to drain her bladder. She said, "What have you done to me that I can no longer pee normally? This is ridiculous and you didn't have permission to do this." The third day following surgery she developed a temperature of 99° F. Nevertheless, she was

*Students are advised to refer to their nursing diagnosis text and identify possible or potential problems.

eager to be released to her home. Everything there was so orderly and predictable. Her home was integral to her self-concept. She found that coping with the hospitalization seemed to make her weaker each day even though she ambulated three times daily and scrupulously followed whatever directions she was given regarding her care and recovery. The morning of the fourth day following surgery the Foley was discontinued and her temperature had returned to 98.6° F. She was released and her daughter took her home. She found that she was dribbling urine everywhere, seemingly having totally lost control. She attributed this to the trauma of surgery and began wearing disposable pads. When she went to the clinic for her postsurgical check, she told the nurse she felt fine except for her inability to control her urine and her fear that her odor repulsed people.

Based on the case study, develop a nursing care plan using the following procedure:*

List comments of client that provide subjective data.

List information that provides objective data.

From these data identify and state, using accepted format, two nursing diagnoses you determine are most significant to this client at this time. List two client strengths that you have identified from data.

Determine and state outcome criteria for each diagnosis. These must reflect some alleviation of the problem identified in the nursing diagnosis and must be stated in concrete and measurable terms.

Plan and state one or more interventions for each diagnosed problem. Provide specific documentation of source used to determine appropriate intervention. Plan at least one intervention that incorporates the client's existing strengths.

Evaluate success of intervention. Interventions must correlate directly with the stated outcome criteria in order to measure the outcome success.

STUDY QUESTIONS/ACTIVITIES

What are the most plausible reasons for Mrs. J's incontinence?

From data available, what would you surmise are important aspects of Mrs. J's personality?

Discuss your thoughts about the effects of being incontinent on Mrs. J's self-concept.

What would you say to Mrs. J about her situation?

What might you recommend to Mrs. J?

Would pelvic floor exercises be beneficial to Mrs. J? Explain your reasoning.

*Students are advised to refer to their nursing diagnosis text and identify possible or potential problems.

RESEARCH QUESTIONS

What percentage of women develop urinary incontinence related to disorders of the reproductive organs?

What are the reasons women refrain from seeking treatment for urinary incontinence?

What are the effects of various systemic diseases on continence; for example, diabetes, hypothyroidism, arthritis, and CHF?

What are the most frequent reasons men experience urinary incontinence? Do they seek treatment more readily than do women?

How closely does the loss of urine control correlate with feelings of loss of control in other aspects of life?

What percentage of elders curtail social activities purely because of incontinence?

How often is urinary incontinence identified as the trigger event that precedes institutionalization?

Do correlations exist among age, decreased tissue elasticity, and the formation of pressure ulcers?

Do individuals at high risk for pressure ulcer development who never develop ulcers have a protective characteristic or factor?

Which risk assessment factors best predict pressure ulcer development in selected subgroups of high-risk patients; for example, frail elderly or critically ill?

Are the parameters used in risk assessment tools common or different in acute care, long-term care, and home care?

How does documentation of pressure ulcers affect prevention of pressure ulcers?

REFERENCES

Abrams BN: Management of diabetes complications: a focus on peripheral neuropathy. Available at *www.ceanytime.com*

Agency for Health Care Policy and Research: Urinary incontinence in adults, pub no (PHS) 96-0682 (no 2), Rockville, MD, 1996, U.S. Department of Health and Human Services.

Allen LH, Casterline J: Commentary: Vitamin B_{12} deficiency in elderly individuals: diagnosis and requirements, *Am J Clin Nutr* 60:12, 1994.

American Diabetes Association: 2000 standards of medical care for patients with diabetes mellitus: position statement, *Diabetes Care* 23(suppl 1), 2000.

American Diabetes Association: 2002 guidelines. 60th Annual Scientific Sessions, 2002, American Diabetes Association. Available at *www.advancefornp.com/npfeatures*

American Nurses' Association: 2000.

American Nursing Association: *Standards of clinical nursing practice,* ed 2, Washington, DC, 2002, American Nurses Publishing.

American Stroke Association: Reducing stroke risk, *Stroke Connection,* Sept–Oct, 2000, p. 6.

American Stroke Association (2002). Abrupt changes in body position can trigger stroke. Meeting report 2/08. American Heart Association. Available at *www.americanheart.org/presenter.jhtml?identifier=3000721*

American Thoracic Society: American Thoracic Society guidelines: targeted tuberculin testing and treatment of latent tuberculosis infection, *Am J Respir Crit Care Med* 161(4 pt 2):S221, 2000.

Anderson MA et al: A rural perspective on home care communication about elderly patients after hospital discharge, *West J Nurs Res* 22(2):225, 2000.

Anthonisen NR, Connett JE, Kiley JP: Effects of smoking intervention and the use of inhaled anticholinergic bronchodilator on the rate of decline of FEV_1: the lung health study, *JAMA* 272:1497, 1994.

Balch PA, Balch JF: *Prescription for nutritional healing,* ed 3, New York, 2000, Avery.

Baldridge D: Diabetes: a crisis for American Indians of all age, *Aging Today* 22(4):1, 2001.

Banerjee DK et al: Underdiagnosis of asthma in the elderly, *Br J Dis Chest* 81:23, 1987.

Bates-Jensen BM: Pressure ulcers. In Sussman C, Bates-Jensen BM, editors: *Wound care,* Gaithersburg, MD, 1998, Aspen.

Beers MH, Berkow R: *The Merck manual of geriatrics,* ed 3, Whitehouse Station, NJ, 2000, Merck Research Laboratories.

Bergstrom N, Allman RM, Alvarez OM: *Treatment of pressure ulcers. Clinical practice guideline no 15,* pub no 95-0652, Rockville, MD, 1994, US Department of Health and Human Services, Public Health Service, Agency for Health Care Policy and Research.

Brain Attack Coalition: *Recommendations for the establishment of primary stroke centers,* 2001, National Guideline Clearinghouse. Available at *www.guideline.gov/VIEWS/summary.asp?guideline=1784&summary_type=brief_su*

Brashears VL: Alterations of cardiovascular function. In McCance K, Huether S, editors: *Pathophysiology: the biologic basis for disease in adults and children,* ed 4, St Louis, 2002, Mosby.

Braunwald E, Grossman W: Clinical aspects of heart failure, *Heart Disease* 16:444, 1992.

Bungard TJ et al: Why do patients with atrial fibrillation not receive warfarin? *Arch Intern Med* 160:41, 2000.

Burrows B et al: Characteristics of asthma among elderly adults in a sample of the general population, *Chest* 100:935, 1991.

Camilleri M et al: Insights into the pathophysiology and mechanisms of constipation, irritable bowel syndrome and diverticulosis in older people, *J Am Geriatr Soc* 48(9):1142, 2000.

Carmel R: Prevalence of undiagnosed pernicious anemia in the elderly, *Arch Intern Med* 156:1097, 1996.

Carpenito LJ: *Nursing diagnosis: application to clinical practice,* ed 9, Philadelphia, 2002, JB Lippincott.

Castro CM, King AC: Telephone versus mail interventions for maintenance of physical activity in older adults, *Health Psychol* 20(6):438, 2001.

Castro JM et al: Home care referral after emergency department discharge, *J Emerg Nurs* 24(2):127, 1998.

Cefalu C: Urinary incontinence. In Ham R, Sloane PD, Warshaw G, editors: *Primary care geriatrics,* St Louis, 2002, Mosby.

Chan PD, Johnson MT: *Treatment guidelines for medicine and primary care,* Laguna Hills, CA, 2002, Current Clinical Strategies Publishing.

Chan TY: Vitamin D deficiency and susceptibility to tuberculosis, *Calcif Tissue Int* 66(6):476, 2000.

Cobb DK, Durfee SM: Involuntary weight loss and pressure ulcers: the role of nutrition and anabolic strategies, *Ann Long-Term Care* (suppl), May 2002.

Colom F: Medication compliance in bipolar disease, *J Clin Psychiatry* 61(8):549, 2000.

Cook CB, Lyles RH, El-Kebbi I: The potentially poor response to outpatient diabetes care in urban African Americans, *Diabetes Care* 24(2):209, 2001.

Corbin JM, Strauss A: *Unending work and care: managing chronic illness at home,* San Francisco, 1988, Jossey-Bass.

Corsini E et al: In vivo dehydroepiandrosterone restores age-associated defects in the protein kinase C signal transduction pathway and related functional responses, *J Immunol* 168(4):1753, 2002.

Cotran RS, Kumar V, Robbins SL: *Robbins pathologic basis of disease,* ed 5, Philadelphia, 1994, WB Saunders.

Coward R, Horne C, Peek D: Predicting nursing home admissions among incontinent older adults: a comparison of residential differences across six years, *Gerontologist* 35(6):732, 1995.

Cravens DD: Case report: a woman who falls, *Ann Long-Term Care* 6(7):230, 1998.

Daly R: Diabetes mellitus. In Adelman AM, editor: *20 common problems in geriatrics,* New York, 2001, Bantam.

Davies PD: Tuberculosis in the elderly. Epidemiology and optimal management, *Drugs Aging* 8(6):436, 1996.

Dunlop MJ: Is a science of caring possible? In Benner P, editor: *Interpretive phenomenology: embodiment, caring and ethics in health and illness,* Thousand Oaks, CA, 1994, Sage.

Dychtwald K, Flower J: *Age wave,* New York, 1990, Bantam.

Eisen SV et al: Assessing behavioral health outcomes in outpatient programs: reliability and validity of the BASIS-32, *Journal of Behavioral Health Services and Research* 26:5, 1999.

Enright P: Underdiagnosis and undertreatment of asthma in the elderly, *Chest* 116(3):603, 1999.

Enright PL et al: Spirometry reference values for women and men 65 to 85 years of age: cardiovascular health study, *Am Rev Respir Dis* 147(1):125, 1993.

Estes MEZ: *Health assessment and physical examination,* Albany, NY, 2002, Delmar.

Farmer JA, Gotto AM Jr: Dyslipidemia and other risk factors for coronary artery disease. In Braunwald E, editor: *Heart disease,* ed 5, Philadelphia, 1997, WB Saunders.

Ferrell BA: Pressure ulcers. In Ham R, Sloane P, Warshaw G, editors: *Primary care geriatrics,* St Louis, 2002, Mosby.

Flanagan S: Stroke rehabilitation: recovery comes with time and patience, *Focus on Healthy Aging* 4(1):1, 2001.

Folstein MF, Folstein SE, McHugh PR: Mini-Mental State: a practical method for grading the cognitive state of patients for the clinician, *J Psychiatr Res* 12:189, 1975.

Fourcroy JL: Overactive bladder, *Adv Nurse Pract* 9(3):59, 2001.

Frenchman IB: Cost of urinary incontinence in 2 skilled nursing facilities, *Clin Geriatr* 9(1):1-4, 2001.

Giger JN, Davidhizar RE: *Transcultural nursing,* St Louis, 1991, Mosby.

Giger JN, Davidhizar RE: Cultural diversity in health and illness. In *Transcultural nursing: assessment and intervention,* ed 3, St Louis, 1999, Mosby.

Grant JS et al: Social problem-solving telephone partnerships with family caregivers of persons with stroke, *Int J Rehabil Res* 24(3):181, 2001.

Guyer B et al: Annual summary of vital statistics: trends in the health of Americans during the 20th century, *Pediatrics* 106(6):1307, 2000.

Halphen M, Blain A: Natural history of colonic diverticulosis, *Review Practicial* 45(8):952, 1995.

Harvard Medical School Health Publications: Strengthening the pelvic floor, *Women's Health Watch* 3(12):2, 1996.
Hazzard WR et al: *Principles of geriatric medicine and gerontology,* ed 2, New York, 1990, McGraw-Hill.
Health and Age: *Preventing diabetes.* News alert no 89, 2002. Available at *www.healthandage.com*
Hemingway S: Putting the telephone into practice, *Mental Health Nursing* 22(3):6, 2002.
Higgins M: Epidemiology and prevention of coronary heart disease in families, *Am J Med* 1(108)(5):387, 2000.
Hill CA: Caring for the aging athlete, *Geriatr Nurs* 22(1):43, 2001.
Holden K: Chronic and disabling conditions: the economic cost to individuals and society, *Public Policy and Aging Report* 11(2): 1, 2001.
Huether S: Structure, function, and disorders of the integument. In McCance K, Huether S, editors: *Pathophysiology: the biologic basis for disease in adults and children,* ed 4, St Louis, 2002, Mosby.
Hunder GG: Treatment of giant cell arteritis, *UpToDate* 10(1):1, 2002. Available at *www.uptodate.com*
Janssens JP, Zellweger JP: Clinical epidemiology and treatment of tuberculosis in elderly patients, *Schweizerische medizinsche Wochenschrift* 129(3):80, 1999.
Johnson M, Maas M, Moorhead S: *Nursing outcomes classification (NOC),* ed 2, St Louis, 2000, Mosby.
Joosten E et al: Prevalence and causes of anaemia in a geriatric hospitalized population, *Gerontology* 38:111, 1992.
Joslin Diabetes Center: *Type II diabetes—treating the progression,* Cincinnati, 2001, Continuing Medical Education, Joslin Diabetes Center.
Kahsai D, Roekens CV: Acute anemia, *eMedicine,* 2001. Available at *www.emedicine.com/emerg/topic808.htm#section~differentials*
Kaltenbach G et al: Influence of age on presentation and prognosis of tuberculosis in internal medicine, *La Presse Medicale* 30(29):1446, 2001.
Katz SJ, Kabeto M, Langa KM: Gender disparities in the receipt of home care for elderly people with disability in the United States, *JAMA* 284(23):3022, 2000.
Kee JL: *Handbook of laboratory and diagnostic tests,* ed 4, Upper Saddle River, NJ, 2001, Prentice Hall.
Kemper P: The use of formal and informal home care by the disabled, *Health Service Res* 27(4):421, 1992.
Kistler JP, Furie KL, Ay H: Treatment of transient cerebral ischemia, *UpToDate,* 2002. Available at *www.uptodate.com*
Klusch L: *Solutions in restorative caregiving,* Des Moines, IA, 1995, Briggs Health Care Products.
Koton S: Abrupt changes in body positions can trigger stroke. American Heart Association Meeting Report, Feb 8, 2002. Available at *www.americanheart.org/presenter.jhtml?identifier=3000721*
Kuzminski AM et al: Effective treatment of cobalamin deficiency with oral cobalamin, *Blood* 92:1191, 1998.
Landi F et al: A new model of integrated home care for the elderly: impact on hospital use, *J Clin Epidemiol* 54(9):968, 2001.
Langsjoen PH et al: The aging heart: reversal of diastolic dysfunction through the use of oral CoQ_{10} in the elderly. In Klatz RM, Goldman R, editors: *Anti-aging medical therapeutics,* St Louis, 1997, Health Quest Publications.
Lapp D: Practical demonstration of cognitive training techniques, *Proceedings of the Third Congress of the International Psychogeriatric Association* 3:84, 1987 (abstract).
Lawrence PF: Diseases of the vascular system. In Lawrence PF, Bell RM, Dayton MT, editors: *Essentials of general surgery,* ed 3, 2000, Lippincott, Williams & Wilkins.
Liu Z, Shilkret KL, Ellis HM: Predictors of sputum culture conversion among patients with tuberculosis in the era of tuberculosis resurgence, *Arch Intern Med* 159(10):1110, 1999.
Lubkin IM: *Chronic illness: impact and interventions,* ed 3, Boston, 1995, Jones & Bartlett.
Mahler DA, Horner A: Clinical measurement of dyspnea. In *Dyspnea,* Mt Kisco, NY, 1990, Futura.
Mandelstam D, Robinson W: Support for the incontinent patient, *Nurs Mirror* 144(15):xix, 1977.
Masterson TM, editor: *A pocketful of prevention: preventive care guidelines adapted from the United States Preventive Services Task Force Report,* McLean, VA, 1998, International Medical Publishing.
Mayo L: *Guides to action on chronic illness,* New York, 1956, National Health Council, Commission on Chronic Illness.
McCloskey JC, Bulechek GB: *Nursing Interventions Classification (NIC),* ed 3, St Louis, 2002, Mosby.
McCrory DC et al: Management of acute exacerbations of COPD: a summary and appraisal of the published evidence, *Chest* 119:1190, 2001.
McCulloch DK: Definition and classification of diabetes mellitus, *UpToDate,* 2002. Available at *www.uptodate.com*
McGee SR, Boyko EJ: Physical examination and chronic lower-extremity ischemia, *Arch Intern Med* 158:1357, 1998.
MDS: MDS 2.0 information site. Available at *http://cms.hhs.gov/medicaid/mds20/default.asp*
Melange M, Vanheuverzwyn R: Eitopathogenesis of colonic diverticular disease: role of fiber and therapeutic perspectives, *Acta Gastroenterol Belg* 53(3):346, 1990.
Melvin J: Rehabilitation in the year 2000. Paper presented at the 10th International Congress of Physical Medicine and Disability, Milwaukee, 1988.
Mikami M, Kawasaki Y: Two step tuberculin testing among elderly Japanese admitted to residential homes, *Tuberculosis* 75(11):643, 2000.
Milne HA, McWilliam CL: Considering nursing resources as "caring time," *J Adv Nurs* 23(4):809, 1996.
Moss SE, Klein R, Klein BE: Long-term incidence of lower-extremity amputations in a diabetic population, *Arch Fam Med* 5(7):391, 1996.
Nadel M: Synopsis of diverticulosis. University of Connecticut Health Center, Pathology Department, 2001. Available at *http://esynopsis.uchc.edu/S203.htm*
National Academy on an Aging Society: 1999.
National Center for Health Statistics: Asthma prevalence, health care use and mortality, 2000-2001. Available at *www.cdc.gov/nchs/products/pubs/pubd/hestats/asthma/asthma.htm*
National Heart, Lung and Blood Institute: *International c onsensus report on diagnosis and management of asthma,* pub no 92-3091, Bethesda, MD, 1992, National Heart, Lung and Blood Institute.
National Heart, Lung and Blood Institute: *Global initiative for asthma: global strategy for asthma management and prevention NHLBI/WHO workshop report,* pub no 95-3659, Bethesda, MD, 1995, National Heart, Lung and Blood Institute.
National Heart, Lung and Blood Institute: Available at *www.nhlbi.nih.gov/health/prof/lung/asthma/as_elder.htm*

National Institutes of Health, NINDS: *Brain basics: preventing stroke*, 2001. Available at *www.ninds.nih.gov/health_and_medical/pubs/preventing_stroke.htm*

National Institutes of Health Panel: Reaching a consensus on incontinence, *Geriatr Nurs* 10:78, 1989.

Newman D: Continence control: vision for the future. Senior Focus, Mills Peninsula Hospitals Conference, San Francisco, Oct 26-27, 1992.

Norton D, McLaren R, Exton-Smith AN: *An investigation of geriatric nursing problems in the hospital,* London, 1962, National Corporation for the Care of Old People.

Novartis Foundation for Gerontology: *Geriatric syllabus 2002.* Available at *www.geriatricsyllabus.com/other/cardio/epide.htm#chap10*

Nursing Interventions Classification: 2001. Available at *www.nursing.uiowa.edu/nic*

Nursing Outcomes Classification: 2002. Available at *www.nursing.uiowa.edu/noc/benefits.htm* (accessed Oct 21, 2002).

Nutrition Screening Initiative: Study shows poor nutrition key cause of pressure ulcers, issue 33, pp 1, 4, Fall/Winter 2001.

O'Conner PJ: *Improving diabetes care,* 2001. Available at *primarycare.medscape.com/ABFP/JABF....041fp140512*

Orem DE: *Nursing: concepts of practice,* ed 2, New York, 1980, McGraw-Hill.

Orem DE: *Nursing: concepts of practice,* St Louis, 1995, Mosby.

Packham S: Tuberculosis in the elderly, *Gerontology* 47(4):175, 2001.

Palmer MH: *Urinary continence assessment and promotion,* Gaithersburg, MD, 1996, Aspen.

Peat JK, Woolcock AJ, Cullen K: Rate of decline of lung function in subjects with asthma, *Eur J Respir Dis* 70:171, 1987.

Peterson PG: *Gray dawn: how the coming age wave will transform America and the world,* New York, 1999, Three Rivers Press.

Piano M, Huether S: Mechanisms of hormonal regulation. In McCance K, Huether S, editors: *Pathophysiology: the biologic basis for disease in adults and children,* ed 4, St Louis, 2002, Mosby.

Rajagopalan S: Tuberculosis and aging: a global health problem, *Clin Infect Dis* 33(7):1034, 2001.

Rajagopalan S, Yoshikawa TT: Tuberculosis in the elderly, *Gerontologie and Geriatrics* 33(5):374, 2000.

Redeker N: Health beliefs and adherence in chronic illness, *J Nurs Sch* 29(1):31, 1988.

Reed RL, Mooradian A: Diabetes mellitus. In Ham R, Sloane P, Warshaw G, editors: *Primary care geriatrics,* ed 4, St Louis, 2002, Mosby.

Resnick B, Fleishell A: Developing a restorative care program, *Am J Nurs* 102(7):91, 2002.

Reuben DB et al: *Geriatrics at your fingertips,* New York, 2002, Blackwell.

Robertson DG: The role of combination therapy in the management of patients with type 2 diabetes mellitus. Kentucky Nurse Practitioner Conference, April 2001, Lexington.

Roseman HM: The treatment of patients at high risk for heart failure. Heart failure 2002: the new staging classification of the ACC/AHA guidelines, July 13, 2002, Louisville, KY (presentation and handout).

Rousseau P, Fuentevilla-Clifton A: Urinary incontinence in the aged, part 1 and part 2, *Geriatrics* 47(6):22, 1992.

Rubio MA: Implications of fiber in different pathologies, *Nutrition Hospital* 17(2):17, 2002.

Sacco RL et al: The protective effect of moderate alcohol consumption on ischemic stroke, *JAMA* 281(1):53, 1999.

Saver J: Highlights from the 27th International Stroke Conference, San Antonio, Feb 7-9, 2002. Available at *Medscape Neurol Neurosurg* 4(1), *www.medscape.com/viewarticle/429908*

Schnack M: Who's running home health? *Adv Nurs Pract* 8(4):10, 1995.

Schuster PM, Wright C, Tomich P: Gender differences in the outcomes of participants in home programs compared to those in structure rehabilitation programs, *Rehabilitation Nurs* 20(2):93, 1995.

Shields E: Personal communication, Sept 23, 1990, Vermillion, OH.

Shoben: Hospitals provide similar care to elderly women and men: Rand study finds differences in quality very small, Rand news release, October 14, 1992.

Short P, Leon J: *Use of home and community services by persons ages 65 and older with functional difficulties,* pub no (PHS) 90-3466, Rockville, MD, 1990, U.S. Department of Health and Human Services, Agency for Health Care Policy and Research.

Sica DA: ACE inhibitors and stroke: new considerations, *J Clin Hypertens* 4(2):126, 2002.

Sleisenger MH, Fordtran JS: *Gastrointestinal disease,* ed 5, Philadelphia, 1993, WB Saunders.

Smith DL: Anemia in the elderly, *Am Fam Physician* 62(7):1565, 2000. Available at *www.aafp.org/afp/20001001/1565.html*

Stabler SP: Vitamin B_{12} deficiency in older people: improving diagnosis and preventing disability, *J Am Geriatr Soc* 46:1317, 1998 (editorial).

Stoller JK: Acute exacerbations of chronic obstructive pulmonary disease, *N Engl J Med* 346:988, 2002.

Stone RI, Murtaugh CM: The elderly population with chronic functional disability: implications for home care eligibility, *Gerontologist* 30(4):491, 1990.

Strauss A, Corbin J: *Shaping a new health care system,* San Francisco, 1988, Jossey-Bass.

Strauss A, Glaser B: *Chronic illness and the quality of life,* St Louis, 1975, Mosby.

Tangalos E: *Geriatric pharmaceutical care guidelines,* Covington, KY, 2002, Omnicare.

The Alexander House Group: Consensus paper on venous leg ulcer, J Dermatol Surg Oncol 18(7):592, 1992.

Thom DH: Variations in estimate of urinary incontinence prevalence in the community, *J Am Geriatr Soc* 46:473, 1998.

U.S. Bureau of the Census: *Statistical abstract of the United States: 2002,* ed 122, Washington, DC, 2001, U.S. Bureau of the Census.

U.S. Department of Health and Human Services: *Healthy people 2000: national health promotion and disease prevention objectives,* pub no (PHS) 91-50212, Washington, DC, 1991, U.S. Government Printing Office.

U.S. Department of Health and Human Services: *Urinary incontinence in adults. Clinical practice guideline,* pub no 92-0038, Rockville, MD, 1992, Agency for Health Care Policy and Research, Public Health Service.

U.S. Department of Health and Human Services: *Healthy people 2000: midcourse review and 1995 objectives,* Washington, DC, 1995, National Institutes of Health.

U.S. Department of Health and Human Services: *Urinary incontinence in adults: acute and chronic management. Clinical prac-*

tice guideline no 2, 1996 update, pub no 96-0682, Washington, DC, 1996, Agency for Health Care Policy and Research.

U.S. Department of Health and Human Services: *Healthy people 2010,* Sudbury, MA, 2000, Jones & Bartlett.

Verbrugge LM, Patrick DL: Seven chronic conditions: their impact on US adults' activity levels and use of medical services, *Am J Public Health* 85(2):173, 1995.

Wada M: The adverse reactions of anti-tuberculosis drugs and their management, *Jpn J Clin Med* 56(12):3091, 1998.

Watson J: *Human science and human care: a theory of nursing,* New York, 1988, National League for Nursing.

Wells T, Brink C: Helpful equipment, *Geriatr Nurs* 1:264, 1980.

Wenger NK: Rehabilitation of the elderly coronary patient. In Frengley JD, Murray P, Wykle M: *Practicing rehabilitation with geriatric clients,* New York, 1990, Springer.

Whitehead JB: An overview of the management of diabetes in the elderly, *Ann Long-Term Care* (suppl), 1-7, March 2002.

Williams RA: *The athlete and heart disease,* Philadelphia, 1999, Lippincott.

Woog P: *The chronic illness trajectory framework: the Corbin and Strauss nursing model,* New York, 1992, Springer.

Woolley DC: Polymyalgia rheumatica. In Ham R, Sloane P, Warshaw G, editors: *Primary care geriatrics,* ed 4, St Louis, 2002, Mosby.

Wooten-Bielski K: HIV and AIDS in older adults, *Geriatr Nurs* 20(5):268, 1999.

Yap I, Hoe J: A radiological survey of diverticulosis in Singapore, *Singapore Med J* 32(4):218, 1991.

Yoshimoto H, Takahashi M, Saima S: Influence of rifampin on antihypertensive effects of dihydropiridine calcium-channel blockers in four elderly patients, *Jpn J Geriatr* 33(9):692, 1996.

Young MA, Hoffberg HJ: Poststroke rehabilitation, *Clin Advisor,* 25-26, 31-32, Feb 2001.

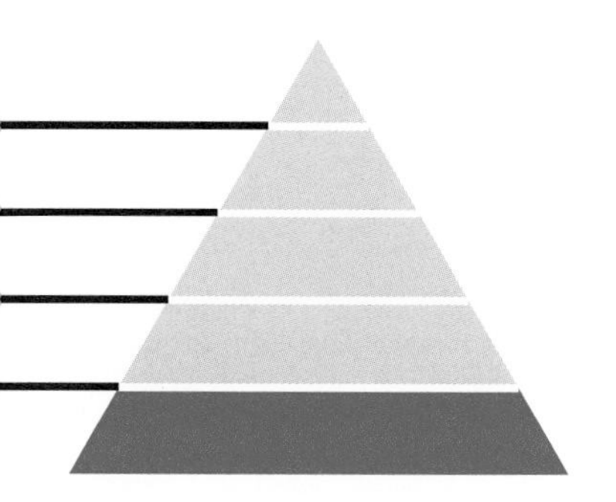

APPENDIX 8-A

Barthel Index

	"Can do by myself"	"Can do with help of someone else"	"Cannot do at all"
Self-Care Subscore			
1. Drinking from a cup	4	0	0
2. Eating	6	0	0
3. Dressing upper body	5	3	0
4. Dressing lower body	7	4	0
5. Putting on brace or artificial limb	0	−2	0 (N/A)
6. Grooming	5	0	0
7. Washing or bathing	6	0	0
8. Controlling urination	10	5 (accidents)	0 (incontinent)
9. Controlling bowel movements	10	5 (accidents)	0 (incontinent)
Mobility Subscore			
10. Getting in and out of chair	15	7	0
11. Getting on and off toilet	6	3	0
12. Getting in and out of tub or shower	1	0	0
13. Walking 50 yards on the level	15	10	0
14. Walking up/down one flight of stairs	10	5	0
15. If not walking: propelling or pushing wheelchair	5	0	0 (N/A)
Barthel total: Best score is 100; worst score is 0.			

Note: Tasks 1-9, the self-care subscore (including control of bladder and bowel sphincters), have a total possible score of 53. Tasks 10-15, the mobility subscore, have a total possible score of 47. The two groups of tasks combined make up the total Barthel Index with a total possible score of 100. From Granger C, Gresham O: *Functional assessment in rehabilitation medicine,* Baltimore, 1984, Williams & Wilkins, p 64.

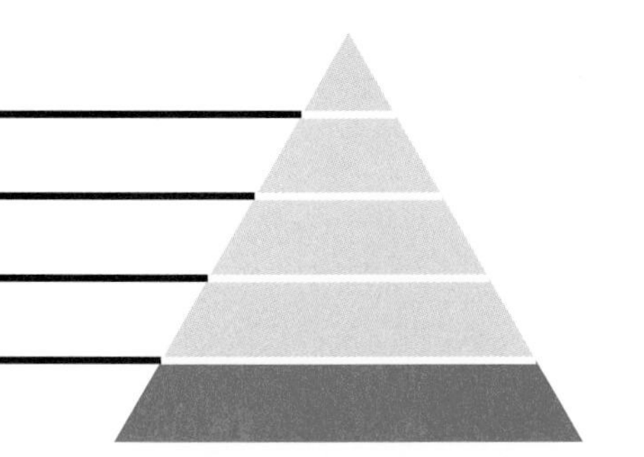

APPENDIX 8-B

Braden Scale for Predicting Pressure Sore Risk

Patient's name:		Evaluator's name:
Sensory Perception Ability to respond meaningfully to pressure-related discomfort	**1. Completely Limited:** Unresponsive (does not moan, flinch, or grasp) to painful stimuli, due to diminished level of consciousness or sedation, OR limited ability to feel pain over most of body surface.	**2. Very Limited:** Responds only to painful stimuli. Cannot communicate discomfort except by moaning or restlessness, OR has a sensory impairment which limits the ability to feel pain or discomfort over $\frac{1}{2}$ of body.
Moisture Degree to which skin is exposed to moisture	**1. Constantly Moist:** Skin is kept moist almost constantly by perspiration, urine, etc. Dampness is detected every time patient is moved or turned.	**2. Moist:** Skin is often but not always moist. Linen must be changed at least once a shift.
Activity Degree of physical activity	**1. Bedfast:** Confined to bed.	**2. Chairfast:** Ability to walk severely limited or nonexistent. Cannot bear own weight and/or must be assisted into chair or wheel chair.
Mobility Ability to change and control body position	**1. Completely Immobile:** Does not make even slight changes in body or extremity position without assistance.	**2. Very Limited:** Makes occasional slight changes in body or extremity position but unable to make frequent or significant changes independently.
Nutrition Usual food intake pattern	**1. Very Poor:** Never eats a complete meal. Rarely eats more than $\frac{1}{3}$ of any food offered. Eats 2 servings or less of protei (meat or dairy products) per day. Takes fluids poorly. Does not take a liquid dietary supplement, OR is NPO and/or maintained on clear liquids or IV for more than 5 days.	**2. Probably Inadequate:** Rarely eats a complete meal and generally eats only about $\frac{1}{2}$ of any food offered. Protein intake includes only 3 servings of meat or dairy products per day. Occasionally will take a dietary supplement, OR receives less than optimum amount of liquid diet or tube feeding.
Friction and Shear	**1. Problem:** Requires moderate to maximum assistance in moving. Complete lifting without sliding against sheets is impossible. Frequently slides down in bed or chair, requiring frequent repositioning with maximum assistance. Spasticity, contractures, or agitation leads to almost constant friction.	**2. Potential Problem:** Moves feebly or requires minimum assistance. During a move skin probably slides to some extent against sheets, chair, restraints, or other devices. Maintains relatively good position in chair or bed most of the time but occasionally slides down.

From Braden B, Bergstrom N: 1988.
NPO, Nothing by mouth; *IV*, intravenously; *TPN*, total parenteral nutrition.

	Date of assessment				
3. Slightly Limited: Responds to verbal commands but cannot always communicate discomfort or need to be turned, OR has some sensory impairment which limits ability to feel pain or discomfort in 1 or 2 extremities.	**4. No Impairment:** Responds to verbal commands. Has no sensory deficit which would limit ability to feel or voice pain or discomfort.				
3. Occasionally Moist: Skin is occasionally moist, requiring an extra linen change approximately once a day.	**4. Rarely Moist:** Skin is usually dry; linen requires changing only at routine intervals.				
3. Walks Occasionally: Walks occasionally during day but for very short distances, with or without assistance. Spends majority of each shift in bed or chair.	**4. Walks Frequently:** Walks outside the room at least twice a day and inside room at least once every 2 hours during waking hours.				
3. Slightly Limited: Makes frequent though slight changes in body or extremity position independently.	**4. No Limitations:** Makes major and frequent changes in position without assistance.				
3. Adequate: Eats over half of most meals. Eats a total of 4 servings of protein (meat, dairy products) each day. Occasionally will refuse a meal, but will usually take a supplement if offered, OR is on a tube feeding or TPN regimen, which probably meets most of nutritional needs.	**4. Excellent:** Eats most of every meal. Never refuses a meal. Usually eats a total of 4 or more servings of meat and dairy products. Occasionally eats between meals. Does not require supplementation.				
3. No Apparent Problem: Moves in bed and in chair independently and has sufficient muscle strength to lift up completely during move. Maintains good position in bed or chair at all times.					
	Total Score				

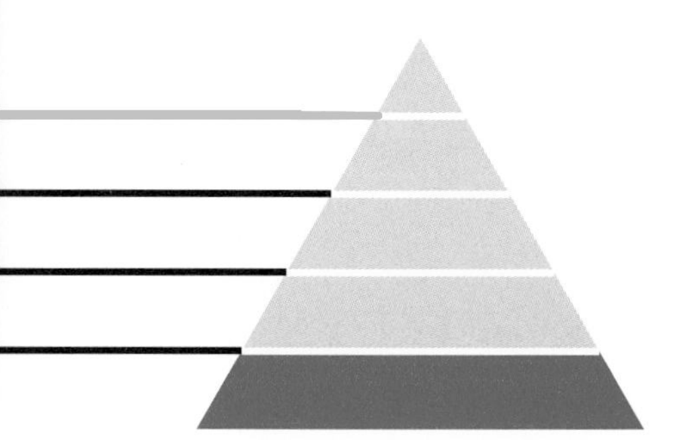

APPENDIX 8-C

Activities of Daily Living and Instrumental Activities of Daily Living

ACTIVITIES OF DAILY LIVING

	Independent	Dependent	
Bathing			Initiation of bath Type of bathing (tub, shower, sponge) Bath preparation Get in/out of tub Ability to wash self Hair washing
Dressing			Clothing selection Putting on garments Doing up buttons, etc. Appropriateness of attire Undressing Laundry
Transfer			From bed to chair From chair to standing
Toileting			Able to find bathroom Able to use toilet appropriately Hygiene
Bowel continence			Frequency and control Constipation
Feeding			Serving self Utensils to mouth Readying food for consumption (buttering, cutting, etc.)

INSTRUMENTAL ACTIVITIES OF DAILY LIVING

	Alone	Assist	Never (N/A)	No longer	
Telephone					Look up number Dial
Medication					Preparation Taking
Outside of home					Organization Getting lost
Driving					Limitations Legal parameters
Housework					Organization Doing (list what able to do)
Food preparation					Planning Shopping Preparing
Finances					Banking Paying bills Balancing checkbook

URINARY CONTINENCE

Does patient have "accidents"? (If "yes," when?) ______
Patient's knowledge of accidents: ______ Frequency: ______
Urgency: ______ Can patient get to bathroom in time? ______
Does patient wet when coughing or sneezing or at other times? ______
Where is center or concern about wetting (patient, family, both)? ______
Other concerns: ______
______

MOBILITY

Walking ability (use of assistive devices): ______
Distance able to walk (and frequency): ______
Gait and posture: ______
Stiffness (morning, after inactivity, evening, where?): ______
______
What does patient do to maximize mobility? ______
Hand dexterity and function: ______
Problems with feet and shoes: ______
Other concerns of patient/family: ______
______

NUTRITION

No. of meals per day: ______ No. of glasses of fluid: ______
Indigestion, nausea/vomiting, change in bowels: ______
Dentition: ______
Appetite: ______ Weight stability: ______
Concerns of family (need for referral to nutritionist): ______
______
______

MEDICATIONS

List medications as prescribed and how they are taken. Note how long patient has been on medication and patient's knowledge of medications (reason for, side effects, precautions).

______
______
______
______
______

Nonprescription medications: ______
______
Allergies (medications): ______ (other): ______
Person responsible for medication administration: ______
Alcohol intake (past/present): ______ Smoking history: ______

SAFETY

Is patient alone at any time? ______ Gets lost? ______
Kitchen safety: ______
Household safety (rugs, cords, railings, stairs): ______
Other concerns: ______
______

CAREGIVER

Name of formal caregiver: ______________________________ Relationship: ____________________

Informal caregiving system: ____

Caregiver's role/function: ____

____

Impact of care giving on caregiver/family: ____________________________________

____

Assessment of stability/security provided in present care environment: ____________________

____

____

SUMMARY

Assessment: ____

____

____

____

____

____

____

Problem list: ____

____

____

____

____

____

____

____

Plan: ____

____

____

____

____

____

Completed by: ______________________________

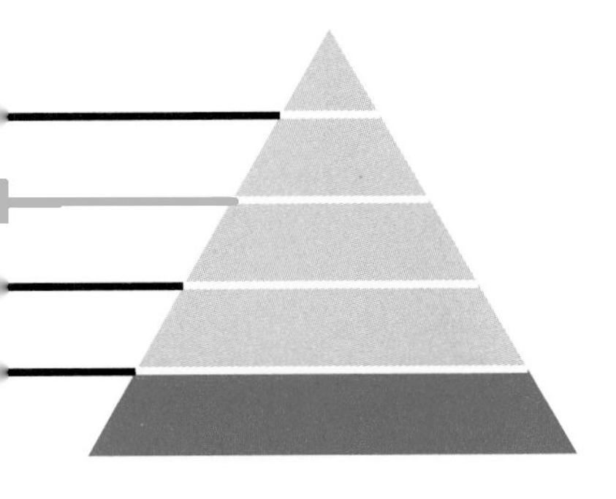

APPENDIX 8-D

Minimum Data Set (MDS) Version 2.0 (Condensed) for Nursing Home Resident Assessment and Care Screening

IDENTIFICATION INFORMATION	Name, gender, birthday, Social Security and Medicare numbers, provider number, reasons for assessment
BACKGROUND INFORMATION	Assessment reference date, date of entry, marital status, payment sources, responsible person, advance directives
DEMOGRAPHIC INFORMATION	Date of entry, situation before admission, occupation, education, language, mental health history and conditions related to MR/DD status
CUSTOMARY ROUTINE	Usual cycle of daily events, eating patterns, functional ability in activities of daily living, social involvement
COGNITIVE PATTERNS	Consciousness, memory, recall ability, decision-making skills, delirium, disordered thinking, changes in cognitive status
COMMUNICATION/ HEARING PATTERNS	Hearing, communication devices/techniques, modes of expression, speech clarity, ability to understand, changes in communication or hearing
VISION PATTERNS	Vision, specific limitations/difficulties, visual appliances
MOOD AND BEHAVIOR PATTERNS	Indicators of depression, anxiety, sad mood, mood persistence, mood changes, behavioral symptoms, changes in behavioral symptoms
PSYCHOSOCIAL WELL-BEING	Sense of initiative/involvement, unsettled relationships, past roles
PHYSICAL FUNCTIONING AND STRUCTURAL PROBLEMS	Activities of daily living (ADL) self-performance: bed mobility, transfer, walking/locomotion, dressing, eating, toileting, personal hygiene, bathing, range of motion, modes of transfers, modes of locomotion, functional and rehabilitation potential, changes in ADL function
CONTINENCE IN LAST 14 DAYS	Self-control categories, bowel continence, bladder continence, bowel elimination pattern, appliances and programs, changes in urinary continence
DISEASE DIAGNOSES	Diseases, infections, other diagnoses
HEALTH CONDITIONS	Problem conditions, pain symptoms, pain site, accidents, stability of conditions
ORAL/NUTRITIONAL STATUS	Oral problems, height and weight, weight changes, nutritional problems, nutritional approaches, parenteral or enteral intake
ORAL/DENTAL STATUS	Oral status and disease prevention, tooth decay, disintegration; buccal cavity examination; dentures, bridges, missing teeth
SKIN CONDITION	Ulcers, type of ulcers, history of unresolved ulcers, other skin problems or lesions, skin treatments, foot problems and care
ACTIVITY PURSUIT PATTERNS	Time awake, time involved in activities, preferred activity settings, general activity preferences, prefers change in daily routines
MEDICATIONS	Number of medications, new medications, injections, days received the following medications (antipsychotic, antianxiety, antidepressant, hypnotic, diuretic)
SPECIAL TREATMENTS AND PROCEDURES	Treatments, procedures and programs; intervention programs for mood, behavior, cognitive loss, nursing rehabilitation/restorative care, devices and restraints, hospital stays, emergency room visits, physician visits, physician orders, abnormal lab values
DISCHARGE POTENTIAL AND OVERALL STATUS	Discharge potential, overall change in care needs
RESIDENT PARTICIPATION IN ASSESSMENT	Resident, family members, significant other

Resident's Name:	Medical Record No.:

1. Check if RAP is triggered.
2. For each triggered RAP, use the RAP guidelines to identify areas needing further assessment. Document relevant assessment information regarding the resident's status.
   - Describe:
     —Nature of the condition (may include presence or lack of objective data and subjective complaints).
     —Complications and risk factors that affect your decision to proceed to care planning.
     —Factors that must be considered in developing individualized care plan interventions.
     —Need for referrals/further evaluation by appropriate health professionals.
   - Documentation should support your decision-making regarding whether to proceed with a care plan for a triggered RAP and the type(s) of care plan interventions that are appropriate for a particular resident.
   - Documentation may appear anywhere in the clinical record (e.g., progress notes, consults, flowsheets).
3. Indicate under the *Location of RAP Assessment Documentation* column where information related to the RAP assessment can be found.
4. For each triggered RAP, indicate whether a new care plan, care plan revision, or continuation of current care plan is necessary to address the problem(s) identified in your assessment. The Care Planning Decision column must be completed within 7 days of completing the RAI (MDS and RAPs).

A. RAP Problem Area	**(a) Check if Triggered**	**Location and Date of RAP Assessment Documentation**	**(b) Care Planning Decision—check if addressed in care plan**
1. DELIRIUM	☐		☐
2. COGNITIVE LOSS	☐		☐
3. VISUAL FUNCTION	☐		☐
4. COMMUNICATION	☐		☐
5. ADL FUNCTIONAL/ REHABILITATION POTENTIAL	☐		☐
6. URINARY INCONTINENCE AND INDWELLING CATHETER	☐		☐
7. PSYCHOSOCIAL WELL-BEING	☐		☐
8. MOOD STATE	☐		☐
9. BEHAVIORAL SYMPTOMS	☐		☐
10. ACTIVITIES	☐		☐
11. FALLS	☐		☐
12. NUTRITIONAL STATUS	☐		☐
13. FEEDING TUBES	☐		☐
14. DEHYDRATION/FLUID MAINTENANCE	☐		☐
15. ORAL/DENTAL CARE	☐		☐
16. PRESSURE ULCERS	☐		☐
17. PSYCHOTROPHIC DRUG USE	☐		☐
18. PHYSICAL RESTRAINTS	☐		☐

B. ______________________________ 2. ☐☐–☐☐–☐☐☐☐ (Month Day Year)

1. Signature of RN Coordinator for RAP Assessment Process

______________________________ 4. ☐☐–☐☐–☐☐☐☐ (Month Day Year)

3. Signature of Person Completing Care Planning Decision

TRIGGER LEGEND

1 —Delirium
2 —Cognitive Loss/Dementia
3 —Visual Function
4 —Communication
5A —ADL-Rehabilitation
5B —ADL-Maintenance
6 —Urinary Incontinence and Indwelling Catheter
7 —Psychosocial Well-Being
8 —Mood State
9 —Behavioral Symptoms
10A —Activities (Revise)
10B —Activities (Review)
11 —Falls
12 —Nutritional Status
13 —Feeding Tubes
14 —Dehydration/Fluid Maintenance
15 —Dental Care
16 —Pressure Ulcers
17 —Psychotropic Drug Use
18 —Physical Restraints

Modified from *Minimum Data Set (MDS)—Version 2.0 for Nursing Home Resident Assessment and Care Screening,* Form 1728HH, Des Moines, IA, 1995, Briggs Corporation.

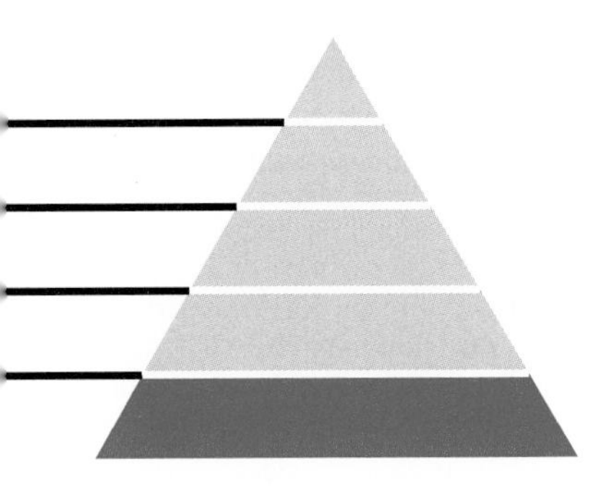

CHAPTER 9

Pain and Comfort

Patricia Hess

Not only degrees of pain, but its existence, in any degree, must be taken upon the testimony of the patient.

Peter Mere Latham (1789-1875), Diseases of the Heart, Lecture XI

LEARNING OBJECTIVES

On completion of this chapter, the reader will be able to:

1. Define the concept of pain.
2. Identify factors that affect the elder's pain experience.
3. Differentiate between acute and chronic pain.
4. Describe data to include in a pain assessment.
5. Identify barriers that interfere with pain assessment and treatment.
6. Discuss comfort measures.
7. Discuss pharmacologic and nonpharmacologic pain management therapies.
8. Discuss the goals of pain management for the elderly.

Comfort seems to be an intrinsic balance of the physiologic, emotional, social, and spiritual essence of the individual and can be perceived as an integral component of wellness. By definition, *comfort* is "a state of ease and satisfaction of the bodily wants and freedom from pain and anxiety." The absence of physical pain is not always sufficient to provide comfort. The aged may have their biologic or bodily needs satisfied but be emotionally distressed. Conversely, physical needs may be the priority and no comfort is possible until need fulfillment is accomplished.

Nurses use the word *comfort* to describe goals and outcomes to nursing measures, but the meaning remains vague and essentially abstract to the person who is the recipient of the nursing intervention. Hamilton (1989) studied the meaning and attributes of comfort from the point of view of the chronically ill elderly hospitalized in a geriatric setting. The questions explored were the elderly's definition of comfort, contributors to and distractors from comfort, and how to increase elders' comfort. The findings identified several themes: disease process (pain, bowel function, and disability); self-esteem (feelings, adjustment, independence, usefulness, faith in God); positioning (if elders could carry out activities in bed, chair, or wheelchair); approach and attitude of staff (relationships, encounters); and hospital life (surroundings and environment—feeling at home, well fed, pleasant surroundings). Table 9-1 summarizes each of these themes and includes contributors to and distractors from comfort and elders' suggestions for facilitating more comfort.

The International Association for the Study of Pain (IASP) and the American Pain Society define *pain* as "an unpleasant sensory and emotional experience associated with actual or potential tissue damage, or described in terms of such damage" (IASP, 1979; The American Pain Society, 1999).

Hamilton (1989) describes comfort as multidimensional "and meaning many things to different people." This description parallels McCaffery's definition of pain, which states: "Pain is whatever the person experiencing pain says it is" (McCaffery and Pasero, 1999). From these interpretations of pain and comfort the question can be raised as to whether there is a way to identify comfort-discomfort zones outside acute or chronic pain in a manner similar to the pain assessment measures presently used. This remains a fruitful area for research.

In this chapter physical pain is the primary focus. Subsequent chapters of the text address psychologic pain (see Chapters 22, 23, and 24).

Table 9-1 Summary of Comfort Findings

Comfort themes	Contributors to comfort	Distractors to comfort	Adds to comfort
Disease process	Achieving relief from pain; regular bowel function	Physical disabilities; being in pain most of time	Better pain management
Self-esteem	Faith in God; being independent; feeling relaxed; feeling useful	Adjust to change; being afraid	Being informed; taking part in decision making
Positioning	Individually adjusted seating; sitting correctly; independent movement in chair	Unsuitable wheelchairs; sitting too long; sliding down in chair; being in unfavorable position in bed	Return to bed when requested; better seating arrangements
Staff approach and attitudes	Friendly, kind people; empathetic nurses; reliable nurses	Lack of caring and understanding; inaccessible nurses	Caring and understanding; encouraging patients to help themselves
Hospital life	Homelike surroundings; social and family contacts; informal pastimes; occupational and physical therapy	Fragmented care; tolerate the system; boredom with activities; lack of privacy Unpleasant meal atmosphere	Staff continuity New content in activities; continuation of personal pastimes; improved patient mealtimes; some privacy

Modified from Hamilton J: Comfort and the hospitalized chronically ill, *J Gerontol Nurs* 15(4):28, 1989.

Pain, whatever its sources, is one of the most common complaints of the elderly. It erodes personality, saps energy, and manifests itself in an ever-intensifying cycle of pain, anxiety, and anguish until the cycle is broken. Pain can evoke depression, sleep disorders, decreased socialization, impaired mobility, and increased health care costs (Thernstrom, 2001; Morley, 2001; Fine, 2002; Jeffery and Lubkin, 2002). The nurse has a definition or an interpretation of pain, as does the patient to whom the nurse ministers. These interpretations are formulated from experiences and are influenced by the unique history of the individual and the meaning ascribed to the pain. It is also important to realize that an individual responds in a certain way to pain because he or she has been taught that this is correct and normal. Likewise, nurses and other caregivers respond based on their own pain experiences. In addition, repeated exposure to the pain of others desensitizes and may make it seem commonplace (Box 9-1).

Meinhart and McCaffery (1983) cite two factors that influence nurses' and other caregivers' responses to a client's pain and discomfort: (1) one's ability to sympathize with another

Box 9-1 **Misconceptions about the Pain Experience**

Misconceptions Held by Elders

Pain is expected with aging
Nothing can be done about it
Pain is punishment for past actions
Asking for medication is too demanding or a personal sign of weakness
Pain medication has bad side effects or causes addiction
Pain means loss of independence
Pain is not harmful
Complaining of pain means the prospect of many tests and serious illness
Medications are too expensive
Chronic pain means death is near
Pain is expected in the hospital

Misconceptions Held by Nurses

Elders have decreased sensation to pain
Elders who are cognitively impaired do not feel pain
A sleeping patient is not in pain
Elders complain more about pain as they age
The elder who asks for pain medication has a low pain tolerance
Elders cannot tolerate pain medications or manage PCA
Narcotics will hasten death
Potent analgesics are addictive
Obvious pathology, test results, and surgery determine the existence or intensity of pain
The elder is not an expert about pain; health professionals are
Patients in long-term care say they are in pain in order to get attention
Elders should expect to have pain in the hospital

Modified from Watt-Watson JH, Donovan MI: *Pain management: nursing perspective*, St Louis 1992, Mosby; Victor K: Properly assessing the elderly, *RN* 64(5):45, 2001; American Medical Directors Association: *Chronic pain management in long-term care settings, clinical practice guidelines*, 1999, AMDA; Fine P: Elder care summit, San Francisco, 2002.

Box 9-2 General and Cultural Factors Influencing Client's Response to Pain

General	Cultural
Pain experience Culture Gender Significance of pain Depression Fatigue Physiologic age changes Altered pain stimulus transmission Decrease in inflammation response	Minimize pain with significant others or use pain to elicit sympathy and support from others Carefully controls the expression of pain (calm or emotional) or is vocal about pain (cries, moans, complains) Withdraws and wants to be alone when pain is severe or seeks attention and presence of others Willingly accepts pain-relief measures or avoids pain-relief measures in the belief that they indicate weakness Wants and expects quick pain relief or accepts pain for long periods before requesting help

Modified from Eland JM: Pain management and comfort, *J Gerontol Nurs* 14(4):10, 1988; Bates MS: *Biocultural dimensions of chronic pain*, 1996, State University of New York Press; Koiser B et al: *Fundamentals of nursing*, Redwood City, CA, 1995, Addison-Wesley; Salerno E, Willens JS: *Pain management handbook*, St Louis, 1996, Mosby.

person, which depends on one's ability to identify imaginatively with the person, and (2) whether one is responsive to hurt in individuals that one does not know. Ethnically diverse responses are based on years of social modeling, group influence on pain tolerance, and the observation of the family when in pain (Bates, 1996; Jeffery and Lubkin, 2002). Thus social learning is extremely influential in the perception of the meaning of and attitudes toward pain, something older adults have had many years to internalize. In American culture a dichotomy exists for some: The practice of self-inflicted pain (in a sense) is seen in professional and amateur sports activities. This infliction of pain is expected in young adults and is a rite of passage, so to speak. Equally significant is that until experiencing body discomfort such as aches and pains, an older person does not perceive himself or herself as old. However, when these manifestations do occur, they become a rite of passage into perceived old age (Box 9-2).

ACUTE AND CHRONIC PAIN

Acute pain is temporary and includes postoperative, procedural, and traumatic pain. It is easily controlled by analgesic preparations. Almost everyone has experienced this type of pain and knows that it is a temporary, time-limited situation with attainable relief. Chronic pain is not that simple. It has no time frame; it is continually persistent at varying levels of intensity, and it manipulates the individual and can manipulate the person attempting to give care (Portenoy, 1995; Salerno and Willens, 1996; Lipman and Jackson, 2000). Table 9-2 compares the many facets of acute and chronic pain. Meinhart and McCaffery (1983) and Lipman and Jackson (2000) note that chronic pain can manifest itself as depression, eating disturbances, or sleep disturbances. Pain is categorized as acute pain, chronic pain of nonmalignant origin, and chronic pain of malignant origin. Intractable nonmalignant pain is the most common pain in elders and erodes an individual's coping ability.

Chronic pain may described as follows (Ferrell, 2000):

1. *Nociceptive pain* such as trauma, burns, infection, inflammation, ischemia, pain from mechanical causes (deformity, pressure, distention), arthropathies (rheumatoid arthritis and osteoarthritis, gout) myalgia, nonarticular inflammatory disorders, and internal organ and visceral pain.
2. *Neuropathic pain* such as *peripheral nervous system* pain (postherpetic neuralgia, trigeminal neuralgia, diabetic polyneuropathy, postamputation, phantom limb). Pain is often described as searing, burning, tingling, pins and needles, electric shock, or shooting pain. This may last for 6 to 12 months, but 25% or more elders experience this type of pain for longer periods of time. *Central nervous system* pain such as poststroke (central pain or thalamic pain), myelopathic, or radiculopathic (spinal stenosis, multiple sclerosis, root sleeve fibrosis). *Sympathetic nervous system* pain such as complex regional pain (causalgia-like syndrome).
3. *Mixed* or *unspecified pain* such as chronic recurrent headaches (tension, migraine) or vasculopathic pain syndrome (vasculitis).
4. *Psychologically mediated pain* such as somatization disorders (hysterical reactions).

Neuropathic pain of peripheral vascular occlusion in people with advanced diabetes often produces a constant burning pain, similar to the pain of frostbite, to the extremities. The aged person who suffers a paralyzing or weakness-inducing stroke with loss of complete sensation on the affected side often experiences deep, boring, crushing sensations, or burning and cold sensations in the face, neck, trunk, leg, or generally over the entire affected side. Movement of the affected side and other sensations such as touch, sound, bright light, and air increase this kind of pain. Feeling in the affected extremity may be perceived as similar to a person being squeezed or twisted. Often the extremity is held in a strange position by the patient.

PAIN IN THE AGED

The prevalence of pain in the elderly who live in the community is known to be twice that of the young and is considered to be extremely high in the long-term care setting. Ferrell (1991), Fine (2002), and Herr (2002) suggest that the incidence of pain in the community is 25% to 50% and as much as 85% in long-term care because of the presence of multiple

Table 9-2 Comparison of Acute and Chronic Pain

	Acute pain	Chronic pain (nonmalignant origin)	Chronic pain (malignant origin)
Source	An event External agent or internal disease	A situation, state of existence Unknown or if known, changes cannot occur or treatment is prolonged or ineffective	Usually associated with terminal disease
Onset	Usually sudden	May be sudden or insidious	Unpredictable
Duration	Hours, days, usually transient, lasting no more than 3-6 mo	Prolonged for months or years	Prolonged, often for the course of the disease or in its later stages
Pain identification	Pain vs. lack of pain Areas generally well defined	Pain vs. lack of pain Areas are less well defined Intensity becomes more difficult to evaluate (change in sensation): intensity varies, may be constant or intermittent	Areas(s) may be well defined or diffuse; pain may be more constant than intermittent
Associated pathology	Present	Often unknown	Usually present
Associated problems	Uncommon	Depression, anxiety, secondary pain issues	Many of the same as chronic nonmalignant pain
Behavior	Typical response patterns with more visible signs: Facial expressions Crying, guarding Guarding, moaning Clenching teeth Biting lower lip Tightly shut eyes Open, somber eyes Involuntary movements Immobility of body part Purposeless body movement Rhythmic body movements, rocking, rubbing Change in speech and vocal pitch (anxiety) Slow monotone (severe pain) Fetal position	Response patterns vary, few overt signs (adaptation): Sleeping Sleep disturbances Confusion Rubbing Stoicism Depression Inactivity Combativeness Inactivity Immobilizing body part or assuming an awkward body position	Response pattern similar to chronic nonmalignant pain: Sleep disturbance Withdrawal Depression Inactivity Slow moving Anger Anxiety Fearful Short tempered or passive
Nerve conduction	Rapid	Slow	Slow
Autonomic system involvement (clinical signs)	Present Elevation of blood pressure Tachycardia Diaphoresis	Generally absent No change in vital signs	May be present or absent
Meaning pattern	Meaningful: informs person something is wrong; self-limiting or readily corrected	Meaningless: person looks for meaning	May have meaning or be meaningless
Treatment	Primary—analgesic drugs	Multimodal: primary behavioral and physical therapy; drugs may be primarily adjunctive	Multimodal: analgesics usually play a major role

Compiled and modified from Karb V: Pain. In Phipps W, Long B, Woods N, editors: *Medical-surgical nursing: concepts and clinical practice*, ed 4, St Louis, 1991, Mosby; Forrest J: Assessment of acute and chronic pain in older adults, *J Gerontol Nurs* 21 : 10, 1995; Lipman AG, Jackson KC: *Use of opioids in chronic noncancer pain*, Stamford, CT, 2000, Power-Pak Communications, Inc., Purdue Pharma LP.

chronic conditions that cause chronic pain such as peripheral vascular disease, diabetic neuropathies, musculoskeletal disorders, trigeminal neuralgia, herpes zoster, and cancer. Osteoarthritis may cause pain in nearly 80% of those over age 65 (Schnitzer, 1998).

In the aged, fear and anxiety generate negative effects that emanate from thoughts that pain will result in crippling, forced dependency or that it will be of such intensity that the ability to cope will be inadequate. Pain weakens and interrupts the individual's relations to self, to others, to the environment, and in time and space.

The aged are at high risk for pain-inducing situations. They have lived longer and have a greater chance of developing degenerative and pathologic conditions through disease or accumulated injury. Several conditions may be present simultaneously, so a single pain-producing condition is overlooked in the complexity of health management. Increased susceptibility to accidents because of medications, cognitive function, or illness affects functional abilities, which contributes to falls. The resultant hip fractures, sprains, and hematomas require a longer time to heal and prolong the pain experience. Loneliness through loss of a spouse, a job, independence, and friends and the presence of boredom and depression decrease the ability to cope with pain. Psychosocial aspects of an elder's life are rarely self-reported because of the associated stigma or stoicism. Chronic pain often results in dramatic lifestyle changes such as altered family relationships and the inability to visit friends. In a study by Ferrell and Ferrell (1990) of 65 elderly patients, 54% experienced impairment of enjoyable activities; 53% experienced impaired ambulation; 49% experienced impaired posture; and 45% and 32% experienced sleep disorders and depression, respectively. In this sample it was apparent that lowered pain tolerance existed.

Clinical speculations that pain perception decreases with age remain unclear. Portenoy (1995) reported pain sensitivity reduction at organ and tissue sites except the joints. Literature has revealed instances of serious abdominal and cardiac conditions that should elicit severe pain but have produced little or no pain in the aged. It is common for acuity of symptoms or severity of pain to be less dramatic than in younger persons (Witt, 1989). Ferrell and co-workers (1991) and Harkins (1996) indicate that there is no consensus on decreased pain sensation among elders. Hoffman and co-workers (1998; cited in Herr, 2002) indicate that insensitivity to pain is basically clinically insignificant. Sensitivity to pain remains subject to individual responses.

Questions continue to arise about how to discern pain in the cognitively impaired and nonverbal elderly. Meinhart and McCaffery (1983) cite behavioral changes or manifestations such as confusion and restlessness as possible indicators of painful stimuli in the aged. The elderly often suffer in silence or attempt to relieve pain with inadequate measures because of the high cost of medical care, consultation, equipment, diagnostic tests, hospitalization, and medications. In addition, the elderly often underreport pain because they consider it a normal part of the aging process. The perceptions of pain by others, including caregivers, influence the elder's pain (Hofland, 1992; Sarvis, 1995; Jeffery and Lubkin, 2002). Nurses must be extremely observant of subtle cues such as guarding a part of the body, wincing, or favoring certain movements rather than projecting their own pain experience on others. Box 9-3 separates fact from fiction.

Pain management and interventions often differ from those of other age-groups because of changes in cognitive function (Fulmer et al, 1996; Jeffery and Lubkin, 2002). In addition, medications are affected by the increase or decrease of absorption time, depending on what other medications are being taken and the individual illness. The ability of elders to swallow pills easily may be impaired because of a dry mouth or ill-fitting dentures. Injectable medication may also be unreliable because of the inadequacy of the elder's circulation. (Refer to Chapter 10 for pharmacokinetics and pharmacodynamics of medications.) A viable alternative to provide pain relief might be rectal or topical administration of pain medication. New forms of medication administration have been and are being developed, among them medication in lollipop form (oral transmucosal) and transdermal patches (Managing pain, 1996). The Agency for Health Care Policy and Research (AHCPR) guidelines (*Acute Pain Management,* 1992; *Management of Cancer Pain,* 1994) were outstanding contributions to pain intervention, but they do not provide specific directions for caregivers of elders who need pain relief.

Box 9-3 Fact and Fiction about Pain in the Elderly

MYTH: Pain is expected with aging.
FACT: Pain is not normal with aging. The presence of pain in the elderly necessitates aggressive assessment, diagnosis, and management similar to that of younger patients.
MYTH: Pain sensitivity and perception decrease with aging.
FACT: This assumption is dangerous! Data are conflicting regarding age-associated changes in pain perception, sensitivity, and tolerance. Consequences of this assumption are needless suffering and undertreatment of both pain and underlying cause.
MYTH: If a patient doesn't complain of pain, there must not be much pain.
FACT: This is erroneous in all ages but particularly in the elderly. Older patients may not report pain for a variety of reasons. They may fear the meaning of pain, diagnostic workups, or pain treatments. They may think pain is normal.
MYTH: A person who has no functional impairment, appears occupied, or is otherwise distracted from pain must not have significant pain.
FACT: Patients have a variety of reactions to pain. Many patients are stoic and refuse to "give in" to their pain. Over extended periods of time, the elderly may mask any outward signs of pain.
MYTH: Narcotic medications are inappropriate for patients with chronic nonmalignant pain.
FACT: Opioid analgesics are often indicated in nonmalignant pain.
MYTH: Potential side effects of narcotic medication make them too dangerous to use in the elderly.
FACT: Narcotics may be used safely in the elderly. Although elderly patients may be more sensitive to narcotics, this does not justify withholding narcotics and failing to relieve pain.

From Ferrell BR, Ferrell BA: Pain in the elderly. In Watt-Watson JH, Donovan MI, editors: *Pain management: nursing perspective,* St Louis, 1992, Mosby.

PAIN CONTROL

Pain control for elders is challenging. Several pain theories have been used to explain pain phenomena and interventions for pain control (Box 9-4).

The *specificity theory* provided the first explanations as to why an individual experiences pain. In essence, this theory proposed that single specialized peripheral nerve fibers were responsible for pain transmission. The discovery of delta-A and C fibers lent credence to this theory (Duff, 1988; Salerno and Willens, 1996).

The *pattern theory* followed later and suggested that excessive stimulation of all nerve endings produces a pattern interpreted as pain by the brain cortex. This implied that there were no specific nociceptive receptors for pain because temperature and pressure elicited similar responses. Pain was thought to come from a combination of intense stimuli and central stimulation of the dorsal horn. A pattern of pain left a memory such as is seen with phantom limb pain. The pain, experienced before amputation of the limb, leaves a memory tracing that is recalled after amputation.

The *gate theory,* introduced by Melzack and Wall (1965) and among the most readily accepted, integrated the specific and pattern theories and proposed that an anatomic gate modulates the pain experience. It was thought that peripheral nerve fibers carrying pain impulses to the spinal cord can have their input modified at the spinal cord before the impulses are transmitted to the brain. Stated another way, the gate theory suggests that pain impulses traveling up the spinal cord can be blocked before they reach the brain by a mechanism that acts like a gate closing. Melzack and Wall's theory helps explain why such interventions as rubbing the skin, acupressure, or acupuncture relieve certain types of pain. The theory also suggests that complex physiologic, psychologic, and cognitive processes, such as anxiety, past experiences, and the meaning of pain, are heavily influenced by sociocultural learning. These experiences affect human pain perception and response, which can influence the opening and closing of the gates (Bates, 1996). The gate control theory is most relevant to pain management of the elderly.

Box 9-4 Four Stages of Pain Phenomenon

Activation or nociception*—The stimulation of nerve endings
Pain—The mind's perception of nerve impulses
Suffering—One's emotional reaction to pain, such as alarm, anxiety, frustration, or depression; varies from person to person based on self-esteem, memory of past pain, family, social and cultural factors
Pain behavior and psychologic changes—Decreased self-worth: invalid, sick role

Modified from Chronic pain: medical essay. *Mayo Clinic Health Letter*, June 1996.
*The process of pain transmission; usually related to a receptive neuron for painful sensations.

Pharmacologic Pain Control

Generally pain relief is accomplished by medication aimed at altering sensory transmission to the cerebral cortex. Various analgesics (nonnarcotic and narcotic agents) are available for use. Nonnarcotic preparations are effective for mild to moderate pain, whereas narcotics should be reserved primarily for moderate to severe pain. General principles of pain control for the aged are the same as those for the young, but dosage adjustment is often required.

Meperidine (Demerol) should *not* be used with the elderly because of altered metabolism and excretion in the elderly. Reduced metabolism and excretion of Demerol metabolites can produce confusion, psychotic behavior, and seizure activity. The same can be said for pentazocine (Talwin) and methadone. Various morphines and codeines are considered safer drugs for use with the elderly (Watt-Watson and Donovan, 1992; Portenoy, 1995; Fine, 2002). It is important to be aware of equianalgesic doses so that oral pain and parenteral pain medication doses possess pain relief power equivalent to another narcotic drug (Box 9-5).

The patient's misbeliefs about pain and its control may include the following (Watt-Watson and Donovan, 1992):
- "Pain is to be expected with treatment and diagnoses such as cancer."
- "I have no control over my pain."
- "Surgery or a pill will fix me up."
- "I should not ask for anything for pain unless I'm desperate."

In addition, Davies (1996) and Sarvis (1995) point out that health care professionals may not ask the elder about his or her pain for the following reasons:
- The health care professional may assume that the individual will spontaneously report pain.
- The elder does not want to bother the physician with pain complaints, considering all the other medical problems he or she may have.
- Many older adults consider pain an expected part of aging.
- Clinicians are hesitant to prescribe analgesics for the elderly because of concern for troubling side effects with polypharmacy.
- Gray (1996) notes that under managed care, the ability to provide appropriate pain relief is limited by removal of more effective but more costly analgesics from hospitals' formularies.
- Use of opioids causes too many problems, such as addiction and associated stigma. Other medications that the physician may prescribe for the elderly may be as effective but less problematic.

When acute pain is severe, as in postoperative recovery, it is prudent to combine a nonnarcotic and a narcotic preparation to achieve maximum pain relief. This combination

Box 9-5

Guidelines to Use of an Equianalgesic Chart

An eqianalgesic chart is helpful when (1) switching from one drug to another or (2) switching from one route of administration to another.

Equianalgesic means approximately the same pain relief.

Individual responses must be observed. Dose and interval between doses are then titrated according to the individual's response.

Based on clinical experience, the intravenous (IV) dose is approximately the same as an intramuscular (IM) dose. Dose adjustments are then made to the individual's response. Some clinicians suggest approximately half the IM dose equals the IV dose.

Equianalgesic Chart Approximate Equivalents to 10 mg Morphine for Analgesic Effect

	Route		
Analgesic	*IM*	*Oral (PO)*	*Comments*
Morphine-like agonist			
Morphine sulfate	10 mg	60 mg (30)	
Dilaudid	1.5 mg	7.5 mg	
Oxycodone	—	30 mg	
Methadone	10 mg	20 mg	
Levorphanol	2.0 mg	4.0 mg	
Fentanyl	0.1 mg	—	Transdermal patch equivalent to 30 mg sustained-release morphine 8 hr
Oxymorphone	1.0 mg	—	
Meperidine	75 mg	300 mg	Not recommended
Mixed agonist/antagonist			
Nalbuphine	10 mg	—	
Butorphanol (Stadol)	2.0 mg	—	
Dezocine	10 mg	—	
Partial agonist			
Buprenorphine	0.4 mg	—	

affects pain response at both the peripheral nerve and central nervous system levels.

When a person is allowed nothing by mouth (NPO; from the Latin, *nil per os*), a nonnarcotic analgesic can be given by suppository along with the injectable narcotic or transdermal patch. An essential point to remember is that the dose of the nonnarcotic analgesic must be sufficiently strong to work synergistically with the narcotic preparation. In addition, medication should be given when discomfort begins, not at the height of pain intensity. Around-the-clock (ATC) medicating schedule has been in the literature since about 1989. It has not been implemented in many instances. This is unfortunate because it is a viable way to provide a more stable therapeutic plasma level of drug and eliminate the extremes of overmedication and undermedication. With this approach to pain control, breakthrough pain allows for an as needed (prn; from the Latin, *pro re nata*) dose of medication (McCaffery and Ritchey, 1992; Sarvis, 1995; Fine, 2002; Herr, 2002). Narcotic use for long-term chronic pain control in the elderly should be convenient, easy to administer, and short acting for ease of dose adjustment; there is less drug accumulation in the body and low incidence of side effects. It is also important that an ATC schedule be considered for older adults with chronic pain, because it will allow for continued involvement in functional activities. Frequently this can be attained with sustained-action pain medications. Box 9-6 lists preferred narcotics and those to be avoided for use with the elderly.

Mild and moderate pain relief may be achieved with nonnarcotic analgesics such as nonsteroidal antiinflammatory drugs (NSAIDs) or acetaminophen. NSAIDs bind with proteins and may induce toxic responses in elders if serum albumin levels are low. In addition, other drugs that elders routinely take compete for the same protein receptor sites and may be displaced by the NSAID, creating unstable therapeutic effects. Drugs that cause central nervous system (CNS) effects should be used with caution in elders sensitive to CNS effects. Box 9-6 identifies preferred NSAID drugs and those to be avoided for use with elders. The following are guidelines for the selection and use of NSAIDs:

- Weigh risks versus benefits in selection.
- Start with a low dose to determine the patient's reaction (e.g., side effects). Increase gradually to a dose that relieves pain, not to exceed the maximum daily dose. The dose may need to be increased one to two times the starting dose.
- If maximum antiinflammatory effect is desired in addition to analgesia, allow adequate trial before discontinuing or switching. With regular doses for 1 week or longer, pain relief may increase.

Box 9-6 Elder Pain Relief Drugs to Use and Avoid

Type of Drug	Preferred	Avoid
Opioids	Tylenol with codeine	Pentazocine
	Oxycodone	Meperidine
	Dilaudid	Methadone
NSAID	Ibuprofen	Indomethocin
	Acetaminophen	Aspirin
	Salsalate	Feldene
	Dolobid	Phenylbutazone
Adjuvant	Trazodone	Amitriptylene
	Prozac	Phenothiazines
	Desipramine	

- If one drug becomes ineffective, but the pain is about the same, try a drug from a different chemical class.
- If the NSAID does not relieve pain when used alone, combine with oral (preferred route), intramuscular, intravenous, or transdermal narcotics for added analgesic effect (McCaffery and Pasero, 1999).

Sharp, shooting, dull, aching, or burning pain that is not responsive to NSAIDs or narcotics alone may respond to adjuvant drug therapy. Some adjuvant drugs help control symptoms and signs associated with pain. Adjuvant drugs are not analgesics; in combination with analgesics they may potentiate or enhance overall analgesic effects. Elders frequently respond well to adjuvant pain regimens. This is especially useful in treatment of chronic pain. However, it is important to remember that many adjuvant drugs have a very long half-life, which increase the plasma concentration in elders. This can lead to adverse or toxic effects. Box 9-6 lists preferred adjuvant drugs and those to be avoided for use in elders. Some guidelines for the administration of adjuvant drugs to the elderly include the following:

- Avoid drugs with potent anticholinergic effects. These may result in urinary retention and subsequent urinary tract infection; constipation; blurred vision, which increases the chance for injury; dry mouth, affecting the ability to eat; and confusion.
- Neuroleptics, if used, should have the least sedating, cardiotoxic, and hypotensive effects.
- Avoid drugs that precipitate or potentiate extrapyramidal symptoms.
- Tranquilizers that produce sedation and have a long half-life should be avoided. Drugs with a short half-life are more suitable.
- Drugs that can cause orthostatic hypotension should be used with caution, especially when there is a preexisting cardiac condition.
- Interactions with other drugs must be monitored carefully because elders take many medications for coexisting conditions (polypharmacy).

A summary of pharmacologic principles in pain management of the elderly appears in Box 9-7.

Nonpharmacologic Pain Control

Nursing staff are often afraid of inducing iatrogenic addiction and thus undermedicate elders. Indeck (1977) considers pain control in the aged to be more effective through the use of various alternative means that include physical methods, such as cutaneous stimulation, and central methods, in which the individual learns to live with his or her pain (e.g., biofeedback, behavior modification, hypnosis, meditation, or variations of these modalities) (Lubkin and Jeffery, 2002) (Box 9-8). It has now been shown that a combination of pharmacologic and nonpharmacologic interventions appears to be most effective in the relief of acute or chronic pain.

Cutaneous Nerve Stimulation. Deep and superficial stimulation of the skin by direct, proximal, or distal application for the purpose of pain relief has been practiced for centuries. Massage, vibration, heat, cold, and ointments have been a part of nursing interventions for years. Heat is effective for musculoskeletal disorders such as rheumatic conditions. It is contraindicated with occlusive vascular disease and in the

Box 9-7 Principles of Pharmacologic Pain Management in Elderly Patients

1. Follow AHCPR guidelines (see Box 9-14).
2. Use a combination of pharmacologic and nonpharmacologic pain management strategies (see Box 9-8 and Figure 9-3).
3. Give adequate amounts of drug at the appropriate frequency to control pain based on constant assessment.
4. Use around-the-clock dosing; avoid prn drug administration and provide for breakthrough pain events; do not wait for a crisis.
5. With all narcotic analgesics, especially with the elderly, start low and increase dose slowly (titrate). This does not mean giving the least amount of the drug that has been prescribed because of fear the elder might not tolerate prescribed dose.
6. Anticipate and prevent side effects common in elders:
   a. Give antiinflammatory drugs with food.
   b. Begin a bowel regimen early to prevent constipation when beginning opioid therapy, not after constipation has occurred.
   c. Be prepared to give an antiemetic medication with narcotic analgesic drugs.
   d. Anticipate some impaired balance and cognitive function with narcotic analgesic drugs.
7. Consult an equianalgesic potency table when changing medications (see Box 9-5).

Modified from Glickstein JK, editor: Managing chronic pain, *Focus Geriatr Care Rehabil* 10(3):6, 1996; McCaffery M, Pasero C: *Pain: clinical manual*, St Louis, 2000, Mosby; Fine P: Elder care summit, San Francisco, 2002.

Box 9-8 Nonpharmacologic Pain Management Strategies

- Distraction
  - Movies
  - Laughter
  - Art therapy
  - Music therapy
- Behavior modification
  - Imagery/meditation
  - Relaxation techniques
  - Biofeedback
  - Hypnosis
- Physical therapy
  - Massage
  - Ultrasound
  - Hot/cold therapies
  - Exercise
- Neurostimulation
  - Transcutaneous electrical nerve stimulation (TENS)
  - Dorsal nerve stimulation (DNS)
  - Acupuncture/acupressure

Modified from Kozier B et al: *Fundamentals of nursing*, Redwood City, CA, 1995, Addison-Wesley; Jeffery JE, Lubkin IM: In Lubkin IM, Larsen PD: *Chronic illness*, ed 5, Boston, 2002, Jones & Bartlett; Perry G: Elder care summit, San Francisco, April 24, 2000.

presence of cancer. In nonexpansive tissue such as bursae, heat may even increase pain. Intermittent cold packs are helpful in low back pain and radicular disturbances. They serve to negate or delay the transmission of pain impulses to the cerebral pain center. Pathophysiologic conditions should be taken into consideration when using heat and cold with the elderly. Care must be taken when applying heat and cold to the skin of the aged to prevent skin damage from extended periods of heat and cold applications.

Transcutaneous Electrical Nerve Stimulation. Another method of cutaneous stimulation is transcutaneous electrical nerve stimulation (TENS), or dorsal column nerve stimulation. Electrodes, taped to the skin over the pain site or on the spine, emit a mild electric current that is felt as a tingling, buzzing, or vibrating sensation. The patient operates the stimulator and starts the electric impulses, which then activate the large nerve fibers that transmit impulses to close the hypothetic gate in the spinal cord and prevent pain signals from reaching the brain. TENS has been helpful in phantom limb pain, postherpetic neuralgia, and low back pain.

Touch. Touch is a natural comfort modality, although its therapeutic properties are still not clearly understood. Sometimes considered a cutaneous stimulation technique, "therapeutic touch" used in experimental laboratory and clinical settings showed that placing hands on or near the body might result in healing or improvement (Kreiger, 1992). Relaxation and proper sensory stimulation decrease anxiety, reduce muscle tension, and help relieve pain. Petrie (1975) found that perceptual tendencies and sensory dimensions influence pain reactions and tolerance. Persons who were sensory deprived exhibited low pain tolerance, but those who received adequate or a high degree of sensory stimulation possessed a high pain tolerance. Laying on of hands employed by Kreiger (1975) and the Touch for Health Movement proved to be beneficial, but the reasons behind its effectiveness have not been fully established.

Fakouri and Jones (1987) demonstrated the positive effects of a 3-minute, slow-stroke back rub on both sides of the spinous processes from the crown of the head to the sacrum as a means of promoting relaxation in the aged. Physiologic effects that occurred were a decrease in heart rate and blood pressure and an increase in skin temperature. Meek (1993) found that slow-stroking back massage increased relaxation as evidenced by decreases in blood pressure and heart rate and an increase in body temperature of hospice patients. No mention was made of its effect on pain. However, it is known that tension and anxiety reduction can contribute to an increase in pain tolerance. Mackey (1995) describes the use of therapeutic touch for pain relief and admits that it was not successful as the sole therapy for pain relief. Peck (1997) and Lin and Taylor (1998) indicate that therapeutic touch is a complementary/alternative therapy with growing scientific evidence that it can reduce chronic or acute pain. It is suggested that it is valuable as an adjunct to pharmacologic therapy.

The Touch Research Institute at the University of Miami has been engaged in numerous projects to determine the effects of massage. Massage is a powerful modality of therapeutic touch. It can induce muscle relaxation, increase circulation, decrease swelling, soften and stretch scar tissue, reduce adhesions, and relieve pain (Kastner, 1994). Pain reduction through touch therapy continues to be an area for additional research.

Acupuncture and Acupressure. Acupuncture and acupressure are complementary/alternative therapies with growing scientific evidence that they are effective for chronic pain (National Institutes of Health, 1990; Berman and Swyer, 1999; Lee, 2000). Acupuncture is an alternative to electric stimulation. Small nerve fibers are stimulated by the twirling of the needles. Acute pain is registered as pain impulses pass through the gate of the spine. The acute pain registers in the brain and signals the central mechanism of the brain to return counter-impulses, which close the gate. Acupuncture points are located near clusters of nerve cell endings. It is thought that acupuncture stimulates these nerves and causes the gate to close or that it triggers the release of the body's own opiate substances, enkephalins (endorphins).

Acupressure is acupuncture without needles. Pressure applied to the traditional acupuncture points with the thumbs, tip of the index finger, or palm of the hand or pinching and squeezing as means of applying pressure stimulate the nerves and close the gate or trigger the release of the body's natural endorphins.

Biofeedback. Biofeedback is a cognitive behavioral strategy. An individual can learn voluntary control over some body processes and alter them by changing the physiologic correlates appropriate to them. Response to certain types of pain can be controlled. Boczkowski (1984) found that biofeedback decreased chronic pain of rheumatoid arthritis. Other studies demonstrated no appreciable effect of biofeedback on migraine headaches in the elderly (Hamm and King, 1984). Training and often time and equipment of some type are needed to learn how to alter one's body response. Biofeedback results have provided conflicting data. In some instances it has proved successful in the reduction or elimination of pain.

Distraction. Distraction is a behavioral strategy that lessens the perception of pain by drawing the person's attention away from the pain and relegating it to the peripheral awareness. In some instances the individual is completely unaware of the pain; in other instances the intensity of pain is significantly diminished. The success of distraction can be explained by the gate theory. Pain messages are slower than diversional messages, therefore the gate closes before the pain signal arrives, and less pain is felt.

Mild to moderate pain responds well to distraction. At times, if an individual concentrates intently on another subject, the acute pain may be relieved. The most common forms of distraction include slow rhythmic breathing, slow rhythmic massage, rhythmic singing or tapping, active listening, guided imagery, and humor (Kosier et al, 1995; Jeffery and Lubkin, 2002). Box 9-8 lists the various forms of distraction.

Relaxation, Meditation, and Imagery. As behavioral strategies, relaxation enables the quieting of the mind and muscles, providing the release of tension and anxiety. Relaxation should be adjunctive to pain medication or other pain-relieving measures because of its indirect manner of pain relief. Meditation and imagery are two methods of promoting relaxation. Imagery uses the client's imagination to focus on settings full of happiness and relaxation rather than on stressful situations. Several studies using guided imagery have shown that there was a decrease in pain perception in foot pain and abdominal pain. It was suggested that a strong image of a pain-free state effectively alters the autonomic nervous system's responses to pain (Hamm and King, 1984; Griffin, 1986; Pearson, 1988; McCaffery and Pasero, 1999).

Hypnosis. Hypnosis, another behavior strategy, has been used to help alter pain perception through positive suggestions. Research has demonstrated that hypnotic analgesia reduces what are called "overreactions" to pain when apprehension and stress are apparent.

Some people have the ability to induce self-hypnosis, and some do not. Most of the population, however, has some capacity for hypnosis and with training can increase their control in this area. There are three recognized modes of hypnosis: (1) spontaneous, which is what most of us do when we daydream; (2) the self-induced trance; and (3) formal hypnosis, which requires the services of a hypnotist.

Intense concentration is required for hypnosis. Hypnosis can be used to alter pain perception, thus blocking pain awareness; to substitute another feeling for a painful one; to displace pain sensation to a smaller body area; or to alter the meaning of pain so that it is viewed as less important and less debilitating (Thomas, 1990; Sarvis, 1995). Table 9-3 illustrates the advantages and disadvantages of specific nonpharmacologic pain relief measures.

PLACEBO

Placebo is defined as "any medication or procedure, including surgery, that produces an effect in a patient because of its implicit or explicit intent and not because of its specific physical or chemical properties" (McCaffery and Pasero, 1999, p. 54). The placebo was an attempt to fool the patient into thinking that he or she is getting the "real thing." Patients whose pain or illness was relieved by placebo were considered "crocks" or "complainers." A placebo is never justified to determine the existence of pain (McCaffery and Ritchey, 1992; Fox, 1994; McCaffery and Pasero, 1999; Fine, 2002).

There is a general misunderstanding about the use and effect of placebos. The "pure" placebo is a sugar pill or saline injection or some other inert substance. "Impure" placebos are active drugs with pharmacologic effects unrelated to the condition being treated; for example, giving vitamin B_{12} injections for fatigue. Despite the fact that a placebo is generally thought to be inert and therefore harmless, reports of adverse effects such as rash, nausea, and thirst have been noted (Todd, 1987). The most common side effects are headaches, depression, and CNS stimulation. This could be considered a nocebo effect. The nocebo effect can occur when one thinks that the outcome of a particular medication, treatment, or intervention will be negative (Pain relief, 1995).

The American Holistic Nurses' Association (2000) refers to the placebo effect in its Standards for Holistic Nursing: "The placebo effect is evidence of the mind's role in disease and healing, and therefore evaluated as a valid healing event." Spiro (1996) reinforces this idea by suggesting that recognition of the placebo effect as a useful tool has reemerged as a result of interest in mind, body, and spirit integration and hypothesizes that perhaps placebos "turn the mind, or the brain, away from recognizing the pain, even while the C fibers are still firing their torment" (p. 7). Although in the past there were more pros than cons on the use of placebos, today there are many more ramifications and strong support by health professionals for not using placebos in the treatment of pain, whether acute or chronic. Many of these reasons follow:

- It is not appropriate for the treatment of pain.
- It may be harmful.
- Placebos cannot be justified to avoid side effects of opioids.
- The deception involved in placebo use harms the relationship between the patient and the health care professional.

Table 9-3 Advantages and Disadvantages of Nonpharmacologic Measures

Therapy	Advantages	Disadvantages
Cutaneous nerve stimulation TENS DNS Touch Acupuncture/acupressure	Pleasurable sensations make it popular with elders Pain decreases during and after stimulation Requires little patient participation Good for those with limited mobility Relaxation and distraction from pain May be feasible for elders with limited income Requires limited energy expenditure Self-administration provides a sense of control	Some elders perceive stimulation as objectionable; odors from creams and ointments intolerable, such as menthol Improper use of heat, cold, etc. may do tissue damage Choice may be limited by cognitive and sensory impairment TENS requires special education and learning
Distraction Tactile, auditory, visual, kinesthetic	Improved mood Easy to learn Relaxation Increased pain tolerance	Lasts only as long as stimulus present
Relaxation	Decreases skeletal muscle tension Decreases anxiety Useful with chronic pain, muscle spasms, sleep loss due to pain	Must be able to understand instructions Takes time and energy to learn Ineffective with depressed or very fatigued Must be practiced daily
Biofeedback	Decreases chronic pain	Requires equipment (moderate to expensive) Time and energy to learn Must be cognitively intact
Imagery	Very simple, uses elder's imagination: may enhance relaxation and distraction; may feel control over pain; may perceive an escape from pain; always available Little or no economic or social impact for elderly	Must be cognitively intact Not all health professionals able to teach it
Hypnosis	Pain relief on a long-term basis without side effects Useful for elders unable to tolerate pharmacologic measures Does not alter mental function (a fear of the elderly)	Feel loss of mental control Must be cognitively intact Requires trained personnel May not be available in remote or small settings May be too expensive

Developed by Patricia Hess.

- Legal and ethical issues exist, such as liability, fraud, malpractice, breach of contract, and negligence.
- It deprives the patient of appropriate assessment and treatment.
- There is no individual or condition for which placebo is a recommended treatment.

State boards of nursing have also issued statements regarding use of placebos for the management of pain. Nurses must know what their respective state says about placebos. For example, the California Board of Registered Nursing states that "use of placebos for the management of pain would not fulfill informed consent parameters" (California Board of Registered Nursing, 1997, p. 12).

PAIN CLINICS

Pain center experience with elders has been limited; however, referral for elders with significant and psychologic impairment in most instances is appropriate when the usual standard measures to relieve pain (particularly chronic pain) are unsuccessful.

The number and types of pain center programs have increased as a response to continued poor pain management by general medical practice. Pain centers may be inpatient or outpatient and are generally one of three types: syndrome oriented, modality oriented, or comprehensive. Syndrome-oriented centers focus on a specific chronic pain problem such as headache or arthritis pain. Modality-oriented centers focus on a specific treatment technique or several treatment techniques such as relaxation, massage, or acupuncture/acupressure. The comprehensive centers tend to be larger and associated with medical centers. These centers include many services that require a thorough initial assessment (physical, mental, and psychosocial). Only then can a comprehensive treatment plan with follow-up be developed. Staff members are usually part of a coordinated, multidisciplinary team consisting of physician, nurse, physical therapist, occupational therapist, massage therapist, rehabilitation specialist, social worker, and patient with family/surrogate.

The goals of pain management at pain centers are to decrease pain intensity to a tolerable level or eliminate it, if possible; improve functionality and activities of daily living; increase involvement in family and social activities; decrease depression; and improve mood. This is accomplished by improving quality and frequency of assessment, improving optimal use of analgesics, assisting in minimizing analgesic adverse reactions, and documenting outcomes associated with treatment and recommendations. Treatment includes a variety of approaches; medical treatment may be oral or topical, which are much preferred over the parenteral route. Because long-term use of potent medications can lead to tolerance or dependency when one has chronic pain, medication adjustment may occur. Medication is used only when absolutely necessary in the management of the patient's pain. Physiologic and cognitive-behavioral modalities are used to reduce or alleviate chronic pain during and after the pain center program. Even though older adults may find these therapies foreign to them, they are good candidates for these treatment programs and their benefits (Saxon and Etter, 1994; Pain—the fifth vital sign, 2001; Fine, 2002). The nurse should be familiar with the types of pain management clinics to provide the patient or family, or both, with the necessary information to make a knowledgeable decision and what to look for in considering a pain center.

NURSE'S ROLE

There is a dilemma in providing comfort. Because bureaucratic policies limit staff, the time that staff members spend with patients is confined to the basic needs of treatment, medications, and physical care. The quality of physical care suffers when the paraprofessional is discouraged from taking time to fulfill comfort needs such as providing a back rub or discussing the patient's concerns. If the caregiver could spend 5 minutes massaging and talking with the older person after a bath or treatment, anxiety, pain, and depression would be reduced. The nurse is in an influential position to make a meaningful contribution to pain relief. Although this text does not discuss the various pain theories in depth, it would be expected that nurses providing care to the aged would have sufficient knowledge of the physiologic condition of pain and the theories currently accepted by the medical community. In addition, nurses must educate themselves about nonpharmacologic and pharmacologic approaches to pain and how they can be used alone or in combination to relieve pain, as well as become proficient in the assessment of acute pain and chronic pain.

The ability to assess pain of another becomes complicated because of differing attitudes and the multidimensional aspects that pain projects. There are no easy answers of how to evaluate, differentiate, or judge the uniquely personal estimates of the quality of pain. Pain experiences are highly individualized, and there is much yet to learn about pain.

Nurses are most familiar and comfortable with acute, temporary pain because it is short lived and amenable to expedient relief. Chronic pain is complex and presents a frustrating situation for the nurse and an intolerable situation for the patient. Nurses expect patients suffering from chronic pain to display behavior characteristics of acute discomfort; an organic basis for pain makes it legitimate. Nurses tend to undermedicate patients with chronic pain because they fear that they will foster addiction or the pain expressed is exaggerated. Often nurses caring for the patient with chronic pain, especially in long-term care situations, become so familiar with the pain that they ignore it as a means of protecting themselves from feeling overwhelmed and powerless in what seems an insurmountable, futile situation. Frequently patients with chronically painful conditions are told they must "just learn to live with it." To the individual experiencing pain, that is a dismal pronouncement and implies a withdrawal of interest and concern.

Assessment

Assessment of pain is the most critical component of pain management. Successful pain management begins with an accurate assessment (Watt-Watson and Donovan, 1992). It includes psychosocial and mental aspects, not just the physical component. Assessment of pain in the elderly is important for several reasons: (1) Pain is the most common symptom in the older adult. Significant pain occurs in 25% to 50% of community-dwelling elders and 83% of elders in long-term care (Ferrell et al, 1995; Morley, 2001). Teno and co-workers (2001) indicate from studying minimum data set (MDS) results that 15% of elders are in severe pain daily, 20% are in pain weekly, and 40% are in severe pain 60 to 180 days later. (2) Accurate assessment leads to an accurate diagnosis and thus appropriate treatment, decreasing the consequences of poorly assessed and managed pain. (3) Assessment facilitates evaluation of the effectiveness of treatment. (4) Assessment can help differentiate acute endangering pain from long-standing chronic pain. Box 9-9 lists the consequences of unrelieved pain.

The characteristic of pain can be described as sharp and throbbing or as sensations of pressure, dullness, and aching. It can manifest itself in acute physical signs. Psychosocial pain or discomfort was identified as occurring from unkindness by caregivers or while awaiting new procedures or staff not taking the client's pain seriously.

Observe the patient for physical and psychologic signs. Acute pain precipitates restlessness, grumbling, and audible moans, groans, and crying, to mention a few manifestations. The individual in chronic or acute pain decreases movement; movements are quiet, controlled, and deliberate. Vital signs may be unstable, or there may be an increase in pulse rate and an elevation in blood pressure; however, if pain persists for some time, vital signs stabilize and are not a reliable

Box 9-9
Harmful Effects of Unrelieved Pain

↑ Heart rate, ↑ cardiac output, ↑ peripheral vascular resistance, ↑ systemic vascular resistance, ↑ coronary vascular resistance, hypertension, ↑ myocardial oxygen consumption, hypercoagulation, deep vein thrombosis
Reduction in cognitive function, mental confusion
↑ Behavioral and physiologic responses to pain, altered temperaments, higher somatization, ↑ vulnerability to stress disorders, addictive behavior, and anxiety states
↑ Adrenocorticotropic hormone (ACTH), ↑ cortisol, ↑ antidiuretic hormone (ADH), ↑ epinephrine, ↑ norepinephrine, ↑ growth hormone (GH), ↑ catecholamines, ↑ renin, ↑ angiotensin II, ↑ aldosterone, ↑ glucagon, ↑ interleukin-1, ↓ insulin, ↓ testosterone
Debilitating chronic pain syndrome: postmastertomy pain, postthoracotomy pain, phantom pain, postherpetic neuralgia
↓ Gastric and bowel motility
↓ Urinary output, urinary retention, fluid overload, hypokalemia
Depression of immune system
Glucogeneogenesis, hepatic glycogenolysis, hyperglycemia, glucose intolerance, insulin resistance, muscle protein catabolism, ↑ lipolysis
Sleeplessness, anxiety, fear, hopelessness, ↑ thoughts of suicide
↓ Flow and volumes, atelectasis, shunting, hypoxemia, ↓ cough, sputum retention, infection

Modified from McCaffery M, Pasero C: *Pain: clinical manual*, ed 2, St Louis, 1999, Mosby.

indicator of pain. Ask questions and discuss the situation you observe (see Table 9-2).

Jacox (1979) noted that 70% of patients studied did not like to discuss their pain with others or were ambivalent when they did talk about it. Two thirds of patients remained calm and did not show their pain experience. No verbal communication occurred until the pain was severe. Accurate assessment includes questioning the patient about pain. Do not rely on the word "pain" alone; use other synonyms: discomfort, sore, ache, hurt, and so on (Watt-Watson and Donovan, 1992). Jacox (1979) found that 80% of patients considered itching (a form of pain) as discomfort.

The cognitively impaired and nonverbal patient is the most difficult to assess and requires astute observation. Marzinski (1991) studied five patients with dementia and pain. She found significant behavior changes during painful experiences. Closs (1994) identified two types of behavior in the cognitively impaired with pain: vocal and nonverbal behavior. It is not wise to extrapolate on limited studies, but the findings might be helpful (Box 9-10). Individuals who moan and groan may become withdrawn and quiet; disjointed verbalization may turn into an accurate description of the location of pain; the quiet and nonverbal person may be observed rapidly blinking with slight facial grimacing; and the friendly, outgoing individual might become agitated and combative. The person who is easily involved in activities may cry easily and withdraw from activities, or the elderly may rhythmically rock back and forth (Matteson et al, 1995). It is important to remember that the inability to interpret or detect pain in elders who cannot and do not communicate can lead to undertreatment of pain (Sengstaken and King, 1993; Epp, 2001; Herr, 2002). At present, the tools for assessing pain in those who are nonverbal are inadequate (Saxson, 1991; Hayes, 1995; Ferrell et al, 1995). Victor (2001) suggests that even when there is cognitive impairment, ask simple questions, asking about the current pain not how the pain has been. Ask if the pain feels burning, sharp, and so on. "Don't underestimate the effect your words, tone of voice and gestures may have on the patient's response" (Victor, 2001, p. 49). It may take longer for the person to comprehend what is being asked in order to respond. Speak calmly and avoid invasion of the individual's personal space; this might be seen as a threat. If necessary, repeat the questions and phrase them with the same words to avoid confusion. Environmental overstimulation is a hazard with some cognitively impaired elders. Administration of assessment tools should be done with the least amount of surrounding distraction, conversation, and noise. It is important to involve the family or caretaker in the assessment of pain and its evaluation in cognitively impaired elders. The development of new methods of pain appraisal is an inviting area for research.

Culture and gender are additional factors that make pain assessment more difficult and complex. Box 9-10 highlights some culturally oriented responses to pain. Study of gender responses to pain is a relatively new area of research. Nurses until now have thought that women should receive smaller doses of narcotic analgesics than men. Nurses believed that gender differences affected sensitivity to pain (Ferrell et al, 1992). It is now thought that gender-related variations in pain perception may be physiologic rather than psychologic differences in willingness to report pain (Vallerand, 1995).

Assessment Tools. Assessment tools have been developed to help both clinicians and researchers measure, document, and communicate clients' pain experience more accurately when patients can communicate their pain. Qualitative tools attempt to describe the client's pain using such tools as pain diaries, pain logs, pain graphs, and observation. The diary and graph are particularly helpful in determining adequacy of pain management. The pain log or diary is a record written and kept by the client. For these methods to be effective, the client should carry a notebook and pencil to record pain as soon as possible after the pain episode. Such items as activity, intensity, and duration of the pain during daily activities, medications taken, and when they were taken should be recorded. The diary should be reviewed with the caregiver to assess the relationship among pain, medication use, and activity. The pain graph provides a visual picture of the highs and lows of

Box 9-10 Pain Cues in Older Adults

Overt Behavior

Aggressive

Striking out: pinching; hitting; biting; or scratching

Physical movements

Restlessness/agitation
Drawing legs up or fetal position
Stretches
Repetitive movements
Clenched fists
Slow movements, cautious movements
Guarding
Trying to get someone's attention

Activities of daily living

Resists care
Change in appetite (decrease)
Altered sleep (decreased)

Sounds

Verbalizations

Says has pain
Antisocial behavior
Complains
Critical
Blames
Silence—does not speak

Sounds—cont'd

Vocalizations

Groans
Moans
Screams
Cries
Babbles
Noisy breathing

Appearance

Facial expression

Expressionless; stares or looks past you
Winces
Pleading
Grimaces: eyes—tighten up or light up; mouth—open or pinched; brows—wrinkled or folded

Body language

Complexion—flushed look

Miserable

Tense

Lacks concentration
Perspires

Modified from Parke B: Gerontologic nurses' way of knowing, *J Gerontol Nurs* 24(6):21, 1998; and McCaffery M, Pasero C: *Pain: clinical manual*, ed 2, St Louis, 1999, Mosby.

the client's pain. The caregiver can assist the client when necessary in the plotting of the pain experience.

Quantitative assessment tools include pain rating, the visual analog scale (VAS), and the verbal descriptor scale (VDS) to help measure pain severity. The McGill Pain Assessment Questionnaire (Melzack, 1975) is a comprehensive tool that is useful for initial intake pain assessments, if the client is not in acute distress. Questions about past pain experience, medications used, other treatments tried, current pain episode, pain effect on activity and work, and quality and location of pain are asked. The tool relies heavily on verbal and cognitive capacity and takes a long time to administer.

An initial pain assessment tool that can be completed by the client or with the help of the caregiver appears in Figure 9-1. Information similar to the McGill questionnaire is evident but developed in a different format. There are several versions of the VAS, including a scale of 0 to 5 and a scale of 0 to 10. The Descriptive Pain Intensity Scale uses the same principle but uses pain descriptions: no pain, mild pain, moderate pain, severe pain, very severe pain, worst possible pain. The scales are usually presented in a horizontal layout. Research, as well as empirical data, has found that elders do better with a vertical rather than a horizontal VAS. Color has also been used to quantify pain. Stewart (1977) designed a color variation scale for children that can be used with adults and elders as well. The scale progresses from yellow-orange to red-black with verbal descriptors, with yellow indicating no pain and black indicating worst pain. Use of colored markers on a body outline is another approach to learning the intensity of a client's pain. Four marker pens or crayons are used to pinpoint the pain on a body outline (Eland, 1981). Each color represents a degree of pain (none, mild, moderate, worst). This is a useful tool for an individual who has difficulty with language.

Using these tools, the nurse can obtain a fairly accurate idea of the degree of discomfort or pain. The Face Pain Scale, used with children for many years, is also useful with older adults. Each facial expression represents a level of pain. The latest tool, the Painometer, a handheld tool developed by Dr. Fannie Gaston-Johanson, incorporates many of the features of existing scales to make it a multidimensional approach. It has been clinically tested and meets current clinical practice guidelines. The Joint Commission on Accreditation of Healthcare Organizations (JCAHO) approved its use in May 2000 with implementation in the accreditation compliance beginning 2001 (Mattson, 2000). The Painometer is being used to assess pain in major cancer centers in the United States (Mattson, 2000). The existing tools for pain assessment should be adapted for the elderly, based on their verbal, physical, and cognitive capabilities (Figure 9-2). McCaffery and Pasero (1999) present a compendium of assessment tools that the nurse may employ in pain assessment. Box 9-11 lists the quantitative and qualitative tools that are available for a complete pain assessment. When the client is unable to tolerate lengthy questioning, a quick assessment should be done, illustrated by the example presented in Box 9-12.

Elements of a complete pain assessment include an accurate history, physical examination (attention to musculoskeletal system and nervous system; palpation of trigger points), functional assessment (one of several available evaluations of activities of daily living), and psychologic assessment (mini mental status examination) (Box 9-13). Leading questions often give the nurse inaccurate information. Patients frequently answer according to what they think the nurse expects to hear. Ask questions that have the patient describe the pain.

Nurses must seek answers to the following questions to intervene most effectively:

1. Is the elder concerned about the pain sensation itself or about the future implications of pain?

Brief Pain Inventory

Date _______ / _______ / _______ Time: _______

Name: _______________ _______________ _______________

Last First Middle Initial

1) Throughout our lives, most of us have had pain from time to time (such as minor headaches, sprains, and toothaches). Have you had pain other than these everyday kinds of pain today?
   1. Yes 2. No

2) On the diagram, shade in the areas where you feel pain. Put an X on the area that hurts the most.

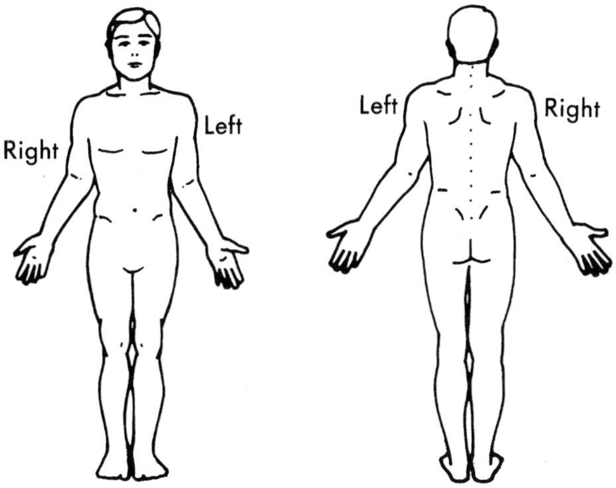

Right Left Left Right

3) Please rate your pain by circling the one number that best describes your pain at its **worst** in the past 24 hours.

0 1 2 3 4 5 6 7 8 9 10
No pain — Pain as bad as you can imagine

4) Please rate your pain by circling the one number that best describes your pain at its **least** in the past 24 hours.

0 1 2 3 4 5 6 7 8 9 10
No pain — Pain as bad as you can imagine

5) Please rate your pain by circling the one number that best describes your pain on the **average.**

0 1 2 3 4 5 6 7 8 9 10
No pain — Pain as bad as you can imagine

6) Please rate your pain by circling the one number that tells how much pain you have **right now.**

0 1 2 3 4 5 6 7 8 9 10
No pain — Pain as bad as you can imagine

7) What treatments or medications are you receiving for your pain?

____

____

8) In the past 24 hours, how much **relief** have pain treatments or medications provided? Please circle the one percentage that most shows how much relief you have received.

0% 10 20 30 40 50 60 70 80 90 100%
No relief — Complete relief

9) Circle the one number that describes how, during the past 24 hours, pain has **interfered** with your:

A. General activity

0 1 2 3 4 5 6 7 8 9 10
Does not interfere — Completely interferes

B. Mood

0 1 2 3 4 5 6 7 8 9 10
Does not interfere — Completely interferes

C. Walking ability

0 1 2 3 4 5 6 7 8 9 10
Does not interfere — Completely interferes

D. Normal work (includes both work outside the home and housework)

0 1 2 3 4 5 6 7 8 9 10
Does not interfere — Completely interferes

E. Relations with other people

0 1 2 3 4 5 6 7 8 9 10
Does not interfere — Completely interferes

F. Sleep

0 1 2 3 4 5 6 7 8 9 10
Does not interfere — Completely interferes

G. Enjoyment of life

0 1 2 3 4 5 6 7 8 9 10
Does not interfere — Completely interferes

Figure 9-1. Brief pain inventory. (Copyright Charles S. Cleeland, PhD, Houston, Texas.)

Box 9-11

Qualitative and Quantitative Pain Assessment and Evaluation Tools

Qualitative (life indicator) tools
- Mini Mental Status Examination (MMSE) or Short Portable Mental Status Questionnaire (SPMSQ)
- Katz ADL Index of activities of daily living
- Instrumental activities of daily living
- Geriatric Depression Screen
- Brief Pain Inventory
- Pain Disability Index
- Multidimensional Pain Inventory
- Chronic Pain Experience Instrument

Quantitative tools
- Visual Analog Scale (VAS)
- Face Pain Scale (FPS)
- Verbal Descriptor Scale (VDS)
- Pain Thermometer*
- Painometer*
- Numeric Rating Scale (NRS)*
- McGill Pain Questionnaire (MPQ) or short form

Compiled by Patricia Hess.
*Best qualitative tools with elders.

2. Is the elder afraid that the pain indicates fatal illness or that the pain does or will deprive him or her of some specific pleasures of life?
3. Does the elder want to be asked about the pain or not be reminded of it?
4. Does the elder want to be alone for fear of showing an emotional response, or does he or she want to be alone because of having one's own method of handling pain?
5. Does the elder want visitors to share the pain or to use visitors as a distraction?
6. Does the elder expect to obtain relief immediately or to suffer a while?
7. Does it matter to the elder if relief is palliative or curative?
8. Does the elder believe that drugs are unnatural pain relief measures or fear the consequences of addictive drugs?
9. Does crying mean that the elder wants immediate pain relief or sympathy, or is it a desire for a demonstration of technical skill?
10. Does the elder view the expression of pain as natural, serving a particular purpose, or indicative of defeat?

In addition, assessment should consider how the pain interferes with the patient's ability to meet needs of security,

Box 9-12

Immediate Help for Assessment

Quick Assessment in Situations Where Patients are Unable to Tolerate Lengthy Questions

Time involved: Reading time, 5 minutes; implementation time, about 10 minutes.

Sample situation: Mr. M., 65 years old, with lung cancer and widespread metastasis, is admitted to your floor. He is not able to concentrate long enough to answer many questions. He grimaces frequently and cries out, saying "It hurts, please give me something." His wife states that he is not swallowing anything by mouth.

Possible solution: Assess pain with minimal number of questions in order to give initial analgesic safely.

Expected outcome: Patient states he is comfortable.

Further pain assessment is completed at a later time so that a detailed plan of care may be implemented.

Tell the patient that you are going to work to get him comfortable as quickly as possible but that you must get some information first:

1. Point (on his body) to where the pain is. Mr. M. points to his lower back.
2. Is this the same location for the pain over the last several days?
   Mr. M. says that this is the same area that has bothered him over the last week, but it has gotten much worse since yesterday evening.
3. On a 0 to 10 scale (0 = no pain, 10 = worst pain), what number would you give your pain right now? Mr. M. becomes very agitated and yells "It is unbearable." This is a good enough answer under the circumstances.
4. What medication were you taking at home, and did it help the pain?
   Mrs. M. tells you that her husband was taking morphine 90 mg q4h with Motrin 800 mg q6h. He has not been able to swallow anything since late last night, so he has had nothing for pain since then. Before this, the medication was keeping the pain well controlled.
   Because of Mr. M.'s condition, it was appropriate to ask only the most essential questions to initiate an analgesic regimen. The above four questions give you important baseline data and establish an initial narcotic dose.
   Using a flow sheet, the immediate goal is to establish pain control quickly. Using Mr. M.'s words ask "Is the pain more bearable now?" Once Mr. M.'s comfortable, additional questions from the initial pain assessment tool may be filled in, and a long-term plan of care may be reviewed with the patient and his wife.

From McCaffery M, Bebee A: *Pain: clinical manual of nursing practice*. St Louis, 1989, Mosby.

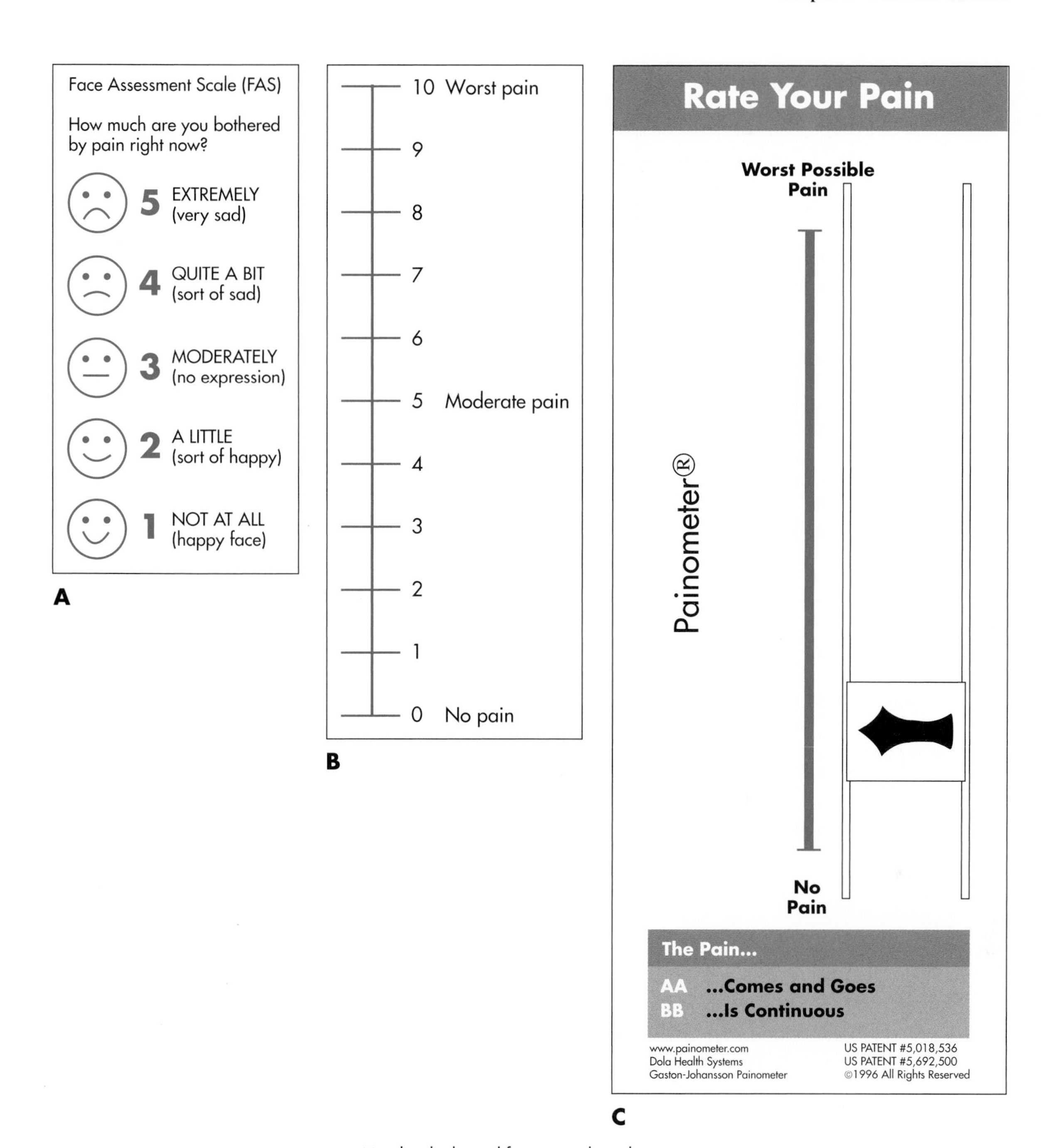

May be duplicated for use in clinical practice.

Figure 9-2. Examples of pain distress scales that are elder-friendly. **A,** Face Assessment Scale (FAS). **B,** Numeric Rating Scale (NRS). **C,** The Gaston-Johansson Painometer. (**A**, Adapted from Philadelphia Geriatric Center Pain Intensity Scale. In Cramer K et al: Philadelphia College of Pharmacy proposed guidelines for the management of chronic nonmalignant pain in the elderly LTC resident, Feb 1988; Jacox A et al: pub no 94-0592, Rockville, MD, 1994, Agency for Health Care Policy and Research (AHCPR), U.S. Department of Health and Human Services; Gaston-Johansson F et al: *Nursing Home Medicine* 4[11]:325, 1996; McCaffery M: *Nursing Home Medicine* 5(4):143, 1997; Bridgeport, CT, HealthCare Center Pain Assessment, created from pain assessment methodologies of the Joint Commission on Accreditation of Healthcare Organizations (JCAHO); **B**, From McCaffery M, Pasero C: *Pain: clinical manual,* ed 2, St Louis, 1999, Mosby; **C**, Copyright 1996 Fannie Gaston-Johansson, Dr. Med Sc., RN, FAAN, Baltimore, MD.)

Box 9-13 Content for Assessing Pain in the Elderly Patient

Pain description: Identify location, quality, intensity (present, worst, best), onset, duration, pattern of radiation or variation, manner of expression pain, relationship to movement or position, time of occurrence, and related motor or sensory complaints.

Observations: Note vocalizations such as grunting or groaning and facial expressions including wrinkled forehead, tightly closed or widely opened eyes or mouth, or other distorted expressions. Observe body movements noting guarding, rocking, pulling legs into abdomen, increased hand/finger movements, inability to keep still, pacing behaviors, or other restrictive motions.

Alleviating or aggravating factors: Explore what intensifies or decreases the pain and what treatments, remedies, or activities relieve the pain.

Impact: Identify any changes in daily activities, gait, behaviors. Note onset of new behaviors such as confusion, irritability, increased activity; accompanying symptoms such as nausea, dizziness, sweating, fatigue; any changes in sleep, appetite, emotions, concentration, physical activity, relationships with others, social interactions, and common routines.

Social history: Explore functional status before onset of symptoms, marital status, family/community resource network, social and leisure activities, and environmental barriers to social activity.

From Herr KA, Mobily RR: Complexities of pain assessment in the elderly: clinical considerations, *J Gerontol Nurs* 17(4):12, 1991.

belonging, socialization, and self-esteem. The person who considers himself or herself strong and courageous may find it humiliating to be forced to whimper or cry out with pain. What does the person want to be able to do? How does the person feel about himself or herself? Is the pain a mask for depression, of which one is unaware? Does the person feel useless, dependent, isolated? Has the pain changed interpersonal relationships? And last, can you, the nurse, help control the pain so that the individual can do what is most important to him or her?

The nurse may not be overtly aware of the influences that the patient's pain experience has on him or her as a participant and observer in the elder's care. If the elder patient is in control of the pain, it has a calming effect on the caregiver who observes and ministers. If the elder patient's pain is uncontrollable, it makes the caregiver agitated and irritated, thus coloring the ability to accurately assess pain. Another impediment to accurate pain assessment is that the patient perceives pain as more severe than do the caregivers, namely, the physicians and nurses. Cultural expectations of the caregiver and preconceived gender expectations also affect the accuracy of assessment. Exploration of one's own pain beliefs and attitudes is necessary before it is possible to understand others' pain (Kosier et al, 1995; Vallerand, 1995; Jeffery and Lubkin, 2002).

Mnemonics to assist with pain assessment are provided in Box 9-14.

Intervention

Approximately half the adults who undergo surgery continue to have pain after surgery as a result of the common practice of prn dosing of intramuscular opioids. The nurse often refrains from giving narcotics to the elderly because of the fear of patient complications, legal pressures, and misbeliefs and lack of knowledge about pain management. Needless suffering takes a toll physiologically and psychologically. These problems were addressed by the World Health Organization (WHO) and reflected in the Agency for Health Care Policy and Research, Department of Health and Human Services guidelines published in 1992. These national guidelines provide direction for pain management strategies. The guidelines should help health care professionals improve the effectiveness of pain management for their patients (Box 9-15). Various authors have adapted the WHO three-step ladder format for the choice of pain medication. A variation of this ladder appears in Figure 9-3.

Pain can be minimized through gentle handling and touch. Use of pillows for support or body positioning, just sitting and holding the patient's hand, or allowing the individual to move at his or her own speed provides pain relief.

Activity can be helpful in several ways. Gaumer (1974) indicates that the less active an individual is, the less tolerable activity becomes. Anyone who becomes inactive will feel more aches and pain than the active person. Distraction through

Box 9-14 Mnemonics for Pain Assessment

Pain is real (Believe the patient!)
Ask about pain regularly
Isolation (psychologic and social problems)
Notice nonverbal pain signs
Evaluate pain characteristics
Does pain impair function?
Onset
Location
Duration
Characteristics
Aggravating factors
Relieving factors
Treatment previously tried

From *Aging Successfully*, Newsletter of the Division of Geriatric Medicine, St Louis University School of Medicine; Geriatric Research, Education and Clinical Centers, St Louis Veterans Administration Medical Center; and the Gateway Geriatric Education Center of Missouri and Illinois, 11(3):6, Fall 2001.

Box 9-15 Agency for Health Care Policy and Research Guidelines

1. A collaborative, interdisciplinary approach to pain control, including all members of the health care team, and input from the patient and the patient's family, when appropriate
2. An individualized proactive pain control plan developed preoperatively by patients and practitioners (because pain is easier to prevent than to bring under control, once it has begun)
3. Assessment and frequent reassessment of the patient's pain
4. Use of both drug and nondrug therapies to control or prevent pain
5. A formal institutional approach to management of acute pain, with clear lines of responsibility

From *Clinical practice guideline: acute pain management*, U.S. Department of Health and Human Services, Public Health Service. Agency for Health Care Policy and Research, no 920032.

the use of activity may help change the behavior of the individual who uses pain to gain attention and sympathy. It is important to identify activities that are compatible with the relief of anxiety. Use of analgesics in conjunction with activity may be necessary. The administration of a medication 20 to 30 minutes before a specific activity that elicits pain or giving an analgesic during activity to lessen or eliminate fear of discomfort after the activity can greatly enhance the individual's capacity for that activity. The nurse should learn the patient's body potential for coping with pain and work within those parameters.

The patient with chronic pain can be involved by keeping a weekly journal that includes an account of pain during the day; the times, type, and dose of medication taken; its effect; and the duration of its benefit. This type of information helps establish patterns that may be useful in improving pain management by adjusting activity, providing medications appropriately, and helping the patient feel useful and in control of some aspect of care. Patient-controlled analgesia (PCA) has not been used as extensively with elders in the acute setting as it has with other adult patients. This may be based on criteria that require the user of PCA to be alert, mentally intact, and able to follow simple directions. In addition, elders with multisystem involvement are at high risk for respiratory and renal complications (Salerno and Willens, 1996). However, many elders meet the PCA criteria but still do not receive pain control with PCA (Matteson et al, 1995). Elders who cannot use or are not treated by PCA should receive ATC analgesia to alleviate pain.

The nurse's involvement in psychologic modulation of pain is in providing understanding and support for patients and learning and practicing relaxation techniques, guided imagery, biofeedback conditioning, TENS, and other psychologic practices that help patient relaxation and coping with pain. Meinhart and McCaffery (1983) suggest the following guidelines for individualizing pain control measures:

1. Use a variety of pain control measures.
2. Institute pain control measures before pain becomes severe.
3. Consider patients' ideas about what they feel is most effective in controlling pain when making the nursing care plan.
4. Consider patients' ability or willingness to participate in their pain control.
5. Listen to how patients describe the severity of pain. Physical signs and perceived severity are not predictably related.
6. Be aware that patients respond differently to different pain control measures. What is effective one day may not be effective the next day.
7. Encourage patients to use a pain control method more than one time. Repeated use may prove effective. A patient's bill of rights for pain appears in Box 9-16.

Whether the pain is brief or long standing, or the anticipated result of diagnostic procedures or surgery, a pain plan should be initiated. This should begin with a discussion between the nurse or physician and the patient of how much pain there might be and how long it might last, along with how it will be treated and what alternatives are available if the initial treatment does not adequately relieve the pain. In addition, for

Box 9-16 Pain Patient's Bill of Rights

I have the right to:

- have my pain prevented or controlled adequately
- have my pain and pain medication history taken
- have my pain questions answered freely
- develop a pain plan with my doctor
- know the risks, benefits, and side effects of treatment
- know what alternative pain treatments may be available
- sign a statement of informed consent before any treatment
- be believed when I say I have pain
- have my pain assessed on an individual basis
- have my pain assessed using the 0 = no pain, 10 = worst pain scale
- ask for changes in treatment if my pain persists
- receive compassionate and sympathetic care
- refuse treatment without prejudice from my doctor
- seek a second opinion or request a pain-care specialist
- be given my records on request
- include my family in decision making
- remind those who care for me that my pain management is part of my diagnostic, medical, or surgical care

Modified from Batten M: Health: take charge of your pain, *Modern Maturity*, 38(1):80, 1995; Cowles J: *Pain relief*, New York, 1994, MasterMedia.

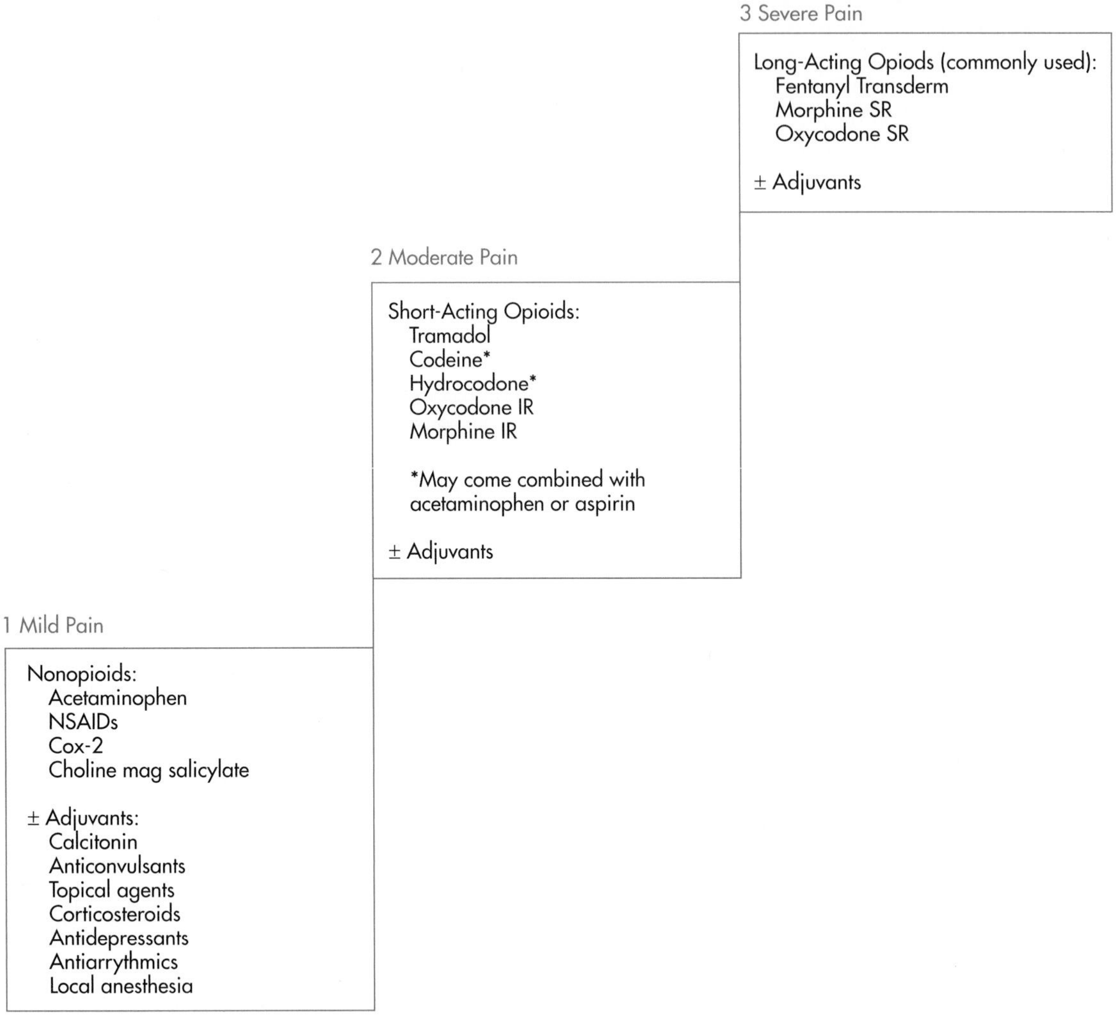

3 Severe Pain

Long-Acting Opiods (commonly used):
Fentanyl Transderm
Morphine SR
Oxycodone SR

± Adjuvants

2 Moderate Pain

Short-Acting Opioids:
Tramadol
Codeine*
Hydrocodone*
Oxycodone IR
Morphine IR

*May come combined with acetaminophen or aspirin

± Adjuvants

1 Mild Pain

Nonopioids:
Acetaminophen
NSAIDs
Cox-2
Choline mag salicylate

± Adjuvants:
Calcitonin
Anticonvulsants
Topical agents
Corticosteroids
Antidepressants
Antiarrythmics
Local anesthesia

Figure 9-3. The ladder of frequently used drugs for pain management. (Compiled from *Operative or medical procedures and trauma—clinical practice guidelines,* Washington, DC, 1992, US Department of Health and Human Services, Public Health Service, Agency for Health Care Policy and Research, Acute Pain Management; Lipman AG, Jackson KC: *Use of opioids in chronic noncancer pain,* Stamford, CT, 2000, Purdue Pharma LP, Power-Pak, Inc.; McCaffery M, Pasero C: *Pain: clinical manual,* ed 2, St Louis, 1999, Mosby; Fine PG: Chronic pain in long-term care: assessment, management, and improvement of quality indicators, Elder Care Summit, San Francisco, 2002.)

those who leave the hospital with pain or have chronic pain (e.g., cancer, arthritis, peripheral neuropathy), the plan should include the medications: when, how many, how often, and how to be taken; medications to be used if there are side effects; actions to prevent complications of medication therapy, such as constipation or nausea; any other pertinent instructions; and important numbers to call if necessary (Glickstein, 1996; Managing pain, 1996; Fine, 2002). Appendix 9-A provides one type of pain control plan.

Evaluation

Evaluation of outcomes requires repeated assessments of the patient's pain status (see Box 9-14). Utilization of the quantitative pain assessment tools is a key part of reassessment. Physical indicators of adequate intervention may include relaxation of skeletal muscles that were tense and rigid during pain. The individual no longer assumes a constricted pain posture. Behavior may reflect an increased activity level and sense of self-worth and the ability to better concentrate, focus, and increase attention span. The individual is more able to rest, relax, and sleep. In fact, the individual may sleep for what might seem like excessively long periods, but this is in response to the exhaustion that pain imposes on the body. Verbal indicators reflect the patient referring to the decrease in pain or the absence of pain during conversation.

Chronic Pain. By age 50, nearly 90% of adults have degenerative abnormalities of the lower spine. One of the most typical is thinning of the intervertebral disks, which can eventually

Box 9-17 Common Nonmalignant Pain Conditions in the Elderly

Temoral arteritis
Osteoarthritis of neck, shoulders, lumbar area, hips, knees, or hands
Rheumatoid arthritis
Lumbar disk disease
Lumbar stenosis
Osteoporosis
Peripheral vascular disease
Trigeminal neuralgia
Herpes zoster
Postsurgical intercostal neuralgia
Postherpetic neuralgia
Peripheral neuropathy
Diabetic neuropathy
Reflex sympathetic dystrophy
Phantom limb pain
Angina
Postmastectomy pain
Hiatal hernia
Irritable bowel syndrome
Chronic constipation
Acute cholecystitis

lead to arthritis and other painful conditions. The most common pain in elders is probably musculoskeletal: Among community-dwelling elders, 66% have joint pain and 28% have back pain; among elders in long-term care facilities, 70% have joint pain, 13% have pain from old fracture sites, and 10% have neuropathic pain (Ferrell, 2000). Box 9-17 lists common nonmalignant pain conditions in elders. Geriatric clients with benign chronic pain from musculoskeletal disorders have generally been treated pharmacologically without consideration of multidimensional, multidisciplinary rehabilitation programs that are frequently offered to younger patients. For some unknown reason many of these rehabilitation programs exclude individuals over 55 years of age. Middaugh and colleagues (1988) debunked the bias that elderly patients do not benefit from such rehabilitation programs. The Middaugh study, using a group of young and old persons with chronic pain, showed that geriatric patients had results as good as, if not better than, those of the younger patients. The study attributes some of the improvement that occurred to a high level of compliance, realistic expectations, and a lack of work-related obligations. Studies indicate that 60% of patients with chronic pain who participate in a multidisciplinary program function better after 1 year of treatment (Eland, 1988). Age should not be a significant factor in the offering of multidisciplinary treatment to patients with chronic pain.

Postherpetic Neuralgia. Nearly 1 million cases of herpes zoster (shingles) occur each year. Shingles affects mostly those between ages 60 and 79. It has been estimated that about 50% of people who live to age 80 will have an attack of shingles (Diamond and Urban, 2002). This may be due to the decrease in cellular immune response to the varicella zoster antigen, which is undetected in up to 30% of previously immune healthy elders over 60 (Chiu, 2000). An attack of shingles can occur when there is reactivation of the varicella virus through immunosuppression, malignancy, trauma, surgery, or local radiation (Gilchrest, 1995). Postherpetic neuralgia (PHN) is a complication that is experienced because of irritation of the nerve roots that leave the spinal cord (thoracic zoster). Ophthalmic zoster causes PHN when the ophthalmic division of the trigeminal nerve is involved. The stinging, burning pain with or without an underlying sharp, jabbing sensation continues for weeks, months, and for some elderly indefinitely after the initial skin lesions have healed. Once PHN is established it is hard to treat. Analgesics provide limited relief from the pain, although codeine is often prescribed. More effective in providing relief is a combination of antiviral medications, steroids, aspirin, and topical anesthetics for pain. The U.S. Food and Drug Administration (FDA) has approved such prescription medications as acyclovir and famciclovir, which shorten the duration of chronic shingle pain but may not prevent PHN. Capsaicin cream (Zostrix), an over-the-counter topical anesthetic, or the anesthetic EMLA patch (Reyes, 1994; Chiu, 2000) may be helpful in relieving PHN pain. The use of TENS and adjuvant therapy such as desipramine (which is considered one of the safer tricyclic drugs for use with the elderly) is effective. Newer neuropathic drugs such as gabapentin and nerve blocks are considered in resistant cases.

Primary prevention of shingles (herpes zoster) and subsequent PHN may be attainable in the future with widespread use of the varicella vaccine. Trials of zoster vaccine are underway, and it is hoped that it will provide a means of prevention in the future (Chiu, 2000). When immunosuppressed individuals with herpes zoster eruptions are treated in the early eruption stage, it prevents or limits the dissemination of vesicles and herpetic pain.

Osteoarthritis. Osteoarthritis is one of the most common forms of joint disease and the most disabling for those persons over age 65. Its prevalence increases into the eighth decade (Ettinger, 2000). Joint pain and stiffness is initially intermittent and then can become constant. Pain is characterized by aching in the joints, surrounding muscles, and soft tissue, usually relieved by rest and exacerbated by activity. The distal and proximal interphalangeal joints, cervical and lumbar spine, hips, knees, and toes are affected. Many older adults have other medical conditions in addition to osteoarthritis, which requires that the total picture be considered when the arthritic pain is treated.

Nonpharmacologic measures are the crux of therapy. Nonpharmacologic pain management includes application of moist heat to relieve pain, spasm, and stiffness; orthotic devices such as braces and splints to support painful joints; weight reduction if the patient is overweight or obesity is a contributing factor; and occupational and physical therapy. Cognitive-behavioral measures are directed at coping skills and self-efficacy and feeling safe with activity. Pharmacologic intervention consists of antiinflammatory preparations such as aspirin; however, this is not recommended for elders because of the effect on the gastric mucosa. NSAIDs are also used, but they too can have an adverse effect on the gastrointestinal lining. Acetaminophen, although not as effective as antiinflammatory preparations, is preferred to salicylates. Effective pain relief can be achieved without the risk of gastric irritation or potential for gastric hemorrhage. Topical capsaicin may reduce osteoarthritis pain, as well as the pain of PHN; however, it is necessary to warn patients to wash their hands after application and to keep their hands away from their eyes. It is also important to tell patients to expect a strong sensation of burning. Severe arthritis with unrelieved pain and extensive disability may require local anesthetics and corticosteroid injections into joints or epidural spaces for lumbar pain, or surgical intervention such as joint replacement for intractable pain.

Terminal Cancer Pain. Terminal cancer pain requires a thorough understanding of the dynamics of pain management. The nurse cannot be caught in the assumption that frequent use of analgesic drugs will create iatrogenic addiction; the real issue is adequate pain relief. Key to this relief is providing medication on time without the necessity of the patient asking for pain medication. Standard narcotic preparations or mixtures are effective. Current medications (see Figure 9-3 for the progression of medications for moderate to severe pain) should be provided on an ATC basis with provision for medications for breakthrough pain. Adjuvant medications are also considered to improve pain control or other symptoms produced by the disease and to temper the level of anxiety. Additionally, invasive anesthetics and neurosurgical or neurostimulating approaches may be used. Newer intraspinal pain relief approaches are used for pain relief below the midthorax. This requires persons with special expertise.

Pain management entails control of not only physical pain but also emotional, psychologic, and spiritual pain of the patient. The concept of the pain, anxiety, and anguish cycle mentioned earlier is crucial to successful management of pain in terminal cancer. Reduction or relief of anxiety can be achieved by allowing the individual some control over the pain situation. Self-medication is one method. Teaching the patient about his or her medication and allowing the patient to administer the medication and keep dosage records eliminate the fear that medication will not arrive on time and that the patient may have to suffer until someone arrives to provide relief. Obviously not all patients can administer their own medication, but the potential is there, and each situation must be assessed on an individual basis.

A flow sheet, kept by the patient or staff to rate pain using one of the pain rating assessment tools, provides the information to individually titrate the medication to the patient's pain need. Studies have shown that effective control of pain (attention to psychologic, emotional, spiritual, and physical distress) in many instances has reduced the amount of medication needed.

The nurse need not look on pain with fear and trepidation. If assessment is correct and the patient is listened to and handled gently and with care, anxiety can be controlled and interventions will prove more effective. Regardless of the type of pain that the nurse encounters with elder patients, but particularly for elders with chronic pain, the following principles should be the rule:

- ATC (not prn) dosing
- Provide rescue doses to avoid pain crisis
- Start low, go slow (titrate dose until relief is sustained)
- Use least invasive route (oral or transdermal)
- Limit or avoid procedures that cause pain, and premedicate sufficiently ahead of time to avoid discomfort
- Reassess frequently

Human Needs and Wellness Diagnoses

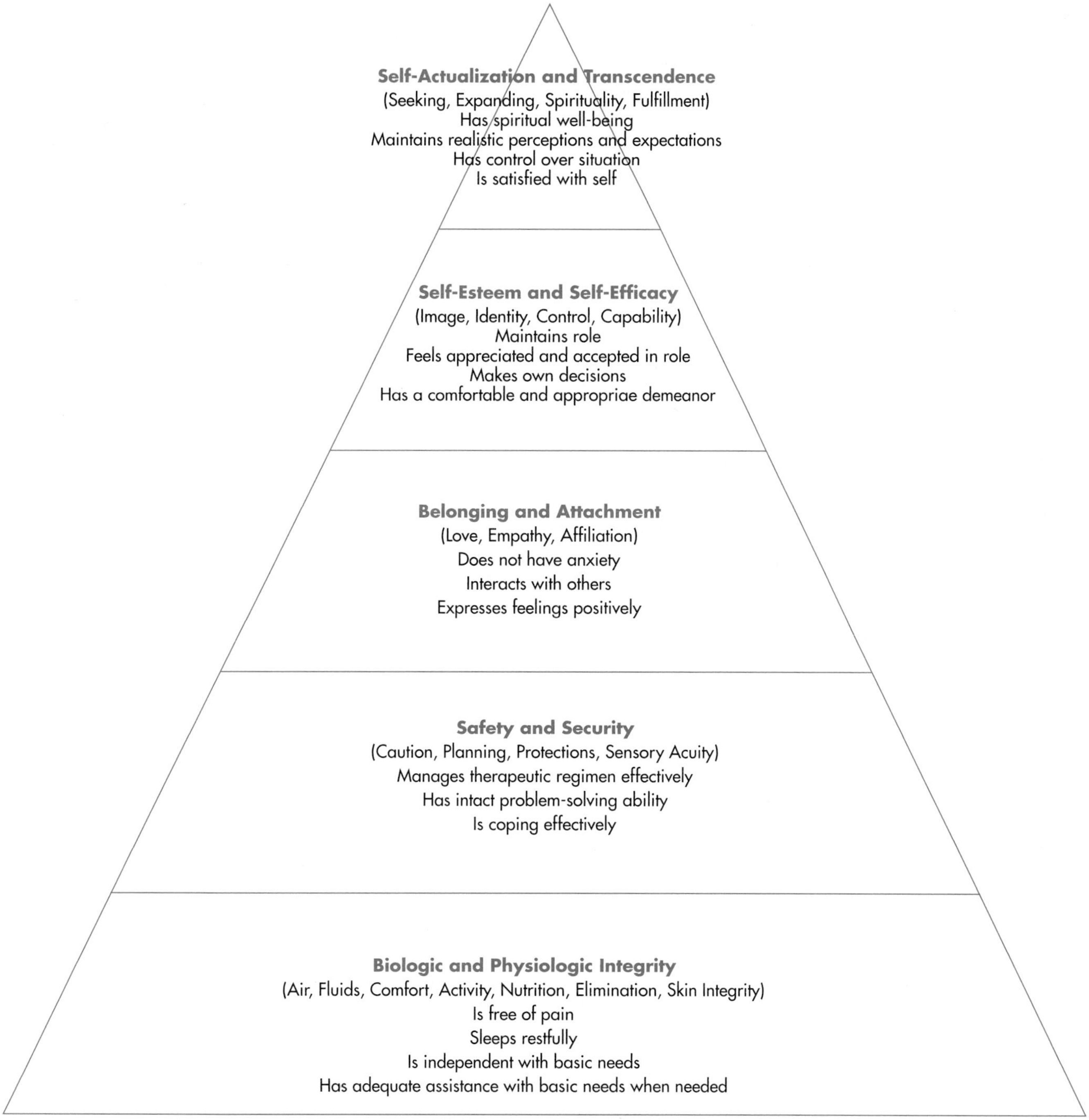

Self-Actualization and Transcendence
(Seeking, Expanding, Spirituality, Fulfillment)
Has spiritual well-being
Maintains realistic perceptions and expectations
Has control over situation
Is satisfied with self

Self-Esteem and Self-Efficacy
(Image, Identity, Control, Capability)
Maintains role
Feels appreciated and accepted in role
Makes own decisions
Has a comfortable and appropriae demeanor

Belonging and Attachment
(Love, Empathy, Affiliation)
Does not have anxiety
Interacts with others
Expresses feelings positively

Safety and Security
(Caution, Planning, Protections, Sensory Acuity)
Manages therapeutic regimen effectively
Has intact problem-solving ability
Is coping effectively

Biologic and Physiologic Integrity
(Air, Fluids, Comfort, Activity, Nutrition, Elimination, Skin Integrity)
Is free of pain
Sleeps restfully
Is independent with basic needs
Has adequate assistance with basic needs when needed

These are not all the possible wellness diagnoses that may be identified. The above are examples of nursing diagnoses that should be considered when planning care for the older adult.

KEY CONCEPTS

- The absence of pain does not necessarily imply comfort. Comfort is a state of ease and satisfaction of the bodily wants and freedom from pain and anxiety.
- The nurse's response to a client's pain is influenced by the degree of ability to imaginatively identify with another and how well the other is known. Nurses, like others, feel less concern for the stranger than for a loved one.
- Culture, ethnicity, family, and individual characteristics all influence one's tolerance and expressions of pain.
- Aged individuals with various degrees of cognitive impairment may demonstrate pain by increased levels of confusion, restlessness, or withdrawal.
- Though sometimes assumed, it has not been shown that pain sensitivity and perception decrease with age.
- Pain is what the elder says it is. The nursing goal is to assist in pain relief. Some pain medications are more appropriate for use with elders than others.
- Acute and chronic pain require different therapeutic approaches. Chronic pain predominates in the life of the aged.
- Various combinations of pharmacologic and nonpharmacologic pain control can be effective but must be individually designed with client decision making.
- Age-related pharmacokinetic and pharmacodynamic changes in the elderly influence the selection of drug therapy; drugs with a short half-life are preferred initially.
- Some elders may find autogenics helpful in pain control, although others may, depending on personal background and expectations, find them totally ineffective.
- Giving a placebo (an inert substance disguised as medication) is never justified to determine the existence of pain.

▲ CASE STUDY

Katy was a 66-year-old diabetic, and, following a stroke, her diabetes rapidly fulminated to uncontrollable fluctuations. Her blood sugar ranged from 20 mEq/ml to 800 mEq/ml. Some of this was due to erratic eating habits, almost no exercise, frequent urinary tract infections, and considerable stress related to her condition and her future. She bumped her toe while being assisted into her wheelchair after occupational therapy. In a few days the bruise had sloughed skin, and an open sore was evident. In spite of the use of local ointments and various dressings, the sore became necrotic and was débrided. Within a few weeks the debridement of necrotic tissue had removed half of her left great toe. Katy, who rarely complained, began to moan while she was sleeping and cry a lot during the day. She complained of a continuous burning sensation and said that it felt as if her toe was "on fire." One day she threw her coffee cup across the room, unable to bear the discomfort without expressing her frustration and anger. Various pain medications were given by mouth on an inconsistent basis, but the relief she experienced was minimal. She began to beg to die. The nurses thought perhaps she was right—after all, her general condition was poor, and life held little satisfaction for her. Maybe she should be allowed to die.

Based on the case study, develop a nursing care plan using the following procedure:

List comments of client that provide subjective data.

List information that provides objective data.

From these data identify and state, using accepted format, two nursing diagnoses you determine are most significant to this client at this time. List two client strengths that you have identified from data.

Determine and state outcome criteria for each diagnosis. These must reflect some alleviation of the problem identified in the nursing diagnosis and must be stated in concrete and measurable terms.

Plan and state one or more interventions for each diagnosed problem. Provide specific documentation of source used to determine appropriate intervention. Plan at least one intervention that incorporates the client's existing strengths.

Evaluate success of intervention. Interventions must correlate directly with the stated outcome criteria in order to measure the outcome success.

STUDY QUESTIONS/ACTIVITIES

Discuss Katy's situation and her probable prognosis.

What could be done, based on the information you have, to improve Katy's condition?

Do you think Katy's focus on pain is realistic or an avoidance mechanism?

What do you think impedes the nurses' understanding of Katy's pain?

Do you believe elders feel the pain of a necrotic (dead tissue) toe in the same degree that you would feel pain if someone cut away half of your toe?

Discuss the reasons for sporadic pain medication and inattention to the patient's signals and requests.

Do you think nurses are concerned about addiction in cases like Katy's?

In what situations do you believe addiction to pain medications is a priority concern?

Discuss issues of power and control related to pain management.

RESEARCH QUESTIONS

How frequently is pain responsible for an elder's expressed desire to die?

Do pain perceptions generally diminish as one ages?

What type of chronic pain do elders find most intolerable?

How do elders describe the pain of arthritis?

Do elders really fear the physical pain that may accompany dying?

What nonchemical means of pain control do elders use most frequently?

What nonchemical means of pain control are effective, and in what circumstances do they provide pain relief?
What are the reliable ways of assessing pain in cognitively impaired elders?
How can pain and pain relief be evaluated in the cognitively impaired?
How effective is PCA use by elders?
For whom and under what circumstances should the various modalities of pain management be used?

REFERENCES

Acute pain management: operative or medical procedures and trauma—clinical practice guideline, Washington, DC, 1992, US Department of Health and Human Services, Public Health Service, Agency for Health Care Policy and Research.

American Holistic Nurses' Association: AHNA standards of holistic nursing practice, Flagstaff, AZ, 2000, American Holistic Nurses' Association. Available online at www.ahna.org

American Pain Society: *Principles of analgesic use in the treatment of acute and cancer pain,* ed 4, Skokie, IL, 1999, American Pain Society.

Bates MS: *Biocultural dimensions of chronic pain,* Albany, NY, 1996, State University of New York Press.

Berman BM, Swyer JP: Complementary medicine treatments for fibromyalgia syndrome, *Baillieres Best Practice Res Clin Rheumatol* 3:487, 1999.

Boczkowski JA: Biofeedback training for the treatment of chronic pain in the elderly arthritic female, *Clin Gerontol* 2:39, 1984.

California Board of Registered Nursing: BRN focus on pain management, *BRN Report* 10(1):12, 1997.

Chiu N: Herpes zoster. In Beers MH, Berkow R, editors: *The Merck manual of geriatrics,* ed 3, Whitehouse Station, NJ, 2000, Merck Research Laboratories.

Closs SJ: Pain in elderly patients: a neglected phenomenon, *J Adv Nurs* 19:1072, 1994.

Davies P: Pharmacological management of pain in the elderly, *Analgesia* 7(1):4, Apr 1996.

Diamond S, Urban G: Coping with postherpetic neuralgia, *Consultant* 42(5):639, 2002.

Duff VG: Pain theories and their relevance to nursing practice, *Nurs Pract* 13:66, 1988.

Eland JM: Minimizing pain associated with prekindergarten IM injections, *Issues Compr Pediatr Nurs* 5:361, 1981.

Eland JM: Pain management and comfort, *J Gerontol Nurs* 14:10, 1988.

Epp CD: Recognizing pain in the institutionalized elder with dementia, *Geriatr Nurs* 22(2):71, 2001.

Ettinger HW: Local joint, tendon, and bursa disorders. In Beers MH, Berkow R, editors: *The Merck manual of geriatrics,* ed 3, Whitehouse Station, NJ, 2000, Merck Research Laboratories.

Fakouri C, Jones P: Slow stroke back rub, *J Gerontol Nurs* 13:32, 1987.

Ferrell BA: Pain management in elderly people, *J Am Geriatr Soc* 39:64-73, 1991.

Ferrell BA: Pain. In Beers MH, Berkow R, editors: *The Merck manual of geriatrics,* ed 3, Whitehouse Station, NJ, 2000, Merck Research Laboratories.

Ferrell BR, Ferrell BA: Easing the pain, *Geriatr Nurs* 11(5):175, 1990.

Ferrell BR, Ferrell BA, Rivera L: Pain in cognitively impaired nursing home patients, *J Pain Symptom Manage* 10:591, 1995.

Ferrell BR, McCaffery M, Rhiner M: Does the gender gap affect your pain control decisions? *Nursing* 92(8):48, 1992.

Ferrell BR, Rhiner M, Cohen MZ, Grant M: Pain as a metaphor for illness (part II), *Oncol Nurs Forum* 18:8, 1991.

Fine PG: Chronic pain in long-term care: assessment, management, and improvement of quality indicators, Elder Care Summit Conference, San Francisco, Apr 24, 2002.

Fox AE: Confronting the use of placebos for pain, *Am J Nurs* 94(9):42, 1994.

Fulmer TT et al: Pain management protocol, *Geriatr Nurs* 17(5):222, 1996.

Gaumer WC: Psychological potentials of chronic pain, *J Psychiatr Nurs* 12:23, 1974.

Gilchrist BA: Skin changes and disorders. In Abrams WB, Beers MH, Berkow R, editors: *The Merck manual of geriatrics,* ed 2, Whitehouse Station, NJ, 1995, Merck Research Laboratories.

Glickstein JK, editor: Managing chronic pain, *Focus Geriatr Care Rehab* 10(3):6, 1996.

Gray BB: Managed care policies affect nurses' ability to provide pain management, *Nurseweek* 9(3):1, 1996.

Griffin M: In the mind's eye, *Am J Nurs* 86:804, 1986.

Hamilton J: Comfort and the hospitalized chronically ill, *J Gerontol Nurs* 15(4):28, 1989.

Hamm BH, King V: A holistic approach to pain control with geriatric clients, *J Holistic Nurs* 11:32, 1984.

Harkins SW: Geriatric pain: pain perception in the old, *Clin Geriatr Med* 12:435, 1996.

Hayes R: Pain assessment in the elderly, *Br J Nurs* 4:119, 1995.

Herr K: Chronic pain challenges and assessment strategies, *J Gerontol Nurs* 28(1):20, 2002.

Herr K: Chronic pain in the older patient: management strategies, *J Gerontol Nurs* 28(2):28, 2002.

Hoffman MT et al: Pain in the older hospice patient, *Am J Hospice Palliat Care* 15:259, 1998.

Hofland SL: Elder beliefs: blocks and pain management, *J Gerontol Nurs* 18(6):19, 1992.

Indeck W: Pain in geriatric patients, *Geriatrics* 32:43, 1977.

International Association for the Study of Pain: *Position statement,* Seattle, 1979.

Jacox AK: Assessing pain, *Am J Nurs* 79:895, 1979.

Jeffery JE, Lubkin IM: Chronic pain. In Lubkin IM, Larsen PD, editors: *Chronic illness,* ed 5, Boston, 2002, Jones & Bartlett.

Kastner M: Researching massage as real therapy, *Massage Ther J* 33(3):56, 1994.

Kozier B et al: *Fundamentals of nursing: comfort and pain,* Redwood City, CA, 1995, Addison-Wesley.

Kreiger D: Therapeutic touch: the imprimatur of nursing, *Am J Nurs* 75:784, 1975.

Krieger D: *The therapeutic touch: how to use your hands to help or heal,* New York, 1992, Prentice-Hall.

Lee TL: Acupuncture and chronic pain management, *Ann Acad Med Singapore* 29(1):17, 2000.

Lin Y, Taylor AG: Effects of therapeutic touch in reducing pain and anxiety in an elderly population, *Integrative Medicine* 1(4):155, 1998.

Lipman AG, Jackson KC: *Use of opioids in chronic noncancer pain,* Stamford, CT, 2000, Purdue Pharma LP, Power-Pak, Inc.

Mackey RB: Discover the healing power of therapeutic touch, *Am J Nurs* 95(4):27, 1995.

Management of cancer pain, clinical guidelines no 9, Rockville, MD, 1994, Agency for Health Care Policy and Research, U.S. Department of Health and Human Services.

Managing pain: medical essay, *Mayo Clin Health Lett* (suppl):1, June 1996.

Marzinski LR: The tragedy of dementia: clinically assessing pain in the confused, nonverbal elderly, *J Gerontol Nurs* 17(6):25, 1991.

Matteson MA et al: Pain in cognitively impaired older adults, 48th Annual Scientific Meeting, Gerontological Society of America, Los Angeles, October 1995.

Mattson JE: The language of pain, *Reflections Nursing Leadership* 26(4, fourth quarter):10, 2000.

McCaffery M, Pasero C: *Pain: clinical manual,* ed 2, St Louis, 1999, Mosby.

McCaffery M, Ritchey KJ: Pain assessment: debunking the myths and misconceptions, *Nurseweek* 5(16):8, 1992.

Meek SS: Effects of slow stroke back massage on relaxation in hospice clients, *Image J Nurs Sch* 25(1):17, 1993.

Meinhart N, McCaffery M: *Pain: a nursing approach to assessment and analysis,* East Norwalk, CT, 1983, Appelton-Century-Crofts.

Melzack R: The McGill pain questionnaire: major properties and scoring method, *Pain* 1:277, 1975.

Melzack R, Wall PD: Pain mechanisms: a new theory, *Science* 150:971, 1965.

Middaugh SJ et al: Chronic pain: its treatment in geriatric and younger patients, *Arch Phys Med Rehabil* 69(12):1021, 1988.

Morley JE: Aging successfully. In *Aging Successfully,* Division of Geriatric Medicine, St Louis University School of Medicine, 11(3):1, 2001.

National Institutes of Health: *Special report on aging,* Bethesda, MD, 1990, Department of Health and Human Services, National Institutes of Health.

Pain—the fifth vital sign. In *Aging Successfully,* Division of Geriatric Medicine, St Louis University School of Medicine, 11(3):1, 2001.

Pain relief, *Univ Calif Berkeley Wellness Lett* 5(11):4, 1995.

Pearson BD: Pain control: an experiment with imagery, *Geriatr Nurs* 13:28, 1988.

Peck SDE: The effectiveness of therapeutic touch for decreasing pain in elders with degenerative arthritis, *J Holistic Nurs* 15:176, 1997.

Petrie A: In Bushman MS: *The roots of individuality—brain waves and perception, an NIMH program report,* Washington, DC, Oct 1975, US Department of Health, Education, and Welfare, Public Service, Alcohol, Drug Abuse and Mental Health Administration.

Portenoy RK: Pain. In Abrams WB, Beers MH, Berkow R, editors: *The Merck manual of geriatrics,* ed 2, Whitehouse Station, NJ, 1995, Merck Research Laboratories.

Reyes KW: Early treatment makes shingles easier to bear, *Modern Maturity* 36(6):79, Nov/Dec 1994.

Salerno E, Willens JS: *Pain management handbook,* St Louis, 1996, Mosby.

Sarvis CM: *Pain management in the elderly,* Sacramento, CA, 1995, CME Resources.

Saxson SV: *Pain management techniques for older adults,* Springfield, IL, 1991, Charles C Thomas.

Saxson SV, Etter MJ: *Physical changes and aging,* ed 3, New York, 1994, Tiresias Press.

Schnitzer TJ: Non-NSAID pharmacologic treatment options for management of chronic pain, *Am J Med* 105(1B):455, 1998.

Sengstaken EA, King SA: The problems of pain and its detection among geriatric nursing home residents, *J Am Geriatr Soc* 41:541, 1993.

Spiro HM: The art and science of placebo, *Science Med* 3(2):6, April/May 1996.

Stewart ML: Measurement of clinical pain. In Jacox A, editor: *Pain: a source book for nurses and other health professionals,* Boston, 1977, Little, Brown.

Teno JM et al: Persistent pain in nursing home residents, *JAMA* 285:2081, 2001.

Thernstrom M: Pain, the disease, *New York Times Magazine,* Dec 16, 2001, p 66.

Thomas BL: Elder care: pain management for the elderly—alternative interventions, part I, *AORN J* 52(6):1268, 1990.

Todd B: The placebo effect: real or imaginary, *Geriatr Nurs* 8:154, 1987.

Vallerand AH: Gender differences in pain, *Image J Nurs Sch* 27(3):235, 1995.

Victor K: Properly assessing pain in the elderly, *RN* 64(5):45, 2001.

Watt-Watson JH, Donovan MI: *Pain management nursing perspective,* St Louis, 1992, Mosby.

Witt JR: Relieving chronic pain, *Nurse Pract* 9(1):36, 1989.

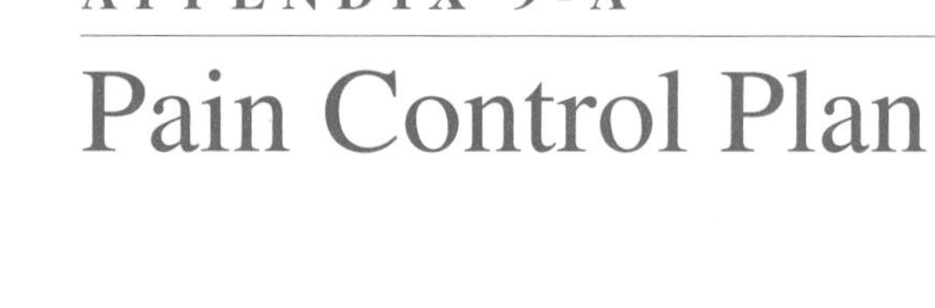

APPENDIX 9-A

Pain Control Plan

Pain Control Plan

Pain Control Plan for ______________________________

At home, I will take the following medications for pain control:

Medication	How to take	How many	How often	Comments

Medicines that I may take to help side effects:

Side effect	Medicine	How to take	How many	How often	Comments

Constipation is a common problem when taking opioid medication. When this happens, do the following:

__________ Increase fluid intake (8 to 10 glasses of fluid per day)

__________ Exercise regularly

__________ Increase fiber in diet (bran, fresh fruit, vegetables)

__________ Use a mild laxative, such as milk of magnesia, if no nondrug pain control methods

____

____

If you do not have a bowel movement in 3 days:

______ Take __________ every day at ________ (time) with a full glass of water.

______ Use a glycerine suppository every morning (this may help make a bowel movement less painful).

Additional instructions:

____

____

Important phone numbers:

Your doctor ____________________ Your nurse ____________________

Your pharmacy ____________________ Emergencies ____________________

Call your doctor or nurse immediately if your pain increases or if you have new pain. Also call your doctor early for a refill of pain medication. Do not let your medication get below 3 or 4 days' supply.

From Agency for Health Care Policy and Research: *Managing cancer pain*, consumer version, Clinical Practice Guide no 9, Washington, DC, 1994, Public Health Service, U.S. Department of Health and Human Services.

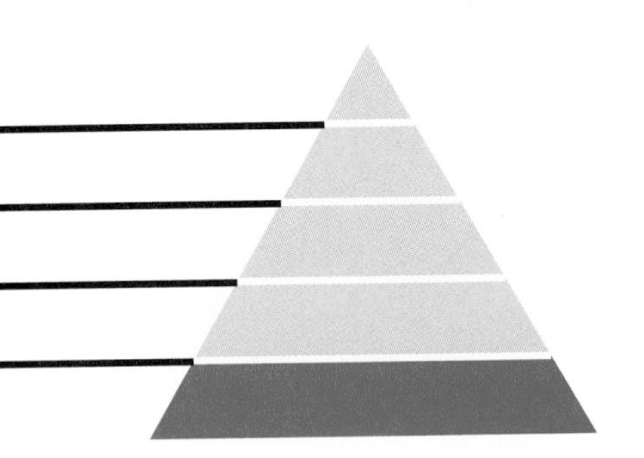

CHAPTER 10
Geropharmacology

Martha Buffum
John C. Buffum

An elder speaks

I was playing golf every day and enjoying my life. The same small amount (5 to 7 mg) of Valium had been working for 30 years in helping me get to sleep, and I saw no need to change that. Gradually, I found I couldn't get out of bed, was unsteady on my feet, slurred my words, drove through stop lights, and certainly had to stop playing golf. My doctor thought I'd had a stroke and scheduled me for an MRI! What happened? My nephew, a pharmacist, questioned me and learned about the Valium and that I was eating a half grapefruit for breakfast. Apparently, that small amount of Valium, appropriate when I was 30 years younger, now was excessive, and the grapefruit, harmless by itself, increased the Valium level. I stopped my grapefruit and, with my doctor, gradually discontinued the Valium. My MRI was negative for stroke and my symptoms cleared. Now I have my life back and am playing golf again.

Anonymous, age 82

LEARNING OBJECTIVES

On completion of this chapter, the reader will be able to:

1. Describe the pharmacokinetic changes that occur in the aged.
2. Identify the altered effects of drugs on the aged.
3. Describe problems associated with drug therapy in elders.
4. Discuss the information that the elderly should know about medication use.
5. Identify medications that may or may not be used by the aged.
6. Describe medications used for behavioral issues.
7. Identify some of the problems associated with antidepressants, antipsychotics, and antianxiety agents in the aged.
8. Explain the factors that affect medication adherence.
9. Discuss the role that the health care professional has in assisting the aged with adherence to their medication regimen.
10. Develop a nursing plan to promote safe medication practices and prevent drug toxicity.

Drugs are powerful agents that can produce miraculous cures and also tragic death. Chronic conditions increase with age, and pharmacologic therapies can prolong life and improve quality of life. Elderly persons make up the largest consumer group of prescription and over-the-counter medications (Salom and Davis, 1995). According to the Food and Drug Administration (FDA), persons over 65 years of age purchase 30% of all prescription drugs and 40% of over-the-counter drugs (Trenter, 1999). The elderly are particularly vulnerable to the effects of drugs because of physiologic aging processes, functional changes, cognitive changes, and social or situational changes. This chapter focuses on all aspects of geropharmacology and includes discussions about trends in health care, pharmacodynamics and pharmacokinetics, problems with drug therapies and prevention strategies, patterns of drug use and their assessment, the use of drugs to control and treat behaviors, and patient education. The role of the nurse in all settings is emphasized, with recommendations for interacting with patients. Many clinical examples exemplify problems, nursing roles, and care planning. Tables and boxes address drug interactions, categories of drugs with monitoring activity and common side effects, drugs that should be avoided in the elderly, dosage guidelines, drugs that should not be chewed or crushed, drugs that cause photosensitivity, and drugs used for behavioral and psychiatric issues. With the continuous expansion of biotechnology and drug therapies, research is needed to determine the safest and most effective geriatric medication utilization.

TRENDS IN HEALTH CARE THAT AFFECT MEDICATIONS IN ELDERS

The biotechnology and pharmaceutical industries have provided a continuously growing number of medications. New drugs have become available for symptoms and conditions such as pain, cancers, arthritis, hypertension, cardiovascular conditions, neurologic conditions, bacterial and viral infections, psychosis, depression, and anxiety. Along with these advances in drugs, marketing has provided information to the public that is often pure advertising. That is, media such as television, radio, and the Internet offer information about indications and side effects for taking medications. This has led increasingly to a public that requests medications and diagnostic tests from providers. Advertising to targeted populations, such as elders, can optimally promote knowledge through critical questioning of medical professionals but can also prompt adverse reactions from mixing too many medications.

Fragmentation of care is a problematic trend in current health care that affects elders' potential for drug problems. Because of disease-specific specialization, for example, patients may see different providers for their different medical conditions. Polypharmacy refers to the prescribing or administering of multiple same-class medications for the treatment of one or more chronic diseases (Schafer, 2001). The result is that no one provider is coordinating care or medications; consequences can include inappropriate medication use, prescriptions for duplicative and interacting drugs, drugs at unsafe dosages, and the development of adverse effects of varying intensity. The prescribing providers may not collaborate with each other, so their knowledge of the patient's medications is limited and relies on patient report. Afflicted by a drug interaction, an elder can suffer cognitive effects and may be deemed demented and then treated inappropriately. Potentially, a patient or family member who has been well educated about all of the medications could participate in preventing such drug problems.

Medication teaching is an important aspect of pharmacotherapy that involves many health care providers. That is, the prescriber—including the physician or nurse practitioner—must begin the education about medical condition and treatment. The pharmacist who dispenses the medication must provide specific information about the medication and the method for administering it. The nurse in any setting—hospital, long-term care, home, clinic, day center—has the opportunity to assess the patient's knowledge about all of the medications and to coordinate the medication regimen in collaboration with the physician. *The nurse's role is of paramount importance because she or he may be the only provider who comes to learn about all of the conditions and treatments.* Hence the nursing role includes assessing the patient's readiness to learn, ability to comprehend, and functional capacity to incorporate lifestyle adaptations for medication management. The patient and family member or caregiver needs to be a collaborative part of the medication teaching.

Another current trend that affects elder's medication management is the high cost of drugs. While politicians are proposing Medicare prescription drug benefits and lawsuits are occurring charging the pharmaceutical industry with keeping generics off the market, many elders are unable to afford the costs of their medicines (Barry, 2002; Carlson and Fleck, 2002; Nicholson, 2002; Pear, 2002). Indeed, persons 65 years and older make up more than 40% of prescription sales. Some of the new drugs differ only in subtle ways from older, and less expensive, therapeutic agents. As new drugs are introduced, advantages of the newer drugs draw attention, obscuring their potential side effects. The tendency to believe that new is better can result in providers prescribing their older patients the newer, and more expensive, medications. Methods of keeping costs down include using generic drugs whenever possible, using scored tablets that could be halved for more numerous doses, using older but equally effective drugs, and subscribing to drug plans that are offered through the American Association of Retired Persons (AARP) or drug companies. Increasingly, elders are utilizing pharmaceutical sources from outside the United States. Canadian, Mexican, Israeli, and Indian pharmacies are all advertising for U.S. patients.

PHARMACOKINETICS

Merriam-Webster's Online Collegiate Dictionary defines *pharmacokinetics* as "the study of the bodily absorption, distribution, metabolism and excretion of drugs" (Merriam-Webster Online, 2003). Simply put, pharmacokinetics is what the body does to the drug.

Pharmacokinetics determines the concentration of drugs in the body. The concentration of the drug at different times depends on how the drug is taken into the body (absorption); where, or to what compartments (vascular, extracellular), the drug goes within the body (distribution); how the drug is broken down by the body (metabolism); and how the body gets rid of the drug (excretion).

Absorption

Drug administration may be oral, sublingual, rectal, topical, transdermal, intramuscular, intravenous, subcutaneous, intra-arterial, intranasal, ophthalmic, intraperitoneal, intrathecal, by inhalation, and auricular (in the ear). How the drug is given greatly influences the amount and rate of absorption. Because of these differences, a dose that is proper for one mode of administration may be inappropriate for another mode.

Drugs given orally pass through the mouth and esophagus and enter the stomach. Most solid oral drug dosage forms (e.g., tablets, capsules, powders, and pills) are designed to dissolve in the stomach. The rate of dissolution of a tablet depends on the amount of liquid in the stomach, the type of coating the tablet has, the extent of tablet compression used in making the tablet, the presence of expanders in the tablet, and the solubility of the drug in the acid environment of the stomach (Wilkinson, 2001). Some tablets are so tightly compressed that they never dissolve and are eliminated whole in the feces. Others, such as Bayer aspirin, break apart so quickly that they may reach the stomach in tiny pieces. Grinding up a tablet or administering a powder yields the same result. Capsules are powdered drugs, with their diluents, encased in a gelatin capsule. Liquid drug dosage forms for oral use come as solutions, suspensions, tinctures, and elixirs. Solutions are the drug dissolved in water. Suspensions are the drug (generally a water-insoluble drug) suspended in some liquid. Tinctures are alcoholic solutions of a drug. Elixirs are semi–water-soluble solutions of drugs held in solution by alcohol. Oral liquid dosage forms are generally absorbed faster than tablets or capsules.

Following oral administration the drug dissolves in the stomach and then passes into the duodenum or small intestine (Wilkinson, 2001). The small intestine has a very large surface area and is efficient at absorbing drugs. Most drugs are absorbed from the small intestine, although some (e.g., alcohol) are absorbed from the stomach. The drug passes from the small intestine into the network of veins surrounding it. These veins, known as the portal system, drain into the portal vein, which enters the liver where the drug may undergo metabolism. Drugs that pass through the liver before they reach the systemic circulation may undergo what is termed *first-pass metabolism.* Drugs that are extensively metabolized as they pass through the liver from the portal system are said to have a large first-pass effect. Drugs with a large first-pass effect usually have a much larger oral therapeutic dose than the same drug given by injection (Wilkinson, 2001). Following passage through the liver, the drug enters the systemic circulation through the hepatic vein and is distributed throughout the body. The percentage of orally administered drug entering the systemic circulation compared with the same amount given intravenously is termed the *percent bioavailability.* Presence of food in the stomach may delay absorption or not. Food may increase, decrease, or delay the total absorption of the drug.

With sublingual administration the drug is absorbed from the oral cavity and passes directly into the systemic circulation (Wilkinson, 2001). This route bypasses the stomach, small intestine, portal system, and liver. As a result, to the extent that the drug can be absorbed sublingually, the drug reaches the systemic circulation much faster and avoids first-pass metabolism by the liver. The buccal mucosa does not have a large surface area, so it is not very efficient at absorbing drugs.

Rectal administration may be useful when the patient cannot tolerate oral medications (Wilkinson, 2001). Drugs absorbed by the rectum pass into the portal system and the liver before reaching the systemic circulation. The rectum does not have a large surface area, so it is not very efficient at absorbing drugs.

Drugs given by injection avoid the first-pass effect and usually require a smaller dose. Intravenous administration has the fastest onset of drug effect and is the most efficient drug delivery method (Wilkinson, 2001). The intramuscular and subcutaneous routes of drug administration result in a slower onset of drug action and depend on the rate of absorption from the injection site. Some drugs that are effective by intravenous administration are poorly absorbed from an intramuscular injection (e.g., phenytoin, diazepam). Drugs given intravenously should be injected slowly so as not to produce toxicity from excessive blood levels. Some drugs must be administered over 1 to 2 hours. Always check with the pharmacy or a good drug reference to find out the safe rate of drug administration before administering a drug by the intravenous route. Drugs given by intramuscular or subcutaneous routes do not have to be given slowly, but one must always make sure the needle is not in a vein or an artery before injecting.

Very few drugs are given by the intraarterial, intraperitoneal, or intrathecal routes (Wilkinson, 2001). Specialized training is required to administer such drugs.

Intranasal, ophthalmic, and auricular drug administration is usually for the purpose of delivering the drug to the site of administration, but systemic absorption may occur (Wilkinson, 2001).

Topical drug administration is for delivering drug to the skin area where it is applied (Wilkinson, 2001). If the area is occluded with a dressing, systemic absorption may occur.

Transdermal administration is the topical application of a drug for systemic use (e.g., clonidine patch, nicotine patch).

Aging has no effect on oral drug absorption; however, there may be reduced absorption of some drugs from intramuscular injection sites (Eddington, 1996; Hammerlein et al, 1998; O'Mahony, 2000).

Metabolism

Metabolism is the process by which drugs and other toxic substances are broken down by the body so that they may be more readily excreted. For purposes of this discussion, metabolism will refer to drug metabolism; however, it should be pointed out that the drug-metabolizing enzyme systems evolved to detoxify natural products ingested as foods.

Some molecules may exist in an ionized (charged) or non-ionized (uncharged) state depending on the pH of the solution they are in. For molecules to move in or out of cells they must pass through the lipoprotein membranes of the cells (Wilkinson, 2001). The non-ionized molecules pass through the membranes whereas the ionized molecules do not. Lipophilic (fat-soluble) drugs pass easily through biologic membranes to their receptor sites. Hydrophilic (water-soluble) drugs do not pass easily through membranes. In general, metabolism chemically changes the lipophilic molecules into hydrophilic metabolites. The kidney is the primary organ of excretion. When a non-ionized or a lipophilic molecule enters the kidney and passes through the cellular membrane into the kidney tubules, it will be mostly reabsorbed because it will pass freely back into the blood through the kidney's lipoprotein basement membrane. In contrast, an ionized or a hydrophilic molecule will not be reabsorbed and will be excreted in the urine (Wilkinson, 2001).

The primary site of metabolism is the liver, although many other organs have metabolizing enzymes (e.g., gut, brain, and lungs). The primary types of metabolism are phase I metabolism, or oxidative metabolism, and phase II metabolism, or conjugation.

The oxidative metabolizing enzymes are known as the cytochrome P450 (CYP450) monooxygenase system. The human CYP450 system is composed of about 50 isoforms, each of which can perform a specific chemical reaction (e.g., CYP3A3/4, CYP2D6, CYP2B6, CYP2C19, CYP1A2, CYP2E1, and CYP2C9) (Wilkinson, 2001). Eight to ten of these isoforms are responsible for the majority of all drug metabolism. These isoforms metabolize the parent compound by adding or subtracting a part of the drug molecule (e.g., adding an oxygen atom or subtracting a methyl group), thereby changing the molecule into a more hydrophilic (polar) compound. The drug molecule may undergo several enzymatic conversions by different CYP450 isoforms before it is hydrophilic enough to be excreted by the kidney. Each CYP450 isoform has an enzymatic affinity for a uniquely different type of molecular structure. Thus different drugs and drug metabolites may be substrates for specific CYP450 isoforms (Hartshorn and Tatro, 2003).

Conjugation reactions primarily convert drugs and their metabolites to glucuronides. Glucuronides are very hydrophilic and are more readily excreted in the urine or bile (Wilkinson, 2001).

A drug may be initially metabolized to one or more different metabolites. Each one of the metabolites may be excreted or metabolized to one or more metabolites. If a blood or urine sample is taken following drug administration, it may contain the parent drug and several of its metabolites. Each metabolite may or may not have the activity of the parent drug. Some metabolites are active at different receptor sites than the parent drug. Usually the drug metabolites are less potent than the parent compounds.

The more lipophilic a drug molecule is, the easier it can pass through the blood-brain barrier. The blood-brain barrier protects the brain from toxic foreign compounds such as drugs. By metabolizing drugs to less lipophilic, more hydrophilic compounds, the enzymes protect the central nervous system (CNS) (Wilkinson, 2001). Other drugs and certain foods can inhibit a metabolic isoenzyme (e.g., grapefruit juice inhibits CYP3A3/4 in the gut). This inhibition of enzymatic metabolism can prevent the normal metabolism of other drugs (e.g., grapefruit inhibits metabolism of calcium channel blockers). Some drugs and foods can induce or increase the action of specific CYP450 isoforms (e.g., rifampin induces CYP3A4 metabolism of estradiol, thereby reducing its contraceptive action). Some drugs autoinhibit their own metabolism (e.g., fluoxetine is both a substrate and an inhibitor of CYP2D6) (Flockhart, 2003). Some drugs autoinduce their own metabolism (e.g., carbamazepine is both a substrate and an inducer of CYP3A4) (Lacy et al, 2003). Drugs with a large first-pass effect are more prone to drug interactions, because more of the parent compound reaches the systemic circulation when another drug or food inhibits its metabolism. These types of drug interactions are covered in greater detail elsewhere in this chapter.

Following a drug's first pass through the liver and entry into the systemic circulation, it may undergo further metabolism. Other organs, such as the brain, lungs, and kidneys, contain drug-metabolizing enzymes. Some of the drug circulates back through the liver via the hepatic artery and undergoes further metabolism. Because the drug concentration has been decreased by its distribution throughout the body, less is metabolized compared with the first pass through the liver.

Several of the CYP450 isoforms demonstrate genetic polymorphism (CYP2D6, CYP2C9, CYP2C19, CYP2A6, CYP2E1, CYP3A5, CYP1A2, and CYP1B1) (Kimura et al, 1998; Lamba et al, 1998; Huang et al, 1999; Zheng et al, 2000; Chou et al, 2001; Leung et al, 2001; Mulder et al, 2001; Omer et al, 2001; van der Weide et al, 2001; Ujjin et al, 2002). Frequently these genetic differences in CYP450 isoforms manifest as differences in the way ethnic populations metabolize drugs. An example of genetic polymorphism would be seen in the fact that there are four types of CYP2D6 metabolizers: poor metabolizers, intermediate metabolizers, extensive metabolizers, and ultrarapid metabolizers (Wilkinson, 2001). In whites of northern European ancestry, 5% to 10% are CYP2D6 poor metabolizers. This contrasts with Asian and black populations, in which poor metabolizers constitute only 1% of the population. The clinical consequence is that when poor metabolizers take codeine for pain, they get no analgesic effect. The reason is that codeine's analgesic action depends on the 7% of the codeine that is converted to morphine by CYP2D6. The morphine is really the analgesic, not the codeine. Concomitant administration of a CYP2D6 inhibitor (e.g., quinine, fluoxetine) can also inhibit codeine's conversion to morphine. In an ultrarapid metabolizer, ingestion of codeine produces an exaggerated effect from the greater amount of morphine formation (Wilkinson, 2001).

Other drug-metabolizing pathways include hydrolysis and conjugation reactions and enzymatic cleavage of proteins and peptides (Wilkinson, 2001).

Disease states affecting the liver can alter drug metabolism. Severe liver damage, such as occurs in hepatitis, cirrhosis, and hepatocarcinomas, can decrease hepatic drug metabolism by 50% to 70% (Wilkinson, 2001). The metabolism of drugs undergoing a substantial first-pass effect is more affected by severe liver damage. These drugs may have greatly increased bioavailability with pronounced increases in blood levels (Wilkinson, 2001).

Disease states affecting the circulation of blood through the liver also affect metabolism. Severe cardiac failure and shock decrease liver perfusion and drug metabolism (Wilkinson, 2001).

Because of the considerable interindividual variability in drug metabolism, it is difficult to ascribe decreased drug-metabolizing capability to increased age. Studies have shown no decrease in either conjugative metabolism or CYP450 system function as a result of age (O'Mahony, 2000). Liver size and hepatic blood flow tend to decrease with advanced age. Because of this decrease in hepatic exposure, drugs that undergo extensive first-pass metabolism are affected by age, whereas non–first-pass drugs are not (Eddington, 1996; Hammerlein et al, 1998; O'Mahony, 2000). These drugs may exhibit decreased metabolism and increased bioavailability (e.g., nalbuphine, propranolol, and lidocaine) (Eddington, 1996).

Distribution

The systemic circulation transports the drug throughout the body. The organs of high blood flow (e.g., brain, kidneys, lungs, and liver) rapidly get the highest concentrations (Wilkinson, 2001). Distribution to organs of lower blood flow (e.g., skin, muscles, and fat) generally occurs more slowly and results in lower concentrations of the drug in the tissues. Lipophilic drugs pass through capillary membranes more easily than hydrophilic drugs, resulting in more rapid tissue distribution and a greater volume of distribution. The volume of distribution, or apparent volume of distribution (V_d), refers to the theoretical fluid volume that would be required to hold all the drug in the body if the concentration of the drug in this theoretical volume was equal to the concentration of drug in the plasma. Lipophilic drugs may concentrate in adipose tissue to a greater extent than in the vasculature or other tissues. As a result of this higher concentration, the V_d of the drug might exceed the total volume of the body. More hydrophilic drugs tend to be held in the vasculature and are therefore more easily metabolized and excreted by the liver and kidneys.

Drugs can bind to plasma proteins. Acidic drugs bind tightly to the albumin, and basic drugs bind tightly to α_1-acid glycoprotein (AAG) (Wilkinson, 2001). The extent of protein binding determines whether a drug is free to interact with its receptor site and exert a pharmacologic action. Protein-bound drugs are not free to exert their effect, nor are they able to be metabolized. Disease states (e.g., hypoalbuminemia due to liver or kidney disease) can decrease the amount of protein-bound drug, resulting in the same dose producing a greater effect (Wilkinson, 2001). Other diseases (e.g., cancer and arthritis) can elevate levels of AAG, increasing the protein binding of basic drugs, thereby decreasing the drug's pharmacologic effect (Wilkinson, 2001). Drugs may compete with each other for protein binding, with the result that the drug with the stronger binding affinity may displace the other drug from the binding protein. This could result in the unbound drug exerting a much greater effect on the body when free of its protein binding. This is covered in greater detail in the section on drug interactions.

Lipid solubility is a major determinant of a drug's passage through the blood-brain barrier into the CNS. Generally, only unbound, non-ionized, and lipid-soluble drugs pass through the uniquely configured capillary endothelial lining into the brain. Drugs may also be actively transported into and out of the brain by specific carrier molecules (Wilkinson, 2001). The blood-brain barrier protects the brain from many drugs and chemicals that are ingested into the body. Certain inflammatory disease states can compromise the integrity of the blood-brain barrier (e.g., meningitis and encephalitis) (Wilkinson, 2001).

Aging is usually accompanied by changes in body fat composition. There is generally an increase in body fat and a decrease in lean body mass and total body water (Eddington, 1996; Hammerlein et al, 1998; O'Mahony, 2000). This would result in a higher V_d for lipophilic drugs (e.g., diazepam and lorazepam) and a lower V_d for hydrophilic drugs (e.g., cimetidine and morphine) (O'Mahony, 2000).

The healthy elderly show no changes in plasma binding proteins. Albumin may be reduced in the sick elderly, due to malnutrition or an acute illness. In contrast, AAG can be increased in the sick elderly. The consequence is that basic drugs (e.g., lidocaine and propranolol) will show increased protein binding and less effect (due to increased AAG), and acidic drugs (e.g., warfarin and phenytoin) will show decreased protein binding and greater effect (due to decreased plasma albumin) (Eddington, 1996; Hammerlein et al, 1998; O'Mahony, 2000).

Excretion

The major organ for drug excretion is the kidney. Drugs are either excreted unchanged or as metabolites (Wilkinson, 2001). A few drugs are eliminated through the lungs, as unreabsorbed metabolites in bile and feces, and in breast milk. Very small amounts of drugs and metabolites can also be found in hair, sweat, saliva, tears, and semen.

Renal drug excretion occurs when the drug is passed through the kidney and involves glomerular filtration, active tubular secretion, and passive tubular reabsorption (Wilkinson, 2001). Glomerular filtration is the passage of the drug from the renal capillaries into the glomerulus and depends on the glomerular filtration rate and the extent of protein binding of the drug (Wilkinson, 2001). The process is passive filtration, and only unbound drugs are filtered. Some drugs (e.g., organic cations and amphipathic* anions) are actively secreted into the proximal renal tubule by way of a carrier-mediated process.

*The term *amphipathic* refers to molecules that have a polar water-soluble group attached to a water-insoluble hydrocarbon chain (e.g., soap, detergent).

Conjugated drugs and metabolites are also actively secreted into the proximal tubule.

Active, carrier-mediated drug reabsorption can also occur in the distal renal tubule. Most tubular reabsorption of drugs is passive and occurs by non-ionic diffusion (Wilkinson, 2001). Non-ionized forms of weak acids and bases undergo pH-dependent tubular reabsorption. The ionized form of the drug or metabolite can pass through the tubular wall from urine into the blood or blood into urine. If the pH of fluid is such that the drug or metabolite becomes ionized when it passes into the fluid, the drug or metabolite cannot pass back through the membrane because the ionic charge prevents passage. This process is known as ion trapping and occurs in the kidney between blood and urine and between the gut or stomach and blood. An example of this process is the ion trapping of amphetamine (a weak base) in acidic urine and barbiturate (a weak acid) in basic urine. Amphetamine will reabsorb in basic urine, and barbiturate will reabsorb in acidic urine.

Aging has a considerable impact on renal drug excretion. Adult renal function declines at a rate of about 1% per year after age 20 (Eddington, 1996; Wilkinson, 2001). There is a decline in glomerular filtration rate, renal plasma flow, tubular function, and reabsorptive capacity (Hammerlein et al, 1998). Creatinine clearance (Cl_{cr}) is a measure of renal function. The doses of many renally excreted drugs are based on the patient's measured or estimated creatinine clearance. The Cockcroft and Gault equation estimates creatinine clearance from age, serum creatinine (S_{cr}), and ideal body weight (IBW) (Cockcroft and Gault, 1976). Doses of some hydrophilic drugs are based on lean body weight rather than IBW.

The estimated Cl_{cr} in milliliters per minute (ml/min) is as follows (Semla et al, 2003):

$$\text{Male} = \frac{(140 - \text{age}) \times \text{IBW(kg)}}{72 \times S_{cr}}$$

$$\text{Female} = \text{Male} \times 0.85$$

$$\text{IBW(male)} = 50 + (2.3 \times \text{Height in inches over 5 feet})$$

$$\text{IBW(female)} = 45.5 + (2.3 \times \text{Height in inches over 5 feet})$$

$$\text{Lean body weight} = \text{IBW} + 0.4(\text{Actual body weight} - \text{IBW})$$

PHARMACODYNAMICS

Pharmacodynamics is "a branch of pharmacology dealing with the reactions between drugs and living systems" (Merriam-Webster Online, 2003). It refers to "the biochemical and physiological effects of drugs and their mechanisms of action" (Hohl et al, 2001). Pharmacodynamics is what the drug does to the body. Drugs do not create their own effects unrelated to body systems. They modulate existing physiologic processes by increasing or decreasing their rates or inhibiting them altogether (Hohl et al, 2001). In the case of antibiotics the action of the drug is not on the physiology of the body but on that of the infectious agents (e.g., bacteria, viruses, or parasites).

Physiologic processes occur as a result of body chemicals interacting with receptors. Receptors are generally specifically configured cellular proteins that, because of their shape and charge distribution, bind to specific chemicals. The body chemical structure has a specific shape and a distribution of charged areas within the molecule. The receptor protein has a specific shape that fits the chemical molecule like a glove to a hand. It also has charged areas within the receptor that are opposite in charge to those of the chemical. This is known as the ligand-binding domain (Hohl et al, 2001). When the chemical binds to the receptor a physiologic process is initiated (e.g., nerve conduction and enzyme inhibition). The location on the receptor where the physiologic effect is initiated is the *effector domain* (Hohl et al, 2001).

Drugs are usually similar in chemical configuration or charge distribution to the body chemical such that they bind to the same receptor sites. When they bind to the receptor sites they may initiate the same physiologic action as the chemical (agonist), or they may occupy the receptor sites and not initiate the physiologic action, thus blocking the action of the body chemical (antagonist). Usually a drug will not bind to only one type of receptor, but will attach to various other types of receptors. To the extent that they produce physiologic effects as a result of binding to the other types of receptors they produce unwanted side effects. Changes in the molecular structure of the drug may cause the drug to bind with greater or lesser affinity to the receptor site. Intermediate compounds called *second messengers,* which catalyze ion movement or an enzymatic process, usually mediate the physiologic and biochemical effect (Hohl et al, 2001).

Continuing to stimulate a receptor with an agonist results in desensitization or down-regulation of the receptor. Continuous blocking of a receptor with an antagonist results in sensitization or up-regulation of the receptor (Hohl et al, 2001). Consequently when a drug is given over an extended period of time the dose may need to be increased to maintain the drug effect, because of the change in receptor sensitivity.

The dose-response curve is important to the understanding of receptor pharmacology. It is a graphic depiction of the drug effect as a function of its concentration at the receptor (Hohl et al, 2001). Different drugs have different dose-response curves. Some have increased action directly proportional to the concentration of the drug at the receptor. Some reach a point of saturation and show no further response beyond a certain concentration. Some begin to decrease after an initial increase when concentration exceeds a certain level. Whereas pharmacokinetics determines what drug level occurs at the receptor, pharmacodynamics determines how the receptor responds to that level.

Aging usually results in decreased receptor density (e.g., muscarinic acetylcholine receptors in brain, α_1-adrenergic receptors in liver, and opioid receptors in brain) (Hammerlein et al, 1998). Decreased muscarinic receptors in the brain are associated with decreased memory. Consequently if any of the muscarinic receptors are blocked with muscarinic antagonists (anticholinergic), the memory is further impaired. The elderly are highly sensitive to anticholinergic side effects of drugs. Aging is associated with decreased sympathetic innervation of the juxtaglomerular cells of the kidney, which results in decreased plasma renin levels and decreased blood and urine aldosterone levels (Hammerlein et al, 1998). Baroreceptor reflex responses decrease with age. This causes increased susceptibility to positional changes (orthostatic hypotension) and volume changes (dehydration). Drugs affecting these systems (e.g., diuretics and α_1-adrenergic blockers) have a greater effect in the elderly (Hammerlein et al, 1998; Crome, 2000).

Age-related increases in sympathetic nervous system activity occur as a result of decreased myocardial sensitivity to catecholamines (e.g., norepinephrine and epinephrine) (Hammerlein et al, 1998). This is due to decreases in the ability to activate adenylate cyclase, an enzyme necessary in the generation of cyclic adenosine monophosphate (cAMP), the second messenger for the β-adrenoceptor, rather than because of any decreases in the numbers of β-adrenoceptors (Hammerlein et al, 1998). This decreased responsiveness of the β-adrenergic system results in decreased sensitivity to β-agonists and β-antagonists (β-blockers). Because of the decreased effectiveness of β-blockers and increased sensitivity to diuretics, thiazide diuretics and not β-blockers are recommended for treatment of hypertension in the elderly (Seventh Report of the Joint National Committee, 2003; Crome, 2000).

PROBLEMS WITH DRUG THERAPY AND THEIR PREVENTION

The elderly tend to have more adverse drug reactions (ADRs) than younger patients (Crome, 2000). In one study, 20% of those over 70 years old developed an ADR (Crome, 2000). ADRs contributed to hospital admission in 24% of patients age 70 and older in another study (Mannesse et al, 1997). In one hospital the average age of the patients who had ADRs was 67 years (Buffum, 2003). In 1994, 2,216,000 hospitalized U.S. patients suffered a serious ADR, almost half (over 1,000,000) of them fatal (Gruchalla, 2000). A large study of elderly, ambulatory Medicare patients found 1523 ADRs. Of those, 421 (27.6%) were preventable (Gurwitz et al, 2003).

Because the elderly tend to have more chronic problems, they take a greater number of drugs. The greater number of drugs predisposes them to more drug-drug and drug-food interactions. As a result of the increasing popularity of dietary herbal supplements, there is also a real probability of drug-herbal interactions (Lambrecht et al, 2000; Shader and Greenblatt, 2000; Izzo and Ernst, 2001; Scott and Elmer, 2002; Valli and Giardina, 2002). More food-drug interactions are also being recognized (Schmidt and Dalhoff, 2002). Checking with the pharmacist or a reference book such as *Drug Interaction Facts 2003* may prevent such interactions (Tatro, 2003).

Age-related pharmacokinetic and pharmacodynamic changes may mean that the elderly should take lower dosages of drugs, especially when starting a drug regimen. When providing care to anyone over 65 years of age, starting drug dosages should be verified as appropriate. Checking with the pharmacist or a reference book such as the *Geriatric Dosage Handbook* is always prudent (Semla et al, 2003).

Adverse Drug Reactions

ADRs can usually be predicted from the pharmacologic action of the drug (e.g., bone marrow depression from cancer chemotherapy and bleeding from warfarin). A lesser number are unpredictable and have nothing to do with the action of the drug (e.g., hives from penicillin and bone marrow depression from methimazole). These reactions may be due to allergic or autoimmune processes.

ADRs that are extensions of the drug's pharmacology may not always be predictable. An elderly patient who is well controlled on a stable dose of a drug may undergo a change in his or her environment such that the relationship with the drug is altered. Changes in diet can have a profound impact on drug regimens (e.g., decreased salt intake causing lithium toxicity and increased leafy green vegetables counteracting anticoagulant effects of warfarin) (Lacy et al, 2003). Some drugs interfere with the body's ability to regulate temperature such that hot weather can lead to heat stroke (e.g., antipsychotics and stimulants) (Semla et al, 2003). Some drugs are photosensitizing, and an increase in sun exposure can lead to sunburn much more quickly than expected (e.g., sulfa drugs and antidepressants) (Semla et al, 2003) (Box 10-1). Elderly patients who decrease their fluid intake because of illness or

Box 10-1 Drugs with Potential for Causing Photosensitivity*

Drug Classes	Individual Drugs
Anticancer agents	Amiodarone
Antidepressants	Atorvastatin
Antihistamines	Benzocaine
Antihyperlipidemics	Captopril
Antimicrobials	Chlordiazepoxide
Antiparasitics	Diltiazem
Antipsychotics	Disopyramide
Antiseizure agents	Enalapril
Diuretics	Estazolam
Hypoglycemics	Estrogen
NSAIDs	Fluvastatin
Saquinavir	Gold sodium thiomalate
Selegiline	Hexachlorophene
Simvastatin	Lovastatin
Zolpidem	PABA
	Pravastatin
	Quinidine

From Semla TP, Beizer JL, Higbee MD: *Geriatric dosage handbook*, ed 8, Cleveland, 2003, Lexi-Comp, Inc.

*These classes of drugs contain specific medications that can increase sensitivity to ultraviolet light. (For specific drugs under these classes, consult *Geriatric Dosage Handbook.*)

inadequate intake during hot weather may become volume depleted and develop increased sensitivity to the orthostatic hypotensive effects of α-blockers (e.g., phenothiazines and terazosin) (Lacy et al, 2003).

More predictable ADRs can occur when a patient is started on a drug at a dose that is inappropriately high, or one that requires laboratory monitoring that is not done. A good example of this is seen in the case of the elderly hypertensive patient (more than 80 years old) started on hydrochlorothiazide (25 mg) for blood pressure control. Within a month the patient came to the emergency department with mental status changes and severe hyponatremia (Buffum, 2003). The recommended starting geriatric dose of hydrochlorothiazide is 12.5 to 25 mg daily (Semla et al, 2003). Because the elderly show an increased susceptibility to thiazide-induced hyponatremia, it may be prudent to either start at the 12.5 mg dose or monitor the patient's serum sodium, or both (Clark et al, 1994).

Another example of inappropriate dosing is the case of a 75-year-old man admitted to an orthopedic ward for a procedure. Because of the man's high level of anxiety about being in the hospital, he was given a total of 20 mg of diazepam over a 12-hour period. The following day the man wandered off the ward and was not seen again until he came to the emergency department with sore feet, 5 days later. He had been wandering the streets with no idea of where he was or how he got there (Buffum, 2003). The elderly man had been given an inappropriate dose of a long-acting benzodiazepine, which had caused delirium and anterograde amnesia. Table 10-1 provides dosages of psychoactive medications for older persons.

Drug-Drug Interactions

The more medications a person takes, the greater the probability that one or more of those drugs will interact with another drug the person is taking. In one study, 50% of the elderly patients (over 65 years old) treated in an emergency department for an adverse drug-related event had an unrelated potential adverse drug interaction (Hohl et al, 2001). About 31% of all the patients had one or more potential adverse drug interactions.

In pharmacokinetic interactions one drug alters the absorption, distribution, metabolism, or excretion of another drug (Hartshorn and Tatro, 2003). In pharmacodynamic interactions one drug alters the patient's response to another drug without changing any of the pharmacokinetic parameters.

Altered absorption can occur when one drug binds another drug (chelation) in the small intestine to form a nonabsorbable compound (e.g., tetracycline and calcium carbonate or ciprofloxacin and iron compounds). Separating the administration of the two drugs by 2 hours or longer can prevent such interactions.

The mechanism for altered distribution may be due to displacement of one drug from its receptor site, from plasma albumin, or from α_1-acid glycoprotein binding by another drug. These interaction rarely cause problems clinically (McElnay and D'Arcy, 1983; Israili and Dayton, 2001; Hartshorn and Tatro, 2003).

Altered metabolism can occur when one drug increases (induction) or decreases (inhibition) the metabolism of another drug (Flockhart, 2003; Hartshorn and Tatro, 2003). Drugs may induce or inhibit the specific CYP450 isoenzymes responsible for metabolizing another drug. One drug may inhibit the metabolism of another drug if they are both substrates for the same metabolic pathway. Table 10-2 shows examples of some of the drugs that are inhibitors, inducers, or substrates of specific CYP450 isoenzymes. These are only a few examples. For a more complete listing see Hartshorn and Tatro's table in *Drug Interaction Facts, 2003* (Hartshorn and Tatro, 2003) or Flockhart's table at *http://medicine.iupui.edu/flockhart* (Flockhart, 2003).

When interpreting CYP450 tables it is important to understand that not all drugs that induce or inhibit a CYP450 isoenzyme do so equally. Some are far more potent than others. A drug may also be a substrate for more than one CYP450 isoenzyme; that is, it may have multiple metabolic pathways. In general, enzyme induction may take time to develop. Enzyme inhibition occurs immediately. Some drugs may induce their own metabolism (e.g., modafinil), and some drugs inhibit their own metabolism (e.g., fluoxetine) (Lacy et al, 2003).

Altered excretion can occur when one drug changes the urinary pH such that another drug is either reabsorbed or excreted to a greater extent (e.g., sodium bicarbonate raises urinary pH, resulting in greater reabsorption of amphetamine and thereby prolonging its half-life) (Hartshorn and Tatro, 2003). Another mechanism may involve one drug increasing or decreasing the active transport in the renal tubules (e.g., probenecid decreases the active transport of penicillin, thereby prolonging its half-life) (Hartshorn and Tatro, 2003).

Pharmacodynamic drug interactions include the additive pharmacologic effects of two or more similar drugs (e.g., additive CNS effects of sedative-hypnotic drugs or anticholinergic drugs used simultaneously) (Hartshorn and Tatro, 2003).

Natural Product–Drug Interactions

The passage of the Dietary Supplement Health and Education Act (DESHEA) in 1994 allowed the marketing of natural herbal supplements without FDA oversight. Unless an herbal product can be shown to be harmful, the FDA has no control over its sale and use (Scott and Elmer, 2002). Many natural products interact with over-the-counter and prescription drugs to produce adverse effects. Because of the lack of regulation, dietary supplement manufacturers are not required to label their products with warnings of side effects or interactions with drugs. See further discussion in Chapter 11.

There may be considerable variation in the content of the active herb between different manufacturers of similar products. This has great bearing on both therapeutic outcome and potential for natural product-drug interactions. The ingredient of St. John's wort responsible for its antidepressant effect is hyperforin (de los Reyes and Koda, 2002). Hyperforin also

Table 10-1 Geriatric Dosages for Common Psychoactive Medications

Category	Drug	Recommended to maximum daily dose for persons older than 65 years	Starting dose in persons with dementia/daily dose
Antipsychotic	Haloperidol	50-100 mg	0.5 mg qd/4 mg
	Fluphenazine	20-40 mg	1 mg qd/4 mg
	Clozapine	25-450 mg	12.5 mg qd/50 mg
	Olanzepine	10-15 mg	2.5 mg qd
	Quetiapine	300-400 mg	12.5 mg hs
	Risperidone	1-16 mg	0.5 mg qd/2 mg
	Ziprasidone	20-80 mg bid (in divided doses, gradually increasing dose) No dosage change for elderly May have antidepressant properties	

Category	Drug	Recommended to maximum daily dose for persons older than 65 years	Starting dose for depression in elderly
Antidepressant	Buproprion	225-450 mg	50-100 mg qd
	Citalopram	20-60 mg	20 mg qd
	Fluoxetine	20-80 mg	10 mg qAM
	Fluvoxamine	100-300 mg	25 mg qhs
	Paroxetine	20-40 mg	10 mg qAM
	Sertraline	50-100 mg	25 mg qAM
	Venlafaxine	75-375 mg	25 mg bid-tid 37.5 mg qd XR (time release)
	Nefazodone	300-600 mg	50 mg bid
	Trazodone	150-600 mg	25 mg hs up to tid
	Mirtazapine	15-45 mg	7.5 mg qhs

Category	Drug	Geriatric daily dosage range	Starting dose in elderly with dementia
Anxiolytic	Alprazolam	0.25-0.75 mg	0.25 mg bid
	Clonazepam	0.5-1.5 mg	0.25 mg bid
	Lorazepam	0.5-2 mg	0.5 mg qd
Sedative/Hypnotic	Triazolam	0.0625-0.125 mg	0.125 mg hs
	Temazepam	7.5-15 mg	7.5 mg hs

Data from Maletta G, Mattox KM, Dysken M: Guidelines for prescribing psychoactive drugs, *Geriatrics* 55(3): 65-69, 2000; Semla TP, Beizer JL, Higbee MD: *Geriatric dosage handbook,* ed 8, Cleveland, 2003, Lexi-Comp, Inc.; Sadock B, Sadock V: *Pocket handbook of psychiatric drug treatment,* ed 3, New York, 2001, Lippincott Williams & Wilkins.

interacts with other drugs through its induction of both CYP3A4 and P-glycoprotein (P-gp) (Scott and Elmer, 2002). P-glycoprotein is a cell membrane-localized protein that functions as a transporter for drug substrates in organs that influence drug absorption, CNS penetration, or excretion (Matheny et al, 2001). One analysis of eight commercial St. John's wort preparations determined that the hyperforin content ranged from 0.01% to 1.89%, almost a 200-fold difference (de los Reyes and Koda, 2002). Another study of eight commercially available German St. John's wort preparations showed a range of less than 0.5 mg to 12.43 mg of hyperforin per dosage unit (a 25-fold difference), with wide variations between different batches from the same company (Wurglics et al, 2001). The lack of standardization increases the possibility of an adverse drug event or interaction. St. John's wort is known to decrease blood levels of indinavir (for treatment of human immunodeficiency virus infection) and cyclosporin (for organ transplants) through induction of CYP3A4 and decrease digoxin levels through induction of P-gp (Scott and Elmer, 2002).

Ginkgo biloba, a nutritional supplement touted for maintaining optimal cognitive function in the elderly, interacts with the anticoagulant warfarin to increase the international normalized ratio (INR; used to monitor warfarin effect) or cause a bleed when it is added to a stable warfarin regimen (Scott and Elmer, 2002; Valli and Giardina, 2002). Many elderly patients take warfarin for thrombosis or for atrial fibrillation. Such patients should not take ginkgo, not only because of the interaction, but also because "ginkgo provides no measurable benefit in memory or related cognitive function to adults with healthy cognitive function" (Solomon, 2002).

Glucosamine, a nutritional supplement touted for maintaining optimal joint function, can cause decreased glucose

Table 10-2 Cytochrome P450 Drug Interactions

CYP450 isoenzyme	Inhibitor	Inducer	Substrate
1A2	Ciprofloxacin	Phenobarbital	Clozapine
	Amiodarone	Rifampin	Caffeine
	Cimetidine	Omeprazole	Ondansetron
	Ticlopidine		Clomipramine
	Fluvoxamine		Zolpidem
	Methoxsalen		Tacrine
2A6	Ketoconazole	None	Ritonavir
	Methoxsalen		Tamoxifen
	Miconazole Ritonavir		
	Pilocarpine		
2B6	Diethyldithiocarbamate	Phenobarbital	Bupropion
	Orphenadrine	Rifampin	Tamoxifen
	Thiotepa	Phenytoin	Ifosfamide
		Primidone	Cyclophosphamide
2C8	Omeprazole	Primidone	Omeprazole
	Diethyldithiocarbamate		Diazepam
	Anastrozole		Isotretinoin
			Diclofenac
			Benzphetamine Isotretinoin
2C9	Amiodarone	Carbamazepine	Ibuprofen
	Teniposide	Ethanol	Diclofenac
	Sulfamethoxazole	Phenytoin	Tolbutamide
	Ritonavir	Secobarbital	Piroxicam
	Trimethoprim	Rifampin	Glipizide
	Isoniazid		Losartan
2C18	Cimetidine	None	Naproxen
			Retinoic Acid
			Piroxicam
			S-warfarin
			S-tetrahydrocannabinol
2C19	Felbamate	Rifampin	Citalopram
	Indomethacin	Prednisone	Lansoprazole
	Fluvoxamine	Carbamazepine	Clomipramine
	Cimetidine	Norethindrone	Omeprazole
	Topiramate		Valproic acid
	Ticlopidine		Nelfinavir
2D6	Fluoxetine	Dexamethasone	Codeine
	Amiodarone	Rifampin(?)	Sertraline
	Methadone		Methamphetamine
	Celecoxib		Tramadol
	Quinidine		Haloperidol
	Carvedilol		Lidocaine
2E1	Diethyldithiocarbamate	Ethanol	Acetaminophen
	Disulfiram	Isoniazid	Ethanol
	Ritonavir		Isoniazid
			Halothane
			Theophylline
			Sevoflurane
3A3	Cimetidine	None	Erythromycin
	Nefazodone		Midazolam
	Ranitidine		
3A4	Erythromycin	Carbamazepine	Alprazolam
	Norfloxacin	Phenobarbital	Nicardipine
	Nefazodone	Dexamethasone	Midazolam
	Fluvoxamine	Rifampin	Erythromycin
	Ketoconazole	Prednisone	Nifedipine
	Nelfinavir	Phenytoin	Triazolam

tolerance by causing increased insulin resistance (Scott and Elmer, 2002). Glucosamine can interfere with the treatment of diabetes.

These interactions represent only a small fraction of the many real and potential nutritional supplement-drug interactions. Because of inadequate labeling requirements, drug interactions may not be listed on the product labels of these herbal supplements. Both patients and prescribers should check to see if a supplement might interfere with the therapeutic action of drug regimens before taking the supplement.

Food-Drug Interactions

Foods may interact with drugs to increase or decrease the effect of the drug. Such interactions may be pharmacokinetic or pharmacodynamic in nature (Gauthier and Malone, 1998; Schmidt and Dalhoff, 2002). Pharmacokinetic interactions may result in increased or decreased absorption, metabolism, or excretion. Pharmacodynamic interactions potentiate or antagonize the action of the drug.

Foods can bind (chelate) to drugs, preventing their absorption. Calcium in dairy products will bind tetracycline and ciprofloxacin, greatly decreasing their absorption (Gauthier and Malone, 1998; Schmidt and Dalhoff, 2002). Other drugs must be taken with food to enhance their absorption. Lovastatin absorption is increased by a high-fat, low-fiber meal (Gauthier and Malone, 1998; Schmidt and Dalhoff, 2002). Saquinavir dissolution and absorption is enhanced by a high-fat meal (Lacy et al, 2003; Schmidt and Dalhoff, 2002).

Certain foods inhibit the metabolism of some drugs whereas other foods induce the metabolism of other drugs. Grapefruit juice contains substances that inhibit CYP3A4-mediated metabolism in the gut (Greenblatt et al, 2001). Blood levels of amiodarone, lovastatin, simvastatin, and buspirone are greatly increased by concomitant administration (within 24 hours) of grapefruit juice (Greenblatt et al, 2001). Broccoli, Brussels sprouts, and char-grilled meat all induce CYP1A2 metabolism (Flockhart, 2003). Because CYP1A2 mediates the major metabolic route of metabolism for both theophylline and clozapine, ingestion of those particular foods might result in subtherapeutic blood levels (Hartshorn and Tatro, 2003).

Certain foods antagonize the therapeutic action of a drug. The vitamin K in leafy green vegetables antagonizes the anticoagulant effects of warfarin (Gauthier and Malone, 1998; Schmidt and Dalhoff, 2002). It is recommended that patients on warfarin ingest a consistent amount of greens and not radically increase or decrease the amount they eat (Lacy et al, 2003).

Some foods greatly increase the action of a drug, sometimes resulting in toxicity. Lithium ions (Li^+) and sodium ions (Na^+) compete for excretion by the kidney. When a person greatly decreases salt (NaCl) intake (low-salt diet) or increases salt excretion through sweating, the kidney attempts to conserve salt by tubular reabsorption. Thus when a patient on lithium carbonate decreases salt intake or increases salt excretion, the kidney stops excreting lithium, resulting in lithium toxicity (Atherton et al, 1990). Spironolactone causes increased potassium (K^+) reabsorption by the renal tubule. If a patient ingests a diet high in potassium (KCl salt substitute, molasses, oranges, or bananas) while taking spironolactone, toxic K^+ levels could occur (Lacy et al, 2003).

Drug Allergy

An allergic reaction to a drug can occur following prior or continuous exposure to the drug. This can happen if the drug or its metabolite is an antigen or combines with an endogenous protein to form an antigenic complex (Klaassen, 2001). The antigen or antigenic complex can induce the development of antibodies in 1 to 2 weeks. When the patient is exposed to the drug again or if exposed continuously, an antigen-antibody reaction may occur, with resultant allergic response.

It is noteworthy that these reactions subside within 1 to 3 weeks after discontinuing contact with the offending irritant.

Coombs and Gell Classification of Allergic Response (Gruchalla, 2000; Choquet-Kastylevsky et al, 2001; Klaassen, 2001).

Type I. Immediate hypersensitivity reactions, characterized by anaphylaxis and urticaria and mediated by IgE antibodies (e.g., penicillin). These subside within a few days after discontinuing the drug.

Type II. Cytolytic reactions, characterized by destruction of cells in the circulatory system and mediated by IgG and IgM antibodies (e.g., cephalosporin-induced hemolytic anemia). These subside within several months after discontinuing the drug.

Type III. Arthus reactions or serum sickness, characterized by skin eruptions, arthralgia or arthritis, lymphadenopathy, and fever and mediated by IgG (e.g., sulfonamides). These subside within 6 to 12 days after discontinuing the drug.

Type IV. Delayed hypersensitivity reactions or contact dermatitis, characterized by an inflammatory skin reaction and mediated by sensitized T lymphocytes and macrophages (e.g., poison oak).

It has been estimated that about 1% to 1.5% of hospitalized patients have an adverse drug reaction that may be allergic or immunologic in nature (Gruchalla, 2000). There are no specific statistics on how many of these may occur in the elderly. The elderly make up a greater percentage of the hospitalized patient population and the elderly are exposed to more drugs, so a disproportionate share of allergic reactions may occur in that population.

Taking an adequate drug and allergy history plays a great role in preventing allergic reactions. Patients should be asked if they have ever had an allergic reaction to a drug or food. They should also be asked if they have ever been given penicillins, cephalosporins, quinolones, sulfas, gentamicin, erythromycin, intravenous iodinated contrast media, local anesthetics, nonsteroidal antiinflammatory drugs (NSAIDs), and opiates. Sometimes a patient will say that he or she is allergic to a drug such as penicillin, but may say that he or she has had another penicillin without a reaction. One such patient developed a rash with intramuscular procaine penicillin but not oral penicillin V. It was determined that this patient was allergic to procaine (Buffum, 2003). Some patients will state that they are allergic to a drug when they became nauseated or vomited after taking it. Such a reaction would be drug intolerance rather than an allergy. Opiates cause histamine release. This is a pharmacologic effect of the drug, not an allergy. *It is important to record the type of allergic reaction the patient had, when the patient had it, how long it lasted, and how it was treated.* It is important to ask about food allergies such as eggs, shellfish, tomatoes, strawberries, dairy products, and nuts. Because of the common presence of latex in the clinic or hospital environment, latex allergy must be asked about. Allergy information should be entered into the patient's chart, on the front of the patient's chart, and into the patient's computerized record.

Drugs and Sexuality

Many drugs can affect human sexual response, for better or for worse. Sexual dysfunction usually has many risk factors associated with its occurrence (Buffum et al, 1988; Buffum, 1992, 1999; Melman and Christ, 2002).

Male Sexual Function. The male sexual response consists of increased sexual desire (or libido), erection, ejaculation, and orgasm. Central nervous system dopaminergic and serotonergic neurons and testosterone mediate sexual desire. Drugs that decrease dopamine (antipsychotics) or increase serotonin (selective serotonin reuptake inhibitors [SSRIs]) may decrease sexual desire (Buffum, 1992). Drugs that increase dopamine (amphetamine, cocaine, or L-dopa) may increase sexual desire (Buffum et al, 1988; Buffum, 1999). Drugs that lower testosterone (ketoconazole and antipsychotics) may decrease sexual desire, whereas testosterone administration may increase sexual desire.

Erection is due to innervation of nonadrenergic, noncholinergic, parasympathetic nerves resulting in dilation of penile (helicine) arterioles and relaxation of smooth muscle of the corpora cavernosa (penile spongy tissue) (Melman and Christ, 2002). These events result in accumulation of blood under pressure within the corpora. The corpora are surrounded with an inelastic sheath so the penis becomes rigid. This process is dependent on normal blood supply and nervous innervation. Penile flaccidity is due to α_1-adrenergic (sympathetic) nervous innervation causing contraction of corporeal smooth muscle with subsequent release of blood from the spongy tissue (Melman and Christ, 2002). Drugs or disease states that interfere with the blood supply (antihypertensives, alcohol, nicotine, or atherosclerosis) or nervous innervation (pseudoephedrine or diabetes) can cause erectile dysfunction (impotence) (Buffum et al, 1988; Buffum, 1992, 1999; Melman and Christ, 2002). Drugs that increase blood supply to the corpora (sildenafil, alprostadil) can enhance erectile function (Melman and Christ, 2002). Priapism, or prolonged painful erection, unaccompanied by sexual desire, may occur following use of α_1-adrenergic blocking agents (trazodone and antipsychotics) (Buffum, 1992). Priapism is a surgical emergency, and patients need to be warned to get to an emergency department should they experience it.

The ejaculatory phase consists of two parts: emission and ejaculation proper. Emission is the movement of seminal fluid through rhythmic contractions of the epididymis, vas deferens, and prostate into the posterior urethra (Buffum, 1992). This is mediated by parasympathetic (cholinergic) and α_1-adrenergic sympathetic innervation. Ejaculation occurs when the internal urethral sphincter closes and the seminal fluid is propelled out of the urethra with rhythmic contractions of the ischiocavernosus and bulbocavernosus muscles at the base of the penis (Buffum, 1992). Drugs that interfere with emission (α_1-adrenergic blockers such as phenoxybenzamine or thioridazine) can decrease or eliminate emission, resulting in orgasm with no ejaculation. Rarely, retrograde ejaculation (ejaculation back into the bladder) can occur when a drug interferes with internal urethral sphincter closure. This is more common following surgical procedures on the prostate (Buffum, 1992).

Orgasm usually accompanies ejaculation in males, although they may occur separately. Orgasm has been described by many but has not been clearly physiologically defined (Mah and Binik, 2001). The process can be described as an intensely pleasurable psychologic and physical event resulting from sexual stimulation. Orgasm and ejaculation are followed by the relaxation phase and penile detumescence.

Drugs alone may not always cause sexual dysfunction. There are usually other risk factors present. Age, diabetes, atherosclerosis, tobacco or alcohol use, illegal drug use, depression, anxiety, or lack of attraction for a partner may all contribute to sexual dysfunction.

Female Sexual Function. The female sexual response consists of increased sexual desire (or libido), clitoral erection with labial engorgement, lubrication, and orgasm. Some women experience ejaculation with orgasm. Sexual desire in women is mediated by central nervous system dopaminergic and serotonergic neurons and testosterone as in men. Drugs that decrease dopamine (antipsychotics) or increase serotonin (SSRIs) may decrease sexual desire (Buffum, 1992). Drugs that increase dopamine (amphetamine, cocaine, or L-dopa) may increase sexual desire (Buffum et al, 1988; Buffum, 1999). Drugs that lower testosterone (ketoconazole and antipsychotics) may decrease sexual desire, whereas testosterone administration may increase sexual desire.

Clitoral erection, labial engorgement, and lubrication are mediated by the same nervous innervation as erection in males. Clitoral erection is due to innervation of nonadrenergic, noncholinergic, parasympathetic nerves resulting in dilation of clitoral arterioles and relaxation of smooth muscle clitoral spongy tissue (Melman and Christ, 2002). These events result in accumulation of blood under pressure within the tissue and erection. The same innervation causes labial and perivaginal engorgement, resulting in vaginal transudation or lubrication

(Buffum, 1992; Melman and Christ, 2002). Drugs and disease states that negatively affect male erection may also decrease the female response (alcohol).

Female orgasm is governed by similar processes as in the male. Vaginal contractions occur, accompanied by intensely pleasurable psychologic and physiologic feelings (Mah and Binik, 2001). Drugs that delay or inhibit ejaculation and orgasm in men may also delay or inhibit orgasm in women (alcohol, amphetamines, and SSRIs) (Buffum et al, 1988; Buffum, 1992; Mah and Binik, 2001).

The risk factors for sexual dysfunction in women are the same as those for men. Because women do not require the same level of hemodynamic functioning that penile erection requires, they may not be as sensitive to those risk factors as men are (Buffum, 1992).

NURSING ROLE AND INTERVENTIONS

The nurse is key as an interdisciplinary member in preventing drug problems. Nurses educate patients about the safe use and administration of medications. Perhaps more visible in institutional care, the nurse is part of an interdisciplinary team and works with the physician, pharmacist, and dietitian to teach, monitor, and promote the actions necessary to prevent drugs from becoming toxic and to treat toxicity promptly should it occur. In all settings, the vital nursing functions in educating patients are ensuring that the patient understands the purpose and side effects of the medications and assisting the patient and family in adapting the medication regimen to functional ability and lifestyle.

Monitoring

The most effective way to prevent or minimize drug effects is by monitoring the patient. Monitoring involves making astute observations and documenting those observations, noting changes in physical and functional status (e.g., vital signs, performance of activities of daily living, sleeping, eating, hydrating, and eliminating), and mental status (e.g., attention and level of alertness, memory, orientation, behavior, mood, emotional display and affect, and content and characteristics of interactions). Some of these observations need to be made in conversation with the patient; if the patient is not able to participate, the nurse should involve a caregiver or someone closely familiar with the patient. Monitoring involves nursing knowledge, an ability to attribute patient changes to signs and symptoms of problems with the drugs. Communication of observations through documentation and physician interaction follows when problematic changes are detected. (See Tables 10-3, 10-4, and 10-5 for monitoring parameters of general and psychiatric drugs.)

Advocacy Role

The nurse acts as advocate in all clinical settings. An advocate functions to support the patient, ensuring that the patient's best interest is reflected in all care planned and given. This is translated into safe medication practices. To be an effective advocate, the nurse has awareness of the elder's overall functioning, and this is usually obtained through personal clinical experience, observation, chart review, and caregiver assistance. With knowledge about the patient's needs, the nurse can have a positive impact on the therapeutic goal setting involved in interdisciplinary treatment planning and can coordinate other providers' activities to keep the focus on the patient and family goals. An example of optimal safe medication monitoring that would apply to some medications is using a blood level to determine whether a therapeutic parameter has been attained. Advocacy for the patient extends to the interdisciplinary team and the patient and family. Box 10-2 illustrates considerations when medicating elders.

PATTERNS OF DRUG USE

In the United States, persons 65 years of age and older are the largest users of prescription and over-the-counter (OTC) medications. In a 1999 survey, 53% of older persons took 3 or more medications, and 33% took 8 or more; these included both prescription and OTC medications (Preventing medication errors in the elderly, 2002). Because of multiple medical conditions, elders are likely to require different medications concurrently. As of 1998, persons in this age-group took concurrently an average of 4.5 prescription medications and 2 OTC medications (Besdine et al, 1998). These authors estimate that the elderly use at least 25% of all OTC medications for their conditions, including arthritis, insomnia, and pain (Besdine et al, 1998). How elders use their prescribed medicines and their OTC drugs depends on many factors related to their own unique characteristics and situations, beliefs and understanding about illness, functional and cognitive status, perception about necessity of the drugs, severity of symptoms, reactions to the medications, finances, access, alternatives, and compatibility with lifestyle. The provider-patient relationship can be a motivating force for some persons to adhere to their medication regimen (Balkrishnan, 1998; Ciechanowski et al, 2001).

Polypharmacy

Polypharmacy occurs when providers prescribe more than one medication of the same class for a condition. The prescription can apply to using several drugs for the treatment of each of several conditions. Polypharmacy also applies to patients' concurrent mixing of OTC, nutritional supplements, or herbal products with their prescription medications for the same conditions. Polypharmacy stems from the prescribing methods of physicians, the beliefs and practices of the elder, and the ever-increasing practice of seeing more than one primary care provider, each of whom prescribes the same or similar class drugs. Polypharmacy leaves aged patients vulnerable to excessive dose, drug interactions, and dangerous adverse reactions.

The practice of polypharmacy is based on a philosophy and belief that individual drug receptors can be affected and

Table 10-3 Determining Whether the Drug Is Working: Monitoring Parameters and Common Side Effects of General Drug Categories

Class of drug	Monitoring activity	Common side effects
Antibiotics and antivirals	Improvement of infection: symptom reduction Take complete prescription	Change in normal flora: yeast infections in mouth or vagina, diarrhea
Antihyperlipidemics	Lipid profile (specific drug is matched to lipid profile) Modify changeable risks: lifestyle changes (exercise, smoking cessation); dietary alterations (decreased fat intake, eliminate trans-fat products); gradual improvement in low-density lipoprotein (LDL) and high-density lipoprotein (HDL) levels, see change within 2-4 weeks Monitor liver function and blood glucose	Statins: muscle weakness, aches Niacin: muscle weakness, aches; flushing (hot flashes); diabetes symptoms
Cardiac medications	Maintenance of baseline (normal) heart rate and rhythm	Mental status change visual changes Bradycardia Fever, chills
Anticoagulants	Clotting times (international normalized ratio [INR], protime)	Bleeding, bruising, blood in stool
Anticonvulsants	Blood levels Decrease seizure activity	Sedation Mental status changes
Antihypertensives	Maintenance of normal blood pressure CNS effects Intake and output Weight	Diuretics: postural hypotension, bradycardia, hypokalemia β-Blockers: bradycardia, hypotension, chest pain, constipation, diarrhea, nausea, mental status changes (insomnia, confusion, depression, lethargy)
Hypoglycemics	Blood glucose	Hypoglycemia, allergic reactions to beef or pork insulin
Antineoplastics	Cancer activity Bone marrow suppression, laboratory values (e.g., white blood cell [WBC] count)	Nausea, vomiting, diarrhea, signs of infection, hair loss, fatigue
Antihistaminics	Relief from allergy symptoms such as rhinitis	Drowsiness, blurred vision, confusion
Antiarthritics	Relief from arthritis symptoms such as pain and inflammation	Gastrointestinal (GI) problems, depression, personality disturbance, irritability, toxic psychoses
Antiparkinsonians	Improved functional status Less visible immobility; improved mobility	Nausea, hypotension, dyskinesia, agitation, restlessness, insomnia
Cholinergic agents (antidementia medications)	Improved mental status in mildly and moderately demented patients	Nausea, diarrhea, anorexia, weight loss, bradycardia, hypotension, headache, fatigue, depression
Analgesics	Improved symptoms of pain and inflammation	NSAIDs: GI distress Opiates: constipation, sedation, confusion, decreased respiration

From Semla TP, Beizer JL, Higbee MD: *Geriatric dosage handbook,* ed 8, Cleveland, 2003, Lexi-Comp, Inc.

stimulated to achieve a desired effect. In reality, most drugs react to many receptors. One of the drugs may inhibit the metabolism of the other drug, or the two drugs may have additive effects. An example of polypharmacy is the concomitant use of two antidepressants. This might happen when a patient complains of the sexual side effects of fluoxetine. Bupropion does not have the same sexual side effects. Hence, the thinking in polypharmacy is that bupropion will counteract the undesirable side effect of fluoxetine. However, both of the drugs affect many different receptors and the drug metabolites may also affect many receptors. Consequently, the desired sexual function may not be affected at all. Further, the concomitant use of both drugs may cause other side effects, such as nervousness, irritability, or anxiety.

A patient can practice polypharmacy without knowing that she or he could cause harm. For example, the concomitant use of a prescribed antidepressant, such as fluoxetine, with an OTC herbal product, such as St. John's wort, can produce synergistic SSRI side effects. A patient or family caregiver may be desperate and despondent in waiting for depression to lift. Because most antidepressants take about 4 to 6 weeks or longer before patients feel the benefits, it would be easy to begin the "natural" product available over the counter. In reality, the two medications are synergistic and can create

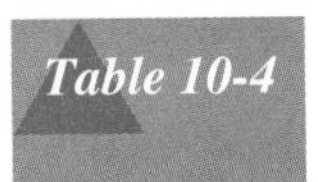

Table 10-4 Drugs That May Cause Psychiatric Symptoms in Elders

Drug category	Examples
Amphetamine-like drugs	Dextroamphetamine
Angiotensin-converting enzyme (ACE) inhibitors	Lisinopril
Anticholinergics	Atropine
Antiepileptics or antiseizure drugs	Phenobarbital, diazepam
Antiparkinsonian drugs	Trihexyphenidyl
Antipsychotics	High risk in anticholinergic antipsychotics: chlorpromazine, clozapine, thioridazine Low risk in less anticholinergic antipsychotics: risperidone
Barbiturates	Phenobarbital
Benzodiazepines	Diazepam
β-Blockers	Propranolol
β-Lactam antibiotics	Cefazolin
Calcium channel blockers	Verapamil
Cholinesterase inhibitors	Donepezil, tacrine
Corticosteroids	Dexamethasone
Fluoroquinolones	Ciprofloxacin
Histamine H_1–receptor blocker	Diphenhydramine
Histamine H_2–receptor blocker	Cimetidine
Monoamine oxidase (MAO) inhibitors	Parnate
Nonsteroidal antiinflammatory drugs (NSAIDs)	Indomethacin
Opioid agonists	Methadone
Salicylates	Aspirin
Selective serotonin reuptake inhibitors (SSRIs)	Fluoxetine, sertraline
Sulfonamides	Sulfamethoxazole
Thiazide diuretic	HydroDiuril
Tricyclic antidepressants (TCAs)	Amitriptyline

Specific drugs known to cause psychiatric symptoms
Caffeine
Amantadine
Bupropion
Chloroquine
Digoxin
Disulfiram
Deet
Clonidine
Isoniazid
Levodopa
Sildenafil
Venlafaxine
Zolpidem
Selegiline
Trimethoprim-sulfamethoxazole
Theophylline
Erythropoietin
Trazodone

Sources: Drugs that may cause cognitive disorders in the elderly, *Medical Letter* 42(1093):111-112, 2000; Drugs that may cause psychiatric symptoms, *Medical Letter* 44(1134):59, 2002.

uncomfortable side effects such as nervousness, irritability, or anxiety, or serious side effects such as delirium and psychosis, as part of the serotonin syndrome.

Polypharmacy should not be confused with the concomitant use of drugs in many conditions. For example, in pain control, different classes of drugs are combined to treat pain as in the case of NSAIDs and opioids. Similarly, asthma is treated with several drugs and often two types of inhalers. This is the case in congestive heart failure also. Different drugs act on the body differently. Polypharmacy is counterproductive because drug mixtures from the same class can be additive or can prevent the action of another, with the end result that it is difficult to determine which drug caused the side effect.

Self-Prescribing of Medications: Prescription, Over-the-Counter, and Herbal Drugs

Despite Medicare, the cost of medications continues to rise. Physician reimbursement for patient visits is low, and the number of physicians who will accept Medicare as total reimbursement continues to decrease markedly. So elders may not seek or obtain medical assistance because of the out-of-pocket cost, or they may not want to bother the physician unless they are very ill. They medicate themselves with former prescriptions, prescriptions borrowed from friends, or OTC drugs. Likewise, self-treatment includes purchasing herbal and nutritional supplements, which may be recommended by acquaintances and are thought to be harmless because they are "natural." See Chapter 11.

Symptoms experienced by elderly persons include pain and discomfort, constipation, indigestion, insomnia, fatigue, and feelings of anxiety or depression; these symptoms are amenable to OTC self-treatment. Use of OTC drugs often enables elders to gain relief from symptoms less expensively than prescription drugs and to obtain sufficient comfort to continue their activities of daily living (Cameron, 1996). An added benefit from purchasing OTC drugs is their accessibility at markets, drug stores and pharmacies, and on-line vendors. OTC items can be obtained more quickly than prescription drugs, which necessitate seeing a physician or nurse practitioner. The use of OTC products extends beyond American borders. In a study of 100 elderly hospitalized patients in the United Kingdom, 78% were reportedly self-medicating with OTC products and less than 1% were recorded in the physician notes (Barnett et al, 2000).

According to the National Council on Patient Information and Education (NCPIE) (2002), the OTC market has more than 100,000 drug products, with 700 of them containing ingredients and dosages that would have required prescriptions 30 years ago. Medication problems can be reduced if elders are well informed about all aspects of their medicines. The many problems with OTC drug availability include excessive dose, drug interactions, adverse reactions, masking or delaying diagnosis of a serious condition, self-medicating, using analgesics and other OTC medicines to promote sleep,

Table 10-5 Determining Whether the Drug Is Working: Monitoring Parameters and Common Side Effects of Psychiatric Drug Categories

Class of drug	Monitoring activity	Common side effects
Anxiolytics	Decreased anxiety Immediate effect Habit-forming	Sedation, confusion, gait disturbances, disinhibition
Mood stabilizers	Blood levels: gradual behavior change based on blood level Lithium: avoid salt restriction; maintain adequate hydration Ensure adequate renal function Decreased hyperactivity, explosive outbursts, mania	Sedation, confusion, tremors
Antidepressants	Dose titration depends on side effects; start with low dose and increase dosage slowly Gradual effect; patient does not usually see early improvement of depression	Tricyclics: dry mouth, blurred vision, constipation, sedation, confusion, urinary retention, orthostatic hypotension SSRIs: restlessness, insomnia, irritability, sexual dysfunction
Antipsychotics	Decreased agitation Immediate response Use lowest possible dose and eliminate medication as soon as possible	Sedation, confusion, dyskinesia, akathisia, extrapyramidal effects, parkinsonian reactions, somnolence
Hypnotics	Nighttime sleep improvement Habit-forming Taper (rebound on withdrawal from those causing decrease in rapid eye movement [REM] sleep)	Daytime drowsiness, hangover, worsening dementia, confusion, hypotension, delirium, depressed respirations

From Semla TP, Beizer JL, Higbee MD: *Geriatric dosage handbook,* ed 8, Cleveland, 2003, Lexi-Comp, Inc.

Box 10-2 Questions to Consider about the Drug and the Specific Patient

1. Is the drug working to improve the patient's symptoms?
   a. What are the therapeutic effects of the drug? (What symptoms are targeted?)
   b. What is the time frame for the therapeutic effects?
   c. Have the appropriate drug and dose been prescribed?
   d. Has the appropriate time been tried for therapeutic effects?
2. Is the drug harming the patient?
   a. What physiologic changes are occurring?
   b. What laboratory values are changing?
   c. What mental status changes are occurring?
   d. What functional changes are occurring?
   e. Is the patient experiencing side effects?
   f. Is the drug interacting with any other medication?
3. Does the patient understand the following?
   a. Why he or she is taking the drug
   b. How the drug is supposed to be taken
   c. How to identify side effects and drug interactions
   d. How to reduce or manage side effects
   e. Limitations imposed by taking the drug (e.g., sedative effects)

and OTC herbal medicines with toxic ingredients (Barnett et al, 2000).

Mixing or combining medications poses problems. For example, Tylenol (acetaminophen), if combined with prescription medications such as Percocet and Vicodin, can lead to liver damage because of an excessive dose of acetaminophen. A not uncommon case is when a patient receives prescriptions for Percocet and Vicodin on two separate occasions. The pain is chronic and bothersome, and the patient takes all of the medications, including the OTC Tylenol. Inadvertently, the patient overdoses on acetaminophen and develops liver failure. No one has been monitoring this patient's pain management.

Another example is when an elderly person is taking a prescription dosage of an antihistaminic allergy medication on a chronic basis. During a bout of insomnia, the person purchases the OTC drug diphenhydramine, thinking it will relieve insomnia. The anticholinergic properties are additive with another antihistamine that had been prescribed; in the elderly, smaller doses are required and cumulatively larger doses can lead to adverse effects. Anticholinergic symptoms include dry mouth, blurred vision, constipation, tiredness, and confusion. A sudden episode of confusion may not be attributed to the combination of medications if no one knew the patient added the diphenhydramine.

Another aspect of OTC medication self-management is the tendency to purchase combination medications. OTC cold and flu remedies that combine analgesic, antihistamine, and antitussive medications can lead to increased risk of side effects. Dosages in the adult range, usually recommended in the labeling, may be too high for elders. As mentioned previously, taking a combination medication with other drugs can lead to side effects. Further, combination medications are usually more expensive than purchasing generic versions of each type of medication.

Drug interactions are another potential danger of self-medicating with OTC medicines. For example, an elder taking warfarin is at risk when purchasing a drug for indigestion. Warfarin is commonly given for anticoagulation for atrial fibrillation. Cimetidine, an OTC product used for indigestion, will interact with warfarin to increase the effects of warfarin. Prolonged bleeding, even hemorrhage, can result (Tatro, 2003). Alternative indigestion aids can be used, but the patient should work with the physician to do so.

New medications are always being added to the OTC market. This trend means that more elders will be treating themselves, particularly if they are unable to afford health care and prescription prices. The nursing role must include communication with the elder and family in assessing what medications—OTC and prescription and herbal or nutraceutical supplements—are included in the patient's self-medication practices and what the patient knows about the drugs she or he is taking. The nurse needs to be aware of possible interactions among the variety of drugs and dosages and to inform the patient of potential dangers. Additionally, the elder's reasons for taking the drugs should be explored because the self-treatment strategies may need medical evaluation. The pharmacist can be consulted and can provide a valuable resource for the nurse, patient, and family.

Herbal Medicines

According to a recent review, the seven top-selling herbal medicines are ginkgo, St. John's wort, ginseng, garlic, echinacea, saw palmetto, and kava (Izzo and Ernst, 2001). The popularity of these herbs is evident in the 1998 U.S. market, as follows: ginkgo, $150 million; St. John's wort, $140 million; ginseng, $96 million; garlic, $84 million; echinacea, $70 million; saw palmetto, $32 million; kava, $17 million. The percentage of increased sales between 1997 and 1998 on all of these herbals ranged from 11% for ginseng to 462% for saw palmetto (Izzo and Ernst, 2001).

Although few interactions have been reported in the literature, there is a growing documentation of the drug-herb interactions; interestingly, these have occurred frequently in persons 65 years and older. In the four interactions with ginkgo, all four cases involved bleeding in elderly persons; interactions were with warfarin, thiazide diuretic, trazodone, and aspirin. In two of four interactions, kava interacted with levodopa in two elderly persons with Parkinson's disease, causing an increase in the frequency of "off" periods. Of 32 interactions with St. John's wort, 11 were in elderly persons; the most frequent interaction was with the SSRI antidepressants, thought to result from a synergism with the serotonin uptake inhibition. Patients experienced dizziness, nausea, vomiting, headache, anxiety, restlessness, irritability, and confusion. Another frequent interaction was with warfarin, causing a decreased INR, and resulting in a decreased anticoagulant effect (Izzo and Ernst, 2001).

In a review article, Gold and colleagues (2001) report that interactions between these same herbals and other drugs have been published in 28 articles (11 articles about St. John's wort, 4 about ginkgo, 5 about kava, 1 about valerian, and 7 about ginseng), most of which describe case reports. More evidence is needed for efficacious use of these herbals, because none of the herbal medicines is free of adverse effects (Ernst, 2002).

The nurse should be aware that herbs commonly used for psychiatric symptoms in the elderly include St. John's wort for depression and for depression associated with early dementia (Gold et al, 2001), kava for anxiety, ginkgo biloba for memory enhancement, and valerian for sleep (Beaubrun and Gray, 2000). A recent study reported that ginkgo was ineffective in elders with normal cognition for improvements such as memory enhancement and attention (Solomon et al, 2002). As mentioned previously, few studies validate the benefits without warning of the potential for adverse effects. Because the herbal medicines are not regulated as drugs by the FDA, their preparation is not regulated. Hence, mixtures that are combinations of the herbs with other ingredients and are formulated as concentrates, extracts, teas, or capsules are not standardized. This means that doses of the actual herb may vary or be impure. In sum, current translation of evidence of efficacy in treating psychiatric illnesses or symptoms with herbal medicines is problematic related to small sample sizes, nonstandardized measures, and variable preparations.

Medications Prescribed for Behavioral and Psychiatric Concerns

Medications may cause and treat psychiatric symptoms or illness. Medications that are known to cause psychiatric symptoms are presented in Table 10-5. The rate of depression in elderly persons living in the community is estimated at 20% and for those living in long-term care is estimated at 50% (Pollock and Reynolds, 2000). Likewise, widowed persons and children and spouse caregivers of patients with dementia have high rates of depression, estimated at about 10% to 20% (Pollock and Reynolds, 2000). Antipsychotics are prescribed for about 23% of geriatric patients for conditions such as dementia, delirium, schizophrenia, delusional disorder, mood disorder with psychotic features, neurologic conditions, substance abuse, and drug-induced psychoses; those with dementia experience psychotic symptoms, agitation, and aggression, which often prompt long-term care placement (Byerly et al, 2001). The antianxiety agents, usually benzodiazepines, are used frequently for a variety of anxiety symptoms and illness. Caution is required in the administration of all of these agents to elderly persons. Table 10-5 depicts effectiveness, monitoring activities, and side effects for psychiatric drugs. Table 10-2 shows the geriatric dosages for common psychoactive medications (e.g., antidepressants, antipsychotics, anxiolytics).

Noncompliance/Nonadherence

Medication noncompliance, sometimes used interchangeably with nonadherence, is one of the biggest issues affecting the health and safety of older persons. The rate ranges between

20% and 70% in community-dwelling elders (Barat et al, 2001). *Compliance,* or *adherence,* is defined as following a prescribed medication regimen. The term *adherence* has become popular because it connotes patient collaboration with the treatment regimen and is less authoritarian than the term *compliance* (Helping patients adhere to medical instructions, 2001). Adhering to treatment can prevent relapses of symptoms of serious illnesses such as diabetes, heart failure, schizophrenia, depression, asthma, and pain. Noncompliance, sometimes considered deliberate misuse of medication, is a source of irritation to health care providers.

Reasons for nonadherence must be assessed. As examples, some elders alter the dose or stop taking a drug because it had been ineffective, they disliked the side effects, they felt they had had enough medication, they wanted to avoid feeling stigmatized (e.g., antidepressants), they wanted some control over their own lives, they had difficulty adapting the regimen to their lifestyle, or they had poor understanding of instructions. Elders may have difficulty adapting the regimen to their lifestyle, as when a person omits a dose of diuretic to prevent the need for toileting. Patients who feel the medications are not necessary are not likely to comply (Horne and Weinman, 1999). Factors that contribute to noncompliance include elders' depression (Ciechanowski et al, 2000), poor cognitive ability (Barat et al, 2001), low educational level (Aljasem et al, 2001), living alone (Barat et al, 2001), more severity of illness (Aljasem et al, 2001), longer number of years with the illness (Aljasem et al, 2001), poor knowledge of the medications (Lowe et al, 1995), no experience with consequences of nonadherence (Aljasem et al, 2001), and larger number of medications and greater frequency of taking doses (Barat et al, 2001). A busy and active lifestyle has been attributed to forgetting to take medicines (Park et al, 1999). On the other hand, experiencing unwanted and inconvenient pain may promote adherence to analgesics if persons learn how to take the medication properly (Edworthy and Devins, 1999).

Characteristics of nonadherence behaviors are described in a 1995 national telephone survey of 874 persons over 50 years old conducted collaboratively by the American Association of Retired Persons, the National Pharmaceutical Council, and the *Pharmaceutical Executive* magazine about prescription drug issues and usage (American Association of Retired Persons Research, 1996). About 40% of the subjects within a 2-year period had chosen not to comply fully with their physicians' prescriptions, as follows: (1) stopped taking the medication before it ran out, (2) took less than prescribed, (3) filled the prescription but decided not to take it, or (4) did not fill the prescription at all. Most said they had not had problems with their medications (86%); only 14% had a problem, the most frequent of which was side effects (80%). The researchers found that those 50 to 64 years of age were more likely not to comply (47%) compared with those age 65 and older (39%), and that women were more likely than men not to comply (49% vs. 35%). Another important finding was that low-income Americans had difficulty paying for their prescriptions; 37% said they had to sacrifice food or heating fuel to pay for a prescription.

Another study revealed that patients' adherence reports differed from what their physicians believed. Of a random sample of 348 persons with a mean age of 75 years, patients disagreed with their physicians' prescriptions (22%), doses (71%), and regimens (66%). Nonadherence was significantly related to decreased knowledge of the drugs, frequency of drug intake per day, the use of three or more drugs, prescriptions from more than one doctor, and probability of dementia (Barat et al, 2001). The message for nurses is clear that adherence must be approached from interactional and educational perspectives in the relationship between the provider and the patient.

The important point for the nurse is that assessment must be done for many aspects of ability: (1) to manage medication scheduling—related to number of other medications and conditions, organizational functioning, and lifestyle adaptability; (2) to understand instructions—related to cognitive functioning, language, and culture; (3) to hear the instructions—related to their hearing or language usage or difficulty with the provider's speech and language; (4) to read written material and labels—related to diminished visual ability or to being non-English speaking; (5) to open medication bottles—related to strength or arthritic changes; (6) to ask questions of the provider; (7) to report side effects; and (8) to interact with the nurse about the impact of the illness or medication. As with all interventions, the nurse has to evaluate the effectiveness of the communication between the nurse and the patient and family.

Applying Theory to Practice

Elderly persons who do not adhere to pharmacologic treatments do so for many reasons, some related to themselves, some related to the environment, and some related to the relationship with the provider. Several theoretical suppositions about predicting adherence are presented in the following paragraphs. Theory can help the nurse understand a patient's nonadherence behaviors, can help the nurse understand his or her own reactions, and can promote critical thinking about interventions. There is no single intervention that will work for all situations.

An innovative hypothesis has been proposed that past trauma from medical illness is related to nonadherence with treatment for that medical illness. Shemesh and colleagues (2001) followed 102 patients with an average age of 61 years who had survived myocardial infarction (MI) for their adherence post-MI up to 1 year. They found that nonadherence to medication (i.e., captopril) was associated with adverse outcome during the first year and that nonadherence was associated with posttraumatic stress disorder symptoms. The authors suggest that patients avoided medication because it reminded them of the MI trauma. The implication is that the trauma symptoms need addressing before adherence interventions can be successful. Because chronic illness is prevalent in elders, this hypothesis should be tested with a larger population.

Patients' beliefs about their capability to adhere, conceptualized as self-efficacy, is theorized to predict adherence (Bandura, 1977). A person's self-judgments reflect his or her beliefs about his or her own ability to practice healthy self-care behaviors (Bandura, 1982; O'Leary, 1985). The self-efficacy theory has been used in an exploratory study of 309 persons with type 2 diabetes. The researchers found from patients' self-reports that greater self-efficacy was predictive of diabetic self-care behaviors that included diet, exercise, frequent blood glucose testing, less frequent omission of medication, and less binge eating (Aljasem et al, 2001). A clinical implication of this study for the nurse in working with elders includes asking patients whether they believe they can (i.e., ability, desire) follow a particular regimen.

The theory of stages of change is another approach to working with patients on medication adherence, particularly in behavior change in addictive disease or adaptation to chronic illness (Prochaska and DiClemente, 1982). Norcross and Prochaska (2002) report 90% accuracy with prediction of adherence outcome. They describe five stages, each of which can be matched to interventions based on a patient's stage of readiness to change. The stages and interventions are as follows:

1. *Precontemplation* is when persons have no serious intention of changing behavior but express a vague wish; the nurse could intervene to provide information through a supportive and nurturing manner.
2. *Contemplation* is when persons are aware of a problem and think seriously about changing but have not yet made a decision; support and nurturance are important, and the nurse might help the person ventilate feelings.
3. *Preparation* is when an attempt has been made to change, was unsuccessful, and action is intended; support is needed and offering of more information or a tour of programs may be helpful.
4. *Action* is when major change occurs and is based on energy already spent and an environment already created to make change happen; encouragement is needed, and active support for action taken will be appreciated. Patients also need the opportunity to express insights and involvement in active participation in a program.
5. *Maintenance* is when the aim is to be proactive to prevent a recurrence of the problem; support and encouragement are needed, and the nurse can provide an opportunity for the patient to express feelings, describe actions, focus on goals, and discuss strategies.

According to Norcross and Prochaska (2002), in an intensive smoking cessation program for cardiac patients 22% of precontemplators, 43% of contemplators, and 76% of those in action or prepared for action at the start were successful in quitting smoking 12 months later. Staging an elder's readiness to change behavior for adapting to a new medication regimen can be useful for determining teaching strategies and providing appropriate interventions.

Attachment theory as applied to the provider-patient relationship has been purported to make a difference in patients' adherence to a diabetes medication regimen. According to Bowlby's attachment theory, individuals develop lifelong interaction styles based on the kinds of interactions they experienced from infancy (Bowlby, 1973). Based on behavior observed in all stages of the life cycle, there are four categories of attachment: secure, dismissing, preoccupied, and fearful (Bartholomew and Horowitz, 1991). The adult who has a secure attachment has a positive view of self and others and is open and trusting. An adult with a dismissing attachment style is compulsively self-reliant, has a positive view of self and a negative view of others, and is distrustful and uncomfortable with others. An adult with a preoccupied attachment has a negative view of self and a positive view of others and is continuously seeking approval. The adult with a fearful attachment style demonstrates a desire for social contact but is inhibited by a fear of rejection.

The attachment theory was applied in a study with 367 diabetic older adults (ages 56 to 63) to determine the impact of patient attachment style on perception of provider communication quality and association with medication adherence (Ciechanowski et al, 2001). Results indicated that patients with a dismissing style of attachment were more likely to rate communication as poor and to have poorer treatment adherence. This study looked only at patient attachment style. Further research is needed to explore the impact of the provider attachment style on the patient's responses and on adherence (Ciechanowski et al, 2001). Nonetheless, implications for practice include evaluating the nurse's communication with the patient, including cultural and language sensitivity. Outcomes to consider include patient satisfaction, knowledge of medications, adherence to appointment attendance, and adherence based on refill lapses.

Considering Provider Behavior: Guidelines for Safe Medication Practices

Providers' roles in contributing to adherence need emphasis. The physician or nurse practitioner prescribes, the pharmacist dispenses, and the nurse helps the patient understand and implement what has been taught by the other disciplines (see Box 10-2). In this role, the nurse actively teaches about medications to reinforce the physician's and pharmacist's teachings, ensures that the patient has knowledge, reinforces the need for the regimen, and assists the patient in adapting the regimen to his or her lifestyle (Box 10-3). Aside from teaching to maximize adherence, the other role of every provider is adherence to guidelines for safe medication practices. Guidelines for safe geriatric medication administration include geriatric dosage guidelines (see Box 10-4 for indications of appropriate and inappropriate medications in elders in facilities), avoidance of inappropriate medications for the elderly (Table 10-6), and guidelines for crushing medications (Table 10-7). As with polypharmacy, providers may not always adhere to guidelines that promote safety. The nursing role involves

Box 10-3 Empowering the Patient for Safe Medication Practices: What Elders Should Know about Taking Their Medications

- What is the name of each drug?
- What is the purpose of each drug?
- What is the dose per administration?
- What is the number of doses every day?
- What is the best time to take the medication?
- How should the medication be taken?
- Can the medication be taken with other drugs?
- Which medications can and cannot be taken together?
- Are any special techniques, devices, or procedures necessary to administer the medication?
- For how long should the medication be taken?
- What are the common side effects?
- If side effects occur: What should the elder do? What changes in administration are necessary? When should the drug be stopped? When should the physician or pharmacist (or both) be called?
- What can be done at home to monitor for a therapeutic drug response?
- What should be done if a dose is missed?
- How many refills are allowed?
- How should the medication be stored?
- What are the nonprescription (OTC) preparations that should not be used with the present drug therapy?
- Take all medications prescribed unless the physician states otherwise.
- Stop taking the medication and report any new or unusual problems such as shortness of breath, nausea, diarrhea, vomiting, sleepiness, dizziness, weakness, skin rash, or fever.
- Never take medication prescribed for another person.
- Do not take any medication more than 1 year old or past the expiration date on the container.
- Store medications in a safe place, preferably the kitchen, rather than the bathroom, where moisture from bathing, especially showers, may affect the medicine.
- Do not keep medicines, especially sedatives and hypnotics, on the bedside stand, because when you are sleepy, you may forget that you have already taken the medication earlier.
- Do not place different medicines in the same container.
- Take a sufficient supply of all medicines in their individual containers when traveling away from home.
- Use a chart to keep track of medications.

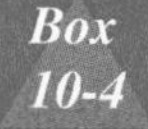

Box 10-4 Defined Indications and Behaviors for Appropriate and Inappropriate Use of Neuroleptics in the Nursing Facility, According to OBRA Guidelines

1. Unnecessary drugs; each resident's drug regimen must be free from unnecessary drugs.
2. Antipsychotic drugs are given only as necessary therapy to treat the following specific conditions as diagnosed and documented in the clinical record:
   - Schizophrenia
   - Schizoaffective disorder
   - Delusional disorder
   - Psychotic mood disorder (mania, depression with psychotic features)
   - Acute psychotic episode
   - Brief reactive psychosis
   - Tourette's disorder
   - Huntington's disorder
   - Organic mental syndromes (dementia and delirium included) with associated psychotic or agitated behaviors (or both)
   - Short-term (7 days) symptomatic treatment of hiccups, nausea, vomiting, or pruritus
3. Behaviors for which antipsychotic medication is appropriate:
   - Agitated psychosis (biting, kicking, hitting, scratching, assaultive and belligerent behavior, sexual aggressiveness) presenting a danger to self or care providers or interfering with ability to provide care
   - Hallucinations, delusions, paranoia
   - Continuous crying out and screaming
4. Behaviors less responsive to antipsychotics; antipsychotic therapy should not be used if one or more of the following is/are the only indication:
   - Repetitive, bothersome behavior (pacing, wandering, repetitious statements or words, calling out, fidgeting)
   - Poor self-care
   - Unsociability
   - Indifference to surroundings
   - Uncooperativeness
   - Restlessness
   - Impaired memory
   - Anxiety
   - Depression (without psychotic features)
   - Insomnia
   - Agitated behaviors that do *not* represent danger to the patient or others

Data from Omnibus Budget Reconciliation Act (OBRA) of 1987, 101 Stat 1330-160; US Health Care Financing Administration: Medicare and Medicaid: requirements for long-term care facilities, *Federal Register* 54(21):5316, 1989; Stoudemire A, Smith DA: OBRA regulations and the use of psychotropic drugs in long-term care facilities: impact and implications for geropsychiatric care, *General Hospital Psychiatry* 18:77, 1996; Semla TP, Beizer JL, Higbee MD: *Geriatric dosage handbook,* ed 7, Cleveland, 2003, Lexi-Comp, Inc.

Table 10-6 Drugs Considered Inappropriate for the Elderly

Drug	Concern
Analgesics	
Propoxyphene and combinations containing propoxyphene	No analgesic advantage over acetaminophen Side effects are similar to narcotics
Indomethacin	Produces the most CNS effects of all NSAIDs
Phenylbutazone	Can produce hematologic effects
Pentazocine	Produces CNS effects more commonly than narcotics, including hallucinations and confusion
Meperidine	Potent metabolite, normeperidine, can accumulate in elderly, causing tremors and seizures
Antiemetic	
Trimethobenzamide	Ineffective as an antiemetic Produces extrapyramidal reactions
Muscle relaxants	
Methocarbamol, carisoprodol, oxybutynin, chlorzoxazone, metaxalone, cyclobenzaprine	Side effect profile high: anticholinergic side effects, sedation, weakness Doses of effectiveness not tolerated well in elderly
Hypnotics	
Flurazepam, diazepam	Long-acting benzodiazepines produce prolonged sedation, increasing fall risk and confusion risk Small doses of short- and intermediate-acting benzodiazepines may be more appropriate
Barbiturates except phenobarbital	More side effects than other sedative/hypnotics Highly addictive Use only for seizure control
Antidepressants	
Amitriptyline	Strong anticholinergic and sedating properties
Doxepin	Strong anticholinergic and sedating properties
Anxiolytic	
Meprobamate	Highly addictive and sedating
Hypoglycemic	
Chlorpropamide	Long lasting, danger of hypoglycemia increased in elderly
Antiarrhythmic	
Disopyramide	May induce heart failure Strongly anticholinergic
Antiplatelet	
Dipyridamole	Causes orthostatic hypotension in elderly Beneficial only in artificial heart valves
Anticoagulant	
Ticlopidine	No better than aspirin in preventing clots More toxic than aspirin in elderly
Antihypertensive	
Methyldopa	May cause bradycardia May exacerbate depression
Reserpine	Poses danger to elderly: depression, impotence, sedation, orthostatic hypotension
Cerebral vasodilators	
Ergot mesyloids, cyclospasmol	Not effective; not to be used for dementia or other conditions
Gastrointestinal antispasmodics	
Dicyclomine, hyoscyamine, propantheline, belladonna alkaloids, clidinium-chlordiazepoxide	Highly anticholinergic, generally cause toxic effects in elderly Effectiveness at doses tolerated by elderly questionable
Treatment/prophylaxis of duodenal ulcers	
Cimetidine	Highly anticholinergic CNS effects: confusion, agitation, headache, fatigue
Antihistamines (prescription and nonprescription)	
Chlorpheniramine, diphenhydramine, hydroxyzine, cyproheptadine, promethazine, tripelennamine, dexchlorpheniramine	Potent anticholinergic properties For elderly, use cold and cough preparations without antihistamines in them Diphenhydramine should not be given for insomnia; only small doses (25 mg) for limited time should be used for allergy

Modified from Beers MH: Explicit criteria for determining potentially inappropriate medication use by the elderly, *Arch Intern Med* 157:1531, 1997; Buffum J: *Geriatric dosage guidelines,* 1996.

Table 10-7 Medications That Should not Be Chewed or Crushed

Type	Rationale	Examples
Extended-release products, with any of the following abbreviations: CR = controlled release CRT = controlled-release tablet LA = long acting SR = sustained release TR = timed release TD = time delay SA = sustained action XL = extended length XR = extended release	Medication is formulated to be slowly released into the body. The drug may be centered within the core of the tablet, and the multiple layers around it are shed. The outer tablet may be waxed, because this melts in the GI tract; this appears as a shiny tablet. An extended-release capsule may have beads within it that will dissolve at different times once ingested.	Potassium chloride: K-Dur, Slow-K Adalat PA, XL Belladenal Spacetab Bellergal Spacetab Bentylol Dospan Wellbutrin SR Tegretol CR Diltiazem CD Choledyl SA Contact C Diamox Sequels Diclofenac tab Dimetapp Extentab Drixoral Tab Duralith Entex LA Inderal LA Indocid SR Macrobid Cap MS Contin Napoxen Nitro-Bid Nitrong SR Norflex Orudis SR Quinidex Entab Theophylline tab
Medications irritating to the stomach or destroyed by stomach acid are enteric coated. These are considered delayed release.	Enteric coating delays release of the drug until it reaches the small intestine.	Enteric-coated aspirin Bisacodyl tab Carters Liver pills Divalproic acid Donnazyme Ecotrin Fe sulphate Lansoprazole Mandelamine Phazyme Pyridium Omeprazole
Foul-tasting medication	If a tablet unpleasant to taste, the manufacturer may coat the tablet in a sugar coating. If crushed, the drug is unpalatable and may lead to noncompliance, but the drug is not altered.	Cefuroxime, chloral hydrate cap, fluoxetine, fluvoxamine, omeprazole, promethazine
Sublingual medication	Absorption is designed for under-the-tongue administration. It is not always easy to distinguish this type of medication; the package should indicate that it is sublingual.	Nitroglycerin SL
Effervescent tablets	Tablets that dissolve in a liquid, yielding a solution. If crushed, the tablets will not dissolve quickly.	

From Spectrum Society for Community Living: Oral drugs that should not be crushed or chewed, 2002. Available at *www.spectrumsociety.org/library/SpectrumMedManual.pdf*; Semla TP, Beizer JL, Higbee MD: *Geriatric dosage handbook,* ed 8, Cleveland, 2003, Lexi-Comp, Inc.

interdisciplinary collaboration, ensuring the safety and appropriateness of the prescribed medication and the evaluation of the patient's response.

Patient Education: A Nursing Role

Nurses have an opportunity to improve treatment outcomes through patient education. In a collaborative process, the nurse works with the elder to provide medication information. Ideally, the nurse is empowering the person to participate fully in goal setting and treatment planning. In providing education, the following tips may be useful for the nurse to implement:

1. Pay attention to the environment where education is occurring. If in the hospital, minimize distraction and avoid competing with television or others demanding the patient's time. The setting should be comfortable for the patient; if at home, the patient may feel more receptive to learning. Timing is important and the patient's needs should have been attended to, because learning occurs best when a person is not hungry, thirsty, tired, too warm or too cold, in pain, or needing to use the bathroom. If the patient requires glasses or hearing aids, those should be in place. The length of time for teaching should be as short as possible, comprehensive yet succinct, using simple and direct language and avoiding jargon. There should be openings so the patient can ask questions.
2. Determine whether it would be helpful to have a family member or caregiver present. Is the patient cognitively impaired? Does the patient rely on a caregiver?
3. Provide memory aids while teaching. Have the medications present so that the patient can see them and begin learning with visual association. Written material in large letters and simple language should be given to the patient to reinforce any verbal directions. Use actual memory aids to illustrate strategies. Pictures of the medications could be used for an instruction sheet, depicting what the drug does and when it is given. If food is required with the medication, a discussion should occur about meal preparation, snack consumption, or convenient management of the requirement. Likewise, pictorial representation can illustrate foods or drugs that interact and should be taken or avoided. Examples of memory aids include the following: a weekly calendar with pockets for medications indicating day, time, and date; a daily tear-off calendar to remind the elder to take daily medication; larger calendars to list all drugs to be taken, and a check can be placed in the date square each time a medication is taken; clear envelopes or sandwich bags containing the medication can be affixed to the dated square on a daily basis, and each envelope or bag should state the name of the drug, dose, and times to be taken that day; commercial drug caddies are available for single or multiple doses by the day, week, or month, and some have alarms; and color coding the medication containers and matching the colors to a clock face.
4. Have the patient repeat back instructions, including names of medications, purposes, side effects, times of adminis-

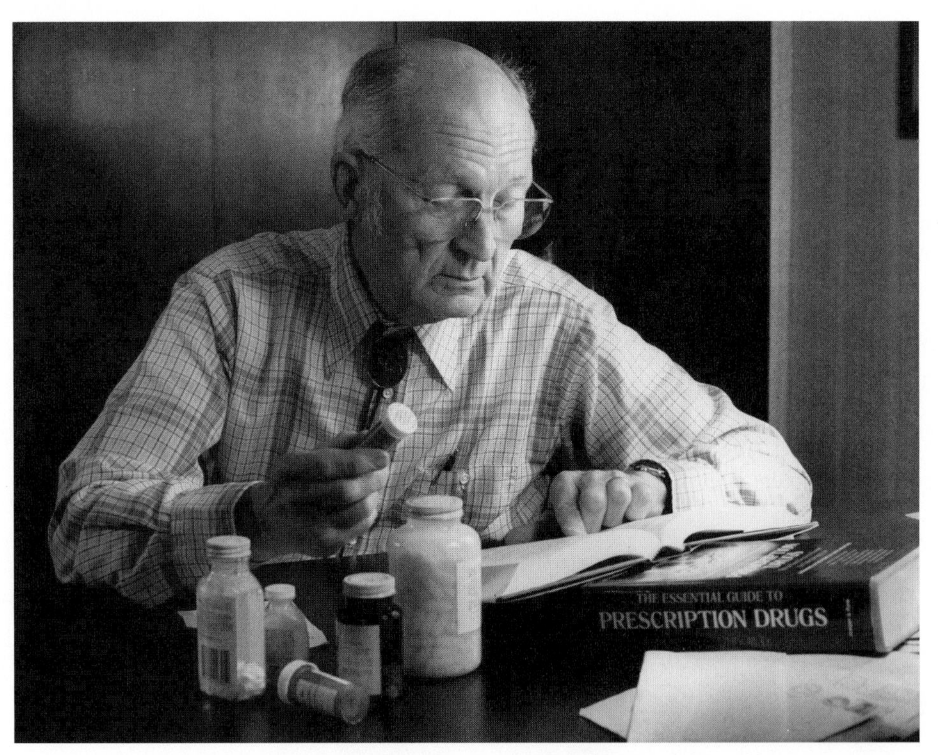

An elder prepares to take his medicine. (Courtesy Rod Schmall.)

tration, and method for remembering to take the medicines and to mark off their ingestion. For example, a strategy is to turn medication bottle upside down once the dose has been taken for the day.

5. Have the patient demonstrate an ability to remove the cap from the bottle. The patient should be taught to request a large cap from the pharmacist if unable to remove the usual or childproof cap.
6. Have the patient demonstrate the procedure for preparing medications. Have the elder read the label and pour the correct amount of medicine. If the person cannot break a tablet in half, the pharmacist needs to know to dispense a smaller dose. If the person cannot read the label, the pharmacist needs to be asked to prepare a larger label.
7. Encourage questions. Patients need to be encouraged to realize their own partnership in their treatment.
8. Consider follow-up medication teaching. After discharge from the hospital, a follow-up phone call can help with assessing functional status and proper medication usage or other problems with medications. A nurse's home visit to patients at high risk for problems, such as those with cognitive deficits or those with many medications for new conditions, could reinforce medication information and provide assessment information.
9. Consider alternative teaching methods when personal contact is not possible. Computer-assisted medication teaching has demonstrated effectiveness for improving medication knowledge, adherence, and clinical outcome when given to older patients with osteoarthritis (Edworthy and Devins, 1999).

Self-Evaluation Questions

How does the nurse know the education was effective? Observing the patient while teaching will provide information about the patient's alertness and interest. Facial expression and body language will demonstrate tension, confusion, anxiety, or comprehension and eagerness to learn. Questions to ask oneself include the following: Did the elder appear to be listening during the teaching? Did the elder ask relevant questions? Could the person repeat the instructions, purpose, and side effects to watch for? Did the person express a desire to improve his or her health and condition? Did the person participate in planning the medication regimen? Is the person motivated to comply with the regimen? How did the patient perform in recalling instructions? In demonstrating procedure? What are the impairments? What does the person need? What type of follow-up should be done to reinforce the patient's learnings? How did we (the patient and the nurse) respond to each other? What was the quality of our communication?

Teaching Safe Practices

Empowering the patient means teaching elders about their medications and how to communicate about their health care and medications with their provider. More specifically, the FDA recommends that elders learn to recognize side effects and learn to report them to their physicians. Some of the symptoms that should prompt physician notification include dizziness, constipation, diarrhea, incontinence, sleep changes, blurred vision, mood changes, and rash (Trenter, 1999). The following additional suggestions should be taught to the elder about safe medication practices (Trenter, 1999):

1. Only take a drug if absolutely necessary. Ask the provider if an alternative, such as diet change or exercise, could work as well.
2. Share with the provider all of the current prescription, OTC, herbal, and nutraceutical medications. If several providers are involved, ask one person to coordinate the drugs (e.g., physician, pharmacist, or nurse). Take all of the medicinals with you to your physician or provider visit.
3. Determine whether your physician is certified for any specialized training in geriatric medicine.
4. Discuss with the physician the chance of being given drugs that could possibly treat more than one condition. For example, some medications could be used for both hypertension and cardiac problems.
5. Be alert to new symptoms. These could be side effects from medications rather than aches and pains of advancing age. Be sure to report these to the provider.
6. Learn about the drugs by asking questions of the physician, pharmacist, and nurse. Learn the names of the drugs, the foods and other drugs they interact with, how to take them properly, and whether there are less expensive generic drugs available. Ask the pharmacist for written information about the drugs. Be sure the instructions are legible and large enough or that you have a magnifying glass.
7. When given a new medication, check the name to be sure you are getting the correct drug. Be sure you can open the container. Ask the pharmacist to explain any questions you have about the drug. For example, if the name differs from what the doctor told you, is it because it is a generic drug? The pharmacist can provide a different cap so you can open it more easily.
8. If you get medication information off the Internet, be sure to discuss what you learn with your provider. Share the Internet sites, because their credibility needs determination. Be cautious when making decisions about drugs based on Internet sites and others' stories.
9. Ask the provider when you can stop taking the drugs. Ask how to tell whether the drugs are working.
10. Read the label and follow the instructions each time you take the medicines. Check that you are taking the correct dose and at the right time.
11. Select a method to help with memory. Helpful tips include using a pillbox with the days marked or a daily calendar for checking off medicines required and already taken. Some persons use watch alarms to remind them to pour medicines. One person described preparing her medications daily and placing them on plates labeled with a designated meal; then she would turn the bottles upside down after the doses had been taken (Trenter, 1999).

DRUG USE ASSESSMENT: THE INTERVIEW

The initial step in ensuring that elders achieve safe and effective drug use is interviewing the patient or caregiver (or both) for a comprehensive drug history. In many cases, a pharmacist does the drug history. Sometimes the physician will do it as part of a physical and history procedure. Whoever is in a position to prescribe should complete this important interaction with the patient. For example, a nurse practitioner or a clinical nurse specialist may be in positions to interview the senior. A bedside nurse, who is not usually optimally situated to do this part of a history-taking, may be asked to complete parts of it.

Good interviewing and communication skills will help the drug history-taker to conduct the interview with the patient or the caregiver. One should start by asking, "What prescription medications are you taking?" A systematic way to gather information is to do a 24-hour medication history. If asking about each system in a review of systems approach, the nurse may ask what medications are routinely used for headache, eye problems, ear problems, and endocrine problems (thyroid, insulin, etc.). Additional information about drug management can be gathered in the interview, such as the medication names, doses, frequency, and purpose.

Open-ended questions should be asked, such as "What do you take for headaches?" and "What do you use for indigestion, or bowels?" The purpose of open-ended questions is for the elder to engage in discussion, and the nurse can ascertain motivation and beliefs concerning the taking of medications. Information the nurse will need to gather includes the following: number and type of current prescriptions, OTC preparations, herbals, and nutraceutical supplements; current administration schedule; the elder's knowledge about his or her medications; medication-related problems such as side effects or nonadherence; number of other remedies used; frequency of visits to the physician or primary care practitioner; level of sensory, memory, and physical disability; ability to pay for prescription medications; use of other drugs such as tobacco or nicotine in either gum, patch, or smoking forms; and the level of use of social drugs such as alcohol and caffeine. Discussion about addictive drugs, illicit drugs, or drugs obtained from others' prescriptions should occur and may require some sensitivity and a nonjudgmental attitude. Patients should be encouraged to ask questions and to learn about interactions between drugs, regardless of prescription status. Included in the discussion should also be any discontinued drugs, because they may be excreted slowly and have relevance to currently prescribed medications.

When the senior does not remember all that he or she is taking, ask that all medications be put in a paper bag and brought in for evaluation. Garner as much information as possible from the individual regarding amount, frequency, reason for taking each drug, known side effects, and method of remembering when to take it.

The nurse who obtains the patient's drug information should be thinking of a plan for intervening. That is, communicating with the interdisciplinary care team is vital for establishing safe medication usage, the patient's cognitive ability, and motivation to adhere to a medication. The nurse should focus discussion on the need for the drug, any side effects from taking it, any interactions with it, and any deficiencies it may be causing, such as dehydration or malnutrition. Ideally, the nurse should know what resources are available for teaching about medications, such as the clinical pharmacist in a hospital or the patient's physician. The nurse is ideally situated to coordinate care, learn about the patient's goals, learn what the patient needs for understanding his or her medications, and arrange for follow-up care to determine outcome of medication teaching.

Outcomes

Reassessment of the elder will determine the outcomes of medication use. Observation of the aged client should be an ongoing process to determine if physical or mental changes have occurred, as well as whether the therapeutic goal or response has been achieved. Listen to the elderly when they describe how they feel or changes that they notice after they have begun a new medication, have had a dose adjustment, or even when they continue to take several medications. Periodically check blood levels of such drugs that have a cumulative effect or are enhanced or diminished by interaction with other medications such as warfarin (Coumadin), digitalis preparations, quinidine, theophylline, phenytoin, carbamazepine, and various antibiotics.

Human Needs and Wellness Diagnoses

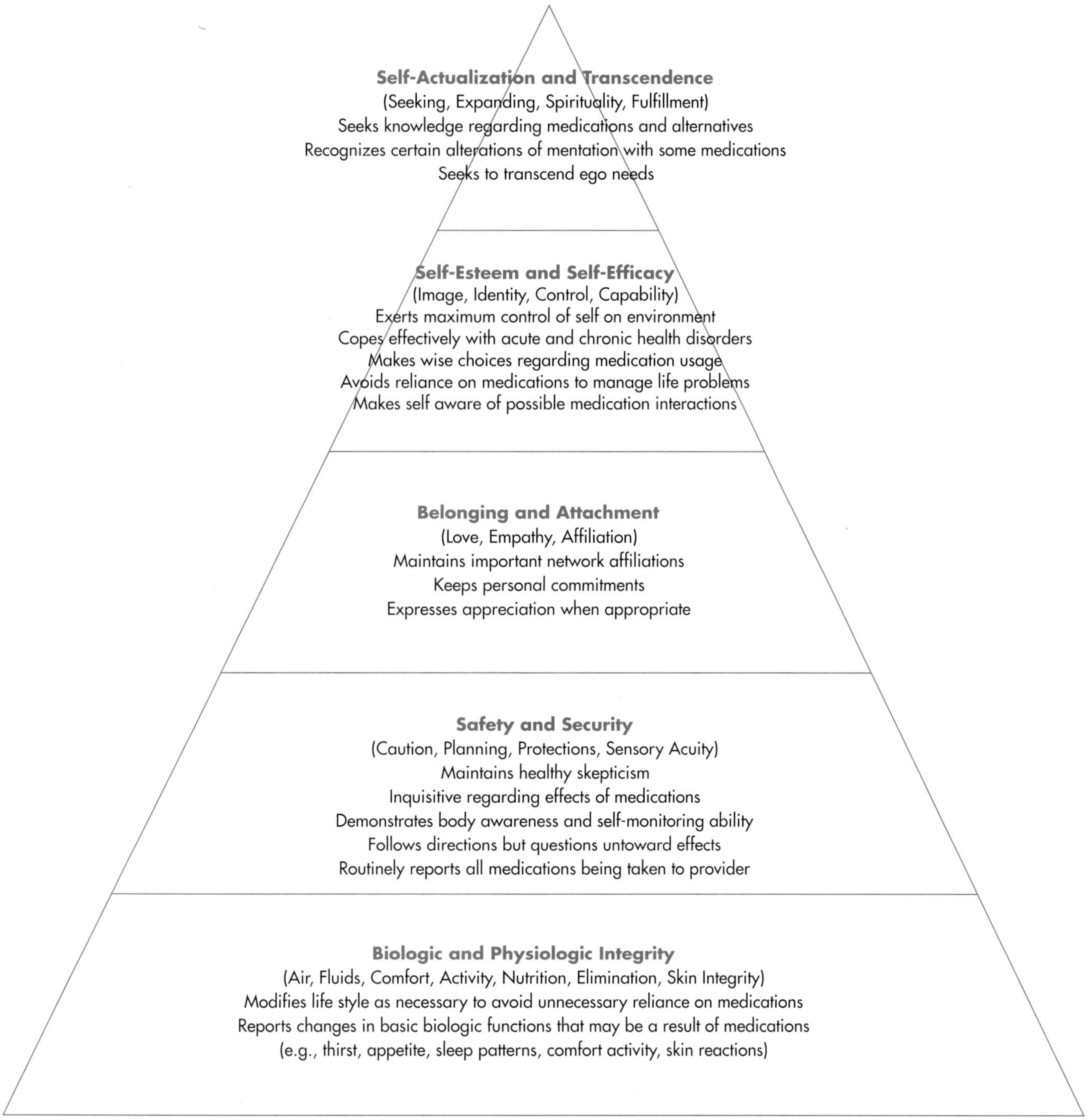

Self-Actualization and Transcendence
(Seeking, Expanding, Spirituality, Fulfillment)
Seeks knowledge regarding medications and alternatives
Recognizes certain alterations of mentation with some medications
Seeks to transcend ego needs

Self-Esteem and Self-Efficacy
(Image, Identity, Control, Capability)
Exerts maximum control of self on environment
Copes effectively with acute and chronic health disorders
Makes wise choices regarding medication usage
Avoids reliance on medications to manage life problems
Makes self aware of possible medication interactions

Belonging and Attachment
(Love, Empathy, Affiliation)
Maintains important network affiliations
Keeps personal commitments
Expresses appreciation when appropriate

Safety and Security
(Caution, Planning, Protections, Sensory Acuity)
Maintains healthy skepticism
Inquisitive regarding effects of medications
Demonstrates body awareness and self-monitoring ability
Follows directions but questions untoward effects
Routinely reports all medications being taken to provider

Biologic and Physiologic Integrity
(Air, Fluids, Comfort, Activity, Nutrition, Elimination, Skin Integrity)
Modifies life style as necessary to avoid unnecessary reliance on medications
Reports changes in basic biologic functions that may be a result of medications
(e.g., thirst, appetite, sleep patterns, comfort activity, skin reactions)

These are not all the possible wellness diagnoses that may be identified. The above are examples of nursing diagnoses that should be considered when planning care for the older adult.

KEY CONCEPTS

- Individuals over 75 years old cannot be expected to react to any medication in the way they did when they were 25 years old.
- Any medication has side effects, and the therapeutic goal is to reduce the targeted symptom without undesirable side effects. Drug-drug, drug-food, and drug-herb incompatibilities are an increasing problem of which nurses must be aware.
- Polypharmacy reactions are one of the most serious problems of elders today and are usually the first arena to investigate when untoward physiologic events occur.
- Drug misuse may be triggered by physician practices, individual self-medication, physiologic idiosyncrasies, altered biodegradability, nutritional and fluid states, and inadequate assessment before prescribing.
- Drug toxicity occurs when the amount of drug taken exceeds the amount necessary to bring about a therapeutic effect. Toxicity can also result from intrinsic patient factors and from drug interactions.
- Many drugs cause temporary cognitive impairment in older persons. These should be discontinued, or if that is not possible the individual needs to be informed in order to forestall fears of Alzheimer's disease. The nurse should educate caregivers, spouses, and family members that worsening cognitive impairment is an adverse reaction and requires immediate attention.
- Nurses must investigate drugs immediately if confusion is observed in an individual who is normally alert and aware. Family members should be made aware of this plan of action.
- Nonadherence with medication regimens is a constant concern among health care professionals. We recommend that the nurse focus on possible reasons. One cannot and will not comply with a prescription or treatment plan when there are incompatibilities that interfere with the practicalities (including economics) of life or are distressful to the individual's well-being or when actual misinformation or disability prevents compliance. In sum, the nurse needs to consider language, cultural, social, economic, psychologic, motivational, and functional factors as possible influences on adherence.
- The provider's responsibility in patient adherence includes ensuring that the drug is necessary, is a safe dose for a geriatric person, will not interact with other medications or supplements the patient will be taking, and will not cause harm. The provider must provide as much drug information as possible and do follow-up reassessment when possible. The provider needs some reassurance that the senior will report side effects or any adverse effect.
- An important aspect of medication administration is developing a reliable plan for administering the appropriate amounts at the correct time. Nurses may be most helpful is assisting the elder with such a plan.
- Drugs can cause and treat psychiatric symptoms. Nurses need to be aware of problems associated with causative agents and the side effects associated with drugs prescribed for psychiatric symptoms.

▲ CASE STUDY

Rose was a 78-year-old woman who lived alone in a large city. She had been widowed for 10 years. Her children were grown, and all were successful. She was very proud of them because she and her husband had emigrated to the United States when the children were small and had worked very hard to establish and maintain a home. She had had only a few years of primary education and still clung to many of her "old country" ways. She spoke a strange mixture of English and her mother tongue, and her children were somewhat embarrassed by her. They thought she was somewhat of a hypochondriac because she constantly complained to them about various aches and pains, her knees that "gave out," her "sugar" and "water" problems, and her heart palpitations. She had been diagnosed with mild diabetes and congestive heart failure. She was a devout Catholic and attended mass each morning. Her treks to church events, to the senior center at church, and to her various doctors (internist; orthopedic, cardiac, and ophthalmic specialists) constituted her social life. One day the recreation director at the senior center noticed her pulling a paper bag of medication bottles from her purse. She sat down to talk with Rose about them and soon realized that Rose had only a vague idea of what most of them were for and tended to take them whenever she felt she needed them.

Based on the case study, develop a nursing care plan using the following procedure:

List comments of client that provide subjective data.

List information that provides objective data.

From these data identify and state, using accepted format, two nursing diagnoses you determine are most significant to the client at this time. List two client strengths that you have identified from data.

Determine and state outcome criteria for each diagnosis. These must reflect some alleviation of the problem identified in the nursing diagnosis and must be stated in concrete and measurable terms.

Plan and state one or more interventions for each diagnosed problem. Provide specific documentation of source used to determine appropriate intervention. Plan at least one intervention that incorporates the client's existing strengths.

Evaluate success of intervention. Intervention must correlate directly with the stated outcome criteria in order to measure the outcome success.

STUDY QUESTIONS/ACTIVITIES

When you are given a prescription for medication, what do you ask about it?

As a nurse visiting the center for a 6-week student assignment, how would you begin to help Rose?
What factors about Rose's probable medication misuse would be most alarming to you?
What aspect of Rose's situation related to medications do you think are common among elders?
Do you think most elders seek adequate information about their medications before taking them?
Who should be responsible for teaching and monitoring medication use in Rose's case? In any case?
Where would you obtain sufficient drug information for persons who speak English as a second language (ESL)?
How can you determine whether medication information is geared to Rose's difficulty with literacy?

▲ CASE STUDY

Mr. G is an 82-year-old man who has recently married after 3 years of widowhood. During the past 2 months, he has become increasingly withdrawn and isolated. From being an active person involved with his photography hobby, he has retreated to bed and spends most days sleeping or watching television. His wife complains about his sudden and progressive change, wondering whether he is depressed. His internist prescribes sertraline 50 mg once daily at bedtime for depression. After 2 days, Mr. G is agitated, suffering from insomnia, and dizzy, and he has a slight tremor. He also complains about being tired, having a dry mouth, and having no appetite. His wife encourages him to take the medicine, but he refuses.
What do you think is causing Mr. G's sudden changes?
What actions would you take with Mr. and Mrs. G? Why?
What interdisciplinary communication needs to occur?
What data will you collect from the Gs to contribute to understanding Mr. G's withdrawal and possible depression?

▲ CASE STUDY

Ms. S is a 65-year-old woman who has been falling asleep lately in the middle of her bridge games at her board and care home. She has been her usual friendly, chatty self lately except for the frequent catnaps. The board and care director says Ms. S has become unsteady on her feet and is fearful that she will fall. Also, occasionally, Ms. S gets confused and forgets which card game she is playing (she keeps yelling "Fish"). She has begun asking someone else to shuffle the cards for her because she says her hands are weak. The only medication she takes is a small amount of Valium to help her sleep at night, so she knows the daytime sleeping, mild confusion, and weakened state are all part of growing old. She does not want to worry anyone by complaining.
What do you think about her attitude toward the changes taking place? What action would you consider taking with Ms. S? Why?

▲ CASE STUDY

Mr. E is a 75-year-old Hispanic man who has difficulty understanding English and is usually very nervous. He has a heart problem for which he takes digoxin and a diuretic to lower his blood pressure. Last week his doctor changed the doses of both medications. Mr. E has been complaining to you of feeling sick to his stomach, occasional vomiting, dizziness, and stumbling a lot. He stopped taking his medications today because he decided they were making him sick.
What do you think about his decision? What action would you consider taking with Mr. E? Why?

▲ CASE STUDY

Ms. J is a 70-year-old retired school teacher who likes to drink a glass of wine with lunch and dinner to calm her nerves. She takes a narcotic pain medication, as needed, for her hip pain. Last month her doctor prescribed a mild sedative to help her sleep at night. She has been using an OTC cough syrup whenever she feels a cough coming on, which seems to be fairly often. Recently she has been more forgetful and sometimes cannot remember where she lives. She continues to insist on a monthly doctor's appointment because she has great faith in modern medicine.
What do you think about the way she is handling her health care? What action would you consider taking with Ms. J?

RESEARCH QUESTIONS

What are the best methods to promote prescribers' adherence to geriatric drug restrictions and dosage guidelines?
What is the prevalence of adverse drug events in elderly living in the community? In nursing homes? In a hospitalized population? What influences these rates?
What do elders know about their medications? What are their sources of information and knowledge?
What symptoms do elders self-treat with OTC and herbal medicines?
What are nursing roles in preventing adverse events in elders?
Among the following three teaching strategies, which works the best: computer-assisted medication teaching, telephone teaching, and in-person medication teaching?
Which elders tend to be given the most adequate information about their medications?
Who provides the most complete information about medications?
How many elders have access to sources for looking up their own medications?
What questions do elders ask before taking prescriptions?
What percentage of elders are not taking any prescribed drugs?
How many elders are aware of possible negative drug interactions?

What symptoms do elders recognize as possible drug reactions?

How do prescribers determine the best antidepressant for individual elders?

REFERENCES

Aljasem L et al: The impact of barriers and self-efficacy on self-care behaviors in type 2 diabetes, *Diabetes Educ* 27(3):393, 2001.

American Association of Retired Persons Research: Survey on prescription drug issues and usage among Americans aged 50 and older, 1996. Available at *wysiwyg://15/http://research.aarp.org/health/mainexec.html*

Atherton JC et al: Lithium clearance in healthy humans: effects of sodium intake and diuretics, *Kidney Int Suppl* 28:S36, 1990.

Balkrishnan R: Predictors of medication adherence in the elderly, *Clin Ther* 20(4):764, 1998.

Bandura A: Self-efficacy: toward a unifying theory of behavioral change, *Psychol Rev* 84:191, 1977.

Bandura A: Self-efficacy mechanism in human agency, *Am Psychol* 37:122, 1982.

Barat I, Andreasen F, Damsgaard S: Drug therapy in the elderly: what doctors believe and patients actually do, *Br J Clin Pharmacol* 51:615, 2001.

Barnett N, Denham MJ, Francis SA: Over-the-counter medicines and the elderly, *Journal of the Royal College of Physicians of London* 34(5):445, 2000.

Barry P: New scramble over drugs, *AARP Bulletin* 43(6):6, 2002.

Bartholomew K, Horowitz LM: Attachment styles among young adults: a test of a four-category model, *J Pers Soc Psychol* 61:226, 1991.

Beaubrun G, Gray GE: A review of herbal medicines for psychiatric disorders, *Psychiatric Services* 51(9):1130, 2000.

Beers M: Explicit criteria for determining potentially inappropriate medication use by the elderly, *Arch Intern Med* 157:1531, 1997.

Besdine R et al: *When medicine hurts instead of helps: preventing medication problems in older persons,* Washington, DC, 1998, Alliance for Aging Research and the American Society of Consultant Pharmacists.

Bowlby J: *Attachment and loss,* vol II, *Separation: anxiety and anger,* New York, 1973, Basic Books.

Buffum J: Prescription drugs and sexual function, *Psychiatr Med* 10(2):181, 1992.

Buffum J: *Geriatric dosage guidelines,* San Francisco, 1996, VA Medical Center.

Buffum J: Appendix: the effects of drugs on male sexuality. In Zilbergeld B, editor: *The new male sexuality,* rev ed, New York, 1999, Bantam Books.

Buffum J: Unpublished data, 2003.

Buffum J, Moser C, Smith D: Street drugs and sexual function. In Sitsen J, editor: *Handbook of sexology,* vol 6, *The pharmacology and endrocrinology of sexual function,* New York, 1988, Elsevier Science.

Byerly M et al: Antipsychotic medications and the elderly, *Drugs Aging* 18(1):45, 2001.

Cameron K: *Nonprescription medicines: new opportunities and responsibilities for self care,* Washington, DC, 1996, United Seniors Health Cooperative.

Carlson E, Fleck C: Bringing down drug costs, *AARP Bulletin* 43(6):7, 2002.

Choquet-Kastylevsky GT et al: Drug allergy diagnosis in humans: possibilities and pitfalls, *Toxicology* 158(1-2):1, 2001.

Chou FC et al: Genetic polymorphism of cytochrome P450 3A5 in Chinese, *Drug Metab Dispos* 29(9):1205, 2001.

Ciechanowski P, Katon WJ, Russo JE: Depression and diabetes: impact of depressive symptoms on adherence, function, and costs, *Arch Intern Med* 160:3278, 2000.

Ciechanowski P et al: The patient-provider relationship: attachment theory and adherence to treatment in diabetes, *Am J Psychiatry* 158(1):29, 2001.

Clark BA et al: Increased susceptibility to thiazide-induced hyponatremia in the elderly, *J Am Soc Nephrol* 5(4):1106, 1994.

Cockcroft DW, Gault MH: Prediction of creatinine clearance from serum creatinine, *Nephron* 16(1):31, 1976.

Crome P: Adverse drug reactions. In Crome P, Ford G, editors: *Drugs and the older population,* London, 2000, Imperial College Press.

de los Reyes GC, Koda RT: Determining hyperforin and hypericin content in eight brands of St. John's wort, *Am J Health Syst Pharm* 59(6):545, 2002.

Drugs that may cause cognitive disorders in the elderly, *Medical Letter* 42(1093):111-112, 2000.

Drugs that may cause psychiatric symptoms, *Medical Letter* 44(1134): 59, 2002.

Eddington N: Pharmacokinetics. In Roberts J, Snyder D, Friedman E, editors: *Handbook of pharmacology of aging,* ed 2, Boca Raton, FL, 1996, CRC Press.

Edworthy S, Devins GM: Improving medication adherence through patient education distinguishing between appropriate and inappropriate utilization. Patient Education Study Group, *J Rheumatol* 26(8):1793, 1999.

Ernst E: The risk-benefit profile of commonly used herbal therapies: ginkgo, St. John's wort, ginseng, echinacea, saw palmetto, and kava, *Ann Intern Med* 136(1):42, 2002.

Flockhart D: *Cytochrome P450 drug interaction table,* 2003, Indiana University Department of Medicine.

Gauthier I, Malone M: Drug-food interactions in hospitalised patients: methods of prevention, *Drug Saf* 18(6):383, 1998.

Gold J et al: Herbal-drug therapy interactions: a focus on dementia, *Current Opinion in Clinical Nutrition and Metabolic Care* 4:29, 2001.

Greenblatt DJ et al: Drug interactions with grapefruit juice: an update, *J Clin Psychopharmacol* 21(4):357, 2001.

Gruchalla R: Understanding drug allergies, *J Allergy Clin Immunol* 105(6 pt 2):S637, 2000.

Gurwitz JH et al: Incidence and preventability of adverse drug events among older persons in the ambulatory setting. *JAMA* 289(9):1107, 2003.

Hammerlein A et al: Pharmacokinetic and pharmacodynamic changes in the elderly: clinical implications, *Clin Pharmacokinet* 35(1):49, 1998.

Hartshorn E, Tatro D: *Principles of drug interaction, drug interaction facts 2003,* St Louis, 2003, Facts and Comparisons.

Helping patients adhere to medical instructions, 2001, Lifeline Connections for the Healthcare Professional. Available at *www.lifelinesys.com/images/summer01.pdf*

Hohl CM et al: Polypharmacy, adverse drug-related events, and potential adverse drug interactions in elderly patients presenting to an emergency department, *Ann Emerg Med* 38(6):666, 2001.

Horne R, Weinman J: Patients' beliefs about prescribed medicines and their role in adherence to treatment in chronic physical illness, *J Psychosom Res* 47(6):555, 1999.

Huang JD et al: Detection of a novel cytochrome P-450 1A2 polymorphism (F21L) in Chinese, *Drug Metab Dispos* 27(1):98, 1999.

Israili ZH, Dayton PG: Human alpha-1-glycoprotein and its interactions with drugs, *Drug Metab Rev* 33(2):161, 2001.

Izzo A, Ernst E: Interactions between herbal medicines and prescribed drugs: a systematic review, *Drugs* 61(15):2163, 2001.

Kimura MI et al: Genetic polymorphism of cytochrome P450s, CYP2C19, and CYP2C9 in a Japanese population, *Ther Drug Monit* 20(3):243, 1998.

Klaassen C: Principles of toxicology and treatment of poisoning. In Hardman J, Limbird L, Gilman A, editors: *Goodman and Gilman's the pharmacological basis of therapeutics,* ed 10, New York, 2001, McGraw-Hill.

Lacy C et al: *Drug information handbook 2003-2004,* Cleveland, 2003, Lexi-Comp, Inc.

Lamba JK et al: Genetic polymorphism of the hepatic cytochrome P450 2C19 in north Indian subjects, *Clin Pharmacol Ther* 63(4):422, 1998.

Lambrecht J, Hamilton W, Rabinovich A: A review of herb-drug interactions: documented and theoretical, *US Pharmacist* 25(8):1, 2000.

Leung AY et al: Genetic polymorphism in exon 4 of cytochrome P450 CYP2C9 may be associated with warfarin sensitivity in Chinese patients, *Blood* 98(8):2584, 2001.

Lowe C et al: Effects of self-medication programme on knowledge of drugs and compliance with treatment in elderly patients, *BMJ* 310(6989):1229, 1995.

Mah K, Binik YM: The nature of human orgasm: a critical review of major trends, *Clin Psychol Rev* 21(6):823, 2001.

Maletta G, Mattox KM, Dysken M: Guidelines for prescribing psychoactive drugs, *Geriatrics* 55(3):65-69, 2000.

Mannesse CK et al: Adverse drug reactions in elderly patients as contributing factor for hospital admission: cross sectional study, *BMJ* 315(7115):1057, 1997.

Matheny CJ et al: Pharmacokinetic and pharmacodynamic implications of P-glycoprotein modulation, *Pharmacotherapy* 21(7):778, 2001.

McElnay JC, D'Arcy PF: Protein binding displacement interactions and their clinical importance, *Drugs* 25(5):495, 1983.

Melman A, Christ GJ: The hemodynamics of erection and the pharmacotherapies of erectile dysfunction, *Heart Dis* 4(4):252, 2002.

Merriam-Webster Online: *Merriam-Webster's collegiate dictionary,* 2003, Merriam-Webster. Available at *www.m-w.com/home.htm*

Mulder AB et al: Association of polymorphism in the cytochrome CYP2D6 and the efficacy and tolerability of simvastatin, *Clin Pharmacol Ther* 70(6):546, 2001.

National Council on Patient Information and Education (NCPIE): *Attitudes and beliefs about the use of over-the-counter medicines: a dose of reality,* Bethesda, MD, 2002, Harris Interactive. Available at *www.harrisinteractive.com*

Nicholson T: AARP taking high costs to court, *AARP Bulletin* 43(6):7, 2002.

Norcross J, Prochaska JO: *Using the stages of change,* Harvard Mental Health Letter, Harvard Health Online, 2002. Available at *www.health.harvard.edu/medline/Mental/M0502c.html*

O'Leary A: Self-efficacy and health, *Behav Res Ther* 23:437, 1985.

O'Mahony S: Pharmacokinetics. In Crome P, Ford G, editors: *Drugs and the older population,* London, 2000, Imperial College Press.

Omer BU et al: Genetic polymorphism of cytochrome P450 2E1 in the Turkish population, *Cell Biochem Funct* 19(4):273, 2001.

Park D et al: Medication adherence in rheumatoid arthritis patients: older is wiser, *J Am Geriatr Soc* 47(2):172, 1999.

Pear R: AARP joins three lawsuits against large drug companies, *New York Times,* May 30, 2002, p A19.

Pollock G, Reynolds CF III: Depression in late life. Harvard Mental Health Letter, Harvard Health Online, 2000. Available at *www.health.harvard.edu/medline/Mental/M0900b.html*

Preventing medication errors in the elderly, HCPro's Patient Safety Monitor's Pick of the Week, Marblehead, MA, April 24, 2002, HCPro. Available at *www.accreditinfo.com/ptsafety/ptsafety_pick.cfm?content_id=21864*

Prochaska J, DiClemente C: Transtheoretical therapy: toward a more integrative model of change, *Pscyhother Theory Res Pract* 19:276, 1982.

Sadock B, Sadock V: *Pocket handbook of psychiatric drug treatment,* ed 3, New York, 2001, Lippincott Williams & Wilkins.

Salom IL, Davis K: Prescribing for older patients: how to avoid toxic drug reactions, *Geriatrics* 50(10): 37, 1995.

Schafer SL: Prescribing for seniors: it's a balancing act, *J Am Acad Nurse Pract* 13(3):108, 2001.

Schmidt LE, Dalhoff K: Food-drug interactions, *Drugs* 62(10):1481, 2002.

Scott GN, Elmer GW: Update on natural product—drug interactions, *Am J Health Syst Pharm* 59(4):339, 2002.

Semla TP, Beizer JL, Higbee MD: *Geriatric dosage handbook,* ed 8, Cleveland, 2003, Lexi-Comp, Inc.

Seventh report of the Joint National Committee on Prevention, Detection, Evaluation, And Treatment Of High Blood Pressure (JNC 7 Express). National Institutes of Health Publication No. 03-5233, May 2003.

Shader RI, Greenblatt DJ: More on oral contraceptives, drug interactions, herbal medicines, and hormone replacement therapy, *J Clin Psychopharmacol* 20(4):397, 2000.

Shemesh E et al: A prospective study of posttraumatic stress symptoms and nonadherence in survivors of a myocardial infarction (MI), *General Hospital Psychiatry* 23:215, 2001.

Solomon P et al: Ginkgo for memory enhancement, *JAMA* 288(7):835, 2002.

Spectrum Society for Community Living: Oral drugs that should not be crushed or chewed, 2002. Available at *www.spectrumsociety.org/library/SpectrumMedManual.pdf*

Stoudemire A, Smith DA: OBRA regulations and the use of psychotropic drugs in long-term care facilities: impact and implications for geropsychiatric care, *General Hospital Psychiatry* 18:77, 1996.

Tatro D: *Drug interaction facts 2003,* St Louis, 2003, Facts and Comparisons.

Trenter ME: *From test tube to patient,* 1999, Food and Drug Administration. Available at *www.fda.gov/cder*

Ujjin PS et al: Variation in coumarin 7-hydroxylase activity associated with genetic polymorphism of cytochrome P450 2A6 and the body status of iron stores in adult Thai males and females, *Pharmacogenetics* 12(3):241, 2002.

Valli G, Giardina EG: Benefits, adverse effects and drug interactions of herbal therapies with cardiovascular effects, *J Am Coll Cardiol* 39(7):1083, 2002.

van der Weide JL et al: The effect of genetic polymorphism of cytochrome P450 CYP2C9 on phenytoin dose requirement, *Pharmacogenetics* 11(4):287, 2001.

Wilkinson G: Pharmacokinetics. In Hardman J, Limbird L, Gilman A, editors: *Goodman and Gilman's the pharmacological basis of therapeutics,* ed 10, New York, 2001, McGraw-Hill.

Wurglics MK et al: Comparison of German St. John's wort products according to hyperforin and total hypericin content, *J Am Pharm Assoc (Wash)* 41(4):560, 2001.

Zheng WD et al: Genetic polymorphism of cytochrome P450-1B1 and risk of breast cancer, *Cancer Epidemiol Biomarkers Prev* 9(2):147, 2000.

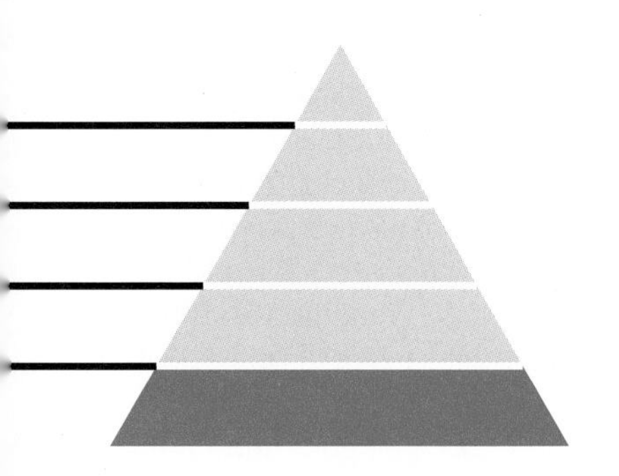

CHAPTER 11

Herbs and Supplements

Dianne Thames

LEARNING OBJECTIVES

On completion of this chapter, the reader will be able to:

1. Identify the legal standards that affect herbal supplement use.
2. Describe the altered effects of herbs on the older adult.
3. Discuss the information that older adults should know about the use of herbal supplements.
4. Discuss the role of the health care professional assisting the older adult who uses herbal supplements.
5. Describe the effects of commonly used herbs on the older adult.
6. Develop a nursing care plan to prevent adverse herbal reactions.
7. Identify the important aspects of patient education related to the use of herbal supplements with the older adult.
8. Describe the effects of herbal supplements on the older adult with chronic disease.
9. Describe the effects of herbal supplements on the older adult who is experiencing altered health conditions.

USES

Herbs

Herbs have been used by humans for hundreds of years to treat illness and more recently as a mechanism for returning to the "natural" way of maintaining health (Gray, 1996). The use of herbs is the most common form of alternative medicine in the United States (Keller and Lemberg, 2001). Most clients who take herbs are "white, highly educated and have higher incomes" (Stuypay and Sivertsen, 2000, p. 57).

The renewed interest in herbal therapies is based in part on the focus of preventing illness (Youngkin and Israel, 1996). Herbs are often used by individuals who want to be more involved in their own health care (Stupay and Sivertsen, 2000). They are interested in having control over their health (Fryback and Reinert, 1997). This aspect of personal health care is supported by Judith Miller's concept of powerlessness and chronic illness: The more an individual feels a sense of control over the outcome of a situation such as his or her health care, the more likely it is that the individual's situation will improve (Miller, 1983). Individuals less than satisfied with the results of their medical treatment often seek alternative medicines.

Older adults who are diagnosed with chronic conditions are more likely to use herbal supplements (Stupay and Sivertsen, 2000). Approximately 15 million consumers use herbs along with prescribed medications each year (Sutherland, 2001). These individuals usually continue their traditional therapies in addition to herbal therapies (Stupay and Sivertsen, 2000).

Herbs are manufactured in several forms: capsules, extracts, oils, pills, salves, teas, and tinctures. Efficacy varies depending on the form of the herb that is used. An extract is a "concentrated form of the herb that is derived when the crude herb is mixed with water, alcohol or another solvent and distilled or evaporated. Extracts may be either fluid or solid" (Skidmore-Roth, 2001).

Oils are found in two forms. Essential oils are aromatic, are volatile, and can be derived from various parts of the fresh plant. To be therapeutic, they are usually diluted (Skidmore-Roth, 2001). Infused oils, on the other hand, are a volatile oil of one herb that is mixed with another oil (Skidmore-Roth, 2001). Herbal oils can be used for massages or aromatherapy (Eliopoulos, 1999).

When an herb has been soaked in a liquid, such as water, alcohol, vinegar, or glycerine, for a specific time, strained, and the plant then disposed of, a tincture has been made. The liquid is used therapeutically at a concentration of 1 : 5 or 1 : 10 (Skidmore-Roth, 2001).

A salve is a type of ointment, a semisolid substance that is used topically. Salves and ointments can be purchased or prepared by "simmering two tablespoons of the herb in 220 grams of a petroleum-based jelly for about ten minutes" (Eliopoulos, 1999, p. 103).

Different parts of an herb can be used for different reasons. For example, the bulb of the garlic is used whereas the leaf of the chamomile is used. Different parts of the herb produce different reactions (Eliopoulos, 1999).

Teas

The manufacture of herbal teas is a million-dollar business, and because there are few if any reports of untoward effects, the consumer may believe that herbal teas are harmless. This may indeed be true in cases where the teas are consumed at a moderate or less rate, but in cases where individuals have consumed more than the suggested amounts of the teas, conditions such as liver disease have been reported. Because of these types of reports, comfrey has been removed from the market (Youngkin and Israel, 1996).

COMMONLY USED HERBS AND TEAS

Chamomile (Matricaria recutita) is also known as *German chamomile* and *Hungarian chamomile* and usually taken in tea form. It is used as an antiinflammatory and an antispasmodic (Youngkin and Israel, 1996). Chamomile relaxes smooth muscles (Stupay and Sivertsen, 2000). It may cause contact dermatitis and hypersensitivity-type reactions and should be used cautiously with clients who report allergies to ragweed, asters, or chrysanthemums (Youngkin and Israel, 1996).

Echinacea (Echinacea angustifolia) is also known as *Sampson root* and *purple coneflower.* It is used as an immune stimulant and is usually taken in tea form, but it can also be used as a tincture. Using echinacea should not exclude using antibiotics. Few allergies have been reported, but it should "not be used by persons with conditions such as tuberculosis, AIDS, collagen diseases or multiple sclerosis" (Youngkin and Israel, 1996). When used as a tea, the dose is 0.5 to 1 g (Scorza, 2002). The usual dosage time is 10 to 14 days, but it should not be continued for more than 6 to 8 weeks (Youngkin and Israel, 1996).

Garlic (*Allium sativum* bulb), also known as *clove garlic,* is thought to protect against stroke and atherosclerosis. Garlic is usually available in oil and tincture form. It is also thought to decrease cholesterol and blood pressure, while prolonging clotting time. Individuals have been known to have allergic reactions to garlic, and consuming more than five cloves a day could lead to heartburn and to increased flatulence (Youngkin and Israel, 1996). Clients taking aspirin or anticoagulants should not ingest large amounts of garlic (Youngkin and Israel, 1996). Clients with peptic and reflux disease should avoid garlic. Using topical preparations can cause a skin irritation (Scorza, 2002). The suggested dose is 600 to 1000 mg/day (Stupay and Sivertsen, 2000). Cooking garlic decreases its effectiveness (Keller and Lemberg, 2001).

Ginkgo (*Ginkgo biloba* leaf abstract) is also known as *maidenhair tree, Asiatic ginseng, Chinese ginseng,* and *wonder of world.* It is the oldest living tree species (Waddell et al, 2001). It is prepared in capsule, extract, and tablet form. Clients taking anticoagulants should not take ginkgo. Bleeding has been reported with patients who take ginkgo while taking aspirin, warfarin, acetaminophen, or preparations containing ergotamine-caffeine (Kuhn, 2002). The German Commission E reported that it is effective in treating vertigo, impaired memory, and mood swings (Youngkin and Israel, 1996). It has been thought by some to improve cognitive function and to increase blood flow to the brain, but the results of research in this area remain controversial (Kuhn, 2002).

Side effects of taking ginkgo include gastrointestinal upset, headache, and hypersensitivity (Waddell et al, 2001). Because one of the side effects of taking ginkgo is headache, the client may want to take an analgesic. Acetaminophen and ibuprofen are recommended because there is no bleeding complication associated with that combination. The combination of aspirin and ginkgo can lead to bleeding of the small blood vessels of the eyes (Waddell et al, 2001). Patients who take ginkgo should be taught to report bleeding, bruising, dizziness, headache, and blurred vision to their health care provider (Kuhn, 2002). Ginkgo seeds can be toxic (Allen and Bell, 2002). Use with monoamine oxidase inhibitors should be avoided. The usual dose varies (Stupay and Sivertsen, 2000).

Ginseng (*Panax schinseng,* a Chinese perennial herb), also known as *American ginseng, five-fingers,* and *five-leafed ginseng,* has no data supporting any clinical benefits. Ginseng is most commonly prepared in capsule, extract, and tincture form. The German Commission E reports that it could be useful in conditions associated with fatigue or poor concentration. The German Commission E also recommends that ginseng be used for no more than 3 months. Adverse effects include difficulty sleeping and diarrhea. Concerns remain over the differences between North American and Chinese ginseng and standardization of the herb itself (Youngkin and Israel, 1996). Ginseng has a hypertensive effect (Eliopoulos, 1999). Clients with hypertension, cardiac problems, or diabetes should use ginseng with caution. The usual dose is 200 to 300 mg daily or twice daily for 2 weeks, then stop for 1 to 2 weeks before starting again (Stupay and Sivertsen, 2000).

Glucosamine is also known as *chitosamine* and *glucosamine sulfate.* It is used as an antiinflammatory and antiarthritic. The dose varies, but glucosamine is usually prepared in capsule and tablet form. Bronchopulmonary complications and interference with insulin secretion have been reported (Youngkin and Israel, 1996). The usual dose is 500 mg three times daily. Research indicates that side effects are similar to those of a placebo (Scorza, 2002).

Hawthorn (Crataegus monogyna, Crataegus iaevigata) is also known as *May bush, May tree, thornapple tree,* and *whitehorn.* It is usually prepared in extract and tea form. It is thought to have positive effects on coronary and myocardial circulation. There are no warnings, but it should be taken only under the supervision of a health care provider. Hawthorn may interact with cardiovascular medications and can affect blood sugar levels (Allen and Bell, 2002). With large doses, hawthorn can cause blood pressure to drop (Eliopoulos, 1999).

St. John's wort (Hypericum perforatum) is also known as *amber, goatweed, Johnswort,* and *Klamath weed.* St. John's wort is commonly used to treat depression and can be used as an astringent. Research indicates that it may also have antiviral properties (Youngkin and Israel, 1996). It is one of the most popular herbs used today. It is known to have few side effects, but it may cause photosensitivity and dermatitis. Other cytochrome P450 enzyme inducers, such as red wine, broccoli, and cigarette smoke, should be used cautiously with St. John's wort (Swanson et al, 2000). The usual dose is 300 mg three times daily or 450 mg twice daily (Waddell et al, 2001). It may take up to 6 weeks for St. John's wort to reach its full effect (Stupay and Sivertsen, 2000).

Thought to act as a selective serotonin reuptake inhibitor (SSRI), St. John's wort should not be taken while taking SSRIs. Patients on SSRIs should wait at least 2 weeks after discontinuing them before beginning the St. John's wort. In addition, patients taking St. John's wort should be careful about their exposure to the sun (Kuhn, 2002). When taking St. John's wort, patients should be warned not to take medications containing monoamines, such as medications for nasal decongestants, hay fever, and asthma, because this combination can cause hypertension (Waddell et al, 2001). Table 11-1 lists commonly used herbs and their recommended dosages.

Table 11-1 Commonly Used Herbs and Recommended Dosages

Herb	Form	Recommended dosage
Chamomile	Capsule: 360 mg	300-400 mg 6 times/day
	Fluid extract	1-2 ml tid
	Tea	2-4 oz prn
	Tincture	3-10 ml tid
Echinacea	Capsule	500 mg-1 g tid
	Fluid extract	1-2 ml tid
	Tea	2 tsp simmered 15 minutes
	Tincture	15-30 drops bid-qid
Garlic	Extract	4 ml qd
	Fresh	4 g qd
	Oil	10 mg qd
Ginkgo	Capsule	80 mg tid
	Extract	80 mg tid
	Tablets	80 mg tid
Ginseng	Capsules	200-500 mg qd
	Extract	200-500 mg qd
	Tincture	1-2 ml qd
Glucosamine	Capsule/tablet	1500 mg and 1200 mg of chondroitin
Hawthorn	Extract	120-240 mg tid
	Tea	1-2 tsp in 8 oz of water for 15 minutes
St. John's wort	Extract	300 mg tid

Adapted from Skidmore-Roth L: *Mosby's handbook of herbs and natural supplements,* St Louis, 2001, Mosby.
bid, Twice a day; *prn,* as required; *qd,* every day; *qid,* four times daily; *tid,* three times daily; *tsp,* teaspoon.

HERBAL INTERACTIONS WITH MEDICATIONS

The study of herbal interactions with medications is one that has many facets and is not well understood. When this type of interaction does occur, the medication, which is usually more pharmacologically active than the herb, is typically the cause. The more herbs that the client is taking, the more likely it is that an interaction will occur (Kuhn, 2002). Patients taking medications that have a narrow therapeutic index should be discouraged from using herbal remedies (Kuhn, 2002).

There are several types of interactions. Those that occur as absorption-type interactions, such as aloe or rhubarb, usually bind to a medication, such as digoxin or warfarin, reducing the effectiveness of the medication. In these cases, the drug should be taken at least 1 hour before the herb (Kuhn, 2002).

Herbs that are more likely to cause a distribution-type interaction may increase the possibility of adverse effects. For example, meadowsweet and black willow may interact with warfarin and carbamazepine. When taken together, the adverse effects of the medications are amplified (Kuhn, 2002).

Metabolism-type interactions may increase or decrease the effectiveness of the medication, depending on the herb and the medication. The action of digoxin is increased in the presence of St. John's wort, whereas the action of corticosteroids is decreased in the presence of licorice. There are also additive-type interactions, such as ginkgo increasing the action of warfarin (Kuhn, 2002).

Table 11-2 lists the interactions between commonly used herbs and selected medications. Complications and nursing actions are also listed.

MISUSE

Most health care providers are aware that many of the more potent medications used today, such as morphine, atropine, and digitalis, are derived from potent plants, but many Americans believe that herbs and supplements are derived from harmless plants (Kuhn, 2002). The old saying, "If it sounds too good to be true—it probably is," could not be more appropriate.

At the present time, the U.S. government has no standards in place to control the quality of herbs or herbal products. Before 1962 all herbs were regarded as medications. During that year, the Food and Drug Administration (FDA) began to require that all drugs be evaluated for safety and efficacy. In

Table 11-2 Herb-Medication Interactions

Herb	Medication	Complication	Nursing action
Garlic	Heparin sodium Ketoprofen Streptokinase Methotrexate Urokinase Warfarin sodium	Risk of bleeding may increase	Teach patient not to take concurrently
	Pioglitazone	Serum glucose control may improve, requiring less antidiabetic medication	Monitor blood glucose levels
	Tolbutamide		
Ginkgo	Acetaminophen Aspirin Heparin sodium Warfarin sodium	Risk of bleeding may occur	Teach patient not to take concurrently
Ginseng	Insulin	Blood glucose levels can be affected	Monitor blood glucose levels; monitor for hyperglycemia and hypoglycemia
	Pioglitazone hydrochloride	Blood glucose levels can be improved, requiring less antidiabetic medication	Monitor blood glucose levels
	Tolbutamide		
	Meperidine	Headaches, tremors, and mania	
	Barbiturates	Decreases the effects of anticoagulants	
Green tea	Warfarin sodium	May alter anticoagulant effects	
Hawthorn	Digoxin	May cause a loss of potassium, leading to drug toxicity	Monitor blood levels
St. John's wort	Amprenavir	May decrease drug level and increase indinavir level	
	Cholestyramine		
	Citalopram	Risk of serotonin syndrome	Advise against use of drug and herb concurrently
	Digoxin	Decreases the effects of the drug	
	Efavirenz	May decrease drug level	
	Indinavir sulfate	May decrease drug level	
	Ketoprofen Sulfamethoxazole Triazolam	Photosensitivity	Advise to use sun block
	Nevirapine	May decrease drug level	
	Olanzapine	May reduce drug blood level Psychotic symptoms may be severe	If blood level is adjusted for taking St. John's wort, stopping the herb may lead to drug toxicity
	Paroxetine hydrochloride	Sedative-hypnotic intoxication	
	Ritonavir	May reduce drug blood level, leading to lower therapeutic effects	If blood level is adjusted, when herb is discontinued toxic blood levels could occur
	Sertraline	May increase serotonin levels	Explain importance of the wash-out period before changing from SSRI to St. John's wort
	Theophylline	Increases metabolism; decreases drug blood level	Monitor drug effects
	Warfarin	May decrease anticoagulant effect	

Source: *NDH pocket guide to drug interactions,* Philadelphia, 2002, Lippincott Williams & Wilkins.

response to this standard, herbal manufacturers decided to label herbs as foods (Youngkin and Israel, 1996).

Under this label, herbs are regulated by the Dietary Supplement Health and Education Act (DSHEA). Under the DSHEA the herb cannot advertise prevention, treatment, or cure of a condition. It may only state an effect on the body (Stupay and Sivertsen, 2000).

The herb must be found to be dangerous and then reported to the FDA before the FDA will investigate the product and possibly remove the herb from the market (Allen and Bell, 2002). To date, the FDA has found only nine herbs to be both safe and therapeutic, leaving approximately 1400 proclaiming unsubstantiated health claims (Youngkin and Israel, 1996).

Because herbs are not typically under the protection of the patent laws, companies are not inclined to participate in trials. The fact that there is no consistency between the methods different companies use to produce different herbal products adds to the lack of research in this area (Allen and Bell, 2002).

In 2000 the FDA ruled that expressed disease claims and implied disease claims could not appear on labels with review by the FDA. Health maintenance and nondisease claims are permitted (Stupay and Sivertsen, 2000).

THE NURSE'S ROLE

One of the most important aspects of the role of the health care provider working with an older adult who is using herbal supplements is distinguishing the reliable data from the unproven claims. Maintaining a sound knowledge base is an ongoing responsibility of the health care provider.

A second and equally important role is that of educator. Facilitating the acquisition of information is an essential facet of assisting the older adult to use herbal supplements to improve the health of the individual.

Assessment

As part of the comprehensive nursing assessment, the nurse should ask the patient about over-the-counter (OTC) medications and complementary treatments. Because patients may consider herbal remedies insignificant, they may not mention them unless specifically asked. These questions should be asked in a nonconfrontational manner, remembering that it may take several interviews to complete the data (Stupay and Sivertsen, 2000).

Diagnosis

Several possible nursing diagnoses are included in the following list. Their applicability to the situation depends on the assessment retrieved during the first phase of the nursing process.

- I. Health maintenance, ineffective
- II. Health-seeking behaviors (specify)
- III. Knowledge, deficient (specify)
- IV. Management of therapeutic regimen, individual, ineffective
- V. Powerlessness
  - A. Etiologies and related factors
    1. Aging process of liver and renal function
    2. Self-medication
    3. Inadequate or misunderstood information related to herbal supplements
  - B. Defining characteristics
    1. Cognitive or emotional difficulties
    2. Effects of polypharmacy
    3. Variability of herbal preparation
    4. Effects of herbs on the aging body
  - C. Knowledge
    1. Therapeutic ranges of herbs
       - a. Side effects
       - b. Toxicity
    2. Safe administration of herbs
       - a. Medication-herb interaction
  - D. Clinical judgments and related skills
    1. Act as a resource for information in the correct use of herbal supplements
    2. Monitor for effectiveness, side effects
    3. Patient teaching

Planning

If there is a beneficial rationale for the client to continue to use the herb(s), the health care provider should continue to assess the situation. A review of the client's health condition, the medications that have been prescribed, possible adverse interactions, the herbs, and any OTC medications is an important part of the planning phase (Stupay and Sivertsen, (2000). It is helpful to know what the client hopes to accomplish by using the herb. Reinforcing the positive effects, as well as the costs, of using the herbs can assist the client to relax and open additional lines of communication.

If the client is using an herb in an inappropriate manner, the goal is to have the client discontinue the use of the herb or use only the recommended amount for a specific condition. This can be accomplished by giving the client the needed information and asking the client to consider the appropriate use of the herb. The client may be willing to bring the herb to the health care provider and discuss better ways to use the herb. Whatever strategy is selected, the assistance of the family or a close friend could prove to be invaluable (Stupay and Sivertsen, 2000). When planning care, the health care provider should remember that for many Asian or Asian American clients, the whole family is included in the decision-making process and should be included in the planning phase (O'Hara and Zhan, 1994).

If it is unclear as to whether or not the herb is beneficial or harmful in the client's condition, the responsibility of informing the client about this belongs to the health care provider (Stupay and Sivertsen, 2000). The health care provider may also observe the placebo effect with clients who are taking herbs. That is, the taking of the herb, and not the action of the herb itself, may produce a positive effect on the client.

Intervention

Important interventions include education, checking for side effects, and checking for interactions between herbs and medications. Health care providers should remain sensitive to the patient's situation. Whether it is a need for additional information about an herbal supplement or including the assessment for side effects and drug-herb interactions, the health care provider must be alert for opportunities to intervene in the patient's behalf.

Evaluation

The review of medication-drug interactions is an important aspect of the evaluation phase. Outcomes of all teaching should be evaluated, as well as the effectiveness of herbs used in selected conditions. In evaluating the outcomes of client goals, the health care provider must discuss and consider the client's condition from a holistic view and the important effect that culture has on the outcomes.

Education

Patient education is one of the most important roles that the health care provider has when working with clients who are taking herbal supplements. Education can occur in a variety of formats. One-on-one teaching sessions are useful, as is the use of written materials. Education could also occur in senior citizen centers. Scientific data should be included, as well as information on the safe use of herbs. Whichever strategy is chosen, follow-up is essential. Just because it says "natural" on the label does not mean that it is healthy for every client. Clients may switch from one harmful herb to another without talking with their health care provider (Stupay and Sivertsen, 2000). The provider must seek the motivation for the use of herbs or supplements in order to provide significant help.

Several issues must be addressed with clients who are taking herbs: (1) There is no standardization among manufacturers, so there is no consistency in the amount of active ingredients per dose between brands. (2) Herbal supplements should be purchased from reputable sources. (3) Herbs are available in different forms, making accurate dosing difficult. (4) Research is lacking on both the side effects and the benefits of herbs. This makes recommending specific herbs difficult. (5) Clients who have allergies to plants may have allergies to herbs.

Clients should be asked to report the use of all herbal supplements to their health care provider. Clients should be encouraged to speak with their health care provider before beginning an herbal supplement for the first time. Clients should use only the supplement that is recommended by the health care provider and only for the time prescribed. If side effects occur within an hour or two of taking the supplement, the supplement should be discontinued immediately. If the side effects continue or worsen, the client should report them to the health care provider. Because older adults may react differently to supplements, health care providers may need to prescribe less than the recommended dose. Herbs taken with other herbs may cause unpredictable effects (Stupay and Sivertsen, 2000).

Patients who are taking platelet activity products, such as vitamin E, excessive garlic, warfarin, aspirin, and low-molecular-weight heparins, should be instructed not to take ginkgo concurrently (Kuhn, 2002).

Patients should not take any herb containing comfrey (Youngkin and Israel, 1996).

As is true in so many facets of life, taking herbal supplements in and of itself is neither a good nor a bad thing; it is neither a healthy nor an unhealthy approach to health care. But taking an herbal supplement requires the patient and the health care provider to be knowledgeable and to continue to seek out the latest information on herbs, OTC medications, prescribed medications, and drug-herb interactions.

SELECTED CONDITIONS

Use by Transplant Patients

As other patients would, transplant patients will often speak with their health care provider about the use of prescribed medications, but may forget to mention herbal products. Recent research indicates that there can be significant drug-herb interactions when clients are taking medications for immunosuppression. Side effects, symptoms of rejection, and other complications are often more difficult to identify. In addition, immunosuppressive agents have a very narrow window of therapeutic effectiveness (Allen and Bell, 2002). Herbs with specific effects on the transplant patient's immune function are listed in Table 11-3.

Table 11-3 Herbs and the Transplant Patient

Herb	Claim	Interactions/contraindications
Echinacea	Stimulates the immune system	Contraindicated with infections, autoimmune disease, immunosuppressants
Ephedra	Used as a decongestant; stimulates central nervous system, decreases appetite	Not to be used by transplant or dialysis patients; may increase blood pressure, heart rate, risk of stroke
Garlic	Decreases cholesterol, triglycerides, and blood pressure; may increase bleeding time	May interact with antiplatelet drugs
Ginger	Prevents nausea and vomiting	May interact with antiplatelet drugs
Ginkgo	Antioxidant	Slows body's ability to metabolize drugs
Ginseng	Used as either stimulant or relaxant; may enhance immunity	Slows drug metabolism; interacts with antiplatelet drugs
St. John's wort	Used to treat depression	Reduces blood levels of cyclosporine

Source: Allen D, Bell J: Herbal medicine and the transplant patient, *Nephrol Nurs J* 29(3):269 , 2002.

Table 11-4 Herbs and the Perioperative Patient

Herb	Perioperative issue	Preoperative discontinuation
Echinacea	Allergic reactions; decreased effectiveness of immunosuppressants	No data
Garlic	Potential for increased bleeding	7 days before surgery
Ginkgo	Potential for increased bleeding	35 hours before surgery
Ginseng	Hypoglycemia; potential for increased bleeding	7 days before surgery
St John's wort	Potential for increased sedation with anesthetics	5 days before surgery

Adapted from Norred CL, Brinker F: Potential coagulation effects of preoperative complementary and alternative medicine, *Alternative Therapies* 7(6):58, 2001.

Hypertension

Four herbs are commonly used in the treatment of hypertension: *Rauwolfia serpentina, Stephania tetrandra, Panax notoginseng,* and *Crataegus* hawthorn extract. Hawthorn has been used as a treatment for hypertension for several years. It acts to inhibit the progress of atherosclerosis. In addition, it decreases heart rate, decreases blood pressure at exercise, and increases circulation to the myocardium. Because therapeutic levels have not been established, overtreatment and undertreatment can occur. Overdose may result in hypotension. Hawthorn may increase the activity of digitalis and therefore should not be used by clients on digitalis. Blood pressure should be monitored (Sutherland, 2001).

Human Immunodeficiency Virus–Related Symptoms

Clients with human immunodeficiency virus (HIV)–related symptoms are known to use a number of alternative therapies, including herbs. Garlic and St. John's wort are used to treat dyslipidemia and depression, respectively. Some research indicates that after 3 months of garlic use, there is a significant reduction in cholesterol levels. Other research shows no demonstrable effects. The efficacy of garlic is still to be determined. Although the mechanism of action for St. John's wort is not known, research indicates a lowered blood level of antiretroviral medications when taken with St. John's wort (Swanson et al, 2000).

Gastrointestinal Disorders

Chronic alcohol-induced and fulminant hepatitis have both been positively affected by the use of milk thistle. Misuse of herbs may cause physical harm, such as liver damage, or delay the client from seeking appropriate traditional health care. Comfrey and chaparral are examples of herbs that may be toxic to the gastrointestinal system (Giese, 2000).

Cancer

In the United States, many herbs have the potential for the treatment of cancer, but none has met the goals for use in biomedicine. Garlic has folk cancer use, but it can be irritating in large amounts. Initial studies on the use of echinacea are encouraging, but it is too early to draw any conclusions. Not much is known about the toxicity of echinacea (Montbriand, 1999).

Claims are often made that a substance or an herb will "cure" or help the cancer patient, even though there are no data to support such claims. Clients and their families may become desperate in an effort to "do something" to help. Health care providers must be sensitive to this situation and work with all concerned to provide the most appropriate care possible.

Alzheimer's Disease

Ginkgo increases blood supply to the brain. Recommended doses vary according to research (Zand et al, 1999), but 120 to 240 mg daily of ginkgo extract for 3 to 6 months has a "small but significant effect on cognitive function in patients with Alzheimer's disease" (Waddell et al, 2001, p. 52). Primarily memory and attention are improved.

Perioperative Assessment

Including herbal remedies in the perioperative assessment is an important aspect of total care. Patients should be told to stop the herbal treatments 5 to 7 days before the scheduled surgery. Patients having emergency surgery should be questioned about the use of herbal remedies. Herbs that affect bleeding and clotting time (e.g., chamomile, garlic, ginkgo, and ginseng) should be especially noted and reported to the surgical team (Kuhn, 2002). Herbs and their perioperative effects are listed in Table 11-4.

Human Needs and Wellness Diagnoses

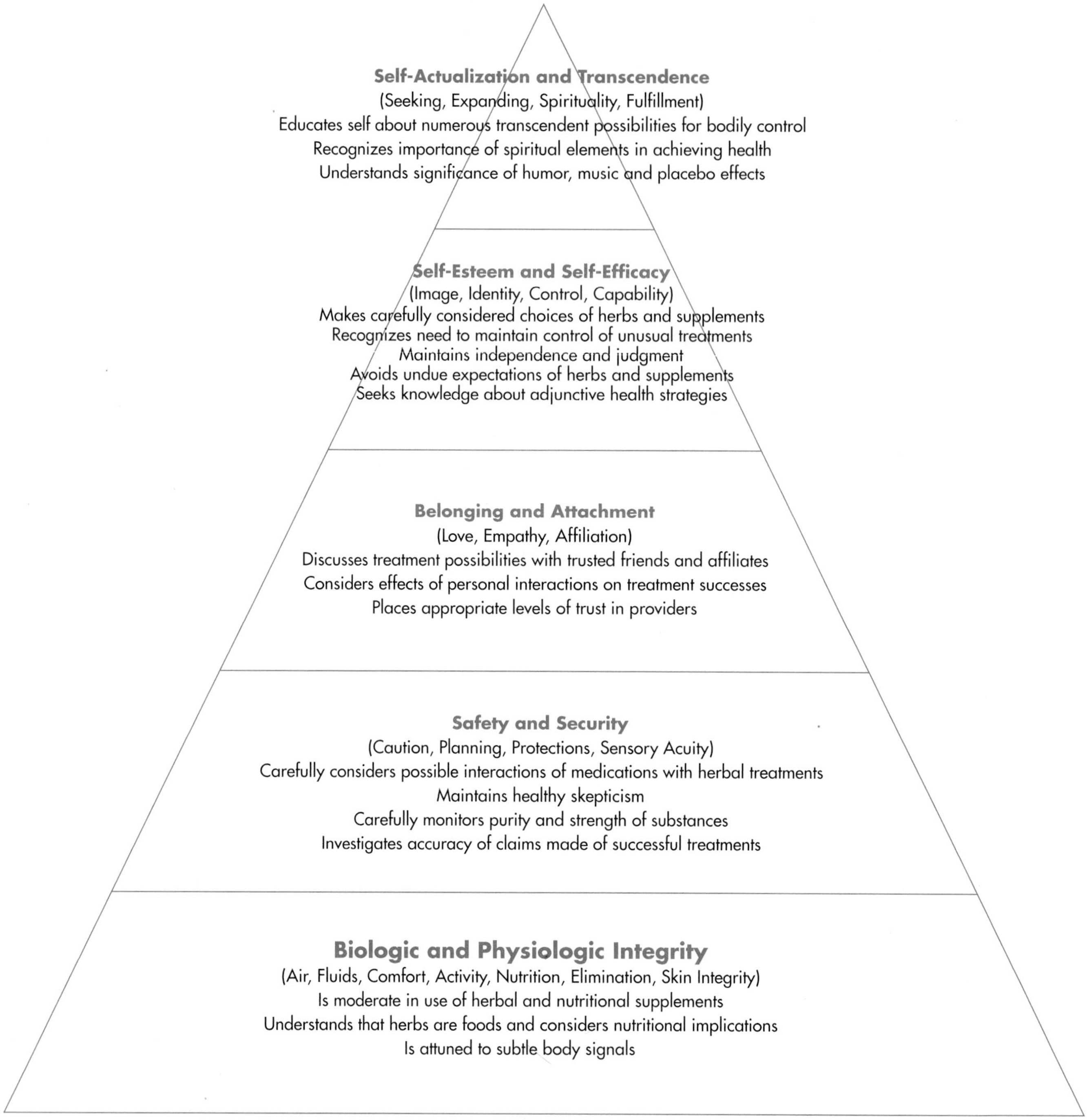

Self-Actualization and Transcendence
(Seeking, Expanding, Spirituality, Fulfillment)
Educates self about numerous transcendent possibilities for bodily control
Recognizes importance of spiritual elements in achieving health
Understands significance of humor, music and placebo effects

Self-Esteem and Self-Efficacy
(Image, Identity, Control, Capability)
Makes carefully considered choices of herbs and supplements
Recognizes need to maintain control of unusual treatments
Maintains independence and judgment
Avoids undue expectations of herbs and supplements
Seeks knowledge about adjunctive health strategies

Belonging and Attachment
(Love, Empathy, Affiliation)
Discusses treatment possibilities with trusted friends and affiliates
Considers effects of personal interactions on treatment successes
Places appropriate levels of trust in providers

Safety and Security
(Caution, Planning, Protections, Sensory Acuity)
Carefully considers possible interactions of medications with herbal treatments
Maintains healthy skepticism
Carefully monitors purity and strength of substances
Investigates accuracy of claims made of successful treatments

Biologic and Physiologic Integrity
(Air, Fluids, Comfort, Activity, Nutrition, Elimination, Skin Integrity)
Is moderate in use of herbal and nutritional supplements
Understands that herbs are foods and considers nutritional implications
Is attuned to subtle body signals

These are not all the possible wellness diagnoses that may be identified. The above are examples of nursing diagnoses that should be considered when planning care for the older adult.

KEY CONCEPTS

- Older adults who are diagnosed with chronic conditions are more likely to take herbs.
- Many individuals continue their traditional therapies in addition to herbal therapies.
- The renewed interest in herbal therapies is based in part on the focus of preventing illness. Herbs are often used by individuals who want to be more involved in their own health care.
- Currently, the U.S. government has no standards in place to control the quality of herbs or herbal products.
- Health care providers should always ask about the use of herbs and supplements when conducting a health interview.
- Health care providers should teach patients to ask about the concurrent use of herbs and medications, both prescribed and OTC.
- Patients should be told to stop the herbal treatments 5 to 7 days before scheduled surgery.
- Whichever educational strategy is chosen, follow-up is essential to determine that instructions are being followed and that the patient is aware of the situation.

▲ CASE STUDY

Anna is an 80-year-old woman who lives with her 83-year-old husband in the suburbs of a large city. They have been married for 57 years and have two grown children, six grandchildren, and five great-grandchildren. Anna is very proud of all of them. Anna taught high school English for 20 years but was raised with many of the "old country" traditions, speaking French for most of her formative years. As part of her background, she would rather use herbs and "home treatments" than prescribed "pills." She has been diagnosed with hypertension, diabetes mellitus, and arthritis. She often complains of symptoms that are related to these chronic conditions, but she refuses to consistently follow her diet or take prescribed medications. Anna attends mass daily and, with her husband, is active in community activities. While accompanying her husband on a visit to his health care provider, she mentions the use of herbal supplements. After some discussion, the nurse realizes that Anna has little information about herbal supplements and has some incorrect assumptions about them.

Based on the case study, develop a nursing care plan using the following procedure:

List comments of client that provide subjective data.

List information that provides objective data.

From these data, identify and state, using an accepted format, two nursing diagnoses that you determine are most significant to the client at this time. List two client strengths that you have identified from data.

Determine and state outcome criteria for each diagnosis. These must reflect some alleviation of the problem identified in the nursing diagnosis and must be stated in concrete and measurable terms.

Plan and state one or more interventions for each diagnosed problem. Provide specific documentation of source used to determine appropriate intervention. Plan at least one intervention that incorporates the client's existing strengths.

Evaluate success of intervention. Intervention must correlate directly with the stated outcome criteria in order to measure the outcome success.

STUDY QUESTIONS/ACTIVITIES

How would you begin your discussion with Anna regarding her knowledge of herbal supplements?

What information would you be especially interested in regarding herbal supplements and each of Anna's medical diagnoses?

How would you prepare Anna should she need surgery?

Prepare a teaching plan for Anna to include the effective use of herbal supplements.

Interview a member of your health care community who recommends the use of herbs along with traditional strategies. How does this individual decide which herbs to use? How does he or she ensure standardization between products?

Tour a local health food store. Read the labels of the more commonly used herbal supplements. Do the labels list the information you expected? How would you make sure that your clients have the necessary information?

Visit a senior citizen center. Talk with members about their use of herbal supplements. Keep track of the more commonly used herbs and the reasons for their use. How did the older adults find out the herbal action?

RESEARCH QUESTIONS

Are older adults aware of possible negative effects of herbal supplements?

What questions do older adults ask before taking an herbal supplement?

What information do older adults need before considering taking an herbal supplement?

What are the rewards versus the costs of using herbal supplements?

What strategies should health care providers use to bridge the gap between herbal remedies and traditional health care?

Why do older adults choose to use herbs?

REFERENCES

Allen D, Bell J: Herbal medicine and the transplant patient, *Nephrol Nurs J* 29(3):269, 2002.

Eliopoulos C: *Integrating conventional and alternative therapies: holistic care for chronic conditions,* St Louis, 1999, Mosby.

Fryback PB, Reinert BR: Alternative therapies and control for health in cancer and AIDS, *Clin Nurse Spec* 11(2):64, 1997.

Giese AA: A study of alternative health care use for gastrointestinal disorders, *Gastroenterol Nurs* 23(1):19, 2000.

Gray MA: Herbs: multicultural folk medicines, *Orthop Nurs* 15(2):49, 1996.

Keller KB, Lemberg L: Herbal or complementary medicine: fact or fiction, *Am J Crit Care* 10(6):438, 2001.

Kuhn M: Herbal remedies: drug-herb interactions, *Crit Care Nurse* 22(2):22, 2002.

Miller JF: *Coping with chronic illness: overcoming powerlessness,* Philadelphia, 1983, FA Davis.

Montbriand MJ: Past and present herbs used to treat cancer: medicine, magic or poison? *Oncol Nurs Forum* 26(1):49, 1999.

NDH pocket guide to drug interactions, Philadelphia, 2002, Lippincott, Williams & Wilkins.

Norred CL, Brinker F: Potential coagulation effects of preoperative complementary and alternative medicine, *Alternative Therapies* 7(6):58, 2001.

O'Hara EM, Zhan L: Cultural and pharmacologic considerations when caring for Chinese elders, *J Gerontol Nurs* 20(10):11, 1994.

Scorza E: *Use of herbal and nutritional supplements.* Paper presented at National Conference of Gerontological Nurse Practitioners, Chicago, 2002.

Skidmore-Roth L: *Mosby's handbook of herbs and natural supplements,* St Louis, 2001, Mosby.

Stupay S, Sivertsen L: Herbal and nutritional supplement use in the elderly, *Nurse Pract* 25:56, 2000.

Sutherland JA: Selected complementary methods and nursing care of the hypertensive client, *Holistic Nurs Pract* 15(4):4, 2001.

Swanson B et al: Complementary and alternative therapies to manage HIV-related symptoms, *J Assoc Nurses AIDS Care* 11(5):40, 2000.

Waddell DL, Hummel ME, Sumner AD: Three herbs you should get to know, *Am J Nurs* 101(4):48, 2001.

Youngkin EQ, Israel DS: A review and critique of common herbal alternative therapies, *Nurse Pract* 21(10):39, 1996.

Zand J, Spreen AN, LaVaeel JB: *Smart medicine for healthier living,* New York, 1999, Avery.

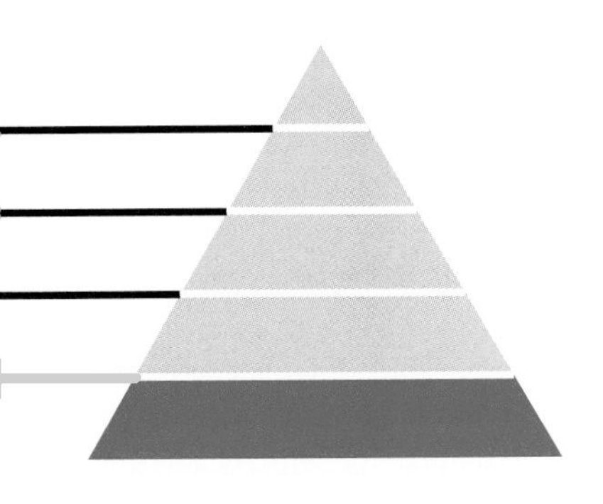

CHAPTER 12

Sensory Function

Ann Schmidt Luggen

A student speaks

During the years I worked as a food server I grew accustomed to waiting on older people. They can't always read the menu, they complain that the lighting in the restaurant is too low, they like their dinner experience to be slower, they can't find their silver when they need it, the soup is never hot enough and the cup of coffee is never full enough. They would yell at me because they could not hear me. It used to make me mad, but now I understand they are just real people experiencing growing old. Yes, they may have problems like losing some of their senses and other physical changes, but in actuality they are the same as me.

Debbie, age 27

An elder speaks

One of the great frustrations is the matter of eyesight. One can get used to large print and hope for black letters on white paper but why do modern publishers seem to prefer the shiny, slick off-white paper and pale ink in miniscule print? And, my new prescription glasses have not restored my ability to cut my own toenails without danger of wounding myself. I find myself wishing for some treatment for incipient cataracts. Please researchers, let's get rid of this scourge of the elderly.

Lyn, age 85

LEARNING OBJECTIVES

On completion of this chapter, the reader will be able to:

1. Identify several sensory changes accompanying aging that alter the perceived world of the aged.
2. Explain changes in the aging system that impair sensation.
3. Relate sensory changes to perceptual and environmental insecurity and behavioral disturbances.
4. Discuss the use of various accoutrements that assist the aged with sensory deficits and how they are best used.
5. Describe several conditions that affect sensory function and awareness.
6. Identify several interventions that enhance sensory function and perceptual integration.
7. Develop a nursing care plan appropriate to the care of an elder experiencing a sensory deficit.

THE SENSORY APPARATUS

The common view is that sensory organs are our windows on the world. Less poetically, the senses are the primary interface with the environment. The senses seem to put boundaries and order into our lives, and when they are understimulated or overloaded, the structure weakens. We rely on our senses to perceive the environment and to enjoy the pleasures of life. Most sensory losses are irreversible but occur gradually so that function is maintained. Although there is great individuality in sensory changes, there is increasing functional dependency and loss of independence.

Appreciation of Sensory Changes

With old age, many of our senses gradually lose their acuity. Although normal changes of aging do not result in an abrupt awareness of sensory loss, the accumulated atrophy of sensory receptors in the eyes, ears, nose, buccal cavity, and peripheral afferent nerves substantially reduces the vividness of environmental impressions. Events no longer alert the nervous system with such clarity as in youth. Habituation to certain sensations may also diminish their impact. When the senses are impaired, the sense of self is altered.

The natural gradual loss of sensory functioning with old age may be pragmatically sound. It lends some credence to the disengagement theory. With age the filters atrophy and the perceptible universe shrinks. This may be a mechanism of gradual withdrawal from the experienced universe. Is it less traumatic to gradually disengage from the impressions of life than to abruptly cease to exist? Perhaps we should consider the possibility of sensory disengagement as well as social disengagement. A world that is not so bright and vivid as that of the child's may not be so hard to leave. Perhaps the muting of sensory detail is an aspect of the development of wisdom. The elder is less distracted from the larger sense and meanings.

The issues of concern to nurses are devising methods to keep the senses functional enough to negotiate the environment effectively: to enjoy the beauty and respond to the pain. Both joy and pain are meaningful; pain perception signals danger but also can be ambivalently mixed with pleasure. Pain and pleasure are often intertwined; both are part of living and experiencing. We must dull excruciating pain but avoid dulling awareness with medications and mechanistic limitations that effectively reduce one's appreciation of pleasure and sorrow.

The caregiver's job is to keep the environment within reach; to supplement sensory loss with additional pleasures to the remaining senses; to provide touching and stroking, color and variety; to refrain from pushing and shoving the elements in haste and irreverence. The sensory environment is to be revered and cultivated. Therein lie many problems. Old age subjects one to decreased appreciation of the environment through drugs, machines, treatments, paresthesias, presbyopia, presbycusis, agnosia, and other factors. Life may be more cautiously sampled. Stored experiences often come to the rescue, and old people remember things they can no longer perceive.

When describing the capacities and changes in the various sensory apparatus, we must understand that they all work in consensus. The senses are tightly interwoven in forming the perceptual base of our world. Possibly the "sixth sense" (intuition, or the power of perception that goes beyond that of the five senses) is really the consensus of all the senses in an acutely aware individual. In some cases a disorder of one of the senses may stimulate the others in a compensatory manner. No one has studied this in the aged, but anecdotally some elders have experienced and described enhancement of the sense of hearing when sight was poor or vice versa.

Personal hardiness and an orderly, meaningful environment contribute in ways yet unidentified to good perceptual processing and high-level functioning. It is not uncommon that elders are thought to be cognitively impaired when, in fact, attention to enhanced sensory function through an adapted environment and well-fitted accoutrements reveal much higher functional levels. General perceptual organization and efficiency are modified by health status, frailty of aging, illness, medications, fatigue, and stress and anxiety.

In this chapter we focus on the normal age-related alterations and the most commonly experienced problems of the major sensory organs. How these affect the individual and his or her ability to successfully negotiate the environment is the nurse's concern. The task is to augment and maximize sensory experiences when senses are diminished and to help design a colorful, rewarding environment that fits the needs and abilities of the individual (Table 12-1).

Alteration in Sensory Experience

The normal gradual diminution of the senses during the aging process is usually well accommodated by experience. We are all subject to alterations in our sensory experience, and with increasing age it is likely that these circumstances will occur more frequently and perhaps be more devastating.

Alterations in sensory input may contribute to increased anxiety in the aged population. When the senses are grossly underloaded or overloaded, perception and reactions are distorted. The world becomes an alien, confusing place. Fear and anxiety increase, or one withdraws into a fabricated world that provides security. Altered sensory experience will affect one's view of self and one's ability to relate to others (Figure 12-1). Isolation and loneliness may be the result. Emotional responses to altered sensory input include boredom,

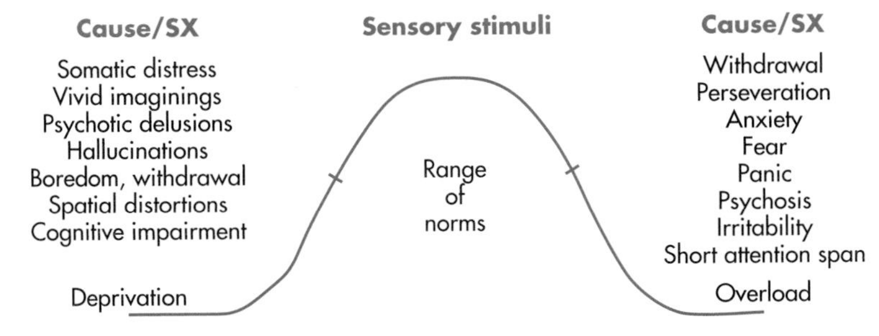

Figure 12-1. Reaction to sensory and environmental alterations. (Illustration by Joseph Pierre.)

Table 12-1 Age-Related Sensory Changes, Outcomes, and Prevention, Health Promotion, and Maintenance Approaches

Age-related changes	Outcomes	Health prevention, promotion, and maintenance
Vision		
Lid elasticity diminishes	Pouches under the eyes	Use isotonic eye drops as needed
Loss of orbital fat	Excessive dryness of eyes	
Decreased tears		
Arcus senilis becomes visible		
Sclera yellows and becomes less elastic		
Yellowing and increased opacity of cornea	Lack of corneal luster	
Increased sclerosis and ridgidity of the iris		
Decrease in convergency ability	Presbyopia	Have eyes examined at least once a year
Decline in light accommodation response	Lessened acuity	Use magnifying glass and high-intensity light to read
Diminished pupilary size	Decline in depth perception	Increase light to prevent falls
Atrophy of ciliary muscle	Diminished recovery from glare	Clip on sunglasses, visors, sun hat, nonglare coating on prescription glasses/sunglasses
Night vision diminishes	Night blindness	Do not drive at night Keep night-light in bathroom and hallway Paint first and last step of staircase and edge of each step between with a bright color
Yellowing of lens	Diminished color perception (blues and greens)	
Lens opacity	Cataracts	Surgical removal of lens
Increased intraocular pressure	Rainbows around lights	Have a yearly eye examination including tonometer testing
Shrinkage of gelatinous substance in the vitreous	Altered peripheral vision	
Vitreous floaters appear		
Ability to gaze upward decreases		
Thinning and sclerosis of retinal blood vessels		
Atrophy of photoreceptor cells		
Degeneration of neurons in visual cortex		
Hearing		
Thinner, drier skin of external ear		
Longer and thicker hair in external ear canal		
Narrowing of auditory opening		
Increased cerumen		Check ears for wax or infection
Thickened and less resilient tympanic membrane		
Decreased flexibility of basilar membrane	Difficulty hearing high-frequency sounds (presbycusis)	Formal hearing test
Ossicular calcification		
Diminished neuron, endolymph, hair cells and blood supply to inner ear and auditory nerve	Gradual loss of sound	Consultation for proper hearing and speaking tone-shouting distorted
Degeneration of spiral ganglion and arterial blood vessels		
Weakness and stiffness of muscles and ligaments		
Smell		
Decreased olfactory cells	Decreased appetite Decreased protection from noxious odors and tainted food	Encourage social dining
Taste		
Possible decrease in size and number of taste buds	Poor nutrition	Nutritional supplementation; use of stronger flavors

diminished concentration, incoherent thoughts, anxiety, fear, depression, lability of affect, delusions, and even hallucinations. Clear and sometimes repetitive data about the environment must be given when perceptions are impaired. Manipulating the environment to reduce demands and enhance sensory function should decrease these symptoms, although studies show that signs may persist for several days.

Significant research on elders' varied adaptations to sensory losses is limited. The assumption of increasing loss of acuity of all senses and the importance of well-designed and well-fitted accoutrements comprise the bulk of attention given to the topic. Adequate input is essential to continued cognitive development.

Sensory Deprivation. There are at least three types of sensory deprivation: (1) reduced sensory capacities, (2) elimination of patterns and meaning from input, and (3) restrictive, monotonous environments. Prisoners, astronauts, and solitary explorers have made the public aware of the effects of isolation from ordinary environmental stimulation. Psychologic and physiologic effects of such situations have been reported through personal accounts and from studies of artificial situations constructed for the express purpose of studying sensory deprivation. None of the natural or laboratory experiences demonstrated the particular significance of age variables. It has been more or less assumed that aged people who are isolated from adequate stimuli by failing sensory organs or reduced environmental variation react with the same symptoms as younger adults. Certain effects thought to be "confusion" or "old age" may arise from sensory deprivation. Box 12-1 summarizes some effects of sensory deprivation. Any situation lacking varied environmental stimuli deprives the senses of adequate material for perceptual integrity.

Common contributors to sensory deprivation in the elderly are altered sensory capacities and restrictive environments. Problems such as poor vision, decreased energy, poor hearing, extended periods in a supine position, debilitating illness and chronic disorders, few pleasant sounds, and limited meaningful contact with others often result in *disorientation.* Late afternoon may aggravate the deprivation if daylight is diminished and there is inadequate indoor lighting. Simple nursing actions will alleviate this barren existence. Open drapes and the window a crack; sights, sounds, and smells of outdoors and life can be enjoyable and reassuring. Turn on lights; raise the head of the bed or assist the person to a chair bolstered comfortably with pillows; bring a flower to the room; sit down; speak, touch, and listen to the client's feelings. Discuss the isolated person's interests; radio, television, computers, books, puzzles, and handicrafts may all amuse the solitary person. It is essential to plan with them, not for them. When these efforts fail, it is because of inadequate assessment. If the individual is concerned about more fundamental issues such as maintaining biologic integrity, comfortable and nondemanding surroundings will be a priority.

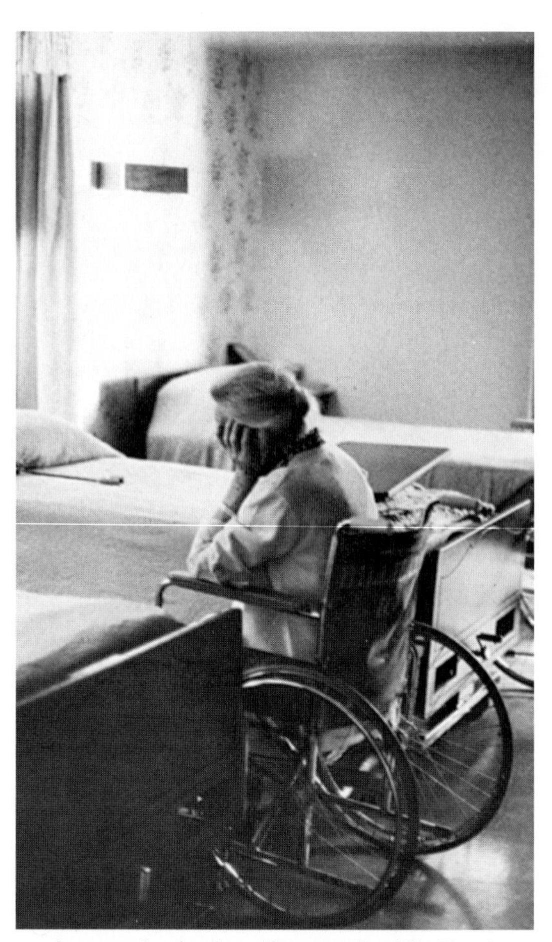

Sensory deprivation. (Courtesy Patricia Hess.)

When the ambiance is one of monotony, even a small stimulus may trigger a strong response. Knowing this makes it easier to understand the overreactions displayed when a routine is interrupted. One lady became extremely upset when a large sign was hung above her bed; another refused to return to her room after it had been rearranged. People are more sensitive to changes of any sort when they feel deprived of control. Following sensory deprivation, there is a good response to gradual environmental enrichment. Rapid increases may produce emotional outbursts. The benefits of orderly, gradual environmental enrichment geared to individual personality and interests are yet to be thoroughly studied.

Sensory Overload. Neuroexcitability and secretion of stimulating neurotransmitters decrease as one ages. Overarousal is most often from abrupt, unexpected environmental change such as accident or hospitalization. These are situations of sensory overload precipitated by actual or perceived environmental demands. Emergency reactions sustained for long periods exhaust the organism's physiologic adaptive mechanisms (Selye, 1956). An individual with marginal adaptation and cognitive decrements is particularly vulnerable. Sensory overload is a highly individual matter, often related to cognitive capacity. It can be recognized by certain

Box 12-1 Effects of Sensory Deprivation

- Sensory deprivation tends to amplify existing personality traits. Vernon and Makowsky (1961) believe sensory deprivation generates a great need for socialization and physical stimulation.
- Perceptual disorganization occurs in visual/motor coordination, color perception, apparent movement, tactile accuracy, ability to perceive size and shape, and spatial and time judgment. Sensory deprivation brings about temporary loss in color perception, motor coordination, and weight loss.
- Affectual changes include boredom, restlessness, irritability, anxiety, and panic.
- Sensory deprivation alters mechanisms of attention, consciousness, and reality testing, resulting in general disorganization of brain function similar to that produced by anoxia.
- Marked changes of behavior occur, such as inability to think and solve problems, affectual disturbance, perceptual distortions, hallucinations and delusions, vivid imagination, poor task performance, increased anxiety and aggression, somatic complaints, temporal and spatial disorientation, emotional lability, and confusion of sleeping and waking states.
- Monotony produces a disruption of the capacity to learn and the ability to think. In the absence of varied stimulation, brain function becomes less efficient; an electroencephalogram shows slowed alpha waves maintained by constant sensory flux.
- Illness often increases the perceptual confusion, particularly among the aged, although studies show that adults of all ages experience distortion and depersonalization when environmental stimuli are bland.

symptoms: thoughts may race, and attention scatters in many directions. People find it difficult to sit still. Aberrant thoughts or actions may occur. Evidences of anxiety are present.

The amount of stimuli necessary for healthy function varies with each individual; relevance and familiarity of stimuli may be more important than amount. Biorhythms are another important consideration. Individuals may be more subject to environmental overload at one time than another. Sensations are generally most acute in the late afternoon when cortisol levels are highest, although effects on the aged have not been established. Sensory overload cannot always be avoided, but when one is extremely stressed and bombarded with adaptive demands, time must be arranged for peacefulness and frequent rest periods. It is often helpful to sit quietly with the person, saying very little, or to engage him or her in a nondemanding repetitive activity that will help focus attention on something that provides security and reduces stress. Walking can be beneficial.

One must be cautious in arbitrarily attributing anxiety, agitation, mood swings, or disorientation to sensory overload. One man was intermittently disoriented for several days following hip surgery. A nursing assistant reported his disorientation and anxiety and concluded that he was suffering sensory overload. She therefore wanted to keep the lights dim, reduce noise, move the patient to a private room, and advise others to disturb him as little as possible. Although these interventions would be useful in one experiencing overload, it would further reduce this man's ability to remain in touch with his surroundings. It is likely he was reacting to medications, dehydration, infection, and the stress of translocation and major surgery. It is best to have a consistent attendant with him to reassure him repeatedly that this is a reaction to surgery and to interpret sounds, actions, and items that are in his present environment.

HEALTHY PEOPLE 2010

Healthy People 2010, begun by the U.S. Surgeon General in 1979, is a national health promotion and disease prevention initiative. The new *Healthy People 2010* contains goals and objectives that relate to sensory problems of older adults (Healthy people 2010: vision and hearing, 2002). The following are some of these objectives:

- Increase the number of persons who have dilated eye examinations at appropriate intervals
- Reduce visual impairment caused by glaucoma and cataracts
- Increase vision rehabilitation
- Increase the number of persons who have hearing examinations at appropriate intervals
- Increase access to hearing rehabilitation services and adaptive devices

VISION

Vision impairment is common in the elderly population. Visual acuity and accommodation normally decrease with age. These changes, particularly presbyopia, begin making themselves felt in the forties for many people. They are not usually great problems but are mainly an inconvenience. Although major aging of the eye (presbyopia) occurs between 45 and 55 years of age, 80% of the aged have fair to adequate vision past 90 years of age. Nearly 95% of adults older than 65 wear glasses (Burke and Laramie, 2000), and 18% also use a magnifying glass for reading and close work (Desai et al, 2001).

According to the Centers for Disease Control and Prevention (Desai et al, 2001), 1.8 million community-dwelling elders report difficulty with activities of daily living because of visual impairment. *Visual impairment* is defined as vision loss that cannot be corrected by glasses or contact lenses. About 2.7 million elderly adults have severe visual impairment. About 27% of elderly men 85 years and older are visually impaired. Women are more visually impaired than men; 33% of women

85 and older report visual impairment. African Americans are twice as likely to be visually impaired as whites of comparable socioeconomic status. Hispanics, who have three times the risk of developing type 2 diabetes as whites, have a higher risk of visual complications (Healthy people 2010: vision and hearing, 2002).

Blindness increases with age. It peaks at about 85 years and occurs in 2.4% of this population (Desai et al, 2001). Visual impairment and blindness are caused by cataracts, age-related macular degeneration, glaucoma, and diabetic retinopathy.

Light and dark adaptation is problematic for aging adults. This may become a great source of insecurity to those older adults who drive. Glare from bright lights causes decreased visual perception. Some elders may continue driving only in daytime while wearing sunglasses. These changes increase the risk of falls and can decrease the elder's social relationships.

Glare is caused by changes in the lens and vitreous humor and an increase of scattering of light (Tumosa, 2001). Many safety factors are obviously attached to visual adequacy, although people with limitations often adapt remarkably well. Dark adaptation problems are due to diminished and slowed response (accommodation) to a change in lighting, such as going into a darkened room from a brightly lit room.

Vertical flashing lights in the temporal (lateral) fields may occur in elderly individuals. This occurs because the vitreous humor, normally clear, develops discrete opacities leading to a general haziness. It undergoes liquefaction with increasing age. As a result, normal eye movements produce intermittent tension at attachment points in the retina, stimulating the peripheral retina and causing the flashing lights (Tumosa, 2001).

Some visual distortions that *require immediate attention* to prevent blindness are closed-angle glaucoma, retinal detachment, stroke, and temporal arteritis. The signs and symptoms of these disorders vary and are discussed later in the chapter.

Presbyopia

The condition of vision in which the normally flexible lens of the eye gradually loses elasticity, affecting the refractive ability of the eye, is *presbyopia.* Usually, it is noticed when one has difficulty reading close up and begins holding reading materials farther away. One notices the blurring of near vision in the midthirties and early forties. It affects everyone, and there is no known prevention. For most individuals the reading lens must be increased in strength every 2 or 3 years after age 45.

For those who are "farsighted" (hyperopic) the presbyopia tends to occur earlier than for the "nearsighted" (myopic—a condition that occurs early in life). As lens opacity increases, some refractive power increases at the same time that accommodation, or lens resilience, decreases. The result is a temporary shift toward myopia and improved close vision. Thus some individuals at 60 or 70 years of age develop better vision in that they can again read without glasses, which they may have used since childhood.

Increasingly, more ophthalmologists are prescribing contact lenses and surgery to correct presbyopia with varying degrees of acceptance and success. It is useful to use a red night-light for those who use a night-light. Also, it may be useful to keep a flashlight at the bedside if one needs to transit to dimly lit areas. If the patient usually gets up during the night, it may be best to keep a light on at all times so that one does not need to enter a dark room.

Dry Eye

Tear production normally diminishes as we age. The condition is termed *keratoconjunctivitis sicca.* It occurs most commonly in women after menopause. There may be age-related changes in the mucin-secreting cells necessary for surface wetting, in the lacrimal glands, or in the meibomian glands that secrete surface oil, and all of these may occur at the same time (Beers and Berkow, 2000). The older person will describe a dry, scratchy feeling in mild cases (xerophthalmia). There may be marked discomfort and decreased mucus production in severe situations.

Medications can cause dry eye, especially antihistamines, diuretics, beta-blockers, and some sleeping pills. The problem is diagnosed by an ophthalmologist using a Schirmer tear test in which filter paper strips are placed under the lower eyelid to measure the rate of tear production. A common treatment is artificial tears, but dry eyes may be sensitive to them because of preservatives, which can be irritating. The ophthalmologist may close the tear duct channel either temporarily or permanently. Other management methods include keeping the house air moist with pans of water in each room, avoiding wind and hair dryers, and the use of artificial tear ointments at bedtime. Vitamin A deficiency can be a cause of dry eye, and vitamin A ointments are available for treatment.

Sjögren's syndrome is a cell-mediated autoimmune disease that has decreased lacrimal gland activity as part of the syndrome and can occur in elderly people. Systemic manifestations that occur in the autoimmune disease include Raynaud's phenomenon, polyarthritis, interstitial pneumonitis, vasculitis, psychiatric manifestations, and loss of exocrine functions (Beers and Berkow, 2000).

Glaucoma

Glaucoma is a chronic, progressive, degenerative disease involving increased intraocular pressure, usually bilateral, that can lead to permanent damage of the optic nerve and blindness. It is a major public health problem in the United States (Healthy people 2010: vision and hearing, 2002). There are several types of glaucoma: primary open-angle glaucoma (more than two thirds of cases); normal-pressure glaucoma; and *acute angle-closure glaucoma, which is an emergency.* It is a group of diseases that are characterized by progressive optic neuropathy. Blacks develop glaucoma at younger ages

Box 12-2 Risk Factors for Glaucoma

- Elevated intraocular pressure (greater than or equal to 22 mm Hg)
- Age greater than 50 years
- African-American race
- Family history
- Associated conditions:
  Diabetes mellitus (strongest association with glaucoma)
  Thyroid disease
  Nearsightedness
  Hypertension
  Cardiovascular disease

From Ralston ME et al: Glaucoma screening in primary care: the role of noncontact tonometry. *J Fam Pract* 34(1):73, 1992. Reprinted by permission of Appleton and Lange.

and with more frequency than whites (15% versus 7%) (Desai et al, 2001). Further, blacks acquire glaucoma at a younger age and are diagnosed with more severe glaucoma (Palmisano et al, 2001). Asians, particularly the Chinese, are prone to develop glaucoma. Other risk factors have been identified and are listed in Box 12-2.

Many drugs that are given to elders, with little or no thought to the ramifications, will exacerbate glaucoma. Drugs with anticholinergic properties or those that cause pupil dilation, including antihistamines, stimulants, vasodilators, clonidine, and sympathomimetics, are particularly dangerous for patients predisposed to angle-closure glaucoma (Table 12-2). Though the etiology of glaucoma is variable and often unknown, the problem occurs when the natural fluids of the eye are blocked by ciliary muscle rigidity or an overproduction of aqueous humor and the buildup of pressure, which damages the optic nerve (Figure 12-2).

Primary open-angle glaucoma accounts for 80% to 90% of the cases and is asymptomatic until very late in the disease, when there is a noticeable loss of peripheral vision causing tunnel vision (Cotter and Strumpf, 2002; O'Neil, 2002). Age is the single most important predictor of glaucoma, affecting about 2% of all Americans older than 40 and 20% of adults older than 60 (Kidd and Robinson, 1999). It is the most common cause of blindness in Americans over age 65. In primary open-angle glaucoma there is obstruction to aqueous flow and increased intraocular pressure.

In acute angle-closure glaucoma, elderly women are afflicted more frequently than elderly men, but in chronic glaucoma there is no gender difference (Kennedy-Malone et al, 2000). It can be bilateral, but more commonly occurs in one eye. An acute attack of angle-closure glaucoma is characterized by a rapid rise in intraocular pressure (IOP) accompanied by redness and pain in and around the eye, severe headache, nausea and vomiting, and blurring of vision. Usually medications such as timolol or pilocarpine can control glaucoma; however, surgery is now an equally effective option (American Academy of Ophthalmology, 2001).

Screening. Glaucoma screening is recommended annually for early detection on everyone with a family history of glaucoma who is older than 40; about 20% of loss of visual fields is found in elders *at diagnosis* (Luggen, 2001). Medicare began paying for annual screening in January 2002, but only in high-risk patients. Referral to an ophthalmologist is prudent in older adults because a funduscopic examination is difficult to perform without using mydriatics (Kennedy-Malone et al, 2000). Normal IOP is between 11 and 20 mmHg. Glaucoma is present when the pressure is greater than 20 mmHg; there is nerve head atrophy, optic cupping, and loss of peripheral visual fields in all types of glaucoma (Reuben et al, 2000). There are no symptoms in the early stages. Presently many elders have undiagnosed glaucoma that has not been screened or evaluated. The "silent thief" will steal vision with no forewarning. Individuals with any of the risk factors identified should be evaluated annually, and those with medication-controlled glaucoma should be examined at least every 6 months.

Cataracts

Another disorder that is prevalent among the aged is the development of cataracts. Cataracts are opaque, cloudy areas in the lens of the eye. They are caused by oxidative damage to lens protein and the deposit of lipofuscin in the ocular lens. When lens opacity reduces visual acuity to 20/30 or less in the central axis of vision, it is considered a cataract. Cataracts are categorized according to their location within the lens and are usually bilateral. They are virtually universal in the very old but may be only minimally visible, particularly in individuals with pale irises. Cataracts are recognized by the clouding of the ordinarily clear ocular lens; the red reflex may be absent or may appear as a black area. Cataracts are normal in the aging process but may be worsened by diabetes, hypertension, kidney disease, poor nutrition, cigarette smoking, high alcohol intake, eye trauma, and long-term exposure to ultraviolet light. The cardinal sign of cataracts is the appearance of halos around objects as light is diffused. Other common symptoms include blurring, decreased perception of light and color (a yellow tint to most things), and sensitivity to glare. Cataracts are the second leading cause of blindness in the United States. Eighteen percent of people between 65 and 74 years of age have cataracts, and 46% of those ages 75 to 84 years have cataracts that impair their daily activities and ability to live independently.

There was a time when cataracts were allowed to "ripen" before surgery was undertaken, and in those cases many elders became virtually blind before cataract removal. Some stories still remain of individuals who were blind until their cataracts were removed, some not even aware that cataracts were the problem. Now aged individuals are considered for elective surgery whenever the visual disturbance becomes an impediment in the individual's daily life. However, Medicare

Table 12-2 Drugs Commonly Prescribed for Elders That Are Contraindicated or Must Be Used with Caution in the Presence of Glaucoma or Prodromal Signs of Glaucoma

Generic name	Trade name*	Generic name	Trade name*
Aminophylline or theophylline with ethylenediamine	Aminophyllin Corophyllin	Lorazepam	Ativan
Amitriptyline hydrochloride*	Amitril Elavil	Loxapine succinate	Daxolin Loxitane
Amyl nitrate*		Mesoridazine	Serentil
Atropine*		Methamphetamine hydrochloride	Desoxyn
Benztropine mesylate*	Cogentin	Nitroglycerin	Nitrostat
Biperiden hydrochloride*	Akineton	Nortriptyline hydrochloride*	Aventyl
Carbamazepine	Tegretol	Orphenadrine citrate	Norflex
Chlorpheniramine maleate	Chlor-Trimeton preparations	Papaverine	Pavabid
Chlorphenoxamine hydrochloride	Phenoxene	Pentaerythritol tetranitrate	Peritrate
Chlorpromazine*	Thorazine	Perphenazine	Phenazine Trilafon
Chlorprothixene	Taractan	Phenylephrine hydrochloride	Neo-Synephrine Tear-Efrin
Clorazepate dipotassium	Tranxene	Prochlorperazine	Compazine Stemetil
Clonazepam	Clonopin	Promazine hydrochloride	Sparine
Cyclobenzaprine hydrochloride	Flexeril	Promethazine hydrochloride*	Phenergan
Cyproheptadine hydrochloride	Periactin	Protokylol hydrochloride	Ventaire
Desipramine hydrochloride*	Norpramin Pertofrane	Protriptyline hydrochloride	Vivactil
Diazepam*	Valium	Pseudoephedrine hydrochloride*	Sudafed
Dimenhydrinate	Dramamine	Succinylcholine chloride	Anectine
Diphenhydramine hydrochloride*	Benadryl	Tetrahydrozoline hydrochloride	Murine Visine
Doxepin hydrochloride*	Adapin Sinequan	Theophylline*	Aerophylline Theo-Dur
Ephedrine sulfate	Efedron	Thioridazine hydrochloride	Mellaril
Epinephrine	Bronkaid mist Primatene mist	Thiothixene hydrochloride	Navane
Fluphenazine hydrochloride*	Prolixin	Trifluoperazine hydrochloride	Stelazine
Glutethimide	Doriden	Trihexyphenidyl*	Artane
Glycopyrrolate*	Robinul	Trimeprazine tartrate	Panectyl
Haloperidol*	Haldol	Tripelennamine hydrochloride	Pyribenzamine
Hydrocodone bitartrate	Hycodan	Triprolidine hydrochloride	Actidil
Imipramine hydrochloride*	Antipres Impril Tofranil	Tropicamide	Mydriacyl
Isopropamide iodide	Darbid	Xylometazoline hydrochloride	Neo-Synephrine II
Isosorbide dinitrate	Isordil	Zinc sulfate	Op-Thal-Zin
Levodopa*	Bendopa Dopar Levopa		

*Multiple trade names not listed.

policies restrict payment for surgery to those unable to function normally without the surgery or those whose problem cannot be corrected with eyeglasses. Preoperative medical clearance is required before surgery for those with private insurance.

Most often cataract surgery involves only local anesthesia and is one of the most successful surgical procedures, with 95% of patients reporting excellent vision after surgery (Tumosa, 2001). The surgery involves removal of the lens and placement of a plastic intraocular lens. If the plastic lens is not inserted, the patient may wear a contact lens or glasses. This is not commonly done because the older adult may have difficulty placing and removing the contact lens, and the glasses would be very thick.

Unfortunately, cataracts and other related eye diseases such as maculopathy, diabetic retinopathy, or glaucoma often occur simultaneously, which complicates the management of each. Individuals who have had cataract surgery are less likely to be surgically treated effectively for glaucoma. The nursing role is to prepare the individual for significant changes in vision and adaptation to light and to be sure the individual has received adequate counseling regarding realistic postsurgical expectations.

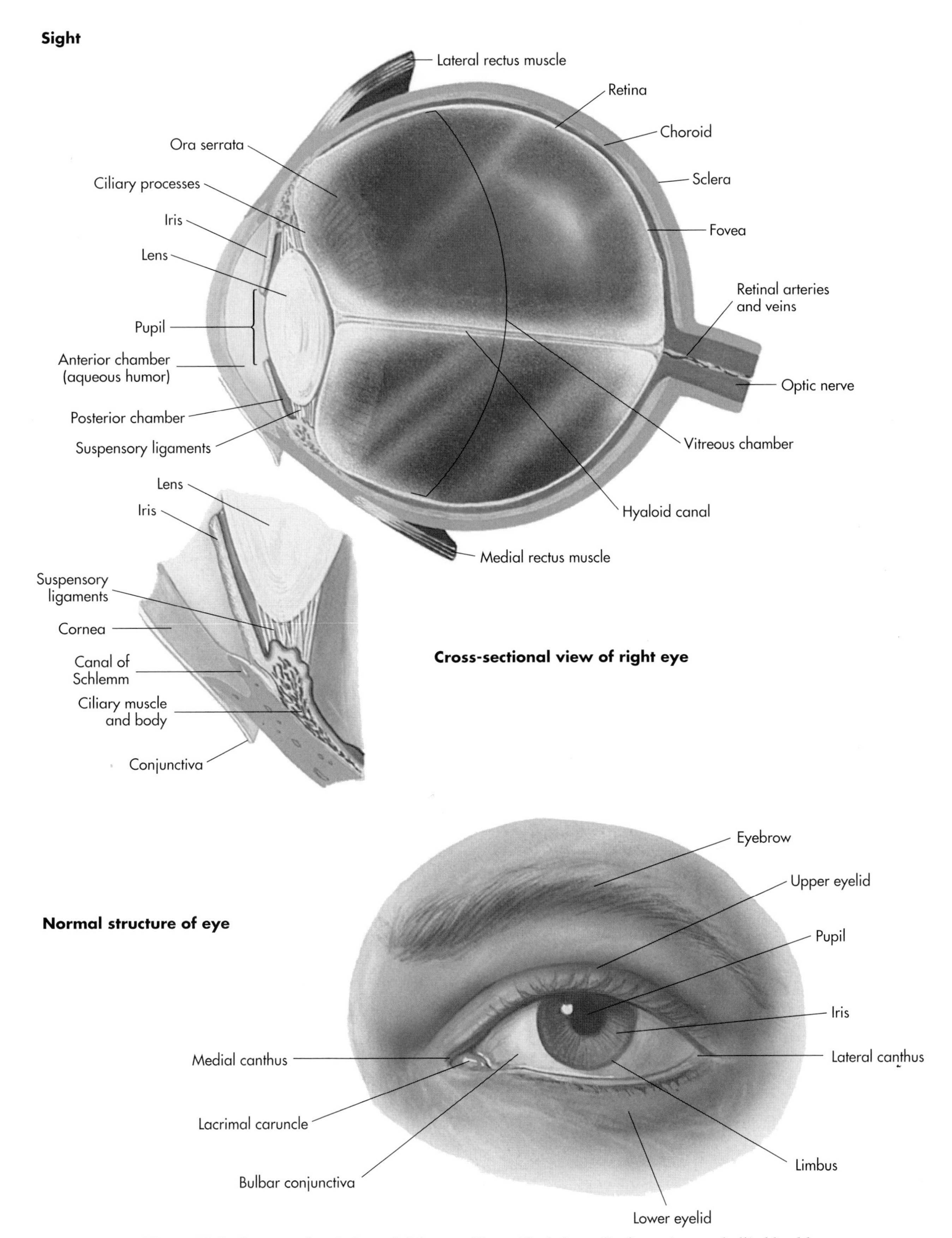

Figure 12-2. Cross-sectional view of right eye. (From *Mosby's medical, nursing, and allied health dictionary,* ed 2, St Louis, 1986, Mosby.)

Diabetic Retinopathy

Some visual disabilities are acquired through the deleterious effects of elevated blood sugar due to diabetes, which creates microaneurysms in retinal capillaries. These are the source of diabetic retinopathy. Because of vascular and cellular changes accompanying diabetes, there is often rapid worsening of other pathologic vision conditions as well. Diabetic retinopathy accounts for 7% of the blindness in the United States, the third leading cause of blindness, and the incidence curves upward abruptly with increasing age (Tumosa, 2001).

There is little to no evidence of retinopathy until 3 to 5 years or more after the onset of diabetes. Early signs are seen in the funduscopic examination and include microaneurysms, flame-shaped hemorrhages, cotton wool spots, hard exudates, and dilated capillaries (Tumosa, 2001). Yearly evaluation by an ophthalmologist is essential, with more frequent consultation after retinopathy is present. Laser treatment can reduce vision loss in 50% of patients. Constant, strict control of blood sugar can slow progress of the disease (Tumosa, 2001).

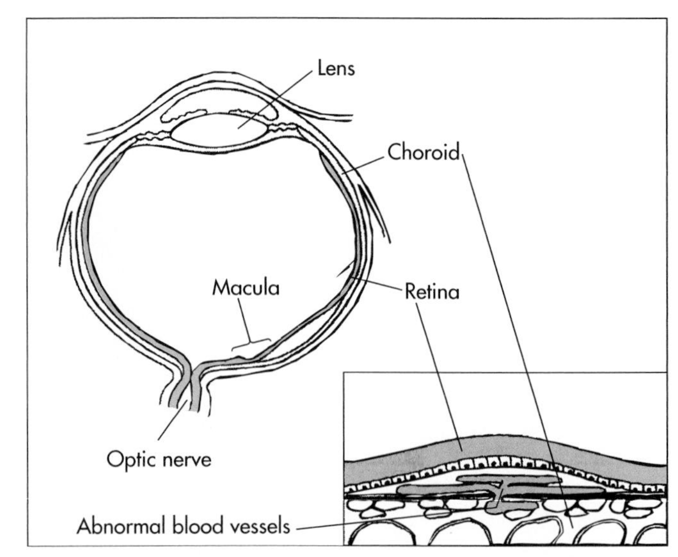

Figure 12-3. Age-related macular degeneration (AMD) results if abnormal blood vessels grow in the choroid layer beneath the retina or if any part of the retina fails to receive proper nutrients. (From Macular degeneration, *Mayo Clinic Health Letter* 8[9]:5, 1990.)

Macular Degeneration

The macula is the central visual point of the retina and is the source of central vision. Age-related macular degeneration (AMD) results from systemic changes in circulation, accumulation of cellular waste products, tissue atrophy, and growth of abnormal blood vessels in the choroid layer beneath the retina. Fibrous scarring disrupts nourishment of photoreceptor cells, causing their death and loss of central vision. This is the "wet" type of AMD, which accounts for 10% of maculopathy cases but 90% of legal blindness cases (Tumosa, 2001). The "dry" type of maculopathy is caused by disintegration of the retinal epithelium and the loss of overlying photoreceptor cells. This type of AMD reduces vision, but not to serious levels (Figure 12-3).

Macular degeneration leads to loss of central visual acuity, but peripheral vision is not affected. The etiology is unknown; however, risk factors are family history of the disease, sunlight, age, and white race (Reuben et al, 2000). It usually occurs after age 60 (Lighthouse International, 1999). Early in the disease an Amsler grid is used to determine clarity of central vision (Figure 12-4). A perception of wavy lines is diagnostic of beginning macular degeneration, and vision loss can

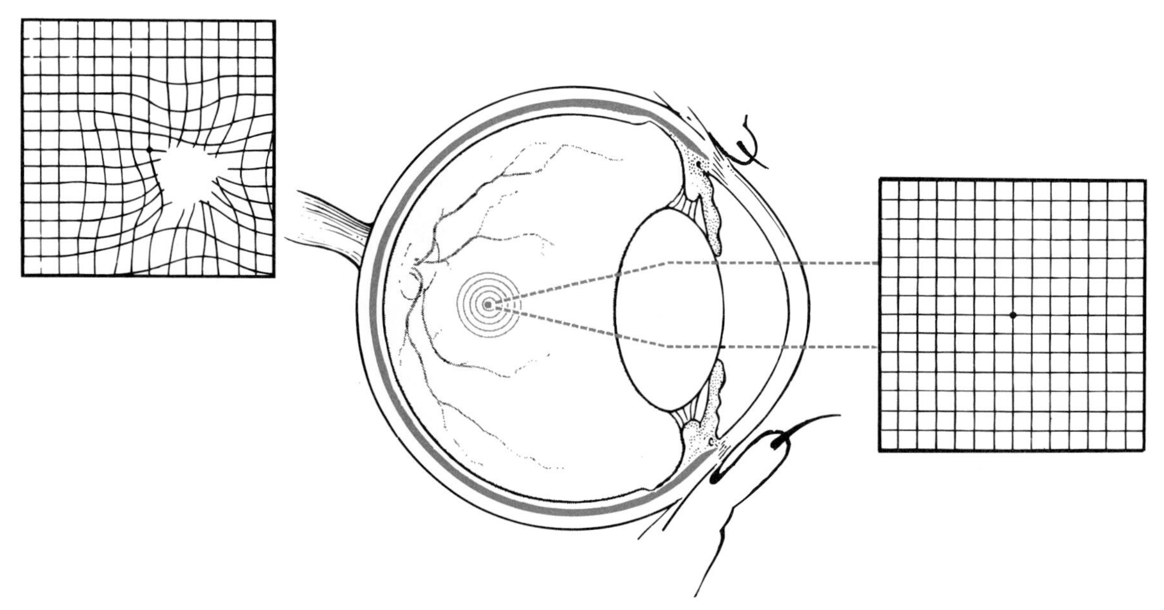

Figure 12-4. Macular degeneration: distortion of center vision; normal peripheral vision. (Illustration by Harriet R. Greenfield, Newton, MA.)

occur in days. There has been no treatment for the more common dry type of macular degeneration until recently. Laser treatment and photodynamic therapy in the wet type will prevent further visual loss for a period of time. After about 5 years, only 20% of elders will have sustained benefit (Tumosa, 2001).

Quality of life can be maintained with the use of devices and services. High-intensity lighting similar to daylight is helpful for reading. Magnifying lenses are especially useful for reading or handwork such as crocheting and knitting. Special telescopes are available for outside travel. There are watches with high-contrast dials. Large-print books and "talking" books are available at many local libraries. There are high-tech options such as video magnification with closed-circuit television and word processing programs with enlarged text and an optical character recognition program that converts text into sound. A 6-year study by the National Eye Institute, published in the October 2001 issue of *Archives of Ophthalmology,* reveals that a specially formulated dietary supplement of vitamins C and E, beta-carotene, zinc, and copper reduced the advancement of the dry form by 25% compared with placebo. The supplement is available from Bausch & Lomb under the name Ocuvite PreserVision (All About Vision, 2001).

Assessment of Vision

The Snellen chart is commonly used by nurses to test for distance vision. Testing the aged should be done in good light and with the bulb shielded to prevent glare. If the 20/40 line on the chart cannot be read, looking through a pinhole in a piece of cardboard should improve vision. If it does improve, that is indication for a change in eyeglass prescription. Gross visual field deficits, or confrontation, can be determined by displaying a wide arc with outstretched arm and noting when the individual no longer detects the moving finger of the nurse's arm. These are superficial assessments and are not meant to replace more thorough examination by an ophthalmologist. Near vision can be evaluated using a book or newspaper or a Rosenbaum chart about 12 to 14 inches away and asking the elder to read several lines. This is an excellent way to assess the need for change of glasses and a more sophisticated evaluation.

Color vision is evaluated using an Ishihara chart, which is a plate with multiple colors in the background. Results are determined by the number of plates identified correctly. This examination is sensitive for red/green blindness but not for blue, which is more common in older adults. This examination is used when taking a driver's license test to determine if the older adult is able to discriminate red from green.

Observation of the retina and optic nerve disc via funduscopy reveals important systemic, circulatory, and vision information, but pupillary constriction and clouding of the vitreous and lens often hamper the eyeground ophthalmologic examination of an older person. One must be cautious because pupil dilation with a mydriatic for the purposes of examination may precipitate an acute attack for those predisposed to angle-closure glaucoma.

Caring for the Elder with Visual Impairment

General principles in caring for the elder with visual impairment include the following: use warm incandescent lighting; control glare by using shades and blinds; suggest yellow or amber lenses to decrease glare; suggest sunglasses that block all ultraviolet light; select colors with good contrast and intensity; and recommend reading materials that have large, dark, evenly spaced printing.

Environmental Lighting. The pupil of the aged eye admits less light to the retina. This is a normal condition known as *senile miosis.* A simple and effective intervention for the visually impaired is often neglected: increased environmental lighting.

In the process of aging, the intensity of illumination must be three times as powerful to produce the same visual capacity. Intensity must be tempered by appropriate diffusion to avoid glare. Sensitivity to glare increases markedly in the aged due to clouding of the lens and vitreous that results in scattering of light as it passes through the lens. This is particularly noticed in night driving or in low levels of illumination when the pupil is slightly dilated (Burke and Laramie, 2000). This may cause eyestrain, fatigue, tension, and actual pain. Individuals are advised to avoid night driving and looking directly at oncoming headlights.

Contrasting Colors. Color contrasts are used to facilitate location of items. Sharply contrasting colors assist the partially sighted. For instance, a bright towel is much easier to locate than a white towel hanging on a beige wall. Boxes 12-3 and 12-4 provide further ideas regarding caring for the visually impaired elder. Most visually impaired people have enough residual vision to use their eyesight with proper aids or training to read, write, and move around safely. Unfortunately, many older persons with serious visual impairments consider themselves blind and are usually treated as if they are. Adequate training in using residual vision can prevent partially sighted older persons from falling into unnecessarily dependent lifestyles.

Low-Vision Devices. Technology advances in the last decade have produced some low-vision devices that may be used successfully in the care of the visually impaired elder. An array of assistive devices are now available for these individuals, such as Microspiral Galilean Telescopes, Telephoto Microscopes, Clear Image Lens, Behind the Lens Telescopes, and the Low Vision Enhancement System. This last device uses tiny cameras to place an enlarged image on a video screen in front of the eyes. This is worn as a headset and can be used for distance viewing, as well as reading. Persons with reduced visual acuity should be encouraged to consider some of these sophisticated aids because severe visual deficits may result in mobility restrictions, as well as create cognitive, sensory, and behavioral disturbances.

Box 12-3 Suggestions for Communicating with and Caring for the Visually Impaired Patient

1. Always identify yourself clearly.
2. Always make it clear when you are leaving the room.
3. Make sure you have the resident's attention before you start to talk.
4. Try to minimize the number of distractions.
5. Whenever possible, choose bright clothes with bold contrasts.
6. Check to see that the best possible lighting is available.
7. Assess you position in relation to the resident. One eye or ear may be better than the other.
8. Try not to move items in the resident's room.
9. Staff members should try to narrate their actions.
10. Try to keep the resident between you and the window, or you will appear as a dark shadow.
11. Use some means to identify residents who are known to be visually impaired.
12. Use the analogy of clock hands to help locate objects.
13. Keep color and texture in mind when buying clothes.
14. BE CAREFUL ABOUT LABELING A RESIDENT AS CONFUSED. He or she may be making mistakes due to poor vision!

From McNeely E, Griffin-Shirley N, Hubbard A: Diminished vision in nursing homes, *Geriatr Nurs* 13(6):332, 1992.

Box 12-4 Caring for the Visually Impaired

- Remember there are many degrees of blindness; allow as much independence as possible.
- Speak normally but not from a distance; do not raise or lower voice, and continue to use gestures if that is natural to your communication. Do not alter your vocabulary; words such as "see" and "blind" are parts of normal speech. When others are present, address the blind person by prefacing remarks with his or her name or a light touch on the arm.
- When entering the presence of a blind person, speak promptly, identifying yourself and others with you. State when you are leaving to make the person aware of your departure.
- Speak descriptively of your surroundings to familiarize the blind person. State the position of people who are in the room.
- Do not change room arrangement without explanation.
- Speak before handing blind person an object. Describe positions of food on plate in relation to clock position (e.g., 3 o'clock, 6 o'clock).
- When walking with a blind person, offer your arm. Pause before stairs or curbs; mention them. In seating, place the person's hand on the back of the chair. Let him or her know position in relation to objects.
- Blind people like to know the beauty that surrounds them. Describe flowers, scenery, colors, and textures. People who have been blind since birth cannot conceive of color, but it adds to their appreciation to hear full descriptions. Older people most frequently have been sighted and can enjoy memories of beauty stimulated by descriptive conversation.

Magnifying lenses are available in many forms in addition to those commonly found in spectacle frames (Figure 12-5). These can be recommended in relation to the use for which they are desired. The most complex of the low-vision devices are telescopes that can be focused at various distances, thus increasing the number of tasks that can be performed. In addition, closed-circuit television magnifying units are available that can enlarge written characters up to 45 times.

Another method of magnification is through the use of a standard copying machine that has magnifying capabilities. One need not buy one of these but only make use of those available to the public. By repeatedly magnifying printed words or images, even small print can be made as large as desired.

Eyeglasses, once heavy and bulky, are now cosmetically appealing. Many also incorporate prismatic lenses that expand the visual field. Sunglasses are designed to filter out ultraviolet rays that may be harmful to sensitive retinas. Some eyeglasses adjust to light source and become darker in the sun. Magnifiers have been redesigned for ease of changing batteries and bulbs, positioning, and grasping. Telescopic lens eyeglasses are smaller, are easier to focus, and have a greater range (Figure 12-6). It is now possible to electronically magnify video- and computer-generated text. Some software converts text into artificial voice output. All of these resources must be considered when attempting to help the visually impaired elder achieve the visual activities that are important to his or her quality of life. Because individual needs are unique, it is recommended that before investing in any of these vision aids, the client be advised to consult with a low-vision center or low-vision specialist.

Orientation Strategies for the Nonsighted

Methods to assist those individuals with total lack of sight are not generally included in nursing curricula. Methods in common use include the following: (1) the clock method, in which the individual is simply told where the food or item is as if it were on a clock face; (2) the sighted guide, in which a companion guides the visually impaired and enables safe mobility; (3) the cane sweep, which encounters obstacles; (4) varied textured surfaces; (5) sound signals, for example, at street crossings; and (6) seeing-eye dogs.

Sighted Guide. Ask the blind person if he or she would like a sighted guide. A strong element of dependency and trust is necessary in this method, and many people would rather manage on their own. Initially, as a person is adjusting to

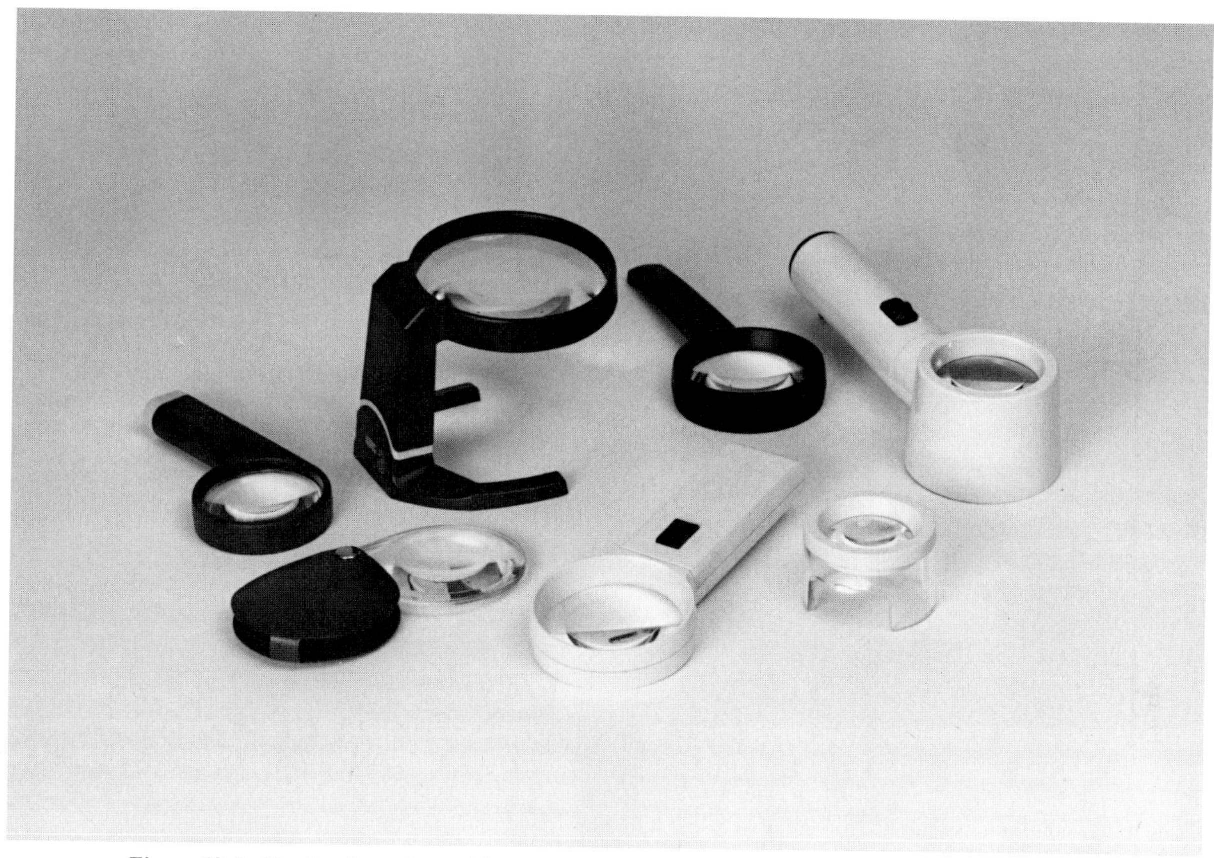

Figure 12-5. Hand and stand magnifiers. (Courtesy The Lighthouse Inc., New York.)

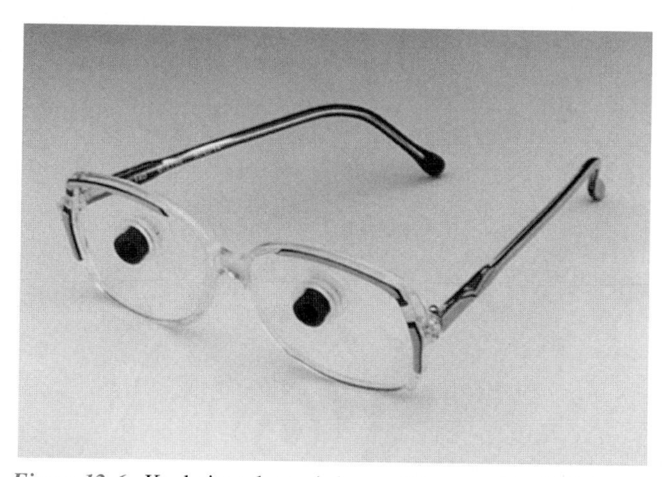

Figure 12-6. Keplerian telescopic lenses. (Courtesy The Lighthouse, Inc., New York.)

blindness, it can be helpful. If assistance is accepted, offer your elbow or arm. Instruct the person to grasp your arm just above the elbow. If necessary, physically assist the person by guiding his or her hand to your arm or elbow.

Go one-half step ahead and slightly to the side of the blind person. The shoulder of the person should be directly behind your shoulder. If the person is frail, place his or her hand on your forearm. With this modified grasp, the person will be positioned laterally to your body. Relax and walk at a comfortable pace. Tell the person when you are approaching doorways or a narrow space.

Cane Sweep. White canes, sometimes called "long canes," are used by about 109,000 persons in the United States to alert others to their presence as a nonsighted person, as well as to signal the blind person to obstacles in the space ahead (All About Vision, 2001). However, an architectural design that includes slanted beams and inverted pyramidal designs can be deceiving. In the early 1970s there were numerous college students who were blind as a result of being exposed at birth to concentrated oxygen in isolettes. One brought to my attention the difficulty he had negotiating the student center with a cane. It was designed with large angled concrete beams from floor to ceiling, and when the path at cane level seemed clear, the beam would surely present a hazard at the level of his head.

Sound Signals. In some U.S. cities and most European and Japanese cities, intermittent sound signals alert the nonsighted when it is safe to cross the street—a simple solution, surprisingly not common in the United States. As nurses become more involved in political activist groups, this would be an area on which to focus federal and state lawmakers' attention.

Varied Textures. Those elders who have been blind for some time have developed hypersensitivity to textural variations. This sensitivity can be incorporated into the environment in numerous ways to assist the blind person.

Guide Dogs. There are guide dog schools in the United States, and about 10,000 persons use dog guides to assist them in mobility. Trained guide dogs are matched to individuals' needs and personalities, and those elders who have guide dogs have had several during the course of their adult years. Each dog becomes a companion, as well as a guide, and the elder grieves on its demise, though no specific studies regarding this could be found. Some altruistic nurses have become involved in raising and training guide dogs.

Driving. Although vision testing is required in all states for original licensure, the states vary on further vision testing. Eleven states do not require additional vision testing; two, Connecticut and Oregon, have age-based periodic vision testing after age 65 and 50, respectively (Coley, 2001).

HEARING AND HEARING IMPAIRMENT IN THE AGED

Oliver Sacks, author of the well-known book *Awakenings* (on which a popular film was based), wrote *Seeing Voices* (Sacks, 1989) to elucidate "a journey into the world of the deaf." Sacks presents a view that blindness may in fact be less serious than loss of hearing because of the interference with communication with others and the interactional input that is so necessary to stimulate and validate. One elderly man said that a great annoyance of hearing loss is in the subtle aspects of living with a partner, who also most probably has a hearing loss as well. "You must often repeat what you say, and in lovemaking, whispering sweet words becomes a gesture for yourself alone." Perhaps Helen Keller was most profound in her expression: "Never to see the face of a loved one nor witness a summer sunset is indeed a handicap. But I can touch a face and feel the warmth of the sun. But to be deprived of hearing the song of the first spring robin and the laughter of children provides me with a long and dreadful sadness" (Keller, 1902).

For those deafened in later life after hearing was well established, the world may remain full of "phantasmal," or imagined, sounds. This is a unique type of imagined sound in which visual experience (movement and speech) is rapidly and unconsciously translated into an auditory correlate. It is thought that special visual-auditory neurologic connections are established (Sacks, 1989).

Today in the United States more than one third of all community-dwelling elders are hearing impaired (Desai et al, 2001). It is estimated that 50% of persons over age 85 have a hearing problem, and the occurrence is as high as 90% among the institutionalized aged. In all age-groups, elderly men are more likely than women to be hearing impaired. Further, white men and women report hearing loss more than blacks. As a review, we have included the anatomy of the ear in Figure 12-7.

Hearing impairments related to aging are numerous. There is drying and sagging of the auricle and elongation of the

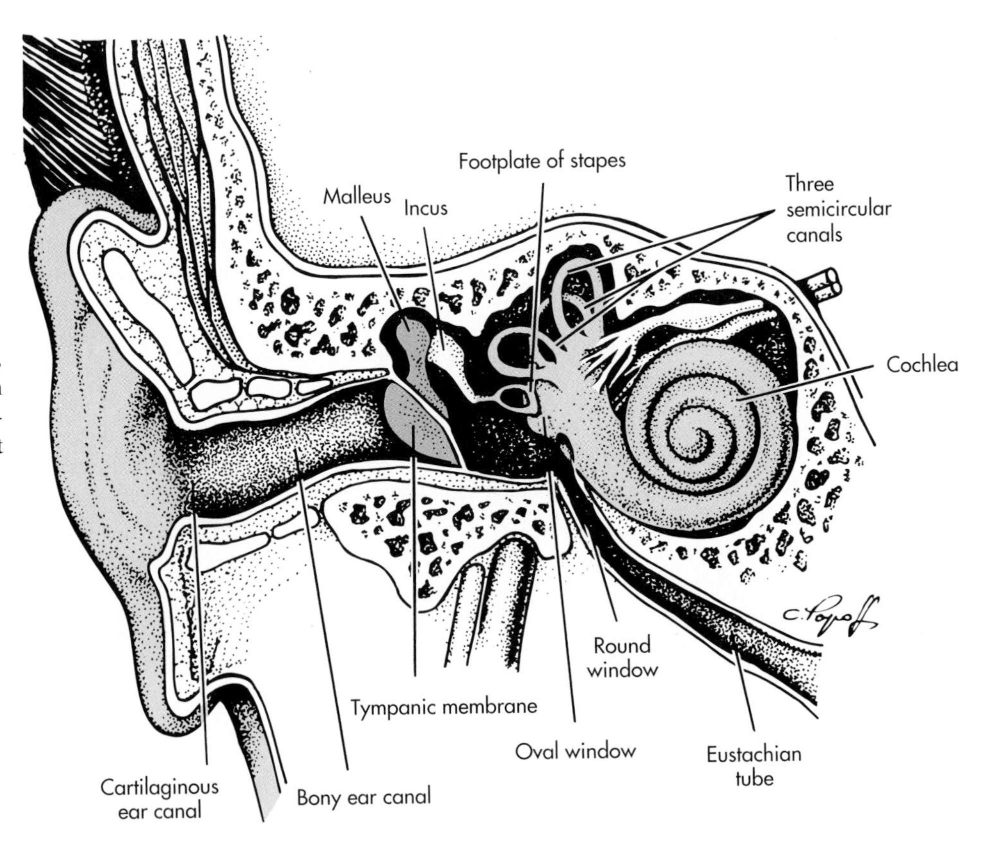

Figure 12-7. External auditory canal, middle ear, and inner ear. (From Malasanos L, Barkauskas V, Stoltenberg-Allen K: *Health assessment,* ed 4, St Louis, 1991, Mosby.)

earlobe, which causes an alteration in the shape of the auditory canal, narrowing it. The tympanic membrane thickens and the bony joints in the inner ear degenerate. Most significant, there is degeneration of the vestibular structure, which affects speech, equilibrium, and sensitivity to sound (Cotter and Strumpf, 2002). Other factors contributing to hearing loss are the accumulation of cerumen in the auditory canal, history of intense noise exposure, and ototoxic drugs such as aspirin, loop diuretics, and certain antibiotics. Like visual impairment, hearing impairment diminishes the quality of life. It may lead to miscommunication, social isolation, confusion, depression, cognitive decline, and decreased mobility (Demers, 2001; Desai et al, 2001).

Presbycusis

Presbycusis is primarily an issue of normal aging in which there is impairment of high-frequency tones, frequency discrimination, sound localization, and speech discrimination and an increase in the sensation of loudness (Burke and Laramie, 2000; Reuben et al, 2000). It is an affliction of individuals over 50 but is not a universal change. When low-frequency sound is impaired, it is more likely due to noise exposure (Cotter and Strumpf, 2002).

Presbycusis is a slowly progressive, symmetric, sensorineural hearing loss. Older adults take longer to process and comprehend information in higher auditory centers and have a great deal of difficulty with people who speak rapidly. In addition, the consonants with high frequencies, such as t, f, and g, present more difficulties (Cotter and Strumpf, 2002).

Older persons are often unaware of hearing loss because of the gradual manner in which it usually develops. Some people are aware of a hearing loss and are disturbed by misperceptions and distortions, often imagining derogatory remarks said about them. However, knowing that one has a hearing loss is not sufficient. Testing must be done to determine the nature of the loss, how much it interferes with communication, whether it is treatable (as may be the case with metabolic alterations or middle ear structural changes), and whether a hearing aid will be useful.

Prelingual Deafness

Reading and writing skills may be impaired. Even though the intelligence of prelingually deaf persons may be normal, they may not have had the common educational opportunities of their cohort. This is thought to be related to the early orientation to signing and lip reading. For these individuals, signing is their first language and English their second. Subtleties of verbal communication may be lost to them, though they often compensate and become extremely alert to nonverbal cues and feelings. At times a certified interpreter, well enmeshed in the world of the deaf, will be needed. For additional information in this regard the reader might contact the National Information Center on Deafness at Gallaudet University (800 Florida Avenue NE, Washington, DC 20002: [202] 651-5051).

Box 12-5 Myths and Assumptions about the Deaf

The deaf elderly should be treated like children.
Congenital deafness is a form of mental retardation.
Deaf people can understand speech through lip reading.
Deaf people can read and write English.
Smiling and head nodding indicate agreement or comprehension.
A hearing aid and talking louder help the deaf person to hear better.
Anger, stubbornness, and uncooperative behavior mean the deaf person is becoming senile.
Consistency of personnel is no more important for the deaf than for anyone else.

See Box 12-5 for myths and assumptions about people who are deaf.

It is often incorrectly assumed that an elder can read lips; more likely it is body language and the context of a situation that clues an elder to words being said. In addition, it seems common to overlook the fact that vision may also be fading, thus impinging on lip-reading ability. Perhaps it is the desire of nursing personnel to believe that lip reading is common rather than face the fact that communication can be extremely difficult for some elders. Some elders become dependent on vision for understanding speech at the same time their vision is becoming compromised. Nurses will need to seek resources appropriate to augment vision to the greatest degree possible in these individuals.

Cerumen Impaction

Cerumen impaction is the most common and easily corrected of all interferences in the hearing of the aged. The reduction in the number of cerumen-producing glands and activity of the glands results in a tendency toward cerumen impaction in the aged. This can be removed and must be before accurate audiometry can be done. A protocol for removal is outlined in Box 12-6. Irrigation is contraindicated if the tympanic membrane has been perforated because it may induce an infection. Cautions are also necessary for those with especially sticky cerumen, which can damage the mechanism of a hearing aid and involve costly repairs.

Long-standing impactions become hard, dry, and dark brown in color. Many elderly admit to using foreign objects to clean their ears. This may compact the cerumen and make the problem more difficult to solve. Some have perforated the tympanic membrane in the process and thus suffered severe hearing loss in the injured ear. Individuals at particular risk of impaction are elderly men with large amounts of ear canal tragi (hairs in the ear) that tend to become entangled with the cerumen, which prevents dislodgment.

A medical student was examining Bob's ear with the aid of an otoscope and was having great difficulty visualizing anything. In the

Box 12-6

Protocol for Cerumen Removal

Assess for ear pain, traumas, abnormalities, drainage, surgeries, or perforations. These or any other unusual findings should be referred to an otolaryngologist.

When aural examination reveals cerumen impaction with no other abnormalities the nurse may irrigate for cerumen removal using the following techniques:

- Carefully clip and remove hairs in ear canal
- Instill a softening agent, such as slightly warm mineral oil, 0.5 to 1 ml twice daily for several days until wax becomes softened
- Protect clothing and linens from drainage of oil or wax by small cotton ball placed in each external ear canal
- When irrigating the ear use handheld bulb syringe, a 2 to 4 ounce plastic syringe or Water Pik with emesis basin under ear to catch drainage; tip head to side being drained
- Use solution of 3 ounces 3% hydrogen peroxide in quart of water warmed to 98 to 100 degrees; if client is sensitive to hydrogen peroxide use sterile normal saline
- Place towels around neck, empty emesis basin frequently, observing for residue from ear; keep client dry and comfortable; do not inject air into client's ear or use high pressure when injecting fluid
- If the cerumen is not successfully washed out begin the process again of instilling a softening agent for several days

Adapted from Webber-Jones J: Doomed to deafness, *Am J Nurs* 92(11):37, 1992.

process she dislodged a hard ball of cerumen that became lodged even farther in the ear. In panic he yelled that she had deafened him. He was immediately taken to his physician, who removed the wax with the aid of an aural speculum and a cerumen spoon. Then Bob was all smiles, saying he hadn't heard so well in years.

Others who may develop excessive cerumen are those who habitually wear hearing aids, those with benign growths that narrow the external ear canal, and those who have a predilection to cerumen accumulation. More commonly, older adults will have less cerumen and dryer cerumen because of a greater amount of keratin present (Maas et al, 2001).

Tinnitus

Tinnitus, or ringing in the ear, may also manifest as buzzing, hissing, whistling, crickets, bells, roaring, clicking, pulsating, humming, or swishing sounds. The most common type is high-pitched tinnitus with sensorineural loss; less common is low-pitched tinnitus with conduction loss such as is seen in Meniere's disease (Dinces, 2001). The sounds may be constant or intermittent.

Tinnitus generally increases over time. It is a condition that afflicts many aged and can interfere with hearing, as well as become extremely irritating. It is estimated to occur in nearly 11% of elders with presbycusis. Approximately 50 million people in the United States have tinnitus, and 12 million people are estimated to have tinnitus to a distressing degree (American Tinnitus Association, 2002). Suicides related to severe tinnitus have been reported (Dinces, 2001).

Tinnitus is associated with otosclerosis, ototoxic drugs, antiinflammatories, sedatives, antidepressants, diabetes mellitus, Meniere's disease, labyrinthitis, severe anemia, temporomandibular joint dysfunction, otitis media, carotid artery atherosclerosis, cervical spondylosis, thyroid problems, auditory canal obstruction, severe hypertension, hypotension, trauma, and tumors (Dinces, 2001; Springhouse, 2001; Cotter and Strumpf, 2002).

In a retrospective review of 84 patients with pulsatile tinnitus in a neurology clinic, 42% were found to have a significant vascular disorder, most often an arteriovenous fistula or a carotid sinus fistula (Dinces, 2001). However, the majority of elders have sensorineural tinnitus. The incidence of tinnitus peaks between ages 65 and 74 (about 11%), is higher in men than in women, and then seems to decrease in men.

Assessment. Tinnitus may be described as pulsatile (matching the beating of the heart) or nonpulsatile (unilateral, asymmetric, or symmetric). Tinnitus may be subjective (audible only to the person) or objective (audible to the examiner). Subjective tinnitus is more common. Objective tinnitus is rare and is frequently due to a vascular or neuromuscular condition. The mechanisms of tinnitus are unknown but have been thought to be analogous to cross-talk on telephone wires, phantom limb pain, or transmission of vascular sounds such as bruits, and they are sometimes hallucinatory.

A thorough history is essential in determining the cause of tinnitus because it is a symptom, rather than a disorder. The history is useful in directing the practitioner to the cause. Many patients suffer insomnia from tinnitus and will have symptoms decreased by treating the insomnia. Patients with pulsatile tinnitus may benefit from vascular surgery.

Cora, 80 years old, was complaining of sounds in her ears that would not go away. A complete physical examination, aural examination, and audiometric testing were prescribed. At the completion of testing the audiometrist asked Cora to describe the sounds. Cora began singing, "I'll Be Loving You Always." Perhaps the first question should have been, "Describe the sounds you hear that won't go away."

Treating tinnitus is usually not successful. However, there are many things for the practitioner to try that may give some relief. To tolerate tinnitus, the practitioner may prescribe vasodilators, tranquilizers, or antiseizure drugs. Biofeedback may be useful. There is a tinnitus masker, or competing sound, that produces a band of white noise of about 1800 Hz, which helps block out tinnitus and does not interfere with hearing (Springhouse, 2001). Hearing aids can be prescribed to amplify environmental sounds to obscure tinnitus, and there is a device that combines the features of a masker and a hearing aid, which emits a competitive but pleasant sound that distracts from head noise. Electrical stimulation has been successful for patients with severe hearing loss and tinnitus (Dinces, 2001).

Because patients with tinnitus exhibit signs of depression, treatment with serotonin reuptake inhibitors may be tried. Tinnitus may be reversible in patients who are taking ototoxic drugs. Stopping the drugs will stop progression even if some damage has already been done. Intravenous lidocaine has been used with some success (50% to 75% improvement for the short term) in elders with the less common low-frequency tinnitus (Dinces, 2001). A number of other therapies have been tried, including electrical stimulation, acupuncture, ginkgo, and niacin; however, none has been demonstrated to be better than placebo (Dinces, 2001).

Nursing actions include discussions with the client regarding times when the noises are most irritating; perhaps suggest a diary in order to identify patterns. There is some evidence that caffeine, alcohol, cigarettes, stress, and fatigue may exacerbate the problem. Assess medications for possible contribution to the problem. Discuss lifestyle changes and alternative methods that some have found effective. Also, refer clients to the American Tinnitus Association for research updates, education, and support groups.

The Hospitalized Hearing-Impaired Person

Hospitalization or internment in a new facility can be very difficult for a hearing-impaired elder. The geriatric nurse can apply a number of supports to ease the process:

- Note on the patient's chart that he or she is deaf.
- Place a sign in a prominent place in the patient's room.
- Determine from the patient or family the most effective way to communicate with the patient.
- If the patient "signs," try to avoid restrictions of arms and hands.
- Use visual aids (charts, models) to explain procedures.
- Ensure good lighting in the patient's room.
- Encourage the use of the patient's hearing, aid and ensure the safety of the hearing aid at night.
- Obtain a certified sign language interpreter for obtaining consent for any procedure. It is essential that the patient understand possible risks and outcomes.

Assessment of Those with Impaired Hearing. Assessment of a hearing disability may be done in a superficial manner by almost any observant health care professional. However, the responsibility for the initial identification of hearing problems usually falls on the nurses, and therefore rapid, reliable, effective screening methods must be available to them. There is an excellent tool to use for screening elders with impaired hearing: the Hearing Handicap Inventory for the Elderly—Screening (HHIE-S), a 5-minute, 10-item questionnaire that assesses how the elder perceives the social and emotional effects of hearing loss (Demers, 2001). Audiologic referral is recommended for those with a score of 10. In addition, the nurse should make a visual inspection of the ear and should obtain the patient's history, which can begin with these questions:

1. In the past 3 months, have you had discharge from your ears?
2. In the past 3 months, have you experienced dizziness (not related to sudden changes in position)?
3. In the past 3 months, have you had pain in your ears?
4. In the past 3 months, have you noticed a sudden or rapid change in your hearing?
5. Have you ever experienced tinnitus, vertigo, or sudden or gradual loss of hearing?
6. How much does this problem interfere with your communications?
7. In which situations do you have difficulty hearing?
8. In the past, have you experienced ear infections, surgery, treatment, or hearing aid use?
9. Has anyone in your family had hearing loss?
10. What drugs have you used or are now using? (Note particularly toxic levels of antibiotics and aspirin.)

It is important that nurses become aware of these considerations. The patient's history and visual inspection require little time to effectively identify subjects who need medical referral. Pure-tone screening is highly reliable but is sometimes difficult to administer to elders. Each elder is entitled to a complete and thorough audiometric examination if there is any doubt about adequate hearing capacity. Early detection of hearing loss often depends on a nurse's observational assessment. The following are useful initial screening observations:

- Does the person often seem inattentive to others?
- Does the person respond with inappropriate anger or irritation when spoken to?
- Does the person believe people are talking about him or her?
- Does he or she lack a movement response to sounds in the environment?
- Does the person have difficulty following clear directions?
- Is he or she withdrawn and alone much of the time?
- Does the person frequently ask to have something repeated?
- Does he or she tend to turn one ear toward a speaker?
- Does the person have a monotonous or unusual voice quality?
- Is speech unusually loud or soft?

Before concluding that any of these signs are evidence of "senility" or other aberrant behaviors, consider the possibility of a hearing problem. When there is any doubt, referral should be made to an otologist or otolaryngologist to identify possible medical conditions and then to an audiologist or a speech-hearing clinic for an audiologic evaluation before contacting a hearing aid representative.

Nurses are reminded that the best judge of adequate hearing capacity will come from the aged individual's own evaluation (Figure 12-8). However, older persons are often unaware of mild to moderate hearing loss because of the gradual manner in which it usually develops.

Hearing evaluation. Few elders have had audiometric testing even though a great many elders over 75 years old have hearing impairment. Nursing service can and should provide initial assessment by investing in a tuning fork, an

Hearing Handicap Scale

Rating:

Always—1 or 2
Frequently—3 or 4
Never—5

Scoring:

Raw score − 29 × 1.25 = %

Scores:

No handicap	0% to 20%
Mild hearing handicap	21% to 40%
Moderate hearing handicap	41% to 70%
Severe hearing handicap	71% to 100%

	Score
1. At 2 to 4 m from radio or television, do you understand speech?	
2. Can you converse on telephone easily?	
3. Can you carry on conversation comfortably when in a noisy place?	
4. Can you understand speech when in a noisy bus, on an airplane, at a movie, on the street corner?	
5. Can you understand a person when seated beside him and you cannot see his face?	
6. Can you understand speech if someone is talking to you while chewing crunchy foods?	
7. Can you understand a whisper when you cannot see a person's face?	
8. Can you carry on conversation across a room when someone speaks in normal tone of voice?	
9. Can you understand women when they talk?	
10. Can you carry on conversation outdoors when it is reasonably quiet?	
11. When in a meeting or a large dinner would you know what speaker said if lips were not moving?	
12. Can you follow conversation at a large dinner or in a small group?	
13. When seated under balcony of a theater or auditorium, can you hear what is going on?	
14. When in church, lodge meeting, or lecture hall, can you hear if speaker does not use a microphone?	
15. Can you hear telephone ring when it is located in another room?	
16. Can you hear warning signals such as automobile horns, railway crossing bells, or emergency vehicle sirens?	
17. Can you carry on conversation in car with windows open?	
18. Can you carry on conversation in car with windows closed?	
19. Can you hear when someone calls from another room?	
20. Can you understand when someone speaks to you from another room?	
21. Can you carry on conversation with someone who speaks quietly?	
22. When you ask for directions, do you understand what is said?	
23. When you are introduced, do you understand the name the first time it is spoken?	
24. Can you hear adequately when conversing with more than one person?	
25. When seated in the front of an auditorium, can you understand most of what is being said?	
26. Can you carry on everyday conversations with family members without difficulty?	
27. When seated in the rear of an auditorium, can you understand most of what is said?	
28. When in a large formal gathering, can you hear what is said if speaker uses a microphone?	
29. Can you hear night sounds, such as dogs barking, distant trains, bells, trucks passing, etc.?	

Figure 12-8. Hearing Handicap Scale. (Modified from High WS et al: *J Speech Disord* 29:215, 1964.)

otoscope, and an audioscope and learning to use them appropriately. An otoscope allows visualization of the ear and discovery of perforated eardrums and cerumen impaction. A tuning fork placed on an individual's forehead will determine the presence of unilateral conductive hearing loss. This is a nonspecific test and does not measure bilateral hearing loss. The audioscope can then be used, following the instructions in Figure 12-9, to determine the frequency range of hearing. Human speech is usually heard below the 2000 to 3000 Hz range. Those who have used the audioscope find it a highly valid screening instrument. Although it should not be used exclusively for determining etiology and degree of hearing loss, it is a simple, fast, and accurate method of screening for hearing loss. Assessment of hearing disorders is done with audiometric and nonaudiometric testing tools. Assessment of structural changes and gross evidence of hearing loss is part

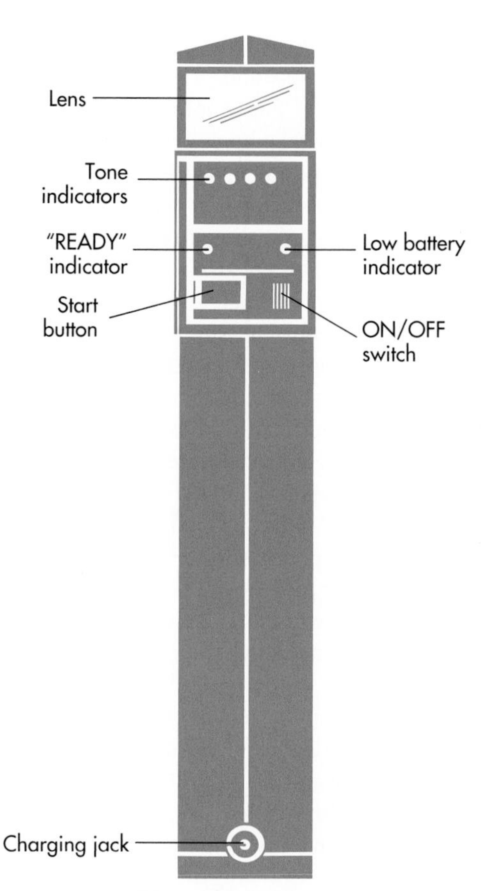

1. Turn on the instrument by sliding the ON/OFF switch up.
2. Inform the client that he/she will hear some faint tones and ask the client to raise the index finger each time the sound is heard.
3. Gently pull the ear canal up and back and then carefully insert the audioscope into the ear canal using the largest ear speculum that can be comfortably inserted into the ear canal.
4. The tip is positioned so that the tympanic membrane is visualized.
5. Depress the start button.
6. The tone indicators illuminate sequentially (with a red light) as each tone is presented to the client for 1.5 seconds.
7. Repeat the same procedure in the opposite ear.

NOTE: Occluding the opposite eardrum does not appear to influence the accuracy of the test results.

Figure 12-9. The audioscope. (From Campbell S: The audioscope: a valuable hearing assessment tool, *J Gerontol Nurs* 12[12]:28, 1986.)

of a physical examination. Audiometry is needed for more precise information.

Because many elders are sensitive about admitting losses, they may be reluctant to share such information. It can best be obtained by first establishing rapport with the elderly person and then proceeding to open interviewing with a comment such as, "Many people have difficulty hearing in certain situations. Have you experienced any difficulty?" "Describe these for me." If friends and relatives have insisted the older person needs hearing evaluation, he or she may be doubly resistant.

Interventions for Those with Impaired Hearing. Physical examination, interview, self-assessment, relative or friend assessment, and audiometric findings are all necessary to arrive at a meaningful recommendation for the hearing-impaired aged person. Counseling includes specific information regarding the problem, encouragement that sensorineural loss (nerve deafness) can often be partially counteracted by a hearing aid, assistance in the adjustment phase of wearing a hearing aid, and work with family members to improve their communication techniques.

Hearing aids. Many factors may influence an individual who refuses to wear a hearing aid. If the person has been taught to use an aid gradually and correctly and yet does not do so, the nurse should attempt to discover the reasons: the appearance of having an infirmity, difficulty manipulating a small object, lack of energy, uncomfortable fit, forgetfulness, anger expressed through passive resistance, cost, or simply self-neglect. In this era of highly sophisticated, personalized, and computerized hearing aids, almost everyone can find some hearing enhancement that is acceptable to them. Hearing aids have changed dramatically in recent years, but many individuals, having tried one several years ago, have decided against using them.

A hearing aid is a personal amplifying system that includes a microphone, an amplifier, and a loudspeaker. The appearance and effectiveness of hearing aids have greatly improved in recent years. Hearing aids have been miniaturized, but the small size may present difficulties for the aged with visual deficits, loss of sensation, or arthritic hands. A recent advance has been the introduction of a remote control device that contains an on/off switch and volume device. There are approximately 50 different manufacturers of hearing aids, and thus the informed consumer has a broad selection from which to choose.

Many ear, nose, and throat specialists have an audiologist and audiologic testing available in the office. Audiologists may favor certain hearing aid models, and it is wise for a client to shop around for fit and sound regardless of what the physician and audiologist recommend. The investment in a good hearing aid is considerable, and a good fit is crucial.

Since 1991 all new telephones are required to be compatible with hearing aids. Hearing aids with a telecoil can be set on "T" to receive the signal from the magnetic coil in the telephone (Beck and Roe-Beck, 2000).

Styles. There are numerous hearing aids and assistive devices to improve hearing (Figure 12-10). The behind-the-ear hearing aid, which looks like a shrimp and fits around and behind the ear, is the most powerful ear-level unit (Beck and Roe-Beck, 2000). This type of hearing aid is used for elders with moderate, severe, or profound hearing loss. There is also a larger version that is custom made to fit the entire external auricular cavity. This type of hearing aid is the most visible and least expensive. It is usually recommended for elders with mild or moderate hearing loss.

In-the-canal hearing aids are smaller and more expensive than in-the-ear hearing aids. They are easily inserted and removed. These aids are used for patients with mild to moderate hearing loss.

There are hearing aids that are built into the frame of eyeglasses. The frame carries the signal from one ear to the other, so there is good amplification in both ears. These are not commonly used because if the hearing aid malfunctions, the elder must go without glasses. Also, if the glasses are misplaced, the hearing aid is lost as well (Beck and Roe-Beck, 2000).

There are now sound amplifiers on the market that fit in a pocket or are worn on the belt and are inexpensive, walkabout-style hearing boosters. Their appearance is similar to that of a Walkman. These are particularly useful for individuals with conductive hearing loss and in situations where background noise is inevitable. The amplifying microphone can be attached to the TV or telephone or clipped on a friend's collar. In situations where a primary sound source is desirable, these devices are ideal. Headsets with small or large earphones are available. Thus amplification of desired sounds is available without the use of a hearing aid (see Figure 12-10, *B*). The receiver is a custom-made clear plastic ear mold in the ear canal and attached to the unit by a wire. This type of hearing aid is used for those with profound hearing loss. It is less esthetically pleasing compared with the other types.

Digitally programmed hearing aids are becoming available that have more than a million different settings from which to select. These are matched to the individual's hearing loss. In most hearing aids today there is a miniaturized computer with a memory chip integrated into the hearing aid that eliminates many of the major problems such as adjustment levels, background noise, and whistling. These aids automatically electronically separate incoming sound without the need to adjust the volume.

With rapidly developing technology, it behooves the hearing-impaired individual to be thoroughly evaluated in an audiologic center that is not marketing specific hearing aids. Many hospitals and health centers have such services and may have dozens of models an individual can try until one is found that is most suitable. The following are guidelines for anyone who is thinking of purchasing a hearing aid:

- Have a complete hearing evaluation by a qualified audiologist.

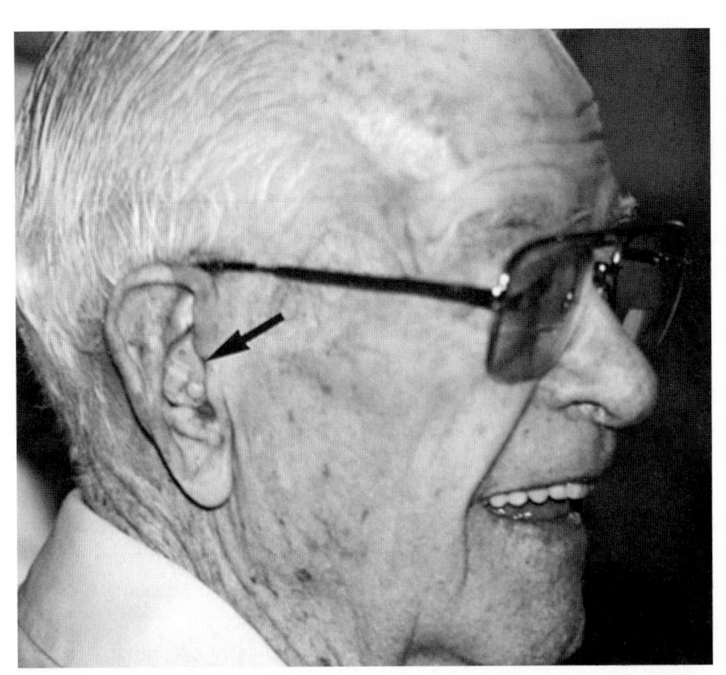

Sensory augmentation of vision and hearing. (From Castillo HM: *The nurse assistant in long-term care: a rehabilitative approach,* St Louis, 1992, Mosby.)

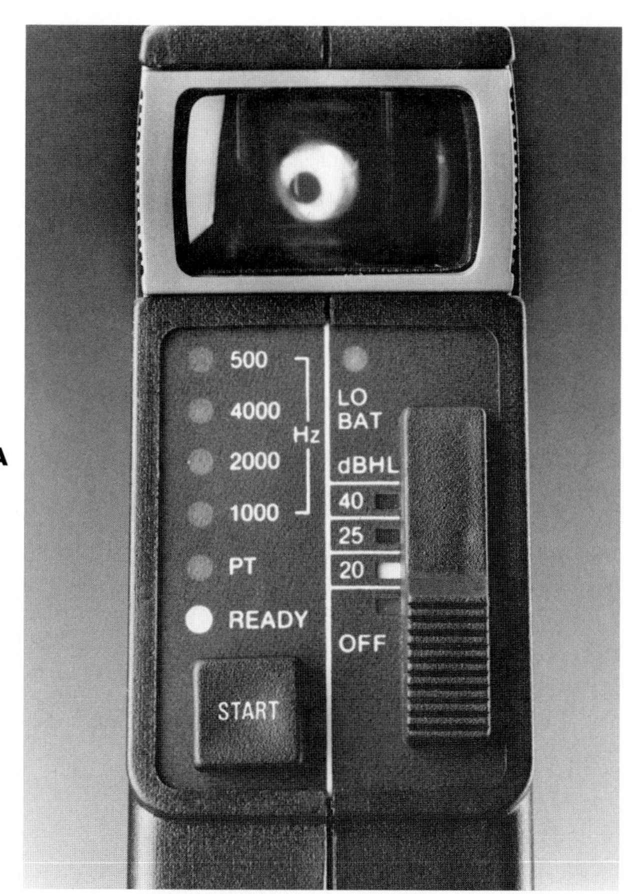

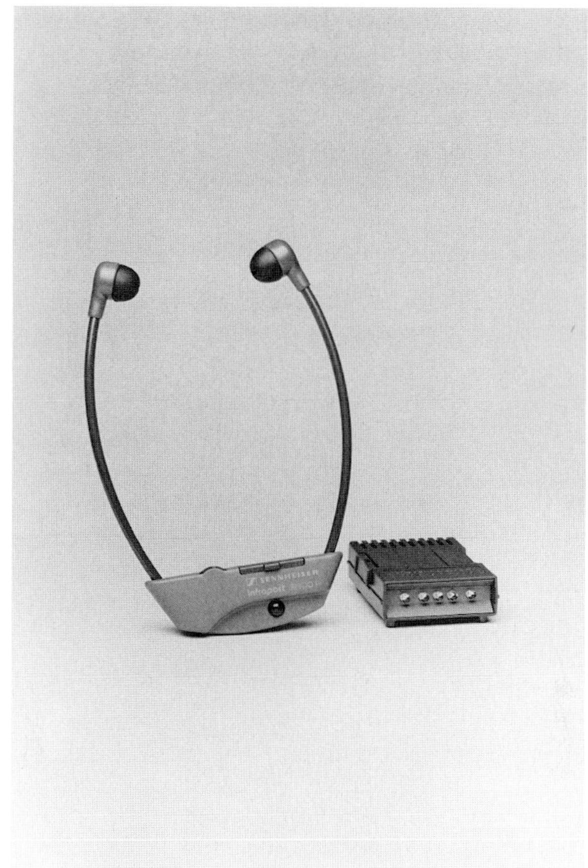

Figure 12-10. **A,** Audioscope. **B,** DirectEar (personal hearing system). (**A**, Courtesy Welch Allyn, Inc., Skaneateles Falls, NY. **B**, Courtesy Sennheiser, Old Lyme, CT.)

- "Nerve deafness" is no longer a reason for not seeking a timely evaluation.
- Hearing aids of whatever type will require individual motivation to adapt and adjust to the aid.

Suggestions for using and caring for a hearing aid are given in Table 12-3. At least a 30-day trial should be given before purchasing a hearing aid. If problems occur during that time, return to the audiologist for assistance. Recent federal regulations have influenced hearing aid manufacturers toward more careful marketing and fitting procedures.

Currently, before a hearing aid can be purchased, medical clearance consisting of a signed waiver from a physician is mandatory, stating that none of the following conditions exist:

1. Visible congenital or traumatic deformity of the ear
2. Active drainage from the ear in the last 90 days
3. Sudden or progressive hearing loss within the last 90 days
4. Acute or chronic dizziness
5. Unilateral sudden hearing loss within the last 90 days
6. Visible evidence of significant cerumen accumulation or a foreign body in the ear canal
7. Pain or discomfort in the ear
8. Audiometric air-bone gap equal to or greater than 15 dB

Nurses can detect the first seven of these conditions on physical examination and advise clients to seek further counseling from an otolaryngologist. They must also advise clients that routine hearing examinations and hearing aids are not paid for by Medicare (Centers for Medicare and Medicaid Services, 2001). Elders can contract for Medicare + Choice plans, which are available in many parts of the United States. There are often extra benefits but also extra rules to be followed. Also, there are 10 standard Medigap insurance policies from which to choose. None provide hearing aids.

Cochlear Implants. In the 1980s cochlear implants became available to profoundly deaf individuals with sensorineural hearing loss who derived little benefit from hearing aids (Beck and Roe-Beck, 2000). These have been refined considerably since then.

The cochlear implant is inserted in the mastoid bone behind the ear and electrically stimulates the eighth cranial nerve, the auditory nerve (Figure 12-11). The device also consists of an external microphone, a transmitter, and the implanted receiver (Springhouse, 2001). The transmitter receives signals from the microphone and sends them to the receiver located near the auditory nerve. The signals travel along an implanted wire to the nerve. The failure rate of the cochlear implant is less

Table 12-3 Care and Use of Hearing Aids

Hearing aid use	Care of the hearing aid
• Initially, wear aid 15 to 20 minutes daily. • Gradually increase time until 10 to 12 hours. • Hearing aid will initially make client uneasy. • Insert aid with canal portion pointing into ear, press and twist until snug. • Turn aid slowly to ⅓ or ½ volume. • A whistling sound indicates incorrect ear mold insertion. • Adjust volume to a level comfortable for talking at a distance of 1 yard. • Do not wear aid under heat lamps or hair dryer or in very wet, cold weather. • Do not wear aid while bathing or perspiring heavily. • Concentrate on conversation, request repeat if necessary. • Sit close to speaker in noisy situations. • Continue to be observant of nonverbal cues. • Be patient with self and realize the process of adaptation is difficult but ultimately will be rewarding.	• Insert battery when hearing aid is turned off. • Store hearing aid in a dry, safe place. • Remove or disconnect battery when not in use. • Batteries last 1 week with daily wearing 10 to 12 hours. • Clean cerumen from tip weekly with the pipe cleaner. • Common problems include switch turned off, clogged ear mold, dislodged battery, twisted tubing between ear mold and aid. • Ear molds need replacement every 2 or 3 years. • Check ear molds for rough spots that will irritate ear. • Avoid exposing aid to excess hear or cold. • Clean batteries occasionally to remove corrosion; use a sharpened pencil eraser and gently scrape.

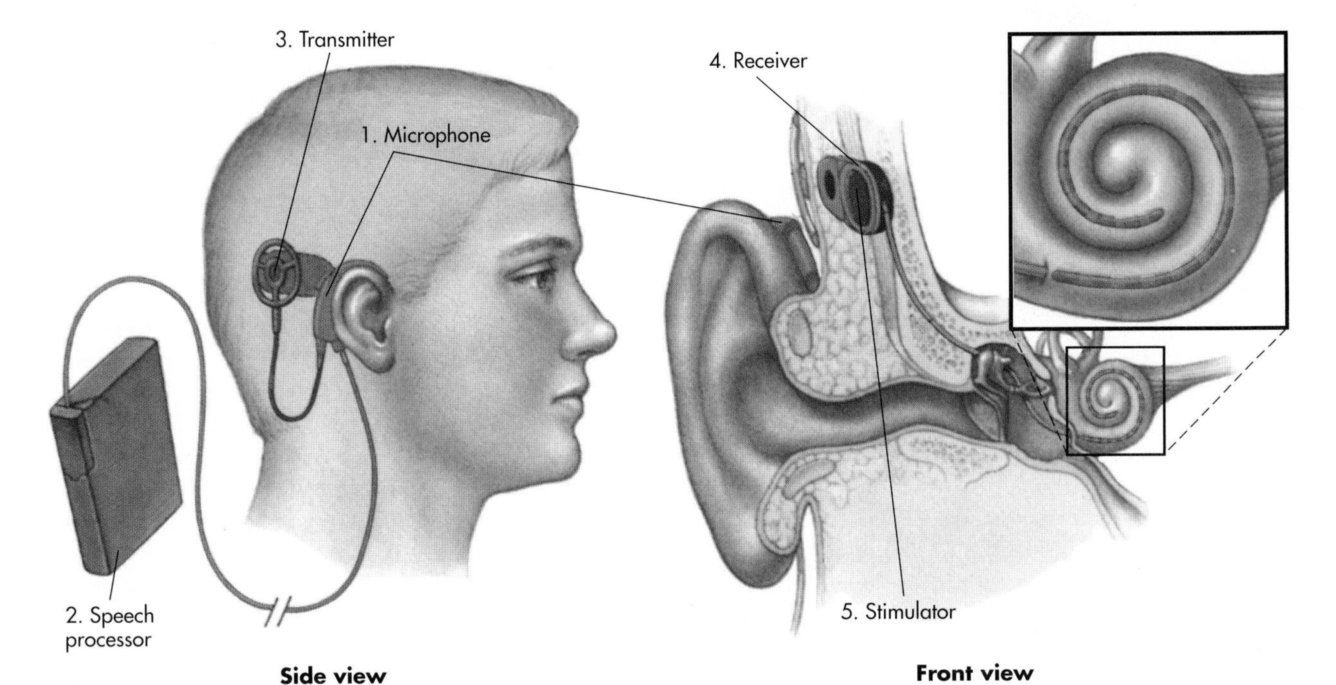

Figure 12-11. How cochlear implants work: A microphone *(1)* picks up sound. The sound travels through a thin cable to a speech processor *(2)*. The processor can be worn on a belt or in a pocket. The processor converts the signal into an electrical code and sends the code back up the cable to a transmitter *(3)* fastened to the head. The transmitter sends the code through the skin to a receiver-stimulator *(4 and 5)* implanted in bone directly beneath the transmitter. The stimulator sends the code down a tiny bundle of wires threaded directly into the cochlea (snail-shaped primary hearing organ). Nerve fibers are activated by electrode bands on this bundle of wires. The auditory nerve carries the signal to the brain, which interprets the signal. (From Cochlear implants, *Mayo Clinic Health Letter* 9[11]:4, 1991.)

than 1% (Beck and Roe-Beck, 2000). One of the *Healthy People 2010* goals is to increase access to hearing rehabilitation services and adaptive devices, including hearing aids and cochlear implants (Healthy people 2010: vision and hearing, 2002).

Adaptive devices. Many devices have been developed to assist the hard of hearing. These include alarm clocks that shake the bed or activate a flashing light; television and telephone amplifiers; and sound lamps that respond with light to sounds such as doorbells, babies crying, telephones, or other noises. The sound on timers, alarm clocks, and smoke detectors can be modified to a signal that is within the hearing range of the particular person. These can be purchased from hearing aid dealers, telephone companies, and electronic and appliance shops, as well as by mail or through the Internet.

Environmental adaptations can be made. Minimizing background noise is helpful, as is eliminating background music (Wharton, 2000). Acoustic materials such as heavy drapes, upholstered furniture, and carpeting will absorb noise. Tight window seals can keep out exterior noise.

Any facility that receives financial aid from Medicare is required by the Americans with Disabilities Act to provide equal access to public accommodations. Such facilities are required to have sign language interpreters, telecommunications devices for the deaf (TDDs), flashing alarm systems, and telecaptioning devices on TVs. Unfortunately, these are seldom seen.

Extensive nursing care plans related to presbycusis can be found in many recent clinical manuals. We suggest that these plans be reviewed for routine management but carefully and thoughtfully modified in relation to the patient's unique needs.

Some highly innovative people have developed ideas and products to enrich the lives of the hearing impaired. One group has recorded music especially for the profoundly hearing impaired that is focused only in the low-frequency cycles that are most easily heard.

Another program that is gaining recognition is Hearing Dogs for the Deaf. There are scores of locations in the United States that train hearing dogs for the deaf. In some locations the Society for the Prevention of Cruelty to Animals (SPCA) trains "shelter dogs." Some dogs are especially bred and raised to be hearing dogs, and in some locations the individual's own dog is trained. Hearing dogs serve to warn the hearing impaired of impending danger, audible signals, phones, fire and smoke alarms, emergencies, and intruders. Although there are other, electronic means of dealing with many of these problems, the hearing impaired most consistently comment on the alleviation of the sense of isolation that so often accompanies hearing impairment. With a hearing dog companion, elders express renewed courage, confidence, and freedom.

Self-help groups. In a small group discussion Dr. Priscilla Ebersole conducted with elders, a portable microphone was brought in and tried by all the participants. After a few moments of play they put it on the table and never used it again during the group. But there was a noticeable difference in how they addressed each other and the level of feedback that was given. They reminded each other when the speaker was mumbling, speaking into his or her own lap, covering his or her mouth, or could not be heard. The auditory consciousness of the group had been raised by a few moments of discussion at the beginning. In years of conducting groups, this was the first time a real discussion of hearing occurred in the group. Dr. Ebersole thought perhaps it was her own consciousness that was raised more than that of anyone else in the group.

In old age, when people have transcended work and have more time to communicate for pleasure, they often develop hindrances to the communication process. When interactions are thwarted by sensory disturbances and motor disabilities, isolation and withdrawal soon follow. However, some people are able to transcend the limitations amazingly well. One very deaf elderly woman remained responsive and warm, often carrying the conversation by sharing her life experiences and observations. The conversation was one sided but enjoyable to those who listened. She was very aware of verbal and nonverbal cues, which encouraged her to continue or to cease sharing.

Health care professionals may need to focus on ability rather than disability and not assume a deaf person does not wish or is not able to talk. The ability to communicate verbally is gratifying to most persons. One aged man said he missed hearing conversations around him almost as much as the ability to comfortably converse. Listening and talking can be comforting, enlightening, and reassuring, particularly for those who may have been surrounded by conversation for most of their lives.

One small group of elders enumerated a few simple suggestions that make a significant difference in their ability to hear:

- Speakers need to keep their hands away from their mouth and project their voices by controlled diaphragmatic breathing.
- Facial and hand expressions used liberally facilitate understanding.
- Careful articulation and moderate speed of speech are helpful.
- Some languages and some cultural levels of verbal expressiveness facilitate understanding more than others; for example, rapid, romance languages are more difficult to understand, and stolid or stoic individuals are more difficult to understand.
- If one has a hearing deficit, wear two hearing aids; in most cases there is a "better ear," but both should be augmented for best results.

Hearing is a binary process and is most effective when both ears are functioning at the maximum. Cost and convenience are factors that hamper many elders from following through on this.

- Face the individual and stand or sit on the same level.
- Gain the individual's attention before beginning to speak.
- Avoid conversations in which the speaker's face is in glare or darkness.
- Avoid speaking from another room or while walking away.
- Enunciate carefully and speak in normal cadence.
- Avoid eating, chewing, or smoking while speaking.
- Realize that the listener will hear less well if ill or fatigued.
- Pause between sentences or phrases to confirm understanding.
- When changing topics, preface the change by stating the topic.
- Provide visual cues to locate noise direction, because there appears to be an age-related deficit in picking up directional cues.
- Restate with different words when you are not understood.
- If paranoia has developed, the individual may not respond well to touch. A handshake is a benign gesture and will signal acceptance or rejection of your efforts to communicate.
- Reduce background noise such as radio or television.

Their mutual problem-solving efforts not only afforded an opportunity for shared concerns but resulted in practical ideas helpful to individuals and their caregivers.

TASTE AND SMELL

Age-related losses of smell and fine taste normally begin in the sixth decade. These senses intertwine to provide links to the environment. They allow appreciation of good tastes and smells and also serve as a warning of environmental hazards (Wharton, 2000). Four basic tastes have been identified (sweet, sour, salty, and bitter), conveyed by approximately 9000 taste buds. Scientists believe there are more yet to be identified and an unknown number of basic and subtle odors. The senses of taste and smell (chemosenses) are intertwined and can provide great pleasure, as well as protection from harm. Fine taste, such as the subtle differences between turkey and chicken, is an olfactory function; crude taste, such as sweet and sour, is dependent on the taste buds. It is thought that there is about a 75% decrement in smell (hyposmia) by age 80 and a 50% loss of taste buds (hypogeusia) by age 60 that accelerates after age 70 (Wharton, 2000).

The senses of taste and smell play an important role in eating behaviors and in the maintenance of health (Maas et al, 2001). The enjoyment of taste is really the totality of the experience of temperature, texture, smell, appearance, and flavors. The sense of smell is affected by aging more than the sense of taste. It is important, then, to identify foods that appeal to the changed senses of smell and taste. Colors and textures may compensate for diminished sensory appeal of foods (O'Neill, 2002).

When dealing with canned foods, older persons should be cautioned to check for bulges in the can and to discard any that are suspicious (Wharton, 2000). Stored foods should be dated and checked for spoilage. Defrosted foods should be used right away because thawing and refreezing significantly affects flavor and texture. Significant, rapid, and noticeable changes in smell or taste may be the result of medication, disease processes, or, in rare situations, hallucination. Gustatory and olfactory hallucinations are danger signals of brain lesions or head and neck cancers and should be immediately suspect.

Diseases that affect taste and smell are numerous. Among them are allergic rhinitis (23% suffer loss of smell), Alzheimer's disease, asthma, cancers, epilepsy, diabetes, liver disease, Parkinson's disease (an early sign), chronic renal failure, viruses, vitamin deficiencies, and zinc deficiency (Luggen, 2001). Drugs affecting taste and smell include many antibiotics, anticonvulsants, antidepressants, antihistamines, antihypertensives, antiinflammatories, beta blockers, bronchodilators, calcium channel blockers, lipid-lowering agents, and vasodilators—all drugs commonly used by elderly persons.

Taste

Taste acuity is at least two thirds dependent on the olfactory sense. Tasting depends on an intact nerve supply (cranial nerves VII [facial] and IX [glossopharyngeal]) (Luggen, 2001). However, it is not only taste but also the sensual aspects of food that are enjoyable. The pleasure of eating comes more from masticating than from the taste buds or the hunger center in the hypothalamus. This knowledge can be important in preparing food for older people.

Taste buds that seem most affected by aging are those for sweet and salty at the tip of the tongue. These supposedly are exposed to more contact and thus may deteriorate slightly. This theory is based on the knowledge that taste buds begin to atrophy and diminish in number in midlife, for some as early as age 40, and the observation that many elders tend to salt and sweeten their foods more than when they were younger. This can be a problem for those with diabetes. Bitterness, located at the very back of the tongue, seems to remain a strong sensation at all ages, and in fact, older persons may experience an increased sensitivity to bitterness, with the resulting complaint that foods taste bitter or sour (Wharton, 2000).

Individuals have varied levels of taste sensitivity that seem predetermined by genetics and constitution, as well as age variations. Comparatively little interest has been demonstrated in studying these differences. Many denture wearers say they lose some of their satisfaction in food, possibly because texture is such an important element in food enjoyment, possibly because mastication is less enjoyable. The sensory pleasure of food and the symbolic nurturance inherent in eating and feeling satiated are important ways one maintains a sense of security. Indeed, when feeling insecure, many people begin to eat compulsively. Difficulties measuring flavor appreciation come from individual variables such as smoking, olfactory sensitivity, attitude toward food and eating, and the presence of moistening secretions. There are also aberrations in flavor sensations caused by certain medications and by viruses, for example, colds.

Assessment. Detailed and meaningful gustatory evaluations are difficult to administer. Assessing taste, especially salty, sweet, sourness, and bitterness, is part of the complete physical assessment examination. Individuals complaining of *dysgeusia* (unpleasant taste in the mouth) should be evaluated for dental disease and dental hygiene, medication side effects, head trauma, upper respiratory disease, and cranial nerve integrity. If these screening procedures are inadequate, the individual may need to be referred to an otolaryngologist for more intensive testing.

There are no known therapies for primary gustatory dysfunction. If all secondary causes have been eliminated, the most useful approach to the client is simply being concerned and supportive. Help the person experiment with various herbs, spices, flavor extracts, and sugar and salt substitutes and identify foods that are most enjoyable (Wharton, 2000). Encourage smokers to refrain from smoking. Do not burden them with a bland, soft, or liquid diet unless it is absolutely essential. They may enjoy the sensations of the food appearance and chewing even if their taste for flavors is not acute.

Olfaction

One of every two persons over the age of 65 has lost some sense of smell, and women are more likely than men to experience such loss (Luggen, 2001). Most people, however, lose some olfactory discriminatory capacity, resulting in a lowered capacity for enjoyment of scents and fragrances and a stronger reliance on texture and visual cues. Smell losses outnumber taste problems. The sense of smell requires an intact cranial nerve I.

A decreased sensitivity to odors may be dangerous for the older person, such as when one may fail to detect the odor of leaking gas, a smoldering cigarette, or tainted food. The loss of smell may also present social problems. We all experience habituation to, and unawareness of, our own body odor. Some elders are unaware that the odor of urine accompanies them even though they have only slight leakage. This particular sensory reduction can be an alienating factor unless attended to. Perfumes may be overused and be overwhelming and offensive to others (Wharton, 2000).

Three causes can explain 60% of the problems with loss of smell: nasal sinus disease that results in obstruction of passages, thereby interfering with odors reaching the smell receptors; repeated injury to olfactory receptors through viral infections (Figure 12-12); and head trauma that results in bleeding into the nasal mucous membrane (least common cause). In the elder, it is more likely that a viral infection will result in permanent changes to the sense of smell. Abrupt loss of the sense of smell may occur after a viral nasal infection, although usually it will not be total loss (anosmia); this requires immediate attention because it could signal a serious disorder.

Exposure to medications and environmental agents affects chemosensation, especially in men and particularly those who have worked in factories. The accumulation of noxious agents over time results in an impaired sense of smell, especially from acid fumes, lead, or cocaine, a growing problem (Springhouse, 2001). Olfactory dysfunction can be among the first signs of Parkinson's disease and may in fact be a preclinical indication of the disease.

Olfactory nerve cells are thought to be the only sensory nerves capable of regeneration (Figure 12-13); however, if the sense of smell has been absent for 6 months or more it is likely to be permanent, indicating destruction of the olfactory nerve (cranial nerve I) or olfactory neuroepithelium (Springhouse, 2001) (Box 12-7).

Assessment. A reliable and easy odor recognition tool is the University of Pennsylvania Smell Identification Test, a prepackaged scratch-and-sniff test that can be done with ease

Box 12-7 Assessing the Nose

- Visually inspect the nose. Note any asymmetry that could interfere with breathing or smell. Expect that the nose will be relatively long and broad because of the ongoing formation of cartilage through the years. Examine the color and texture of the surface of the nose. Diffuse redness, papules, pustules, and dilated venules can signal excess alcohol intake.
- Palpate the nose. Feel for raised bumps along the frontal bone at the base and hard nodes in the cartilage. Note any frontal bone depression suggesting nose fracture in the past.
- With an otoscope, look inside the vestibule of each nare. With age, nasal hair becomes coarser and thicker. Inspect the base of the hairs for signs of irritation or infection caused by clipping the hairs too close. Examine the nasal mucosa: Is it moist and intact? Or dry and broken? With age, the mucosa becomes fragile and easily broken. A smooth, shiny membrane with engorged turbinates is a sign of vasomotor rhinitis. Check the arterior septum and note whether it appears straight or deviates to the left or right of the columella separating the nares. At least a mild degree of septal deviation is common in adults.
- Occlude each nostril, one at a time, and ask the person to close his mouth and breathe through the open nostril. Note whether both nostrils are patent.
- Test olfactory nerve function by asking the person to identify various smells: Nerve fibers in the olfactory bulb decline at a rate of about 1% per year, which may account for a decreased ability to recognize or distinguish smells with age.
- Palpate the paranasal sinuses to detect swelling or any sign of tenderness that may indicate sinusitis or postnasal drip.

From Knapp MT: A rose is still a rose: how does losing the sense of smell affect an elder's life? *Geriatr Nurs* 10(6):290, 1989.

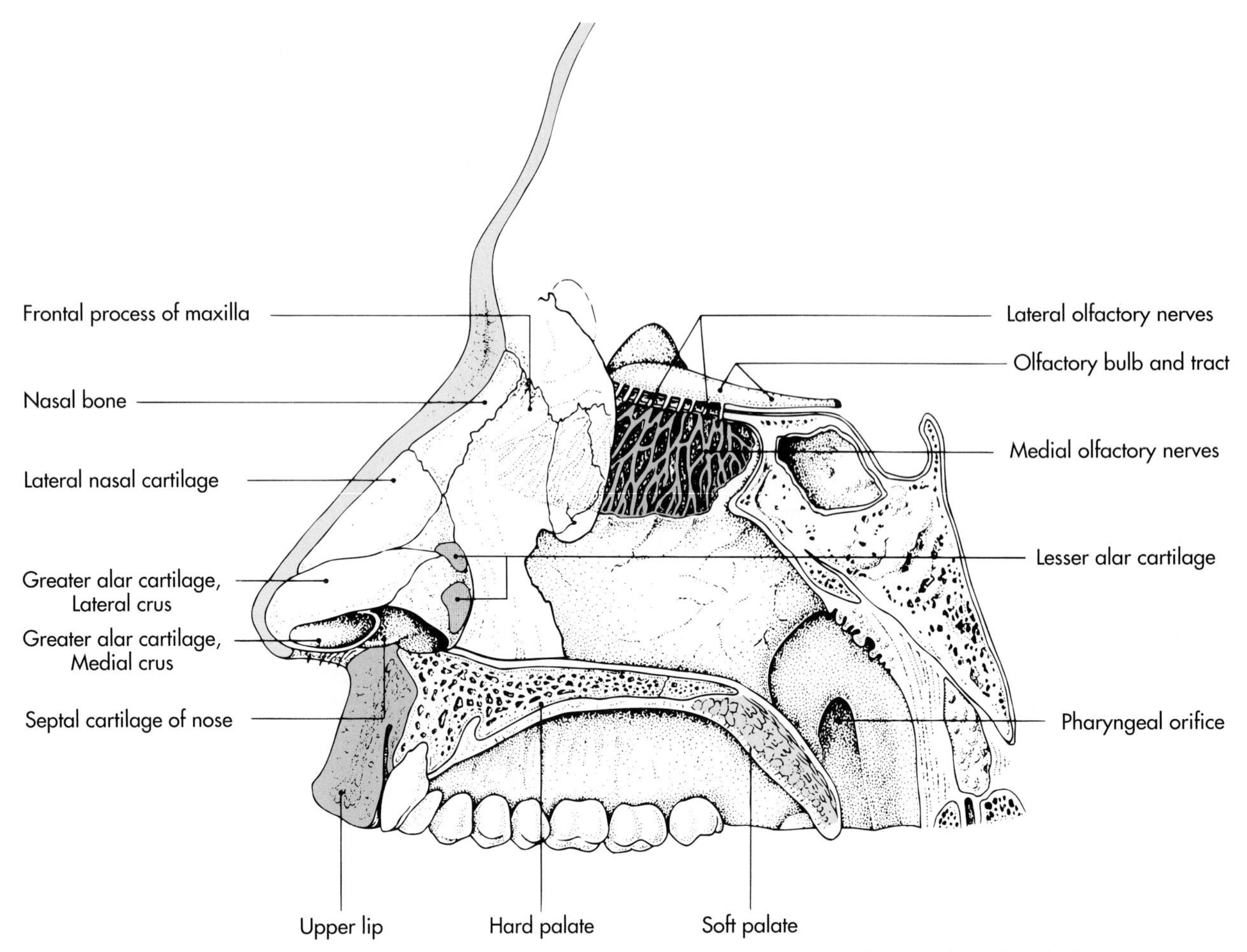

Figure 12-12. Key structures of the nose. (From Knapp MT: A rose is still a rose: how does losing the sense of smell affect an elder's life? *Geriatr Nurs* 10[6]:290, 1989.)

in any setting. *Dysosmia* (the sensation of unpleasant smell) may be individually idiosyncratic. For example, one woman found a particular incense nauseating; others are repelled by certain perfumes.

The practitioner will want to check the nose for swelling of the mucous membranes. It is important to look for polyps, which may be obstructive. Assess hydration. Ask about smoking and past viral infections. Sinusitis and rhinitis are major causes of loss of smell and taste.

PERCEPTUAL ORGANIZATION

Perception arises from the integration of sensory signals into percepts that give meaning to raw data. Perception depends on sensations and experience. An old person has a wealth of experience to draw from when interpreting data, but at times the sensation is incomplete or experience distorts the present reality. When this happens, we may label the person "confused." *Confusion* is a term that is frequently misplaced. It often refers to the nurse as much as the client. When nurses are confused, they need more data. When clients are confused, nurses need to find out the specific source and limits of their data. The terms *confusion* and *disorientation* are sometimes used synonymously, although "confusion" is a catchall diagnosis of unexplained symptoms whereas "disorientation" can be highly specific. For thorough understanding we recommend *Confusion: Prevention and Care* (Wolanin and Phillips, 1981). It is the classic work on this subject. Disorientation and illusions most frequently have an organic base. Hallucinations may be organic or functional in origin.

Disorientation

Thoreau (1946, p. 285) said, "If a man does not keep pace with his companions, perhaps it is because he hears a different drummer." When people are disoriented, they are listening to a different drummer in another time or place, but the beat is uneven and the impulses disquieting. Following their inner drummer brings insecurity and uncertainty. Sensory

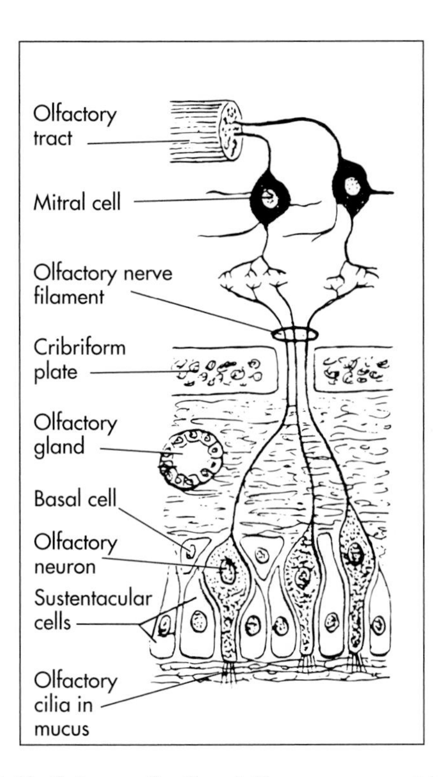

Figure 12-13. Scheme of cell and fiber arrangement in olfactory epithelium. (From *Mosby's medical, nursing, and allied health dictionary,* ed 2, St Louis, 1986, Mosby.)

impressions are confusing and disconnected rather than intermingling in the subtle manner necessary for integration and accurate perception.

Perception of Time. The first level of disorientation to emerge is often related to timing of events. Being unclear about time measurement puts one out of step with the world at large and subject to an altered sense of linear time. Time orientation is evidence of a personal organization and structure and is somewhat more subjective in the old than in the young. It is the first level of individual awareness to be distorted by stressful circumstances, monotonous environments, or altered awareness. Illness, loss, and crises are frequently accompanied by an expanded, contracted, or muted sense of time passage. Keeping track of time requires attention, devices, and interest; all of these are easily diverted by biologic, psychologic, and sociologic disruption. When stress is severe enough, personal time may remain out of synchronization with the world of clocks and dates or become totally submerged. Widows often move in slow motion for several weeks after the spouse's death. People in these major crises are preoccupied and experience sensory distortion. This kind of reaction has important implications for caregivers. When the world is perceived as threatening and chaotic, we must attempt to move slowly and patiently to restore order.

Elderly persons in monotonous environments who lack contrasting events and experiences that mark progression in most peoples' lives eventually lose interest and pay little attention to the flow of time. Organic impairment most often produces disorientation toward recent events such as whether the last meal was lunch or breakfast. It is difficult for the individual with physiologic disturbance in cerebral function to focus attention or to remember events.

In these situations our interventions are aimed toward capturing the elderly person's attention by direct, personalized communication and through provision of cues in the form of cards, name tags, calendars, clocks, reality boards, and schedules. Daily living patterns should remain as constant as possible. Meaningful stimulating events introduced into a consistent supportive atmosphere may produce improved client affect and function.

Some clients experience time disorientation of multiple origins: organic impairment, personal crises and loss, and colorless and boring environment. These are the clients whose time sense is likely to be most profoundly impaired.

Perception of Place. The second level of orientation is interrupted when a person is uncertain of territory. At this time we will explore the internal perception of placement. Distortion of perception relating to one's place usually occurs following translocation. It seems as if one's subconscious lends itself toward establishing security. An individual will perceive characteristics in the environment that relate to previous life experiences; for example, "Did you hear that ringing? It must be the trolley going by," or "What kind of hotel is this? I can't find the bar." Misconceptions of the environment are intensified by poor lighting, intercoms, and room transfers.

Frequently an individual is disoriented toward time and place; most often the aged slip into the security of the familiar past; for example, "I heard the clattering pans and thought Mother would call me for breakfast any minute." The nurse who responds with, "Mr. Jones, this is a hospital and it will soon be lunchtime," is listening and assessing on a most superficial level. It would be far more useful to sit with the client for a few moments, ask about his remembrance of breakfast when he was a child, note the strange noises that disturb one's rest in the hospital, and ask if the client may have been dreaming about a time that was more comfortable and secure.

The nurse will recognize themes of dependence, fears, unfamiliar expectations, and pain. All these commonly expected reactions to illness and hospitalization may be exacerbated by medications, lying in bed (alters perceptions), and slipping from waking to dozing state and states of reverie. If the client consistently insists that he or she is not in the place he or she should be or repeatedly calls for someone who is not there, interventions aimed toward increasing security and orientation may be helpful.

1. Gear activity to client level and reduce or increase stimulation toward a more normal range because either extreme will increase psychologic stress and the need to hold onto delusion.

2. See the client frequently, introduce yourself each time, and explain what you would like to do.
3. Obtain some objects that provide comfort or familiarity; for example, pictures or sentimental objects. If the client has no family, find out comfort routines; for example, a glass of warm water with lemon before breakfast, a spread carefully folded on the foot of the bed, or a particular brand of toothpaste or denture cleanser on the nightstand. In long-term care situations it is imperative to alter the environment toward personalization.

Perception of Person. The third level of disorientation is to person and often is closely tied to confusion about one's whereabouts. A patient who believes he or she is at home may expect a family member to enter the room. Often health care personnel resemble a significant person in a client's past and are believed to be that person. Sometimes it is not disorientation but rather longing that precipitates identity confusion. One aged man wandered the halls of a nursing home calling his wife's name toward the backs of departing female patients. This phenomenon is not limited to the old. Younger people also sometimes imagine they see a dead loved one.

Disorientation regarding one's identity is the most profound insecurity. Even stuporous patients will usually give some response to their own name. Standing very close to a comatose patient, holding the hand firmly but gently, and calling the patient by name close to his or her ear may bring a flicker of recognition.

Disorientation Resulting from Traumatic Treatments. It is common to encounter patients who have transient periods of disorientation related to abrupt or massive interference with body integrity. Cardiac surgery can be a precipitant of disorientation and hallucinatory experiences. Cataract surgery in the past was considered a threat to orientation because of sensory deprivation resulting from eye patches and the general stress of hospitalization, medications, and surgery. With the rapidity of same-day surgery and home recovery, this problem is now seldom seen.

Perception of Space. In old age certain changes occur in total body awareness (proprioception) that affect one's sensorium. Reaction time increases and movement decreases steadily after 20 years of age. Psychomotor slowing seems to be related to four central nervous system processing factors: (1) functional neuron loss reduces signal strength and processing capacity, (2) an increase in random neural activity creates "noise" interference in processing, (3) reconstitution after neural activity takes longer, and (4) arousal levels are diminished. Some people find natural ways to stimulate vestibular function and movement integration. Perhaps old people rock frequently in response to a subliminal need for body movement.

When a patient has been bedridden for some time, it is important for the nurse to alert the patient to unfamiliar environmental sensations and support the patient as he or she regains upright bearings. The patient is in fact seeking navigational bearings to reorient himself or herself, just as a sailor develops sea legs and must adapt to the feel of the land again. An old person is particularly vulnerable to this disorientation because the sensory/spatial body systems do not reintegrate as quickly as in youth. Both physical support and psychologic support are necessary as older persons regain strength and movement.

Touch Sensitivity. A significant amount of vestibular stimulation, information, and sensual gratification come about through touching. Touch is used for awareness and protective responses. Touch intensifies bonding and defines boundaries of self. Those who have visual and hearing impairment often compensate by cultivating the sense of touch to a high degree. Touch is often lacking in the older person's environment, which can contribute to a diminishing sensorium (Wharton, 2000).

Little research has been done on the sense of touch. Although it varies in individuals, it is believed that it diminishes with aging (Wharton, 2000). Many of the losses of this sensitivity are due to disease processes; for example, diabetes mellitus causes peripheral neuropathy and the loss of light touch in the extremities. Loss of sensitivity to hot and cold, or thermal sensitivity, predisposes the elder to burns and hyperthermia and frostbite and hypothermia.

Degenerative changes in Meissner's corpuscles on the hand and foot result in diminished sensitivity of the palms and soles (not on hairy areas) (Wharton, 2000). This may cause a decrease in reaction time when stepping on a sharp object or touching the burner on the stove. Less obvious is the deprivation of tactile senses. Introducing texture, for example, textured upholstery and very soft blankets, into the elder's environment can enhance tactile input and contribute to safety.

Nursing to Integrate Sensory Stimuli

Throughout this chapter we have examined the aged person's communication with the environment through the senses and perceptual organizational processes. These factors are fundamental to the maintenance of safety and security. When in disorder, these limitations hinder one's ability to obtain what is needed from the environment. Many of the aged rely on devices to assist them in this process. Those most frequently used to facilitate environmental contact are hearing aids, spectacles, wheelchairs, dentures, canes, and crutches. The nurse's presence in the environment provides a lighthouse to those running aground in their perceptual storms. Here our goal has been to increase the nurse's understanding of how one may assist an aged person to effectively negotiate and make meaning of the personal environment, using all capacities to an optimum level.

Human Needs and Wellness Diagnoses

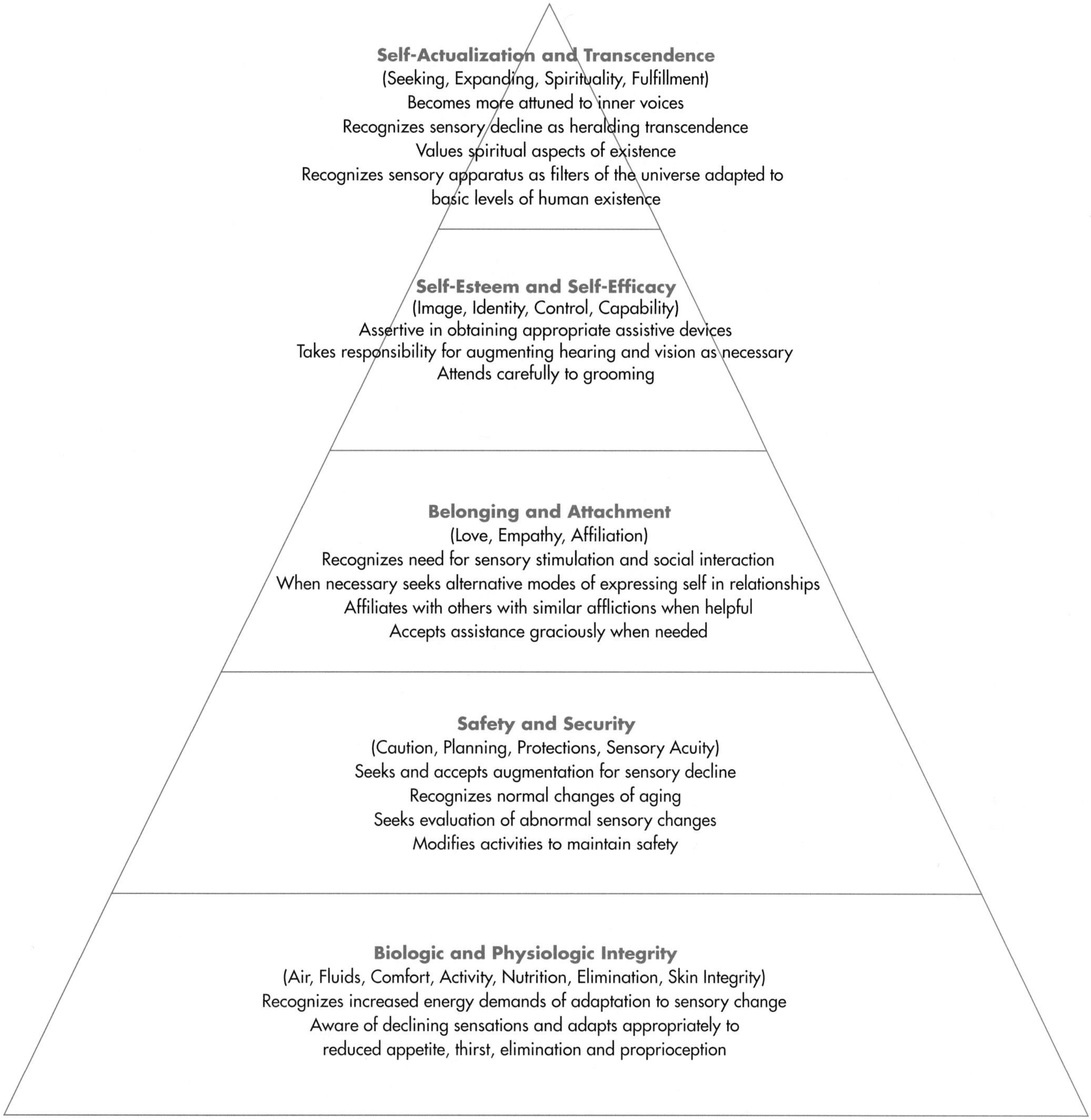

Self-Actualization and Transcendence
(Seeking, Expanding, Spirituality, Fulfillment)
Becomes more attuned to inner voices
Recognizes sensory decline as heralding transcendence
Values spiritual aspects of existence
Recognizes sensory apparatus as filters of the universe adapted to basic levels of human existence

Self-Esteem and Self-Efficacy
(Image, Identity, Control, Capability)
Assertive in obtaining appropriate assistive devices
Takes responsibility for augmenting hearing and vision as necessary
Attends carefully to grooming

Belonging and Attachment
(Love, Empathy, Affiliation)
Recognizes need for sensory stimulation and social interaction
When necessary seeks alternative modes of expressing self in relationships
Affiliates with others with similar afflictions when helpful
Accepts assistance graciously when needed

Safety and Security
(Caution, Planning, Protections, Sensory Acuity)
Seeks and accepts augmentation for sensory decline
Recognizes normal changes of aging
Seeks evaluation of abnormal sensory changes
Modifies activities to maintain safety

Biologic and Physiologic Integrity
(Air, Fluids, Comfort, Activity, Nutrition, Elimination, Skin Integrity)
Recognizes increased energy demands of adaptation to sensory change
Aware of declining sensations and adapts appropriately to reduced appetite, thirst, elimination and proprioception

These are not all the possible wellness diagnoses that may be identified. The above are examples of nursing diagnoses that should be considered when planning care for the older adult.

KEY CONCEPTS

- The sensory apparatus all lose some degree of acuity in the aging process; hearing is the most prevalent loss.
- The importance of cerumen removal is frequently overlooked and often greatly improves hearing.
- Those with hearing impairment often find it difficult to adapt to hearing aids. If they have not recently been to a certified audiologist they should do so. Many improvements have recently been made, and a proper assessment is essential in order to obtain a recommendation for the most appropriate hearing aid.
- The loss of vision is greatly feared by many elders. However, vision impairment is only one third as common as hearing loss, and total loss of vision is rare and due to pathologic processes rather than aging per se.
- When working with the visually impaired, announcing your presence and vivid, detailed descriptions of surroundings are usually greatly appreciated.
- Some believe that the "sundowner's" confusion is magnified by sensory impairment and that all experiences of confusion and illusion are magnified by sensory losses.
- Many stimuli in the environment are not perceived within the narrow parameters of the human sensory equipment. Therefore we may sometimes "sense" things that are not clearly discerned by the senses. Some of these may be labeled intuition, paranormal phenomena, or extrasensory perception. These would be an area of fruitful investigation with the aged.
- Environments and environmental changes have major effects on the sensory input available to elders.
- Environmental sensory deprivation may have seriously disorienting consequences for the elderly.
- Sensory overload when individuals are physically depleted by illness may cause behavioral disturbances and great anxiety. Maintaining a quiet and peaceful environment allows for the use of healing energies toward recovery.

▲ CASE STUDY

Sonya is a 66-year-old high school nurse/consultant. She retired from the Army Nurse Corps with an officer's rank after having served 20 years, much of it in the Korean conflict with heavy exposure to shelling in the early part of her career. She became aware of hearing loss at about age 45, and by age 55 it had become severe. While in the service she had considerable assistance from noncommissioned personnel and functioned very well. When she entered civilian life, it became more difficult for her to manage, but she was unwilling to admit to others her major hearing deficit. During those years she simply attempted to cover it as much as possible, and some of her co-workers felt she was rather obtuse—others suspected her deafness. When she took the position with the school district, she was involved with three high schools, numerous faculty, and students, and interpersonal communication was a major aspect of her position. When she was evaluated at the end of the first year, it was pointed out that feedback indicated she was inattentive. She did then admit her hearing problem and was advised to get hearing aids. She said, "I've known several people over the years that have hearing aids, and none of them were really satisfied with them. I guess that is why I have not gotten them before now." She complied but, after a few weeks, rarely wore them. The personnel officer of the school board, after hearing several more complaints of inappropriate communication, told her she must wear the hearing aids if she wished to continue in her position. Sonya knew that hearing aids were essential, not only for communication but for safety—she had almost been hit by a car while walking because she simply didn't hear it coming. Yet she didn't want to go back to the audiology clinic, because they didn't seem to know what they were doing, and each time she saw someone they gave her different information. She tried three different types of aids that seemed of little help. She lost confidence in her ear, nose, and throat specialist because he had been unable to help her resolve the ringing in her ears. Now her school district had contracted with a health maintenance organization, and she wasn't even sure which health care provider she should see.

Based on the case study, develop a nursing care plan using the following procedure:*

List comments of client that provides subjective data.

List information that provides objective data.

From these data identify and state, using accepted format, two nursing diagnoses you determine are most significant to this client at this time. List two client strengths that you have identified from data.

Determine and state outcome criteria for each diagnosis. These must reflect some alleviation of the problem identified in the nursing diagnosis and must be stated in concrete and measurable terms.

Plan and state one or more interventions for each diagnosed problem. Provide specific documentation of source used to determine appropriate intervention. Plan at least one intervention that incorporates the client's existing strengths.

Evaluate success of intervention. Interventions must correlate directly with the stated outcome criteria in order to measure the outcome success.

STUDY QUESTIONS/ACTIVITIES

What are some of the possible reasons Sonya suffered severe hearing loss at so young an age?

Discuss the stigma of hearing loss and hearing aids.

---

*Students are advised to refer to their nursing diagnosis text and identify possible or potential problems.

Obtain a "hearing aid loaner." Instruct students to wear it for several hours and report their reactions in writing. List difficulties experienced.

How would you advise Sonya if you were her nurse/friend?

Discuss the various kinds of hearing aids and how they differ.

Discuss reasons why Sonya may have discontinued wearing her hearing aids.

What might you suggest that would be helpful in adapting to the wearing of a hearing aid?

What are some of the options you would discuss with Sonya?

Which of the various sensory/perceptual changes of aging would you find most difficult to cope with?

Discuss the meanings and the thoughts triggered by the student's and elder's viewpoints expressed at the beginning of the chapter. How do these vary from your own experience?

RESEARCH QUESTIONS

How frequently is cost a factor that prohibits elders from the use of eyeglasses or hearing aids?

Does participation in simulated experiences of sensory loss change a provider's attitudes toward these losses in the aged?

What environmental hazards are most detrimental to hearing?

What percentage of older individuals are troubled by tinnitus (ringing or other internally generated sounds)?

What methods are most effective for reducing the interference of tinnitus?

Which sensory losses are elders most aware of experiencing?

Do aged individuals who grew up in urban/industrial cities experience sensory losses earlier in their life span than those individuals from a more pastoral environment?

Are there distinct cohort differences in the types and degrees of sensory loss older individuals experience?

How many elders are aware of the specific sensory/perceptual changes that occur with the use of certain medications?

What assistance is most commonly sought for hearing impairment and tinnitus, and is satisfaction obtained?

REFERENCES

All About Vision: Slow or prevent vision loss for AMD, 2001. Available at *www.allaboutvision.com*

American Academy of Ophthalmology: *Initial study results indicate that medicine or surgery may be equally effective treatments for newly diagnosed open-angle glaucoma,* 2001. Available at *www.aao.org/aaoweb1*

American Tinnitus Association: *Information about tinnitus,* Portland, OR, 2002, American Tinnitus Association.

Beck D, Roe-Beck B: Hearing loss. In *Merck manual of geriatrics,* 2000. Available *at www.merck.com*

Beers MH, Berkow R: The Merck manual of geriatrics, ed 3, Whitehouse Station, NJ, 2000, Merck Research Laboratories.

Burke MM, Laramie JA: *Primary care of the older adult: a multidisciplinary approach,* St Louis, 2000, Mosby.

Centers for Medicare and Medicaid Services: *Medicare and you 2002,* pub no HCMS-10050, Baltimore, Sept 2001, U.S. Department of Health and Human Services.

Coley M: Older driver relicensing laws: the state of the states, *Public Policy and Aging Report* 11(4):3, Summer 2001.

Cotter VT, Strumpf N: *Advanced practice nursing with older adults,* New York, 2002, McGraw-Hill.

Demers K: Hearing screening: try this, *Hartford Institute for Geriatric Nursing,* no 12, July 2001. Available at *www.hartfordign.org*

Desai M et al: *Trends in vision and hearing among older Americans. Aging trends no 2,* Hyattsville, MD, 2001, Centers for Disease Control and Prevention, U.S. Department of Health and Human Services.

Dinces EA: Tinnitus. *Up-to-date,* 2001. Available at *www.uptodate.com*

Healthy people 2010: vision and hearing, 2002. Available at *www.health.gov/healthypeople/document/html./volume2/28vision.htm*

Keller H: *The story of my life,* Garden City, NY, 1902, Doubleday.

Kennedy-Malone L, Fletcher K, Plank LM: *Management guidelines for gerontological nurse practitioners,* Philadelphia, 2000, FA Davis.

Kidd PS, Robinson DL: *Family nurse practitioner certification review,* St Louis, 1999, Mosby.

Lighthouse International: Macular degeneration, 1999. Available at *www.lighthouse.org*

Luggen AS: Sensory problems. In Luggen A, Meiner S, editors: *NGNA core curriculum for gerontological nursing,* ed 2, St Louis, 2001, Mosby.

Maas ML et al: *Nursing care of older adults: diagnoses, outcomes, and interventions,* St Louis, 2001, Mosby.

O'Neill PA: *Caring for the older adult: a health promotion perspective,* Philadelphia, 2002, WB Saunders.

Palmisano P, Hynes M, Mueller L: *Glaucoma and race: a case for screening in Connecticut,* 2001, Connecticut State Medical Society. Available at *www.medem.com*

Reuben D et al: *Geriatrics at your fingertips,* New York, 2002, Blackwell.

Sacks O: *Seeing voices: a journey into the world of the deaf,* Berkeley, 1989, University of California Press.

Selye H: *The stress of life,* New York, 1956, McGraw-Hill.

Springhouse: *Signs and symptoms,* ed 3, Springhouse, PA, 2001, Springhouse.

Thoreau HD: *Walden XVIII, conclusion,* New York, 1946, Dodd, Mead.

Tumosa N: Aging and the eye. In The Merck manual of geriatrics online, 2001. Available at *www.merck.com/pubs/mm_geriatrics*

Wharton MA: Environmental design: accommodating sensory changes in the elderly. In Guccione AA, editor: *Geriatric physical therapy,* ed 2, St Louis, 2000, Mosby.

Wolanin MO, Phillips LRF: *Confusion: prevention and care,* St Louis, 1981, Mosby.

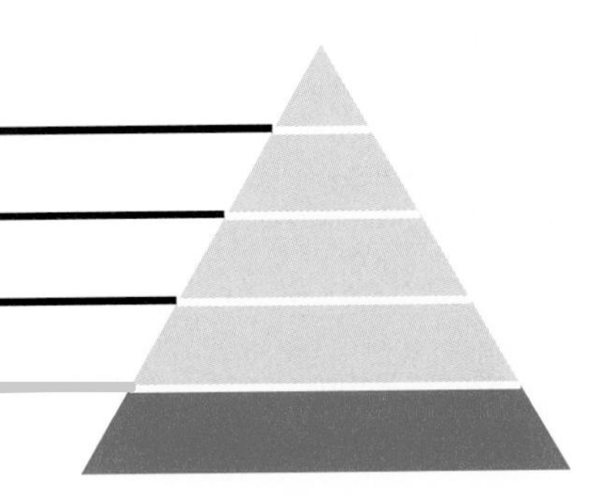

CHAPTER 13

Mobility

Ann Schmidt Luggen
Catherine Hill

A student speculates

The thought of needing someone to help me shower and dress and transfer me from a chair to bed requires more acceptance than I have ever had to muster. I'm very good at making the best out of a bad situation, but somehow adapting to something like never walking again cannot be equated with a "bad situation." It is permanent, and it is the sacrifice of my precious independence. I was born on Independence Day! Thinking about these things overwhelms me with sadness.

Holiday, age 22

An elder speaks

I hate to have the family see me like this. You know, I was a military man. I took pride in the way I marched . . . or just stood at attention. I never imagined a time when I wouldn't be able to walk without assistance.

Jerry, age 78

LEARNING OBJECTIVES

On completion of this chapter, the reader will be able to:

1. Describe age-related changes in bones, joints, and muscles that may predispose the individual to falls and accidents.
2. Discuss the effects of impaired mobility on general function and quality of life.
3. Discuss risk factors for impaired mobility.
4. Discuss factors that increase vulnerability to falls.
5. Describe the effects of restraints and alternative measures of protection.
6. Describe assessment measures to determine gait and walking stability.
7. Enumerate several measures to prevent falls and identify those at high risk.
8. Develop a nursing care plan appropriate to an elder at risk of falling.
9. Consider the impact of available transportation and driving in relation to independence.

Mobility is the capacity one has for movement within the personally available microcosm and macrocosm. In infancy moving about is the major mode of learning and interacting with the environment. In old age one moves more slowly and purposefully, sometimes with more forethought and caution. Throughout life, movement remains a significant means of personal contact, sensation, exploration, pleasure, and control. Movement is integral to the attainment of all levels of need as conceived by Maslow. Needs identified by elders include pride, maintaining dignity, social contacts, and activity (Wright and Aizenstein, 1993). All of these are facilitated by mobility. Thus, in terms of Maslow's hierarchy and the needs identified by elders, maintaining mobility is an exceedingly important issue.

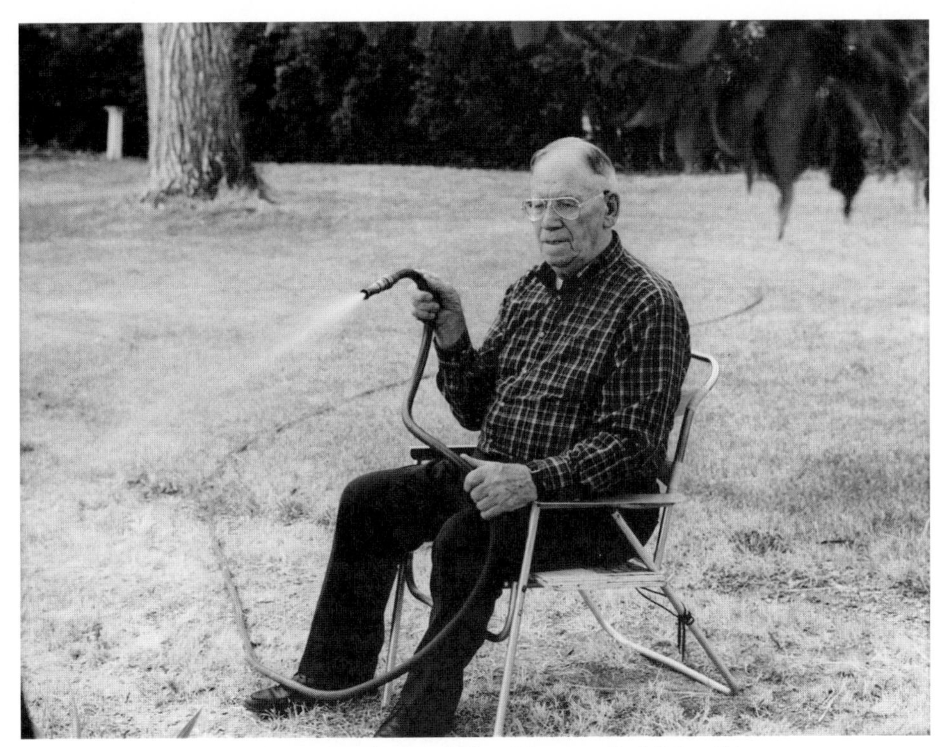

Adapting to impaired mobility. (Courtesy Rod Schmall.)

This chapter focuses on maintaining maximum mobility in health and in the presence of various disorders, the assessment of gait and mobility status, the effects of restraints and immobility, risk factors related to falls and preventive actions that nurses may take to reduce the risks, and aids and interventions that are useful when mobility is impaired. Also included are transportation and driving as essential aspects of environmental mobility.

Mobility and comparative degrees of agility are based on muscle strength, flexibility, postural stability, vibratory sensation, cognition, and perceptions of stability. Aging produces changes in muscles and joints, particularly of the back and legs. Strength and flexibility of muscles decrease markedly; endurance decreases to a somewhat lesser extent, especially if there is a diminution of activity as one ages. Movements and range of motion become more limited. Normal wear and tear reduces the smooth cartilage of joints. Movement is less fluid as one ages, and joints change as regeneration of tissue slows and muscle wasting occurs. Some normal gait changes in late life include a narrower standing base, wider swaying when standing, slowed responses, a greater reliance on proprioception, diminished arm swing, and increased care in gait. Steps are shorter and with a decreased stepping motion. These changes are less pronounced in those who remain active and at a desirable weight.

Inappropriate clothing may hinder mobility. Fitted, back-closing, or knee-length clothing is not comfortable for persons confined to wheelchairs, those with limited range of motion, or those who require catheters or prosthetic devices. Elders living alone have no one to help them button or zip the back of clothing. This can make dressing and undressing a time-consuming and frustrating experience. Adaptive fashions have been designed to facilitate easy or independent dressing and include features such as back and side openings, Velcro front openings, raglan sleeves, and cape-styled clothing. Slacks, with front flaps or extra room in back, or longer skirts are helpful. The fabric should be chosen for comfort, durability, attractiveness, and ease of laundering. Other items to facilitate moving about include wheelchair bags, catheter bags, and carefully chosen footwear.

Various degrees of immobility are often the temporary or permanent consequences of illness. On a broader scale, elders frequently have limited environmental mobility because of lack of transportation or loss of driver's license. On the most personal level, some elderly are immobilized by the fear of falling. In summary, many normal and abnormal changes affect the fluidity and comfort of movement and the capacity for involvement with surroundings. Limitations in mobility for whatever cause have serious consequences.

DISORDERS AFFECTING MOBILITY

Common conditions that accompany the normal changes of aging, as well as disorders that occur more frequently in the elderly, merit special attention. Such disorders or orthopedic impairments significantly impede the aged. Osteoporosis, gait disorders, Parkinson's disease, accidents, and fear of falling must be considered. Rheumatoid arthritis, osteoarthritis, and osteoporosis markedly affect movement and functional capacities. Mobility may be limited by paresthesias; hemiplegia; neuromotor disturbances; fractures; foot, knee, and hip problems; and illnesses that deplete one's energy. All of these conditions are likely to occur more frequently and have more devastating effects as one ages. Many elders in later years have some of these afflictions, with women significantly outnumbering men in this respect. There may be some difficulty among elderly men and women in accomplishing mobility-related tasks (Table 13-1).

Falls

The incidence of falling increases with age (Centers for Disease Control and Prevention [CDC], 1999). In the community

Table 13-1 Percentage of Women Reporting Difficulty in Mobility-Related Tasks and Level of Difficulty Reported[a,b]

		Age group			Disability level	ADL difficulty	
Task and level of difficulty	Total (N = 1002)	65-74 (N = 388)	75-84 (N = 311)	85+ (N = 303)	Moderate[c] (N = 343)	Receives no help (N = 478)	Receives help (N = 181)
Stooping, crouching, or kneeling[d]	82.6	84.5	82.1	78.1	68.2	89.5	93.1
Level of difficulty[e,f]							
A little	10.3	11.7	9.8	7.5	14.4	8.4	7.1
Some	14.0	17.3	12.3	8.9	16.6	15.2	5.2
A lot	20.7	23.9	20.4	11.8	16.0	25.2	17.6
Unable to do	37.5	31.6	39.6	49.4	20.9	40.7	63.2
Doing heavy housework such as washing windows, walls, or floors[g]	81.6	80.4	82.8	82.0	77.1	79.7	96.4
Level of difficulty[e,f]							
A little	6.4	8.4	5.5	2.7	10.5	5.4	0.7
Some	9.2	11.5	8.5	4.0	11.0	10.1	2.7
A lot	11.1	15.6	8.5	4.6	15.7	10.4	3.5
Unable to do	54.8	44.6	60.3	70.1	39.9	53.7	89.0
Walking for a quarter of a mile, that is, about 2 or 3 blocks[h]	74.4	69.7	76.5	82.4	66.0	75.4	89.0
Level of difficulty[e,f]							
A little	13.7	12.9	16.4	9.1	20.0	12.5	4.2
Some	14.8	14.8	16.3	11.1	17.5	13.9	11.8
A lot	19.1	20.7	19.6	13.3	17.2	22.6	13.6
Unable to do	26.3	21.0	24.3	47.4	11.2	25.9	58.8
Walking up 10 steps without resting[h]	51.9	49.3	53.3	55.3	37.2	53.5	77.6
Level of difficulty[e,f]							
A little	8.4	6.6	10.8	7.2	8.9	9.2	5.2
Some	15.0	17.4	13.7	11.7	14.8	15.4	14.3
A lot	15.1	16.6	13.8	14.4	9.4	17.1	21.4
Unable to do	13.2	8.8	15.1	21.5	4.1	11.6	36.7
Walking across a small room[d]	25.5	19.4	25.2	44.1	7.2	26.6	60.0
Level of difficulty[e,f]							
A little	4.4	2.5	4.4	9.8	3.0	5.1	5.3
Some	8.4	6.2	8.5	14.8	3.3	10.6	13.1
A lot	5.4	4.8	4.7	9.3	0.9	5.7	14.0
Unable to do	7.0	5.6	7.6	9.4	0.1	4.8	27.2

Women's Health and Aging Study, screening and baseline interviews, 1992-1995. From Guralnik JM et al: *The Women's Health and Aging Study: health and social characteristics of older women with disability*, NIH pub no 95-4009, Bethesda, MD, 1995, National Institute on Aging.

[a]All variables have less than 2% missing data. Results are based on nonmissing data.

[b]Descriptive statistics are based on weighted data.

[c]No ADL difficulty; disabled in two or more domains.

[d]The question is in the form "By yourself, that is, without help from another person or special equipment, do you have any difficulty . . .?"

[e]How much difficulty do you have?

[f]The percentages of participants reporting their levels of difficulty may not add up to the percentage reporting difficulty due to (1) rounding and (2) level of difficulty not reported.

[g]The screener question is the form "Because of a health or physical problem, do you have any difficulty . . .?" The presence of the condition was confirmed in the baseline interview.

[h]The screener question is in the form "By yourself, that is, without help from another person or special equipment, do you have any difficulty . . .?" The presence of the condition was confirmed in the baseline interview.

setting, more than 30% of elders fall at least once every year and 50% fall repeatedly (Coleman and Fox, 2002). For those elders between 65 and 84, falls are the second leading cause of injury-related death and are the leading cause in elders older than 84. There is also a significant morbidity associated with falls. Many elders fall and are taken to the emergency department from home or long-term care settings. Hospitalization is common, and the stay may be prolonged. More than 90% of hip fractures are related to falls (Mahoney, 1998), but other injuries occur as well. These include injury to soft tissue, dislocated joints, and subdural hematomas, to name a few.

Causes or risk factors for falling are multifactorial and include increasing age, weakness, limitations in function, hazards in the home or community environment, psychoactive medications, and a history of falls (CDC, 1999). Several years ago the CDC made falls a central focus of attention and produced *Check for Safety,* a home fall prevention checklist for older adults (CDC, 1999).

FALLS: CAUSES AND CONSEQUENCES

Falling is one of the most serious and frequent problems associated with the aging process. Falls are a symptom of a problem, although they become the focus of the problem when they occur. Because falls may indicate neurologic, sensory, cognitive, medication, or musculoskeletal problems, it is important for nurses to evaluate each older client's biopsychosocial vulnerability to falling (Table 13-2). Intrinsic changes in the capacities of the aged (see Chapter 15 for a discussion of frailty), disease processes, psychologic factors, and extrinsic factors all contribute to a greater vulnerability to falls as one ages.

The CDC (1999) estimates that each year one third of all persons age 65 and older who live at home fall, and about half of those fall repeatedly. Falls and the consequent broken hips cause 40% of nursing home admissions annually, according to the NIA. Up to 20% of hospitalized patients and 45% of those in long-term care facilities will fall. Fall-related mortality rate increases with advanced age, and death rates of elders 65 years and older are 10 to 150 times greater than those of younger age-groups (Tideiksaar, 1998). The problem is particularly prevalent in the very old and is the leading cause of accidental death in men and women over 85.

Factors Contributing to Falls

Falls are generally classified as extrinsic (related to environment), intrinsic (related to host factors), or iatrogenic (related to treatment factors). After age 65 individuals fall most frequently because of external reasons; however, with increasing age, internal and locomotor reasons become increasingly prevalent. Fall risk factors that increase proportionally as one ages are disturbances in visual acuity, postural hypotension, and cardiac arrhythmias. Declines in depth perception, proprioception, vibratory sense, and normotensive response to postural changes are important factors, although the

Table 13-2 Fall Factors

Psychogenic	Physiologic	Environmental
Dementia Alterations in gait and vitamin B_{12} level; poor evaluation of ability and environment Depression Disinterest in surroundings, no concern for safety, subliminal suicide Fear/anxiety Distraction, scattered perceptions	Neurologic Dementias Somnolence Normal pressure hydrocephalus Neurosensory and visual deficits: loss of proprioception; peripheral neuropathy; vestibular dysfunction; dizziness; vertigo; syncope; seizures, brain tumors, or lesions; Parkinson's disease; cervical spondylosis Cardiovascular disorders Cerebrovascular insufficiency, strokes and TIAs, carotid sinus syncope, vertebral artery insufficiency Arrhythmias: Stokes-Adams Valvulopathies Congestive heart failure Hypotension: postural hypotension, postprandial drop in blood pressure, medication induced, male micturition when urethral obstruction present, hypovolemia (dehydration, hemorrhage), impaired venous return (venous pooling, valsalva), impaired vasoconstriction (autonomic disorders, vasovagal) Metabolic disorders: anemia, hypoxia, hypoglycemia, hyperventilation Debilitating disease: cancer, pulmonary disease, immunosuppressant disorder	Slippery floor: urine or fluid on the floor, loose throw rugs Uneven and obstructed walking surfaces: electrical cords, furniture, pets, children, uneven door steps or stair risers, loose boards, cracked sidewalks Inadequate visual supports: glaring; low wattage bulbs; lack of night-lights for bathroom, stairs, and halls; poor marking of steps and other hazards Inadequate construction: absence of railing, lack of grab bars on shower or tub, poorly designed stairs and walkways

majority of falls occur in individuals with multiple medical problems (Tideiksaar, 1998).

In long-term care facilities the most prevalent causes of falling are stroke, parkinsonism, blindness, drug-related hypotension, and arthritis. Those who fall more often are women, more functionally impaired, and taking more medications.

Vision Problems. Sudden unexpected visual problems become major fall risks; visual changes may be transient, a symptom of other problems such as hypotension, cardiac arrhythmia, temporal arteritis, or vertebrobasilar artery insufficiency. Additionally, new glasses or recent cataract surgery may be impediments. The more gradual and progressive visual changes become serious fall risks when they interfere with depth perception.

Balance Problems. Vertigo and dizziness are the result of dysfunction in balance control systems and vestibular apparatus. Benign positional vertigo is the most common form experienced by the elderly. Ear infection and head trauma are common precipitants. Labyrinthitis is an infectious or toxic process that results in dizziness and gait ataxia. Drug toxicity causes tinnitus and hearing loss, which may become permanent. Treatment of the infection, discontinuation of the drug, or removal of cerumen impaction often resolves the problem. Disequilibrium may arise from many disorders, including Parkinson's disease, Alzheimer's disease, peripheral neuropathy caused by pernicious anemia, alcoholism, or diabetes. Patients experience unsteadiness and a tendency to fall. They often need an assistive device for walking and a medication evaluation. Contributing factors are summarized in Box 13-1.

Interruption of Cerebral Oxygenation. Transient ischemic attacks (TIAs) affect the perfusion of the brain and cause intermittent dizziness. It is estimated that up to 25% of falls are due to drop attacks associated with TIAs. The individual may not have a loss of consciousness but will feel as if the legs gave way. Patients subject to these attacks should wear cervical collars to prevent backward flexion of the head.

Syncope, or a brief loss of consciousness caused by cerebral ischemia, has many causes. Vasodepressor syncope typically occurs during emotional upset, injury, excessive fatigue, or prolonged standing in a warm environment. Orthostatic syncope is a compensatory response to rapid rising to a standing position when depletion of body fluids or medications interfere with rapid venous return and dynamic homeostatic responses. Postprandial reductions in blood pressure may also occur sufficiently to produce syncope.

Many elders are susceptible to orthostatic hypotension. Paradoxically, age-related elevations in blood pressure increase the risk of hypotension. Baroreflex responses mediate both hypertension and hypotension, and in old age the efficiency of this function progressively declines; thus the aged are more vulnerable to episodes of cerebral ischemia with rapid changes of posture.

Box 13-1 Fall Risk Factors for Elders

Conditions

Female or single (incidence increases with age)
Sedative and alcohol use, psychoactive medications
Previous falls, unsteadiness, dizziness
Acute and recent illness
Pathologic conditions, drop attacks
Cognitive impairment, disorientation
Disability of lower extremities
Abnormalities of balance and gait
Foot problems
Depression, anxiety
Decreased vision or hearing
Fear of falling
Terminal drop (dies in following year to 2 years)
Skeletal and neuromuscular changes that predispose to weakness and postural imbalance
Acute and severe chronic illness, debilitation
Functional limitations in self-care activities
Women (75 years and older)
Multiple disorders and medications
Wheelchair-bound
Sensory deficits
Impaired locomotion
Predisposing physiologic and psychologic conditions
Preoccupation with stressors
Anxiety related to previous falls
Confusion, dementia

Situations

Urinary urgency, particularly nocturia
Environmental hazards
Recent relocation
Assistive devices needed for walking
Inadequate or missing safety rails, particularly in bathroom
Poorly designed or unstable furniture
Low stools
High chairs and beds
Floor surfaces
Glossy, highly waxed floors
Wet, greasy, icy surfaces
Inadequate lighting
General clutter
Pets that inadvertently trip an individual
Electrical cords
Loose or uneven stair treads
A detailed discussion of these can be found in Chapter 14.

Data from Tinetti et al (1988), Craven and Bruno (1986), Kaufmann (1985), Barbieri (1983), and Fife et al (1984).

Carotid sinus syncope occurs frequently in older people who have sinus node disease. This hypersensitivity to pressure or mechanical obstruction makes the individual vulnerable to syncope when applying pressure to the carotid while shaving, turning the head sharply to one side, or wearing tight collars.

Unusual and rarely mentioned is micturition syncope, which occurs immediately following voiding in some elderly men with bladder outlet obstructions (often prostatic hypertrophy). The loss of consciousness is due to vagal bradycardia. These individuals should sit during urination.

Cardiac arrhythmias are a common cause of syncope, particularly supraventricular tachycardias. Heart monitoring for 24 to 48 hours is often necessary to reveal these bradyarrhythmias or tachyarrhythmias.

Fatigue Factors. Postural training for individuals has many benefits. Few individuals realize that fatigue may result from, or be more pronounced because of, poor posture. In addition, poor posture contributes to the incidence of falls. Physiotherapists should be engaged to teach nurses and clients correct postural habits.

Fear of Falling. Fear of falling may actually be a more pervasive problem than falling, and the fear that becomes obsessional can become detrimental and limiting. Fear can result in avoidance phobias that continually and gradually restrict the environment until one is confined to bed. Fear of falling is an important predictor of general functional decline.

Mr. W was a sprightly 83-year-old widower, the son of an immigrant laundry worker. He had lived in San Francisco's Chinatown all his life. He hurried about in the crowded area and bartered with the market vendors for his fresh vegetables and other needs. He tripped and fell one day for no known reason and suffered shoulder contusions and a mild concussion. After an examination and thorough radiographic studies, he was released from the emergency department with the physician's warning, "Be careful, you are an old man." Gradually Mr. W began to believe this and slowed his pace, carefully watching the ground to see that there was nothing to trip him. He began to shuffle rather than walk. All of this was so gradual that it was a year before his family realized he was not leaving his room very often. In deference and respect they did not interfere until during a surprise visit they discovered he had no food in his flat, dirty clothes were heaped about, and it appeared that he rarely left his bed. He had obeyed the physician.

Tinetti (1989) studied 300 community-residing people over age 65 to determine their fall propensity and frequency. A quarter of the people who fell restricted their activities following the fall. The fear of falling became a psychosocial impediment, even limiting performance of activities of daily living (ADLs). Tinetti and colleagues (1990) developed the Falls Efficacy Scale (FES), an instrument to measure fear of falling based on self-perceived ability to avoid falls during normal nonhazardous ADLs. It was found that anxiety, depression, and slowed walking pace were correlates of the fear of falling. The FES proved useful in predicting functional decline based on limitations induced by fear. Health care providers thought that getting dressed, getting on and off the toilet, preparing meals, and taking baths or showers were the most demanding activities. Elderly individuals named activities they most avoided because of fear of falling as reaching into cabinets or closets, taking a bath or shower, walking around the house, and getting in and out of bed. These data may be useful because home health nurses may assess these particular activities and suggest ways the individual can alter activities and feel more secure.

There is a correlation between fear of falling and actual falls. Individuals tend to stiffen their posture when afraid of falling, and this actually induces more falls. Postural changes cannot unequivocally be attributed to fear of falling, and therefore the current trend to measure postural sway and one leg stance as evidence of fall potential should be interpreted carefully when used with apprehensive individuals.

Drop Attacks. When an elderly person falls "just because my leg went out from under me," we often call these *drop attacks*. These falls cause hip trochanter cracks or femur fractures, sometimes both. This is thought to be due to osteoporotic bone erosion that accompanies old age and that, in some women with a high-risk profile, reaches pathologic proportions. When osteoporosis of this magnitude occurs, the bone can no longer bear the weight of the individual in walking. It is sometimes difficult to determine whether the fall creates the fracture or the fracture creates the fall. It is of little consequence which precedes the other. In fact, numerous conditions may precipitate a drop attack. Many neurologic disorders may lead to syncope or drop attacks. Seizures, sleep and arousal disorders, vagotonic disorders, and several other central autonomic disorders are sometimes culprits; even psychogenic seizures should be considered. Cerebrovascular disorders account for a high incidence, and some metabolic disorders, such as hypophosphatemia, may cause muscle weakness and periodic paralysis. Regardless of cause, the end result is often immobility, restrictions in movement, institutional living, and all of the physical ailments that tend to follow immobility, especially in very old and frail elders (Box 13-2).

Box 13-2 Types of Falls

1. Slips and trips: The patient may falsely attribute the fall to these causes when in reality it is due to a physical deficit.
2. Falls while attempting a difficult maneuver (such as climbing over a bed rail).
3. Syncope: The loss of consciousness immediately precedes the fall, and may, itself, be preceded by a brief interval of giddiness or unsteadiness.
4. Seizure: The loss of consciousness accompanies the fall. It may be preceded by an aura. It may or may not be accompanied by clonic movements and incontinence.
5. Drop attack: Sudden loss of muscular tone without loss of consciousness.
6. Vertigo: The patient experiences true dizziness (the room seems to spin) and falls to one side or the other.
7. Sliding off furniture: Caused by weakness or somnolence.

From Wieman H, Calkins E: Falls. In Calkins E et al, editors: *The practice of geriatrics*, Philadelphia, 1986, WB Saunders.

In summary, numerous situations and conditions make elderly people susceptible to falls:

- Transient ischemic attacks with vertigo, syncope, or stroke
- Muscle weakness
- Diminution or interference with balance
- Poor eyesight and faulty evaluation of spatial relationships, often resulting from neural deficiencies
- Urinary frequency and urgency leading to unsafe maneuvering at toileting
- Unsteady gait because of pain, fatigue, arthritic changes, or osteoporosis
- Improper footwear or podiatric difficulties
- Improper clothing such as long nightclothes or robes
- Improper use of wheelchairs and walkers, especially on transfer
- Mental confusion and faulty judgment
- Incontinence and dribbling of urine

Assessment. Patients who fall present a complex diagnostic challenge to physicians and nurses. It is helpful to classify a fall in order to better understand the origins, as well as the management. Premonitory falls are those that are secondary to a medical problem, are multifactorial in nature, and are preceded by a symptom. These are subject to treatment. Prodromal falls are those that precede and predict the onset of disease. Extrinsic falls are related to environmental factors. The fall may be accidental or intentional. Isolated falls are those rare occurrences that might be considered "freak" accidents. Cluster falls describe a situation in which an individual falls frequently at a particular time or place.

Any patient with an unexplained fall should have postural pulses and blood pressures taken, a rectal examination for stool guaiac, and a hematocrit. Nursing observations may be essential to establishing an accurate diagnosis. The nurse may be the only professional who has been in the home and seen the elder function in a familiar setting; the nurse may be the one who has knowledge of the elder's usual lifestyle and needs; the nurse is the one most likely to view the elder holistically and to advocate for protection from unnecessary diagnostic testing. Box 13-3 provides assessment information.

Interventions. Environmental (extrinsic) factors require modification for safety. Psychosocial (intrinsic) factors such as confidence and feelings of self-efficacy are seen to reduce the fear of falling (Tinetti et al, 1994). Proprioception and visual acuity contribute markedly to dynamic balance. Therefore any interventions that enhance sensory function and spatial awareness will reduce falls. The aged can adapt well to changes in the environment and reduced sensory input if they occur gradually, although the very old do not. All aged persons should be cautioned against sudden rising from sitting or supine positions, particularly after eating.

As a general principle, any action that increases the individual's confidence and ability to relax is likely to decrease the propensity toward falls. Actions to increase patient safety include:

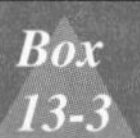

Box 13-3 Assessment of Fall Risk

Obtain history of previous falls and precipitants
Evaluate for orthostatic hypotension (increases with age)
Evaluate visual acuity: peripheral, depth, and color vision
Determine presence of arrhythmias
Massage carotid bulb for carotid sinus sensitivity
Rotation of neck to assess vertebrobasilar artery involvement
Observe movements and evaluate muscle strength and balance:
- Test functional reach (Duncan et al, 1992)
- Rising from chair
- Performing deep knee bend
- Walking 10 feet in a straight line, turning full circle
- Climbing and descending stairs
- Romberg test for increased sway
- Standing on tiptoes and reaching upward
- Bending down to pick up object from floor
- Raising feet while walking; tandem walking

Check feet for abnormalities that affect gait
Evaluate mental status and medication regimen, particularly note psychoactive drugs
Observe ease of routine daily mobility maneuvers
All of these evaluations must be carried out with sufficient support and encouragement to avoid activities threatening to the individual's sense of security or that are potentially dangerous

Data complied from Tideiksaar R: Falls in the elderly: etiology and prevention. In Bosker G et al, editors: *Geriatric emergency medicine*, St Louis, 1990, Mosby; Tinetti M, Speechley M, Ginter S: Risk factors for falls among elderly persons living in the community, *N Engl J Med* 319(26):1701, 1988.

1. Individualize care planning in terms of the patient's level of disorientation.
2. Consistently make efforts to reduce anxiety and uncertainty in new residents. Fear and agitation create clumsiness at any age.
3. Early case finding of the accident-prone individual and concerted efforts by the entire team to minimize unsafe activities and behavior are essential.
4. Review of medications, especially tranquilizers, as to need, dosage, and side effects must be continuous.
5. Adequate staffing, especially at the most dangerous hours, is important.
6. A safe environment, especially for all ambulatory residents, must be maintained.
7. Attempt to deal with confused and agitated individuals through reality therapy, behavior modification, and tender loving care.
8. Residents should be taught the safe use of wheelchairs and walkers.
9. The ambulatory resident should be observed for signs of weakness or fatigue and be assisted as necessary.

10. Continue to gather further information to initiate a program of accident prevention.

The consequences of falls are more serious for old people, and the mortality rate for various types of accidents rises dramatically. To prevent accidents, assess mobility impairments and individual strengths (Box 13-4).

Education regarding hazards may reduce fears of falling. Other suggestions include encouraging the elder to be matter of fact about using a cane or walker to help maintain balance and advising the elder not to hurry to answer phones or doorbells. Haste can be dangerous. Gait training, postural reminders, evaluation of home hazards, and modification of environment have all been effective in reducing fall rates. With training and increased awareness comes a sense of competence and confidence that may obviate the fear of falling.

Risk of Falling

Acute illness is associated with functional impairments that tend to increase the risk of falling. Confusion, generalized weakness, postural instability, and foreign environment are major contributors to falling when hospitalized. Loss of proprioception in the legs because of disuse is also an important factor. Bed rest, understaffing, serious illness, and rapid hospital discharge have contributed to an unknown number of falls. There is an increased vulnerability if the individual has a history of falls, is receiving intravenous therapy, has impaired mental status, or needs assistive devices to walk.

Assessment of the Environment. In the home, look at the floor and the position of furniture (Centers for Disease Control and Prevention, 1999). If you have to walk around furniture, it is hazardous. Look for throw rugs; they may be slippery. Are there objects on the floor, such as shoes, newspapers, books? Keep the floor clear. Look for the cords and wires from lamps and telephones; these should not be in a walking path. Check the stairs for objects, lighting, and the position of the switch at top and bottom of stairs; an electrician can put in a glowing switch in both places so that lighting is not a problem. Make sure the handrails are strong and on both sides of the stairs for going up and going down. Check the carpet to be sure it is firmly attached and not slippery. In the kitchen, see that commonly used objects are not out of reach on high shelves so that a footstool is needed. If a footstool is used, is it steady? Does the elder use a chair for reaching objects placed high? In the bedroom, is the light near the bed and within reach? Is there sufficient light at night to see the way to the bathroom? Is the light sufficient? It should be a minimum of 60 watts. Is the shower floor slippery? Is there a support for getting in and out of the shower or tub and for the toilet?

Other areas of assessment include the amount and the regularity of exercise the elder may participate in each week. Examine the medications taken, including over-the-counter (OTC) drugs. Are there any that may cause drowsiness or dizziness? How often is vision checked? An incorrect glasses prescription can increase the risk of a fall. Watch the elder rise from a chair. Does he or she get up slowly? Examine the elder's shoes; they should not be slippery or have too thick a sole. Doorsills can be painted a different color to prevent tripping, or reflecting tape can be used on the sill or step. Make sure that emergency phone numbers are accessible. Consider an alarm device to wear if the elder is frail or has a number of serious chronic illnesses.

Assessing Balance and Gait. Balance and gait assessment may be the single best predictor of fall risk (Schneider and Mader, 2002). Many studies report that the velocity of walking decreases with age (Howe and Oldham, 2001), and although gait varies widely among elders, often a gait pattern may be seen. The mean stride length of men is 89% of their height when young, and 79% of their height at age 80. Women's stride length also is reduced. Because balance diminishes with increasing age, there is a compensating increase in stride width and angle of the feet. The double stance is the most stable phase of gait, and more time is spent in this phase in elders. The swing phase of gait is a vulnerable time because only one foot is in contact with the ground (Table 13-3).

Balance disorders may result from arthritis, stroke, Parkinson's disease, diabetic neuropathy, cardiac disease, and deconditioning. Elders who have spent much time in bed or at rest can become deconditioned in a very sort time. Balance may be tested in the clinical or home setting. Inability to perform the test indicates increased risk of falling. See Box 13-5 for balance assessment tests.

Box 13-4 Actions to Prevent Falls

Regular testing for vision and hearing; aids if needed; keep glasses clean and ears free of cerumen and infection
Seek evaluation and modification of medications (e.g., diuretics, nitrates, hypnotics, antidepressants, antianxiety agents, antihypertensives, and hypoglycemics) that affect balance, coordination, and cardiovascular sufficiency
Limit alcohol intake
Rise slowly from bed or chair to avoid sudden drop in blood pressure; avoid sudden changes in position
When outdoors watch for wet or slippery surfaces; use extra care getting into and out of vehicles, negotiating curbs and crowds
Ask for assistance when needed
Reduce hazards in home
Stay physically and socially active; increase activities gradually
Wear appropriate footwear; avoid high heels and slippery soles
Use assistive devices for ambulation
Consult with physician if feeling unsteady or ill

Data compiled from Tideiksaar R: Falls in the elderly: etiology and prevention. In Bosker G et al, editors: *Geriatric emergency medicine*, St Louis, 1990, Mosby; Tinetti M, Richman D, Powell L: Falls efficacy as a measure of fear of falling, *J Gerontol* 45(6):239, 1990.

Table 13-3 Gait Changes in Aging

Factor	Aging effect
Velocity	Decreases
Length of step	Decreases
Length of stride	Decreases
Width of stride	Increases
Steps per minute (cadence)	Decreases or changes little
Double stance phase of walking	Increases
Rotation of hip	Increases
Rotation of trunk	Decreases
Ankle movement	Decreases
Toe clearance	Decreases

Adapted from Howe T, Oldham JA: Posture and balance. In Trew M, Everett T, editors: *Human movement,* ed 4, St Louis, 2001, Mosby.

Box 13-5 **Balance Assessment Tests**

1. Get up from an armchair, walk about 10 feet, turn around, walk back to the chair, and sit down (get-up-and-go test). If this can be done in less than 20 seconds and there is no staggering when turning and no need to hold onto something or someone, balance is very good.
2. A variation on the get-up-and-go test is to rise from the armchair without using hands, walk about 10 feet, turn around, walk back to the chair, turn, and sit down (no time frame). Watch for smooth motion, deviation from the walking path, and smooth turns.
3. Put one foot directly in front of the other (heel to toe). Hold position for 30 seconds.
4. Stand on two feet; close eyes. Hold a steady position for 15 seconds.
5. Bend down to pick up an object from the floor; retrieve the object within 5 seconds.
6. Stand with eyes open, placing feet together as closely as possible. For safety, have another person stand behind the elder. Touch or nudge the elder's chest on the sternum with enough gentle force to cause imbalance. The appropriate response is to stretch out one's arms to the front to compensate and possibly take a step backward.

Interventions. If the elder appears unstable, a physical therapy evaluation is a good option. The physical therapist can instruct the elder on strengthening exercises, as well as balance exercises such as tai chi, or prescribe assistive devices with training. Tai chi has been associated with a 25% reduction in falls in one study (Province, 1995).

Gait Disorders

Gait disorders make one vulnerable to tripping and falling. In addition, they impede activity and increase anxiety in the elder who is aware of instability in gait. More than 2.5 million individuals over 65 years of age in the United States (almost 1% of the total population) need assistance to walk. Given the magnitude of this problem, routine examination of the elderly should include not only gait but also postural assessment (Box 13-6). Normal gait involves the vestibular system of balance, proprioception (sensitivity to body in motion), neurophysiologic integrity, and vision.

Box 13-6 **Gait Disorders**

Ataxia
Wide-based gait with-frequent side-stepping

Normal Pressure Hydrocephalus
Step height reduced, shuffling gait as if feet stuck to floor; short steps, unsteady speed, and ataxia

Parkinson's Disease
Stooped posture, short rapid shuffling gait, uncontrollable propulsion or retropulsion, "freeze" walk when feet abruptly halt while body continues to move forward

Spondylotic Cervical Myelopathy
Spastic, shuffling gait, deep tendon reflexes below level of compression increase muscle tone; sometimes nonspecific, e.g., "clumsy feet," "legs gave way"

Senile Gait
Associated with stooped posture, hip and knee flexion, diminished arm swing, stiffness in turning, broad-based, small steps with poor gait intention

Hemiplegia
Poor arm and leg swing, affected limb does not bend at knee; ankle fixed and inverted as leg swings in wide circle; foot tends to drag

Osteomalacia
Ill-defined skeletal pain, pain on weight bearing, unstable waddling gait

Arthritis of the hip, the knee, and especially the foot is a common cause of instability. Arthritis of the knee may result in ligamentous weakness and instability, causing the legs to give way or collapse. Muscle weakness is often experienced in hyperthyroidism and hypothyroidism, hypokalemia, hyperparathyroidism, osteomalacia, and hypophosphatemia, and in some cases it is brought on by various medications. Diabetes, alcoholism, and vitamin B deficiencies may cause neurologic damage and resultant gait problems (Resnick et al, 2001). Vestibular dysfunction causes unsteadiness in walking and listing to one side or the other when the eyes are closed. The individual cannot focus well on a fixed target while moving, or on a moving object while standing still. Some elders experience dizziness, unsteadiness, and light-headedness. Postural instability increases and is exacerbated by some medications. Extrapyramidal symptoms produce a shuffling gait in some individuals taking psychotropic medications and in those who have Parkinson's disease or parkinsonian symptoms. Postural reflex impairment occurs with aging, and postural sway, forward and backward, can be observed when an individual stands still. A cane or supportive device may be essential to provide a sense of security.

Assessment. The get-up-and-go test is a practical assessment tool for elderly people and can be conducted in any setting (Resnick et al, 2001). The client is asked to rise from a straight-backed chair, stand briefly, walk forward about 10 feet, turn, walk back to the chair, turn around, and sit down. Performance is graded on a 5-point scale from 1 (normal) to 5 (severely abnormal). The quality of the movement is assessed for impaired balance. A score of 3 or higher suggests high risk of falling. Gait speed and agility have been found to correlate well with functional level. Marked gait disorders are not normally a consequence of aging alone but are more likely indicative of an underlying pathologic condition.

Investigation of gait disorders in elderly people is a complex issue, and it is important that nurses recognize and advocate for proper and thorough assessment and diagnosis. Nurses are the most likely providers to observe gait disturbances. A guide nurses can use for gait and balance problem descriptions is provided in Box 13-7. The Tinetti Balance and Gait Evaluation is precise and has been tested for validity and reliability (Tinetti, 1986) (see Appendix 13-B). A number of tests may need to be ordered to discover the cause of the gait disorder. These include x-ray and computed tomography (CT) of the cervical spine to assess for a cervical myelopathy; electromyography and nerve conduction studies for peripheral neuropathies; laboratory tests, including thyroid, vitamin B_{12}, folate, complete blood count (CBC), electrolytes, and liver function; CT of the head for normal-pressure hydrocephalus or stroke or tumor; lumbar puncture for infection or amyotrophic lateral sclerosis (ALS); and electrocardiogram (ECG) for arrhythmias and cardiac events (Resnick et al, 2001).

Interventions. Well-fitting shoes, canes, leg braces, pain relief, handrails, or walkers may improve mobility status. The nurse is responsible for initial assessment of gait disturbance and gaining appropriate professional consultation for prostheses and gait training. Rehabilitative specialists are usually responsible for teaching gait training to patients, but nurses must understand concepts and specific methods because they will assist the patient to carry out correct procedures on a daily basis. A complete analysis of gait patterns and characteristics requires special equipment and expertise, but simple gait observation by nurses can yield valuable information. In most gait disturbances, nervousness or anxiety aggravates the condition. Nurses may assist by gently holding the arm on the unaffected side and supporting the client's efforts.

Box 13-7 Gait Description and Assessment

Pain in back and lower limbs	Antalgic gait; short steps flexed toward affected side
Contracture or ankylosis	Short-leg gait; wide outward swing of affected side, unaffected knee flexed and body bent forward
Foot deformities	Loss of spring and rhythm in step, toes inward or outward bilaterally or unilaterally
Footdrop	Foot slap heard due to knee raised higher than usual
Gluteus medius weakness	Waddle gait; drop and lag in swing phase of unaffected side, seen in osteomalacia and senile gait in women
Stroke	Wide, open, flinging foot on affected side, uncoordinated
Cerebroarteriosclerosis	Bilateral involvement manifested by extremely short steps
Parkinsonism	Festinating gait; short, hurried, often on tiptoe, or rigid, tremorous, slow, tends toward retropulsion, mincing
Etat lacunaire	Similar to Parkinson's gait, irregular footsteps
Dementia	Slow, shuffling, apraxic, short steps
Peripheral neuropathy	Difficulty lifting feet, stumbles easily
Subdural hematoma	Ataxic, prominent feature is gait disturbance
Cerebellar ataxia	Staggering, unsteady, irregular, wide-based gait, inappropriate foot placement
Vitamin B_{12} deficiency	Paresthesias, unsteadiness, foot dragging
Endocrine disorders	Gait ataxia, particularly with hypothyroidism
Medications	Ataxia, parkinsonian gait, imbalance

Important interventions for those at risk include patient and family teaching, assessment and management of the environment to make it fall resistant, and assessing and changing medications that may cause falls. Placement of side rails in the hospital may be a needed intervention, although these can be a source of injury as well. Keeping call lights at hand is important in this setting, as well as other items of convenience on the bedside table. One intervention that is useful in a facility is to identify those at risk for falls and make a notation or color code for them, on the chart or at the bedside. Further, a bed sensor is useful for those who may try to get out of bed without the needed assistance. Nurses must attend to call lights in order to prevent injury to those who would hurry to the bathroom without assistance if none is forthcoming when needed, often urgently. This is vital when elders are on diuretics such as furosemide (Lasix). The American Geriatric Society (2001) published a guideline for the prevention of falls in older persons; this is available for free at *www.americangeriatrics.org*. Every facility should maintain fall rates for quality control and management.

Osteoporosis

Osteoporosis (OP) is a major medical, economic, and social health problem in the United States. It results in significant pain, loss of function, suffering, and mortality.

Definition. Normally there is a gradual, continual loss of cortical bone (the outer shell of a bone and 80% of the skeleton) and trabecular bone (the spongy meshwork inside the bone and 20% of the skeleton) in both men and women as they age (Thorndyke, 2001). Osteopenia and osteoporosis are metabolic bone diseases in which bone resorption occurs faster than bone formation. There is increased porosity in the trabecular bone and thinning of the cortical bone. Osteoporotic bones fracture easily.

Osteopenia, or low bone mass, is defined as bone mineral density −1 to −2.5 standard deviations (SD) below that of the normal adult woman, age 30, and is a risk factor for osteoporosis. Osteoporosis, "porous bone," is bone mineral loss at least 2.5 SD below peak bone density, represented by a T score of −2.5 or lower. OP is further defined as primary or secondary. Primary OP is more common and occurs postmenopausally and in elderly people. Secondary OP occurs in men and women when bone resorption and formation are diminished and parathyroid hormone is elevated (Thorndyke, 2001) and is usually caused by an underlying medical condition (e.g., thyroid disease).

Epidemiology. Eighty percent of Americans with osteoporosis are women (Davidson and DeSimone, 2002). One of every two women older than 50 years of age will have an osteoporosis fracture in her lifetime. A woman who has had a fracture before age 50 has a 74% increased risk of another. One in eight men will have osteoporosis. This OP is usually secondary and related to alcoholism, smoking, and previous therapy for prostate cancer (androgen suppression, which accelerates bone loss). Elders who take thyroid replacement therapy are at higher risk for bone loss.

Causation and Pathophysiology. Bone mass peaks at age 20 to 25 and remains stable until menopause (Maricic, 2001). The dynamics of bone loss are complex, involving the interrelationship of dietary mineral metabolism, parathyroid, vitamin D, hormones, and growth factors, including cytokines (interleukins, tumor necrosis factor, and transforming growth factor) (Davidson and DeSimone, 2002). Gastrointestinal age-related changes and the inadequacy of dietary calcium of older adults are among the factors that put elders at risk for osteoporosis.

Risk Factors for Osteoporosis. The amount of bone mass one has as a young adult and the rate at which it is lost as one ages determine risk for osteoporosis (Arthritis Foundation, 2000). Other areas of risk that should be a part of any nursing assessment of an elder include both modifiable and nonmodifiable factors. Nonmodifiable risk factors include the following (Petak, 2001; Curry and Hogstel, 2002) (Box 13-8):

- Personal history of fracture as an adult
- History of fracture in a first-degree relative
- Caucasian race
- Ancestry—northern European and Asian
- Advanced age
- Dementia
- Female sex
- Poor health/frailty

Potentially modifiable risk factors include the following (Arthritis Foundation, 2000; Petak, 2001; Curry and Hogstel, 2002):

- Low body weight, underweight
- Estrogen deficiency from early menopause (before age 45) or bilateral ovariectomy
- Low calcium intake
- Lack of sun exposure and insufficient vitamin D, which is needed to process calcium
- Inadequate physical activity, sedentary lifestyle, or prolonged bed rest
- Current cigarette smoking—causes rapid calcium loss in the urine
- Inflammatory arthritis—produces substances causing bone loss
- Steroid use
- Increased alcohol or coffee intake, which causes diuresis and calcium excretion
- Poor health/frailty

Risk of hip fracture is important to estimate because it is associated with excessive morbidity and a mortality rate of about 20% (Davidson and DeSimone, 2002). This risk rises after age 45 and doubles with every 5 years of increased age (Maricic, 2001). It is even higher for men with hip fracture. It is imperative to identify those at risk for osteoporosis and hip fracture and at risk for fall because 90% of hip fractures occur with a fall. Hip fractures occur later in life in those age 75 or older.

Vertebral fractures are common within about 10 years of menopause because trabecular bone is lost before the cortical bone (as in the hip). These fractures can be extraordinarily painful. Vertebral fractures are the most common, followed by hip (proximal femur) fractures and distal forearm or wrist fractures.

Box 13-8 Risk Assessment for Osteoporosis

Yes		Heredity
[ ]		Family history of osteoporosis
[ ]		Thin, petite, small muscled
[ ]		Fair skin or thin skin
		Hormones
[ ]	[ ]	Surgical removal of ovaries
[ ]	[ ]	Early menopause
[ ]	[ ]	Menopausal
[ ]	[ ]	Never pregnant
		Calcium
[ ]	[ ]	Unsure of amount calcium getting daily
[ ]	[ ]	Avoids milk and dairy products
[ ]	[ ]	Avoided milk as a child
		Physical Activity
[ ]	[ ]	Physically inactive
[ ]	[ ]	Muscles weak and poorly toned
[ ]	[ ]	Seldom exercises
		Lifestyle
[ ]	[ ]	Drinks or smokes heavily
[ ]	[ ]	Taking medications
[ ]	[ ]	Diet contains a large amount of caffeine, salt, protein
Signs of Osteoporosis (Height equals arm span, except for black people, whose arm span is generally greater than height)		
[ ]	[ ]	Lost height
[ ]	[ ]	Upper back curves forward
[ ]	[ ]	Have fractured a wrist, spine, or hip or lost teeth lately
		Living Safely with Osteoporosis
[ ]	[ ]	Wears high-heeled shoes
[ ]	[ ]	Does a lot of bending and lifting
[ ]	[ ]	Takes tranquilizers or drugs that cause drowsiness or dizziness
[ ]	[ ]	Safety hazards exist in home
		TOTAL NUMBER OF RISK FACTORS

Modified from *Osteoporosis*, presentation, Daly City, CA, April 1985, Krames Communications.

Bone Mass. Early identification of diminished bone density is essential for prevention of OP and its subsequent morbidity. The dual-energy x-ray absorptiometry (DEXA) scan of the hip and vertebral column is the standard, and its cost is covered by Medicare. DEXA scans have low radiation exposure. Other screening devices, such as heel or wrist scans done at malls and health fairs (and lists of risk factors), do not give an accurate picture of the bone density in all areas of the body. One area, such as the heel, may be normal, but the vertebrae may be osteoporotic.

Assessment. The loss of bone with OP is silent, without symptoms, until a fracture occurs. Some of the outward signs that identify a history of OP are a loss of height (perhaps 3 to 5 inches since young adulthood) and "dowager's hump," or kyphosis, which is curvature of the thoracic spine, usually with the presence of a bulging abdomen (all indicative of vertebral fractures) (Figure 13-1).

Assess the patient's diet for calcium and vitamin D; a diet that is low will need to be supplemented. Assess lifestyle for risk factors, such as sedentary habits or excessive alcohol intake.

Prevention and Management. Prevention of OP must begin in the teen years. As women increasingly live into their eighties and nineties, the treatment of OP is becoming more important.

Preventive measures include a diet that includes calcium and calcium supplements because most diets contain less than 600 mg/day. About 1500 mg/day is needed in postmenopausal women not taking hormone replacement therapy (HRT) and all women older than 65; 1000 mg/day is recommended for postmenopausal women using HRT (Thorndyke, 2001). Calcium can be taken as calcium carbonate, calcium phosphate, or calcium citrate. Calcium carbonate requires an acid environment for absorption, and many elders do not have this if they are taking proton pump inhibitors or histamine-2 receptor blockers for gastroesophageal reflux disease. Calcium citrate should be taken between meals. Ideally, calcium is taken in small amounts throughout the day. Vitamin K is also necessary. Low vitamin K intake results in increased bone fragility and an increased risk of hip fracture (Grosch, 2002).

Pharmacologic treatments now available are by prescription. The bisphosphonates risedronate (Actonel) and alendronate (Fosamax) are both available in once weekly doses, a great convenience. Calcitonin (salmon) nasal spray (Miacalcin) is less effective than the bisphosphonates but has fewer side effects such as esophagitis or gastric symptoms. HRT in combination with risedronate is known to have a more favorable effect than HRT alone, especially in the femoral neck (hip fractures) and radius (Harris et al, 2001).

Personal safety should be addressed to prevent falls in elders who have OP. Shoes with good support should be worn. Handrails should be used, and walking in poorly lighted areas should be avoided. Basic body mechanics such as not bending or lifting heavy objects should be learned. Use of step stools or chairs for reaching things in high places should be discouraged. Home safety should include good lighting, railings, and other aids as needed. Walkways should be kept free of obstacles; loose rugs and electrical cords should be arranged so that they do not cause falls.

Living with Osteoporosis. Nonpharmacologic management of OP includes good nutrition—the elder must not be underweight (a risk factor for OP). Regular weight-bearing

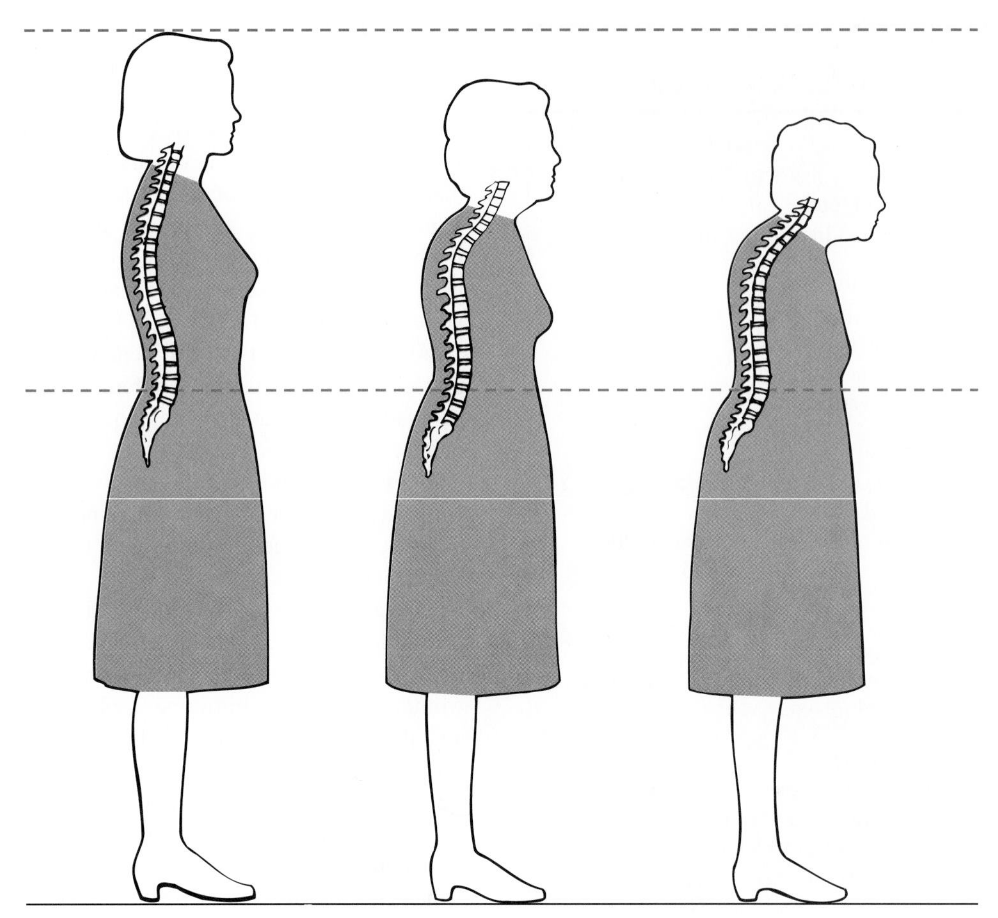

Figure 13-1. Osteoporosis spine alignment.

exercise 20 minutes a day, 5 days a week is helpful in strengthening bones and maintaining flexibility and balance, although this may not be possible for some elders with severe osteoarthritis, especially in the hips and knees. Elders with severe OP should consider the use of hip protectors when up and about during the day, especially if they have suffered a fall in the past. Consider a walker or cane if balance is problematic. Elders who live in long-term care settings will be especially at risk for disease progression unless they are participating actively in daily exercise programs and walks. Immobilization causes rapid loss of bone. Muscle-building exercises help maintain skeletal architecture by improving muscle strength and flexibility. Some evidence indicates that muscle building also helps strengthen bone.

A diet adequate in calcium and vitamin D is essential and is necessary when taking pharmacologic agents for OP. The pharmacologic agents will need to be taken indefinitely, possibly for life. Educating the elder to this need is necessary. There will be follow-up DEXA scans to evaluate improvement, probably 1 to 2 years after starting therapy. This may also help the client with medication and exercise compliance.

Complications. Fractures are common in elders with osteoporosis. Vertebral fractures are the most common. They may be "silent" or be extremely painful with paravertebral muscle spasms and radiation of pain because of nerve root compression (Thorndyke, 2001). There are estimated to be about 1.3 million new OP fractures each year; one half are vertebral, one fourth are hip, and the remainder are forearm and other sites (Russell and Dawson-Hughes, 1999). Hip fractures are associated with increased mortality rates.

In elderly men with fractures, look for a family history of fractures and measure urine calcium levels, because "renal leak" of calcium is often the cause. Hypogonadism is another cause and can be treated with testosterone unless the client has benign prostatic hypertrophy, which is aggravated by testosterone.

Vertebral fractures are often not recognized by clinicians or by the radiologist when an elder has back pain (Watts, 2001). It is suggested that any patient with height loss have a spinal x-ray and obtain lateral spine imaging. Quality of life is greatly impaired with vertebral deformities because they have been shown to limit activity and increase days at bed rest. Further, history of fracture is an additional risk for another fracture; 20% of women will fracture again in less than a year. Treatment of these fractures can be with nonsteroidal antiinflammatory drugs (NSAIDs) if there is osteoarthritis in the area of fracture. Narcotics should be avoided if possible because of the sedation and increased risk of falls. Newer treatments

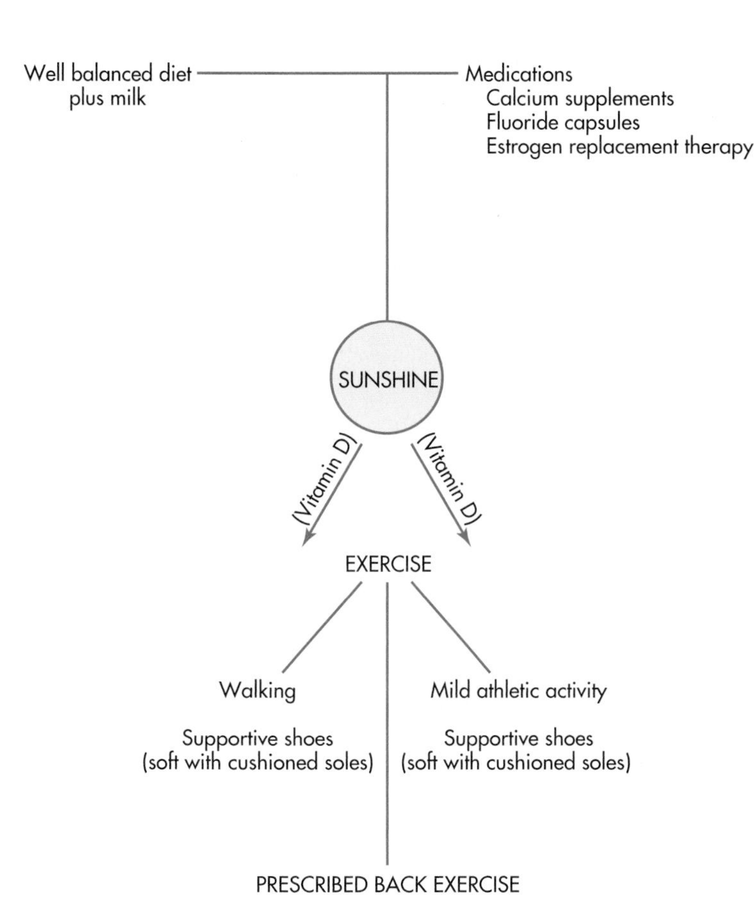

Figure 13-2. Treatment of osteoporosis.

with vertebroplasty and kyphoplasty may be considered in those with continued pain (the average is 2 weeks to 3 months) or severe pain (Lesley, 2002). Usual therapy is bed rest, with variable success and the possible complications of deep vein thrombosis, pneumonia, and further bone loss; fixation surgery, which has a high failure rate because of weakened bone foundation; and analgesics. Vertebroplasty is the percutaneous injection of a cement into the affected vertebral body. It is done under local anesthetic with conscious sedation and is an outpatient procedure. The elder is able to walk within 2 to 24 hours and usually has immediate pain relief (Lesley, 2002).

Nursing Interventions. Intervention, like prevention, should be directed toward educating clients about their medical regimen, assisting them in adapting to their disease, and preventing disease progression. Medical interventions of which the nurse should be knowledgeable include the various types of therapies used in the treatment of osteoporosis (Figure 13-2).

Nursing interventions for the individual with osteoporosis who is not hospitalized should focus on teaching and assisting the individual to maintain a positive approach toward the disease and prevention of its progression or complications. Interventions include:

1. Teach the client about nutritionally balanced calcium-rich diets including milk, or milk substitutes for those who are lactose intolerant.
2. Teach the client to take 1500 mg of calcium daily through diet, calcium supplements, or both.
3. Teach the client about the factors that inhibit calcium absorption, such as excess protein or salt, and calcium excretion enhancers, such as caffeine; excess fiber; phosphorus in meats, sodas, and preserved foods; and the influence of the body's response to stress (decreased calcium absorption and increased excretion of calcium in the urine).
4. Discuss the pros and cons of HRT.
5. Ensure understanding of medication and adjunct regimens.
6. Encourage women to maintain a daily schedule or alternate-day schedule of weight-bearing exercises such as walking, low-impact aerobics, workout machines, swimming, or a combination of activities.
7. Check the medicine cabinet. Determine if the elder is taking any kind of drug that might compromise mentation and be responsible for falls.
8. If the client has an acute vertebral fracture, a short period of bed rest may be tried. Place a pillow under the head and under the knees to decrease the stress on the vertebrae. Apply heat or cold for pain and gentle massage if there are muscle spasms (Neyhart and Gibbs, 2002). Effective pain management will allow early mobilization. Calcitonin may be useful in pain relief.

Much remains to be done in preventing OP. Young women must be taught preventive measures to forestall the development of OP and reduce the enormous cost of osteoporotic fractures and the painful disability and discomfort to the individual.

Rheumatic Diseases of Older Adults

Arthritis is the most common of the afflictions that disable elders. It is estimated that there are 100 different types of arthritis that arise from various combinations of heredity, overuse, obesity, and infections (American College of Rheumatology, 2000). Arthritis affects 45 to 60 million individuals in the United States, young as well as old, and includes disorders of joints and connective tissues throughout the body (Callahan and Jonas, 2002). These disorders create pain, depression, immobility, and functional and self-concept disturbances. Arthritis, though the most prevalent disorder of aging, is by no means equally distributed throughout the elderly population by age, gender, race, socioeconomic group, or geography. *Healthy People 2010* specifically addresses goals of additional research, mutual planning of care and therapy, and implementation of treatment plans for arthritis, osteoporosis, and chronic back problems. A number of rheumatic disorders occur in older adults; some of these are bursitis, polymyalgia rheumatica, gout, rotator cuff tears, tendinitis, frozen shoulder, low back pain, acute disk herniation, chronic disk degeneration, lumbar spinal stenosis, rheumatoid arthritis, osteoarthritis, and many others (Reuben et al, 2002). Because of space considerations, and because management and nursing care are similar in some of these disorders, we highlight the most common.

Osteoarthritis

Definition. Osteoarthritis (OA) is a joint disorder that affects at least 20 million Americans. It was previously thought to be a normal consequence of aging that had no cure (Kalunian and Brion, 2002). However, it is now known that OA results from a complex interplay of many factors, including genetic predisposition, local inflammation, joint integrity, mechanical forces, and cellular and biochemical processes. Clinically, it causes pain that is increased with activity and relieved by rest (Concoff, 2002). As the disease advances, there is pain with little activity, occurring at rest and at night. Episodic pain increases, and inflammation suggests synovitis, which is caused by trauma or crystalline disease. OA has been thought to be noninflammatory, but this is not so. (Figure 13-3 demonstrates changes in the joint with OA.) Physiologically, there is bony growth of osteophytes and joint space narrowing from loss or destruction of cartilage; there may be inflammation of the synovium lining the joint.

Nearly 90% of Americans older than 40 have x-ray evidence of OA, and the incidence increases with increasing age. Native Americans have high prevalence of OA and Asians and Pacific Islanders have low prevalence.

Risk factors. The risk factors for OA include:

- Increased age
- Obesity
- Family history
- Repetitive use of joint
- Trauma

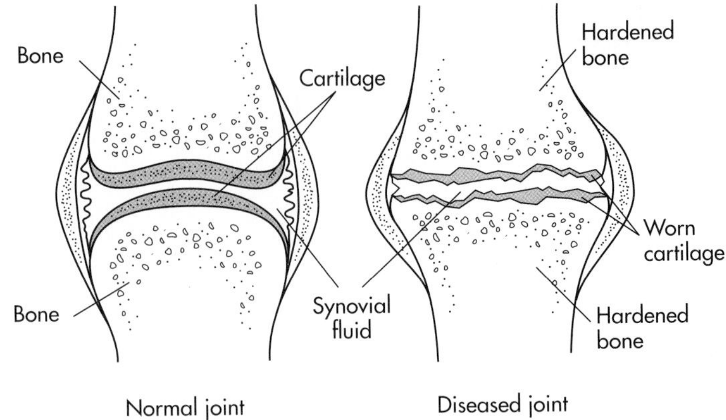

Figure 13-3. Normal joint and diseased joint.

Classification. OA is classified as idiopathic or secondary. Idiopathic OA is localized or generalized disease. Localized OA affects the hands, feet, knee, hip, and spine and less often the shoulder, temporomandibular, sacroiliac, ankle, and wrist joints. Generalized OA is that which involves more than three joints. It can also be classified by anatomic involvement, but this is a description of the disease at only one point in time, and disease manifestations are likely to change a great deal over time.

Assessment. The diagnosis of OA is made clinically; there are no laboratory tests to confirm the diagnosis. The history will reveal a gradual onset of joint pain and stiffness that worsens with activity and is relieved at rest. Morning stiffness is common and lasts less than 30 minutes; however, it may occur again during the day with periods of rest (this is called "gelling"). Weather appears to aggravate symptoms. As the disease advances, more joints become involved. There may be joint instability, and crepitus may be felt or heard in the knees. The joint will enlarge and range of motion diminish. Occasionally, a client will complain of hip pain, but it may be a chronic bursitis of the greater trochanter (Concoff, 2002). With hip arthritis, there will be decreased range of motion, which is not present with bursitis.

Spinal involvement occurs most commonly at C5, T8, and L3, areas of greatest flexibility. Osteophytes (bony outgrowths) in the lumbar region can become spinal stenosis if encroaching in the foramina and spinal cord and result in a radiating low back pain. The *National Guideline on Low Back Pain* is available at *www.guideline.gov* (revised in 2001).

Various assessment tools have been developed to assess patients with arthritis. X-rays are highly insensitive to OA, especially early OA (Concoff, 2002). They may reveal nonpalpable findings such as narrowed joint space, osteophytes, and subchondral cysts. One tool measures joint movement limitations. Grip and the pinch gauge measure strength. Range of motion (ROM) and pain in hands and fingers demonstrate movement limitations. Overhead lift of weight and shoulder rotation test strength and ROM of shoulder. Knee extensor and hip flexion measure ROM, strength, and discomfort. Pain should be assessed at every meeting with the elder. Nursing assessment also should focus on assessing difficulties in living. Assess comfort in walking, cooking, bathing, dressing, using the toilet, and performing household chores (Agency for Healthcare Research and Quality, 2002a). Assess changes in social activities, exercise, and income (i.e., diminished). Look for depression.

Physical assessment may reveal crepitus (a crunching sound) on movement of the joint, indicating loss of a smooth articulating surface, and joint effusion, fluid in the joint. Effusions may be large and hinder movement so that aspiration is needed for relief. In the hands there may be Heberden's nodes or Bouchard's nodes, which are bony enlargements on the distal and proximal interphalangeal joints. Heberden's nodes are thought to have a hereditary component.

Interventions. The goals of intervention and management of OA are to control pain, minimize disability, and educate the client.

Pain management is most important because exercise and ROM exercises will not be done if they cause severe pain. Pharmacologic management is usually necessary, and acetaminophen is useful for pain. The COX-2 inhibitors (Vioxx and Celebrex) have a lower incidence of gastrointestinal (GI) problems, such as bleeding, than the traditional NSAIDs, which work very well but can be dangerous. Misoprostol and proton pump inhibitors such as Prilosec have been recommended for management of an elder with GI risks (Fauci, 2000). Tramadol, used for moderate to severe pain, is not a controlled substance but acts somewhat like one. It is thought to have NSAID-sparing properties (Lozada and Altman, 2001). It can cause nausea and vomiting and should be started in very low doses and increased very slowly to avoid these side effects. Codeine and other opiates can be used for moderate to severe pain, with a bowel regimen.

Glucosamine appears to be useful for pain relief and for slowing the progression of OA (Horstman, 2000). Other touted remedies include cartilage or collagen from sharks, bovines, or chickens (!), as well as bromelain (from pineapples), chondroitin sulfate, collagen hydrolysate (gelatin), devil's claw (root of an African plant), ginger root, green tea, and many others (information is available from the Arthritis Foundation via Arthritis Today at *www.arthritis.org*). There are little or no human data to support their use, and many can be hazardous with unsupervised use.

Other pharmacologic agents often used in OA management include capsaicin from pepper plants available OTC in two strengths. It becomes effective after several days of use. Menthol and aspirin creams are also useful and are preferred by many elders.

Intraarticular therapy of corticosteroids can give long-lasting relief for some OA problems, especially when the synovium is involved and is inflamed (Lozada and Altman, 2001). It can be used in periarticular tissue problems such as bursitis and tendinitis. A newer therapy, hyaluronan derivatives or hyaluronic acid, is said to reduce pain and improve mobility, but a series of injections is necessary.

Temperature. The use of heat and cold is well known for management of pain. Patient preference is important, but cold usually works best for an acute process, using cold packs that decrease muscle spasm, decrease swelling, and relieve inflammatory pain. Heat may be applied superficially or deep; either works well (Lozada and Altman, 2001). Ultrasound provides deep heat. Hot packs, hydrotherapy, and radiant heat provide superficial heat. A recent device available for prolonged heat application is ThermaCare, which is a band applied to the affected area (e.g., neck, lower back, abdomen) and lasts for 8 to 12 hours. It is available OTC and can be worn under clothing throughout the day.

Physical activity. This is important in OA management. More than 70% of elderly people are sedentary (Feldt, 2002). Resnick (2002) studied 175 older adults in a continuing care retirement community and found that the elders initially performed 0 hours of moderate exercise weekly. Resnick (2002) states that education of elders should include (1) the anticipated benefits of exercise—decreased joint stress, pain, risk of falls, improved mood and sleep; (2) anticipated responses of increased heart rate and awareness of heartbeat, increased breathing rate, sweating, and mild muscle aches; and (3) the warning signs of excessive exercise—severe dyspnea, wheezing, coughing, chest pain or discomfort, dizziness, and marked fatigue. With this preparation, elders are better able to start a program. A resource for exercise promotion is available at the University of Iowa's College of Nursing (email: *research-dissemination-core@uiowa.edu*). Exercise programs are linked with pain reduction and functional improvement (Lozada and Altman, 2001). Choose exercises that maximize muscle strengthening and minimize stress on affected joints. Swimming and bicycle riding are known to be good for OA patients; however, some OA is worsened by these activities—for example, chondromalacia patella is worsened by bicycle riding, and lumbar facet OA is worsened by hyperextension of the spine, as in swimming. A specialist should be consulted before the client begins any exercise regimen.

Physical therapy may improve clinical outcomes. Elderly patients usually should be referred to a rehabilitation specialist or physical therapist. Improvement in flexibility and muscle strength helps support the affected joints, reduce pain, and improve function (Brion and Concoff, 2002). Preventive occupational therapy has been shown to improve personal and social relationships in the Well Elderly Study (Agency for Healthcare Research and Quality, 2002b).

Supports. There are devices that unload joints, decrease pain, and improve balance (Lozada and Altman, 2001). Canes, crutches, walkers, collars, shoe orthotics, and corsets are such devices. A cane can unload a hip by 60%. A shoe lift can improve lumbar pain. A knee brace is useful for tibiofemoral OA, especially if there is lateral instability (the knee "gives out").

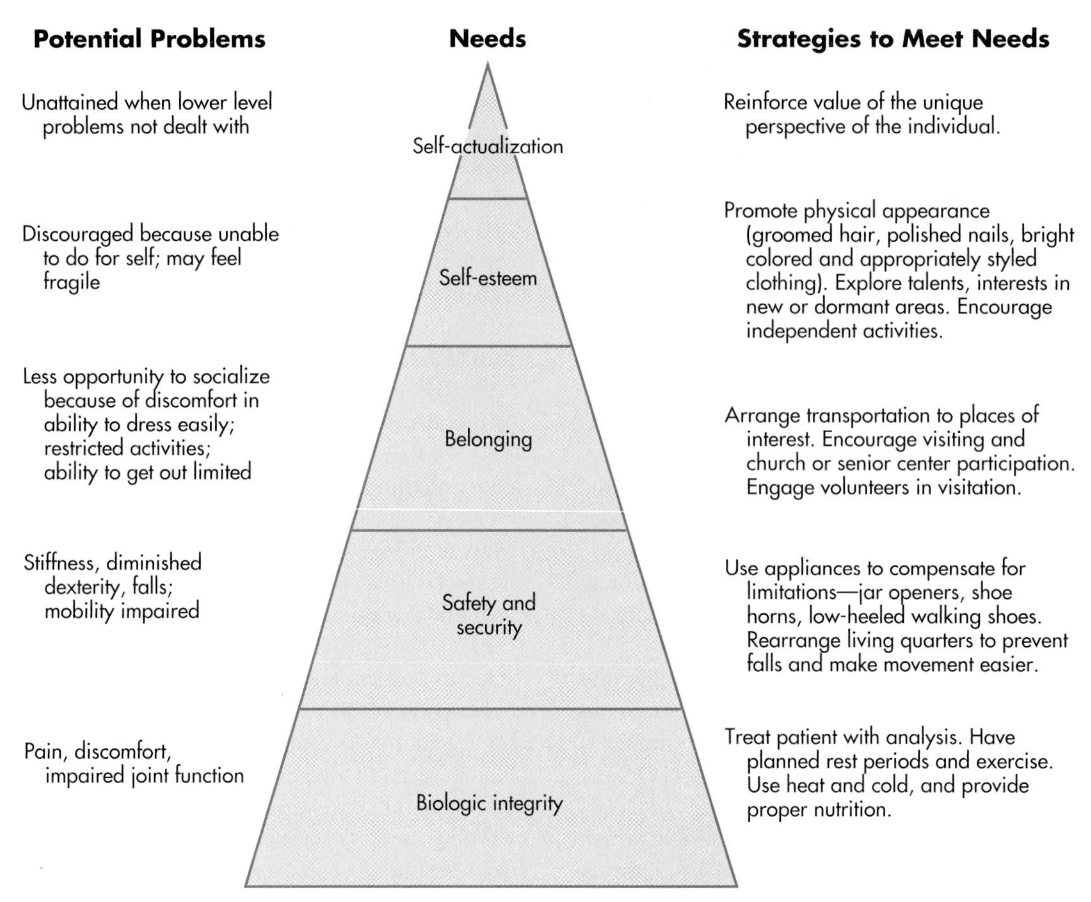

Figure 13-4. Osteoarthritis wellness perspective.

Diet. It is clear that obesity aggravates the symptoms of OA of the knee. Therefore the first positive action an individual might take in self-management is weight reduction. There is disagreement in the literature about the wisdom of walking any more than necessary with an osteoarthritic knee. The value of walking may be in morale and weight control, as well as weight bearing and movement. Figure 13-4 illustrates management of OA from a wellness perspective. Management guidelines for osteoarthritis of the hip are listed in Box 13-9.

Surgery. Total joint arthroplasty (surgical replacement of hips and knees) brings relief from intractable pain and functional limitations. Consideration must be given to the potential for wound healing, rehabilitation, and psychosocial factors. Changes in synovium, cartilage, and soft tissues must be assessed before opting for surgical options such as synovectomy, arthroplasty, arthrodesis, bone grafting, and others. Outcomes depend on the timing of surgery; the number of procedures that the surgeon and the hospital have to their credit; and the patient's medical status, perioperative and postoperative management, and rehabilitation. Nearly twice as many females as males have joint replacements, and over 60% of all joint replacements are in individuals over 65 years of age. The Well Elderly Study found that elderly people report better quality of life, less pain, and better physical function after knee replacement surgery (Agency for Healthcare Research and Quality, 2002b).

Rheumatoid Arthritis

Definition. Rheumatoid arthritis (RA) is a chronic, systemic inflammatory disorder of unknown cause. It is considered an autoimmune disease and is characterized by symmetric polyarticular pain and swelling, morning stiffness lasting longer than 30 minutes, and malaise (Gornisiewicz and Moreland, 2001). Its natural course is variable, with remission and exacerbations. The disease may be unremitting, with continuing progression, disability, and death, or a remitting (rare) disease. Nearly one half of those affected are disabled within 10 years (Luggen, 2003).

Classification. RA is classified as seropositive or seronegative; about 80% of people with RA are rheumatoid factor antibody positive. This is associated with a more severe and progressive course, with a reduced life expectancy of 10 to 15 years (Luggen, 2003). Elders who have seronegative RA may become seropositive.

Epidemiology. RA occurs worldwide but is thought to be more common in northern rather than southern areas and less

Box 13-9 Management of Patients with Osteoarthritis of the Hip

Nonpharmacologic Therapy

Patient education
- Self-management programs (e.g., Arthritis Self-Help Course)
- Health professional social support via telephone contact
- Weight loss (if overweight)
- Physical therapy
  - Range-of-motion exercises
  - Strengthening exercises
  - Assistive devices for ambulation
- Occupational therapy
  - Joint protection and energy conservation
  - Assistive devices for ADLs and IADLs
- Aerobic aquatic exercise programs

Pharmacologic therapy
- Nonopioid analgesics (e.g., acetaminophen)
- Nonsteroidal antiinflammatory drugs
- Opioid analgesics (e.g., propoxyphene, codeine, oxycodone)

From Hochberg MC et al: Guidelines for the medical management of osteoarthritis. L. Osteoarthritis of the hip, *Arthritis Rheum* 38:1535, 1995.
ADLs, Activities of daily living; *IADLs*, instrumental ADLs.

common in Asia and Africa. RA may occur at any age, but it tends to occur more frequently in women (3:1) than men, with increasing age—it rises until age 45, stabilizes, and then declines, but it may occur in the very old. About 1% of adults older than 65 have RA. There is increased risk of mortality with RA compared with a non-RA population, especially from GI problems and cardiac deaths, as well as hematologic, respiratory, and infectious causes (Gornisiewicz and Moreland, 2001). There may be some acceleration in atherosclerosis in RA (Van Doornum et al, 2002). It may be that the inflammatory basis of RA and atherosclerosis is the mechanism for this.

Pathophysiology. The pathophysiology of RA has been studied extensively. Its pathogenesis is likely to be multifactorial, and susceptibility is related to heredity. Probably exposure to environmental factors (as yet unknown) increases susceptibility (Gornisiewicz and Moreland, 2001).

Risk factors. Polymorphism in the genes for T cell receptors or for immunoglobulins is one known risk factor. Severity of disease may be predicted by a shared epitope on HLA-DRB chains (Luggen, 2002). Other risk factors and protective factors include (Luggen, 2003):
- If one twin has RA, the other twin has an eightfold increased risk for development of RA.
- People with allergies have a lower incidence of RA.
- A woman who bears more children may increase her risk of severe illness with RA.
- Oral contraceptives may be protective.
- Those with lower education levels have higher morbidity and mortality rates.
- Postmenopausal women who smoke may be at high risk for RA.
- No risk is associated with silicone breast implants.
- There is a negative association between gout and RA.
- No relationship is known to exist between diet and RA.

Assessment. Early diagnosis is important because irreversible destruction of affected joints may occur within 1 to 2 years after onset. Early signs include generalized fatigue, malaise, stiffness with swelling, erythema, and warmth over affected joints. Weight loss and anemia are common. Usually joint involvement is symmetric rather than asymmetric as in osteoarthritis. Elevated rheumatoid factor and erythrocyte sedimentation rate are most suggestive of rheumatoid arthritis. The American College of Rheumatology has established criteria for the diagnosis of RA (Luggen, 2002):
- Morning stiffness lasting longer than 1 hour (and present for 6 weeks)
- More than three of the following joints are involved: proximal interphalangeal (PIP), metacarpophalangeal (MCP), wrist, elbow, knee, ankle, and metatarsophalangeal (MTP) (for 6 weeks)
- Arthritis of the wrist, MCP joint, or PIP joint (for 6 weeks)
- Joint involvement is symmetric (for 6 weeks)
- Presence of rheumatoid nodules
- Positive serum rheumatoid factor (up to 50% are false positive at age 80)
- X-ray changes such as erosions, bone decalcification (localized in or adjacent to the involved joints)

No one test is necessary to confirm the diagnosis of RA; in some patients all tests will be normal. On the other hand, elderly patients who have a number of other chronic illnesses may have many positive tests that confuse and confound the diagnosis. For instance, a positive rheumatoid factor is often present in older smokers (Gornisiewicz and Moreland, 2001).

A baseline assessment should include subjective data from the elder. Ask about stiffness, joint pain, fatigue, and function. Ask about activities the client is no longer able to do. In the physical examination, note the tender and swollen joints, as well as any deformities present. Assess for depression because this is a common component of RA.

Systemic manifestations. RA is a systemic disease and affects many organ systems in addition to the joints. Rheumatoid nodules may arise within tendons or ligaments and can cause rupture or joint dysfunction (Gornisiewicz and Moreland, 2001). They can also occur (less often) in the lungs, the sclera, and the vocal cords. About 15% of people with RA develop Sjögren's syndrome, which, in addition to RA, has dry eyes (sicca) and oral secretions (xerostomia), Raynaud's phenomenon, vasculitis, and erythema. Many elders develop dry eyes and xerostomia without having RA, thus confusing the diagnosis. Other manifestations include scleritis of the eyes, a serious problem requiring regular ophthalmologic examinations. Pulmonary involvement can occur as interstitial lung disease, or pleurisy with or without effusions; this occurs in about 70% of RA patients. The heart may be involved, with pericarditis or pericardial effusion. Felty's syndrome occurs mainly in older adults with RA. This syndrome is the triad of neutropenia, splenomegaly, and severe RA. The client may have recurrent bacterial urinary tract and pulmonary infections.

Interventions. Many new biologic agents have been developed and found to be helpful in treating RA. Anakinra, infliximab, and etanercept are three recently developed biologic response modifiers that have shown remarkable efficacy in RA management. They work by either blocking tumor necrosis factor or blocking the action of interleukin-1, a cytokine that plays a key role in inflammation (Arthritis Foundation, 2001).

In RA, the management goals are to decrease pain, prevent and control joint damage, and prevent loss of function (American College of Rheumatology, 2002). Further, we have the goals of maintaining normal physical, social, and emotional function and the capacity to do work (Gornisiewicz and Moreland, 2001). As in OA, it is necessary to decrease the pain and inflammation of RA in order to manage the disease, and work with the patient to prevent deformity. It is important that the elder understand the nature of this disease and that the care prescribed must be followed to prevent the pain, deformity, and disability that is the natural course.

NSAIDs are often used to reduce pain and inflammation but are not good choices in the older adult, nor is aspirin, because the incidence of GI events is high in this population. The COX-2 inhibitors are a better choice for elderly patients with RA because there is less likelihood of a GI bleed. Available on the market at this time for RA are celecoxib, rofecoxib, and meloxicam. Corticosteroids may also be used, especially in the acute inflammation of a joint. A short, intense course of therapy is often helpful in quickly reducing the inflammation (and pain). Chronic use of corticosteroids results in osteoporosis, which must be kept in mind by the practitioner. Hormone replacement therapy and bisphosphonates can be given to prevent osteoporosis. Disease-modifying antirheumatic drugs (DMARDs) are often used in management of RA but have no analgesic effect and only some antiinflammatory effect (Gornisiewicz and Moreland, 2001). Methotrexate is the DMARD most often used because of its efficacy, predictability, low cost, and low toxicity, and because it can be taken over many years. It is given at low doses and yet has immunosuppressive and antiinflammatory effects.

Protein A immunoadsorption (Prosorba column therapy) is a new approach in the treatment of those with moderate to severe RA who have not responded to DMARDs (Arthritis Foundation, 2001). Prosorba column therapy removes antibodies that are found in plasma and associated with RA. Side effects include a flulike syndrome with chills, fever, and transient fatigue.

Some of the antimicrobials that have been examined as potentially useful in RA include rifamycin, minocycline, ceftriaxone, ampicillin, and amantadine. Some of these are promising but require more study.

Herbals. Herbal and alternative remedies thought to provide benefit for RA include a Chinese herb, Tripterygium wilfordii Hook f. *(Celastraceae).* It is said to have immunosuppressive activities (Panush, 2002). Zinc (oral) was a benefit to some RA patients in one study. Copper salts are thought by many to be of benefit, but there have been many adverse effects and they are not used as therapy. Acupuncture should not be used in RA patients, is not effective, and is not risk free; one review study reported 2 deaths and 90 pneumothoraxes. Laser therapy using new low light sources has been useful for RA in the hands. Glucosamine and chondroitin are under study by the National Institutes of Health at this time.

Nutrition. The Arthritis Foundation has stated that "there is no scientific evidence that any food has anything to do with causing arthritis and no evidence that any food is effective in treating or curing it" (Panush and Lane, 1994); however, scientists continue to look for relationships. In one client, all RA symptoms disappeared when she was placed on a 3-day fast and returned when she was given milk (Panush, 2002). Cod liver oil is thought to be of benefit; taking 20 ml per day (or 20 capsules of fish oil) provides the appropriate amount of omega-3.

Rest is as important as exercise in RA. For many years it was thought that people with RA should rest only their joints to protect them from damage; however, both rest and exercise are necessary. In terms of rest, this may be resting the particular affected joint, such as a hand or wrist, or total body rest. Therapeutic exercise programs are designed to help maintain or improve the ability to do ADLs. Even a warm, inflamed joint should be given ROM exercises to maintain movement in the joint. A physical or occupational therapist should be consulted for developing a program of rest and exercise.

Self-help. Elderly patients with rheumatoid arthritis have been helped by a self-management program that relied largely on the efficacy of six 2-hour sessions in a self-help group for arthritics. In a 4-year follow-up it was found that knowledge of the disorder had increased and pain had decreased even though the physical disability had progressed (Lorig et al, 1985). Though this is an old study, it would seem to indicate that feelings of self-efficacy, induced by increased knowledge and feelings of control, may have highly positive outcomes even in the presence of increasing debilitation. Replication of these data is needed.

Providing classes in specially designed exercises, relaxation, and pain management techniques has been useful. Participants are also given general information about their disease and taught to use medication wisely. Based on the success of this effort, the National Arthritis Foundation offers courses throughout the United States. Many medical centers and senior care centers have arthritis clinics, and these should be sought for a thorough evaluation and individualized treatment program.

Environmental modifications are often necessary for elders with RA. Zipper pulls and Velcro closures on clothing are two practical measures. Book holders, chairs to sit on while preparing foods, light switch changes, and secure stair railings are more. An online database, ABLEDATA *(www.abledata.com/sire_2/default.htm),* sponsored by the National Institute on Disability and Rehabilitation Research, lists more than 25,000 assistive devices that are available.

In addition to the physical management of RA are the consequences of RA and the management of these. The practitioner should look for and treat problems such as depression, anxiety, poor coping strategies, learned helplessness, cognitive changes, and impaired self-efficacy (Callahan and Jonas, 2002). These problems are associated with poor outcomes and increased use of health care services.

Bursitis and Tendinitis. These disorders are known as soft tissue rheumatic syndromes and become more common with aging. They cause pain, swelling, and inflammation around joints and in the tissues and structures such as ligaments, tendons, bursae, and muscles. Because the problem is so near a joint, it is often confused with arthritis (Arthritis Foundation, 1999).

Pathophysiology. Bursae are closed sacs lined with a membrane, resembling synovium, that secrete and absorb fluid from the bursa (Reginato and Reginato, 2001). This provides a gliding mechanism between two musculoskeletal structures (muscle over muscle or tendon over bone). There are about 150 in the body. Adventitious bursae may develop at pressure points, for example, bunions or Baker's cysts. Inflammation of a bursa can be deep (popliteal) or superficial (elbow, shoulder) and is common in older adults.

Tendinitis refers to inflammation of the tissues or synovial sheaths around a tendon (tenosynovitis). It usually occurs from overuse, unaccustomed activity, or exercise (Reginato and Reginato, 2001).

Bursitis occurs with repetitive physical stresses. It occurs mainly in subacromial bursae (shoulder) and olecranon bursae (elbow). In the lower extremity, it occurs in the trochanteric, prepatellar, gastrocnemius-semimembranosus, and anserine bursae. Inflammation may cause rupture of the bursa, for example, Baker's cyst. Pain is usually described as deep, aching discomfort. Bursitis can occur due to RA and gout.

Hand and wrist tendinitis may exhibit as Dupuytren's contracture. This is a fibrous thickening of the palmar fascia (Reginato and Reginato, 2001). It occurs mainly in middle-aged men and elders of Northern European descent. It is an inherited trait and is associated with tobacco smoking, diabetes mellitus, local trauma, alcohol abuse, and long-term use of epileptic medications. It is usually bilateral. As it progresses, there is contracture of the MCP and PIP joints. Ring and little fingers are often involved. This disorder is associated with "trigger finger" (inflammation causing a popping sound when extending the trigger finger), carpal tunnel syndrome, lateral epicondylitis, and frozen shoulder. Surgical correction is the only treatment and is not curative.

Carpal Tunnel Syndrome. This is a common compression neuropathy caused by impingement of the median nerve at the carpal tunnel. It is seen often in RA, menopause, diabetes mellitus, and trauma. Patients have paresthesias and pain in the thumb, index finger, and middle finger. The whole hand can be numb. Any activity in which the wrist is flexed causes numbness. Management is with NSAIDs, preferably the COX-2 inhibitors to reduce the inflammation and swelling, and a splint, easily obtainable over the counter. Injection of corticosteroids is effective. Surgery should be considered only if symptoms become permanent and conservative measures are ineffective.

Shoulder problems are common in elderly patients. Many joints may be affected, including the acromioclavicular, sternoclavicular, glenohumeral, and scapulothoracic muscular joints (Reginato and Reginato, 2001). Often the problem is caused by bursitis, RA, or pseudogout. Pseudogout is a microcrystalline arthritis associated with calcification of hyaline and fibrous cartilage, often in the shoulder in elders (Beers and Berkow, 2000). It begins in the late fifties, and hypothyroidism is a predisposing factor. Elders with subacromial bursitis often awaken at night with severe pain when they turn to the affected shoulder. It radiates in the C-5 dermatome. Rotator cuff tears are common in elderly people. They may be acute or chronic and full or partial thickness. They cause severe dysfunction because of the pain. These are best diagnosed by magnetic resonance imaging and treated with analgesics, steroid injection, and exercise for the weakness that occurs with disuse. Surgical treatment is necessary if conservative management fails.

Parkinson's Disease

Definition and epidemiology. Parkinson's disease (PD) affects more than one-half million people in the United States older than age 50 and costs $20 billion annually (Swantek, 2002). It occurs in approximately 2% of those older than age 70. It is the most common cause of neurologic disability in people older than age 60 (Boss, 2002). PD is a progressive disease of the basal ganglia (corpus striatum) and involves the dopaminergic nigrostriatal pathway. This type of disorder produces a syndrome of abnormal movement called parkinsonism that leads to difficulty with mobility (Miller, 2002). PD is a clinical syndrome that consists of the following: bradykinesia (slow movement), resting tremor, cogwheel rigidity, impaired erect postural stability, and deficiency of the neurotransmitter dopamine. Box 13-10 lists symptoms of PD.

Pathophysiology. The pathogenesis is unknown. Epidemiologic data suggest genetic, viral, and toxic causes. In more than one half of those with PD, atrophy and neuronal loss are found (Boss, 2002). The main feature is degeneration

Box 13-10 Primary Symptoms of Parkinson's Disease (PD)

Resting Tremor
- Occurs in approximately 50% to 75% of all PD patients and is often the initial symptom
- Affects mainly hands and feet but may also involve the head, neck, face, lips, tongue, or jaw
- Appears regular and rhythmic; approximately four to six beats per second

Rigidity
- Sustained muscle contractions; often mistaken for common stiffness or achiness
- Walking with arms held stiffly at the sides (rather than swinging naturally)
- Most common types include
  - Cogwheeling: muscles move in a series of short jerks
  - Lead-pipe: muscles move smoothly, yet stiffly
- May affect breathing, eating, swallowing, and speech

Bradykinesia—Slow (*brady*) movement (*kinesia*)
- Slowing of ordinary movements, such as walking, sitting down, and getting dressed
- Reduction in semiautomatic gestures, such as crossing the legs or scratching
- Reduction of spontaneous facial movements, resulting in masklike stare
- Handwriting begins large and becomes smaller as patient fatigues
- Voice may become soft and trail off

Postural Instability
- Difficulty maintaining balance when walking or standing
- Leans forward in an effort to maintain center of gravity
- May result in injuries from frequent falls

From The American Parkinson Disease Association, Inc., 60 Bay Street, Staten Island, NY 10301.

of the neurons of the substantia nigra. Lewy bodies and intracytoplasmic eosinophilic inclusions are found in those neurons remaining in the substantia nigra. The severity of PD is associated with the degree of neuron loss and the reduction of dopamine receptors in the basal ganglia.

Clinical signs. Symptoms occur after 60% to 80% of nigral neurons are lost. Classic signs of PD are (1) tremor at rest, (2) rigidity (stiff muscles), (3) akinesia (poverty of movement), and (4) postural abnormalities. PD has such an insidious onset that it is very difficult to diagnose. In the early stages, senses, mental status, and reflexes are normal (Boss, 2002). The most conspicuous sign is the tremor, an asymmetric, regular, rhythmic, low-amplitude tremor. It disappears briefly during voluntary movement. It can occur in the leg, but the arm is more commonly involved. Rarely is the head involved. All tremors are increased with stress and anxiety. Tremor is a minor part of the clinical picture. It is not present during sleep, and when present, is a pill-rolling movement. A greater cause of disability is the rigidity and slow movements and postural instability. Other signs include soft-spoken voice, a whisper, little facial animation, infrequent blinking, restless legs, and greasy skin (Miller, 2002). The gait is called *festination* and consists of very short steps and minimal arm movements. Turning is difficult and may require many steps. If off balance, correction is very slow so that falls are common. Other clinical signs include sleep difficulties (up at night, sleeping all day), constipation, fatigue, excessive salivation, loss of smell, visual disturbances, psychosis, seborrhea, sweating, and hypotension, which is a considerable problem in PD and with the medications used to treat PD.

Rigidity impedes passive and active movement. It is a state of involuntary contraction of all skeletal muscles. There may be severe muscle cramps in the toes or hands. On examination, a limb may exhibit "lead pipe" resistance during passive movement. The most crippling symptom is akinesia and is often overlooked. All of the striated muscles in the extremities, trunk, ocular area, and face are affected, including the muscles of mastication (chewing), deglutition (swallowing), and articulation. Micrographia (small handwriting) is present. Akinesia produces a feeling of being "wooden" and causes rapid fatigue. The symptom of akinesia is bradykinesia (slow movement). The elder with PD will sit for long periods of time, or lie motionless with few shifts in position. The patient has difficulty initiating movement. "Freezing" is a common problem and may be precipitated by trying to move, turning, or initiating tactile and visual contact.

There is a loss of postural reflexes. The elder will have involuntary flexion of the head and neck, a stooped posture, and a tendency to fall backward.

Management. Typically, individuals are maintained on a combination of carbidopa and levodopa (Sinemet), which are dopamine precursors. Sinemet loses effectiveness as the amino acid L-dopa competes with other amino acids for absorption at both the intestinal wall and the blood-brain barrier. Restricting dietary protein is sometimes effective. Other medications useful in management include the dopamine agonists pergolide, bromocriptine, cabergoline, lisuride, pramipexole, ropinirole, and apomorphine (Swantek, 2002). Inhibitors and anticholinergics used for management include tolcapone, entacapone, deprenyl, trihexyphenidyl, and benztropine mesylate (Cogentin). Amantadine (Symmetrel) is often used. The medications used to treat PD are not without serious side effects. Hypotension is a problem, as are dyskinesias, dystonia, end-of-dose deterioration, and the on-off phenomenon. Medications also cause hallucinations, as does PD. The Parkinson's Disease Foundation and these authors warn that patients with PD *must* be maintained on their medication even during acute illness because if they are deprived of their antiparkinsonian medication, they can die within days. There is a trial at this time using a skin patch to treat PD (Kieburtz, 2002). The study is using a new drug, rotigotine, that is experimental and not yet available to patients.

Depression must be managed in elders with PD. Currently, selective serotonin reuptake inhibitors (SSRIs) such as venlafaxine are used. Buproprion, sertraline, paroxetine, trazodone, and mirtazapine are also used. Antipsychotics that may be required should be those with the least anticholinergic effects. Clozapine is probably best but has serious side effects in the bone marrow, requiring frequent laboratory testing (Swantek, 2002).

Exercise and balance work needs to begin early in the course of PD. Later, the elder becomes weaker and less responsive to medications, and each illness that occurs further weakens the individual, so that a backward trend begins. Early in PD, patients may continue to live at home and need care from a spouse or helping other. Late in PD, the elder is completely debilitated and may have no ability to do any ADLs and require an immense amount of care. Further, many late-stage patients have a Lewy-body dementia that often accompanies PD, and nursing home placement must be considered.

Because of the slow progression of the disease, with increasing disability over 20 to 25 years, individuals experience a change in role, activities, and social participation. The expressionless face, slowed movement, and soft, monotone speech may give the impression of apathy, depression, and disinterest and discourage others who might otherwise be social. A sensitive nurse is aware that the visible symptoms produce an undesired facade that may hide an alert, intelligent, and responsive individual who wishes to interact and generate interest. Persons with PD experience great functional problems in mobility, communication, and ADLs. Suggestions for coping with symptoms of PD include:

1. Movement of the limbs decreases the tremors; when walking, swing the arms.
2. Holding an object helps control the tremors; have the patient hold something in his or her hands when sitting quietly.
3. Skin must be kept dry and clean and oil-free lotion applied to avoid seborrhea and skin breakdown; air mattresses and sheepskins are advisable for beds and chairs.
4. Constipation may be avoided by high fluid intake, a high-residue diet, and exercise (as much as the elder is willing and able to do).
5. Speaking and reading aloud should be encouraged to enhance communication; sometimes speech therapy is warranted.
6. Depression, which is common with PD, and low self-esteem may be partially countered by direct discussion of feelings about changes in self-image, sexuality, and functional ability.
7. Support system encouragement and information about the disease are essential if the family is to cope with the slow responses, clumsiness, and poor communication of the afflicted individual.
8. Self-help groups are often helpful, because the members solve their problems collectively.

The Sickness Impact Profile (SIP) is a useful tool that can be used by nurses to determine problems most troublesome from the client's perspective (Table 13-4).

General Interventions to Manage Gait and Balance Disorders

A thorough physical and medication review is essential to identify, describe, and assess causes of gait and balance disorders. The physical examination must include vision, blood pressure, range of motion, muscle strength, balance, posture, podiatric examination, and neurologic and cognitive assessment.

Exercise produces improvements in gait and balance. Older persons actively engaged in exercise develop strength in lower limbs, faster walking pace, longer strides, and improved ankle dorsiflexion strength. Exercise can also benefit individuals with arthritis, increase bone density in osteopenia, and enhance cognitive function. The interventional issue is not only to "educate" the individual but also to identify ways to motivate the elderly to routinely exercise in a manner designed to facilitate health. We must remember that the very problems exercise may affect are the ones that may cause the individual to avoid participation: lack of strength, fear of falling, and lethargy. Creating security and confidence in movement includes encouraging the elder to employ the following strategies:

1. Participating in home exercise programs
2. Wearing carefully fitted, low-heeled, rubber-soled shoes
3. Walking with a companion on smooth ground as a form of exercise and muscle strengthening
4. Asking bystanders for help in navigating high curbs or other hazards to walking
5. Participating in gait training
6. Remembering good posture
7. Evaluating and modifying home hazards

Care of the Feet. Care of the feet is an important aspect of mobility, comfort, and a stable gait and one that is often neglected. Some aged persons in the hospital have been unable to walk comfortably, or at all, because of neglect of corns, bunions, and overgrown nails. Other causes of problems may be traced to loss of fat cushioning and resilience with aging, ill-fitting shoes, poor arch support, excessively repetitious weight-bearing activities, obesity, or uneven distribution of weight on foot. As many as 35% of persons living at home may have significant foot disability that goes untended. The following are common disorders:

1. Arthritic foot disorders resulting from rheumatoid arthritis, osteoarthritis, and gout
2. Atrophy of the plantar pad that leads to loss of shock absorption and metatarsalgia with increased difficulty in walking
3. Onychogryphosis, or overgrown, clawlike toenails that cause walking pain, immobility, and falls
4. Corns that cause pain and may reduce mobility

Table 13-4 Items in the Sickness Impact Profile (SIP) Endorsed by a Third or More of Patients with Parkinson's Disease*

SIP category	SIP item	Percent (no.) of PD patients endorsing item	Percent (no.) of controls endorsing item
Ambulation	I walk more slowly.	59 (26)	30 (13)
Body care and movement	I move my hands or fingers with some limitation or difficulty.	39 (17)	11 (5)
	I dress myself, but do so very slowly.	46 (20)	9 (4)
Mobility	I stay home most of the time	50 (22)	7 (3)
Emotional behavior	I act nervous or restless.	43 (20)	30 (13)
Social interaction	I am going out less to visit people.	50 (22)	14 (6)
	I am doing fewer social activities with groups of people.	50 (22)	27 (12)
	My sexual activity is decreased.	61 (27)	16 (7)
Alertness behavior	I have more minor accidents, drop things, trip and fall, bump into things.	46 (20)	14 (6)
	I forget a lot, for example, things that happened recently, where I put things, appointments.	36 (16)	25 (11)
Communication	I am having trouble writing or typing.	75 (33)	14 (6)
	I often lose control of my voice when I talk, for example, my voice gets louder or softer, trembles, changes unexpectedly.	41 (18)	2 (1)
	I do not speak clearly when I am under stress.	52 (23)	5 (2)
Sleep and rest	I sit during much of the day.	41 (18)	27 (12)
	I lie down more often during the day in order to rest.	34 (15)	16 (7)
	I sleep less at night, for example, wake up too early, don't fall asleep for a long time, awaken frequently.	46 (20)	25 (11)
Home management	I do work around the house only for short periods of time or rest often.	41 (26)	23 (10)
	I am doing *less* of the regular daily work around the house than I would usually do.	59 (26)	25 (11)
	I am not doing *any* of the maintenance or repair work that I would usually do in my home or yard.	39 (17)	11 (5)
	I have difficulty doing handwork, for example, turning faucets, using kitchen gadgets, sewing, carpentry.	39 (17)	9 (4)
	I am not doing heavy work around the house.	48 (21)	23 (10)
Recreation and pastimes	I do my hobbies and recreation for shorter periods of time.	43 (19)	18 (8)
	I am going out for entertainment less often.	43 (19)	32 (14)
	I am cutting down on *some* of my usual physical recreation or activities.	46 (20)	30 (13)

*Patients are instructed to endorse those items that apply to themselves and are related to their health.

5. Hallux valgus that may cause little difficulty unless ulceration or bursitis sets in
6. Foot surgery, which may give rise to severe walking difficulty for several months

Do not do the following after surgery for fractured hip or foot:

1. Turn toes in
2. Bend over too far
3. Cross legs when sitting
4. Lie on side in bed without a pillow between legs
5. Lean forward in bed
6. Forward flex when sitting up or down on a chair or toilet that is too low
7. Keep operated leg planted when turning
8. Have foot rest too high on wheelchair or chair
9. Cross foot of operated hip over the other leg

Falls and fractures often produce periods of immobility. The complications of immobility include the following:

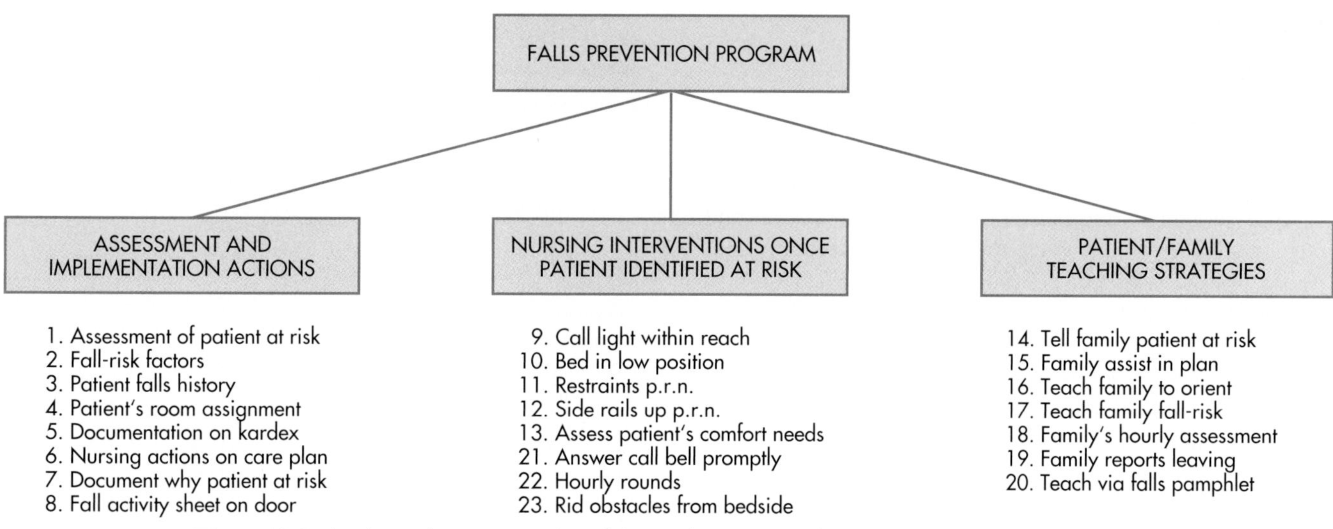

Figure 13-5. A schematic representation of the nursing measures in each major section of the patient falls prevention program. *Note:* The numbering of the interventions in this figure parallels the numbering of the nursing interventions in part A of the study instrument. (From Kaufmann M: *A patient falls prevention program—do nurses perceive it to be an effective intervention?* Unpublished master's thesis, Case Western Reserve University, Cleveland, OH, 1985.)

- Dehydration
- Bronchial pneumonia
- Contractures
- Constipation
- Pressure sores
- Hypothermia
- Iatrogenic complications
- Disability
- Institutionalization
- Loss of independence
- Isolation and depression

Repeated falls are a major precipitant to long-term care admission, and even in a protected setting 25% of these persons continue to fall.

Functional Restoration

Promoting functional restoration and maintenance is more beneficial to the elderly patient than applying restraints to prevent the risk of injury. We suggest the following considerations that have proved beneficial in reducing falls and increasing self-esteem among the fall-prone elderly:

1. Immediately on admission to the hospital conduct a fall assessment risk analysis and, if necessary, institute a fall prevention program.
2. Analyze the effectiveness of each intervention in the fall prevention program. Determine whether the interventions are primarily for the protection of the patient or the institution.
3. Institute a written policy regarding the management of the fall-prone client. Discuss the policy regarding the use of restraints with the family, client, doctor, and nursing staff. Document the conversation regarding the wishes of the family and the client. This must be signed by the family and the client.
4. Purchase beds that are as low to the floor as possible; possibly invent beds that are safe.
5. Increase muscle strength through carefully designed exercise programs.
6. Recognize and reduce fatigue factors.
7. Teach walking exercises in which the client learns to lift up the feet rather than shuffling them.
8. Provide appropriate shoes and slippers that have nonskid soles and broad heels of a height comfortable to the individual.

Prerequisite to a fall prevention program is a thorough assessment of persons who have fallen, including a detailed history and physical examination and assessment of risk of falling (Figure 13-5).

RESTRAINTS

Restraints have been used historically for the "protection" of the client and for security of the client and the staff.

Physical and Chemical Restraints

Stilwell's (1988) definition of physical restraints was developed as a part of her investigations as an expert witness and remains the clearest and most inclusive. Physical restraints are devices, materials, and equipment that (1) are attached to or are adjacent to the patient's body; (2) prevent free bodily movement to a position of choice (standing, walking, lying, turning, sitting); and (3) cannot be controlled or easily removed by the patient. Temporary immobilization of a part of the body for the purpose of treatment, such as casts, splints, and arm boards, is not included in this definition.

The problems of restraint usage were first brought to the forefront of nursing attention by a request from Doris Schwartz, one of the pioneer gerontic nurses, for information from practicing nurses regarding their observations and concerns about restraint usage. In the intervening time, and largely through efforts of her friends and herself, the use of restraints has been drastically reduced (Evans and Strumpf, 1989).

Early studies (Tinetti, 1989; Tinetti et al, 1990, 1991, 1992) clearly have shown that mechanical restraints are associated with serious injuries, such as higher mortality rates, injurious falls, longer hospital stays, nosocomial infections, incontinence, immobility and contractures, and decubitus ulcers (pressure sores). Characteristics of those who were restrained included the following: older, disoriented, dependent for help with dressing, unsteady, disruptive, agitated, and wanderers. Those who were restrained most frequently seemed to have higher levels of need and interactional desires. When unrestrained, they used fewer antidepressants and participated to a greater extent in social activities. It may be that the quiet, noninvolved, nondemanding patients are simply restrained less frequently. The difference in personality types and activity levels is an area needing further nursing research. Factors that increase the likelihood of restraint application are cognitive impairment, severe limitation in ADLs, depression, wandering, and dementias.

Rather than augmenting patient care, restraints often increase agitation and attempts to free oneself from uncomfortable catheters, tubes, and lines. Strumpf and Evans (1988), leaders in the move to untie elderly patients, found that restrained elders responded with anger, fear, humiliation, demoralization, discomfort, and resignation. Even though physical restraints are used to prevent falls, patients who are restrained are more likely to be injured than those who are not. Reports of deaths as a result of restraints emphasized the fact that restraints were not safe.

Many nurses believe that the use of restraints is directly related to a lack of sufficient personnel, and they must be used to prevent falls, injuries, and wandering. However, with the restrictions on restraint usage dictated by the Omnibus Budget Reconciliation Act (OBRA), the reliance on them has been markedly reduced, and other safety measures have proved more effective.

Chemical restraints have come under careful scrutiny, legal and ethical, in recent years. This is the misuse of psychotropic medications and can be considered a potential form of elder abuse (Scott and Guccione, 2001) since OBRA expanded the rights of long-term care residents. Drugs most involved as chemical restraints are antipsychotics, antianxiety drugs, minor tranquilizers, sedatives, hypnotics, and antidepressants. Inappropriate use is when chemical restraints are give under any of the following conditions (Tideiksaar, 1998):

- Given without specific indications
- Given in excessive doses affecting functioning
- Used as sole treatment without using behavioral interventions
- Administered at the convenience of staff

Electronic devices are available to alert nurses when an individual is attempting to get out of bed; these are becoming much more frequently used as human rights are more rigidly enforced. Nursing skills are often needed far more than restraints or electronic devices. Communication and creative planning can reduce the anxiety and agitation in the client. Questions the nurse needs to address include the following: What is frightening the patient? Is there anything in the environment that is familiar to provide security for the client? Is the client cognitively impaired? Is the client isolated, or can contact with the environment be more constant? Information given in measured quantities and frequent brief interactions may reduce the anxiety and agitation to manageable levels.

Some alternatives to restraint use are enumerated in Table 13-5. The methods are limited only by the creativity of the nurse. When the safety and agitation of the client cannot be managed with any known methods, it is the nurse's obligation to insist that the family or facility engage a sitter or companion for the individual.

In the past, the quality of nursing care and specific requirements for facilitating individual mobility of the aged in long-term care was a concern mainly of a few enlightened nurses and administrators. Today, OBRA, the National League for

Table 13-5 Alternatives to Restraint Use

Type of method used	Chronic	Acute
Pain relief	34%	54%
Other comfort measures (e.g., repositioning)	69%	71%
Reality orientation	62%	86%
Pet therapy	3%	0%
Music therapy	36%	14%
Therapeutic touch	31%	11%
Reminiscence	24%	3%
Behavior modification	66%	26%
Companionship	55%	60%
Crafts	21%	6%
Active listening	34%	26%
Clear pathways	31%	11%
Increased lighting	21%	43%
Placement of patient near nursing station	86%	80%
Beds lower to floor	21%	43%
Accessible call light	66%	29%
Regular routine	52%	31%
Defusing agitated behavior	66%	29%
Diversional activities	62%	46%
One-on-one supervision	69%	69%
Other	14%	0%

From Bryant H, Fernald L: Nursing knowledge and use of restraint alternatives: acute and chronic care, *Geriatr Nurs* 18(2):57, 1997.

Box 13-11 Statements on Use of Restraints and Abuse

The resident has the right to be free from any physical or chemical restraints imposed for purposes of discipline or convenience, and not required to treat the resident's medical symptoms. The resident has the right to be free from verbal, sexual, physical, and mental abuse, corporal punishment, and involuntary seclusion.

The facility must develop and implement written policies and procedures that prohibit mistreatment, neglect, and abuse of residents.

The facility must ensure that the resident environment remains as free of accidental hazards as is possible, and that each resident receives adequate supervision and assistance devices to prevent accidents.

From *Federal Register* (V56187), Step 26, 1991, p. 48825.

Nursing, and the Joint Commission on Accreditation of Healthcare Organizations all have specific requirements by which outcome criteria and goal achievement can be measured. No longer can facilities be casual about the requirements of OBRA and the accrediting bodies. There has been a proliferation of materials related to the development of measurable outcomes. All long-term care facilities must comply with statements from the *Federal Register* (1991) that relate to restraints and abuse in order to receive Medicare licensure (Box 13-11).

Environmental Restraints

Intentional environmental impediments may be effective in limiting movement and in some cases may avoid the more devastating alternative of applying physical restraints. Doors may be locked, or chairs may be difficult to rise from. These effectively limit individual movement.

In institutions it is sometimes deemed easier to encourage the use of a wheelchair or "geri-chair" than to modify the environment to increase safety and reduce hazards. Hiding an individual's clothing to prevent venturing away or wandering aimlessly is an infringement on personal rights and is often an unsuccessful deterrent. Recognizing the impact on self-esteem when one is discouraged from the use of maximum capacities should alert the caregiver to provide the aged with more opportunities for independence. If the individual decides to conserve energy by using a wheelchair, it must be a personal decision rather than one imposed for the convenience of others. Attending to individual desire and capacity is a message of affirmation to one who may feel an impending loss of independence in many spheres.

Environmental barriers often discourage ambulation among persons in various settings. In the outer environment, steps and curbs may be too high. Buses, subway trains, elevators, revolving doors, and escalators may move too rapidly for the slow-moving elderly person to enter and exit comfortably. Thus the individual may find the interactional world gradually shrinking because of factors that are unintentional. Fortunately, in the last two decades there has been a concerted effort by government to encourage the elimination of environmental barriers for the disabled, and this has had a beneficial effect on the elderly as they negotiate the environment.

Wanderers. Wandering is one of the most difficult management problems encountered in institutional settings. Each year some residents wander away from a facility and are later found injured or dead. Media attention and litigation may suggest that staff has been lax in allowing this to happen. Some elders are obsessed with the thought of leaving a facility.

Ambulation, in and of itself, is necessary, and sufficient opportunities to do so in areas that are not hazardous are necessary in institutional settings. Individuals whose lifestyle has included great amounts of ambulation are particularly in need of opportunities to continue this behavior. The rate or amount of ambulation may seem excessive, but if it is not inherently dangerous, it should be allowed without interference. The pattern and route of ambulation, as well as the point at which it terminates, are significant. There are many possible patterns and causes for wandering behavior. Some of the most predominant include the following:

- Akathisia-induced ambulation, which is usually a result of long-term use of neuroleptics and is associated with other signs of akathisia, such as inability to sit still, repetitive movements, and other extrapyramidal symptoms. Antiparkinsonian medication may reduce motor restlessness. Usually these persons will not do anything dangerous if made aware of the hazards.
- Self-stimulatory behavior that takes the form of ambulation. This is often seen in advanced dementia and is associated with other stereotyped actions, such as furniture rubbing, hand clapping, and repetitive vocalizations. Little has been done to deal effectively with stereotypy—the persistent, inappropriate mechanical repetition of actions or verbalizations. These may be a form of self-stimulation in the absence of stimulation that is more meaningful. Providing other forms of stimulation such as paper, cloth, or stuffed toys to manipulate may reduce the meaningless repetitive behavior. Continuous self-stimulation may indicate a lack of external sensory stimulation in the environment.
- Modeling, which occurs when a severely demented client shadows an ambulator and will follow him or her everywhere. Engagement in other activities has proved useful to deter the shadowing.
- Exit-seeking behavior, most often exhibited in recently admitted patients on locked wards. The behavior is accompanied by statements reflecting a desire to go home. Distracting activities may be temporarily useful. Exit-seeking behavior is highly motivated and may persist until the individual finds some gratifications in the present environment that reduce the desire to leave. It may be useful to bring some significant items from the home to help the

individual feel more comfortable in the unfamiliar setting. It is important for the nurse to determine how actively the individual was involved in the decision to move to the institution and whether there was adequate orientation to the move.

The first two of these are secondary forms of wandering that are not motivated by the primary desire to move about and are, in fact, evidence of neurologic or cognitive disorders. The interruption of these behaviors may cause more distress for the client and is usually not necessary. When any behavior is negated or discouraged, it is important to provide something to take its place. It is most productive to modify the environment so that the wandering is not likely to be hazardous.

For example, in one facility it was noted that a client always tended to walk out of her room and turn right, toward the exit. By recognizing this pattern and changing her room so that a right turn led her to the lounge area, her tendency to wander outside was abated. Past patterns undoubtedly had something to do with her penchant to make a right turn whenever leaving her room. We might assume that in her home the kitchen was to the right of her bedroom. Alert staff were able to realize this pattern and intervene effectively.

Stimulus for wandering arises from many internal and external sources. Many wanderers have a specific pattern that gives clues as to their needs. When the need is met, the wandering abates. Three psychosocial factors are correlated with types of wandering: previous work roles, lifelong patterns of coping with stress, and the search for security. Attention to the wanderer's nonverbal behavior, past coping strategies, and present mood is essential. Before attempting to manage wandering behavior, the nurse needs answers to the following questions:

What is being sought?

When does the behavior most frequently occur?

What would be done if the person were 20 years old instead of 80?

Is the present setting too restrictive?

How dangerous is the wandering?

What psychologic need or energy process causes the wandering?

Discussion of these questions with caregivers and the wanderer may help arrive at intervention that will diminish the need to search. The following interventions may be helpful:

- Care plans that include past coping styles and work orientation
- Memory training group sessions for wanderers
- Assistance to residents in building cognitive maps
- Interesting activity programs to meet varied needs
- Interpersonal contact with significant people
- Availability of items to meet basic needs (e.g., food, drinks, blanket)
- Activities that dissipate energy
- Continuity of personnel
- Group relationships and meetings to establish feelings of connection
- Established territory and cognitive maps
- Music, exercise groups, and dances to provide opportunities to move in an integrated manner
- Massage to reduce generalized tension
- Imagery exercises to take mental trips to places one enjoyed
- Nature walks outside the facility to provide relief from the institutional setting
- Visits to places of importance such as work sites and homes

Most important, on admission the patient and family should discuss the hazards of wandering versus the hazards of confinement and make a deliberate decision about when and if an individual should be restricted. Electronic ankle bracelets embedded in plastic, for comfort and ease of bathing, can be put on individuals who have been identified as "wanderers." These will activate alarms that are installed at exits. A lighted panel alerts staff to the exit one has crossed. This system allows others to enter and leave the facility at will and eliminates the need for locked exits. There are other electronic tracking devices that are being used to follow the wanderings of some individuals.

A particularly appealing method of dealing with the wandering patient is to form a buddy system with an individual who is willing and able to provide companionship for varying periods and can account for the patient's presence. This might increase the socialization of each, protect the wanderer, and enhance the ego of the "buddy." The "buddy" must not be coerced into such an arrangement. The "buddy" relationship may form spontaneously. Following this plan reinforces the nurse's interest in the patient's feelings and needs and may relieve distress. It seems that tone of voice and eye contact may provide sufficient focus, somewhat like a radar beam, that keeps an individual on course. Perhaps the personal attention filled the empty restlessness that activated the wanderer.

A wanderer's lounge was developed in a nursing home in Long Beach to provide beneficial activities for confused residents and respite for staff and the more alert residents who were annoyed by the intrusions of the wanderers (McGrowder-Lin and Bhatt, 1988). The lounge was made safe, and everything in it could be touched by the residents. Each day just before 3 PM, the time when these residents seem to become the most confused and agitated, a small group of 15 to 20 residents is taken to the designated area. The group members are introduced to each other daily and involved in simple exercises and activities. Refreshments are served. The program employs music, exercise, sensory stimulation, nourishment, and dancing each day. Activities vary from day to day and may include entertainers, poetry readings, sing-alongs, cosmetic sessions, and reminiscing. The program lasts for about 90 minutes.

An activity coordinator, a nursing assistant, and a registered nurse are involved in designing and administering the activities. The nurse evaluates the individual's ability and status during the program, the nursing assistant attends to individual problems such as aggression, and the activity director guides and leads the exercises. Staff members maintain positive attitudes and are not allowed to say "no." Residents are allowed to wander about during the planned activities and to do anything they wish that is not harmful to themselves or others. The observed benefits of this program have been increasing communication among the group members, fewer aggressive episodes, ability to eat finger foods without assistance, and improved nighttime sleep.

Nursing home residents who participated in a 3-week walking regimen outside the nursing home reported that they felt significantly less fatigued. It was suggested that regular outdoor walking programs be instituted as a standard intervention for all nursing home residents who are ambulatory, even if canes and walkers are necessary. In urban settings where traffic and crime may present special problems, internal courtyards may be created or special routes selected for elements of safety. It might also be possible to transport groups to more pleasant settings for walking. Staff accompaniment is usually necessary for the walking group, but in certain cases individuals may be encouraged to walk in pairs or small groups without staff accompaniment. Visitors can also be encouraged to take residents for walks outside a facility.

Reducing environmental hazards, keeping an individual moving about to increase endurance and function, and identifying persons most at risk of falling are methods that may be used to avoid accidents and falls and maintain mobility. Thoughtful, clear communication, creative planning, and nursing skills can obviate the need for restraints. Nurses in many settings are working together to solve the problems inherent in restraint use, but there is still much to be done.

MOBILITY AIDS

Assistive Devices

In ancient times the cane or staff was a symbol of authority. The caduceus is the one with which we are most familiar; it is the symbol of the Greek god Hermes and the Roman god Mercury. It conveys the authority and distinction of Caducifer's staff with the sacred serpents of wisdom entwined on it and is the emblem of the U.S. Army Medical Corps. In Victorian times a walking stick was essential to a gentleman's attire. Canes and walkers are now designed to be functional.

Ella had a lovely gnarled, hand-carved, and highly polished wooden walking stick. It was an assistive device, but because of its beauty it was much more. It represented her defense, her power, and her distinctive personality. It provided her security and independence.

Arthritic hips and knees cause considerable pain. To relieve the pressure, the use of a cane on the uninvolved side is helpful. When both sides are involved, a walker may relieve the pressure equilaterally. Many devices are available that are designed for specific benefits (Figure 13-6).

When helping someone select a walking assistance device, begin with correct shoes. In 1993 it was estimated that sales of walking devices, excluding special shoes, totaled $177 million. Marketers are always ready to sell. If you think your client could benefit by an assistive device, consult specialists and rehabilitation therapists. Physicians who are not specialists in orthopedic or physical medicine are not likely to be much help. Assist your client in obtaining a written prescription from the appropriate therapist because Medicare may cover up to 80% of the cost of the device if this is done; other insurance coverage is variable.

When the correct device is obtained, the client will need assistance in learning to use it correctly. This, again, should be taught by specialists in physical therapy. In general, the following principles should be observed:

- Move the assistance device first, then the weaker leg, and finally the stronger leg.
- Always wear low-heeled, nonskid shoes.
- When using a cane on stairs, step up with the stronger leg and down with the weaker leg. Use the cane as support when lifting the weaker leg. Bring the cane up to the step just reached before climbing another step. When descending, place the cane on the next step down, move the disabled leg down, and then move the good leg down.
- When using a walker, stand upright and lift the walker with both hands. Place all of its legs down at a comfortable distance. Step toward it with the weaker leg and then bring the stronger leg forward. Do not climb stairs with a walker.
- Every assistive device must be adjusted to individual height; the top of the cane should align with the crease of the wrist.
- Choose a size and shape of cane handle that fits comfortably in the palm; like a tight shoe, it will be a constant irritant if it is not properly fitted.
- Cane tips are most secure when they are flat at the bottom and have a series of rings. Replace tips frequently because they wear out and a worn tip is insecure.

Wheelchairs

Josie glides about the center in her motorized chair, forward and back, negotiating sharp turns, and all the time sitting straight, appearing totally at ease and quite regal. There is no hint of impairment in her bearing.

We have come a long way with assistive devices, but because of maldistribution and sparse budgets there are still places in which the old wooden wheelchairs can be found in use.

Wheelchairs are a necessary adjunct at some level of immobility. These can be used in a healthful way and without demeaning the individual. The various types of motorized chairs can be handled with ease and do not leave the impression of an individual encased in metal trappings. Some are quite attractive. There are frequently opportunities to buy them secondhand from those who no longer can use them.

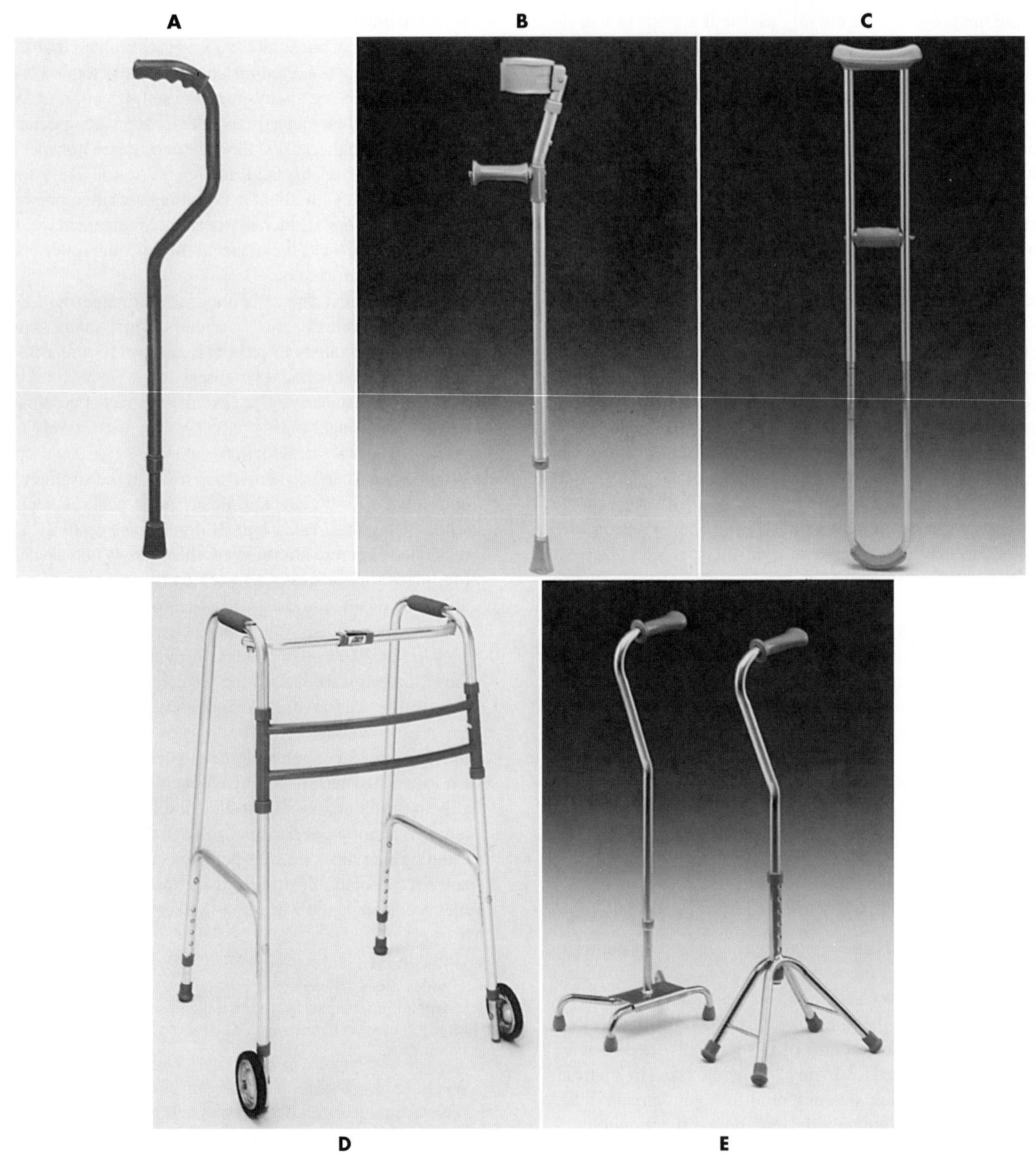

Figure 13-6. Assistive devices. **A,** Standard ortho cane with swan neck. **B,** A forearm crutch stabilizes your elbow while you walk. **C,** "Rolling crutch" provides smoother contact with the ground. **D,** Walker with front wheels allows constant contact with the ground. **E,** Quad cane offers more support than a single-stem walker. (Courtesy Lumex, Inc., New York.)

Transportation

Even though one is physically able to move about, there may be many hindrances to full use of public space. Available transportation is a critical link in the ability of the elderly to remain independent and functional. The lack of accessible transportation may contribute to other problems, such as social withdrawal, poor nutrition, or neglect of health care. Even when municipal transportation service is available, elders may not use it. Urban buses and subways not only are physically hazardous but are often dangerous. A "crisis in mobility" exists for many aged people because of the lack of an automobile, an inability to drive, limited access to public transportation, health factors, geographic location, and economic considerations. Older minority people may experience more difficulty getting around than older whites, and rural residents may experience more difficulty than urban residents. Add to that being female (increased poverty levels), and severe mobility problems exist.

Aged individuals may desire increased contact with other people, particularly relatives; however, even more crucial is the need to reach medical services, shopping areas, and service agencies. If mobility is hampered, both security and the sense of belonging to the mainstream of society may be blocked. The emphasis on a "barrier-free" (structurally revised) transportation system and reduced fares has been helpful to many aged, but some cannot avail themselves of public transportation because of physical disability or residence in a high-crime area. County, state, or federally subsidized transportation is being provided in certain areas to assist aged people in reaching social services, nutrition sites, health services, emergency care, medical care, recreational centers, mental health services, day care programs, physical and vocational rehabilitation, continuing education, and library services.

Although transportation can often be found for special needs, it is virtually impossible to locate transportation for pleasure or recreation. Nurses working with the aged find themselves in a dilemma. Interest and concern may suggest that we, acting as private citizens, provide transportation. Aside from liability considerations, this solution presents other problems. Small cars rarely have space for wheelchairs; access to buildings must be checked before an outing; and institutionalized aged may need permission from families, as well as administration. Finally, the aged should not need to depend on the available time of a few people of good will and compassion.

Some effective local transportation programs include the following services:

- Reduced fares
- Informal, volunteer drivers
- Demand-response transit vehicles
- Specially constructed vehicles for the handicapped
- Door-to-door minibuses requiring advance reservations
- Use of subsidized taxicab services
- Radio-equipped response vehicles
- Demand-response vehicles with a large pool of volunteer drivers (many of them aged)
- Dial-a-ride
- Charter bus trips to special events

The greatest problems in transportation still exist among the rural aged, and this deficit needs increased attention.

Automobiles and Older People

Driving is one of the instrumental activities of daily living for most elders because it is essential to obtaining necessary resources for those individuals who live in rural and suburban areas. Assessments of functional capacities often neglect this important activity. We should evaluate whether an individual can drive, feels safe driving, and has a driver's license.

Changes in vision, reaction time, and physical agility make driving hazardous for some elders. Accident rates have increased 43% for drivers 65 and older since 1980 (Sims and Ball, 2002). Further, automobile accidents are the leading cause of death from injury for those 65 to 74 years of age. Some of the problems that tend to precede driving cessation include visual deficits such as cataracts, glaucoma, and loss of peripheral vision; cognitive deficits; musculoskeletal problems such as low back pain, arthritis, bursitis, and foot problems; medications such as hypnotics, some antidepressants, sedating antihistamines, and alcohol; depression or psychosis; limited ability to walk; falls; and a diagnosis of cardiac or pulmonary disease, diabetes, Alzheimer's disease, stroke, or sleep apnea. Unfortunately, when judgment is impaired, the individual may believe and insist that he or she retains the capacities for safe driving even though objective assessment shows that this is not true. Giving up the mobility and independence afforded by driving one's own car has many psychologic ramifications, as well as inconveniences. With the rapid increase in the elderly population, this is clearly going to be a priority for intervention.

When Maury had a stroke, his doctor told him he could no longer drive. He had been an auto addict all of his adult life and found his major pleasures behind the wheel of the new car that he would buy each year. As a young man, having an auto was a major status symbol because few teenagers owned a car in 1935. Driving was much more than a means of transportation for him.

At this time it is often the physician who determines when an individual should no longer drive. In some states physicians are liable if they have allowed an individual to continue driving when it is dangerous. However, there are systematic and comprehensive performance-based road tests that can identify older drivers who are hazardous on the road. Sims and Ball (2002) report a new test, the Useful Field of View (UFOV) test, a measure of visual processing speed and attention that predicts driving competence, falls, and other measures of processing speed. The test is highly sensitive and specific and is a good predictor of crash incidence. (See Box 13-12 for a self-test of driving adequacy.)

Box 13-12 Driving Skills Quiz

If you answer yes to one or more of the following questions, you may want to limit your driving or take steps to improve a problem.

If you answer yes to most of the questions, it may be time to consider letting someone else do your driving for you.

The quiz is based in part on an American Association of Retired Persons publication.

- Does driving make you feel nervous or physically exhausted?
- Do you have difficulty seeing pedestrians, signs, and vehicles?
- Do cars frequently seem to appear from nowhere?
- At night, does the glare from oncoming headlights temporarily "blind" you?
- Do you find intersections confusing?
- Are you finding it harder to judge the distance between cars?
- Do you have difficulty coordinating your hand and foot movements?
- Are you slower than you used to be in reacting to dangerous situations?
- Do you sometimes get lost in familiar neighborhoods?
- Do other drivers often honk at you?
- Have you had an increased number of traffic violations, accidents, or near-accidents in the past year?

From Mayo Foundation for Medical Education and Research: Driving: how safe are you behind the wheel? *Mayo Clinic Health Letter* 14(7):7, 1996.

To the 10 million people over 65 years of age who drive automobiles, freedom and independence are equated with keeping a "clean" driving record and their driver's license. Some avoid freeways and take circuitous routes to reach their destination. Their concerns are realistic. Accidents involving the elderly increase insurance rates and are twice as likely to be fatal as compared with younger drivers. These considerations tend to make them overly cautious, which is often dangerous.

Most states require special testing before reissuing licenses to those over 70 years old. Some people have limited licenses that restrict driving to specific areas and distances. Good insurance coverage is imperative and can be obtained through the American Association of Retired Persons (AARP). AARP also provides a course, "55 Alive/Mature Driving," that is helpful and in some cases will qualify one for lower insurance rates.

The older person, if continuing to drive, should be advised to do the following: plan the route beforehand; bring someone to act as navigator when possible; allow plenty of room between cars; avoid night driving; wear hearing aids and glasses to augment sensory awareness; avoid driving under the influence of medications or alcohol; avoid driving in fog, heavy rain, snow, and ice; plan relief periods or relief drivers for long distances; and keep the car in good repair. These tips are particularly critical for older drivers.

In summary, the capacity to move about, on two legs, horses, and wheeled vehicles, has been portrayed from the earliest recorded time. The nurse can be significant in facilitating this most fundamental human need, to assist our patients to maintain independence, preserve autonomy, and move as far as their reach extends and as far as the imagination will allow.

Human Needs and Wellness Diagnoses

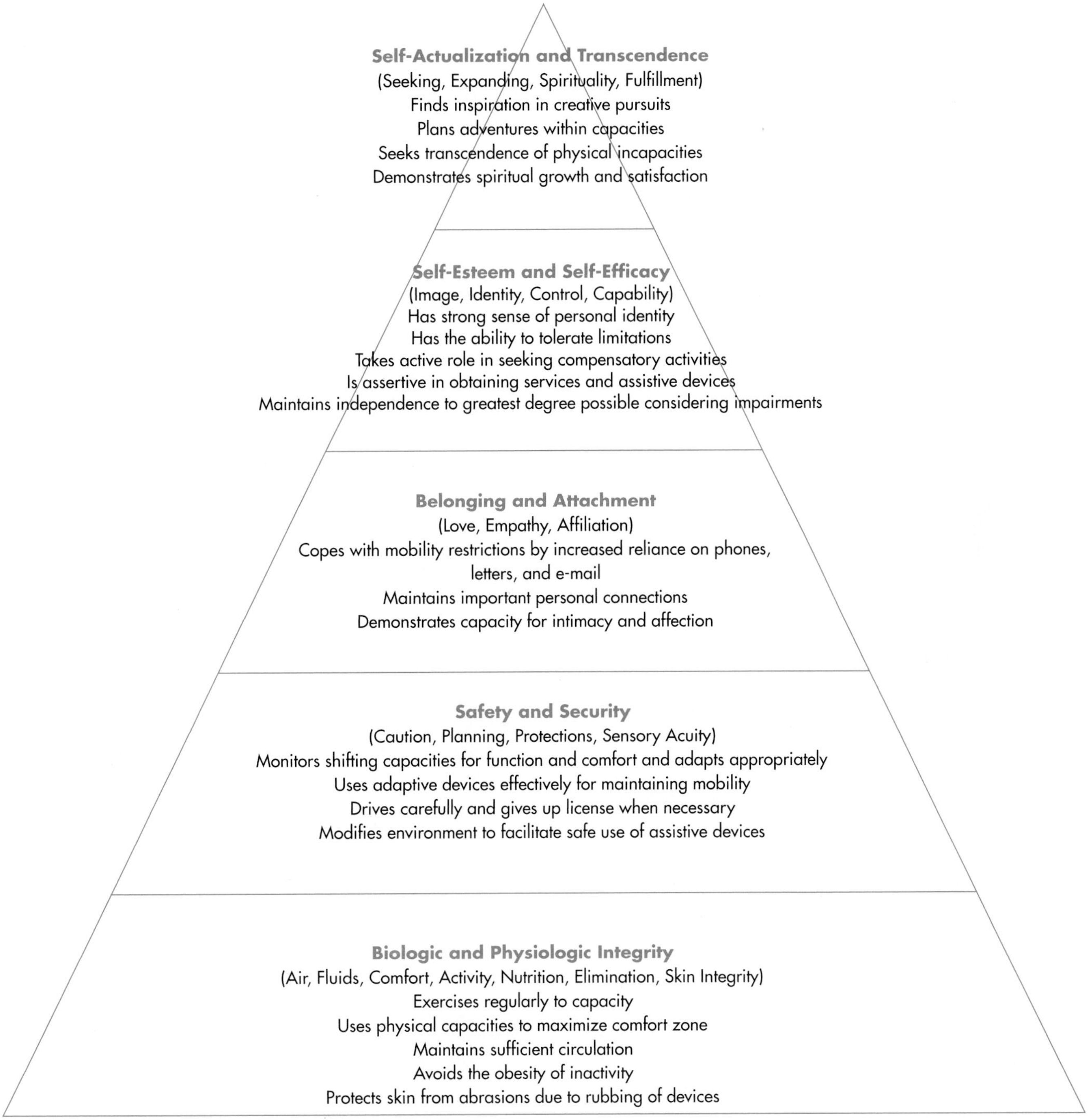

Self-Actualization and Transcendence
(Seeking, Expanding, Spirituality, Fulfillment)
Finds inspiration in creative pursuits
Plans adventures within capacities
Seeks transcendence of physical incapacities
Demonstrates spiritual growth and satisfaction

Self-Esteem and Self-Efficacy
(Image, Identity, Control, Capability)
Has strong sense of personal identity
Has the ability to tolerate limitations
Takes active role in seeking compensatory activities
Is assertive in obtaining services and assistive devices
Maintains independence to greatest degree possible considering impairments

Belonging and Attachment
(Love, Empathy, Affiliation)
Copes with mobility restrictions by increased reliance on phones, letters, and e-mail
Maintains important personal connections
Demonstrates capacity for intimacy and affection

Safety and Security
(Caution, Planning, Protections, Sensory Acuity)
Monitors shifting capacities for function and comfort and adapts appropriately
Uses adaptive devices effectively for maintaining mobility
Drives carefully and gives up license when necessary
Modifies environment to facilitate safe use of assistive devices

Biologic and Physiologic Integrity
(Air, Fluids, Comfort, Activity, Nutrition, Elimination, Skin Integrity)
Exercises regularly to capacity
Uses physical capacities to maximize comfort zone
Maintains sufficient circulation
Avoids the obesity of inactivity
Protects skin from abrasions due to rubbing of devices

These are not all the possible wellness diagnoses that may be identified. The above are examples of nursing diagnoses that should be considered when planning care for the older adult.

KEY CONCEPTS

- Mobility provides opportunities for exercise, exploration, and pleasure and is the crux of maintaining independence.
- Changes in bones, muscles, and ligaments affect one's balance and gait as one ages and increase instability.
- Ease of mobility is thought to be the most visible measure of one's overall health and survival capacity.
- Muscle weakness must be investigated because it is often a result of reversible problems such as endocrine imbalances, particularly hypothyroidism, or medication reactions.
- Gait disorders are often the obvious indexes of systemic problems and should be investigated thoroughly.
- A thorough nursing assessment must include descriptions of gait and mobility patterns.
- Prevention of falls is one of the most important proactive considerations to preserve health and function for the elderly.
- Each institutionalized individual should be assessed for fall risk factor to which one is exposed or inclined.
- Paradoxically, fear of falling and extreme caution actually increase falling propensity in the elderly.
- Physical restraints are to be used only under highly specific conditions, with a doctor's order, and for a very limited time until a better solution can be found. They are not appropriate for "safety" and are not allowed under OBRA guidelines except in highly specific situations.
- Elders who continue to drive may be tested more frequently and may be given restricted licenses.
- Transportation for the elderly is critical to their physical, psychologic, and social health.

▲ CASE STUDY

Osteoporosis

Maude was a small woman, barely 5 feet tall, weighed nearly 100 pounds, and was 73 years old. She had retired from a position as manager of the marketing department of a telephone company in a major U.S. city. She had been active socially and involved in numerous political causes and campaigns. She was known as a dynamo, often working 12 to 14 hours a day and so intensely involved she would forget to eat. During her menopausal years she blithely ignored the whole process and was only slightly aware of vasomotor instability (hot flashes). When her friends argued the pros and cons of estrogen therapy, she said that it was unnatural and she was not interested. And when discussing nutrition, she said, "Milk! You must be kidding—my diet is cigarettes and coffee." When she fell from a stool and braced herself with her right hand, her wrist swelled terribly but was not extremely painful. The bruise extended over the palm of her hand and up her forearm. After several days the pain increased and she went to see a doctor, a member of a preferred providers organization (PPO) of physicians to which she had belonged through her employment. She was very surprised to find that her wrist was broken. She had always climbed about and done whatever she wished with little concern for safety. When the physician casted her wrist, he told her she might have osteoporosis. She usually gave little thought to her physical status, but she began to worry about her bones. She knew that she could manage whatever came along, as she always had, but she wanted to know exactly what her future might hold in relation to osteoporosis and the possibility of broken bones. To reassure herself regarding the integrity of her bone structure, she called the PPO to schedule an evaluation. You are the advanced practice nurse that she will see initially to determine her need for follow-up.

Based on the case study, develop a nursing care plan using the following procedure:*

List comments of client that provide subjective data.

List information that provides objective data.

From these data identify and state, using accepted format, two nursing diagnoses you determine are most significant to this client at this time. List two client strengths that you have identified from data.

Determine and state outcome criteria for each diagnosis. These must reflect some alleviation of the problem identified in the nursing diagnosis and must be stated in concrete and measurable terms.

Plan and state one or more interventions for each diagnosed problem. Provide specific documentation of source used to determine appropriate intervention. Plan at least one intervention that incorporates the client's existing strengths.

Evaluate success of intervention. Interventions must correlate directly with the stated outcome criteria in order to measure the outcome success.

STUDY QUESTIONS/ACTIVITIES

What characteristics put one at risk for osteoporosis?

How would you evaluate Maude regarding risk of developing osteoporosis?

Discuss lifestyle changes that you would suggest to Maude.

What do you imagine her internist will do to determine her propensity for osteoporosis?

What ideally should have been done for Maude, or what should she have done for herself?

RESEARCH QUESTIONS

Compare the accuracy and expense of the various methods of measuring bone density.

What remedial measures have produced the best results in slowing or stopping bone deterioration?

What is the earliest age at which it is possible to detect bone resorption and to predict osteoporosis?

---

*Students are advised to refer to their nursing diagnosis text and identify possible or potential problems.

Has the incidence of osteoporosis decreased in particular geographic areas where fluorides have been added to drinking water?

Does the condition of dentition have any correlation with the condition of skeletal bones?

CASE STUDY

Rheumatoid Arthritis

Marilou is a devout Southern Baptist African American woman who developed rheumatoid arthritis in her early sixties. She learned to manage the pain fairly well, but as she neared 70 years old, the combination of rheumatoid arthritis and the "wear and tear" of osteoarthritis had created deformities and pain that restricted her movement considerably. She could no longer move her arms in positions above her chest, and her shoulders felt stiff. She found it difficult to twist jar lids and to open containers. It was particularly difficult to climb the stairs to her bedroom. Sometimes a soak in a hot tub, a heating pad, or ice packs would bring relief. She often prayed for relief and usually felt better afterward. She tried to keep active by walking her dog every morning, but she was becoming discouraged and depressed, and said, "It upsets me that I never know whether I'm going to have a good day or a bad day." She sometimes found herself tempted to try some of the "miracle cures" that she knew were probably fraudulent but seemed to offer some hope.

Based on the case study, develop a nursing care plan using the following procedure:*

List comments of Marilou that provide subjective data.

List information that provides objective data.

From these data identify and state, using accepted format, two nursing diagnoses you determine are most significant to this client at this time. List two client strengths that you have identified from data.

Determine and state outcome criteria for each diagnosis. These must reflect some alleviation of the problem identified in the nursing diagnosis and must be stated in concrete and measurable terms.

Plan and state one or more interventions for each diagnosed problem. Provide specific documentation of source used to determine appropriate intervention. Plan at least one intervention that incorporates the client's existing strengths.

Evaluate success of intervention. Interventions must correlate directly with the stated outcome criteria in order to measure the outcome success.

STUDY QUESTIONS/ACTIVITIES

Describe the differences between rheumatoid arthritis and osteoarthritis.

Discuss Marilou's lifestyle and beliefs as they may affect her arthritis. What are some of the modifications in her activities that might be useful? How would you incorporate her beliefs into a care plan?

Discuss the meanings and the thoughts triggered by the student's and elder's viewpoints expressed at the beginning of the chapter. How do these vary from your own experience?

RESEARCH QUESTIONS

What factors predispose one to osteoarthritic changes?

What types of alternative comfort measures are sought and used by sufferers of arthritis?

What do elders say reduces the discomfort of arthritis?

What aspects of arthritis cause most distress for elders?

What do demographic comparisons reveal about the geographic, gender, and age distribution of arthritis?

What is the potential for use of vaccines to prevent rheumatoid arthritis?

FURTHER STUDY QUESTIONS/ACTIVITIES

List all of the risk factors in your home that may contribute to falls.

Discuss psychosocial and physiologic issues that affect mobility.

List five hazards of immobility in old age and discuss the effects on an elder's health and function.

Spend 30 minutes in a shopping mall observing older individuals, and identify as many types of gait disorders and mobility assistive devices as possible.

Enumerate and discuss the reasons that falls increase in frequency as one ages.

What are some of the practical tips you would give an elder to prevent falls?

Discuss concerns you have about falling now. What do you think your concerns will be when you are 80 years old?

Discuss the reasons why restraints may be necessary to apply when you are caring for an aged person who is confused, is hospitalized, has a Foley catheter, and is receiving an intravenous infusion.

Discuss the reasons you would avoid applying restraints.

Identify several alternatives to restraint use.

Work with a partner and take turns restraining each other in a chair with soft restraints. Leave the restrained individual alone for 20 minutes, and after both have experienced this discuss your thoughts and feelings.

What are some of the ways that older individuals could be assisted to drive safely? What criteria would you use to deny an individual a driver's license?

FURTHER RESEARCH QUESTIONS

What types of gait disorders trigger falls and in what situations?

---

*Students are advised to refer to their nursing diagnosis text and identify possible or potential problems.

What activities and exercises are most useful in maintaining mobility in the aged?
What are the psychologic reactions of elders to the use of assistive devices for ambulation?
What factors in the institutional environment induce immobility?
What factors outside home and institution (in the community) are most hazardous for the mobility of elders? Where do the most falls occur?
How does a new environment affect mobility? Is there a higher incidence of falls in the first few weeks of adaptation to a new environment as compared with later?
How does obesity affect agility and mobility?
Does obesity predispose one to falling?
How often and in what circumstances are falls precipitated by the distractions or actions of another individual?
How effective are hip pads in reducing fractures?

REFERENCES

Agency for Healthcare Research and Quality: Managing osteoarthritis, helping the elderly maintain function and mobility, *Research in Action,* issue 4, 2002a. Available at *www.ahrq.gov/research/osteoria/osteoria.htm*

Agency for Healthcare Research and Quality: AHRQ research has improved OA management, 2002b. Available at *www.ahrq.gov/research/osteoria/osteoria.htm*

American College of Rheumatology: Recommendations for the medical management of OA of the hip and knee, *Arthritis Rheum* (Internet), 2000. Available at *www.rheumatology.org/research/guidelines/oa-mgr*

American College of Rheumatology: Guidelines for the management of rheumatoid arthritis, 2002 update, *Arthritis Rheum* 46(2):328, 2002.

American Geriatric Society: *Guideline for the prevention of falls in older persons,* May 2001, National Guideline Clearinghouse. Available at *www.american_geriatrics.org*

Arthritis Foundation: *Bursitis, tendonitis and other soft tissue rheumatic syndromes,* Atlanta, 1999, Arthritis Foundation.

Arthritis Foundation: *Osteoporosis,* Atlanta, 2000, Arthritis Foundation.

Arthritis Foundation: *Rheumatoid arthritis,* Atlanta, 2001, Arthritis Foundation.

Barbieri EB: Patient falls are not patient accidents, *J Gerol Nurs* 9(3):171, 1983.

Beers MH, Berkow R: *Merck manual of geriatrics,* ed 3, Whitehouse Station, NJ, 2000, Merck Research Laboratories.

Boss BJ: Alterations in neurologic function. In McCance KL, Huether SE, editors: *Pathophysiology: the biologic basis for disease in adults and children,* ed 4, St Louis, 2002, Mosby.

Brion PH, Concoff AL: Nonpharmacologic therapy of osteoarthritis, *UpToDate,* 2002. Available at *www.uptodate.com*

Bryant H, Fernald L: Nursing knowledge and use of restraint alternatives: acute and chronic care, *Geriatr Nurs* 18(2):57, 1997.

Callahan LF, Jonas BL: Arthritis. In Ham RJ, Sloane PD, Warshaw GA, editors: *Primary care geriatrics: a case-based approach,* ed 4, St Louis, 2002, Mosby.

Centers for Disease Control and Prevention: *A toolkit to prevent senior falls,* Atlanta, 1999, Centers for Disease Control and Prevention.

Coleman EA, Fox EP: Translating evidence-based geriatric care into practice: lessons from managed care organizations. Part II. Falls and medication-related complications, *Ann Long-Term Care* 10(10):42, 2002.

Concoff AL: Clinical manifestations of osteoarthritis, *UpToDate* 10(1), 2002. Available at *www.uptodate.com*

Craven R, Bruno P: Teach the elderly to prevent falls, *J Gerontol Nurs* 12(8):27, 1986.

Curry LC, Hogstel MO: Osteoporosis, *Am J Nurs* 102(1):26, 2002.

Davidson M, DeSimone ME: Osteoporosis update, *Clinician Reviews* 12(4):75, 2002.

Duncan P et al: Functional reach: predictive validity in a sample of elderly male veterans, *J Gerontol* 47(3):93, 1992.

Evans L, Strumpf N: Tying down the elderly: a review of literature on physical restraint, *J Am Geriatr Soc* 37:65, 1989.

Fauci AS: American College of Rheumatology guidelines for the medical management of OA of the hip and knee, *Harrison Online,* 2000. Available at *www.medscape.com/HOL/articles/2001/01/hol76/hol76.html*

Federal Register (V56187), p 48825, Sept 26, 1991.

Feldt KS: Increasing physical activity in frail, older adults: guidance for clinicians. Presentation. American Geriatrics Society 2002 Annual Scientific Meeting, May 8-12, 2002, Washington, DC.

Fife D, Solomon P, Stanton M: A risk/falls program: code orange for success, *Nurs Manage* 15(11):50, 1984.

Gornisiewicz M, Moreland LW: Rheumatoid arthritis. In Robbins L, editor: *Clinical care in the rheumatic diseases,* ed 2, Atlanta, 2001, Association of Rheumatology Health Professionals.

Grosch M: Bone-ing up on vitamin K, *Advance for Nurse Practitioners Online,* 2002. Available at *www.advancefornp.com/npfeature1.html*

Harris ST et al: Effect of combined risedronate and hormone replacement therapies on bone mineral density in postmenopausal women, *J Clin Endocrinol Metab* 86(5):1890, 2001.

Horstman J: Glucosamine: the truth about the talk. In *Arthritis today,* Atlanta, 2000, Arthritis Foundation.

Howe T, Oldham JA: Posture and balance. In Trew M, Everett T, editors: *Human movement,* ed 4, St Louis, 2001, Mosby.

Kalunian KC, Brion PH: Classification and diagnosis of osteoarthritis, *UpToDate* 10(1), 2002. Available at *www.uptodate.com*

Kaufmann M: *A patient falls prevention program—do nurses perceive it to be an effective intervention?* Unpublished master's thesis, Case Western Reserve University, Cleveland, OH, 1985.

Kieburtz K: Skin patch for PD proves effective in large study, *Grapevine* 17(1):9, 2002.

Lesley WS: Osteoporotic compression fractures and treatment with vertebroplasty. Available at *www.cyberounds.com/conferences/ge. . .rics/conferences/current/conference.html*

Lorig K, et al: Outcomes of self-help education for patients with arthritis, *Arthritis Rheum* 28:680, 1985.

Lozada CJ, Altman RD: Osteoarthritis. In Robbins L, editor: *Clinical care in the rheumatic diseases,* ed 2, Atlanta, 2001, Association of Rheumatology Health Professionals.

Luggen AS: Rheumatoid arthritis. In Luggen AS, Meiner S, editors: *Care of the older adult with arthritis,* New York, 2002, Springer.

Luggen AS: Management of arthritis in older adults, *Advance for Nurse Practitioners*, 2003.

Mahoney J: Immobility and falls, *Clin Geriatr Med* 14(4):699, 1998.
Maricic MJ: Osteoporosis. In Robbins L et al, editors: *Clinical care in the rheumatic diseases,* ed 2, Atlanta, 2001, Association of Rheumatology Health Professionals.
Mayo Foundation for Medical Education and Research: Driving: how safe are you behind the wheel? *Mayo Clinic Health Letter* 14(7):7, 1996.
McGrowder-Lin R, Bhatt A: A wanderer's lounge program for nursing home residents with Alzheimer's disease, *Gerontologist* 28(5):607, 1988.
Miller JQ: Parkinson's disease. In Ham RJ, Sloane PD, Warshaw GA, editors: *Primary care geriatrics: a case-based approach,* ed 4, St Louis, 2002, Mosby.
Neyhart B, Gibbs LM: Osteoporosis. In Ham RJ, Sloane PD, Warshaw GA, editors: *Primary care geriatrics: a case-based approach,* ed 4, St Louis, 2002, Mosby.
Panush RS: Complementary and alternative remedies in rheumatic disorders. *UpToDate,* 2002. Available at *www.uptodate.com*
Panush RS, Lane N: Exercise and the musculoskeletal system, *Gaillieres Clin Rheumatol* 8:79, 1994.
Petak SM: *Managing osteoporosis. Part 4. Update in client management,* Chicago, 2001, American Medical Association.
Province M: Effects of exercise on falls in elderly patients, a preplanned meta analysis of the FICST trials, *JAMA* 273(17):1341, 1995.
Reginato AM, Reginato AJ: Periarticular rheumatic diseases. In Robbins L, editor: *Clinical care in the rheumatic diseases,* ed 2, Atlanta, 2001, Association of Rheumatology Health Professionals.
Resnick B: Seven step approach to motivate older adults to exercise. Abstract of the American Geriatric Society 2002 Annual Scientific Meeting, May 8-12, 2002, Washington, DC.
Resnick B, Corcoran M, Spellbring AM: Gait and balance disorders. In Adelman AM, Daly MP, editors: *Twenty common problems in geriatrics,* New York, 2001, McGraw-Hill.
Reuben DB et al: *Geriatrics at your fingertips,* Malden, MA, 2002, American Geriatric Society/Blackwell.
Russell RM, Dawson-Hughes B: Nutrition and osteoporosis, 1999. Available at *www.cyberounds.com/conferences/nutrition/conferences/0199/conference.html*
Schneider DC, Mader SL: Falls. In Ham RJ, Sloane PD, Warshaw GA, editors: *Primary care geriatrics: a case-based approach,* ed 4, St Louis, 2002, Mosby.
Scott R, Guccione AA: Ethical and legal issues in geriatric physical therapy. In Guccione AA, editor: *Geriatric physical therapy,* ed 2, St Louis, 2001, Mosby.
Sims RV, Ball K: The older adult driver. In Ham RJ, Sloane PD, Warshaw GA, editors: *Primary care geriatrics: a case-based approach,* ed 4, St Louis, 2002, Mosby.
Stilwell E: Use of physical restraint on older adults, *J Gerontol Nurs* 14:42, 1988.
Strumpf NE, Evans LK: Physical restraint of the hospitalized elderly: perceptions of patients and nurses, *Nurs Res* 37(3):132, 1988.
Swantek SS: Medical comorbidities in older patients. American Association for Geriatric Psychiatry, 15th Annual Meeting. Available at *www.medscape.com/viewarticle/430712* (accessed June 27, 2002).
Thorndyke L: Osteoporosis. In Adelman AM, Daly MP, editors: *Twenty common problems in geriatrics,* New York, 2001, McGraw-Hill.
Tideiksaar R: *Falls in older adults,* Baltimore, 1998, Health Professions Press.
Tinetti M: Performance oriented assessment of mobility problems in elderly patients, *J Am Geriatr Soc* 34:199, 1986.
Tinetti M: Instability and falling in elderly patients, *Semin Neurol* 9(1):39, 1989.
Tinetti M et al: Risk factors for falls among elderly persons living in the community, *N Engl J Med* 319(26):1701, 1988.
Tinetti M et al: Falls efficacy as a measure of fear of falling, *J Gerontol* 45(6):239, 1990.
Tinetti M et al: Mechanical restraint use among residents of skilled nursing facilities: prevalence, patterns, and predictors, *JAMA* 265(4):468, 1991.
Tinetti M et al: Mechanical restraint use and fall related injuries among residents of SNFs, *Ann Intern Med* 116(5):369, 1992.
Tinetti M et al: Fear of falling and fall-related efficacy in relationship to functioning among community-living elders, *J Gerontol* 49(3):M140, 1994.
Van Doornum S, McGoll G, Wicks IP: Accelerated atherosclerosis: an extraarticular feature of rheumatoid arthritis? *Arthritis Rheum* 46(4):862, 2002.
Watts N: Pharmacologic therapy provides long-lasting fracture risk reduction in postmenopausal women with osteoporosis. Presentation at 2001 Annual Meeting of the Endocrine Society, August 2001.
Wright B, Aizenstein S: Behavioral diagnoses of an elderly nursing home population: how a multi-disciplinary team named behaviors, *Geriatr Nurs* 14(1):30, 1993.

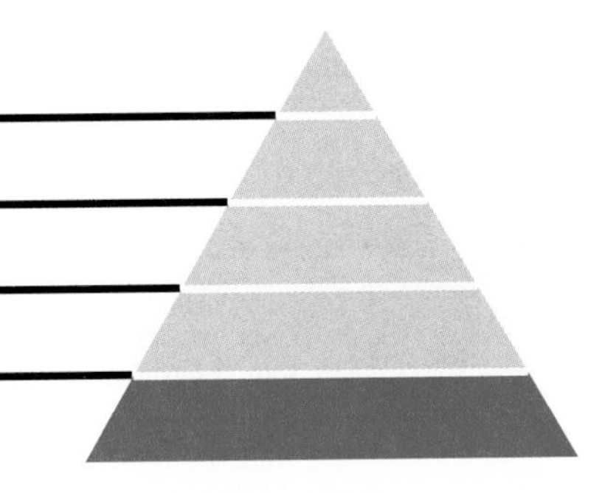

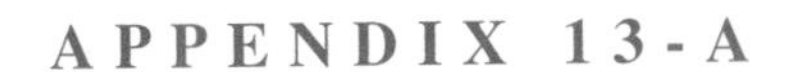

APPENDIX 13-A

Osteoporosis Functional Disability Questionnaire

The osteoporosis functional disability questionnaire was developed as a specific instrument to measure disability in several domains; feelings of adequacy, comfort, mood, activities of daily living, instrumental activities of daily living, and social activities. Self-evaluation of impairment (on a Likert scale 1-5 indicating frequency and/or severity of problems) provides information for designing and planning self-care and supportive activities.

Motivation and need for participation in therapeutic regiments and exercise programs is evaluated by the following indications:

Please indicate in degrees of 1 (good) to 5 (poor) your estimation of your general health aside from your osteoporosis ___________

Please indicate in degrees of 1 (no difficulty) to 5 (very difficult) any problems meeting your financial commitments in the following areas.

Housing ___________
Food ___________
Personal expenses ___________
Transportation ___________
Medical expenses ___________
Other ___________

Please indicate in degrees of 1 (least) through 5 (most) items below that are of most concern related to your osteoporosis.

Pain ___________
General health ___________
Appearance ___________
Interferes with social activities ___________
Interferes with work ___________
Other ___________

Mark in degrees of 1 (least) through 5 (most) the organizations or groups of importance to you that you are hindered from enjoying because of your osteoporosis.

Church ___________
Job related ___________
Recreational ___________
Fraternal ___________
Civic/political ___________
Other ___________

Indicate by numbers 1 (least) through 5 (most) the intensity/frequency of feelings you have experienced in the past week.

I was bothered by things that usually don't bother me. ___________
I did not feel like eating; my appetite was poor. ___________
I was unable to shake off the blues even with help from family and friends. ___________
I felt I was just as well off as other people. ___________
I had trouble keeping my mind on what I was doing. ___________
I felt depressed. ___________
I felt as if everything I did was an effort. ___________
I felt hopeful about the future. ___________
I thought my life had been a failure. ___________
I felt fearful. ___________
My sleep was restless. ___________
I was happy. ___________
I talked less than usual. ___________
I felt lonely. ___________
People were unfriendly. ___________
I enjoyed life. ___________
I had crying spells. ___________
I felt sad. ___________
I felt that people disliked me. ___________
I could not get going. ___________

Indicate by numbers 1 (unable) through 5 (independent) your ability to accomplish the following activities without assistance.

Get in and out of bed ___________
Use the toilet ___________
Bathe yourself ___________
Dress yourself ___________
Put on your shoes ___________
Cut your toenails ___________
Prepare light meals ___________
Prepare meals for family or entertainment ___________
Wash the dishes ___________
Do laundry ___________

Do light housework ___________
Do your vacuuming ___________
Do heavy housework ___________
Go shopping ___________
Go on social outings ___________
Walk around your house ___________
Climb stairs ___________
Walk down stairs ___________
Hold a book to read ___________
Walk outdoors for over 15 minutes ___________
Board a bus ___________
Drive an automobile ___________
Do gardening ___________
Bend down ___________
Reach overhead ___________
Sit down and get out of chair ___________

Ideally, this self-evaluation tool should be used before and after program interventions.

Modified from Helmes E et al: A questionnaire to evaluate disability in osteoporotic patients with vertebral compression fractures, *J Gerontol* 50A(2):M91, 1995.

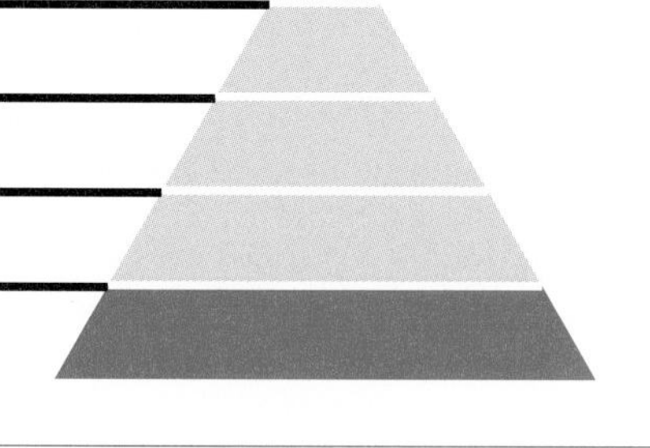

APPENDIX 13-B

Tinetti Balance and Gait Evaluation

Balance

Instructions: Subject is seated in a hard, armless chair. The following maneuvers are tested:

1. Sitting balance
   0 = Leans or slides in chair
   1 = Steady, safe
2. Arise
   0 = Unable without help
   1 = Able but uses arm to help
   2 = Able without use of arms
3. Attempts to arise
   0 = Unable without help
   1 = Able, but requires more than one attempt
   2 = Able to arise with one attempt
4. Immediate standing balance (first 5 seconds)
   0 = Unsteady (staggers, moves feet, marked trunk sway)
   1 = Steady but uses walker/cane or grabs other object for support
   2 = Steady without walker or cane or other support
5. Standing balance
   0 = Unsteady
   1 = Steady, but wide stance (medial heels > than 4″ apart) or uses cane/walker or other support
   2 = Narrow stance without support
6. Nudge (subject at maximum position with feet as close together as possible. Examiner pushes lightly on subject's sternum with palm of hand 3 times.)
   0 = Begins to fall
   1 = Staggers, grabs, but catches self
   2 = Steady
7. Eyes closed (at maximum position #6)
   0 = Unsteady
   1 = Steady
8. Turn 360°
   0 = Discontinuous steps
   1 = Continuous steps
   0 = Unsteady (grabs, staggers)
   1 = Steady
9. Sit down
   0 = Unsafe (misjudged distance falls into chair)
   1 = Uses arms or not a smooth motion
   2 = Safe, smooth motion

/16 BALANCE SCORE

Gait

Instructions: Subject stands with examiner. Walks down hallway or across room, first at his/her usual pace, then back at a "rapid but safe" pace (using usual walking aid such as cane/walker).

10. Initiation of gait (immediately after told "go")
    0 = Any hesitancy or multiple attempts to start
    1 = No hesitancy
11. Step length and height (right foot swing)
    0 = Does not pass L. stance foot with step
    1 = Passes L. stance foot
    0 = R. foot does not clear floor completely with step
    1 = R. foot completely clears floor
12. Step length and height (left foot swing)
    0 = Does not pass R. stance foot with step
    1 = Passes R. stance foot
    0 = L. foot does not clear floor completely with step
    1 = L. foot completely clears floor
13. Step symmetry
    0 = R. and L. step length not equal (estimate)
    1 = R. and L. step length appear equal
14. Step continuity
    0 = Stopping or discontinuity between steps
    1 = Steps appear continuous
15. Path (estimated in relation to floor tiles, 12 inches wide. Observe excursion of one foot over about 10 feet of course.)
    0 = Marked deviation
    1 = Mild/moderate deviation or uses a walking aid
    2 = Straight without walking aid
16. Trunk
    0 = Marked sway or uses walking aid
    1 = No sway but flexion of knees or back or spreads arms out while walking
    2 = No sway, no flexion, no use of arms and no walking aid
17. Walk stance
    0 = Heels apart
    1 = Heels almost touching while walking

/12 GAIT SCORE

/28 TOTAL MOBILITY SCORE (BALANCE AND GAIT)

From Brady R et al: Geriatric falls: prevention strategies for the staff, *J Gerontol Nurs* 19(9):26, 1993. Reprinted with permission, Mary Tinetti, M.D.

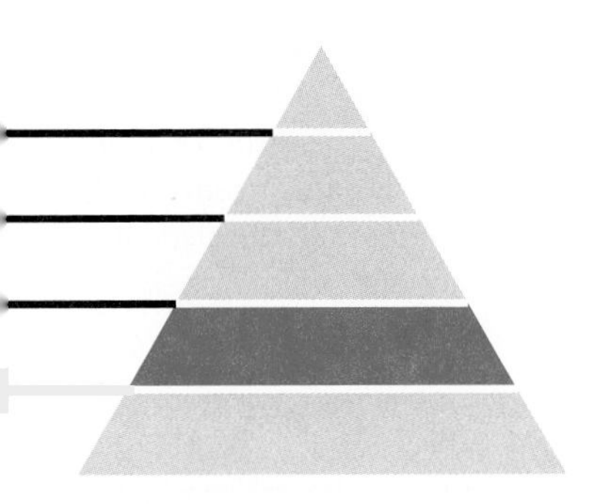

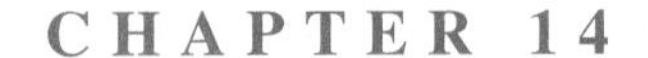

CHAPTER 14

Environmental Safety and Security

Barbara J. Holtzclaw

A student learns

My client during the community nursing experience decided to stay in her own home in spite of being barely able to shuffle around. The state gave a homemaker a small sum each month to provide a few hours of assistance on a daily basis. She had to rely on the goodwill of neighbors when the budget for those services was discontinued. She wants so much to remain in her own home. I worry about her but don't know what I should do.

Jennifer, age 24

An elder speaks

I have been in my home for 50 years and widowed for 25 of those 50. The upkeep on my home is expensive and my resources are limited. I'm hoping I can manage to remain here, but I need some modifications to make it safe and I really don't know how to go about getting assistance to make the necessary changes.

Esther, age 79

LEARNING OBJECTIVES

On completion of this chapter, the reader will be able to:

1. Identify interactions of intrapersonal, interpersonal, geographic, economic, and health factors that influence environmental safety and security for older adults.
2. Discuss the effects of declining health, reduced mobility, relocation, isolation, and unpredictable life situations on the older adult's perception of security.
3. Explain the underlying vulnerability of older adults to effects of extreme temperatures and identify actions to prevent and treat hypothermia and hyperthermia.
4. Define strategies and programs designed to prevent, detect, or alleviate crime, abuse, and neglect aimed at older persons.
5. Characterize factors, predictors, and protective strategies related to rising suicide rates among the elderly.

FEELING SECURE AS ONE AGES

Feeling secure in one's environment surpasses the need for physical safety and freedom from crime or violence. It involves sensing an identity with one's personally significant space, whether that is a home or a tiny cubicle in a care facility. Feelings of security as one ages also depend on the perceived familiarity and predictability of the life-space in which one moves or interacts. The idea of having personal items brought in to make a new location "one's own" is an effort to restore identity and mark one's personal space. Reminiscence therapy is sometimes an effective approach to restoring a connection to the familiar and reducing feelings of isolation for older adults in a new day care or residential community (Pittiglio, 2000). Anxiety and insecurity increase when situations and conditions become unpredictable, whether they are geographic, economic, health, or time related. In addition, these perceptions induce stress-related responses or agitation that can threaten comfort and quality of life. Perceptions of security and feeling safe are strongly influenced by cognitive capabilities and ability to problem solve. Even simple forgetting tends to make a person feel less confident in carrying out daily tasks. Nurses can encourage older persons to participate in steps to organize their environment, use reminders and calendars to gain greater control over time, and create simple maps to outline the "territory" in which they expect to move. Promoting feelings of environmental security in persons with dementia is a more complex challenge because as memory fades one's sense of identity, as well as location, becomes fragmented. Authorities suggest that heightened feelings of fear, insecurity, and inconsolable loss often underpin disruptive behaviors (Woods, 2001). These dynamics are discussed further in Chapter 23. Helping caregivers, both professional and family, understand that these dynamics may redirect interventions aimed at behavioral outbursts toward those promoting comfort and feelings of safety. Efforts to preserve privacy and periphery in one's personal space will help restore pattern, order, and environmental predictability. This, in turn, will promote feelings of safety and security.

INFLUENCES OF CHANGING HEALTH AND DISABILITY ON SAFETY AND SECURITY

Physical Vulnerability

Vulnerability to environmental risks and mistreatment by others increases as people become less physically or cognitively able to recognize or cope with real or potential hazards. Aging itself does not necessarily bring about failing health or disease, yet some physical changes can be anticipated in all body systems. These changes occur at varying rates among older people and are dependent on genetic, immunologic, and general systemic health factors. Older adults are able to learn about these changes and take precautions to avoid risks of unsafe behaviors and situations. Many healthy older adults are also able to share responsibility for maintaining a healthy lifestyle that includes exercise, adequate nutrition and hydration, avoidance of temperature extremes, reduction of environmental hazards, and protection from crime and violence. In teaching about risk reduction, it is important to emphasize the strong influence of stress, whether it is physical, emotional, mental, or spiritual in nature. Stress affects cognitive awareness and vigilance while influencing visual acuity, thirst, and hormonal release. (See Chapter 22 for further discussion of stress-related influences.) This, in turn, makes the older adult more vulnerable to distraction, falls, fatigue, and criminal assault. Physical activity is known to improve mobility, balance, and muscle strength, even among frail and very old adults (Butler et al, 1998). Therefore such activities as walking, stretching, and gardening help improve the strength and stability: factors important to preventing falls and physical injuries. These factors are discussed more fully in Chapters 7 and 13. Helping the older person be vigilant about hazardous surroundings includes offering suggestions for adequate lighting, placement of furniture and rugs, markings on sidewalks and steps, and precautions against accidentally locking oneself out of one's dwelling. Sensory deficits, whether visual, auditory, or olfactory, reduce the individual's ability to detect dangerous conditions or imminent threats. Tactile or neurosensory impairment raises the risk of tissue injury from burns, pressure, or beginning inflammation that escapes the person's awareness. Box 14-1 lists factors that put elders at risk for accidents or injury in the home. Box 14-2 provides a home safety checklist.

Box 14-1 Assessment of Potential Risks for Accidents in the Home

- Activities of daily living (level of function)
- Cognition and emotional state (memory, depression)
- Clinical findings (health history)
- Incontinence
- Drugs (complete inventory)
- Eyes, ears, and environment (sensory deficits)
- Neurologic deficits (gait, balance)
- Travel history (driving ability)
- Social history (alcohol, drugs)

From Escher JE et al: *Geriatrics* 44:54, 1989. Copyright by Advanstar Communications, Inc. Advanstar Communications retains all right to this article.

Box 14-2 Home Safety Checklist

All Living Spaces

1. Remove throw rugs.
2. Secure carpet edges.
3. Remove low furniture and objects on the floor.
4. Reduce clutter.
5. Remove cords and wires on the floor.
6. Check lighting for adequate illumination at night (especially the pathway to the bathroom).
7. Secure carpet or treads on stairs.
8. Avoid waxing floors.
9. Ensure that the telephone can be reached from the floor.

Bathroom

1. Install grab bars in the tub/shower and by the toilet.
2. Use rubber mats in the tub/shower.
3. Pick up floor mats when the tub/shower is not in use.
4. Install a raised toilet seat if the seat is too low.

Outdoors

1. Repair cracked sidewalks.
2. Install handrails on stairs and steps.
3. Trim shrubbery along the pathway to the house.
4. Install adequate lighting by doorways and along walkways leading to doors.

Modified from Yoshikawa TT, Cobbs EL, Brummel-Smith MD: *Ambulatory geriatric care,* St Louis, 1993, Mosby.

Individuals with neurologic disorders may be at risk for falls because of impaired balance and spatial relationships. For example, Alzheimer's disease is known to alter structure and motion perception, causing difficulty in navigating and recognizing objects in relative motion and posing safety risks for walking and driving (Rizzo and Nawrot, 1998). These visuospatial alterations are not necessarily correlated with the level of semantic impairment in Alzheimer's disease and may sometimes occur before the onset of semantic changes (Caine and Hodges, 2001).

Vulnerability to Environmental Temperatures. Given the nation's growing problems with supply and costs of energy, many older adults are exposed to temperature extremes in their own dwellings. Environmental temperature extremes impose a serious risk to older persons with declining physical health. Preventive measures require attentiveness to impending climate changes, as well as protective alternatives. Early intervention in extreme temperature exposure is crucial because excessively high or low body temperatures impair further thermoregulatory function and can be lethal.

Considerable attention to protecting elders from heat loss during surgical procedures has emerged from observations that, in a cool environment, anesthesia alone can sometimes lower body temperatures to hypothermic levels (Holtzclaw, 1997). Concern for older persons' vulnerability to temperature extremes at home or in nursing homes has, unfortunately, been prompted by adverse events that have retrospectively placed the blame on inattention or neglect. In geriatric care, the rising consciousness about thermal vulnerability has centered on heat loss, yet there should be equal attention to problems of overheating. To be vigilant or aware of elders at risk, it is important to understand the basis of thermal vulnerability. A decline in thermoregulatory responsiveness to temperature extremes as one ages is well documented, yet these changes vary widely among individuals and are related more to general health than age (Pandolf, 1994; Wladkowski and Kenney, 1998). The susceptibility to lose or gain heat during extreme temperature changes depends more on the person's physiologic and behavioral coping defenses against transient heat exchange than it does on how old the person is.

Healthy people of all ages have body temperatures that range above and below the level of 37.5° C (98.6° F) and yet are considered "normal" basal temperatures. Large studies of elders show that basal body temperature declines with advancing age (Fox et al, 1973). The delicate equilibrium required to maintain thermal balance at any age involves the generation or replacement of body heat at about the same rate as heat is lost to the environment. A number of physiologic changes associated with aging affect heat generation, distribution, and conservation. Heat conservation is especially affected by changes in body density, water content, and insulation that accompany old age. Circulatory impairment and changes in vascular responsiveness affect the distribution of heat carried by blood. Thermoregulatory sensitivity declines with age, and both cooling and warming responses appear to be blunted (Kramer et al, 1989; Wongsurawat et al, 1990). In addition, many older persons complain of "feeling cool," whether or not their actual body temperatures are lower (Fox et al, 1973). These neurosensory changes tend to delay or diminish the older person's awareness of temperature changes and may impair behavioral and thermoregulatory responses to dangerously high or low environmental temperatures. Many of the drugs taken by older people affect thermoregulation by affecting ability to vasoconstrict or vasodilate, both of which are thermoregulatory mechanisms. Other drugs suppress metabolic heat generation or inhibit neuromuscular activity, a significant source of kinetic heat production. Alcohol is notorious for inhibiting thermoregulatory function by affecting vasomotor responses in either hot or cold weather. Table 14-1 lists drugs and substances that can pose hazards to an older adult's thermoregulatory ability, particularly if underlying physical or environmental conditions predispose him or her to thermal challenges.

Economic, behavioral, and environmental factors may combine to create a dangerous thermal environment where older persons are subjected to temperature extremes they cannot escape from or change. Caretakers and family members should be aware that persons are vulnerable to environmental temperature extremes if they are unable to shiver, sweat, control blood supply to the skin, take in sufficient liquids, move about, add or remove clothing, adjust bedcovers, or adjust the room temperature. Economic conditions often play a role in this vulnerability, such as when an older person cannot afford air conditioning or adequate heating. During winter months, the older person may try using little or no room heat to either reduce or eliminate high cost of fuel. Fear of unsafe neighborhoods in some urban areas prompts many elders to keep doors and windows bolted throughout the year. However, in hot summer months, dwellings without air conditioning or ventilation may hold hazardously high room temperatures. A particularly drastic heat wave in the midwestern United States left nine elderly residents dead from heat exposure (Smith and Schremp, 2001). At least one woman who died had refused to use her air conditioner (Smith and Schremp, 2001). Growing attention to this hazard has motivated local community agencies throughout the United States, such as local gas and electric companies, Rotary clubs, and fire departments, to provide electric fans to elders during summer months and assistance in meeting heating bills in winter. Less encouraging are findings of neglect and subsequent lawsuits in the region of the heat wave mentioned earlier, where at least four deaths in nursing homes were attributed to hyperthermia (Hollinshed and O'Connor, 2001; O'Connor, 2001). Because most deaths and injuries related to temperature extremes are preventable, caretakers and the public at large must work together to educate the community. In turn, greater vigilance by authorities and citizens is imperative.

Hyperthermia. When body temperature increases above normal ranges because of environmental or metabolic heat loads, a clinical condition called *heat illness,* or *hyperthermia,*

Table 14-1 Drug-Related Thermoregulatory Alterations and Outcomes*

Drug group	Examples	Thermoregulatory impairment	Thermal outcome
Sympathomimetics	Cocaine, amphetamines	Raise synaptic concentrations of norepinephrine, dopamine, and serotonin, increasing heat production	Hyperthermia
Antidepressants	Phenothiazines	Blockade of muscarinic acetylcholine receptors impairs sweating	Hyperthermia
Tricyclic antidepressants	Imipramine, doxepin, amitriptyline	CNS depression, vasodilation, suppressed shivering, decreased heat production; anticholinergic and antimuscarinic effects; impaired sweating	Hypothermia
Centrally acting antihypertensives	Clonidine	Decreased heat production	Hypothermia
Anticholinergics	Oxybutynin	Blockade of muscarinic acetylcholine receptors impairs sweating	Hyperthermia
Diuretics	Bumetanide, furosemide, chlorothiazide, hydrochlorothiazide	Hypohydration and hyponatremia; dehydration reduces body water, impairs sweating	Hyperthermia
Beta-blockers	Metoprolol, atenolol, and propranolol	Reduced cutaneous blood flow	Hyperthermia
Mood stabilizers	Lithium	Decreased heat production	Hypothermia
Opiates	Heroin, morphine, codeine, meperidine	CNS depression, decreased heat production, increased cutaneous blood flow, blunted behavioral responses to cold	Hypothermia
Barbiturates	Phenobarbital, secobarbital, pentobarbital	Decreased heat production	Hypothermia
Vasoconstrictors	Ephedrine, phenylephrine	Reduced cutaneous blood flow	Hyperthermia
Antihistamine (toxic dose)	Diphenhydramine	Blockade of muscarinic acetylcholine receptors impairs sweating	Hyperthermia
Ethanol	All alcoholic beverages	Diuresis reduces body water; blunted behavioral responses to heat	Hyperthermia
Ethanol	All alcoholic beverages	CNS depression, decreased heat production, increased cutaneous blood flow, blunted behavioral responses to cold	Hypothermia
Methylenedioxymethamphetamine	Ecstasy	Hyperactivity	Hyperthermia
Concomitant use of selective serotonin reuptake inhibitor and monoamine oxidase inhibitor	Nefazodone, venlafaxine, fluvoxamine, sertraline, or paroxetine with tranylcypromine, phenelzine	Serotonin syndrome, increased muscle rigidity	Hyperthermia

*Drugs and chemical substances can dramatically influence an elderly person's thermoregulatory ability. Depending on underlying physical and environmental conditions, drugs can either promote heat loss or inhibit heat dissemination. In some cases, such as with ethanol, the same drug may have effects that contribute to both hypothermia and hyperthermia.
CNS, Central nervous system.

develops. Recognizing that heat illnesses tend to follow a continuum (Table 14-2), beginning with mild heat strain and ending with the potentially fatal heat stroke, makes it imperative to assess hyperthermia quickly and appropriately. Heat exhaustion is an early stage of heat illness that is characterized by water or salt depletion (or both), usually accompanied by circulatory abnormalities, such as rapid pulse, falling blood pressure, diminished superficial blood flow, clammy skin, and disorientation. Body temperature is generally high, above 38° C (100.4° F). The person usually has lost considerable amounts of sodium in heavy sweating (Horowitz and Hales, 1998). Diuretics and low intake of fluids exacerbate fluid loss and can precipitate the onset of heat exhaustion in hot weather. Medical attention is necessary to prescribe necessary fluid replacement and determine the extent of heat illness present, because heat exhaustion is part of a continuum that leads to heat stroke. Heat stroke, the most serious form of heat illness, is a medical emergency that usually arises from failure of normal body-cooling mechanisms to cope with extremely high environmental heat or humidity. Heat stroke affects the hypothalamic thermoregulatory center and impairs the ability to sweat or lose heat by vasodilation. This condition can quickly

Table 14-2 Hyperthermia

Illness	Causes	Symptoms	Treatment
Heat stroke	Breakdown of body's cooling system	Hot and dry skin, high temperature (106° F), rapid pulse, nausea, hypotension, headache, dizziness, syncope	Move patient to shade, wrap in wet sheet, call for emergency equipment, and give fluids
Heat exhaustion	Loss of fluid and sodium; often follows heavy exertion and precedes heat stroke	Fatigue, giddiness, elevated temperature, muscle cramps, delirium, cold and clammy skin	Have patient lie down away from source of heat and keep feet elevated, give cold fluids with 1 teaspoon of salt per liter, and wrap in cold, wet towels
Heat syncope	Sudden exertion or sudden exposure to unusual heat	Dizziness, lower than usual blood pressure, slowed pulse, sudden fainting, cool and sweaty skin	Get patient out of the sun, put head between knees, and have patient drink fluids

lead to death unless treated, and rising core temperatures above 40° C (104° F) increase the likelihood of irreversible brain damage. Preexisting conditions such as neurologic disorders, alcohol use, and use of atropine-containing drugs make the elder more susceptible to heat stroke by affecting heat loss mechanisms. In addition, alcohol consumption contributes to dehydration, a condition often preexisting in elders. Dehydration increases serum osmolality and reduces circulatory volume. Both of these conditions act to raise body temperature and make the body more vulnerable to thermal stress (Morimoto and Itoh, 1998). High humidity interferes with the ability of sweat to evaporate and cool the body. Hyperthermia requires active cooling and fluid replacement by caregivers. Early treatment includes actively cooling to reduce core body temperature by means of a conductive cooling blanket, until core temperatures drop to levels below 40° C (104° F) to avoid risk of neurologic damage. Because hyperthermia induces loss of thermoregulatory control, caregivers must monitor temperature closely to avoid inducing hypothermia. Concern for skin protection and comfort during cooling procedures makes it prudent to wrap extremities before application of the cooling blanket. It is also an effective measure to suppress shivering and other warming responses (Abbey et al, 1973). Parenteral fluids and electrolytes are given to improve circulation, restore deficits, and promote heat loss from skin. In cases of heat stroke and heat exhaustion, when appropriate action is taken to restore fluids and stabilize body temperature for several hours, there is often remarkable restoration of thermoregulatory ability.

Hypothermia. Hypothermia is a medical emergency requiring comprehensive assessment of neurologic activity, oxygenation, renal function, and fluid and electrolyte balance. The term *hypothermia* literally means "low heat," but it is used clinically to describe core temperatures below 35° C (95° F). During cold weather, two situations tend to produce hypothermia: (1) when exposure involves a healthy individual in severely cold environmental conditions for a prolonged period; or (2) when exposure involves a person with impaired thermoregulatory ability in room temperature without protection. The more severe the impairment or prolonged the exposure, the less able are thermoregulatory responses to defend against heat loss. The elderly are particularly predisposed to hypothermia because the opportunity for heat loss frequently coexists with the decline in heat generation and conservation responses. Such coexistence occurs frequently among persons who are homeless or cognitively impaired, those injured in falls or from trauma, and persons with cardiovascular, adrenal, or thyroid dysfunction. Other risk factors include excessive alcohol use, exhaustion, poor nutrition, inadequate housing, and use of sedatives, anxiolytics, phenothiazines, and tricyclic antidepressants. Box 14-3 lists risk factors for hypothermia.

Under normal temperature conditions, heat is produced in sufficient quantities by cellular metabolism of food, friction produced by contracting muscles, and the flow of blood. Paralyzed or immobile persons lack ability to generate significant heat by muscle activity and become cold even in normal room temperatures. Persons who are emaciated and with poor nutrition lack insulation, as well as fuel for metabolic heat-generating processes, so they may be chronically mildly hypothermic. Box 14-4 lists factors that may induce low basal body temperatures in elders. When exposed to cold temperatures, healthy persons conserve heat by vasoconstriction of superficial vessels, shunting circulation away from the skin where most heat is lost. Heat is generated by shivering and increased muscle activity, and a rise in oxygen consumption occurs to meet aerobic muscle requirements. Circulatory, cardiac, respiratory, or musculoskeletal impairments affect either the response to or function of thermoregulatory

Box 14-3 Factors That Increase the Risk of Hypothermia in the Elderly

Thermoregulatory Impairment

Failure to vasoconstrict promptly or strongly on exposure to cold
Failure to sense cold
Failure to respond behaviorally to protect oneself against cold
Diminished or absent shivering to generate heat
Failure of metabolic rate to rise in response to cold

Conditions That Decrease Heat Production

Hypothyroidism, hypopituitarism, hypoglycemia, anemia, malnutrition, starvation
Immobility/decreased activity (e.g., stroke, paralysis, parkinsonism, dementia, arthritis, fractured hip, coma)
Diabetic ketoacidosis

Conditions That Increase Heat Loss

Open wounds, generalized inflammatory skin conditions, burns

Conditions That Impair Central or Peripheral Control of Thermoregulation

Stroke, brain tumor, Wernicke's encephalopathy, subarachnoid hemorrhage
Uremia, neuropathy (e.g., diabetes, alcoholism)
Acute illnesses (e.g., pneumonia, sepsis, myocardial infarction, congestive heart failure, pulmonary embolism, pancreatitis)

Drugs That Interfere with Thermoregulation

Tranquilizers (e.g., phenothiazines)
Sedative/hypnotics (e.g., barbiturates, benzodiazepines)
Antidepressants (e.g., tricyclics)
Vasoactive drugs (e.g., vasodilators)
Alcohol (causes superficial vasodilation; may interfere with carbohydrate metabolism and judgment)
Other: methyldopa, lithium, morphine

From Worfolk JB: Keep frail elders warm, *Geriatr Nurs* 18(1):7, 1997.

Box 14-4 Factors Associated with Low Body Temperature in the Elderly

Aging

Increases risk of thermoregulatory dysfunction.
Increases risk of acute and chronic conditions that predispose to hypothermia.

Low Environmental Temperature

Risk of hypothermia increased below 65° F.

Thinness/Malnutrition

Very thin people have less thermal insulation, higher surface area–to–volume ratios
Prolonged malnutrition can decrease the metabolic rate by 20% to 30%.

Poverty

Increases risk of thinness/malnutrition, inadequate clothing, low environmental temperature secondary to poor housing conditions and inadequate heat.

Living Alone

Associated with poverty, delayed detection of hypothermia, delayed rescue if person falls.

Nocturia/Night Rising

Associated with falls; if rescue delayed and person lies immobilized for a long time, hypothermia may develop as heat is conducted away from the body to the cold floor.

Orthostatic Hypotension

An indicator of autonomic nervous system impairment; dizziness and postural instability are associated with falls.

From Worfolk JB: Keep frail elders warm, *Geriatr Nurs* 18(1):7, 1997.

mechanisms. Elderly persons with some degree of thermoregulatory impairment, when exposed to cold temperatures, are at high risk for hypothermia if they undergo surgery, are injured in a fall or accident, or are lost or left unattended in a cool place. At brain temperatures below 20° C (68° F), all thermoregulatory ability is lost. This condition, called *poikilothermia,* is potentially lethal if untreated because body temperatures fall to levels incompatible with life. All body systems are affected by hypothermia, although the most deadly consequences involve cardiac arrhythmias and suppression of respiratory function. A less well known effect of hypothermia and cold stress is immunosuppression. Low body temperature is known to suppress immune reactions in laboratory animals (Wang-Yang et al, 1990). Clinical studies have shown significant correlations between hypothermia and infection in hospital admissions (Darowski et al, 1991) and effects of warming body temperature during surgery to reduce postsurgical infections (Kurz et al, 1996). Unfortunately, this topic has been virtually overlooked in keeping elders healthy in home or nursing home care. The potential risk of hypothermia and its associated cardiorespiratory and metabolic exertion make prevention important and early recognition vital.

Detecting hypothermia among home-dwelling elderly is sometimes difficult, because unlike in the clinical setting, no one is measuring body temperature. For persons exposed to low temperatures in the home or the environment, confusion and disorientation may be the first overt sign. As judgment becomes clouded, a person may remove clothing or fail to seek shelter, and hypothermia can progress to profound levels. For this reason, regular contact with home-dwelling elders during cold weather is crucial. For those with preexisting alterations in thermoregulatory ability, this surveillance should include even mildly cool weather. Guidelines for hypothermia prevention for elders include the following:

- Keep aware of the temperature inside and outside the home (know the local weather phone number and place a room thermometer in the home).
- Dress in layers in cold weather to add insulation. Use multiple layers of bed covers at night.
- Large amounts of body heat are lost from the head and neck, so wear a warm hat and scarf to help retain body heat.
- Do not drink hot liquids or alcohol when exposed to cold weather, because both cause blood flow to superficial tissues and loss of heat from the skin.
- Being locked out of your own dwelling can leave you out in the cold. Keep a house key on a chain or shoelace around your neck whenever you leave the house.
- Heat is lost by radiation through any window, despite warm temperatures inside a room. Avoid leaving an immobile or paralyzed person in a bed or wheelchair next to an outside window for prolonged periods in cold weather.
- Always carry a cell phone or enough change to place a phone call when you are out shopping, going to church, or running errands in cold weather. If you are unable to get home or are locked out of the facility for shelter, call the local police for assistance.

EFFECTS OF CHANGING LIFE SITUATIONS

Change is usually stressful, regardless of whether the change is perceived as positive or negative. Advancing age may make a change in residence necessary or even desirable for some persons who wish to live closer to remaining family members, medical facilities, or provision sources. Changing life situations for the older adult can affect safety and security by posing unfamiliar routes, routines, and persons in the environment. Different locations for finding essential resources often present a stressful distraction that contributes to "getting lost," becoming fearful, and straying into unsafe areas of a town or city. These problems are not limited to large metropolitan areas. The Federal Interagency Forum on Aging-Related Statistics has documented continued social activity of older adults as a key indicator for successful aging. Persons who continue to interact with others tend to be physically and mentally healthier than persons who become socially isolated. Friends and family interactions provide emotional, social, and practical support to elders that can reduce the need for formal health care services and possibly enable them to remain in the community longer (Federal Interagency Forum on Aging-Related Statistics, 2000). Conversely, relocation may erode security because of loss of familiar faces and places.

Auto Safety

A factor that often contributes to feelings of isolation for older adults is the decision, sometimes imposed by others, to give up one's driver's license and no longer drive. These decisions are often instigated by automobile accidents, growing feelings of insecurity about driving, failing health, and the influence of family and friends (Johnson, 1995). Finding and navigating public transportation may be a challenge when there are no willing friends or relatives to drive the older person. Losing one's orientation in any area can be frustrating and exhausting, and it may contribute to an elder's vulnerability to injury or crime. Uneven terrain, varying heights of curbs, and one-way traffic in unfamiliar areas increase the chance of stumbling, tripping, or falling. An older person may also have impaired sight and less energy, and may appear to be an easy target for a pickpocket or purse snatcher. One cannot assume that persons living in rural areas have greater difficulty finding transportation or locating health care because they lack public conveyances. Although rural dwellers may have fewer agency supports, they often have strong social supports sustained through family, church, and neighbors. Older urban dwellers, on the other hand, may not have formed a neighborhood network of persons willing or able to provide needed social support, such as transportation or assistance in seeking health care. They may find available public transportation difficult and unsafe to navigate, particularly when they are ill or frail. Neighborhood networks promoted through churches, volunteer service organizations, community agencies, merchants, and health care providers can improve social support for older persons. Community aids in the form of meals-on-wheels, shopping assistance, and volunteer transportation to senior centers and health care facilities are among some of the services provided. Key referrals to these networks come from nurses, social workers, neighbors, and home care providers. Safe driving tips are provided in Box 14-5.

Box 14-5 Safe Driving Tips

- Plan your travel route in advance and carry a map of your area.
- Wear your seat belt.
- Keep your eyes on the road.
- Avoid distractions. If you have to use your car phone, pull over at a convenient place first.
- Follow the 4-second rule when following.
- Obey traffic and motor vehicle laws, signs, and signals.
- Adjust your speed to the road and weather conditions.
- Drive with doors locked and windows rolled up.
- Park your car in a visible, well-lighted area.
- Expect the unexpected and always drive defensively.

From Leahy L: Automobile safety, *Home Health Focus,* 3(4):27, September 1996.

Neighborhood Security

The idea of *neighborhood* is a smaller concept than *community* and is more attuned to the convenience and friendliness of daily contacts. Nine blocks roughly corresponds to the size of most neighborhoods. As social factors or disability shrinks the geographic area in which a person moves, the neighborhood becomes smaller. The neighborhood commonly includes the corner grocery, the newspaper stand, the mail carrier, small cafes, barbershops, the church or synagogue, and, ideally, the clinic or health care provider one uses. This network of contacts may provide informal surveillance of people and activities that can serve as an alert system for neighbors in need. The availability of this network to monitor situations out of the ordinary often points the way to emergency intervention, crime detection, or social services. Low morale and isolation are inversely correlated with one's sense of having a "neighborhood." The neighborhood seems to be a most important environmental unit for the elderly. The character of a neighborhood may be an important source of satisfaction or alienation. Many older people who once belonged in their neighborhood have been left behind by migration to the suburbs and find themselves in a neighborhood that has evolved into an alien and often frightening place. A significant contributor to fear of crime among the elderly is the socioeconomic deterioration of the neighborhood and loss of neighbors.

CRIMES AGAINST THE ELDERLY

Risks and Vulnerability

Older individuals share many of the same fears about violent crime held by the rest of the population, but they may feel more vulnerable because of frailness or disability. In reality, statistics show that violent crime against persons age 65 and older declined from the 1978 rate of 9 per 1000 to the 1998 rate of 3.7 per 1000 (U.S. Bureau of the Census, 2001). Instead, the elderly are more likely to be victims of petty crime, property crime, and being taken advantage of in scams that include telemarketing fraud and undelivered services.

Several crime prevention programs for the elderly have been established through combined efforts of agencies. In 1988 the American Association of Retired Persons (AARP), the Law Enforcement Assistance Administration, the Community Services Administration, the Department of Housing and Urban Development, the International Association of Chiefs of Police, and the National Sheriffs' Association signed a cooperative agreement to work together to reduce both criminal victimization and unwarranted fear of crime affecting older persons (Broome, 2000). The project, called TRIAD, has a senior advisory council, sometimes called Seniors and Law Together (SALT), to act as an advocacy or advisory group. This provides a forum for the exchange of information between seniors and law enforcement. Participants working together involve persons selected by police, sheriffs, older leaders, the AARP, the Retired Senior Volunteer Program (RSVP), the Agency on Aging, and the ministerial association. Local TRIAD projects have formed across the United States and are publicized by local police departments, sheriffs' groups, and AARP affiliates. They are easily found on the Internet by entering *TRIAD elderly crime prevention* on any World Wide Web search engine. Recently, RadioShack, in support of the National Crime Prevention Council, produced a brochure explaining TRIAD and how senior citizens can protect themselves against crime. These brochures can be printed out from the websites of many participating TRIAD police and law-enforcement agencies (National Crime Prevention Council, 2002).

Community-centered projects have shown the effectiveness of neighborhood crime prevention networks, public education in self-protective measures, avoidance of fraudulent schemes, community safety inspection programs, security advice in homes, and civic and organizational assistance in obtaining security devices and escort services. In some instances, elderly volunteer peer counselors provide support and counseling to elderly victims of crime and violence. Strategies for promoting security-conscious behaviors among elders are aimed at decreasing vulnerability to criminal victimization and playing a role in self-protection. Nurses can be instrumental in reducing fear of crime and assisting elders in exploring ways they may protect themselves and feel more secure. The following are important ideas to convey to older persons concerning potential criminal threats:

- Purse and wallet snatchers are usually not interested in injuring anyone. You are less likely to be hurt when accosted if you hand over purse or wallet readily.
- Carry only a little money and personal items in a wallet or purse. Keep your house keys, larger amounts of money, and credit cards in an inside pocket of clothing. Women may need to sew a special pocket inside a coat or jacket.
- Some older persons believe that there is safety in numbers and travel about in groups of three.
- Some people wear a small police whistle around their neck.
- Some people find that a cane or an umbrella provides a deceptive weapon of defense.
- The Social Security payment is a prime target of muggers. Instead of carrying it to the bank or risking its theft from mailboxes, have your check mailed directly to your bank.
- Keep alert to stories and coverage of fraud, bogus schemes, and protective actions on the news media.
- Never let anyone you do not know into your home uninvited. If someone wants to gain entrance by showing identification, always phone the agency involved (before allowing the person to enter) to verify the authenticity of the identification.
- Support and encourage increased police surveillance of areas that you frequent.
- Take advantage of self-defense courses, public awareness programs, and youth escort services in your neighborhood. (Box 14-6 provides other suggestions.)

Fraudulent Schemes against Elders

Fraud against elders ranges from solicitations from seemingly worthwhile charities to requests for a cash deposit to win a nonexistent prize. Trusting elderly persons may be duped into

Box 14-6 Crime Reduction Suggestions

- Do not wear flashy jewelry in public places or carry deadly weapons.
- Identify police and security personnel that are available in high-risk areas.
- Institute informal surveillance agreements by tenants to increase security.
- Receive a home security check by police and follow through on their security suggestions.
- Attend a crime prevention program.
- Keep doors locked, install deadbolt locks, and choose locks that you can easily manipulate. If key is lost, or if you move, have locks replaced. Do not attach ID tag to key ring.
- Use peephole (install one if necessary). Confirm authenticity of a service person's ID by calling that service agency before opening the door. Never open doors to strangers or let them know you are alone.
- Lock windows. Get fire department–approved grates put on ground floor/fire escape windows. Keep all hidden entries locked (e.g., garage, basement, roof). Draw curtains and blinds at night.
- Protect valuables:
  Keep money and securities in a bank.
  Have Social Security pension check deposited directly to your account.
  Mark all valuables with Social Security number, record serial numbers.
- Beware of phone tricks.
  Hang up on (and report) nuisance callers.
  Do not give any information to strangers over phone.
- Consider a pet. A dog—even a small one—can provide excellent protection and good company if you are willing to care for one.
- Organize a buddy system.
  Neighbors can watch out for each other, go to basement/laundry room together, and so on.

giving money to pen pals, phony religious causes, or new acquaintances who "need help." Attractive prices of fraudulent door-to-door contractors, who offer services the older adult cannot perform, may entice a substantial cash outlay. For example, an urban senior recently gave $1000 in cash to a man who came to her door and offered to roof her house. He convinced her that he needed money to buy roofing supplies to complete the job, but he disappeared with the money and was never found. According to the Internal Revenue Service (IRS), every year impersonators swindle vulnerable taxpayers out of thousands of dollars by posing as IRS agents. Elderly people are often targets of these frauds. Scams may involve announcements that they have won a large cash sweepstakes that requires payment of taxes before the prize is delivered. Other IRS impersonators have called on widows or widowers to pay the "back taxes" owed by their deceased spouse. These abuses often go unpunished because the older person waits too long to report the fraud or feels embarrassment at having been taken in. Several key precautions should be shared with those at risk for fraud from IRS impersonators:

- All IRS employees carry identification and are required to show it to taxpayers when visiting a home or office.
- All citizens can obtain an IRS office address in their local telephone directory, or call the national IRS directory number at 1-800-829-1040 to find its location.
- No check should ever be made payable to an IRS employee. Checks for federal taxes should be made payable to the Internal Revenue Service, not IRS; spelling out the full name makes it more difficult for criminals to alter the check.

Medical fraud is another serious type of fraud that affects older citizens on a national scale. Medical supplies and equipment delivered to homes by various suppliers have either been grossly overpriced or charged for but never received by the client. In response to this growing trend, the Health Care Financing Administration (HCFA) established offices to inform Medicare and Medicaid beneficiaries of ways to avoid fraud, and national agencies have combined forces to bring about reform. In a fact sheet issued by the Centers for Medicare and Medicaid Services (CMS), formerly HCFA, several new reforms were identified (Centers for Medicare and Medicaid Services, 1999). In 1995 the U.S. Department of Health and Human Services launched Operation Restore Trust, a groundbreaking and ongoing antifraud project aimed at coordinating federal, state, local, and private resources in targeted areas. HCFA/CMS imposed a 4-month moratorium in 1997 on the enrollment of new home health care providers in the Medicare program while new regulations to screen providers entering the program were developed. HCFA/CMS continues to develop payment systems for home health services that offer incentives for providing efficient care and avoidance of unnecessary visits. In his fiscal year 2000 budget proposal, President Clinton introduced an antifraud and antiabuse legislative package that could save Medicare another $2.9 billion over 5 years. New HCFA/CMS regulations also doubled the number of home health audits and increased claims reviews by 25%. HCFA/CMS also now requires home health agencies to be more accountable for the care they provide and to conduct criminal background checks on the aides they hire. The expectation is that reduction of the expense of these enormous abuses will ultimately preserve the integrity of the Medicare and Medicaid systems (U.S. Department of Health and Human Services, 1995).

FIRE SAFETY FOR ELDERS

Risk Factors for Elders

A number of factors predispose the older person to fire injuries. In home-dwelling elders, economic or climatic conditions may promote the use of ill-kept heating devices. Attempts to cook over an open flame while wearing loose-fitting clothing or inability to manage spattering grease from a frying pan can often start a fire from which the elder cannot escape. Those living in apartment dwellings are often at the mercy of cluttered wooden buildings and the careless behaviors of others. Failing vision can contribute to an elderly person's setting a cook-top burner, heating pad, or hot plate too high and resulting in fire or thermal injury. According to the U.S. Fire Administration, people who are over age 65 are one of the groups at highest risk of dying in a fire. In the United States, 1200 persons over age 65 die each year in fires. Fire-related mortality rates are three times higher in people over age 80 than in the rest of the population. The risk of injury during a fire is greater if medication or illness slows response time or decision making and if help is not available to contain the fire and help the person escape. Most fires occur at home during the night, and deaths are attributed to smoke injury more often than burns. A 6-year study of fire fatalities in New Jersey showed that the most common sources of ignition for residential fires were smoking materials (Barillo and Goode, 1996). Fire-related deaths are more common among men than women, which may be related to higher incidence of smoking and alcohol consumption. Plastic articles and other synthetics can produce noxious fumes that are deadly, particularly to persons with preexisting respiratory disorders. Even flame-retardant garments have been linked to noxious fume release when burned, and therefore they are a possible hazard to elders. Specific fire prevention guidelines for elders appear in Box 14-7.

Reducing Risks in Group Residential Settings. Residents of institutional settings, such as nursing homes or assisted living facilities, are particularly vulnerable to fire because of the high numbers of frail or immobilized elderly. Activities to promote a fire-safe institutional environment include use of noncombustible building materials, sprinkler systems, smoke detectors, closed air spaces, written fire procedures, orientation of personnel, and assessment of environment by fire prevention officials. Nurses are in a position to ensure familiarity of personnel with fire safety procedures and evacuation protocol and also to report or remove any potential fire hazards. Personnel protocols should address these issues:

1. Predetermined staff members should be given specific duties and posts.
2. Notification procedures for fire department and personnel should be clearly described.
3. Management of exit maneuvers should be assigned and specifically described.

Reducing Fire Risks at Home. The following practical suggestions should be practiced by nurses personally and used to educate patients in home safety:

1. When you smell smoke, see flames, or hear the sound of fire, evacuate everyone in the house before doing anything else.
2. Use normal exits unless blocked by smoke or flame. Never use elevators during fire evacuation.
3. Stay near the floor because gases and smoke collect near the ceiling.
4. In a high-rise apartment, remain in room with doors and hall vents closed unless smoke is in your apartment. Open or break a window to obtain fresh air.
5. Define and discuss evacuation plans with other residents of the building.
6. Home fire alarm systems and smoke detectors should have a label indicating Underwriters' Laboratories (UL) approval. Smoke detectors should be installed outside of each sleeping area, at the top of the basement stairs, in the bedroom of smokers, and in all levels of the house. Do not install a smoke detector too near a window, door, or forced-air register, where drafts could interfere with the detector's operation; do not install a smoke detector within 6 inches of where walls and ceilings meet, because air is less likely to circulate smoke to the alarm.
7. Rehearse what to do: If clothing catches fire, do not run; lie down, and then roll over and over ("stop, drop, and roll"). If someone else's clothing is burning, smother the flames with the handiest item, such as a rug, a coat, a blanket, or drapes.

Reducing Home Fire Hazards. A number of potentially hazardous substances are found in most homes and should be surveyed regularly. In cases where the substance is rarely or never used, it is prudent to eliminate it from the home. Some elderly persons may have kept old bottles and cans of hazardous materials in their garage or shed for decades and should be assisted in having them discarded in acceptable reception sites. A local fire department can give instructions regarding where flammable or combustible substances can be taken. Survey of a home's fire hazards should include the following: (1) flammable liquids (e.g., gasoline, acetone, lacquer thinner); (2) combustible liquids (e.g., lighter fluid, kerosene, turpentine); (3) gas leaks; (4) rubbish and trash stored near

Box 14-7 Measures to Prevent Fires and Burns

Do not smoke in bed or when sleepy.
When cooking, do not wear loose-fitting clothing (e.g., bathrobes, nightgowns, pajamas).
Set thermostats for water heater or faucets so that the water does not become too hot.
Install a portable hand fire extinguisher in the kitchen.
Keep access to outside door(s) unobstructed.
Identify emergency exits in public buildings.
If you consider entering a boarding or foster home, check to see that it has smoke detectors, a sprinkler system, and fire extinguishers.
Wear clothing that is nonflammable or treated with a permanent fire-retardant finish. Fabrics of animal hair, wool, or silk are less flammable.
Use several electrical outlets to avoid overloading.

stove, water heater, or furnace; (5) Christmas trees and tree lights that are frayed or poorly insulated; (6) smoking in bed or discarding burning cigarettes; and (7) overloaded or worn electrical systems.

RISK FOR SUICIDE AND SELF-NEGLECT

Perceptions of failing health and isolation can threaten an older person's sense of security and satisfaction with life. Feeling out of control often accompanies declining physical and cognitive abilities. Risk factors for suicide and self-neglect are increased among elders when they feel a loss of meaning and connection with life. Self-neglect is commonly noted as elders lose spouses, decrease interpersonal contact with others, and find self-care more burdensome. Suicide risk for older adults receives less attention than that for teens and young adults, yet the rate is proportionately higher. For example, people over 65 represent 13% of Americans, but ended life in 19% of suicides in 1999 (Centers for Disease Control and Prevention, 1999). Suicide rates increase with age, are higher among whites than other races, and are more than four times higher among males than females (Centers for Disease Control and Prevention, 1996). In general, elderly men with suicidal intent are more determined to die, use more definitive methods, and seem less prone to communicate their suicidal intentions. The most common method of suicide in later life is by gunshot wound. In a recent study, having an accessible firearm in the home significantly increases the risk of suicide (Conwell et al, 2002). Suicides from handguns were higher than those from long guns, and gun locks and gun safes lowered the risk. Study findings support the potential suicide prevention benefit of restricting access to handguns and recommend education programs for elders, family members, and health care providers. Another study makes similar recommendations to heighten caregiver awareness about suicides among the elderly from drug ingestion (Spicer and Miller, 2000). These include limiting quantities of prescription drugs, particularly sedatives and narcotics, and prescribing drugs with lower toxicity to elders (Spicer and Miller, 2000).

Few prospective studies of suicides among elderly exist, but a 10-year, longitudinal, community-based prospective study of aging revealed several predictors for suicidal outcomes (Turvey et al, 2002). This study of 14,456 persons over age 65 surveyed medical status, perceived health, depressive symptoms, presence of a relative or friend to confide in, alcohol use, and sleep quality. In the 21 persons who committed suicide in later years, suicide was not predicted by alcohol use, medical condition, or physical impairment. Instead, significant predictors of suicide were depressive symptoms, perceived health status, poor sleep quality, and absence of a relative or friend to confide in. The rising suicide rates among elders deserve concern by communities and caregivers. Depressive symptoms, complaints of worthlessness, and loss of contacts with others should be followed up with efforts to engage the elder in social or cognitively stimulating activities.

In summary, security and safety of elders should be of utmost importance in priorities for families, care providers, communities, and community agencies. These concerns go beyond simply providing a safe physical environment and freedom from violence and crime. It is abundantly clear that declining health and limited mobility erode the older person's perceptions of security, provide a source of stress, and contribute to depression and self-neglect. Of paramount importance are older persons' connections with the world outside themselves. In this respect, the need is apparent for new "neighborhoods" of contacts and resource people when older persons must relocate to other surroundings. The need for ongoing observation of elders living alone is particularly important during temperature extremes, when dangers of thermoregulatory problems increase. Assisting the older person to keep his or her home environment uncluttered and free of hazardous materials also helps avoid possible injuries from falls, fires, or exposure to danger. Several strategies and programs have been successful across the United States in providing key resources to elders. Enabling the community to become the good neighbor to older citizens provides mutual benefits to all who are involved.

Human Needs and Wellness Diagnoses

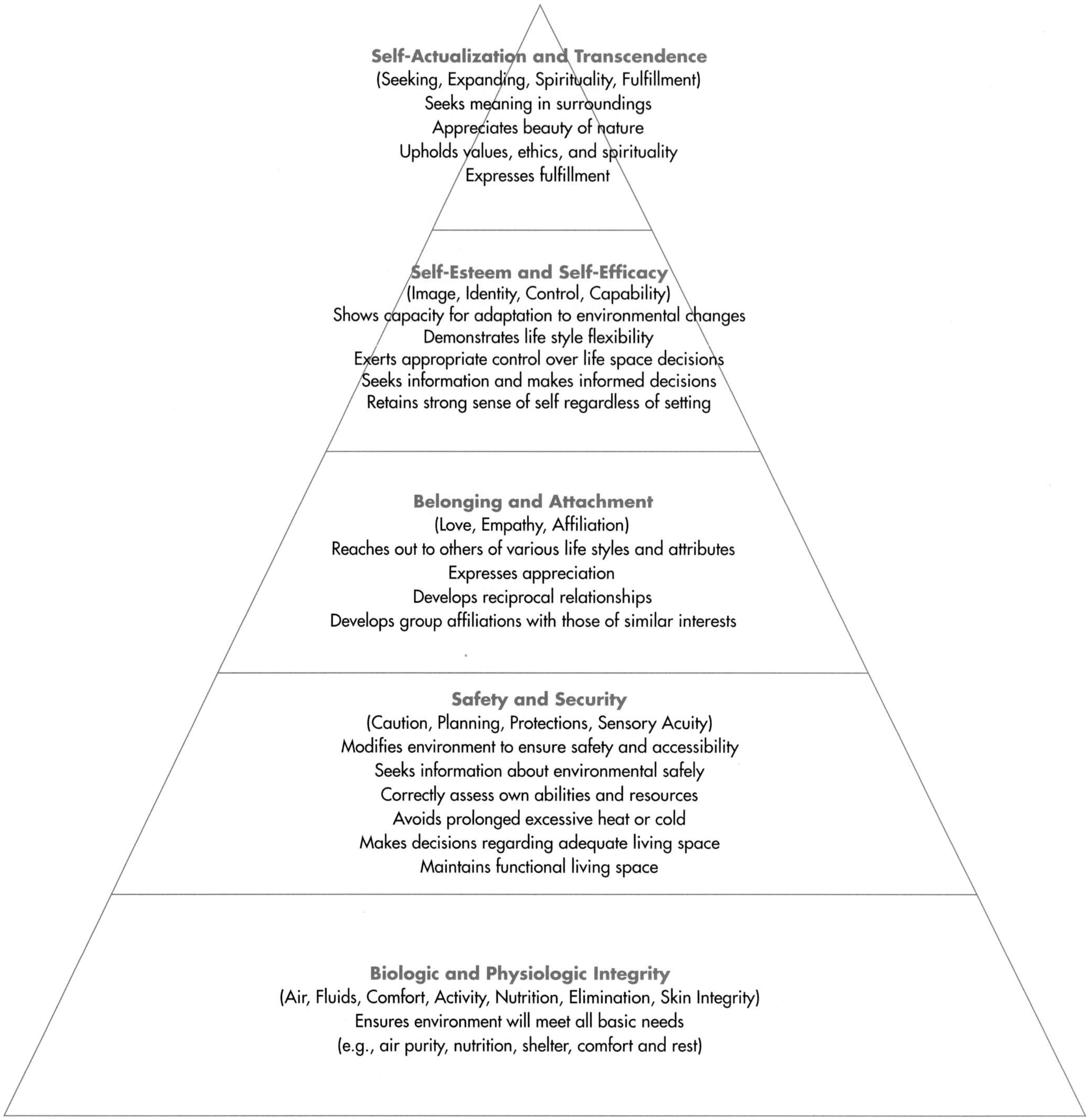

Self-Actualization and Transcendence
(Seeking, Expanding, Spirituality, Fulfillment)
Seeks meaning in surroundings
Appreciates beauty of nature
Upholds values, ethics, and spirituality
Expresses fulfillment

Self-Esteem and Self-Efficacy
(Image, Identity, Control, Capability)
Shows capacity for adaptation to environmental changes
Demonstrates life style flexibility
Exerts appropriate control over life space decisions
Seeks information and makes informed decisions
Retains strong sense of self regardless of setting

Belonging and Attachment
(Love, Empathy, Affiliation)
Reaches out to others of various life styles and attributes
Expresses appreciation
Develops reciprocal relationships
Develops group affiliations with those of similar interests

Safety and Security
(Caution, Planning, Protections, Sensory Acuity)
Modifies environment to ensure safety and accessibility
Seeks information about environmental safely
Correctly assess own abilities and resources
Avoids prolonged excessive heat or cold
Makes decisions regarding adequate living space
Maintains functional living space

Biologic and Physiologic Integrity
(Air, Fluids, Comfort, Activity, Nutrition, Elimination, Skin Integrity)
Ensures environment will meet all basic needs
(e.g., air purity, nutrition, shelter, comfort and rest)

These are not all the possible wellness diagnoses that may be identified. The above are examples of nursing diagnoses that should be considered when planning care for the older adult.

KEY CONCEPTS

- Feelings of security are generated from within an individual and are related to stability of inner drives and convictions.
- With increasing age and dependency, the environment becomes a larger factor in maintaining a sense of security.
- Anxiety and insecurity increase when situations and conditions become unpredictable.
- Feelings of insecurity may result in behaviors that are disruptive or inappropriate.
- Sensory deficits increase feelings of insecurity and uncertainty in the environment.
- Because of declining thermoregulatory mechanisms in the aged, extremes of heat and cold must be avoided.
- Severe hypothermia and hyperthermia are medical emergencies and may result in death if not properly attended.
- Changing living situations may result in deterioration of function for some elders.
- Unavailable or inappropriate transportation considerably reduces an elder's life space.
- Neighborhoods change over the years, and long-term dwellers may find themselves in dangerous or crime-ridden areas as they age.
- Elders are often targets of fraud and deception.
- A fire inspection of an elder's living space is essential for safety.
- Reducing fire hazards is essential to feelings of security.
- Self-neglect, abuse, and suicide (subliminal or overt) may be the result of chronic insecurity.
- A familiar and comfortable environment allows an elder to function at his or her highest capacity.

▲ CASE STUDY

Ethel had lived in one home for all of her married life, but when her husband died her children worried about her safety being alone in a big home. She could fall and lie undiscovered to die of hypothermia, the deteriorating neighborhood was no longer considered safe, and she could no longer drive so was limited in her ability to get around. They convinced her to move to a community in Phoenix near them.

They were able to find a suitable apartment that she could afford. For a while they visited her each week, but each visit became more depressing for them as she continually talked about her old home, old friends, old furniture, old priest; everything old. Their visits became less frequent. She called them faithfully each morning but detected their urge to get off the phone and on with their lives. One morning she called her daughter, Gladys, and said, "I'm so sick! Yesterday I walked outside and I swear I saw my friend Rose from the old neighborhood getting on the bus, but she didn't see me. I was so disappointed but managed to make it home, then couldn't find the key to my apartment so finally had to call 911 for help. They were really irritated with me when I said I had lost my key. I want to go back to Detroit. I know how things work there." After a family conclave they found a nice place in assisted living for her and were much relieved. Ethel said, "I don't know where I am anymore. Seems I bounce around like a rubber ball." She seldom left her room except for meals, and soon meals needed to be brought to her. Last week she wandered out and when found had suffered a serious case of heat stroke.

Based on the case study, develop a nursing care plan using the following procedure:*

List comments of the client that provide subjective data.

List information that provides objective data.

From these data identify and state, using accepted format, two nursing diagnoses you determine are most significant to this client at this time. List two client strengths that you have identified from the data.

Determine and state outcome criteria for each diagnosis. These must reflect some alleviation of the problem identified in the nursing diagnosis and must be stated in concrete and measurable terms.

Plan and state one or more interventions for each diagnosed problem.

Provide specific documentation of source used to determine appropriate intervention. Plan at least one intervention that incorporates the client's existing strengths.

Evaluate success of intervention. Interventions must correlate directly with the stated outcome criteria in order to measure the outcome success.

STUDY QUESTIONS/ACTIVITIES

Locate low-cost housing in your area and assess for convenience and safety.

Are purse snatching and mugging of elders commonplace in your city?

What resources are available to prevent or assist those who may be vulnerable to attack?

Discuss how you would assist your parents in making a decision regarding a change in living situations as they become increasingly disabled and unable to care for themselves.

List several aspects of your environment that are important to you and discuss their significance.

Discuss relocation stress and the significance it has to aged individuals.

Discuss housing options that would be most suitable and feasible for you if you were unable to get around without the assistance of a walker.

Discuss the meanings and the thoughts triggered by the student's and elder's viewpoints expressed at the beginning of the chapter. How do these vary from your own experience?

---

*Students are advised to refer to their nursing diagnosis text and identify possible or potential problems.

Make a plan for assistance to your elderly parents when they are no longer able to fully care for themselves. Discuss the signals that will let you know they are insecure in their environment.

RESEARCH QUESTIONS

What criminal activities are of most concern to the aged?

What percentage of major cities or states have crime victimization programs in place?

What environmental safety factors are most frequently neglected by the aged?

What home safety factors most frequently cause trouble for the aged?

What have proved to be the most effective crime stoppers in relation to protecting the aged from victimization?

What is the geographic distribution and incidence of hypothermia and hyperthermia in the United States?

What are the most frequent causes of fires among elders?

Survey a group of elders and determine what they most fear in their environment.

Survey the homes of elders you are serving in your clinical practice for the presence or absence of safety features.

REFERENCES

Abbey J et al: A pilot study: the control of shivering during hypothermia by a clinical nursing measure, *J Neurosurg Nurs* 5(2):78, 1973.

Barillo D, Goode R: Fire fatality study: demographics of fire victims, *Burns* 22(2):85, 1996.

Broome C: Newly formed TRIAD will help fight crime against seniors, *Coastal Senior,* Sept 25, 2000. Available at *www.coastalsenior.com/archives/november2000/COMtriad.html*

Butler RN et al: Physical fitness: benefits of exercise for the older patient, *Geriatrics* 53(10):46, 1998.

Caine D, Hodges J: Heterogeneity of semantic and visuospatial deficits in early Alzheimer's disease, *Neuropsychology* 15(2):155, 2001.

Centers for Disease Control and Prevention: Suicide among older persons—United States, 1980-1992, *MMWR Morb Mortal Wkly Rep* 45:3, 1996.

Centers for Disease Control and Prevention: Mortality patterns—United States, *MMWR Morb Mortal Wkly Rep* 48:664, 1999.

Centers for Medicare and Medicaid Services: *Fact sheet: fighting fraud, waste and abuse in Medicare and Medicaid: CMS Office of Public Affairs,* Baltimore, 1999, Centers for Medicare and Medicaid Services.

Conwell Y et al: Access to firearms and risk for suicide in middle-aged and older adults, *Am J Geriatr Psychiatry* 10(4):407, 2002.

Darowski A et al: Hypothermia and infection in elderly patients admitted to hospital, *Age Aging* 20:100, 1991.

Federal Interagency Forum on Aging-Related Statistics: Older Americans 2000: key indicators of well-being, 2000. Available at *www.agingstats.gov/chartbook2000/healthrisks.html* (accessed Aug 30, 2002).

Fox RH, Woodward PM, Exton-Smith AN: Body temperatures in the elderly: a national study of physiological social and environmental conditions, *BMJ* 1:200, 1973.

Hollinshed D, O'Connor P: Suit is filed in death at U. City care home: victim's daughter alleges negligence, malpractice in heat-related death, *St Louis Post-Dispatch,* May 17, 2001, p B-4.

Holtzclaw B: Perioperative problems: threats to thermal balance in the elderly, *Semin Perioper Nurs* 6(1):42, 1997.

Horowitz M, Hales JRS: Pathophysiology of hyperthermia. In Blatteis CM, editor: *Physiology and pathophysiology of temperature regulation,* River Edge, NJ, 1998, World Scientific.

Johnson J: Rural elders and the decision to stop driving, *J Community Health Nurs* 12(3):131, 1995.

Kramer MR, Vandijk J, Rosin AJ: Mortality in elderly patients with thermoregulatory failure, *Arch Intern Med* 149:1521, 1989.

Kurz A, Sessler DI, Lenhard R: Perioperative normothermia to reduce the incidence of surgical-wound infection and shorten hospitalization, *N Engl J Med* 334:1209, 1996.

Morimoto T, Itoh T: Thermoregulation and body fluid osmolality, *J Basic Clin Physiol Pharmacol* 9(1):51, 1998.

National Crime Prevention Council: How can senior citizens protect themselves against crime? National Crime Prevention Council/RadioShack, 2002. Available at *www.lapdonline.org/pdf_files/bsc/senior_citizens.pdf* (accessed Sept 20, 2002).

O'Connor P: Two more families sue nursing home where heat killed four: federal officials also are investigating deaths at U. City facility, *St Louis Post-Dispatch,* June 21, 2001, p B-1.

Pandolf K: Heat tolerance and aging, *Exp Aging Res* 20(4):275, 1994.

Pittiglio L: Use of reminiscence therapy in patients with Alzheimer's disease, *Lippincott's Case Management* 5(6):216, 2000.

Rizzo M, Nawrot M: Perception of movement and shape in Alzheimer's disease, *Brain* 121(pt 12):2259, 1998.

Smith B, Schremp V: Nine deaths in area are linked to heat: the most recent victim, a woman, 85, refused to use her air conditioner: cooler weather is expected, *St Louis Post-Dispatch,* Aug 10, 2001, p B1.

Spicer RS, Miller TR: Suicide acts in 8 states: incidence and case fatality rates by demographics and method, *Am J Public Health* 90(12):1885, 2000.

Turvey CL et al: Risk factors for late-life suicide: a prospective, community-based study, *Am J Geriatr Psychiatry* 10(4):398, 2002.

U.S. Bureau of the Census: *Statistical abstract of the United States: 2002,* ed 122, Washington, DC, 2001, U.S. Government Printing Office.

U.S. Department of Health and Human Services: HCFA opens first health care fraud satellite office, Health Care Financing Administration Press Office, 1995, U.S. Department of Health and Human Services. Available at *www.hhs.gov/news/press/1995pres/950901a.html*

Wang-Yang MC et al: Temperature-mediated processes in immunity: differential effects of low temperature on mouse T helper cell responses, *Cell Immunol* 126:354, 1990.

Wladkowski SL, Kenney WL: Fat-free mass and hypothermia in the elderly, *Med Sci Sports Exerc* 30(5, suppl):285, 1998.

Wongsurawat N, Davis BB, Morley JE: Thermoregulatory failure in the elderly, *J Am Geriatr Soc* 38:899, 1990.

Woods R: Discovering the person with Alzheimer's disease: cognitive, emotional and behavioural aspects, *Aging Ment Health (England)* 5(suppl 1):S7, 2001.

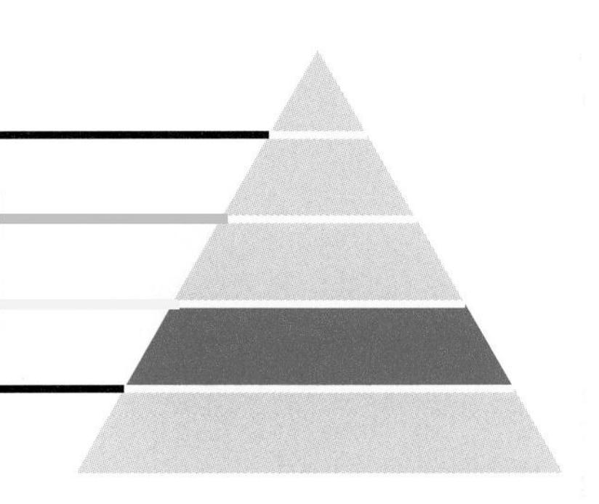

CHAPTER 15

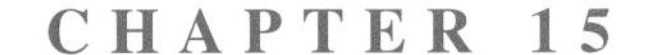

Economic, Health Care, and Legal Issues

Alice G. Rini

A student speaks

I never thought about Social Security or Medicare before I came to nursing school. Now I feel that I will need to be a part of their reform or there will be no way to pay for health care and retirement, if I can ever retire. Everyone needs to be more responsible for themselves.

Sandy, age 22

An elder speaks

Some of the people in my club are finding that their doctors are leaving Medicare or that some specialists are not taking Medicare patients. My doctor told me that Medicare doesn't pay her adequately and has decreased her reimbursement this year even though everything is more expensive. She will keep seeing me, but I fear that if this keeps up, there won't be any doctors for us. I always thought Medicare was good for us seniors, but now I am not sure. Nobody ever planned for so many of us to live so long.

Margaret, age 79

LEARNING OBJECTIVES

On completion of this chapter, the reader will be able to:

1. Explain the fundamentals of Medicare and Medicaid sufficiently to assist elders in obtaining needed information.
2. Briefly explain the history of Social Security and some of the anticipated challenges.
3. Specifically explain legal issues of concern to elders.
4. Define the characteristics of a managed care organization.
5. List several types of long-term care and the various means of financing.
6. Discuss several types of housing for elders.
7. Define various types of elder abuse.
8. Describe the role of the nurse-advocate in relation to legal, health, and economic issues of concern to the aged.

Health care and the law interact intimately in the organization of American health care. The health care system is huge in size and in its consumption of money. More than $1 trillion are spent on health care each year, greater than 15% of the Gross National Product (Blevins, 2001). Health care encompasses a wide variety of services, providers, products, and institutions. Each has its own interest groups, patterns of work, method of financing, and set of laws and regulations. Services, providers, products, and institutions all interact with each other and are therefore influenced by each other and the laws that govern them. Complex federal and state laws affect health care in many areas, many of which are common to all participating in the health care system, and some of which are specific to older adults. Moreover, health care and its systems are undergoing profound change, including the rise of managed care organizations, integrated delivery systems, and changes in the roles of health care providers.

Complicating much of the functioning of the health care system is the fact that the issues affecting the legal environment are unsettled. Fundamental policy questions remain unresolved. The regulation versus competition issue and the tension surrounding the locus of health care decision making—whether centralized in either professional or governmental hands or devolved authority to consumers and their agents—remain undetermined.

Economic factors are always a consideration in the health care system, regardless of who pays. In the United States, there is a complex system of health care providers, payers, insurers, and beneficiaries. For persons over 65 years old, Medicare is the health insurer. Since its inception in 1965, Medicare has exceeded its cost projections and in 2000 spent more than $221 billion on health care for its beneficiaries (Blevins, 2001). Current estimates predict that disbursements will surpass income in 2007.

Medicare is the largest individual payer for health care in the United States. In 2000, Medicare covered health care services for 34 million persons over 65 years of age and 5 million disabled persons under 65 years of age (Board of Trustees, Federal Hospital Insurance Trust Fund, 2001).

Economic conflict exists in several areas: (1) between generations—younger workers, who pay Social Security and Medicare taxes, and elderly retired persons, who use the greatest amount of health care dollars toward the end of their lives; (2) between providers, particularly physicians, who find that reimbursement for care has decreased significantly, and regulators, who are struggling with cost containment; and (3) between Medicare beneficiaries, who are constrained by rules limiting the care for which Medicare will pay, and legislators, who understand the power of the elder voter.

Currently there are more than 35 million persons over age 65 in the United States, accounting for 12.4% of the U.S. population. One in eight persons is more than 65 years old, the age at which the census labels a person as an older adult (U.S. Bureau of the Census, 2001). This is an interesting but probably outdated categorization, given that the image of a 65-year-old is quite different from what it was 25 years ago. Sixty-five was *the* retirement age, arbitrarily determined. Retirement is different today. Some people retire before the usual retirement age, the age at which one can collect Social Security, and go on to pursue a second career. Others, no longer forced to retire at 65, remain productively employed, particularly in professional positions, well into what used to be considered retirement age. Recent statistics reveal that Caucasian women reaching 65 years now have an average additional life expectancy of about 19.2 years; men have 16.1 years. For African Americans, men have 14.3 more years and women 17.3 more years after age 65 (U.S. Bureau of the Census, 2001).

Even more significant for practicing nurses and other health care providers is the rate of change in age-group demographics. Between 1990 and 2000, the number of persons age 1 to 65 years increased by 13.3%, and the number of persons over 65 years increased by 12%. Among those over 65 years, the numbers are even more revealing. Persons 65 to 74 years have increased eight times since 1900, those 75 to 84 years increased 16 times during the same period, and those 85 and older increased 34 times (U.S. Bureau of the Census, 2001). Women live longer than men; in 2000 there were 20.6 million women and 14.4 million men age 65 or older (Table 15-1).

As Table 15-1 shows, women consistently outnumber men at all age levels, becoming more pronounced in the oldest age groups. A close reading of the table, however, reveals that in future decades the differences will diminish (according to current projections).

During the next 30 to 40 years, there will be a significant increase in the number of older adults, particularly the oldest aged, a sharp increase in the percentage of elderly persons in the general population, and changes in the overall age composition of the older adult population. These changes will be brought about mainly by historical and prospective shifts in birth rates and declines in death rates, particularly at the older ages. It is also likely that there will be increases in the numbers of some vulnerable groups, such as the oldest old living alone (especially women), elderly racial minorities living alone and with no living children, and unmarried elderly persons with no living children or siblings (Administration on Aging, 1996).

A small study by Luggen and Rini (1995) also found that the older adults most at risk of isolation, and therefore more likely to be vulnerable, were those who had never had children, or who had no contact with any of their living children.

These data concerning older adults are important factors in determining how society and individuals will cope with the changes expected. Government entitlement programs, developed with apparently good intentions, are at risk because the premise on which they are based is not sustainable—primarily because of the changing demographics of the population, but also because the premise itself is faulty.

This chapter is intended to explain and clarify the legal, political, and economic issues that nurses in all gerontologic practice situations must understand in order to be effective in providing care, education, guidance, and referrals to appropriate resources.

Table 15-1 Ratio of Women to Men by Age Group: 1990-2050

	65-69	70-74	75-79	80-85	85+
1990	1.23	1.34	1.55	1.88	2.59
2000	1.18	1.26	1.39	1.63	2.33
2010	1.16	1.21	1.31	1.49	2.04
2020	1.14	1.19	1.27	1.42	1.91
2030	1.12	1.16	1.24	1.37	1.78
2040	1.13	1.16	1.21	1.31	1.68
2050	1.11	1.14	1.20	1.28	1.60

Compiled by Administration on Aging. From U.S. Bureau of the Census, 2001.

LEGAL AND ECONOMIC NEEDS AND CONCERNS OF OLDER ADULTS

Everyone has a need for legal advice and guidance at some time in his or her life. For older adults, the scope of requirements is expanded or at least enhanced because of the changes that occur with aging. Although nursing has long recognized the need for specialization, the law and lawyers have not always done so, with the exception of a few categories. It is interesting to note that the National Elder Law Foundation (NELF) is one of the few specialty organizations that certifies lawyers who have demonstrated knowledge pertinent to the needs of older adults in several categories. These are outlined in Box 15-1.

These categories of need relate to both legal and economic concerns of older adults and are not very different from those with which nurses deal as they care for their elderly clients, something they have been doing for many years. Gerontologic nursing as a specialty has been evolving and has become more important as the population of older adults has increased and their health care and other needs have been identified, acknowledged, and codified. Nurses who are consulted by clients about legal issues should not attempt to provide legal advice, but should refer their clients to an attorney, preferably one who is certified by NELF. The state or local bar association is able to assist nurses and their clients with this information.

It is somewhat arbitrary to assign a legal or economic label to any of these concerns that older adults may have about their health care and related problems. All of them have elements of both issues. It should be understood that any advocacy for the elderly seeks to preserve their health, independence, dignity, and assets to the extent possible.

HEALTH AND PLANNING FOR CARE

Historical Background

Care of older adults was not very different from that of other persons for many years. When people grew old and unable to live alone or to care for themselves, they were usually cared for by family members. The theory was one of moral responsibility and reciprocity, which was supported by the culture and law (Bohm, 2001). In the early 1900s, almshouses and poor houses emerged to provide care for indigent elderly persons who did not have family available or able to care for them. Most of these facilities were supported by charitable organizations. Later, the government became involved, and when the primary population in almshouses was the elderly, many essentially became public nursing institutions. In some places the law supported the use of public monies for a formerly private purpose—the care of elderly persons—and local governments were authorized to purchase land and erect facilities for the care of the elderly and could tax its citizens to maintain them (*Mason County Infirmary v. Smith's Comm.*, 1901). Public monies usually are not permitted to be used for private purposes; however, in the early 1900s it was determined that the care of indigent elderly could be construed to be a public responsibility (*Maydwell v. Louisville*, 1903).

Because the concept of personal responsibility continued to exist, poor persons who were admitted to care facilities were required to contribute any property they owned that could be used to help pay for the care and maintenance provided (Nacev and Rettig, 2002, p. 142, fn. 26).

Box 15-1 Legal and Economic Needs of Older Adults

- Health and personal care planning
- Residents' rights in long-term care
- Housing issues
- Litigation and administrative advocacy
- Fiduciary representation
- Retirement planning
- Legal capacity
- Income, estate, and gift taxes
- Public benefits
- Insurance matters

From National Elder Law Foundation: *Becoming a certified elder law attorney.* Available at www.nelf.org.

Social Security

Considered by many to be one of the most successful federal programs, Social Security was established in 1935, in the depths of the Great Depression. The primary function of the program was to provide benefits to elderly needy persons and to prevent destitution and dependency in older age (Weinberger, 1996). The program has been managed on what is called a pay-as-you-go system. Payroll taxes collected from employees and employers are immediately distributed to retirees and other beneficiaries. As long as there were more workers contributing than retirees collecting, the program remained solvent. *Solvency* means the ability to pay current debts from current revenues. At the time of its inception the system was constructed to transfer funds from those believed to be relatively well off, workers, to those believed to be relatively poor, retirees. There was probably much truth in that belief at the time.

Another feature of Social Security is something called the Social Security Trust Fund. It has long been known that there is really no "fund" as most people might define it. Instead the federal government treats the Social Security Trust Fund differently than a typical retirement fund that one may have with an employer. Private retirement or pension funds are invested in private sector financial instruments such as stocks, bonds, or real estate holdings, or perhaps government treasury notes. Those funds are held for the beneficiary and may become part of his or her estate if the beneficiary dies before collecting the pension. Some private retirement annuities provide for several choices for receipt of funds after retirement. The retiree could elect to take his or her pension based on his or her own life only, or based on the retiree's and a spouse's life. The amount received is actuarially determined based on the life expectancy of one or two beneficiaries and whether a guaranteed minimum number of years is selected. In all cases, a private pension will cover the actual retiree for his or her lifetime. Social Security funds, although individually deposited by employees, are not reserved for that individual. No one has an account set aside in his or her name. All funds that are not immediately paid out to beneficiaries are used by the federal government for regular operating expenses. The government then puts government bonds, reflecting the debt of the government to Social Security, into the "trust fund." There are no specifically identified funds with which to pay back those borrowed monies to Social Security (Weinberger, 1996).

Financing Social Security. The cost of Social Security is the largest portion of the federal budget, amounting to 22%, more than all other entitlement programs combined, excluding Medicare (Congressional Budget Office, 2002). When the federal government has to pay those claims, in the fairly near future, the only way it will be able to get the monies to do so is to raise taxes or issue additional debt by borrowing from other areas in the economy. This imposes a burden on future generations of workers *and* retirees. The trustees of the Social Security Trust Fund have for many years reported that the fiscal integrity of the fund is in jeopardy and that reform is needed (Friedman, 1999). The 1994 trustees' report expressed concern that if reform and change were not instituted quickly, the magnitude of the changes needed would be great and would threaten the existence of the program (Social Security and Medicare Boards of Trustees, 1994).

Despite the urgent early warnings of the trustees and other analysts, little has been done to address the problems identified. It is widely believed that pressure from certain interest groups, and the belief that the problems are a long way off, have made action politically impossible or deferrable. Steuerle and Bakija (1994) noted that Social Security has possibly lost sight of its primary mission of helping to avoid destitution and dependency among older Americans and changed to an intergenerational money transfer program that ignores need. Furthermore, despite assurances to the contrary, many older persons do not trust the government to make changes that will not hurt the beneficiaries; organizations that represent the elderly are vocal in opposing any change. Eight years after the 1994 predictions and warnings, calculations predicted that the Social Security Trust Fund will be insolvent by 2017—that is, fewer dollars will be paid in compared with what will need to be paid out. Much of this will be due to the influx of the so-called baby boomers, who will begin to retire in 2010 and increase the rate at which the fund is depleted. Funds are predicted to be exhausted by 2029 (Annual report, 2002). To prevent these events the government could raise Social Security taxes, reduce the benefits, or issue new debt. It has already raised the retirement age to as high as 67 for those born after 1960.

The primary causes of the projected growth in Social Security are not factors that Congress can control, although it has been aware of them for many years. The program's growth is influenced by the aging of the population and the percentage of persons in the older age groups, an increasing cost of living, and a higher standard of living (as reflected in higher wages). These factors will place a substantial burden on the economy and the social programs that were designed originally to provide a safety net for the needy. Social Security will not be sustainable in its current form at existing funding levels (OASDI Trustees Report, 2002). Weinberger (1996) asserted that "policymakers have four choices: alter the benefit formula, increase funding for the program, balloon the deficit to meet existing obligations, or restructure the program to allow individuals to save money in private accounts that yield higher returns than the current system."

It is instructive to peruse the OASDI Trustees Reports for the past several years. Although the full documents are lengthy, the summary, *Status of Social Security and Medicare Programs, 2002,* is very readable. These documents are available on the Internet in a user-friendly format at *www.ssa.gov/OACT/TR/index.html* and *www.ssa.gov/OACT/TRSUM/trsummary.html.*

Changing the Face of Social Security. Some proposals for change in Social Security have already been suggested. The most promising, but not without its detractors, is partial privatization, which permits certain persons participating in the Social Security program to invest a portion of their Social Security taxes in a private pension fund. In May 2001, President George W. Bush appointed a bipartisan committee to study and report specific recommendations to preserve Social Security for seniors while building wealth for younger Americans. The committee was asked to make recommendations to modernize and restore fiscal soundness to Social Security, using six guiding principles (President's Commission to Strengthen Social Security, 2001):

- Modernization must not change Social Security benefits for retirees or near-retirees.
- The entire Social Security surplus must be dedicated only to Social Security.
- Social Security payroll taxes must not be increased.
- The government must not invest Social Security funds in the stock market.
- Modernization must preserve the Social Security disability and survivors' insurance programs.
- Modernization must include individually controlled, voluntary personal retirement accounts, which will augment Social Security.

A poll conducted in July 2002 by Zogby International and the Cato Institute Social Security Project found that 68% of those questioned expressed total support of a privatized program. More than half of poll participants 65 and older were in favor of privatization, and the greatest support (82%) was among those under 30. The survey also looked at political and ethnic demographics; there was greater support for than against in all groups (Polling on Social Security, 2002).

Medicare

Medicare, established in 1965 after a tortuous history dating from the time Social Security was proposed, is a federal program that provides mandatory health insurance for persons over 65 and certain disabled persons under 65.

Medicare's Origins. In 1934 President Franklin D. Roosevelt appointed the Committee on Economic Security (CES) to craft a Social Security bill. The original report included a health insurance plan, but there was a great deal of opposition to it, so Roosevelt decided to defer the health insurance part of the bill so as not to lose Social Security (Corning, 1969). The American Medical Association opposed any national program of health insurance, believing it to be "socialized medicine," and made efforts to prevent its implementation (Goodman, 1980). *Fortune* magazine polled the American public in 1942 and found that 76% of those polled opposed government-financed medical care (Cantril, 1951).

Because there was significant opposition to compulsory national health insurance for all, some in Congress recrafted their proposal to provide medical care for the aged, which would cover hospital and nursing home care (Twight, 1997). In 1960, Congress passed the Kerr-Mills bill (P.L. 86-778), which established a needs-based program of medical assistance for poor aged persons. The Kerr-Mills law was believed to be the way to provide care for those who were too poor to pay for it themselves, while avoiding a broader program that would permit government involvement in the general medical care market (Twight, 1997).

Although there continued to be opposition to a broad program of medical care for the aged, Medicare was signed into law in July 1965 by President Lyndon Johnson. Because its supporters knew of the opposition and believed it would not pass Congress alone, it was packaged with a 7% increase in Social Security benefits to all current beneficiaries, grants for maternal and child services, and increased disability coverage (Twight, 1997). Before the final bill was passed, other bills were proposed. One provided for an insurance plan that covered hospital and physician services and medicines; it was a voluntary program. The bill that passed and was signed into law covered only hospital care and provided an optional medical care supplement, but virtually no outpatient medications. It covered persons over age 65 and eligible for Social Security or Railroad Retirement benefits. Twight (1997), in her detailed chronology of the origins of the Medicare program, describes how in Senate and House hearings, some legislators described the Medicare program as a step that would continue to destroy independence and self-reliance and would tax the poor and middle class to subsidize the health care of the wealthy.

Like Social Security, Medicare was designed as a pay-as-you-go system; that is, taxes collected from employers and employees are used for payment of current Medicare beneficiaries and are not placed in a fund earmarked for taxpayers' future medical expenses. Medicare is not means tested; it covers everyone over 65 years old. It is a politically popular program, which is why most legislators have been reluctant to suggest any changes. Few, if any, Medicare beneficiaries alive today know any other way of insuring against unforeseen medical expenses. Most were covered by their employer's health insurance before retirement and have had the expectation of Medicare coverage after retirement.

Medicare is administered by the Centers for Medicare and Medicaid Services (CMS), formerly the Health Care Financing Administration, and is a part of the Department of Health and Human Services, a special entity created to improve the administration of the programs.

Traditional Medicare Today. Today Medicare is the largest single payer for health services in the country. More than 12% of the federal budget is expended for the Medicare program. Forty million persons over age 65 and certain disabled persons younger than 65 were covered by Medicare in 2001. Medicare has two parts:

1. Part A—Hospital Insurance (HI): Covers inpatient care in hospitals, critical access facilities in rural areas, hospice, skilled nursing facilities, and some home care. There is no additional premium for HI other than the Medicare taxes one paid during one's work years. Most people are automatically enrolled in Medicare HI when they reach 65 if they have paid Medicare taxes during their work years. Some of those who did not pay the tax or are eligible for Railroad Retirement may also enroll in Medicare. Those persons who have fewer than 30 quarters of Medicare-covered employment must pay a premium of $316 per month; those with 30 to 39 quarters must pay $175 per month. There is a deductible of $840 in 2003 per benefit period of 60 days for inpatient care. Care that exceeds 60 days incurs a coinsurance cost of $210 per day for days 61 through 90, and $420 for days 91 through 150. The coinsurance for a skilled nursing facility is $105 for days 21 through 100.
2. Part B—Supplemental Medical Insurance (SMI): Covers expenses for physician and nurse practitioner care, as well as some other providers, outpatient hospital care, physical and occupational therapists, and some home care. These services are covered only when medically necessary. There was a premium of $58.70 per month in 2003. Part B is a voluntary enrollment program. However, if one does not enroll within a 7-month period starting 3 months before reaching age 65, there may be a permanent increase of 10% in the premium for the rest of the retiree's life. There is an annual deductible of $100 and 20% coinsurance for covered services.

All Medicare Part A and Part B information is available on the Internet at www.medicare.gov/basics/whatis.asp and www.medicare.gov/amounts2002.

Supplemental or Medigap Insurance Policies. In addition to the original Medicare provisions described earlier, eligible persons may also purchase a supplemental insurance policy, commonly known as a Medigap policy, to help pay for the deductibles and coinsurance not paid by traditional Medicare. The Medigap policies feature standardized benefits, and there are generally several different policies from which to select in each state. Persons searching for an appropriate Medigap plan can peruse the Medicare website for their state or request a print copy of the standard plans (available at *www.medicare.gov/*). Standard plans are designated A through J and all include the basic benefits of Medicare Part A coinsurance, the cost of an extra 365 days of hospital care after the Medicare Part A benefit ends, Medicare Part B coinsurance or copayment, and the first three pints of blood each year. Plans A through J cover increasing benefits and therefore have increasing costs as the number of benefits increases. In some areas, beneficiaries may choose a Medigap Select policy, which restricts enrollees to certain doctors, hospitals, and other providers. Medigap Select policies tend to be less costly (Centers for Medicare and Medicaid Services, 2002b).

Medigap insurance policies cover only the deductibles and part of the 20% coinsurance amounts based on Medicare-approved amounts contracted with providers. It is important to understand that the Medigap policy does not cover 20% of the amount a provider may charge for a service, but only that amount approved by Medicare for that service. Physicians and other providers who agree to accept the Medicare assignment amount will not charge a patient any additional amount beyond the amount unpaid by Medicare and the Medigap policy. Physicians and other providers who do not accept Medicare assignment are paid 75% of the Medicare-approved amount for the service; the provider may then charge the patient the balance up to the approved amount plus 15% (U.S. Department of Health and Human Services, Centers for Medicare and Medicaid Services, 2002b). Patients can save money by asking providers if they accept Medicare assignment or if the provider will waive the 15% surcharge. The patient will still owe the difference between what Medicare actually pays for the service and the total approved amount (Table 15-2).

Medicare + Choice. Established within the Balanced Budget Act of 1997, the Medicare + Choice program was initiated to provide additional choices for beneficiaries and to encourage enrollment in private insurance plans. It was hoped that up to 25% of all beneficiaries would join the Medicare + Choice plans by 2002 (Blevins, 2001). The Balanced Budget Act provided for health maintenance organizations (HMOs), preferred provider organizations (PPOs), medical savings accounts (MSAs), and provider sponsored organizations (PSOs). Although there were no restrictions on the number of persons who could opt for three of these private plans, limitations were placed on MSAs. Only 390,000 persons out of 39 million possible enrollees (1%) were permitted to choose an MSA. By the end of 1998, 346 plans had contracted with Medicare to provide health insurance benefits to Medicare enrollees. By 2000 there were fewer than 260, and in many areas of the country, only one Medicare + Choice plan is available. As of 2001, only 174 Medicare + Choice plans were available, enrolling 14% of possible beneficiaries (Blevins, 2001).

According to the CMS website, only 60% of possible beneficiaries have access to a Medicare + Choice plan, down from 74% in 1998. Plans with prescription coverage are also declining; only 50% of possible beneficiaries have access to such a plan, even with an additional premium. Recently, several more plans have withdrawn from the Medicare + Choice program, and at least 24 will reduce their coverage areas by the end of 2002 (Middleton, 2002). Much of this is related to economic problems in running the plans. Medicare law provides for a 2% increase in premiums to Medicare + Choice plans, but health care costs are increasing at double-digit rates, so they are not cost-effective (Middleton, 2002). Up to 200,000 beneficiaries may lose their Medicare + Choice plan and will have to find another, if possible, or go to traditional, government-run Medicare (Medline Plus, 2002).

Medicare + Choice plans operate by contracting with private insurers who agree to provide all the basic Medicare benefits, plus any additional benefits the plan chooses, to all of its enrollees. The plan is paid a fixed fee each month by Medicare, which is a percentage of the average cost for a

Table 15-2 Examples of Traditional Medicare Transactions with and without Medigap Policy

Amount charged by physician	Amount approved/paid by Medicare	Amount paid by Medigap policy	Amount patient must pay
$1000	$620/$496 at 80%	$99.20 at 80% of balance	$24.80
$2500	$1400/$1120 at 80%	$0 (no Medigap policy)	$280
$1500 (nonparticipating physician)	$850/$680 at 80% less 5% (for nonparticipating) = $646 (usually paid directly to patient)	$130.56 at 80% of balance (if Medigap policy covers nonparticipating physician)	$977.50 (15% above Medicare-approved amount) less $646 from Medicare = $331.50 (possibly partially paid by Medigap policy)

Note: All figures are based on situations where patient has already paid $100 deductible.

Medicare patient in the geographic area; there are high-cost areas and lower-cost areas in the United States. Managed care organizations (MCOs) or HMOs, the most common Medicare + Choice plans, generally have a panel of physicians, hospitals, laboratories, and other providers who agree to provide care and services to the HMO's enrollees for a set fee, either capitated or per service. HMOs use many different reimbursement patterns. Many MCOs/HMOs offer additional services such as vision care, preventive care, and physician or nurse practitioner visits. There is no additional premium for what would normally be covered under traditional Medicare Part A services. Physician and other medical services require the usual Part B premium and some copayment at the time of the office visit. Generally copayments are minimal for primary care practitioners and somewhat higher for specialists. Some insurers require primary care practitioner referrals to specialists. Many MCO/HMO insurers provide prescription drug coverage for an additional premium, often limited in scope, and generally requiring the use of generic drugs (U.S. Department of Health and Human Services, Centers for Medicare and Medicaid Services, 2002a). Box 15-2 provides definitions for various terms related to health care payments and benefits.

MCOs are required to provide information on the incentive arrangements affecting the MCO's physicians to any person receiving Medicare (i.e., a "beneficiary") who requests the information. The following pieces of information must be provided, on request, to current, previous, and prospective enrollees (Centers for Medicare and Medicaid Services, 2002a):

- Whether the MCO's contracts or subcontracts include physician incentive plans that affect the use of referral services
- Information on the type of incentive arrangements used
- Whether stop-loss protection is provided for physicians or physician groups
- If the MCO is required by the regulation to conduct a customer satisfaction survey, a summary of the survey results

CMS has approved 33 applications for PPO plans to be available in 23 states starting in January 2003. Although PPO plans have always been an option, few insurers have used them. This will be a 3-year demonstration project to determine if the Medicare + Choice payment system will work with the PPO. The new plans will be available to any Medicare beneficiaries eligible for Medicare + Choice plans. The plans will establish a provider network that beneficiaries will be encouraged to use, but there will be an out-of-network option (Center for Medicare Advocacy, 2002). See Table 15-3 for a comparison of Medicare plans.

Medicaid. Medicaid is a health insurance program jointly funded by federal and state governments using tax dollars collected into the general funds of each. It provides health services for low-income and other needy persons, including older adults. Medicaid was created in 1965 as part of Title XIX of the Social Security Act at the same time as Medicare. It makes payments for health care provided to Medicaid recipients directly to health care providers. Because it is a joint program, CMS administers the program at the federal level, and there is a state agency in each state that administers at the state level (Nacev and Rettig, 2002).

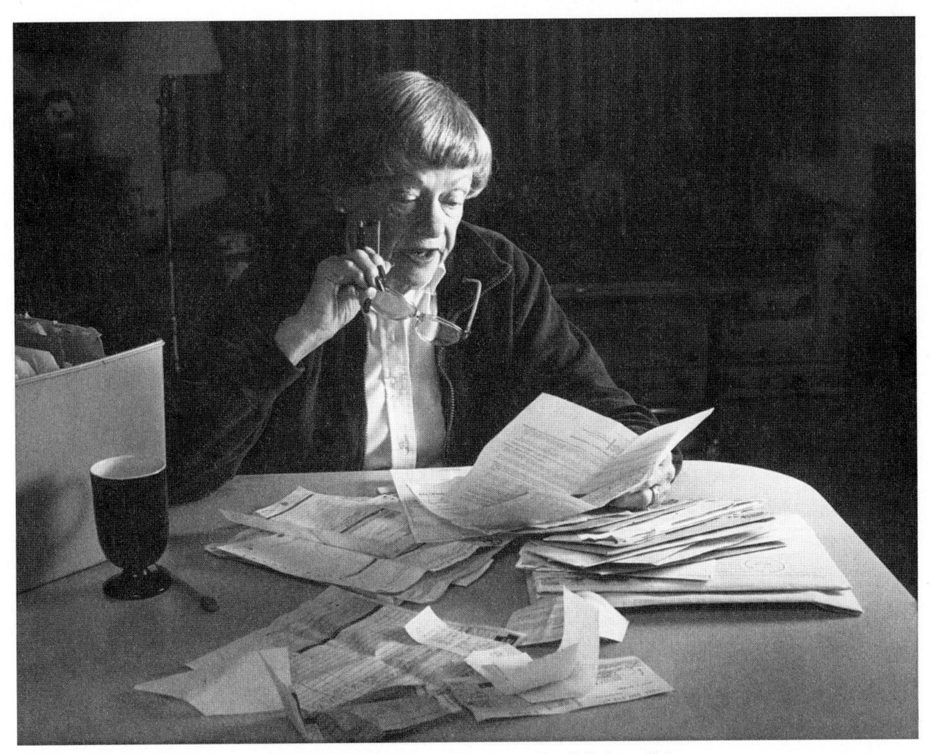

Filling out forms. (Courtesy Rod Schmall.)

Box 15-2 Terms

Managed care organization (MCO): A for-profit or not-for-profit company that manages a system of health care delivery in which patients agree to use health care providers from a panel of physicians, nurse practitioners, therapists, hospitals, pharmacies, and home care agencies, among others designated by the MCO. The MCO monitors the cost of care provided to patients in order to control the cost of care.

Integrated delivery systems: A group of individual entities such as a hospital and physicians that join together into a single entity to provide integrated health care services to contracted clients/patients.

Payers: In the health care context, payers are the entities who pay for health care on behalf of persons who have paid premiums or fees to the payer or, in the case of some government programs, on behalf of persons who are unable to pay themselves.

Providers: One who provides something; a generic term referring to all persons and agencies that provide health care.

Insurer: An individual or organization that underwrites an insurance risk and which agrees to pay compensation or benefits to the insured according to a contract. The insured is the person covered by the insurance contract; with a health insurance contract, the insured is the patient.

Beneficiary: A person who derives a benefit from something; in health care, the person who is a subscriber to an MCO or HMO or who is receiving benefits through Medicare is said to be a beneficiary of those organizations since the person receives medical benefits from his/her association with the organizations.

Preferred provider organization (PPO): A health care delivery system through which providers contract to offer medical services to benefit plan enrollees on a fee-for-service basis at various reimbursement levels in return for more patients and/or timely payment. Enrollees may use any provider in the PPO or outside of the PPO, but they have a financial incentive (e.g., lower coinsurance payments) to use providers within the PPO.

Health maintenance organization (HMO): A health insurance company to which subscribers (patients) pay a predetermined premium or fee in return for a range of medical services from physicians and other health care providers who are approved by the organization. Premiums or fees may also be paid by employers and other organizations on behalf of their employees or members.

Federal law requires states to provide a certain minimum level of service, and states may add other coverage such as prescription drugs, vision care, dentures, prostheses, case management, and other medical or rehabilitative care provided by a licensed health care practitioner. Among the services provided to older adults is nursing home–based care and some home care to eligible persons who cannot afford to pay for their own care. Eligibility for Medicaid is based on income and assets, categorical need, and lack of ability to afford, even with Medicare, the medical care required. There is also a medical need that arises when an older adult requires nursing home care that is not covered by Medicare.

A single adult without a dependent child must contribute all income and assets to pay for nursing home care except for a small personal needs allowance and authorized amounts for medical expenses. If there is a community-dwelling spouse, the spouse is permitted to keep up to $89,000 in assets, the Community Spouse Resource Allowance (CSRA), the family home, a car of any value, and personal property and can have income up to the federal Minimum Monthly Maintenance and Needs Allowance (MMMNA). Realistically, few Medicaid recipients have much in assets or income.

Because there have been instances of transfer of funds by people who need or believe they will soon need nursing home care, in order to become eligible for Medicaid and avoid using their own funds for that care, laws have been enacted to preclude ineligible person from defrauding government programs. Some transfers are permitted, such as to a spouse or a disabled, dependent child. Any other transfer, to another person or to a trust, is considered an improper transfer and will be invalid for the purpose of qualifying for Medicaid. When a person applies for Medicaid, there is a "lookback period" to determine if there have been transfers of funds that would normally be available to the applicant. Transfers to recipients other than a trust have a lookback period of 36 months; transfers to a trust have a lookback period of 60 months. This results in a period of ineligibility for Medicaid until the amount transferred is equal to what the cost of a private-pay stay in a nursing home would cost. For example, a person who transfers $100,000 and is in a nursing home where the monthly rate is $4000 would be ineligible for Medicaid for more than 2 years ($4000 times 24 months = $96,000). Sometimes it is difficult or costly to try to detect transfers guided by devious financial planners, but these costs have become high, and the government will make examples of consumers and professionals who commit fraud.

LONG-TERM CARE

Long-term care consists of a variety of care and services and takes place in many different locations. Long-term care may be chronic care or maintenance care in a nursing home, adult day care, mental health care in a specialized facility, assisted living, home care, subacute care, respite care (which is generally shorter term), and residential care (Teske, 2000). Long-term care is costly, averaging more than $40,000 per year. Teske (2000) identifies three problems with financing long-term care:

1. Cost: An aging population and actual cost increases will quadruple inflation-adjusted costs of long-term care in the next 30 years.

Table 15-3 A Comparison of Medicare Plans

	Original Medicare plan	Medicare + Choice plans	
		Managed care plan (e.g., health maintenance organization)	Private fee-for-service plan
Costs (total out-of-pocket costs)	High	Low to medium	Medium to high
Extra benefits (in addition to Medicare-covered benefits)	None	Most (e.g., prescription drugs, eye examinations, hearing aids, or routine physical examinations)	Some (e.g., foreign travel or extra days in the hospital)
Physician choice	Widest (can choose any physician or specialist who accepts Medicare)	Some (usually must see a physician or specialist who belongs in your plan)	Wide (can choose any physician or specialist who accepts the plan's payment)
Convenience	Varies (available nationwide)	Varies (available in some areas; may require less paperwork and have phone hotline for medical advice)	Varies (available in some areas; may require less paperwork and have phone hotline for medical advice)

From U.S. Department of Health and Human Services, Centers for Medicare and Medicaid Services: *Medicare and you 2002,* pub no CMS-10050, Baltimore, 2002, U.S. Government Printing Office.

2. Reliance on Medicaid: Even the middle and upper middle classes, consciously or not, rely on Medicaid to pay the bulk of nursing home and other long-term care costs.
3. Financing shortfall: Inadequate funds will be available to pay for what has become an entitlement program for those other than the poor, for whom Medicaid was originally intended.

Few people consider how they will live in older age. Although more and more people are planning for financial retirement, rarely has the need for long-term care been included. Because of the failure to plan, and the intention to use government programs, older adults who need long-term care resort to Medicaid. Teske (2000) notes that average Medicaid spending for persons over 65 years is more than six times the spending for younger persons. Older adults make up 10% of the Medicaid population but use 28% of its disbursements. Adults younger than 65 and children make up about 75% of Medicaid recipients but use only 25% of its disbursements. Teske (2000) contends that these differences are almost entirely due to the cost of long-term care.

The federal government has attempted to slow the flow of Medicaid monies to pay for nursing home and other care for the nonpoor by a series of laws enacted to require people to pay as much as they can from their own funds. Examples include the following:

- The 1993 Omnibus Budget Reconciliation Act (OBRA) permitted states to recover the costs of nursing home care from a deceased person's estate.
- The 1996 Health Insurance Portability and Accountability Act (HIPAA) reduced the allowable methods of hiding or transferring monies before needing or entering long-term care.
- The 1997 Balanced Budget Act targeted lawyers and other estate planners, holding them responsible for attempting to circumvent laws that required persons to pay for their own long-term care (Teske, 2000).

To make things worse, long-term care facilities such as nursing homes have been enduring decreases in reimbursement amounts, including a 10% cut in 2002, while regulations regarding the quality of care, quantity of care, and caregiver mix have increased the cost to provide care (Middleton, 2002). A report by the Center for Long Term Care Financing, *The Long Term Care Triathlon* (2000), states that the stakeholders, other than recipients of care, are generally dissatisfied with the long-term care environment and that the current system, if there is one, is not functioning well. Many nursing homes have declared bankruptcy, and many home care agencies have gone out of business. Assisted living communities are not attracting residents in the numbers expected. Stock prices for publicly held long-term care companies are low, and it is difficult to find and keep caregivers.

In the Long Term Care Triathlon study (Center for Long Term Care Financing, 2000), respondents expressed concern that government financing, or its inadequacy, was primarily responsible for the current problems in long-term care. Government financing led the public, uncomfortable with considering the frailties of aging, to avoid responsible planning for long-term care. This reliance on public financing has impeded the development of private financing, and, although some public financing is still necessary for the needy elderly, long-term care insurance is the most promising solution to the future long-term care needs of currently middle-aged and younger people. How to get the public to see this is the hard question.

Long-Term Care Insurance

Only a small percentage of working people and the elderly have long-term care insurance. Part of the reason is the short time frame that legitimate insurance policies have been available. However, most people have not believed that they needed such insurance. Long-term care insurance benefits pay for care in nursing homes, home care, adult day care, and sometimes in assisted living communities. Policies vary in their benefits, and those purchasing them should carefully investigate the insurer company and the contract before buying any policy.

Changing the Long-Term Care Financing Paradigm. Moses and Rosenfeld (2000) suggest a plan to change the paradigm of long-term care financing. People must either save enough to pay for long-term care for a certain time period or buy insurance covering the risk of long-term care. Failing either of these solutions, a person would be required to sign a "long-term care contract" that explicitly acknowledges that one's estate is at risk for the cost of long-term care before government assistance will become available. This policy is no different than the spend-down liability presumed to exist already but which in fact does not.

Another possibility is a federally backed line of credit on a person's estate to enable older Americans to purchase the care they need. This loan would need to be repaid after the death of the borrower's last surviving exempt dependent relative, such as a spouse or disabled child.

Also needed is an improvement of Medicaid and Medicare financing of long-term care by providing more and better home care, assisted living, day care, nursing home care, and other venues not yet established. If fewer Americans are dependent on Medicaid and Medicare for long-term care, it will be easier to help those who are truly needy to obtain adequate care.

Insurance Policies. Long-term care insurance policies typically cover not only nursing home care, but a comprehensive array of care in a variety of settings. Generally one can insure at a specific dollar figure per day with a lifetime maximum. The insured amount is provided if one is a resident in a nursing home, and lesser amounts are available for home care, day care, and other care sites. Generally the insurance policy is triggered if a person needs help with two or three activities of daily living or has a mental or emotional problem that precludes living or staying alone.

As can be seen from Table 15-4, the cost of 1 year of insurance premiums is less than the cost of 1 month in a nursing home at all levels of insurance and at any age. Further, the person who begins paying premiums for the $150/day level at 62 years old will pay $22,440 in 10 years, less than the cost of 1 year in a nursing home or 1 year of home care at 4 hours of care per day; the person who begins paying premiums for the unlimited-duration $150/day level at 52 years old will pay $40,560 in 20 years, again less than the cost of 1 year of nursing home care; the person who begins very early at 45 years old for the $150/day level will pay $34,200 in 30 years. The evidence is strong for the value of long-term care insurance at any age. Generally, insurers will not accept persons over age 65 as an initial insured. Most policies have a waiting period before benefits can be collected. Table 15-4 provides information on premiums for policies that have a 90-day waiting period, meaning that a person needing care will pay the first 90 days from his or her own funds.

Table 15-4 Cost of Long-Term Care Insurance

Age at start of policy	$100/Day for 3 years, $109,500 lifetime limit	$150/Day for 5 years, $274,000 lifetime limit	$150/Day, no limit
45	$52/month	$95/month	$131/month
52	$67/month	$123/month	$169/month
62	$102/month	$187/month	$254/month

Calculated from Federal Employees Long Term Care Insurance Program.

Rights in Long-Term Care

Residents in long-term care facilities have rights under both federal and state law. Care agencies must inform residents of these rights and protect and promote their rights. Because rights are not lost if a resident is incapable of exercising those rights, the person designated by law, such as a guardian, a conservator, or an attorney-in-fact, or the next of kin may exercise these rights. The rights to which residents in long-term care are entitled should be conspicuously posted in the facility. Most laws and rules concerning rights include the following:

- The right to voice grievances and have them remedied
- The right to information about health conditions and treatments and to participate in one's own care to the extent possible
- The right to choose one's own health care providers and to speak privately with one's health care providers
- The right to consent to or refuse all aspects of care and treatments
- The right to manage one's own finances if capable, or choose one's own financial advisor
- The right to be transferred or discharged only for appropriate reasons
- The right to be free from all forms of abuse
- The right to be free from all forms of restraint to the extent compatible with safety
- The right to privacy and confidentiality concerning one's person, personal information, and medical information
- The right to be treated with dignity, consideration, and respect in keeping with one's individuality
- The right to immediate visitation and access at any time for family, health care providers, and legal advisors; the right to reasonable visitation and access for others

Note: This list of rights is a sampling of federal and several states' lists of rights of residents or participants in long-term care. Nurses should check the rules of their own state for specific rights in law for that state.

HOUSING FOR OLDER ADULTS

The large majority of older adults own the homes in which they live. Of the 21.4 million households headed by older persons in 1999, 80% were owners and 20% were renters. The median family income of older homeowners was $22,502. The median family income of older renters was $12,566. In 1999, 39% of older householders spent more than one fourth of their income on housing costs, compared with 36% for homeowners of all ages. For homes occupied by older householders in 1999, the median year of construction was 1962 (it was 1969 for all householders) and 6% had physical problems. In 1999 the median value of homes owned by older persons was $96,442, compared with a median home value of $108,300 for all homeowners. About 76% of older homeowners in 1999 owned their homes free and clear (American Housing Survey, 1999).

According to the U.S. Bureau of the Census (2001), the ownership numbers were similar in 2000. A survey by the American Association for Retired Persons (AARP) completed in 2000 found that 89% of Americans 55 years old and older want to live in their own homes in old age. For those age 75 or older, 94% want to continue to live in their own homes. Rather than move people who need minor help, it is often better to provide such help in the home than resort to institutionalization, for the well-being of the older person as well as financial issues. A good example of such a program is Hope House in New Jersey, a not-for-profit service organization that provides free or low-cost light housekeeping, minor home repair, help with shopping, and other services that help seniors remain living in their homes (Bruno, 2002). Americans are a mobile society, and families do not often all live in the same place. Many younger families have two-worker situations, making it difficult to help with older members of the family, who may be living alone, and perhaps not in close proximity.

Where Older Adults Live

Although older adults overwhelmingly want to live in the homes they own, many express loneliness if they live alone (Bruno, 2002). Even couples seem to need contact with the outside. Many communities offer low- or no-cost centers where seniors can participate in activities that are fun and healthy, such as card-playing, dance and exercise, films, and meals. Older adults tend to stay in the communities with which they are familiar, probably for safety and security reasons, but also because they know other people.

Although many older people are staying in a single-family home, some are looking for smaller or more convenient housing such as town houses or condominiums where maintenance needs, particularly outdoor needs, are eliminated or minimized. Many seniors do not want to continue to care for a large home, or they may not want to have enough space for children, perhaps with grandchildren, to move back home, according to Edward Bloustein of Rutgers University School of Planning and Public Policy (O'Dea, 2002). Bloustein predicts that the most influential "baby boomers" are also shaping the housing market of the future, which is likely to be "empty nester"—type housing, smaller, but not necessarily lower in quality.

It is also important to understand that many current seniors who wish to change housing arrangements are caught in a situation where organized senior housing is too expensive for middle-class and lower-middle-class citizens, but they have too much in income and assets to qualify for subsidized housing.

There are also seniors who, by choice or by need, wish to move into some type of senior housing. Such housing ranges from independent living where people live much as they did in their single-family homes, only with many optional services available and little or no maintenance requirements, through assisted living in its various forms, to skilled nursing facilities. There are many different models of senior housing in each.

Independent Living. Housing facilities for independent-living older adults are planned, designed, and managed to provide for their common housing needs. This housing arrangement varies in types of services offered. Some may provide only an age-segregated environment and an opportunity for socialization. Others provide services such as meals, housekeeping, and in-facility activities. All support the goal of assisting the individual resident to function independently. Resident units may be rented or purchased for ownership. They vary from single-family dwellings, to condominiums, to apartments of various sizes. Usually, children are not permitted to live in senior-designated housing.

Senior housing facilities that have been developed or subsidized through federal programs are monitored by the Federal Department of Housing and Urban Development. Rents vary according to the size of the apartment, the services offered, and the income group the facility is designed to serve. Government subsidies enable some facilities to serve low-income individuals.

Some independent living facilities are luxurious and have gourmet restaurants available for the residents; others are simpler, providing unpretentious but comfortable environments and simple food. Prices are consistent with level of luxury and extent of services.

Assisted Living. Assisted living is a residential long-term care choice for seniors who need more than an independent living environment can offer. They do not, however, need the skilled nursing care and constant monitoring of a skilled nursing facility. There are often several levels of assisted living, or one can purchase the care needed and live relatively independently otherwise. Assisted living provides security with independence and privacy, and it supports physical and social well-being with the health care supervision it provides.

The average age of residents in assisted living facilities in 2000 was 80 years, age ranged from 66 to 94, and more than two thirds were women. The typical assisted living resident is mobile, but needs assistance with approximately two activities of daily living. The most commonly needed help was with housekeeping and medication administration (National Center for Assisted Living, 2000).

Assisted living is more expensive than independent living and less costly than skilled nursing home care, but it is not inexpensive. Costs vary by geographic area, size of a unit, and relative luxury. Cost can range from a low of $1200 to a high of $5000 per month. Most assisted living facilities offer two or three meals each day, light weekly housekeeping, and laundry services, as well as optional social activities at various times of the day.

Assisted living is less strictly regulated than nursing home care; however, several states have enacted statutes that address issues in such facilities. For example, in Kentucky, assisted living laws address what the facility must provide and who the clients of such residences may be (Mitchie, 2001). This prevents the residence from accepting an inappropriate client merely because the person can afford it and protects the vulnerable senior from residing in a place that might be unsafe.

Nursing Homes. Nursing homes are the most regulated of all health care industries and have changed much in the past 20 years. They vary in quality from minimally meeting the regulations to being excellent. However, the evolution of nursing homes and societal needs has necessarily made many changes in service delivery. Most have several levels of care, including assisted living units, subacute care, and rehabilitation. Out-of-pocket costs can be devastating because few patients are covered by Medicare, and then only for limited periods of time and under certain conditions. When used appropriately, nursing homes fill an important need for families and elders. It is highly advisable for individuals to protect themselves and their families with long-term care insurance as they age.

Life Care Retirement Communities. These organizations, also called *continuing care retirement communities*, are residential communities for retired people that provide long-term access to different levels of health care and other services in a single location. Levels of care available include independent living, assisted living, and several degrees of skilled nursing care. Most of these communities provide access to these levels of care for a community member's entire remaining lifetime. Having all levels of care in one location allows community members to make the transition between levels without life-disrupting moves. For married couples in which one spouse needs more care than the other, life care communities allow them to live nearby in a different part of the same community. This industry is maturing. More than 200 such communities are accredited by the Continuing Care Accreditation Commission (CCAC), a national, private, nonprofit organization founded in 1985 and sponsored by the American Association of Homes and Services for the Aging (Life care guide, 2000). Most life care communities charge an entrance fee, which can range from $75,000 to more than $400,000, that covers and reflects the cost of the residence in which the member will live, the possible future care needed, and the quality and quantity of the community services. More information about life care communities is available from the American Association of Homes and Services for the Aging (www.ahasa.org) and the CCAC.

Populations with Special Needs. Gay and lesbian seniors face several problems in housing for their older years. They often have little family support and face some discrimination in housing options. A survey of New York gay persons revealed that two thirds of them lived alone, a much higher number than heterosexual persons of the same age, and were at greater risk for isolation. The need for assisted living may be higher for this population than for others, but many gay and lesbian seniors say that they do not feel welcome at such residences. Those who wish to live together are discouraged from doing so by some organizations. The result has been to design and build assisted living and other care facilities specifically for the gay population. Many of these are small or not yet ready for occupancy, so senior housing remains limited (Human Rights Campaign, 2002).

There is some ambivalence about segregated communities for gay populations. Many gay persons want to remain in their regular communities, much as any other senior. Therefore the market for gay-only retirement housing may not be very large. Some evidence exists that small groups of gay persons have purchased or built homes or rented all the apartments in a building owned by one or more of the group so that they have established their own "community" (Human Rights Campaign, 2002). Nurses should be aware of this heretofore invisible group of aging persons who need access to welcoming resources.

Financial Concerns about Housing

For most housing, older adults must manage for themselves, unless they enter a nursing home, in which case Medicaid may pay for that care. However, most older persons will not need nursing home care; only a small percentage of people will ever need skilled nursing care in a residential setting. Therefore seniors will need to provide for their own living arrangements. The varying possibilities described previously can be costly. To address the need for liquidity in assets for older adults who need cash more than they need the equity in a residence, certain financial vehicles have been established in law to assist them to remain in their home and have money to provide for their needs.

Reverse Mortgages. The greatest asset most middle- and lower-middle-income people have is their house. The increase in the value of much real estate has contributed to the equity many people have that is not being used to provide for life expenses. The reverse mortgage is a mechanism for converting the equity in a house to cash. Lenders who participate in such transactions are bound by federal truth-in-lending laws. Such lenders include banks, private lenders, and the federal government, the latter through the Home Equity Conversion Mortgage (HECM). HECM was established in 1987 and is administered by the Department of Housing and Urban Development (HUD) (O'Reily, 2002). To be eligible for a reverse mortgage, an individual must be at least 62 years old, occupy at least one unit in the residence subject to the reverse mortgage, be able to service the mortgage, receive appropriate and adequate counseling concerning the transaction, and have a very low or no mortgage balance (Nacev and Rettig, 2002).

ADVOCACY

Advocacy consists of arguing on behalf of, supporting, and defending a client or his or her cause. The advocate can be any person, including family members, professional nurses, attorneys, physicians, and other health care personnel. Some advocates are hired for that function alone, such as patient/client/resident care representatives in health care facilities or ombudsmen in any kind of industry who investigate complaints and problems for the consumers of the services or products produced by the industry. Ombudsmen can also assist in achieving fair solutions. Advocacy includes many different actions:

- Represent people with legal needs in administrative and court proceedings so that their rights are protected
- Act as and provide legal briefs as *amicus curiae* (friend of the court) for certain issues affecting the elderly
- Investigate complaints of abuse of any kind or of neglect-related injury or death in institutions
- Provide information personally and publicly to older adults concerning their legal and other civil rights and how to enforce those rights
- Provide referrals to sources of help that the advocate cannot personally provide
- Provide technical support and education or training to clients and families so that they will be better able to manage their own needs

In a health care situation, advocacy is acting for or on behalf of another in terms of pleading for and supporting the best interests of that other person in terms of choice, provision, and refusal of health care. Nurses act as advocates of their clients when they act to support the person as a free agent who has autonomy in the health care situation (Rini, 1998).

Powers of Attorney

There are two types of power of attorney—regular, or general, power of attorney and durable power of attorney. General power of attorney grants specific power to an attorney-in-fact, and this power ends at the disability or death of the principal or grantor. Durable power of attorney survives any subsequent disability or incapacity of the principal. A written document is necessary to appoint an attorney-in-fact, and for a durable power of attorney to attach, it must so state by indicating that the power is not affected by disability or incapacity or lapse of time. Attorneys-in-fact owe their fiduciary obligations to the grantor or principal only, not the court (Nacev and Rettig, 2002). Those holding durable powers of attorney may make health care decisions for a principal consistent with the principal's wishes. Often these wishes are expressed in a living will or advance directive.

Guardians and Conservators

A guardian is an individual, agency, or corporation appointed by the court to have care, custody, and control of a disabled person and manage his or her personal or financial affairs (or both). *Disabled* in this sense means legally, not medically, disabled, meaning the person is unable to manage personal and financial business. Such a disability includes an inability to make informed decisions about personal matters and lack of capacity to provide for one's physical health and safety, including, but not limited to, health care, food, shelter, and personal hygiene. If a person needs assistance only with financial assets, the court will appoint a conservator. If a person is deemed by a court to be partially disabled only, the court will appoint a limited guardian or limited conservator. The court will act in the best interests of the disabled person.

In terms of deciding who or what entity would be best appointed, the court will recognize someone who already has power of attorney from the principal, now disabled, and seek to select someone who was the principal's original preference unless there is a reason not to do so. In any case, the appointed guardian or conservator has a responsibility to the court, as well as the principal or ward. Guardians must be aware of guardianship law in the state of appointment and adhere to it strictly. The guardian must take custody of the ward, establish safe shelter, provide for care and maintenance, provide appropriate consent for medical or other professional care, manage financial resources carefully, protect and ensure the rights of the ward, and file an annual report with the appointing court (Nacev and Rettig, 2002). If the principal had appointed an attorney in fact, and the court later appoints a guardian or conservator, the power of attorney effectively terminates with respect to the duties assigned by the court to the guardian or conservator.

A guiding principle in guardianships is to accomplish the care and protection needed in the least restrictive way; this is not so different from the care nurses provide in long-term care and home care situations. The law supports the idea that a person has a right to as much autonomy as he or she can manage without sacrificing safety. It is, of course, sometimes difficult for a limited guardian to protect a ward completely from acts of bad judgment. The possibility of an elderly, somewhat incompetent man being seduced by a younger woman seeking his wealth is not uncommon. If, however, the man is not considered incompetent enough to withhold his freedom to spend some of his money, the guardian may not be able to stop it. The guardian can go to court to expand the scope of guardianship in such cases; however, if it appears that the only reason is to preserve the assets for heirs, sometimes courts will permit the ward to spend to some degree as he sees fit.

The guardian may also make decisions about end-of-life care. In a major decision the Kentucky Supreme Court permitted a court-appointed guardian, who happened to be the mother of the ward, to terminate artificial nutrition and hydration (*DeGrella v. Elston,* 1993). In this case the ward had not made an advance directive and the court permitted a guardian and next of kin to substitute her judgment for that of the ward on a showing that the ward would have chosen to terminate had he been able to do so.

Consent

Consent is a concept that arises from the idea of human self-determination and autonomy. In the health care situation, consent is related to accepting or refusing care and treatments and is expressed in the legal doctrine of informed consent. Informed consent requires the disclosure of information about a proposed treatment that might be material to a client's decision about consenting to the treatment. State law generally specifies the extent of information to be disclosed. Most courts have upheld providing information that a reasonable health care provider would disclose in the same or similar circumstances, or that which a reasonable client would consider material to his or her decision.

Consent for treatment is based on decision-making capacity of the client. Such capacity is determined by the provider(s) proposing the care or treatment and intending to carry it out. It means that the client is able to understand the nature and purpose of the procedure and appreciate its possible risks and benefits. There is a presumption of decisional capacity in adults, elderly persons, and others unless there is a reason to believe the person cannot understand the provided information or is unable to make an informed decision. Providers then need to seek consent from guardians, attorneys-in-fact, or family members (Rini, 1998). Consent for research participation is a more detailed and extensive process, because treatments provided in such circumstances may not necessarily directly benefit the client.

Competency, in contrast, is a legal judgment rendered by a court on the basis of evidence presented in a hearing in which the person to be judged may testify. Competency means the ability to transact business or sign legally binding documents. If a person is judged incompetent, usually a guardian or conservator is appointed.

Advance Directives

Advance directive is an all-encompassing term used to describe living wills, durable powers of attorney for health care, and health care surrogate appointments. Advance directives are a creation of state law, arising from the federal Patient Self-Determination Act of 1991. The advance directive is a written document executed by a competent declarant who, in advance of need, establishes his or her preferences regarding acceptance or refusal of treatments under certain circumstances, should the declarant be unable to make such decisions at the time. The directive may have elements of the living will in that it specifies what type of life-sustaining care is acceptable or which should be avoided or withdrawn. It may also stipulate a surrogate health care decision maker who would be authorized to make treatment decisions when the declarant is no longer able to do so. The surrogate's decisions are expected to be consistent with the preferences stated in the directive. Advance directives become effective when the declarant is terminally ill and cannot make informed decisions, is in a persistent vegetative state, or is permanently unconscious as defined by state law (Rini, 1998).

Additional Requirements for Effective Advance Directives. In some states declarants will have either a living will or a surrogate decision maker or both in separate documents. Form and process for the execution of any of these documents must be done according to state law so that they are recognized at the time they are needed. Although an attorney is not necessary for the preparation of advance directives, it is often wise to consult one so that all necessary elements are included for the protection of the declarant and any person appointed to make decisions for him or her. Some states provide a standard form for advance directives. Most important is that the declarant's signature is witnessed by the appropriate number of objective persons. Most states prohibit witnesses to be beneficiaries of any will or trust or principals or employees of a residence in which the declarant lives; such restrictions prevent any perception of impropriety. Anyone can be a surrogate, although this is frequently a family member or a trusted attorney for someone without family. Anyone associated with the health care facility in which the declarant is receiving care may not be a surrogate.

Revoking Advance Directives. A declarant may revoke an advance directive at any time either verbally or in writing. The declarant may also indicate revocation by tearing, burning, or destroying the document, preferably with witnesses. Directives may also be amended; the original formal language is not necessary, and declarants can add items in writing or cross out unwanted passages. If the declarant becomes incompetent, revocation is no longer possible.

ELDER ABUSE

Federal definitions of elder abuse, neglect, and exploitation appeared for the first time in the 1987 Amendments to the Older Americans Act. These definitions were provided in the law only as guidelines for identifying the problems and not for enforcement purposes. Elder abuse is defined by state law, and state definitions vary considerably from one jurisdiction to another in terms of what constitutes the abuse, neglect, or exploitation of the elderly (National Center on Elder Abuse, 2002). Abuse of elderly persons can take place at home, in institutions, or by self-neglect. If the abuser or neglectful person is a caretaker, the caretaker is subject to tort litigation; that is, he or she can be sued for the injuries to the elderly person and may have to pay monetary damages. If the abuse or neglect is of such a nature that it rises to a criminal act or if the abuse has to do with theft or conversion of property or money, the caretaker will be subject to criminal prosecution. Many states have reporting statutes that require certain persons who become aware of abuse, neglect, or exploitation to report it to appropriate authorities. Who that authority is can be found in state laws (Nacev and Rettig,

2002). The actual incidence of abuse of all types is probably underreported and underestimated, and therefore it is not well documented.

Physical Abuse

Physical abuse is the use of physical force that may result in bodily injury, physical pain, or impairment. It includes, but is not limited to, acts of violence such as striking (with or without an object), hitting, beating, pushing, shoving, shaking, slapping, kicking, pinching, and burning. The inappropriate use of drugs and physical restraints, force-feeding, and physical punishment of any kind also are examples of physical abuse (National Center on Elder Abuse, 2002). Any unexpected injury, bruise, or change in behavior of the elderly person may be a sign that requires further investigation.

Sexual Abuse

Actually a form of physical abuse, sexual abuse is considered separately because there are so many subtle considerations. Many older people are sexually active and desire closeness and intimacy with a partner. The question that professionals need to answer is whether the sexual contact was consensual or if the person is able to consent. Sexual abuse of elders is nonconsensual sexual contact of any kind with an elderly person. Sexual contact with any person incapable of giving consent is also considered sexual abuse. It includes but is not limited to unwanted touching and all types of sexual assault or battery, such as rape, sodomy, coerced nudity, and sexually explicit photographing (National Center on Elder Abuse, 2002). Nurses and other health care providers may observe injuries from rough or forceful sexual activity; however, sometimes there may not be injury, but certain behaviors may be revealing. Fear of certain persons, resistance to touch in the genital area, or reports of sexual contact should not be ignored.

Emotional and Psychologic Abuse

Emotional and psychologic abuse includes but is not limited to verbal assaults, insults, threats, intimidation, humiliation, and harassment. Treating an older person like a child; isolating an elderly person from his or her family, friends, or regular activities; and enforced social isolation are examples of emotional and psychologic abuse (National Center on Elder Abuse, 2002). This kind of abuse is often a deliberate effort to dehumanize the elderly person, sometimes to mitigate the guilt of providing poor care or abusing the person emotionally (Rini, 1998).

Neglect

Neglect is passive abuse not characterized by physical violence. It may include withholding food, medication, medical treatment, and personal care necessary for the well-being of the elderly person. It also includes behavior that ignores the elderly person's obvious needs even though the caretaker is present. Sometimes this neglect can be the result of feeling overwhelmed by the responsibilities of caregiving; however, this dilemma does not excuse or justify the abuse. The possibility of respite care may be a consideration before taking major legal action if there is a possibility of remedying the situation.

Financial Exploitation

Financial or material exploitation is the illegal or improper use of an elder person's funds, property, or assets. The persons most likely to commit such acts are family members and other caregivers. Exploitation may be accomplished by force, such as demanding that the elderly person sign checks or other documents with the threat of withholding care. It can also be done with stealth through deceit, misrepresentation, fraud, or undue influence, such as cashing an elderly person's checks without authorization or permission, forging a signature, or misusing or stealing an older person's money or possessions. There can also be the improper use of conservatorship, guardianship, or power of attorney. Whereas other forms of abuse have external signs, it is often difficult to detect financial exploitation. Care is costly, and much of the elderly person's assets may be gone before it is noted that far more has been used than seems to be needed. Changes in banking practices, failure to pay medical or other care bills, unexpected changes in a will, and finding personal valuable items missing are all evidence of possible financial exploitation and should be reported to proper authorities.

Self-Neglect

Self-neglect is behavior of an elderly person, usually a function of diminished physical or mental capacity, that threatens his or her own health or safety. Self-neglect generally manifests itself in an older person as a refusal or failure to provide himself or herself with adequate food, water, clothing, shelter, personal hygiene, medication (when indicated), and safety precautions. Situations in which a mentally competent older person, who understands the consequences of his or her decisions, makes a conscious and voluntary decision to engage in acts that threaten his or her health or safety is a matter of personal choice. It is an ethical question as to how much health care professional should intervene in these situations unless it can definitely be determined that the person lacks capacity or competence.

Nursing Intervention

Nurses should be aware of whether they are in mandatory or permissive reporting states so that they can act appropriately in situations where some type of abuse is observed. If the elderly person's life is in danger, however, health care professionals must act to protect the vulnerable person. Nurses who have close relationships with their clients are likely to note subtle changes in physical or emotional condition, behavior, and financial condition early enough to forestall a critical situation. Clients are also more likely to confide in professionals with whom they feel trust.

If nurses report some type of abuse and have to testify in court, it is wise to seek counsel for themselves before responding to subpoenas or court orders so that they know their own rights as witnesses, as professionals, and in relation to the client's information that may be disclosed. This does not mean that the nurse will be excused from testifying; a court order may not be ignored. Nurses are generally protected from liability for breaking confidentiality when responding to a court order; however, the law for a particular state is best interpreted by one's own attorney.

Human Needs and Wellness Diagnoses

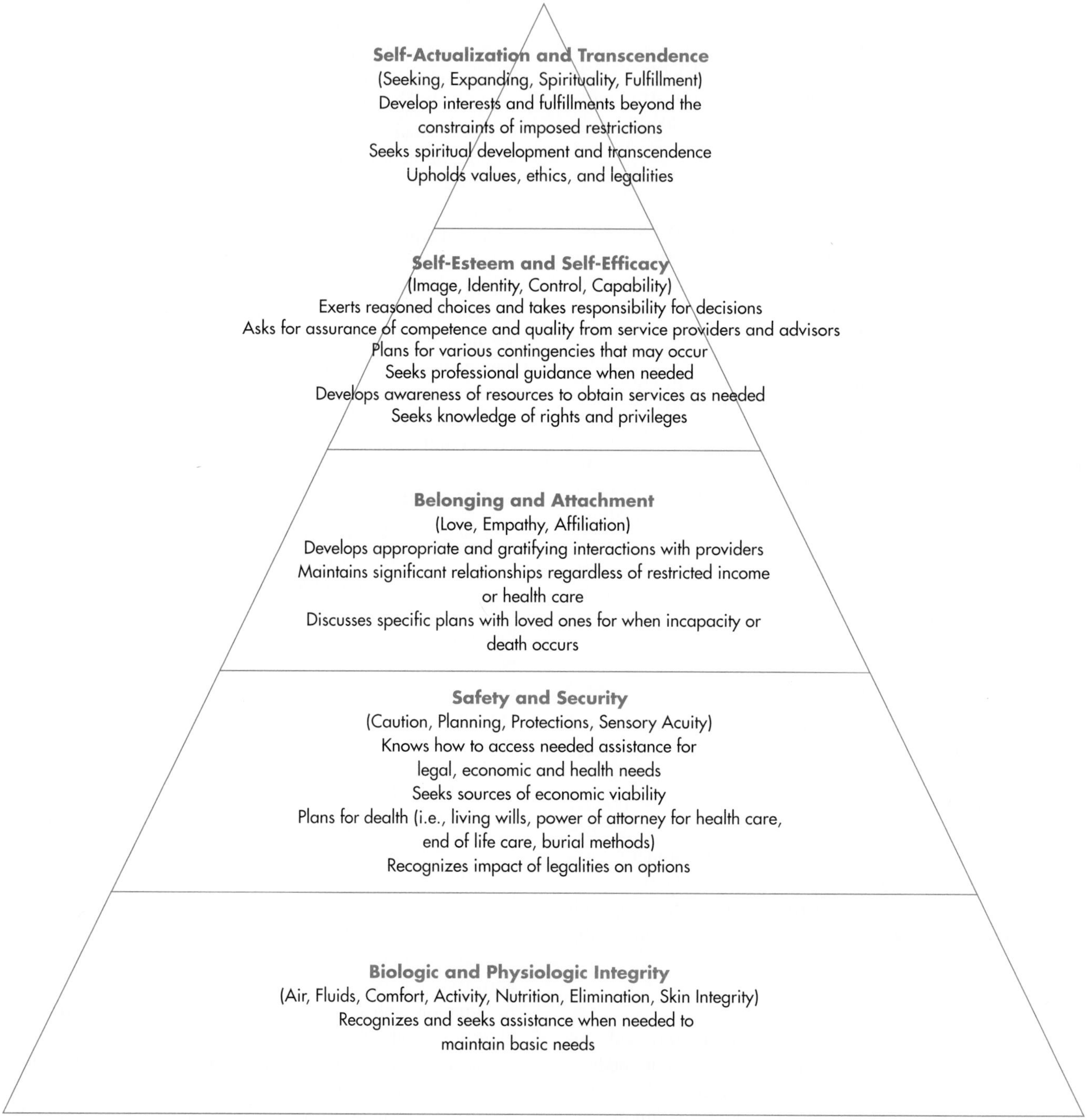

Self-Actualization and Transcendence
(Seeking, Expanding, Spirituality, Fulfillment)
Develop interests and fulfillments beyond the constraints of imposed restrictions
Seeks spiritual development and transcendence
Upholds values, ethics, and legalities

Self-Esteem and Self-Efficacy
(Image, Identity, Control, Capability)
Exerts reasoned choices and takes responsibility for decisions
Asks for assurance of competence and quality from service providers and advisors
Plans for various contingencies that may occur
Seeks professional guidance when needed
Develops awareness of resources to obtain services as needed
Seeks knowledge of rights and privileges

Belonging and Attachment
(Love, Empathy, Affiliation)
Develops appropriate and gratifying interactions with providers
Maintains significant relationships regardless of restricted income or health care
Discusses specific plans with loved ones for when incapacity or death occurs

Safety and Security
(Caution, Planning, Protections, Sensory Acuity)
Knows how to access needed assistance for legal, economic and health needs
Seeks sources of economic viability
Plans for death (i.e., living wills, power of attorney for health care, end of life care, burial methods)
Recognizes impact of legalities on options

Biologic and Physiologic Integrity
(Air, Fluids, Comfort, Activity, Nutrition, Elimination, Skin Integrity)
Recognizes and seeks assistance when needed to maintain basic needs

These are not all the possible wellness diagnoses that may be identified. The above are examples of nursing diagnoses that should be considered when planning care for the older adult.

KEY CONCEPTS

- Health care and its systems are undergoing profound changes, including the rise of managed care organizations, integrated delivery systems, and changes in the roles of health care providers, and all these changes affect the care of the older adult.
- Since its inception in 1965, Medicare has exceeded its cost projections and in 2000 spent more than $221 billion on health care for its beneficiaries. Current estimates predict that disbursements will surpass income in 2007.
- During the next 30 to 40 years, there will be a significant increase in the number of older adults, particularly the oldest aged, a sharp increase in the percentage of elderly persons in the general population, and changes in the overall age composition of the older adult population.
- The fiscal integrity of the Social Security Trust Fund is in jeopardy, and reform is needed. If reform is not instituted quickly, the magnitude of the changes needed will be great and may threaten the existence of the program.
- Few people consider how they will live in older age. Although more and more people are planning for financial retirement, the need for long-term care is rarely included.
- Medicare has been a popular program, but it too continues to sow the seeds of its own destruction. Significant reform is needed, but few seem willing to tackle the chore.
- Elder abuse has not diminished even with more laws and mandatory reporting. With a larger number of frail elderly persons and fewer people to care for them, there is concern that this will likely escalate, as well as concern about how professionals will deal with it.
- Nurses should always be aware of and exercise their own legal rights and responsibilities.

▲ CASE STUDY

Mr. and Mrs. J, ages 62 and 60, respectively, have been married for 35 years. Mr. J was a midlevel executive with a flourishing company. With company stock options and an attractive pension plan, their future looked bright. They owned their home, a split-level, four-bedroom house in a lovely suburban community located on the bay. Their small cabin cruiser gave them a great deal of pleasure, and they also frequently took commercial cruises. Their lifestyle was geared to their upper-middle-class income, as were their friends. When Mr. J was 58 years old, the company was sold to a multinational corporation based outside the United States, and Mr. J no longer had a position with the new company. The stock dropped in price, the pension plan was inadequate if drawn on early, and there was a penalty for drawing on tax-deferred funds before age 59½. It appears the pension funds were poorly invested and may not bring the expected returns. Though their health is presently good, they are concerned about the future of Medicare, managed care, and whether to buy long-term care insurance. Mrs. J had never worked outside the home and had no salable skills. What they had thought to be a very comfortable retirement became one of serious concern. They had saved a considerable amount in their middle years, but it was soon depleted as it was used for general expenses. Now Mr. J has begun to draw on his Social Security at a reduced benefit rate, and Mrs. J is collecting Social Security based on her husband's benefits. Combined, their retirement income is about $2800 per month. This is insufficient to maintain the style of living to which they are accustomed. They are able to get by, but their income will not be adequate for maintaining and repairing their 35-year-old house, maintaining their boat, or their present social life. In addition, taxes keep going up as property values continue to rise. Mrs. J says, "We really don't know what to do to ensure that we will have sufficient income for our needs 20 years from now. I'm really frightened about our future."

▲ CASE STUDY

Jake had retired after 20 years as a sergeant in the U.S. Army. For several years he did odd jobs, often as a mechanic in a nonunion shop or helping friends with home and mechanical repairs. He simply never found his niche after leaving the service. Some thought his war experiences had created serious psychologic problems for him. His wife, a successful nursing faculty person, had a good retirement plan. When his wife realized she was dying of cancer, she selected spousal survivor benefits in her retirement and insurance policies. After her death, Jake was financially secure though grief stricken because he had depended on his wife's practical and emotional support. Two years later Jake met Jane and soon realized he wished to marry her but found that his spousal retirement and Social Security benefits would be terminated if he married. Jake contacted a friend of his deceased wife to discuss his feelings and thoughts with her. He said, "I will not be content unless I marry Jane, but without the benefits I now receive I won't be able to manage. I wonder what I should do?"

Based upon one of the case studies, develop a nursing care plan using the following procedure:*

List comments of client that provide subjective data.

List information that provides objective data.

From these data identify and state, using accepted format, two nursing diagnoses you determine are most significant to this client at this time. List two client strengths that you have identified from data.

Determine and state outcome criteria for each diagnosis. These must reflect some alleviation of the problem identified in the nursing diagnosis and must be stated in concrete and measurable terms.

Plan and state one or more interventions for each diagnosed problem. Provide specific documentation of source used

*Students are advised to refer to their nursing diagnosis text and identify possible or potential problems.

to determine appropriate intervention. Plan at least one intervention that incorporates the client's existing strengths.

Evaluate success of intervention. Interventions must correlate directly with the stated outcome criteria in order to measure the outcome success.

STUDY QUESTIONS/ACTIVITIES

What would be the focus of your first interaction with Mr. and Mrs. J?

Discuss various options that may provide them more economic security. Compare the benefits they might obtain from a reverse annuity mortgage with the benefits of selling the home and entering a life-care community. Discuss the pros and cons. How would you initiate such a discussion?

Discuss the limitations of Medicare and the out-of-pocket costs elders experience.

How common is a situation such as the Js'?

What major economic and legal issues are a concern of yours as you contemplate your old age?

Discuss the pros and cons of managed health care.

Do you believe it is acceptable to spend the great majority of our health dollars on the very old when several million children have no health care?

Is age a valid criterion for denial of certain medical services?

Discuss the meanings and the thoughts triggered by the student's and elder's viewpoints expressed at the beginning of the chapter. How do these vary from your own experience?

Discuss Social Security with an older relative and its effectiveness for him or her.

Consider Jake's dilemma and propose various solutions, remembering his personal history and cohort.

How have your parents' expenditure patterns changed as they age?

What do you believe the "baby boomers" should do about their future economic situation and health care?

RESEARCH QUESTIONS

What do elders find most helpful about Medicare? Least helpful?

How would elders like to see Medicare changed?

What are elders' thoughts and attitudes about managed care?

Whom do elders most frequently contact when they need legal and economic advice?

How many elders feel secure about their economic future?

What are the current average out-of-pocket costs for elder health care?

How do elders feel about the rationing of health care based on age or survivability?

Are the poverty-inducing effects of widowhood and retirement different in specific ways in various ethnic groups?

What are the prevalent attitudes of the aged persons with whom you are acquainted regarding their economic future?

REFERENCES

Administration on Aging: *Special report: aging in the 21st century,* 1996. Available at *www.aoa.gov*

American Housing Survey for the United States in 1999, Current Housing Reports H150/99, Washington, DC, Department of Housing and Urban Development. Available at *www.census.gov/hhes/www/ahw.html*

Annual report of the Board of Trustees of the Federal Old-Age and Survivors Insurance and Disability Insurance Trust Funds, March 2002. Available at *www.ssa.gov/OACT/TR/TR02/index.html*

Blevins SA: *Medicare's midlife crisis,* Washington, DC, 2001, Cato Institute.

Board of Trustees, Federal Hospital Insurance Trust Fund: *Annual report of the Board of Trustees of the Federal Hospital Insurance Trust Fund,* 2001. Available at *cms.hhs.gov/publications/trusteesreport/default.asp*

Bohm D: Striving for quality in American nursing homes, *DePaul Journal of Health Care Law* 4:317, 2001.

Bruno L: Senior living can be lonely, *Daily Record,* March 24, 2002, Morris County, NJ. Available at *www.dailyrecord.com/news/wherewelive/series1/32402seniorliving.htm*

Cantril H: *Public opinion 1935-1946,* Princeton, NJ, 1951, Princeton University Press.

Center for Long Term Care Financing: *The long term care triathlon,* 2000. Available at *www.centerltc.org/pubs/triathlon.pdf*

Center for Medicare Advocacy: Medicare + Choice PPO Demonstration Programs, 2002. Available at *www.medicareadvocacy.org/Medicare+Choice%20%PPO%20Demonstration.htm*

Centers for Medicare and Medicaid Services: *Guidance on disclosure of physician incentive plan information for Medicare beneficiaries,* Baltimore, 2002a, Centers for Medicare and Medicaid Services.

Centers for Medicare and Medicaid Services: *Choosing a Medigap policy,* pub no CMS-02110, Baltimore, 2002b, U.S. Department of Health and Human Services. Available at *www.medicare.gov/Publications/Pubs/pdf/guide.pdf*

Congressional Budget Office: The impact of trust fund programs on federal budget surpluses and deficits, *Long Range Fiscal Policy Brief #5,* 2002. Available at *www.cbo.gov/showdoc.cfm?index=3974&sequence=0*

Corning P: *The evolution of Medicare: from idea to law,* research report no 29, Washington, DC, 1969, U.S. Department of Health, Education and Welfare, Social Security Administration, Office of Research and Statistics, U.S. Government Printing Office.

DeGrella v. Elston, 858 S.W.2d 698 (KY 1993).

Friedman M: Speaking the truth about Social Security reform, *Cato Briefing Paper,* no 46, Apr 12, 1999. Available at *www.socialsecurity.org/pubs/articles/bp-046es.html*

Goodman JC: The regulation of medical care: is the price too high? *Cato Public Policy Research Monograph No. 3,* San Francisco, 1980, Cato Institute.

Human Rights Campaign: Aging: senior housing, 2002. Available at *www.hrc.org/familynet/chapter.asp?article=390*

Life Care Guide, 2000. Available at *www.lifecareguide.com*

Luggen AS, Rini AG: Assessment of social networks and isolation in community based elderly men and women, *Geriatr Nurs* 16(4):179-181, 1995.

Mason County Infirmary v. Smith's Comm., 1901 KY Lexis 234 (KY 1901).

Maydwell v. Louisville, 76 S.W. 1091, 92 (KY 1903).

Medline Plus: Medicare health plan withdrawals confirmed, *Reuters Health News,* 2002. Available at *www.nlm.nih.gov/medlineplus*

Middleton C: Give back this entire price control scheme, *Health Policy Prescriptions* 1(10), October 2002.

Mitchie: KRS 194A.700 et seq., 2001.

Moses SA, Rosenfeld DM: *The myth of unaffordability,* Center for Long Term Care Financing, 2000. Available at *www.centerltc.com/pubs/myth%20Report.pdf*

Nacev AN, Rettig J: A survey of key issues in Kentucky elder law, *Northern Kentucky Law Review* 29(1):139, 2002.

National Center for Assisted Living: *About assisted living,* 2000. Available at *www.ncal.org*

National Center on Elder Abuse: 2002. Available at *www.elderabusecenter.org*

National Elder Law Foundation: Becoming a certified elder law attorney. Available at *www.nelf.org*

OASDI Trustees Report, 2002. Available at *www.ssa.gov/OACT/TR/TR02/index.html*

O'Dea C: Demand is high for low-cost housing, *Daily Record,* March 24, 2002, Morris County, NJ. Available at *www.dailyrecord.com/news/wherewelive/series1/32402lowcosthousing.htm*

O'Reily T: New choices in long term care, *Daily Record,* March 26, 2002, Morris County, NJ. Available at *www.dailyrecord.com/news/wherewelive/series1/032502choices_business.htm*

Polling on Social Security: Cato Institute/Zogby International, 2002. Available at *www.socialsecurity.org/zogby/zogby-2002.pdf*

President's Commission to Strengthen Social Security, May 2001. Available at *www.csss.gov/index.html*

Rini AG: Legal and ethical issues, section VIII. In Luggen AS, Travis SS, and Meiner S: *NGNA core curriculum for gerontological advanced practice nurses,* Thousand Oaks, CA, 1998, Sage Publications.

Social Security and Medicare Boards of Trustees: *Status of the Social Security and Medicare programs: a summary of the 1994 annual reports,* Apr 1994, p 13. Available at *www.ssa.gov/history/reports/trust/1994/1994.pdf*

Steuerle CE, Bakija JM: *Retooling Social Security for the 21st century,* Washington, DC, 1994, Urban Institute.

Teske R: How to cope with the coming crisis in long-term care, *Heritage Lecture #658,* April 2000. Available at *www.heritage.org/Research/HealthCare/h1658.cfm*

Twight C: Medicare's origin: the economics and politics of dependency, *Cato Journal* 16(3), 1997.

U.S. Bureau of the Census: *Statistical abstract of the United States: 2002,* ed 122, Washington, DC, 2001, U.S. Government Printing Office.

U.S. Department of Health and Human Services: The new Centers for Medicare and Medicaid Services, June 14, 2001. Available at *www.hhs.gov/news/press/2001pres/20010614a.html*

U.S. Department of Health and Human Services, Centers for Medicare and Medicaid Services: *Medicare and you 2002,* pub no CMS-10050, Baltimore, 2002a, U.S. Department of Health and Human Services.

U.S. Department of Health and Human Services, Centers for Medicare and Medicaid Services: *Medicare and you: does your doctor or supplier accept assignment?,* Pub no 10134, Baltimore, 2002b. Available at *www.medicare.gov/Publications/Pubs/pdf/10134.pdf*

Weinberger M: *Social Security: facing the facts,* Washington, DC, 1996, Cato Project on Social Security privatization. Available at *www.socialsecurity.org/pubs/ssps/ssp3.html*

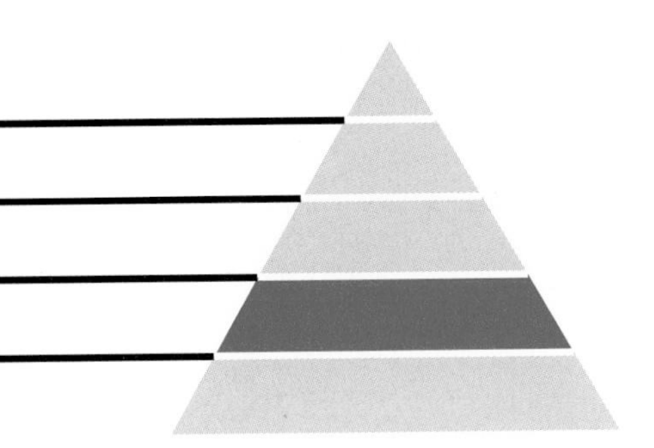

CHAPTER 16

Frailty, Vulnerability, Neglect, and Abuse

Priscilla Ebersole

A student speculates

I really can't believe I will ever feel frail or unable to care for myself. I value my independence. I will never let that happen to me!

Ashley, age 20

An elder speaks

When I was young I was so strong and capable, and I must say, successful. I took care of my in-laws and my wife as she became older and ill. Now there are so many things I find it hard to do and so few things I can eat without unpleasant consequences. Even a glass or so of champagne can put me under. There are times when I feel I just can't keep up with everything, but I won't give up.

Fred, age 88

LEARNING OBJECTIVES

On completion of this chapter, the reader will be able to:

1. Explain concepts of frailty and vulnerability.
2. Identify attributes of the frail old and the hardy old.
3. Specify problems that are characteristic of the frail and vulnerable old.
4. Enumerate several important considerations in caring for the mentally frail older person.
5. Develop a nursing care plan addressing comprehensive needs of a frail elder.
6. Discuss situations that tend to result in neglect and abuse.
7. Name some of the indications of undue influence.
8. Recognize potential risk and signs of abuse.

Chronologic age, ethnicity, lifestyle, health, and socioeconomic status all affect the manner in which an individual ages. Given these considerations and the course of aging, many older people will become frail and vulnerable and subject to abuse or neglect. The normally wide parameters of mental and physical homeostasis in youth narrow until the oldest-old are treading a narrow path of vulnerability. Frailty and vulnerability cannot be judged by external appearance. Older adults are often less vulnerable than they physically appear to be, and many are more vulnerable. Outward appearance gives little information about the capacities or the reserve of an individual. Some very old individuals maintain their capacities because of being genetically, physically, functionally, emotionally, and spiritually sturdy. These people are the hardy individuals who gain considerable attention from researchers who study longevity and envy from less fortunate elders. In this chapter, we are concerned about the less fortunate, frail individuals, of whatever chronologic age, who may need considerable legal, economic, and physical and psychologic support in their later years. Chapter 15 is a prelude to this examination because it addresses many of these issues from the perspective of available resources and entitlements. Nurses are in a position to notice the impending debility that an elder, or the family, may wish not to confront. Nurses can begin to provide appropriate supports to shore up the strength of the individual and the system in which they find themselves. Felton and Hall (2001) discovered that some women over age 85 had amazing resilience and were able to regain physical and emotional health after devastating experiences. The authors thought this resilience was influenced by the degree of frailty, determination, previous life experience, family support, and ability to care for self and others. Felton and Hall recommend considerable more attention be given to these resilience factors.

HARDINESS

Hardiness must be mentioned as that which is at the opposite end of the continuum from frailty and vulnerability. We know little about hardiness except that much of it may be related to genetics and lifestyle. Hardiness is important in assessing the adaptation and survival of the very old. Defined as a personality style, hardiness is characterized by three elements: feelings of control, deep commitment to something or someone, and enjoyment of challenge (Bowsher and Keep, 1995; Pappas, 1995). The fundamental concept developed by Kobasa (1979, 1982) is based in the existential belief that stressors provide the impetus for making choices and taking responsibility for actions. Challenge is perceived as normal and beneficial, and these personality characteristics function as a resource in the face of adversity. We think hardiness often incorporates a sense of humor, an optimistic outlook, and a broad perspective on life. These special old folks have great survival capacity, and little is understood at present of the elements of their endurance. Is it love of life, courage, determination, stubbornness? Perhaps a bit of each.

VULNERABILITY

Vulnerability is a difficult concept to define clearly because all humans are vulnerable at all times and in numerous events and situations, much of the time entirely out of our awareness or control. We have become much more conscious of our vulnerability after the terrorist events. However, in addressing the vulnerability of elders, we are particularly concerned about their susceptibility to abuse, fraud, illness, accident, and debilitation. Older adults are not only vulnerable to physiologic disturbance, but they are also socially vulnerable to various abuses, mentally vulnerable to stressors, and spiritually vulnerable to deprivation of meaning in living and of altruistic opportunities. Recognition of this vulnerability and proactive interventions are the key to longer periods of healthy survival and shorter periods of disability before death. The most important issue in facilitating shortened morbidity, conceptualized as the "rectangularization" of the survival curve (Fries, 1993; Yashin et al, 2001), is to be aware of the vulnerability of the very old and to strengthen their support systems and enhance their adaptive capacities, even when they appear competent in all ways. The key concern of vulnerable elders is remaining in charge of their own lives (Kunzmann et al, 2002). Maintaining a social support network of interdependent caring and exchange is often the critical factor.

Physical Vulnerability

Physical vulnerability afflicts all elders to some degree; energy wanes, sensory, immune, and environmental competence decrease, and falls and infectious processes become more common, as do the effects of detrimental lifestyles. Older adults are subject to fatigue and depression (Martin et al, 2002). The degree of emotional support given and received tends to decrease as the individual becomes more focused on self and survival (Keyes, 2002). Quite often, physical vulnerability is given more attention than other aspects of vulnerability. These issues are examined in depth throughout the text.

Bone and Joint Problems. Problems with osteoarthritis are almost universal by the eightieth birthday. Mobility is greatly decreased in the oldest-old, largely because of degenerative joint disease (osteoarthritis) and osteoporosis (see Chapter 8 for further discussion). These conditions are often accompanied by severe discomfort. Because osteoarthritis

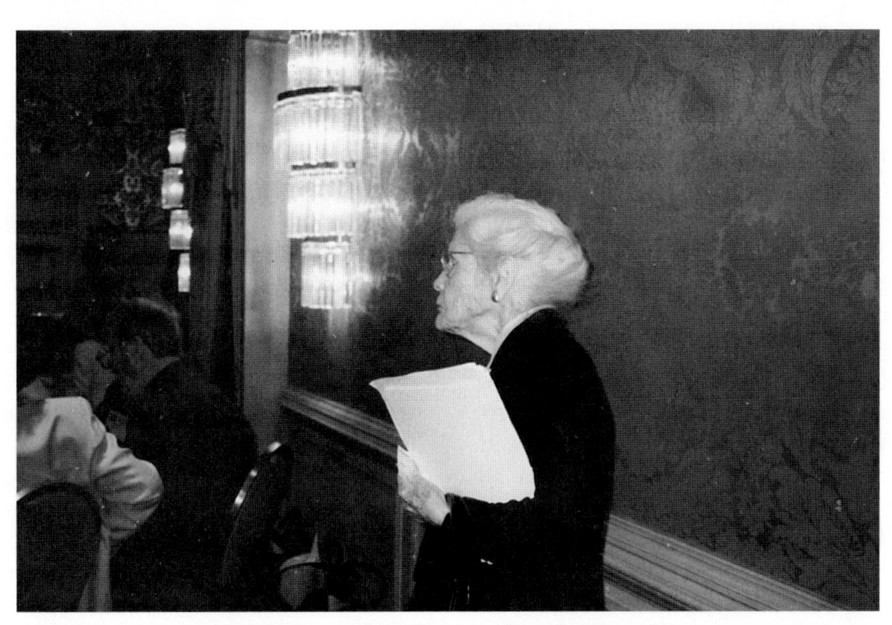

Frail but powerful. (Courtesy Priscilla Ebersole).

affects weight-bearing joints and the spine, it is a key factor in instability and falls. Osteoporosis is another problem that is rampant among older women and increasingly among older men (Birchfield, 2001; Vance, Frampton, 2002). Ninety percent of women over 75 years of age have some degree of osteoporosis. Fractures, falls, pain, and restricted mobility result.

Falls are a serious risk for the oldest-old because of chronic disorders, cognitive clouding, multiple medications, and difficulties with balance and proprioception. These factors are discussed in Chapter 13. A fall may presage immobility, decline, and death.

Visual and Hearing Problems. One half of the oldest-old report having trouble with their vision, even with glasses. Approximately 21% have a lot of trouble seeing, and 12% report blindness in one or both eyes. Most very old elders have hearing loss that has not been adequately assessed. Sensory appraisal and augmentation, when possible, is critical to maximizing function and prevention of accidents (see Chapter 12).

Cognitive Impairment. Cognitive impairment increases gradually but significantly in very old age. Among the oldest-old, 35% report that "senility" causes limitations. Statistics vary, but several sources agree that approximately 35% of people 85 years and over who are living in the community are cognitively impaired, and 40% of these are severely impaired (see Chapter 21). Personality shifts occur as well toward more caution and suspiciousness (Martin et al, 2002).

Energy Allotment. One of the issues with the frail old is their decreasing energy levels, often seen only as a fatigue factor. Wells (1986) discusses energy expenditure from an enlightened perspective:

> An elderly individual may be able to walk but prefers to use a wheelchair in order to travel a greater distance in less time and have more energy remaining. Although the ability to walk should be maintained, the desire to be more mobile should be respected and a wheelchair provided to permit a wider range of social opportunities . . . a person may prefer the privacy of self-toileting and may wish to use considerable energy in that activity but may request assistance in dressing. (p. 21)

The opportunity for choice in energy expenditure may be ignored if we have an all-or-none approach to the dependencies of the aged. Interdependence for the aged is a dynamic concept that implies that they are not helpless recipients, nor are they thrown into the expectation of variations of self-care that may be individually inappropriate. The goal of maximizing function and delaying decline while using and building on personal strengths and desires is the goal of wellness-oriented rehabilitation from our perspective. Unless we have a holistic understanding of the individual, we may ruthlessly and inappropriately press for self-care.

Economic Vulnerability

Living on the edge, economically, becomes more likely with every year of old age. Mary, a widow, had thought of herself as well set economically, had invested wisely, and lived in an upscale life-care facility. As she approached 85 years of age, Mary's resources had not kept pace with inflation, and she found herself "poor but proud." She would not admit that she was no longer able to afford to go shopping with the girls or go to the theater, and soon she would be unable to afford her medications. Because the life care facility had made a commitment to maintain her throughout the remainder of her life, Mary was secure in her apartment and meals but had nothing to spare. This story is only one of many scenarios. Very old African American women subsisting on a pittance of supplemental security income are among the most economically desperate (Table 16-1).

Ethnic Minorities and their Vulnerability

The cumulative effects of poor education, poverty, and discrimination have made many elders particularly vulnerable. Minority people of great old age have been severely disadvantaged and have learned to cope with a lifetime of stress and inadequate resources. Although these patterns are changing as the population becomes more diverse and more opportunities are made available to minority groups, much remains to be accomplished for these neglected groups.

These very old survivors of discrimination and disadvantage merit serious study. Risk taking and abusive behaviors in minority communities, which may include substance abuse, high-risk sex, accidents, and violence, have destructive effects on elders who have managed to maintain residence in these communities (Castro et al, 1995). In addition, these problems in their youth have residual effects that may mar old age for people who manage to survive. Although poverty and ill health are often addressed as problems of the ethnic aged, the psychologic ramifications of a lifetime of exclusion, danger, and fear have scarcely been addressed at all. Frequency of abusive situations is unknown. Additional discussion of elders' diversity and ethnicity can be found in Chapter 19.

Vulnerability to Fraud

The factors that make a person most vulnerable to fraud are many. At present, the telemarketers and Internet have opened even more possibilities to fraud. In each part of the country, schemes vary, but some are so well organized by groups that they capture trusting participants nationwide. Most schemes extract money from gullible and unsuspecting people, but some are designed to drain federal funds, such as Medicare or Medicaid. In California, attorney general Bill Lockyer (California Department of Justice, 2002) filed suit against a major Medi-Cal fraud ring organized in a multistate scheme to steal health care funds.

Individual older people must be especially wary of signing anything that they do not fully understand. A recent experience with an elder involved in signing a paper indicating that a trusted home health aide was injured while working in her home reemphasized that everyone must be extremely circumspect. Fraudulent schemes are also addressed in Chapter 15.

Table 16-1 Assessment of Elderly Vulnerability

General assessment	Specifics
Physiologic	Diminished endurance, weakness
	Decreased mobility, ambulation, range of motion, unstable ambulation
	Bruises easily, often evidence of ecchymosis
	Decreased cardiac output
	Ineffective airway
	Shortness of breath interferes with activities of daily living (ADLs)
	Unstable blood glucose
	Inability to speak
	Altered vision
	Poor nutritional or fluid intake
	Incontinence
	Fragile skin integrity (breaks in skin or potential for)
	Potential infection
	Unable to see wound
	Numbness
	Dizziness
	Dysphagia
Environmental	Factors which create safety concerns in and outside the home
	Potential for falls
	Injuries from various sources in and outside of home
Cognitive	Knowledge deficit
	Signs of brain dysfunction, poor memory
	Confusion
Psychosocial	Lacks confidence in self-care abilities
	Absence of social supports
	Loneliness
	Overwhelmed by treatment
	Anxiety about caregiver's health
	Depression
Caregiver	Dependence on caregiver with limited physical abilities
	Dependence on caregiver with limited mental abilities
	Need for caregiver respite
	Nonacceptance of caregiver
Other	Need for physical assistance
	Self-care deficits
	Inability to adhere to medication or treatment regimens

Modified from Frost MH, Willette K: Risk for abuse/neglect: documentation of assessment data and diagnosis, *J Gerontol Nurs* 20(8):37, 1994.

Spiritual Vulnerability

Toward the end of life, individuals may become preoccupied with the meanings, significance, and consequences of the events of life. Some people are burdened with great sorrow and desire to redo events or make restitution. These feelings are discussed more fully in Chapters 24 and 25. Nurses need to be aware that intense preoccupation with spiritual issues and the gravity of unresolved disappointments may sap the energy of an individual, especially when little time or energy is left to make amends.

FRAILTY

Frailty is an elusive concept and conceptually rather vague, though the term is commonly used to indicate that an aged person is usually able to carry out important practical and social activities of daily living but may have little resilience to loss, change, and illness. Frailty is a normal consequence of aging if the person lives long enough. We believe that frailty of the very old is conveyed in words such as fragile, delicate, brittle, tender, easily disturbed, and confused. Buchner and Wagner (1988) describe frailty as follows:

> A state of reduced physiologic reserve associated with increased susceptibility to disability. Reduced physiologic capacity in neurologic control, mechanical performance, and energy metabolism are the major components of frailty. Although disease is an important cause of frailty, there is sufficient epidemiologic and experimental evidence to conclude that frailty is also due to the additive effects of low-grade physiologic loss resulting from a sedentary life style and more rapid loss due to acute insults (illness, injuries, major life events) that result in periods of limited activity and bed rest. The pathogenesis of frailty involves a complicated interaction of factors that block recovery from rapid physiologic loss. To some extent, frailty is preventable. Approaches to prevention include (1) the periodic monitoring of key physiologic indicators of frailty, (2) the prevention of physiologic loss and acute and subacute episodes of physiologic loss, (3) the prediction of episodes of physiologic loss and the reduction of frailty prior to the loss, and (4) the removal of obstacles to recovery once physiologic loss has occurred. (p. 1)

Anderson and Johnson (1996) say, "In any practice that includes elderly patients, you'll find frail, older individuals teetering on the edge of decline" (p. 16B). The authors also find that 46% of community-dwelling elders over age 85 are frail, meaning that they have significant functional loss in the neurologic, musculoskeletal, and energy metabolism domains. These individuals are at risk of a rapid downward spiral when any acute insult, physiologic or psychologic, is added to the existing chronic, low-grade physiologic losses and changes of aging. The likelihood of returning to the person's previous functional baseline after any acute episode is minimal.

Individuals may be mentally or physically frail or both. Frailty is evidenced by increased susceptibility to disease and accident, diminished physiologic function, and compromised host-defense mechanisms. Blumenthal (1999) attributes this state to mechanisms such as lifelong exposure to unhealthy circumstances, repeated injuries and insults to the body, and the weakening of defense mechanisms. The author also notes that some disorders have a long latency period that appears only in late life.

Mental Frailty

Mental frailty is often the first evident sign of physical frailty. Mental frailty can be conceptualized as the narrowing of the sense of self as the trappings of identity are eroded by loss, changing appearance, and insufficient physiologic reserve to support the lifestyle that has formed an individual's persona. Wolanin (1996) conceptualizes mental frailty as the increasing difficulty in the later years of maintaining the "continuity of self" that characterizes a person's identity and capacity for personal integration. Changes may require more residual energy than an individual can muster in a particularly challenging situation. Anxiety, confusion, and paranoia may be signals that indicate the inability to adapt to the changing demands. Wolanin contends that mental frailty is a normal consequence of aging, and a return to baseline function is to be expected after appropriate intervention.

Splinting is important in this regard. Splinting is another concept that Wolanin was developing and is continuing in the work of Virginia Burggraf and myself (Ebersole) (2001). When an elder has exceeded adaptive ability and is psychologically distressed, the presence of a trusted person and routine activities is essential until the individual regains psychic balance. Couples often function in a splinting manner as they lean on each other for stability but cannot function adequately without the partner.

The study of frailty is complicated by the fact that many individuals who would have died of various disorders have been kept alive through sophisticated medical technology. Therefore among the very old, we find two distinct groups: those hardy souls genetically meant to endure for a century and the extremely frail who have walked the tightrope between survival and death for several decades. In general, people who are most frail present with atypical symptoms, most usually confusion and delirium, regardless of the disorder or problem, and will need attentive and specialized care (Guthrie et al, 2002).

Failure to Thrive

Failure to thrive (FTT) is a rather indiscriminate diagnosis. FTT generally describes a person with unexplained weight loss, nutritional deficits, decline in physical and cognitive function, and depressive symptoms such as remaining in bed, isolating of self, giving up, and feeling helpless (Kimball, Williams-Burgess, 1995).

Periodically, we have wondered whether similarities exist between marasmus babies, studied by Spitz (1945), who were unable to survive without human stimulation, interaction, and caressing and the very old, isolated, frail aged, who lack companionship and caring. Braun and colleagues (1988) found that FTT in adults had many corollaries with those of infants and symptomatically presented a mirror image. Many possible causes have been suggested for these symptoms, therefore they must be evaluated carefully. Gaffney (1995) suggests that FTT is the result of a "downward spiral" similar to that conceptualized by Hess in 1985 (Figure 16-1).

Smeeding (2001) suggests the necessity of a thorough nutritional assessment because many of the symptoms of FTT may be related to serious malnutrition. Certain ongoing chronic disorders are contributing factors (Nutrition Screening Initiative, 2001). Mental assessment must be made to determine cognitive and depressive status.

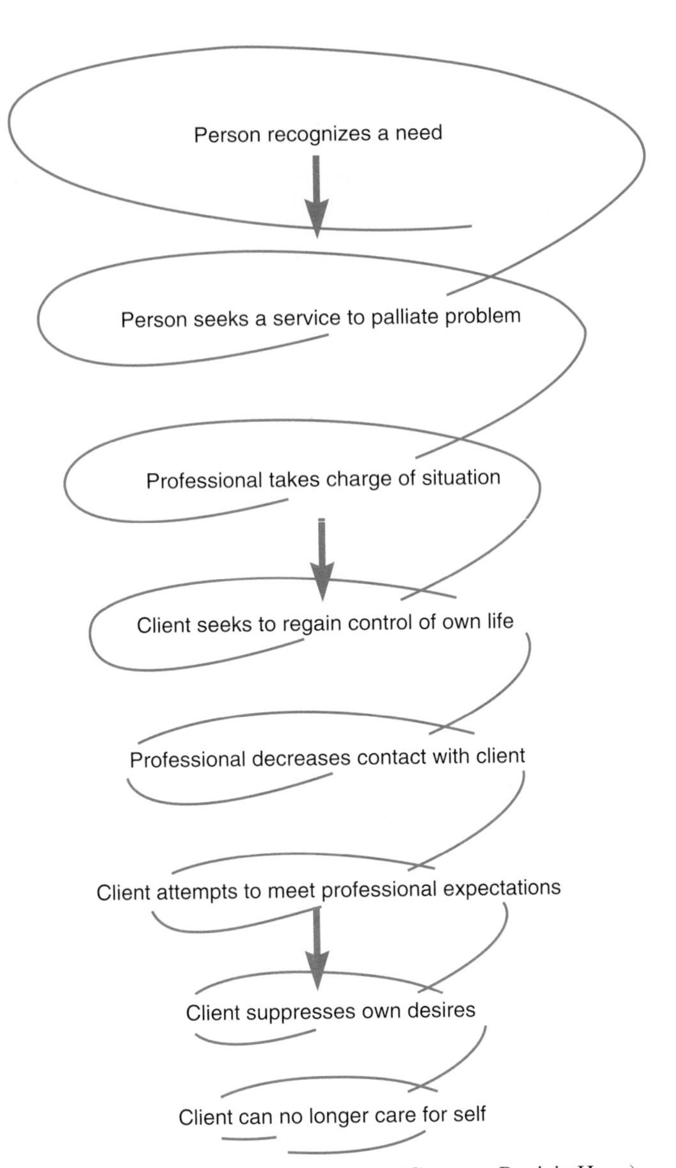

Figure 16-1. Spiral of dependency. (Courtesy Patricia Hess.)

For people suspected of FTT, interventions include physical stimulation through stroking, touching, rocking, and assisting to reestablish personal and social ties. Little is really known about FTT in the aged, and questions must be asked as to whether the issue is a lack of meaning in the person's existence and whether a spiritual deficit is the core problem (see further discussion in Chapters 17 and 25). Bergland and Kirkevold (2001) found that some frail elders thrive well in nursing homes. The authors posit that this relatively healthy state is the result of the resident's earlier growth and development, as well as psychologic and physical health. However, the authors also suggest that a need exists to learn more about factors that make for a sense of well being in these frail elders who may be vulnerable to FTT.

ELDER MISTREATMENT

Elder mistreatment is the term used to include factors such as elder neglect, elder abuse or domestic abuse, exploitation, and abandonment of the elderly (Fulmer, 2002, Fulmer et al, 1999; Hudson, 1988). Elder mistreatment refers to events or situations, caused by others, that can have serious or fatal consequences. Dyer and colleagues (2000) and other investigators have found that individuals over 75 years of age who are diagnosed with depression or dementia are the most likely to be mistreated. Victims are most likely to be female and living in a household with family members. The perpetrators are often younger men (Pavlik et al, 2001). Pillemer and colleagues (1998) found that abusers had a high prevalence of arrests, psychiatric hospitalizations, violent behaviors, and health problems. These individuals were often dependent on the elder for basic needs (Box 16-1 and Table 16-2).

Neglect

Neglect accounts for the majority of the cases of elder mistreatment (Fulmer et al, 2000). Neglect is seen as an act of omission or withholding needed goods and services. The act can be passive neglect based on ignorance or stress of caregivers, or it can be active neglect that is deliberate and malicious (Quinn and Tomita, 1997, 2003). Neglect of self and neglect by caretakers are often difficult to define because they are intertwined with energy, lifestyle, and resources. Nurses must be cautious in setting specific boundaries around neglect. However, when basic needs go unmet, intervention may be required. Physical neglect is the most common and obvious occurrence and may be indicated by FTT (discussed earlier in the chapter), untreated medical conditions, badly neglected grooming, malnutrition, and dehydration (Quinn and Tomita, 1997). Neglect by a caregiver may occur for many reasons.

Table 16-2 Theoretical Definitions by Delphi Panel of Elder Mistreatment Experts

Level I	Violence involving older adults	
Level II	Elder mistreatment	Destructive behavior that is directed toward an older adult occurs within the content of a relationship connoting trust and is of sufficient intensity and/or frequency to produce harmful physical, psychologic, social and/or financial effects of unnecessary suffering, injury, loss and/or violation of human rights and poorer quality of life for the older adult.
	Personal or social relationship	Persons in close personal relationships with an older adult connoting trust and some socially established behavioral norms (e.g., relatives by blood or marriage, friends, neighbors, any "significant other")
	Professional or business relationship	Persons in a formal relationship with an older adult that denotes trust and expected services (e.g., physicians, nurse, social worker, nursing aides, bankers, lawyers, nursing home staff, home health personnel, landlords).
Level III	Elder abuse	Aggressive or invasive behavior/action(s), or threats of same, inflicted on an older adult and resulting in harmful effects for the older adult.
	Elder neglect	The failure of a responsible party(ies) to act so as to provide, or to provide what is prudently deemed adequate and reasonable assistance that is available and warranted to ensure that the older adult's basic physical, psychologic, social, and financial needs are met, resulting in harmful effects for the older adult.
Level IV	Intentional	Abusive or neglectful behavior or acts that are carried out for the purpose of harming, deceiving, coercing, or controlling the older adult so as to produce gain for the perpetrator (often labeled "active" abuse/neglect in the literature).
	Unintentional	Abusive or neglectful behavior or acts that are carried out, but NOT for deceiving, coercing, or controlling the older adult, so as to produce gain for the perpetrator (often labeled "passive" abuse or neglect in the literature).
Level V	Physical	Behavior(s)/action(s) in which physical force(s) is used to inflict the abuse; or available and warranted physical assistance is not provided, resulting in neglect.
	Psychologic	Behavior(s)/action(s) in which verbal force is used to inflict the abuse; or available and warranted psychological/emotional assistance/support is not provided, resulting in neglect.
	Social	Behavior(s)/action(s) that prevents the basic social needs of an older adult from being met; or failure to provide available and warranted means by which an older adult's basic social needs can be met.
	Financial	Theft or misuse of an older adult's funds or property; or failure to provide available and warranted means by which an older adult's basic material needs can be met.

From Hudson, MF: Delphi Study of elder mistreatment: theoretical definitions, empirical referents and taxonomy, 1988, *Dissertation Abstracts International*, 50 (UMIPUZ8909673).

Box 16-1 Evaluative Components of Mistreatment

- Safety of the elder: Is the elder in immediate danger?
- What can be done immediately to increase safety?
- Are there barriers to reaching the elder (cognitive, family interference, emotional)?
- Are adequate physical, social, and financial resources available to properly care for the elder?
- What medical problems may make the elder particularly vulnerable to abuse and neglect?
- What type of mistreatment has occurred, how frequently, and of what severity?

Box 16-2 Signs of Elder Neglect and Abuse

Agitation
Decubitus
Dehydration
Fear
Poor hygiene
Weight loss
Unexplained injuries
Bruises from hand marks, especially on upper arms
Restraint abrasions

Adapted from Fulmer T: Our elderly-harmed, exploited, abandoned, *Reflections*, 3rd Quarter, Indianapolis, 1999, Sigma Theta Tau; Quinn MJ, Heisler CJ: The legal system: civil and criminal responses to elder abuse and neglect, *Public Policy and Aging Report,* Policy Institute of GSA 12(2):8, 2002.

However, some acts of neglect occur because of incompetence, unawareness of importance of the neglected care, no legal requirement to give such care, unavailability of resources, or exhaustion. The caregivers' own frailty and advanced age are often mitigating factors. Passive neglect—simply ignoring or not attending to needs—is most prevalent (Box 16-2).

Self-Neglect

The National Association of Adult Protective Service Administrators defines self-neglect as, "the result of an adult's inability, due to physical and/or mental impairments or diminished capacity, to perform essential self-care tasks . . ." (Duke, 2001, p. 2). Self-neglect may be associated with increasing severity of physical or mental impairments but may also reflect a lifestyle of alcoholism and drug abuse (Quinn, Tomita, 1997). Prescription drug abuse may be intentional or unintentional misuse.

Undue Influence

"Undue influence is the substitution of one person's will for the true desires of another . . . such influence often entails fraud, duress, threats or other deceits and pressures. Undue influence takes place when one person uses his or her role and power to exploit the trust, dependency or fear of another to gain psychologic control over the weaker person's decision-making, usually for financial gain" (Quinn, 2002, p. 11). Undue influence may occur in an insidious way because the victim is isolated from friends and family and convinced that the only one who cares is the caretaker; or, a younger person attempts to defraud a lonely widow or widower of assets through romance and marriage. In these cases, intervention is difficult because the victim has developed trust and reliance on the abuser. Quinn has developed guidelines for nurses attempting to identify signs of undue influence (Box 16-3).

ABUSE

Abuse is intentional and may be sexual, physical, financial, psychologic, or violation of a person's rights. Physical, financial, and emotional abuse are common; unfortunately family members are those most likely to be perpetrators. Psychologic abuse is the most prevalent form of mistreatment, followed by physical abuse and material abuse (Pavlik et al, 2001). An elder abuse and neglect assessment is provided in Figure 16-2; also see the discussion in Chapter 15. These problems need to be assessed by well-trained teams of providers, reported when identified, and addressed by legal action. All states have procedures for health care personnel for reporting elder mistreatment, although protocols specific to each institution may need to be developed (LTC Exchange, 2002). Legalities regarding civil and criminal responses must be considered (Quinn and Heisler, 2002).

Problems may arise because of the uncertainty of an outright abusive situation versus signs and symptoms of co-morbid conditions, medications, and certain therapies, as well as unintentional injury, the reluctance of the victim to report, and the manipulations of the perpetrator. On examination, geriatricians most often found the presence of bruises, physical trauma, and neglected appearance, often accompanied by malnutrition and dehydration (Harrell et al, 2002). Problems may arise when emergency room personnel do not have specific protocols for dealing with abuse and neglect (Fulmer et al, 2000) (Box 16-4).

Prevention of abuse and neglect is often directly related to policy variances (Fulmer, Paveza, and Guadagno, 2002) and the availability of resources and respite from the burdens of constant care. Discussion of caregivers can be found in Chapter 18. Abuse is sometimes domestic violence "grown old" (Pillemer and Wolf, 1986), that is, abused children who have grown into abusive adults. In addition, an important point to recognize is that abuse of aging caregivers by their care recipients is not uncommon (Ayers and Woodtli, 2001). Quinn and Tomita have written the classic texts (1997 and 2003, in press) on the subject, and nurses in situations that may indicate abusive or neglectful behaviors should consult these sources. Chapter

Box 16-3 Signs and Symptoms of Undue Influence

Elder takes actions inconsistent with his or her life history. Documents and actions run counter to the person's previous long-time values and beliefs. For instance, one competent man bought a horse farm within a year after his wife died. Neighbors, who later were tried and convicted of using undue influence, told the man it was a good investment. They encouraged him to think of it as a silent investment. The neighbors arranged the purchase using their realtor and the man's money. When a nephew (a lawyer) pointed out to his uncle that the property was not in his name, the neighbors changed the title to joint tenancy, thereby ensuring they own the property, buildings, and horses when the 86-year-old man dies. The man never had anything to do with horses before becoming involved with his new neighbors.

Elder makes sudden changes with regard to financial management. Examples include cashing in insurance policies or changing titles on bank accounts or real property.

Elder changes his or her will and previous disposition of assets.

Elder is taken to practitioners different than those he or she has always trusted. Examples include bankers, stockbrokers, attorneys, physicians, and realtor.

Elder is systematically isolated from or is continually monitored with others who care about him or her.

Someone suddenly moves into the person's home or the elder is moved into someone's home under the guise of providing better care.

Someone attempts to get income checks directed differently than the usual arrangement.

Documents are suddenly signed frequently as the elder nears death.

A history of mistrust exists in the elder's family, especially with financial affairs, and the elder places unusual trust in newfound acquaintances.

Someone promises to provide lifelong care in exchange for property on the elder's death.

Statements of the elder and the alleged abuser vary concerning the elder's affairs or disposition of assets.

A power imbalance exists between the parties in matters of finances or health.

Someone shows unfairness to the weaker party in a transaction. The stronger person unduly benefits by the transaction.

The elder is never left alone with anyone. No one is allowed to speak to the elder without the alleged abuser having a way of finding out about it.

Unusual patterns arise in the elder's finances. For instance, numerous checks are written out to "cash," always in round numbers, and often in large amounts.

The elder reports meeting a "wonderful new friend who makes me feel young again." The elder then becomes suspicious of family and begins to avoid family gatherings.

The elder is pressed into a transaction without being given time to reflect or contact trusted advisors.

From Quinn M: Undue influence and elder abuse: recognition and intervention strategies, *Geriatr Nurs* 23(1):11–16, 2002.

Box 16-4 Actions to Address in Reporting Abuse

You may want to include the following items in a facility policy and procedure (P&P) manual that addresses abuse. The language can be adapted as appropriate.

- Take immediate action to prevent further incidents pending the investigation.
- Notify the administrator, director of nursing, medical director, attending physician, and resident's family or legal representative.
- Investigate immediately.
- Document any injuries with photographs, who committed the alleged abusive act, the nature of the alleged abuse, where and when it occurred, and action taken.
- Expand the investigation to see if others have been affected in a similar manner.
- Review documentation of the investigation. After the review, the administrator, medical director, and director of nursing may extend the investigation through further interviews and medical and personnel records.
- Notify the corporate legal department and chain of command for additional determination that actual abuse occurred.
- Use the information gathered in the investigation process to determine if abuse has occurred. The administrator holds the ultimate responsibility for the decision.
- Maintain all documentation collected during the investigation, such as interviews with personnel, witness statements, and so forth in a confidential file in the administrator's office.

From LTC Exchange: Putting the brakes on abuse: how the team takes action, *LTC Exchange* 4(1):4, 2002.

15 discusses the legalities in such situations (Boxes 16-5, 16-6, and 16-7).

Elder Violence in Domestic Settings

Domestic violence is often thought to occur most frequently between young women and men in rather psychologically codependent relationships. However, physical and mental codependency among older men and women is very common and often results in domestic violence, particularly if one partner has some degree of dementia and poor behavioral concerns. Suggestions from Davey and Davey (1996) that are applicable to these situations are listed in Box 16-8.

In December of 2001, the first National Summit on Elder Abuse was held to identify future directions in the protection of abused elders (National Center on Elder Abuse, 2002). Selected recommendations from the summit meeting include:

1. Creation of a National Elder Abuse Act
2. Modification of laws that are barriers to appropriate investigation and prosecution of perpetrators
3. Improved training of professionals in detection, reporting, intervention, and prevention

1. **General Assessment**	Very Good	Good	Poor	Very Poor	Unable to Assess
a. Clothing					
b. Hygiene					
c. Nutrition					
d. Skin integrity					
Additional Comments:					

2. **Possible Abuse Indicators**	No Evidence	Possible Evidence	Probable Evidence	Definite Evidence	Unable to Assess
a. Bruising					
b. Lacerations					
c. Fractures					
d. Various stages of healing of any bruises or fractures					
e. Evidence of sexual abuse					
f. Statement by elder re: abuse					
Additional Comments:					

3. **Possible Neglect Indicators**	No Evidence	Possible Evidence	Probable Evidence	Definite Evidence	Unable to Assess
a. Contractures					
b. Decubiti					
c. Dehydration					
d. Diarrhea					
e. Depression					
f. Impaction					
g. Malnutrition					
h. Urine burns					
i. Poor hygiene					
j. Failure to respond to warning of obvious disease					
k. Inappropriate medications (under/over)					
l. Repetitive hospital admissions due to probable failure of health care surveillance					
m. Statement by elder re: neglect					
Additional Comments:					

4. **Possible Exploitation Indicators**	No Evidence	Possible Evidence	Probable Evidence	Definite Evidence	Unable to Assess
a. Misuse of money					
b. Evidence					
c. Reports of demands for goods in exchange for services					
d. Inability to account for money/property					
e. Statement by elder re: exploitation					
Additional Comments:					

5. **Possible Abandonment Indicators**	No Evidence	Possible Evidence	Probable Evidence	Definite Evidence	Unable to Assess
a. Evidence that a caretaker has withdrawn care precipitously without alternate arrangements					
b. Evidence that elder is left alone in an unsafe environment for extended periods without adequate support					
c. Statement by elder re: abandonment					
Additional Comments:					

6. **Summary**	No Evidence	Possible Evidence	Probable Evidence	Definite Evidence	Unable to Assess
a. Evidence of abuse					
b. Evidence of neglect					
c. Evidence of exploitation					
d. Evidence of abandonment					
Additional Comments:					

Figure 16-2. Abuse and neglect assessment. (From Fulmer T: *Elder abuse and neglect assessment. Try this: best practices in nursing care to older adults,* Hartford Institute for Geriatric Nursing, #15, May 2002.)

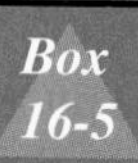

Box 16-5 Profiles of Abused and Abusers

Abused Elders
Woman age 80 or older
Lives alone or with abuser
Mental or physical disability
Dependency on abuser

Abusers
Middle-aged male sibling or offspring
Mental health and substance abuse problems
Financially dependent on abused
History of abuse and being abused

Adapted from Utley R: Screening and intervention in elder abuse, *Home Care Provider* 4(5):198, 1999.

4. Increased awareness in the justice system of the prevalence of abuse and neglect
5. Improved mental health and substance abuse assessment and outreach to victims and perpetrators
6. Increased support and funding of adult protective services

The entire text can be found on the National Center on Elder Abuse website at *www.elderabusecenter.org*.

Principles of Working with Frail and Vulnerable Elders

Working with older adults who are having serious difficulty coping with their lives demands a great deal from the nurse; sensitivity is needed to determine the exact difficulty. Because of reasons of pride or because of mental impairment, older people may not state their problem or problems directly. Although nurses may experience an overwhelming need to assist, our professional obligation is to ask, "What kind of help will make it possible for you to do the things that are important to you?" Clark (1995) contends that professionals are becoming more cognizant that the patient must define the means and ends of care and that the restructuring of health care around the uniqueness of the individual has been a distinct shift in medical practice. The emphasis on basic values and meanings in each health care encounter must fit in relation to the individuals' life goals. The relinquishment of professional control to the individual activates the person's inherent power, accountability, and courage (Kunzmann et al, 2002). These qualities may be more inwardly than outwardly oriented when a person perceives himself or herself as vulnerable. Reinforcing control, mastery, and commitment can be expected to restore the highest level of wellness in the frail and vulnerable elder.

Tolerance and patience may be required to tease out the issues; a great deal of trust must often be present before an abused or vulnerable elder will confide in a nurse. Perhaps several visits will be needed. Working with this group of older people simply takes more time, and the nurse will often need to form a genuine relationship with the client to be effective. This relationship must include sincere caring and concern. The client will also care about the nurse, worry, and possibly want to give gifts of some sort. This gesture may be the older person's way of feeling less dependent and needy, an attempt to still have some control over the situation. An important point to always remember is that these older adults are survivors, people who have lived through major world wars, social upheavals, and personal hardships.

Box 16-6 Identification and Subsequent Action for Elder Abuse

Team

- BASE: *Brief Abuse Screen for the Elderly:* Screens abuse; specifies types, sources of abuse, urgency for treatment.
- Abuse Checklist.
- The Intervention Team's *Home-Care Team:* Trained Basic Intervention Unit: Screens using the Tool Package, intervenes.
  Multidiciplinary Team: About three to five home care team members: confirm/disconfirm abuse (using the BASE); brainstorm, plan, monitor, and evaluate intervention strategies (using the AID).
- *Empowerment Support Group:* Victims discuss problems, strengths, solutions, resources, appropriate responses.
- *The Community Senior Abuse Committee:* An independent group of volunteers: arrange programs and publications to educate/sensitize the community to abuse; advocacy functions; liaison with home care team members.

Interventions

1. Abuse cases are tagged. The initial intervention strategies are planned and implemented.
   Screens abuse; specifies caregiver/care-receiver indicators for intervention focus.
2. Home care team members make initial home visits to further assess and make written (AID) plans. They brainstorm the case with the multidisciplinary team and consult with the expert consultant team for specialized advice and help. They enlist specialized advice and additional assistance as needed (e.g., buddies, empowerment group). They improve and continue the planned (AID) intervention strategies.
3. Empowerment group works to improve self-esteem, active responding, personal control, and empowerment of victims.
4. Committee refers clients, volunteers to the intervention; provides community involvement in combating abuse.

Modified from Reis M, Nahmiash D: When seniors are abused: an intervention model, *Gerontologist* 35(5):667, 1995.

Box 16-7

Nursing Actions in Support of Elders

Support family in adapting to major changes in lifestyle.
Recognize personal losses that make elders vulnerable.
Facilitate adjustment to physical and psychological changes.
Discuss risk factors with elder and family related to declining function.
Recognize elder abuse and have knowledge of reporting procedures.
Explore factors influencing ability to cope.
Promote continued socialization and communication.
Provide time to interview elder alone.
Discuss a safety plan with threatened elder, provide phone numbers of resources.
Ask about history of violence in the family.
Make note of any evidences of neglect or abuse.

Adapted from: Wilber KH, Nielsen EK: Elder abuse: new approaches to an age-old problem, *Public Policy and Aging Report,* Policy Institute of GSA 12(2):1, 24, 2002; LTC Exchange: Creating an abuse free environment, *LTC Exchange* 4(1):4, 2002.

Box 16-8

Elder Violence in Domestic Settings

Signs and Signals

Obvious physical signs of violence
Feeling of the victim that he or she has done something wrong
Large differences in size and physical strength
Isolation from others outside the couple relationship
Restriction of partner's contact with others
Perpetrator easily irritated or agitated and demonstrates poor control of anger
Verbalized threats toward partner

Actions to Be Taken

Assess the presence of physical danger
Identify appropriate options:
- Seek legal advice
- Get a protective order
- Have the abuser arrested
- Support victim's decision to leave or stay
- Develop a workable safety plan

Reestablish contact with family and friends
Identify emergency actions that will assist the victim:
- Give specific information on places of sanctuary

Modified from Davey P, Davey D: Domestic violence: a clinical view, *Home Health Focus* 2(10):78–79, 1996.

Frail and Vulnerable Aged and their Future

The home is now and will continue to be the principal site of care for the frail elderly. Family members, who may or may not be willing to assume the care, most often provide this care. Home health care is discussed in considerable detail in Chapter 18.

Home visitation by physicians and nurses is expanding for the following reasons: (1) to assess needs of patients and families within the context of daily living, (2) to enhance the use of multidisciplinary teams in the home, (3) to avoid premature institutionalization, (4) to provide more personalized and humane care, and (5) because much of the care has been priced out of the hospitals.

The needs of patients who have been discharged "quicker and sicker" are of the most sophisticated and complex nature, particularly for the frail older adult. Not only the treatment related to the disease from which he or she is recuperating, but also the personal and human needs must be attended if the individual is to recover necessary functions.

The hospital has, in large part, moved into the home. Some of the advantages include (1) assessment of patients and families within the context of daily living, (2) increased use of multidisciplinary teams in the home, (3) avoidance of premature institutionalization, and (4) the provision of more personalized and humane care. The disadvantages of home health care are that more sophisticated knowledge is expected of caregivers and that a higher probability may occur of inadequate care and serious errors in caregiving, fragmentation and overlap of services, medical neglect, and financial abuse.

In addition, very old ladies living alone are particularly subject to self-neglect, abuse, and exploitation by hired caregivers. This problem is expected to increase.

Nurses may be the first to gain admittance to the home and to recognize a problem. Advocacy for individual rights and protections require considerable expertise. Consequently, nurses will need to avail themselves of legal and financial consultation (see Chapter 15 for further discussion). The importance of multidisciplinary collaboration in these situations is critical while maintaining the highest level of concern for the autonomy and rights of the individual.

The number of frail and vulnerable elderly being kept alive by advanced medical technology and experiencing more functional deficits will continue to increase. To meet the needs of these individuals and maintain a stable economy, several trends have been identified. Multiple alternatives to institutional placement will be developed in communities. Current thinking holds that alternatives to institutionalization are cost-effective when offered in the context of comprehensive, coordinated health care that includes respite, home health care, domiciliary, and day-care components in combination with social supports in a case management model. Some of the alternatives to institutional care include:

- Self-help education
- Geriatric crisis outreach
- Neighborhood support networks
- Community nursing centers
- Telephone peer networks
- Adopt-a-grandparent programs
- Foster family care
- Adult residential day care

Telecommunication Health Care Management

Coordinated systems of comprehensive care delivering multiple services to the vulnerable elderly have been effectively demonstrated by the Alternative Health System in Georgia, the Mt. Zion Hospital and Medical Center in San Francisco, the On-Lok Senior Health Center in San Francisco, the Hebrew Rehabilitation Center for the Aged in Boston, and the Programs for All-Inclusive Care for the Elderly (PACE) models throughout the nation. These model demonstration projects have shown that a full range of services reduces inappropriate institutional placement and mortality and increases functional status. Frail and vulnerable elders need the availability of an advocate who can function in a flexible enough manner to serve the client's needs and desires. Such a capability should extend to the provision of funds to purchase this presence when necessary.

Nurses are the ideal advocates for the frail elderly and may assist them in actual provision or help them find suitable services to meet their needs. The need for help with daily activities increases sharply as people grow older, especially among the very old. Less than 10% of people who are 65 to 74 years of age need help, compared with 40% who are 85 years or older.

Approximately 80% of care currently provided to older adults is given by informal caregivers, usually family members. Federal policies have historically been unsupportive of these families, denying the most minimum assistance and providing very little support or recognition of their major contribution to the care of the frail elderly in our society. However, the Administration on Aging (AOA) has recently made funds available for projects and services to assist caregivers in the care of elders (Greene, 2002). In the future, institutional costs and financial incentives to families may further increase the number of older adults cared for at home.

Nurses need to be particularly cognizant of legislative trends, political realities, and, as the greatest mass of professional caretakers, our potential for influencing national aging policy. We can expect an increased recognition of our pivotal role in providing long-term care services, clinical research, and assessment data. Nurses are rapidly becoming the primary case managers for the frail aged.

Priorities for the long-term care of the frail and vulnerable elderly include the following:

1. Supporting functional independence
2. Emphasizing prevention at all ages
3. Assisting families caring for elders
4. Seeking increased public financing for long-term care and home-based care
5. Involving physicians, nurses, social workers, aides, and others, and providing incentives for these workers to master geriatric skills
6. Encouraging continuity of professional surveillance
7. Providing adequate quality and cost controls for in-home care
8. Ensuring equal access to publicly funded benefits, regardless of economic status

It has been said that the progress of civilization can be judged by the total fraction of human beings who achieve longevity while maintaining a life of meaning and purpose. In the care of the very old who are frail and vulnerable, subject to the whims of social policy and potential abuses and neglect, human progress (or lack of it) is most visible. Thoughtful examination of social needs and deficiencies is a form of progress if we follow up with appropriate action. If not, we will reap the effects of our neglect. We urge nurses to look at the individual and beyond as we attempt to create a world in which it is safe to depend on the good will and compassion of others.

Human Needs and Wellness Diagnoses

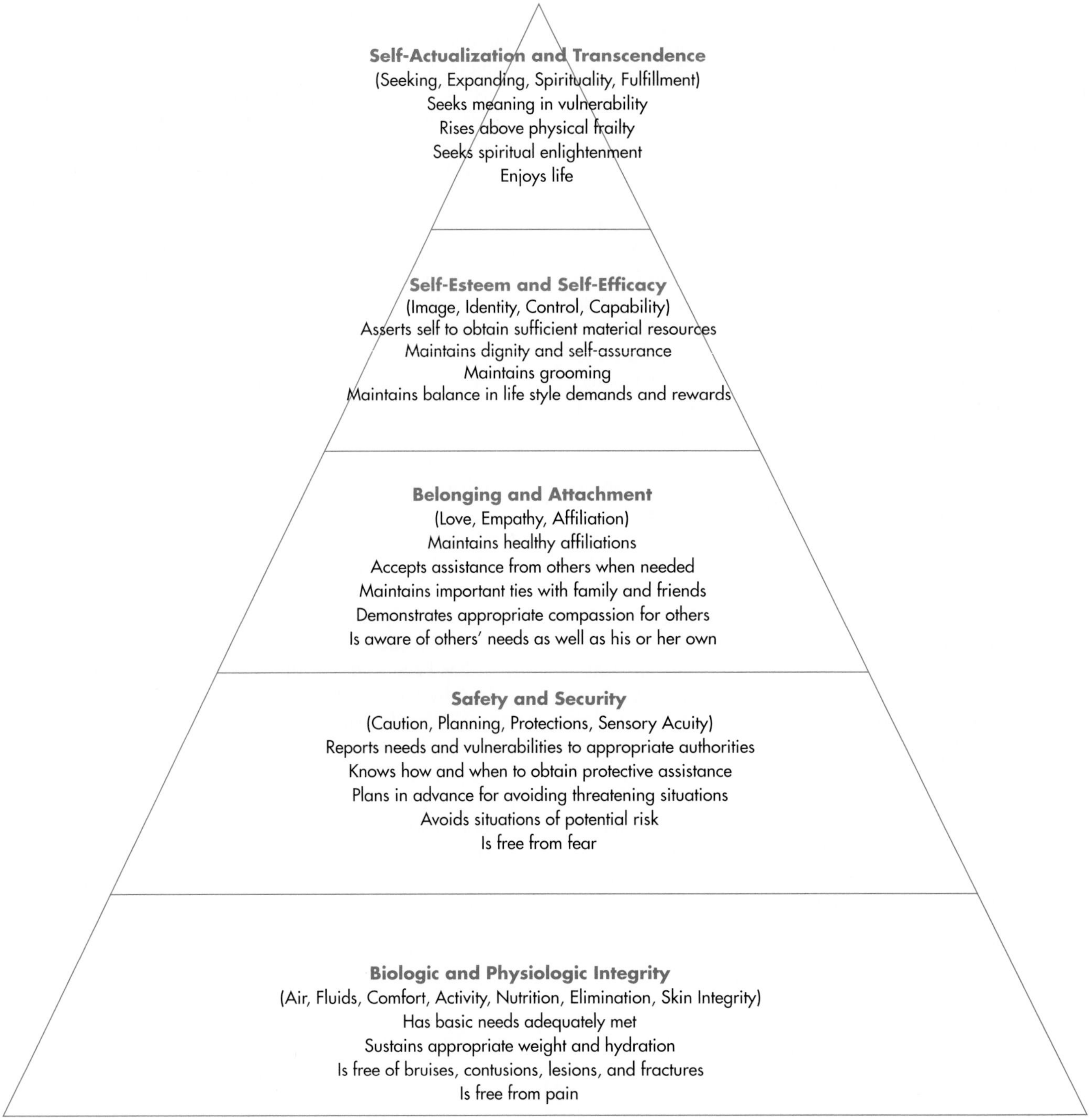

Self-Actualization and Transcendence
(Seeking, Expanding, Spirituality, Fulfillment)
Seeks meaning in vulnerability
Rises above physical frailty
Seeks spiritual enlightenment
Enjoys life

Self-Esteem and Self-Efficacy
(Image, Identity, Control, Capability)
Asserts self to obtain sufficient material resources
Maintains dignity and self-assurance
Maintains grooming
Maintains balance in life style demands and rewards

Belonging and Attachment
(Love, Empathy, Affiliation)
Maintains healthy affiliations
Accepts assistance from others when needed
Maintains important ties with family and friends
Demonstrates appropriate compassion for others
Is aware of others' needs as well as his or her own

Safety and Security
(Caution, Planning, Protections, Sensory Acuity)
Reports needs and vulnerabilities to appropriate authorities
Knows how and when to obtain protective assistance
Plans in advance for avoiding threatening situations
Avoids situations of potential risk
Is free from fear

Biologic and Physiologic Integrity
(Air, Fluids, Comfort, Activity, Nutrition, Elimination, Skin Integrity)
Has basic needs adequately met
Sustains appropriate weight and hydration
Is free of bruises, contusions, lesions, and fractures
Is free from pain

These are not all the possible wellness diagnoses that may be identified. The above are examples of nursing diagnoses that should be considered when planning care for the older adult.

KEY CONCEPTS

- Elders experience an increased narrowing of their physical and psychic adaptability as they age.
- Vulnerable elders are easily influenced and subject to catastrophic responses to changes or demands of their environment.
- The common changes of aging result in increasing susceptibility to injury and discomfort.
- Energy reduction that occurs naturally in the aging process often requires changes in habits and lifestyle.
- Because of a lack of resources throughout life, ethnic minorities are particularly vulnerable to the changes of aging and neglect of health.
- Frail elders must have basic needs met and supportive networks available to maintain physical and psychologic function.
- Failure to thrive (FTT) in elderly people is poorly understood but is likely a deprivation of caring individuals and the downward spiral of dependency.
- Elder mistreatment is an umbrella term that covers abuse, neglect, exploitation, and abandonment.
- Availability of comprehensive resources and coordinated care can keep frail and vulnerable elders functional and independent longer.

▲ CASE STUDY

Harold has lived alone in a luxurious home since being widowed 5 years ago. He is a bright, wealthy, successful, and well-functioning elder approaching his ninetieth birthday. Harold says, "I really miss Melba (his wife), especially in the evening when we would have dinner, summarize the events of the day, and just laugh and talk. I have no one now who really cares or is even interested in me." Harold was married for 60 years and admits that he still desires intimacy. However, when he said something about his desire to his grandson, Harold was told that was "disgusting." When the grandson brought Jane, an attractive young lady that the grandson was dating, to visit his grandfather, it was apparent that there was some mutual attraction between the grandfather and the young lady. Harold later said to his grandson, "I sure wish I was 40 or so years younger. She is such an interesting person." A few weeks later, the young lady dropped in with a bag of homemade cookies because it seemed Harold was lonely. Soon, the visits became a weekly routine. Then, the two began having dinners together. The grandson was rather pleased that his grandfather approved of Jane and announced one evening that he thought she was the one for him and planned on marrying her. Grandfather said, "You can't do that! You must be able to support a wife before you can marry." The grandson became furious and stalked out. That evening, Harold was upset and called Jane to see if she would join him for dinner and talk through this problem with his grandson. When Jane arrived, she found Harold confused and slumped in a chair with a highball glass on the table beside him.

▲ CASE STUDY

Jenny is a rather obese 75-year-old woman and is severely crippled with rheumatoid arthritis, which became apparent when she was in her early 30s. Jenny has been admitted to the hospital after a fall out of her wheelchair, which apparently rolled down some steps when she forgot to set the brake. She has sustained a broken arm, wrist, and ankle, as well as many bruises, even on her face. The breaks have been casted and splinted, and she has been kept in the hospital for observation for several days. A student nurse has become quite friendly with her because she seems so lonely and always wants the nurse to "stay and talk for a while." In the course of conversation, Jenny remarks that she is fortunate to have inherited quite a sum of money from her father because her husband is then able to stay home with her, given that she needs considerable help. On the day she is to be discharged, Jenny confides in the student that "I'm so afraid this might happen again, and next time I might not be so lucky." The student carefully observes the husband when he comes to get Jenny, and they seem to interact in an appropriate way, though not particularly warm. What should the student nurse do?

Based upon one of the case studies, develop a nursing care plan using the following procedure*:

List comments of patient that provide subjective data.

List information that provides objective data.

From these lists, identify and state, using accepted format, two nursing diagnoses you determine are most significant to this client at this time.

List two client strengths that you have identified from the data.

Determine and state outcome criteria for each diagnosis. These criteria must reflect some alleviation of the problem identified in the nursing diagnosis and must be stated in concrete and measurable terms.

Plan and state one or more interventions for each diagnosed problem. Provide specific documentation of source used to determine appropriate intervention. Plan at least one intervention that incorporates the client's existing strengths.

Evaluate success of intervention. Interventions must correlate directly with the stated outcome criteria so as to measure the outcome success.

STUDY QUESTIONS/ACTIVITIES

Discuss the meanings and the thoughts triggered by the students' and elders' viewpoints expressed at the beginning

*Students are advised to refer to their nursing diagnosis text and identify possible or potential problems.

of the chapter. How do these vary from your own experience?

Discuss your concept of frail aged and develop a definition that provides clear distinctions.

What are the physiologic principles that best explain the concept of frailty in aging?

Discuss various legal mechanisms for protecting the frail aged.

What is the distinction between frail and vulnerable as they are used in connection with the aged?

Refer to the chapter on relationships (Chapter 18), and describe factors in a spousal relationship that may be functional or detrimental to the frail aged.

What are your responsibilities in reporting elder abuse in your state?

RESEARCH QUESTIONS

What is the distribution of symptoms in the FTT syndrome in the aged?

What is the demographic and sociocultural profile of elders who develop FTT?

How do health care agencies define frail elderly?

Which agencies offer services specifically designed for the aged, and what are these services?

What proportion of individuals over 80 is considered frail and based on what criteria?

Is the increasing population (over 85 years of age) shifting toward more durability or increasing frailty in recent decades?

How many elders have been victimized economically and legally by family members?

When is it appropriate to intervene?

Study individuals who appear to be thriving in nursing homes and explore their life patterns and satisfactions.

REFERENCES

Anderson SJ, Johnson MA: Caring for patients on the edge of decline, *Am J Nurs* 96(12):16B, 1996.

Ayers MM, Woodtli A: Concept analysis: abuse of aging caregivers by elderly care recipients, *J Adv Nurs* 35(3):326, 2001.

Bergland A, Kirkevold M: Thriving—a useful theoretical perspective to capture the experience of well-being among frail elderly in nursing homes, *J Adv Nurs* 36(3):426, 2001.

Birchfield PC: Osteoarthritis overview, *Geriatr Nurs* 22(3):124, 2001.

Blumenthal HT: A view of aging and disease relationship from age 85, *J Gerontol* 54A(6):B255, 1999.

Bowsher JE, Keep D: Toward an understanding of three control constructs: personal control, self-efficacy, and hardiness, *Issues Ment Health Nurs* 16(1):33, 1995.

Braun JV, Wykle MH, Cowling RW: Failure to thrive in older persons: a concept derived, *Gerontologist* 28(6):809, 1988.

Buchner D, Wagner E: Preventing frail health, *Clin Geriatr Med* 8(1):1, 1988.

Burggraf V, Ebersole P: *Elderly couples splinting,* 2001, paper in development.

California Department of Justice: *News release,* June 26, 2002.

Castro FG et al: Risk taking and abusive behaviors among ethnic minorities, *Health Psychol* 14(7):622, 1995.

Clark PG: Quality of life, values, and teamwork in geriatric care: do we communicate what we mean? *Gerontologist* 25(3):402, 1995.

Davey P, Davey D: Domestic violence: a clinical view, *Home Health Focus* 2(10):78-79, 1996.

Duke J: *A national study of self-neglecting Adult Protective Services clients,* San Antonio, 2001, National Association of Adult Protective Services Administrators.

Dyer CB et al: The high prevalence of depression and dementia in elder abuse and neglect, *J Am Geriatr Soc* 48(2):205, 2000.

Felton BS, Hall JM: Conceptualizing resilience in women older than 85: overcoming adversity from illness and loss, *J Gerontol Nurs* 27(11):46, 2001.

Fries JF: Compression of morbidity 1993: life span, disability, and health care costs. In Vellas B, Albarede JL, Garry PJ, editors: *Facts and research in gerontology*, vol 7, New York, 1993, Springer.

Fulmer T: *Elder abuse and neglect assessment. Try this: best practices in nursing care to older adults,* Hartford Institute for Geriatric Nursing, #15, May 2002.

Fulmer T: Our elderly-harmed, exploited, abandoned, *Reflections,* 3rd Quarter, Indianapolis, 1999, Sigma Theta Tau.

Fulmer T, Paveza G, Guadagno L: Elder abuse and neglect: policy issues for two very different problems, *Public Policy and Aging Report*, National Academy on an Aging Society, Policy Institute of GSA 12(2):15, 2002.

Fulmer T et al: Elder neglect assessment in the emergency department, *J Emerg Nurs* 26:436, 2000.

Fulmer T et al: Prevalence of elder mistreatment as reported by social workers in a probability sample of adult day health care clients, *J Elder Abuse Neglect* 11(3):25, 1999.

Gaffney D: Commentary on failure to thrive: the silent epidemic of the elderly, *APNSCAN* 6:10, August, 1995.

Greene R: Presentation regarding changes in AOA regulations, given at ANA convention, June 2002.

Guthrie PF, Edinger G, Schumacher S: Twice: a NICHE program at north memorial health care, *Geriatr Nurs* 23(3):133, 2002.

Harrell R et al: How geriatricians identify elder abuse and neglect, *Am J Med Sci* 323(1):34, 2002.

Hess P: Crisis, stress, depression and control. In Ebersole P, Hess P, editors: *Toward healthy aging: human needs and nursing response,* ed 2, St Louis, 1985, Mosby.

Hudson MF: Delphi study of elder mistreatment: theoretical definitions, empirical references and taxonomy. Dissertation Abstracts International 50 (UMIPUZ8909673), 1988. In Fulmer T, Paveza G, Guadagno L: Elder abuse and neglect: policy issues for two very different problems, *Public Policy and Aging Report*, National Academy on an Aging Society, Policy Institute of GSA 12(2):15, 2002.

Keyes CLM: Exchange of emotional support with age and its relationship with emotional well-being of the aged, *J Gerontol* 57B(6):B518, 2002.

Kimball MJ, Williams-Burgess C: Failure to thrive: the silent epidemic of the elderly, *Arch Psychiatr Nurs* 9(2):99, 1995.

Kobasa SC: Stressful life events, personality, and health: an inquiry into hardiness, *J Pers Soc Psychol* 37(1):1, 1979.

Kobasa SC, Maddi S, Kahn S: Hardiness health: a prospective study, *J Pers Soc Psychol* 42(1):168, 1982.

Kunzmann U, Little T, Smith J: Perceived control: a double-edged sword in old age, *J Gerontol* 57B(6):P484, 2002.

LTC Exchange: Creating an abuse free environment, *LTC Exchange* 4(1):4, 2002.

Martin P, Long MV, Poon LW: Age changes and differences in personality traits of the old and very old, *J Gerontol* 57B(2):P144, 2002.

National Center on Elder Abuse: National Summit on Elder Abuse, December 2001. Available at *www.elderabusecenter.org*

Nutrition Screening Initiative: The role of nutrition in chronic disease, *Geriatr Nurs* 22(1):46, 2001.

Pappas SH: Creating an environment to support hardiness and quality patient care, *Semin Nurse Manag* 3(3):115, 1995.

Pavlik VN et al: Quantifying the problem of abuse and neglect in adults—analysis of a statewide data base, *J Am Geriatr Soc* 49(1):45, 2001.

Pillemer KA et al: Practice concepts. Building bridges between families and nursing home staff: the partners in caregiving program, *Gerontologist* 38:499, 1998.

Pillemer KA, Wolf RS: *Elder abuse: conflict in the family,* Dover, ME, 1986, Auburn House.

Quinn M: Undue influence and elder abuse: recognition and intervention strategies, *Geriatr Nurs* 23(1):11, 2002.

Quinn MJ, Heisler CJ: The legal system: civil and criminal responses to elder abuse and neglect, *Public Policy and Aging Report*, Policy Institute of GSA 12(2):8, 2002.

Quinn M, Tomita SK*: Elder abuse and neglect: causes, diagnoses and intervention strategies*, ed 2, New York, 1997, Springer Series on Social Work.

Quinn M, Tomita SK*: Elder abuse and neglect: causes, diagnoses and intervention strategies*, ed 3, New York, 2003 (in press), Springer Series on Social Work.

Smeeding SJW: Nutrition, supplements and aging, *Geriatr Nurs* 22(5):219, 2001.

Spitz R: Hospitalism: an inquiry into the genesis of psychiatric conditions in early childhood. In *The psychoanalytic study of the child,* vol 1, New York, 1945, International Universities Press.

Utley R: Screening and intervention in elder abuse, *Home Care Provider* 4(5):198, 1999.

Vance J, Frampton K: Revising AMDA's osteoporosis guideline, *Caring for the Ages* 3(10):26, 29, 2002.

Wells T: Major clinical problems in gerontologic nursing. In Calkins E, Davis P, Ford A, editors: *The practice of geriatrics*, Philadelphia, 1986, WB Saunders.

Wilber KH, Nielsen EK: Elder abuse: new approaches to an age-old problem, *Public Policy and Aging Report*, Policy Institute of GSA 12(2):1, 24, 2002.

Wolanin MO: *Mental frailty*, personal communication, February 20, 1996.

Yashin AL et al: Have the oldest old adults ever been frail in the past? A hypothesis that explains modern trends in survival, *J Gerontol* 56(10):B432, 2001.

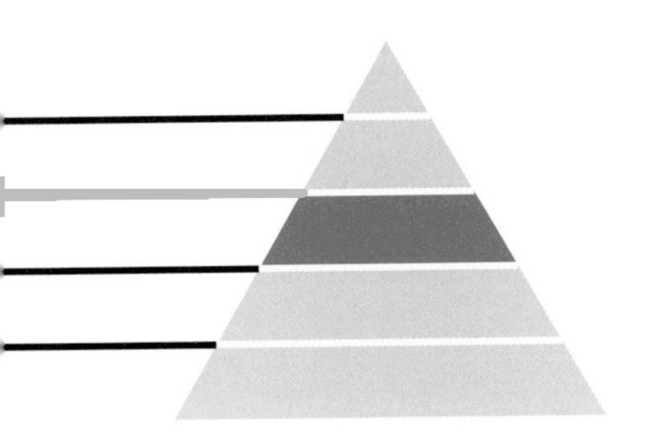

CHAPTER 17

Intimacy, Sexuality, and Aging

Patricia Hess

An elder speaks

These early morning hours are terribly lonely . . . that's when I have such a longing for someone who loves me to be there just to touch and hold me . . . and to talk to.

Sister Marilyn Schwab (From Schwab M: *A gift freely given: the personal journal of Sister Marilyn Schwab,* Mt Angel, OR, 1986, Benedictine Sisters.)

LEARNING OBJECTIVES

On completion of this chapter, the reader will be able to:

1. Define sexuality.
2. Describe the various approaches to sexuality assessment that may reduce nurse-client anxiety in discussing a sensitive area.
3. Discuss the physiologic alterations that affect the older adult's sexual function.
4. Collect data related to sexuality of the aged individual.
5. Identify the risks to sexual integrity.
6. Formulate and validate appropriate nursing diagnoses.
7. Discuss elders' need for closeness, touch, warmth, and sharing.
8. Discuss interventions that foster sexual integrity.

TOUCH

Touch affects almost anything we do. It is the oldest, most important, and most neglected of our senses. Touch is 10 times stronger than verbal or emotional contact. All other senses have an organ on which to focus, but touch is everywhere. Touch is unique because it frequently combines with other senses. An individual can survive without one or more of the other senses, but no one can survive and live in any degree of comfort without touch. In the absence of touching or being touched, people of all ages can become sick and become touch starved (Ackerman, 1995). "Touch is a way to define self and experience the world . . . touch triggers a variety of responses that affect physiology, emotions, and behavior" (Miller, 1992, p. 3).

Mythology, magic, folklore, primitive medicine, and religion all affirm, through the centuries, the importance of touch in healing, destruction, communication, and personal power (Barnett, 1972a). The human yearning for physical contact is embedded in our language in such figurative terms as "keep in touch," "handle with care," and "rubbed the wrong way" (Huss, 1977). We will focus on touch as an overt expression of closeness, intimacy, and sexuality. We believe an individual must recognize the power of touch and its intimacy to fully comprehend sexuality. Touch and intimacy are integral parts of sexuality, just as sexuality is expressed through intimacy and touch. Together, touch and intimacy can offer the aged a sense of well being.

Touch is the first sensory system to become functional. Throughout life, touch provides emotional and sensual knowledge about other individuals—an unending source of information, pleasure, and pain. In all human cultures, gently touching another person conveys affection and friendliness (Barnett, 1972b).

Thayer (1982) describes touch as follows: ". . . like all nonverbal behavior, it rarely has unitary, unequivocal meaning. The message depends upon a host of factors" (p. 266).

We love and are loved by virtue of our skin sensation and appearance. How our skin is arranged affects others' willingness to touch us. Even though beauty is said to be only skin deep, skin is significant. The wrinkled skin of the old person shows the beautiful lines of hard work and experience. Old hands and old faces tell much of the bearer's capacity for intimacy. Sensations of old skin, clean, dry, and powdered or cologned, linger in the remote memories of many individuals who were held by a grandmother or grandfather. These features provide our foundation for intimacy with the old.

In the cases of the isolated or institutionalized aged, higher death rates are more related to the quality of human relationships than they are to the degree of cleanliness, nutrition, and physical disabilities on which our attentions are focused. Montagu (1986) noted that "tactile hunger" becomes more powerful in old age when other sensuous experiences are diminished and direct sexual expression is often no longer possible or available. Furthermore, Montagu believes the cause of illness may be greatly influenced by the quality of tactile support received.

Ackerman (1995) equates touch to be as essential as sunlight. Colton (1983) cites tactile touch or touch hunger as analogous to malnutrition. Malnutrition results from the lack of adequate nutrients for body survival. Touch stimulates chemical production in the brain, which feeds blood, muscles, tissues, nerve cells, organs, and other body structures. Without this stimulation, similar to nutrients in food, the individual would be deprived of sustenance and would starve.

Intimacy Levels of Touch

Patterns. Jourard's cursory observation (1964) of touch in a hospital study revealed no physical contact during 2-hour observation periods. Barnett (1972b), in a similar study, found that senior nursing students did not touch patients at all, but that after graduation when they assumed the role of a registered nurse, touch was used as one means of communication. The absence of touch, or distancing, by the student nurses was thought to be their interpretation of professionalism. Barnett's study showed that women were touched more than men; the hands, forehead, and shoulders were touched, whereas the fingers, toes, ankles, and genitalia were not. The age group least touched was people 66 to 100 years of age, and those in their late teens to 25 years of age were touched the most.

Thayer (1982) describes five types of touch, the first of which, functional-professional touch, reflects Barnett's observations. In this mode, people in their special roles (e.g., nurse, technician, aide) perform a task in which verbal, vocal, or kinesthetic signals of sexuality or disrespect are absent. Social-polite touch is formal or cordial. Friendship-warm touch allows physical demonstrations such as hugs, kisses, and handholding. The touch of love-intimacy reflects strong affection and intimacy and touching in areas that elicit vulnerability. Sexual arousal is touch of the most physical and intimate form in a sexual context.

Cosgray and Davidhizar (1988) defined six types of touch that nurses can use in the care of psychogeriatric patients: procedural, friendly, aggressive, limit setting, meeting own needs, and inappropriate touch. The authors found the vast majority of touch was procedural or related to limit setting. Friendly touch ranked third. No aggressive or inappropriate touch was observed. Many nursing implications can be drawn from these observations.

Response to Touch. Touch may calm or stimulate anxiety, fear, love, comfort, or rage. The subtleties of touch that convey these varied messages are learned early in life. Some people respond warmly to a firm touch and others to a light or casual touch. Useful information may be obtained through a handshake. Does the individual grasp firmly or hesitate? Does he or she relinquish quickly or hold on? Are the fingers intertwined or held together? Is the hand limp, passive, or responsive, or is it tremulous, sweaty, or cold?

Touch, except during illness, injury, or sexual encounters, may be unacceptable to an individual. The use of touch by nurses should be based on the following considerations: Nurses should recognize the influence of their own personality, cultural expectations, and early exposure to touching. Everyone has definite feelings and opinions about touch based on his or her own life experience. Touch only if it is comfortable. Individuals quickly discern the discomfort of another if touch is not an integral part of behavior. An important point to remember is that the comfort of touching depends on the location one is touched, the situation, social status, and age.

Caring touch has been used systematically in a nursing home setting as a cost-effective means of improving communication and quality of life of residents. Staff members were trained to use caring touch frequently as a means of becoming sensitive to the interaction between professional and client. The training model was based on the focusing technique of Gendlin (Sakauye, McDonald, 1987). The results not only showed significant increases in patient satisfaction, but also had a positive impact on staff morale.

Touch Zones. Hall (1969) identifies different categories of touching—expanding or contracting zones around which every individual extends the sensory experience of touching, smelling, hearing, and seeing. Entering the zone of intimacy, which is identified as being in an area within an arm's length of the individual's body and is the space used for comforting, protecting, and lovemaking, is part of the nurse's function (Figure 17-1). Illness, confinement, and dependency seen in institutionalization are stresses on the intimate zone of touch. Just as caregivers enter a room without knocking, so they often intrude into the intimate circle of touch without asking. The parameters of the intimate zone of touch are examined in this chapter to emphasize the importance of understanding behavior that might occur when the nurse enters this arena.

The social zone includes the areas of the body that are the least sensitive or embarrassing to have touched and that do not necessarily require permission to be handled. The consent zone requires the nurse to seek out or ask permission to touch or initiate procedures to these areas. The vulnerable zone is highly sexually charged and will be protected. The most intimate area, the genitalia, is the most personally protected area of the body and causes the most stress and anxiety when approached, touched, and viewed by the caregiver.

A test of the person's readiness to be touched is to initiate a hand clasp or handshake. The person can feel the tension or the welcoming relaxation that occurs. Later, a massage of tired

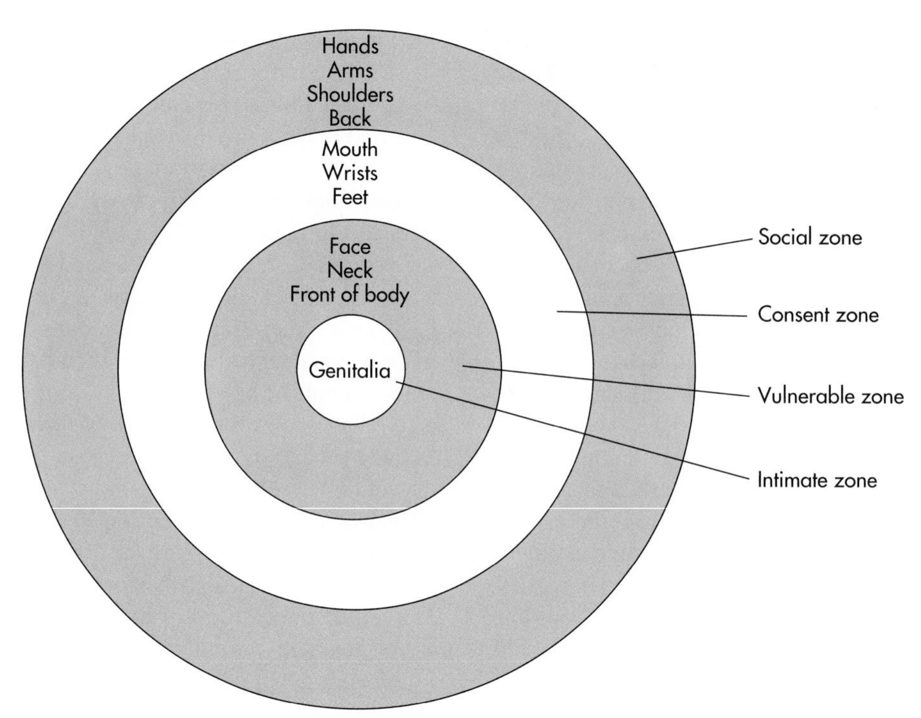

Figure 17-1. Zones of intimacy or sexuality.

neck or back muscles, hands, or feet will take the nurse into a closer area of intimacy. You will recognize in touching the front of the body, face, and the neck that these areas are sexually charged zones. Stroking the temples is a soothing intervention; stroking cheeks usually produces anxiety.

Fear of Touching. Many times a nurse will touch in a condescending way, a pat on the head or a tweak of the toe, or in a circumscribed nursing treatment. Of all health care professionals, nurses have the most frequent opportunities to provide gentle, reassuring, renewing touch. However, the use of touch involves risk and may be misinterpreted by the nurse or patient. The intimacy of nurse-patient contacts may influence a nurse to be overly circumspect. Stirring sexual feelings, if that is a response to gentle touching, is a human response that need not frighten.

Old women and men have stated they miss the touching and holding of their earlier lives. These older adults may seek such comfort by sexually provocative behaviors. Nurses need not encourage such overt behavior but must be cognizant of the underlying needs of intimacy.

Nurses sometimes respond negatively to a breach in the "status" of touch. A status system of touch exists that is significant to health care. A person of higher status may touch an individual of an inferior status, but the reverse is discouraged. Similarly, name familiarity may be used by an individual in a superior position but is greatly resented if the lower-ranking person presumes the same liberty. Because this notion is embedded in many hierarchic structures, treating everyone with respect regarding their name and propensity for touch is prudent. Instant familiarity is seldom useful (Hall, 1969). When a patient reciprocates with the same level of intimacy as the nurse initiates, it should not be surprising.

Touch Deprivation

Do old people suffer touch deprivation? Many elders do if they are separated from caring others. Old men, in particular, may find it hard to reach out to others for stroking and fondling. The previous lifestyles of these men often mitigated against this activity, except in the intimacy of sexual contact, which may no longer be available to them (Montagu, 1986). For old men to be wrongly accused of sexual offenses because they dared to give a child an affectionate pat on the head or on the buttocks is common. Old women are allowed considerably more freedom to touch, although they may lack the opportunity.

Adaptation to Touch Deprivation. People can survive extreme sensory deprivation as long as the sensory experiences of the skin are maintained. An outstanding feature of touch according to Ackerman (1995) is that it does not have to be performed by a person or other living thing. Some sustenance or peace for the old may be gained from the self-contained stimulation of a rocking chair or slowly stroking an animal's fur or wearing something that provides sensory stimulation. Thayer (1982) describes these activities as self-adapters.

Self-adapters are movements not intentionally used to communicate with others but that facilitate or block sensory input. For the aged, rocking in the chair or stroking oneself, the fur of a pet, or a child's silky hair may be self-adapters for touch. Emotionally disturbed people are often found rocking as if the motion is somehow soothing. People rock when grief stricken or when needing comfort. Montagu (1978) believes rocking stimulates and eroticizes skin through a complex series of motions and that it is a self-comforting measure. Perhaps the aged compensate for the lack of touch and closeness by using their rocking chair.

Music, perceived through the skin as well as the ears, may be another source of touch stimulation that is self-induced. Skin touched by the vibrations of music is enveloped and caressed. Music and dancing seem to be two important mechanisms of enjoyment of the aged. In later years, older adults often return to dancing after decades of ignoring the pleasurable activity. Perhaps this desire is a response to the need for more touch.

Therapeutic Touch

Touch is a powerful healer and a therapeutic tool that nurses can use to satisfy "touch hunger" of the aged. Nursing has recognized the importance of touch and has the social sanctions to touch the body in the intimate and personal care of a person, an opportunity too often not fully used for the betterment of the aged person's adaptation to environment and location in time and space. Barnett (1972b) points out that touch can serve as a means of providing sensory stimulation, reduction of anxiety, reality orientation, relief of physical and psychologic pain, and comfort in dying, as well as sexual expression.

Thayer (1982) cites the additional purposes of touch as relief of stress, cleansing, expression of joy, beautification, and sexual pleasure. As the sense of isolation, sensory deprivation, dependency, lack of self-esteem, and fear of death increases, the need for touch will also increase. Conversely, if the need for privacy and distance is great, then the less the person should be touched.

Kreiger's experiments with therapeutic touch (1975) demonstrate physiologic and psychologic improvement in patients who are exposed to consistent "doses" of touch. "Laying on of the hands" and the power of touch to heal had largely disappeared with the scientific revolution. Before that time, divine powers of healing through touch were attributed to priests, religious leaders, and kings. Touch for healing remained a practice in many religions and was used in conjunction with prayer. The phenomenon has reemerged as "touch for health," "laying on of hands," and "therapeutic touch" movements.

Massage has gained acceptance as a touch therapy. Massage stimulates circulation, dilates blood vessels, relaxes tense muscles, and cleans toxins out of the body through the flow of lymph. Many nurses are convinced of the efficacy of touch to restore health and comfort and have thus incorporated it into their care.

SEXUALITY

Sexuality provides the opportunity to express passion, affection, admiration, and loyalty. Sexuality is an affirmation that the individual's body functions well, maintains a strong sense of self-identity, and provides a means for self-assertion. Sexuality also allows a general affirmation of life (especially joy) and a continuing opportunity to search for new growth and experience (Lewis, 1995; Butler, Lewis, 2002).

Sexuality, similar to food and water, is a basic human need, yet it goes beyond the biologic realm to include psychologic, social, and moral dimensions. The constant interaction between these spheres of sexuality work to produce harmony. The linkage of the four dimensions composes the holistic quality of an individual's sexuality.

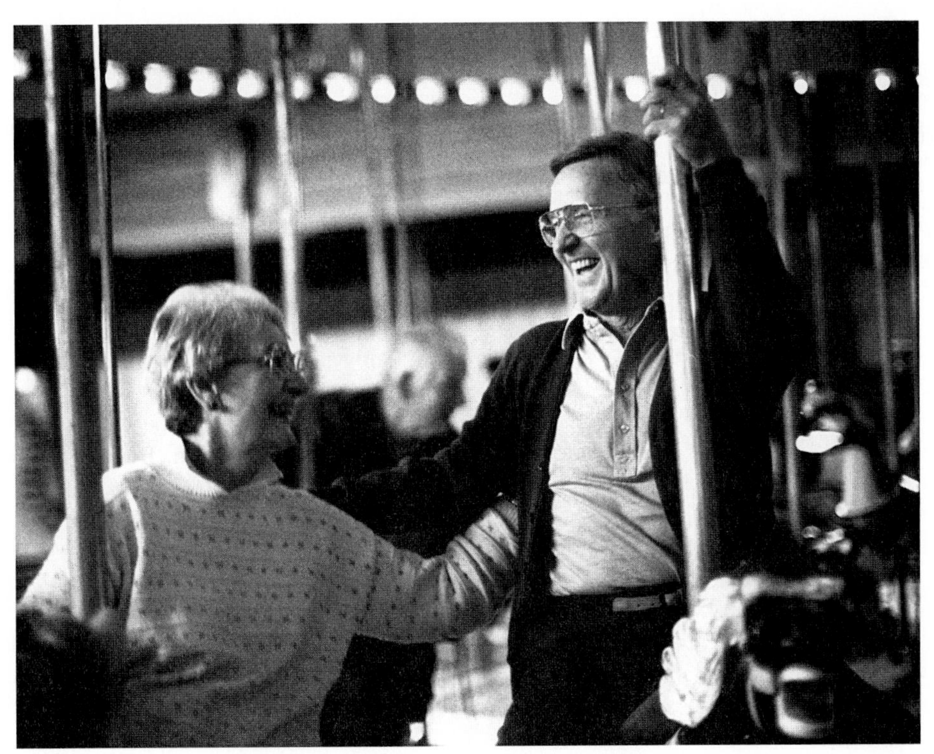

A special togetherness. (Courtesy Rod Schmall.)

The social sphere of sexuality is the sum of cultural factors that influence the individual's thoughts and actions related to interpersonal relationships, as well as sexuality related to ideas and learned behavior. Television, radio, literature, and the more traditional sources of family, school, and religious teachings combine to influence social sexuality. The belief of that which constitutes masculine and feminine is deeply rooted in the individual's exposure to cultural factors.

The psychologic domain of sexuality reflects a person's attitudes, feelings toward self and others, and learning from past experiences. Beginning with birth, the individual is bombarded with cues and signals of how a person should act and think about the use of "dirty words" or body parts. Conversation is self-censored in the presence of or in discussion with certain people.

The moral aspect of sexuality, the "I should" or "I shouldn't," makes a difference that is based in religious beliefs or in a pragmatic or humanistic outlook.

The final dimension, biologic sexuality, is reflected in physiologic responses to sexual stimulation, reproduction, puberty, and growth and development. Because of the interrelatedness, these dimensions affect each other directly or indirectly whenever an aspect of sexuality is out of harmony. Figure 17-2 illustrates the interrelationship of the sexuality dimensions.

Sexuality has become an important theoretic issue of concern in the care of the aged. Kass (1979) has shown that caregivers agree that sexuality is important. Although caregivers support this idea in theory, their actions do not.

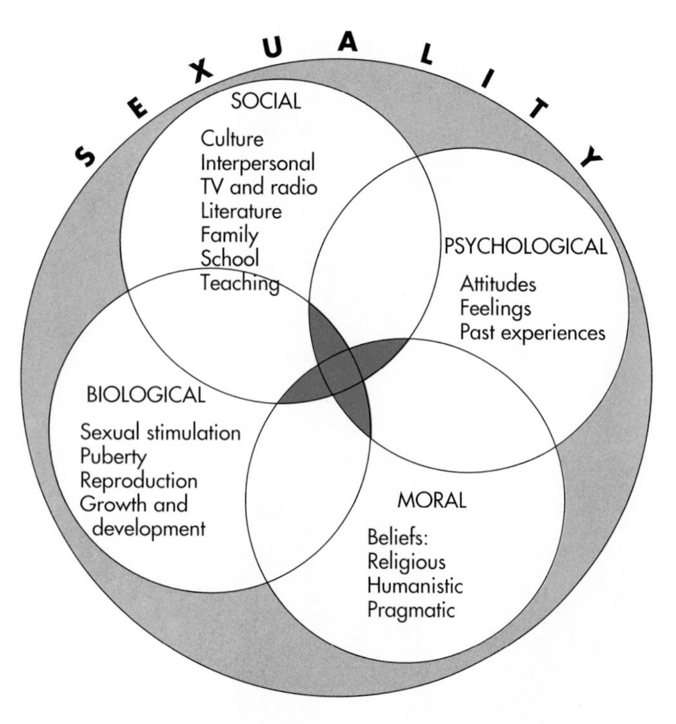

Figure 17-2. Interrelationship of dimensions of sexuality.

Health care professionals rarely treat aged people in congregate living facilities (nursing homes, acute hospitals, homes for the aged, extended care, mental institutions, and other total care facilities) or in the residents' own home as sexual beings.

Sexuality is a vital aspect to consider in the care of the aged person regardless of the setting. Sexuality exists throughout life in one form or another in everyone. All of the aged have a need to express sexual feelings, whether they are healthy and active or frail individuals. Sexuality is linked with the person's personality and identity and has a significant role in promoting better life adaptation (Billhorn, 1994; Wiley, Bortz, 1996; Butler, Lewis, 2002). At a time when the usefulness of the aged is questioned by others and by the aged themselves, this portion of an individual's identity can give meaning to life and bolster security, belonging, and esteem. Sexuality can be envisioned as part of Maslow's hierarchy of needs, with physical reproduction the lowest level and a progression to the higher levels with increased communication, trust, sharing, and pleasure with or without a physical action. Figure 17-3 focuses on the hierarchy of sexuality.

Acceptance and Companionship

Sexuality validates the lifelong need to share intimacy and have that offering appreciated. Sexuality is love, warmth, sharing, and touching between people, not just the physical act of coitus. Margot Benary-Isbert in her book, *The Vintage Years* (1968), expresses the essence of sexuality most eloquently:

> Let us not forget old married couples who once shared healthy and happy days as they now share the unavoidable limitations of old age and grow even closer together in love and patience. When they exchange a smile, a glance, one can guess that they still think each other beautiful and loveable. (p. 200)

Benary-Isbert continues ". . . as long as we live with our companion all these seem worthwhile because each one desires to make life as easy as possible for the other" (Benary-Isbert, 1968, pp. 201-202). *The Hite Report* (Hite, 1977) identified touching at night, listening to the breathing and the heart beat, and open talking that occurs in bed as important features of sexuality expressed by older women; a study by Nay (1992) confirms this contention. Berlin concludes: "Sexuality can mean anything which gives sexual or emotional pleasure, excitement, or comfort" (1978, p. 2).

Femininity and Masculinity

Males and females possess characteristic behavioral traits, which Jung refers to as the *anima* (female) and *animus* (male) (Fordham, 1970; Jacobi, 1973). Past social pressures did not often allow the appearance of sensitivity, gentleness, and

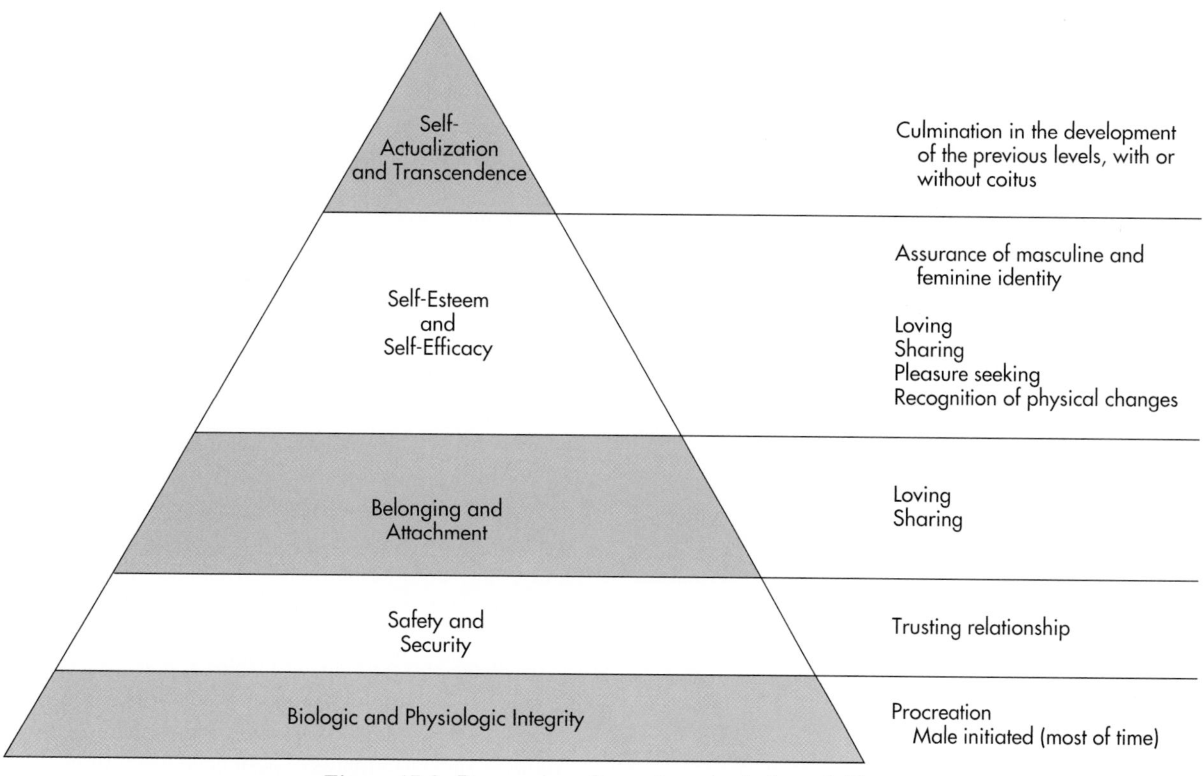

Figure 17-3. Progression of sexual emphasis through life.

sentimentality in most men. Men were expected to be strong, to be in control of situations, and to handle their emotions. Similarly, women were not viewed as aggressive or the major decision makers.

Often seen and perpetuated among older adults are socially accepted standards characteristic of masculine and feminine behavior, which reflect male and female role models dominant in their formative years. Jung's work has shown this view to be so, indicating that strong attitude types (male and female) and roles and functions associated with these attitudes are developed as adaptations of the person to the demands of the environment.

Man believed that repressing his feminine traits was virtuous; and woman, until recently, repressed her animus. Both men and women, however, are not consciously aware that they possess the opposite sexual identity. Goldblatt (1972) contends that neither gonads nor chromosomal sex are determinants of sexual behavior. Money and Tucker (1975) in their work, *Sexual Signatures,* believe that social stimulation provides gender identity and limits the individual's concept of self. In essence, society expects men to be men and women to be women.

In the later part of life, self-knowledge deepens. People tend to discover traits in their nature that were previously suppressed or heretofore remained in the unconscious. At this time, the emergence of the anima (in men) and animus (in women) may be seen. Jung identified this experience as the expression of the psyche that in the first half of life was turned inward. In later life, directed outward, this expression becomes indicative of the capacity for fuller living. Men become more comfortable with tenderness and women with assertiveness. The person's ability to accord his or her other nature its due recognition will enhance sexuality (Box 17-1).

Sexual Health

The World Health Organization defines sexual health as "the integration of somatic, emotional, intellectual, and social aspects of sexual being, in ways that are positively enriching and that enhance personality, communication, and love" (Woods, 1979, p. 75). According to Maddocks (1975) and Denny and Quadango (1992), sexual health is a realistic phenomenon that includes four components: personal and social behaviors in agreement with individual gender identity, comfort with a range of sexual role behaviors and engagement in effective interpersonal relations with both sexes in a love or long-term commitment, response to erotic stimulation that produces positive and pleasurable sexual activity, and the ability to make mature judgments about sexual behavior congruent with one's beliefs and values.

These interpretations speak of the multidisciplinary nature of the biologic, psychosocial, cultural, and spiritual components of sexuality and imply that sexual behavior is the

Box 17-1 Sexuality and Aging Women: Common Myths

- Masturbation is an immature activity of youngsters and adolescents, not older women.
- Sexual prowess and desire wane during the climacteric, and menopause is the death of a woman's sexuality.
- Hysterectomy creates a physical disability that results in the inability to function sexually.
- Sex has no role in the lives of the elderly, except as perversion or remembrance of times past.
- Sexual expression in old age is taboo.
- The elderly are too old and frail to engage in sex.
- The young are considered lusty and virile; the elderly are considered lecherous.
- Sex is unimportant or over.
- Elderly women do not wish to discuss their sexuality with professionals.

Adapted from Morrison-Beedy D, Robbins L: Sexual assessment and the aging female, *Nurs Pract* 14(12):35, 1989.

capacity to enhance self and others. However, these meanings, if literally applied, indicate that people who are neurologically impaired, celibate, transsexual, or ill are not sexually healthy. Taken in its broadest sense, the absence of criteria expressed in these definitions should not automatically mean that one is sexually unhealthy. The aged, in the context of these criteria, may not seek the erotic constancy or prowess of the young and might be considered as experiencing poor sexual health. In truth, these definitions must be considered as guidelines, not rules that govern all healthy sexual behavior. Sexual health is individually defined and wholesome if it leads to intimacy (not necessarily coitus) and enriches the involved parties. Old people may have a limited sexual life by some definitions, but the criterion of assessment and evaluation is their satisfaction. Sexual health also requires sexual fitness. "At any age sexual function is dependent on adaptation between physical capacities, societal mores, and individual desires" (Kass, 1979, p. 372). Attention to exercise (strengthening upper and lower abdominal muscles, improving back muscles, and for women using Kegal exercises), nutrition (proper weight maintenance, limiting intake of alcohol, and keeping teeth in good repair), and adequate rest enhances sexual desire and performance (Butler and Lewis, 2002).

Age Variables

Expectations. A large number of cultural, biologic, psychosocial, and environmental factors influences sexual behavior of the aged. The aged may be confronted with barriers to the expression of their sexuality by reflected attitudes, health, culture, economics, opportunity, and historic trends (Butler and Lewis, 2002).

The aged often internalize the broad cultural proscriptions of sexual behavior in late life that hinder the continuance of sexual expression. A person learns early in life that permission for certain sexual behaviors is given and that what is acceptable and not acceptable changes with age. Permission for social and sexual initiative comes with maturity, status, and wealth. Much sexual behavior stems from incorporating other people's reactions. Anderson and Newton (1966), Jarvik and Small (1988), and Butler and Lewis (1990) indicate that old people do not feel old until they are faced with the fact that others around them consider them old. Similarly, older adults do not feel asexual until they are continually treated as such.

Erikson and colleagues (1986) found a large number of female octogenarians in their study to have been strongly influenced by the prudish, Victorian atmosphere of their youth. Many of the participants experienced difficult marital adjustments and serious sexual problems early in their marriages. Many of the couples found their old-age intimacy had transcended the painful differences they felt when they were young. Few elders acknowledged disharmony within their present marital relationship. People who did so were unhappy at the increased dependency of an ill spouse and, in a sense, were grieving the loss of the patterns and expectations that had become comfortable in the relationship and were now disrupted by illness and incapacity.

Incongruent needs and expectations may cause distress in older couples. These needs and expectations often arise from discordant aging processes: the man may desire to be sexually active, and the woman has lost interest, or vice versa. One couple who had long sustained a satisfactory sexual relationship was unable to imagine engaging in the alternative modes of sexual expression (cunnilingus, mutual masturbation, and repositioning) suggested when the wife developed severe osteoarthritis. The old gentleman brought the worn and dog-eared illustrative pamphlet back to the nurse in the health clinic. "She just won't go for it, nurse!" In such cases, the most well-meant advice may not be useful. To resolve such incompatible needs, the nurse may best counsel the most sexually active and liberal partner in ways to achieve orgasm while still remaining sexually comforting for the other partner.

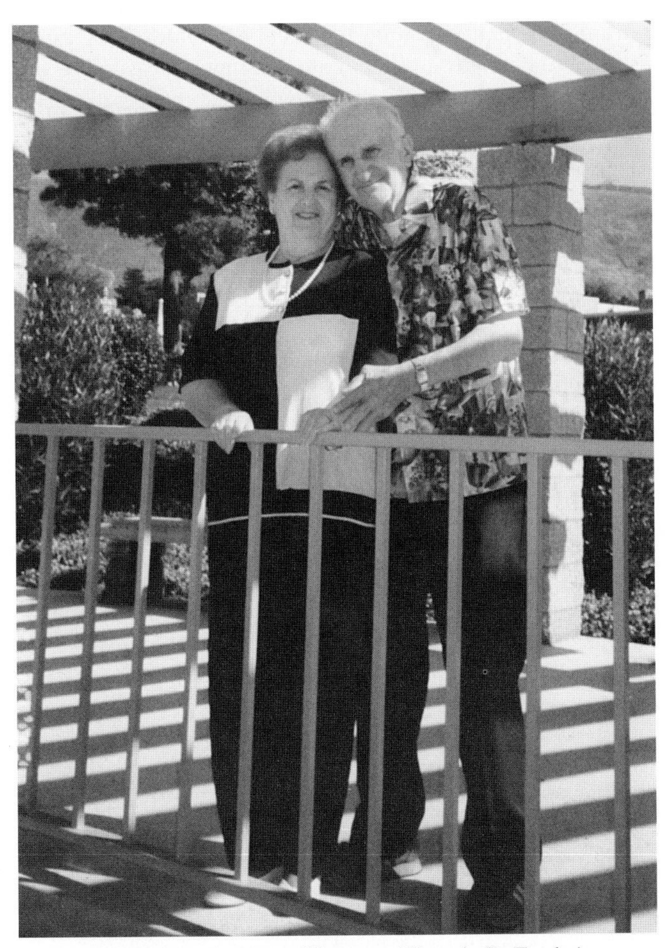

Redefining pleasures. (Courtesy Victoria DeZordo.)

Redefinitions. Sexuality in the aged shifts its focus from procreation to an emphasis on companionship, physical nearness, intimate communication, and a pleasure-seeking physical relationship. Some researchers have coined the phrase "from procreation to recreation," which refers to this change in sexual emphasis. This redefinition of sexuality within Maslow's hierarchical framework simply means the most basic level of function might be male-initiated sex for the purpose of reproduction, and the more complex levels involve a relationship of greater communication, trust, love, sharing, and the giving of pleasure with or without coitus. This change in sexual emphasis is also a reaffirmation of DeNigola and Peruzza's (1974) view that sexuality serves a comprehensive function in adaptation and can be fulfilled in many healthy ways.

Sex can be a way of preventing social disengagement in old age. Sexual activity can also be a means of promoting intergenerational understanding. Both young and old share some of the same fears, insecurities, and pleasures afforded by sex. Sex can be a safe and valuable form of physical exercise. Sex can be a way of maintaining a healthy self-image in old age, and it can be a support in managing personal anxieties by serving as an outlet to defuse anxieties and by providing psychologic refueling and energizing. Sex may even be an escape from depression (Walz, Blum, 1987). The changing emphasis and the totality of sexual behavior of later life is incorporated into the framework of Maslow's hierarchy (see Figure 17-3).

Activity Levels. No national comprehensive surveys of sexuality have been done for any specific age group. Historical and limited data of early studies of sexual behavior by Kinsey in the 1940s and 1950s and Masters and Johnson in the 1960s contained small samples of older adults from which to draw conclusions. These studies did suggest that older people continued to enjoy sexual relations into late life. The Duke Longitudinal Study and the Baltimore Longitudinal Study on Aging were questionnaires (conducted by mail) of self-reported sexual activity. These studies showed that a little more than 50% of the aged couples in the studies were sexually active. After the age of 75 years, sexual activity tended to drop significantly. This cessation was primarily caused by illness of one or both partners or the death of one of the spouses. The studies also revealed that women tended to be less sexually active than men. Even though many old women retain a strong drive, the population imbalance of the sexes limits opportunity to engage in coitus. In 1998, 46% of women age 65 and older were widowed, and 0.5% men were widowers. Aged women have been viewed by themselves and society (Burke, Knowlton, 1992; Nay, 1992) as sexually unattractive and are left out. Old women outnumber old men and thus have fewer opportunities. Statistics show that by the age of 85, there are 83 men for every 100 women in the United States (over 50% widows, 7% never married, 2% divorced, and 60% without spouses, in contrast to 20% elderly men) (Butler, Lewis, 2002). The ratio of old men to old women becomes 1:4.

Men, on the other hand, remain relatively unscathed by social sanction and have none of the limitations imposed on them that women have. In fact, older men become newsworthy when they father a child in their later years. Older men tend to remarry sooner than do their female counterparts after the death of a spouse. Men marry an average of 3 years after the death, whereas women who remarry take an average of 7 years after widowhood (Burke and Knowlton, 1992).

Although her sample of aged women was a small segment of the total study, Hite (1977) helps emphasize that sexuality and the capacity to experience sexual pleasure are lifetime attributes for women. Comments such as the following were recorded: "I am 67, and find that age does not change sex much, circumstances determine it" (p. 510). A septuagenarian commented, "At my age and without responsibility I do not want matrimony but I have a continuing sex drive which keeps me looking 15 to 20 years younger than my chronological age" (p. 509).

Starr (1985; Butler and Lewis, 2002) recognized that elderly individuals' sexual activity and interest are consistent with those in early adulthood. For many people, sexual response improves. The change in perception of the sexual activity of the aged is based on more recent studies of elderly sexual activity that have included an individual's experience and perception rather than just the physiologic and statistical changes characteristic of earlier studies.

Cohort Attitudes. History has shown that basic attitudes toward sexual expression have been the subject of hostility, or they have been venerated or openly accepted. American society continues to struggle with open acceptance of sexual expression for the young but continues to remain hostile to the attempts of the aged to do the same. Sex interest and activity in the elderly are regarded as deviant behavior and described in such terms as "dirty old man," "lecher," and "old biddy." The same activity attempted by a younger person would be viewed as appropriate. The boomer, as they find themselves experiencing sexuality beyond the age they had assigned to their elders, may alter this perception.

Biologic Changes with Age. Acknowledgement and understanding of the age changes that influence coitus may partially explain alteration in sexual behavior to accommodate these changes and facilitate continued pleasurable sex. Appendix 4-A discusses the various physical changes that occur in men and women with age. Table 17-1 summarizes physical alterations that affect coitus in aging people. Physical alteration is one variable in the total picture of sexuality and is therefore included as one of the main factors that influence the act of intercourse. Many texts explain biologic changes in depth.

Biologic factors include (1) adequate circulation to the genital area to support the vasocongestion that takes place; (2) functional neurologic pathways to conduct motor, sensory, and reflex impulses; (3) adequate and appropriate hormone availability to influence the integrity of the genital structure and function; and (4) intactness of the genitalia.

Aging individuals who do not understand the physical changes that affect sexual activity become concerned that their sex life is approaching its natural conclusion with the onset of menopause or, for men, when they discover a change in the firmness of their erection or the decreased need for

Table 17-1 Physical Changes in Sexual Responses in Old Age

	Female	Male
Excitation phase	Diminished or delayed lubrication (1 to 3 min may be required for adequate amounts to appear) Diminished flattening and separation of labia majora Disappearance of elevation of labia majora Decreased vasocongestion of labia minora Decreased elastic expansion of vagina (depth and breadth) Breasts not as engorged Sex flush absent	Less intense and slower erection (but can be maintained longer without ejaculation) Increased difficulty regaining an erection if lost Less vasocongestion of scrotal sac Less pronounced elevation and congestion of testicles
Plateau phase	Slower and less prominent uterine elevation or tenting Decreased muscle tension Decreased capacity for vasocongestion Decreased areolar engorgement Labial color change less evident Less intense swelling or orgasmic platform Less sexual flush Decreased secretions of Bartholin glands	Decreased muscle tension Nipple erection and sexual flush less often No color change at coronal edge of penis Slower penile erection pattern Delayed or diminished erectal and testicular elevation
Orgasmic phase	Fewer number and less intense orgasmic contractions Rectal spincter contractions with severe tension only	Decreased or absent secretory activity (lubrication) by Cowper gland before ejaculation Fewer penile contractions Fewer rectal sphincter contractions Decreased force of ejaculation (approximately 50%) with decreased amount of semen (if ejaculation is long, seepage of semen occurs)
Resolution phase	Observably slower loss of nipple erection Vasocongestion of clitoris and orgasmic platform quickly subsides	Vasocongestion of nipples and scrotum slowly subsides Very rapid loss of erection and descent of testicles shortly after ejaculation Refractory time extended (time required before another erection ranges from several to 24 hours, occasionally longer)

Data compiled from Miller CA: *Nursing care of older adults,* Glenview, IL, 1990, Scott Foresman/Little Brown, Higher Education; Shippee-Rice R: Sexuality and aging. In Fogel C, Lauver D, editors: *Sexual health promotion,* Philadelphia, 1990, WB Saunders; Saxon SV, Etten MJ: *Physical changes and aging,* ed 3, New York, 1994, The Tiresias Press, Inc.

ejaculation with each orgasm or when the refractory period is extended between episodes of intercourse. Morning intercourse is often more satisfying because many aging men experience erection early in the morning. However, couples must find the time of day that works best for them.

Psychologic Factors. Given the gradual biologic changes in genital structures, a potential exists for continued performance of the sex act among older adults. However, psychologic factors such as guilt, depression, monotony, unresolved grief, anger, performance anxiety, and self-doubt may inhibit function (Box 17-2). The client or patient most often believes inhibition is a biologic failure. Many health care professionals also conclude that inhibition is age appropriate, without considering a psychologic base.

Environmental Factors. Environmental barriers result predominantly from the lack of privacy available to the older individual. Lack of privacy can occur when the aged person lives with adult children. If a parent has a suitor in to visit, they rarely have a place to go by themselves without other family members around. Institutions tend to separate the sexes (less today than in past years, but this practice still exists), married and single elderly men from single women. Intimacy of unmarried people in nursing homes to just hold hands, hug, kiss, or any combination is discouraged, even if consenting adults chose to do so. Specific places are available for mixed company to congregate, and rules dealing with male residents going into women's rooms and vice versa are made. Medicaid, however, stipulates that married couples have the right to be housed together (Brier and Rubenstein, 1977). Jacob Reingold, vice president of the Jewish Home for the Aged in the Bronx, New York, established the first policy and procedure in a long-term care institution that clearly stated the residents' rights and also addressed inappropriate expression.

Caregivers are surprised and become moralistic and, at times, angry with the elderly resident who is found in bed with another resident or who is sexually acting out or masturbating. Stevenson and Courtenay (1982) found that nurses' aides who were extremely religious had the most difficulty in accepting the sexual expression of older adults in nursing homes. Hearing a staff member talk to the aged person who has committed an indiscretion (in the staff member's eyes) as if he or she were a child, reprimanding the elder for the behavior, is common.

Staff members themselves sometimes unknowingly provoke a sexual response from the resident or patient. Comments about looking handsome or "Are you going to be my date?" seem harmless and "cute." However, for the elderly man who still has sexual desires but little opportunity to express them, this question may initiate behavior that the staff finds offensive (e.g., sexual statements, grabbing to fondle a staff member) and that results in a reprimand to or punishment of the aged person. The same is true with the aged woman in an institutional setting.

Comments made by male staff members about her appearance or about relationships with male residents can stimulate expressions of sexuality that are dealt with jokingly.

Box 17-2 Psychologic Factors in Elderly Sexuality

- Misinterpretation of physical changes
- Monotony or boredom with repetitious sexual relationship
- Mental and physical fatigue
- Increased expectations on retirement
- Loss of role
- Poor self-image
- Fear of rejection
- Freedom from fear of pregnancy
- Freedom from scheduled activities

Compiled from Steffl BM: *Handbook of gerontologic nursing,* New York, 1984, Van Nostrand; Ham RJ, Sloane PD: *Primary care geriatrics,* St Louis, 1992, Mosby; Lewis MI: Sexuality. In Abrams WB, Beers MH, Berkow R: *The Merck manual of geriatrics,* ed 2, Whitehouse Station, NJ, 1995, Merck Research Laboratories.

Alternative Sexual Lifestyles

Lesbian, Gay, Bisexual, and Transgender (LGBT). Considering the restrictive attitudes within which many elderly people were raised, it is understandable that any alternative sexual behaviors may be unacceptable to the old. Young people may be more accepting of peer variation but are still intolerant of the same behavior in the older people. Estimates suggest that gays and lesbians comprise 10% of the population in the United States; approximately the same proportion of the entire elder population is homosexual, however, no accurate figures are available. The numbers are definitely no lower and may in fact be higher (Lewis, 1995; Freedman, 1995; Butler and Lewis 2002).

Older gay men and lesbians are as diverse as the remainder of the heterosexual elder population. Many gay men and lesbians age successfully, are healthy, and are active with satisfied lives. Some gay and lesbian people are coupled, have children, are open about their sexual orientation, and some are not. Some of these individuals have only recently "come out"; others have been "out" most of their lives; and some find themselves isolated in the larger society. Information about the aged homosexual continues to be limited except for the major works by Berger, *Gay and Gray: The Older Homosexual Man* (1995), and Kehoe's study of lesbians (1988), which provides major insight into the lifestyles of gay males and lesbians.

The studies of Kelly (1977, 1980) found homosexual activity of aged men varied from a low to moderate degree, depending on individual desire. By 65 years of age, sexual satisfaction was still maintained, but the number of friendships had diminished. Both gays and lesbians used a self-selection process to establish friendships or friendship networks (Raphael and Robertson, 1980; Slusher et al, 1996).

Quam and Whitford (1992) noted that over one half of the lesbians in their study reported most of their closest friends were lesbian, but only 27.5% of the gay men reported that their closest friends were gay men. Sixty five percent of the study population indicated that their closest friends were a mix of gay and nongay men and women; about one third of the lesbian women described their friendships to be comparable. In the absence of kinship bonds, gays and lesbians develop homosexual friendship networks.

Lesbians over 60 years of age live with the triple threat of being women, elderly, and having a different sexual orientation (Deevey, 1990). These women tend to keep a very low profile, although conservative estimates are that over 2 million now reside in the United States, preferring rural settings, whereas the gay men prefer urban areas. An intensive study of 100 lesbians between 60 and 86 years of age found that most lived alone, were retired from helping professions, and had college or advanced degrees. Nearly one half were overweight and considered themselves restricted by health problems, although 72% considered themselves healthy, and 82% considered themselves emotionally healthy. Eighty-four percent felt positive about being lesbian, and almost one half had, at one time, been married. Many of these lesbians described themselves as lonely, presently celibate, and desiring a relationship with a woman within 10 years of their own age. The majority desired special senior centers or retirement communities for lesbians (Kehoe, 1988).

Older lesbians have often practiced serial monogamy throughout life and, in late life, continue to anticipate the finding of a new mate if the need arises. According to Robertson (1979), lesbians who consider themselves feminists reject the monogamous love relationship. An interesting note is that approximately one third of the lesbians "come out" after the age of 50. Before this time, lesbians often feel unable to deal with familial and societal pressures. Most lesbians married, raised children, divorced, and lead double lives (Butler and Lewis, 2002).

Gay men until the ages of 46 to 55 years have been found to have had multiple liaisons. However, with the impact of acquired immunodeficiency syndrome (AIDS) on this population, a decrease in multiple liaisons has become evident. Berger (1995) notes that sexual patterns tend to remain consistent over a lifetime. After 46 to 55 years of age, partnerships are nearly nonexistent. The situation has been attributed to several factors: the death of a loved one and rejection of the idea of a single lifelong partner (Kelly, 1977).

Reports indicate that gays and lesbians have less difficulty adjusting to aging because they have already faced difficult adjustments such as coping with the stigma of homosexuality. Adelman (1990) found adjustment to aging was related to the lifestyle of being gay and satisfaction with being gay; the early developmental sequence of gay events correlated with high life satisfaction, low self-criticism, and few psychosomatic problems. Lesbians were found not to fear the prospect of being alone or isolated in old age. Conversely, older gays expressed fear of loneliness and isolation in later life because of too few role models for growing old in partnerships or singleness. Some research indicates that more concern for the loss of youth and change in physical appearance occurred with gay men than with either lesbians or heterosexuals (Raphael and Robertson, 1980; Freedman, 1995). Problems that confront the aged LGBT are similar to those that face any aged person: loss of important people, presence of a stigma associated with being aged, and fear of institutionalization.

One problem unique to the aged LGBT is the lack of the economic, emotional, and physical security that occurs in most heterosexual relationships. Laws and rules governing life insurance and estate benefits discriminate against the lover liaison. Even with a legally recorded will that states that benefits should go to the lover, family members may successfully contest in probate hearings. In addition, health support services do not meet the needs of gay and lesbian elders (Slusher et al, 1996; Flaxman, 1996; Butler and Lewis, 2002).

LGBT elders living in metropolitan areas may find organizations particularly designed for them, such as Senior Action in a Gay Environment (SAGE), (SAGE-Net is now in nine states and Ontario, Canada); Gay and Lesbian Outreach to Elders (formerly GLOE, San Francisco) but is now called New Leaf Outreach to Elders); Rainbow Project (Los Angeles); Gay and Lesbians Older and Wiser (GLOW, Ann Arbor, Michigan); and the Lesbian and Gay Aging Issues Network (LGAIN).

Health care providers lack sufficient information and sensitivity when caring for older LGBTs is considered. This sensitivity is of utmost importance when attempting to obtain a health history. Using open-ended questions such as "Who is most important to you?" or "Do you have a significant other?" is much better than asking "Are you married?" This form of the question allows the nurse to look beyond the rigid category of family. Euphemisms are frequently used for a life partner (roommate, close friend). Asking individuals if they consider themselves as primarily heterosexual, homosexual, or bisexual is also better. This question conveys recognition of sexual variety. An older lesbian woman in a health care situation may refer to herself indirectly by saying "people like us." Nurses need to become more aware of these nuances and try to understand the fear of discovery that is apparent in the older gay man and lesbian woman. These elders are of a generation in which they were and may still be closeted because of the homophobic experiences they had through their younger years.

Better support and care services for gays and lesbians by care providers should include working through a person's homophobia and discomfort discussing sexuality, learning about special issues facing older gay men and lesbians, and becoming aware of the gay and lesbian resources in the community. Finally, a facility or agencies already in the community need to be assessed from the perspective of the client, patient, or resident who may be gay or lesbian.

LGBTs among older adults continues to be a subject ripe for research, because so little is known about these elders. LGBT communities are moving toward research directed toward looking at gay male couples and lesbian couples, bisexual and transgender coupling, the gay widow, and the single older LGBT.

Procreation has been considered the sanctioned reason for sex and then only between people who were socially approved (married). Throughout the world, many older adults still believe this injunction. For older women—single, divorced, or widowed—the only liaison permitted is with socially sanctioned partners. Women are less free to seek sexual alternatives than are men.

Widowhood. The widow too may have an alternative lifestyle. The sexual life of widows is a matter of great concern because so many older women will be widowed. Beresford and Barrett (1982) and Hooyman and Kiyak (1996) found that sexually active widows tended to be younger, widowed for a longer duration, and more liberal in their attitudes than sexually nonactive widows. Most widows indicated a desire for male companionship but possessed an ambivalent attitude toward remarriage. Widows report that they miss sexual relations with their husbands, but they have a great need for nongenital touching. Friends and family often fail to meet these needs.

AIDS and the Elderly

The compromised immune system of an aged individual makes him or her even more susceptible to human immunodeficiency virus (HIV) or AIDS than a younger person. As the geriatric population increases, so will the geriatric AIDS cases increase.

AIDS is not exclusively a young person's disease, but it is frequently underreported in the elderly because the symptoms of fatigue, weakness, weight loss, and anorexia are common to other elder disease conditions. In addition, the idea that elders are not sexually active limits physicians' and other care providers' objectivity to recognize HIV-AIDS as a possible diagnosis.

The Centers for Disease Control and Prevention (CDC) reported in September 1993 that more than 34,000 people over age 50 had full-blown AIDS, a number that had more than doubled since January 1991 (Baker and Crowley, 1994; Goodroad, 2003). Currently, estimates suggest that 10% of the individuals over age 50, 3% over age 60, and 0.7% over age 70 have AIDS (Fletcher, 1995; Fletes, 1995). AIDS is rising faster among the older population than it is in those age 24 and younger (Goodroad, 2003).

Contrary to popular belief, HIV-AIDS in the elderly population is not the result of blood transfusions alone. Research shows that elders are sexually active and thus at risk for HIV-AIDS. A study at the University of California, San Francisco, of 3200 predominantly heterosexual Americans over age 50 found that approximately 10% had at least one risk factor for HIV infection. Butler and Lewis (2002) indicate that 10% over age 50 have active AIDS, one fourth of those are over age 60, and 4% are over age 70. People over 50 years of age were one sixth as likely to use condoms during sex and one fifth as likely to have been tested for HIV (Some older Americans not practicing safe sex, 1993). AIDS is appearing in retirement communities. Though Diokno and colleagues (1990) found that the frequency of sexual activity declined with age, a majority of people over 60 remained sexually active (66.6% of the older men and 31.7% of older women). Homosexuality, bisexuality, and intravenous drug use are not exclusive to the younger population (Schuerman, 1994). The risk factors for the older age group include pre-1985 blood product recipients, spouses of those recipients, and people who participate in unprotected anal and vaginal intercourse outside a monogamous relationship. Because procreation is not an issue with elders, they are least likely to use condoms. Elderly gay men who have spent a lifetime hiding their true sexual orientation may be reluctant to speak frankly with a health care provider. People who know that they are HIV positive may hide the fact for fear of negative judgment from family, friends, and caregivers (Baker, Crowley, 1994).

Physicians do not usually ask sexually active elders about their sexual activity and health. Moreover, elders do not usually confide in a health care provider or friends, because they are uncomfortable admitting to sexual activity "at their age." Elders have bought into the myth that old people do not have sex. Older women who are sexually active are at high risk for HIV-AIDS from an infected partner resulting in part from normal age changes of the vaginal tissue—a thinner, drier, friable vaginal lining. Older men may frequent prostitutes (a potentially high-risk group for HIV-AIDS). Gay men may increase their risk of HIV exposure after the death of a long-term mate by turning to a more available younger partner, who may be more likely to have HIV. In general, elders lack adequate knowledge about HIV-AIDS and believe that HIV-AIDS *"just does not happen in their generation."* This view places elders at high risk for HIV and AIDS.

AIDS in older adults has been called the "Great Imitator." In addition to the vague signs mentioned earlier, symptoms include dementia with increased neurologic abnormalities and unexplained diffuse encephalopathy that is demonstrated in progressive and chronic dementia. Elders may be misdiagnosed as having Alzheimer's disease (AD) (Schuerman, 1994; Whipple and Scura, 1996) instead of AIDS—the actual problem. AIDS dementia is rapid in onset, as opposed to the slow progressive decline associated with AD. Confusion and other cognitive difficulties may wax and wane. Aphasia, which is seen in AD, is usually absent in AIDS dementia. Extrapyramidal symptoms suggestive of parkinsonism may occur but without the tremors and ataxia. Leg tremors, peripheral neuropathy with progressive weakness, and a positive Babinski reflex may also be seen when diagnosing AIDS.

Other AIDS problems that the elder might exhibit include opportunistic infections, malignancies, *Pneumocystis carinii* pneumonia (PCP), tuberculosis, esophageal or recurrent genital candidiasis, toxoplasmosis, non-Hodgkin's lymphoma, Kaposi's sarcoma, or herpes zoster. Women may develop candidiasis or human papilloma virus infections as a first sign of AIDS (Schuerman, 1994; Whipple and Scura, 1996; Butler and Lewis, 2002; Goodroad, 2003). An important point to keep in mind is that conditions that persist or reoccur should be suspect for HIV-AIDS and that the elder should be tested given that the incubation period for AIDS may be as long as 10 years. Other people, however, who have tested positive for HIV have shown no symptoms after 14 years.

Elders need to get the message that they are at high risk for HIV-AIDS. As of 1999, 78,000 people over the age of 50 developed AIDS. This number is ten times that of the decade before. Educational materials and programs need to be developed that include information about what HIV-AIDS is and how it is and is not transmitted, the need to use condoms for protection when engaging in sexual activity, symptoms of which to be aware, and the treatments that are available. Physicians, nurse practitioners, and other health professionals need to become comfortable taking a complete sexual history and talking about sex with the elderly. In addition, the myth that elders do not engage in sexual activity must be put to rest.

The aged are different from other groups at risk for HIV-AIDS in that they have multiple acute and chronic illnesses and still can be highly functional. When hospitalized for multiple diagnoses, few health professionals consider them at risk for HIV. Well known is that the time between acquiring HIV infections and the diagnosis of AIDS is shorter for elders, as is the time between diagnosis and death from AIDS.

Although no substantive research is available, an underlying assumption holds that many elders in nursing homes may be HIV positive. A limited number of long-term care facilities knowingly accept patients with AIDS, and among those that do, the geriatric patient with AIDS competes for extended care services with nongeriatric patients with and without AIDS. Finding appropriate services and facilities may be difficult, although in places in which this care is available, reports are positive. A major concern is that the needs of young people dying of AIDS may be quite different from those of the older adult. If younger and older people are indiscriminately mixed in long-term care settings, neither group is likely to have its needs met.

Because most communities do not have resources to establish separate systems for the aged and the patients with AIDS who have some similar needs, long-term care providers must address these issues.

Sexual Dysfunction

Sexual dysfunction, which occurs in both men and women, has a physiologic or psychologic base or a combination of both. Psychologic dysfunction is more common than physical impairment (Ham, 1997; Butler and Lewis, 1990, 2002). A major problem confronting the aging man is the fear of or the actual occurrence of impotence, now called *erectile dysfunction* (ED). What men generally call *impotence* is diminished potency and frequency of sexual activity. Impotence, according to Ham (1997), is a psychogenic or organic pathologic condition that has its origins in excessive use of alcohol, preoccupation with work problems, monotony in the relationship, anger, fatigue, or neurologic or vascular conditions. Sexual dysfunction in women has not been accorded the same intensive research as has dysfunction in men.

Sexual function in women is as much a quality-of-life issue as it is in men. Drug-related sexual dysfunction is sometimes hard to distinguish from depression or disease. The use of medication by both men and women may also cause a decrease in libido. Sex may be disrupted by acute illness, whereas energy is directed toward regaining and maintaining homeostasis rather than toward physical sex. The fact that disuse decreases the ability of the aged to engage in sex is true, but when a person has maintained regular sexual function before illness, sexual desire begins to return during convalescence.

Male Dysfunction. Impotence or ED is defined as the inability to achieve and sustain an erection sufficient for satisfactory sexual intercourse in at least 50% or more attempts. ED has become recognized as a common problem among men over the age of 50 (Moon, 2000; Butler and Lewis, 2000). Until recently, ED had been a neglected area of health that is fraught with myths and superstition. ED transiently occurs to men of all ages at least once in their life; however, the prevalence of ED increases with age. Butler and Lewis estimate that 70% of men over 50 experience some form of chronic erectile problem.

Nearly 95% of men over the age of 70 who have medical problems such as diabetes mellitus will experience ED. An erection is governed by the interaction among the hormonal, vascular, and nervous systems. A problem in any of these systems can cause ED. Of course, multiple causes exist for this problem in older men (Box 17-3). These factors include psychologic causes such as multiple losses of cohorts (spouse or friends), which can lead to depression. Common medical causes include hypogonadism, thyroid dysfunction, and diabetes. Nearly one third of ED is a complication of diabetes. Alcoholism, medications, and zinc deficiencies are also causes of ED in older men.

Various medications that affect the sympathetic and parasympathetic nervous system interfere with the man's capacity to have an erection or to ejaculate. Adrenergic agents block impulses that affect contractility of the prostate gland and seminal vesicles and depress or interfere with

Box 17-3 Causes of Erectile Dysfunction

Vascular problems
Endocrine problems
Neurologic problems
Structural abnormalities of the penis
Depression
Zinc deficiency
Alcoholism
Diabetes mellitus
Medications
Psychologic problems

Compiled from Gerchafsky M: Impotence: the problem men don't talk about, *Ad Nurse Pract* 3(3):13, 1995; Buczny B: Impotence in older men: a newly recognized problem, *J Gerontol Nurs* 18(5):25, 1992; Butler R, Lewis M: *The new love and sex after 60,* New York, 2002, Ballantine Books.

ejaculation. The anticholinergic preparations affect penis erection by vasocongestion in the venous channels. The ganglionic blocking agents possess properties of both the adrenergic and anticholinergic preparations and affect both penis erection and ejaculation (Jarvik, Small, 1988; Sherman, 1992; Butler and Lewis, 2002).

A few medications have been found to increase sexual desire. The phenothiazines and testosterone increase the libido in the aged woman, and L-dopa heightens sexual desire in the aged man (Sherman,1992; Butler and Lewis, 2002). This situation can be extremely distressful to the individual and the caregiving staff if the person is institutionalized. Table 17-2 lists many drugs that alter sexual function.

Environmental agents, including industrial chemicals and exposure to electromagnetic fields used by some industries, can induce impotence. The effects of inadequate housing, lack of privacy, and feelings of psychologic inferiority are also contributory factors to impotence.

Most men who undergo surgical procedures such as transurethral resection and other types of prostatectomies, Y-V-plasty of the bladder neck, resection of the colon for cancer, or a sympathectomy may find to their dismay that they have acquired ED or that they have retrograde ejaculations, the result of interference with autonomic innervation in the pelvis (Boyarsky, 1983; Butler and Lewis, 2002). Particularly after a prostatectomy, a space remains where the enlarged prostate had been. The principle that fluid travels the path of least resistance applies here. At the point of ejaculation, the semen moves backward into the bladder rather than forward through increased resistance, which produces a retrograde, or dry, ejaculation. Ignorance regarding this physiologic change further convinces men that their sexual activity is over, when, in fact, it is not. Erection can be attained and orgasmic pleasure achieved. Any surgery that involves the male perineum has a high risk of causing ED resulting from potential nerve damage in that area.

Most research on sexual dysfunction has been conducted by men on older men. Less knowledge of female sexual dysfunction is known, particularly drug effects.

Female Dysfunction. Female dysfunction is considered "persistent impediment to a person's normal pattern of sexual interest, response, or both" (Kaiser, 2000, p. 1174). Female sexual function can be influenced by factors such as culture, ethnicity, emotional state, age, and previous sexual experiences, as well as changes in sexual response with normal aging. For the most part, women worry more about youthfulness than they do about problems of sexual performance. For heterosexual women, frequency of intercourse is more dependent on the age, health, and sexual function of the partner or the availability of a partner rather than on their own sexual capacity. However, women may experience pain on intercourse (dyspareunia) because of the thinning of the vaginal wall and the lack of lubrication. In many instances, using water-soluble lubricants such as K-Y, Astroglide, Slip, HR lubricating jelly can resolve the difficulty. Women can experience arousal disorders resulting from drugs such as anticholinergics, tricyclic antidepressants, and chemotherapeutic agents, as well as lack of lubrication from radiation, surgery, and stress. A decrease in libido often occurs because of worry, increased prolactin, and a decrease in testosterone, estrogen, or both. Drugs such as serotonin-specific reuptake inhibitors and anticancer drugs are also libido depressants. Orgasmic disorders may result from drugs used to treat depression.

Radiation to the pelvis is another factor in orgasmic dysfunction as is anorgasmia resulting from decreased libido. Unlike ED, studies of vascular insufficiency are less clear in women with sexual dysfunction. Dyspareunia (painful intercourse or pain with attempted intercourse) occurs in one third of women over age 65 resulting from inadequate lubrication, irritation, dryness, and altered anatomic structure, as well as intromission (the altered angle of intercourse penetration). Vaginismus (a problem related to dyspareunia), is the involuntary, forceful, and painful spasms of the lower vaginal muscles caused by vaginal infection, vaginal mucosal irritation, and fearing the loss of control or being hurt during intercourse (Kaiser, 2000; Barnes, 2000; Butler and Lewis, 2002).

Although hormone replacement therapy (HRT) has been an option for maintaining vaginal integrity, controversy continues regarding the benefits versus the potential danger of induced endometrial or breast cancer (Schiff, 1995). Prolapse of the uterus, rectoceles, and cystoceles can be surgically repaired to facilitate continued sexual activity.

Assessment of ED includes a history and screening for major psychologic problems of the man and spouse, if possible. Physical examination is generally less revealing than a history but can detect structural problems. Testing for levels of testosterone, luteinizing hormone, zinc, thyroid function, alcoholism, and medication side effects is important. A workup for

Table 17-2 Potential Medication Effects on Sexual Function

Drug or drug category	Parameters of effect	
	Physiologic	Psychologic
Antidepressants Tricyclics Amitriptyline Desipramine Doxepin Imipramine Nortriptyline Phenelzine Trazodone	Central nervous system depression Impotence Inhibited ejaculation Orgasmic difficulty	Increased libido if depression reduced
Antihistamine and H_2 blockers	Central nervous system depression Decreased vaginal lubrication H_2 blockers—impotence	Decreased libido Decreased erection ability
Antihypertensives Clonidine Enalapril Guanethidine Hydralazine Methyldopa Prazosin Reserpine Spironolactone Verapamil	Peripheral blockage of innervation of sex organs Decrease/absence of ejaculation Retrograde ejaculation	Decreased libido
Beta-blockers Atenolol Labetalol Metoprolol Propranolol Timolol	Orgasmic difficulties Breast tenderness Gynecomastia	Decreased libido
Antipsychotics Phenothiazines Chlorpromazine Haloperidol Thioridazine Thiothixene Trifluoperazine	Dry ejaculation Erectile difficulty Gynecomastia Decreased vaginal lubrication Spontaneous milk flow from breasts	
Diuretics	Impotence Gynecomastia Breast tenderness	
Antispasmodics	Vasoconstriction Ganglionic blockage of innervation of sex organs Impotence Decreased vaginal lubrication	Decreased libido
Antiparkinsonism Amantadine Benztropine Bromocriptine L-dopa Selegiline	Increased erectile function	Improvement of well being—may be responsible for increased libido
Other drugs		
Cytoxin		Decreased libido
Androgens	Antiandrogenic effect Virilization of female	Decreased libido
Digoxin	Erectile failure Gynecomastia	Decreased libido
Lithium		Increased libido
Opiates	Central nervous system depressant	Reduced inhibitions
Morphine Codeine	Impotence	Decreased sexual enjoyment

diabetes is also necessary. Once the assessment has identified the possible cause or causes, intervention is prescribed, which may take the form of sex therapy or psychosexual counseling (reeducation). Because society views sexual desires as unnatural in the elderly population, older people may feel guilt or shame when they experience these desires. This condition is called geriatric sexuality breakdown syndrome. Therapy redirects and develops graded sexual experiences and is helpful as an adjunct to treatment when medical causes or a combination of causes are identified (Buczny, 1992).

Many therapies are available for ED, including the newest sildenafil citrate (Viagra) (Box 17-4). Before the availability of Viagra, pharmacotherapy such as injections or the intracavernosal injection with drugs papaverine and phentolamine, a vasoactive agent that reduces resistance of arteriolar and cavernosal smooth muscle tissue of the penis, were used. This agent leads to increased arterial flow and subsequent venous trapping, facilitating an erection (Butler et al, 1994; Beers, 1995; Moon, 2000; Butler and Lewis, 2002). Trial and error determines the dose of the drug. The injections seem to help individuals with moderate vascular disease, which is most common in 80% of older men who are impotent. For other men, with psychologically based impotence, the injections seem to bolster self-confidence, and after a few injections, therapy is no longer needed.

Penile implants of the semirigid, adjustable-malleable, or hinged and inflatable types are available when impotence does not respond to other treatments or is irreversible. The hinged and inflatable types, which are inserted in the testicular area, are the most popular. Still evolving is penile

Box 17-4 Viagra: Contraindications and Side Effects

Contraindications

Individuals who:

- Take nitrates
- Have blocked or constricted arteries
- Experience angina or chest pain when not taking nitrates
- Lack the capacity to have safe sex
- Use poppers (amyl nitrate)

Should not be used with other erectile dysfunction treatments

Side Effects*

Headache
Flushing
Stomach upset
Nasal congestion
Transient sensitivity to light
Transient color vision disturbance (seeing blue)

*Most occur at the highest dosages; most are mild and self-limiting. *Nausea, chest pain, and dizziness should be reported to a physican immediately.*

revascularization surgery (the shifting of blood vessels to restore normal blood circulation to the penis). Candidates for this type of surgery would be those with arteriosclerosis and other peripheral vascular conditions, as well as for those with trauma or accidents to the penis and surrounding area. This type of surgery requires extraordinary surgical skill and is only for men who meet the criteria of localized, identifiable lesions (Beers, 1995; Butler and Lewis, 2002).

The geriatric nurse working with clients who have ED serves as a client advocate, advises about assessment, and instructs in the use of prosthetic devices. The nurse's most important role is to provide support and guidance for this touchy subject and provides information and resources (see website for resources).

Chronic Conditions and Sexuality

Sexual activity depends, under most circumstances, on the state of sex drive and performance before the illness or chronic conditions, on the function of the heart, and on response to treatment.

Although pain, fatigue, and joint stiffness and limitation that occur with arthritis may interfere with sexual activity, they need not curtail enjoyment of sexual intercourse. Sexual activity may, in fact, enhance some arthritis therapies and be beneficial because it stimulates the release of cortisone, adrenalin, and other chemicals that are natural pain relievers. Theories also suggest that the act of intercourse is not only good exercise, but also a beneficial means of psychologic and physical tension reduction.

Individuals with heart disease or those who have suffered a stroke often reduce their sexual activity because of fear and lack of knowledge about their condition. Caregivers often fail to discuss sexual matters with the aged person during recovery. The energy expenditure needed for intercourse is comparable to briskly climbing two flights of stairs or walking several blocks rapidly. If the individual can perform this task without adverse effects, he or she can resume normal sexual activity. Participation in a medically supervised exercise program can reduce oxygen requirements during sexual activity and improve the quality of sexual life.

Strokes should not be a cause for stopping sexual activity. Unless the stroke has resulted in severe brain damage, sexual desire is usually unimpaired, although sexual performance may be affected (some men experience ED; some do not). The unaffected side should be the focus of lovemaking.

Diabetes often leads to ED (two to five times greater in this group than in the general population), though interest and desire is still present. When diabetes is properly controlled, ED may disappear in some individuals. Loss of sexual function does not seem to be a problem with females who have diabetes.

Many false beliefs abound about the aftermath of a prostatectomy. If these ideas are not clarified and corrected, the psychologic effect may contribute to ED. Dry orgasms (retrograde ejaculation) are normal after prostatic surgery.

After hysterectomies, the woman's abdomen may feel sore for 3 to 4 months and may interfere with resumption of normal sexual activity. The individual usually abstains from intercourse for 6 to 8 weeks after surgery. A decrease in lubrication and sensation can occur in the lower genital tract, or sensation can be lost if the cervix was a source of stimulation by the penis. If the ovaries are removed with or without the removal of the uterus, sexual desire is lost. Table 17-3 presents common conditions that can affect sexual function. Suggestions for interventions are also given.

HRT continues to be controversial. HRT carries with it the possible side effects of headache, fluid retention, weight gain, vaginal discharge, breast swelling, and the possibility of endometrial and breast cancer. Although HRT has been used to control hot flashes and to maintain vaginal tissue integrity, serious questions regarding its use have been raised by the current findings of the Women's Health Initiative Study that HRT resulted in a significant risk of breast cancer (Kolata, 2002). The study used standard dosage of HRT. Whether this risk would be present using lesser doses or combination patches, which many women also use, was not addressed and raises additional questions.

The controversy over HRT benefits and potential dangers will continue for some time. A possible connection between HRT and ovarian cancer surfaced in 2001 from a study by the University of California, San Francisco (Torassa, 2002). The study also questions whether some of the benefits attributed to HRT, such as protection from heart disease, old age, and bone loss, may not be significant enough for continued HRT

Table 17-3 Chronic Illness and Sexual Function: Effects and Interventions

Condition	Effects/problems	Interventions
Arthritis	Pain, fatigue, limited motion Steroid therapy may decrease sexual interest or desire	Advise patient to perform sexual activity at the time of day when least fatigued and most relaxed Suggest use of analgesics and other pain relief methods prior to sexual activity Encourage use of relaxation techniques before sexual activity such as a warm bath or shower, application of hot packs to affected joints Advise patient to maintain optimum health through a balance of good nutrition, proper rest, and activity Suggest that he or she experiment with different positions, use pillows for comfort and support Recommend use of a vibrator if massage ability is limited Suggest use of water soluble jelly for vaginal lubrication
Cardiovascular disease	Most men have no change in physical effects on sexual function; one fourth may not return to pre-heart attack function, one fourth may not resume sexual activity Women do not experience sexual dysfunction following heart attack Fear of another heart attack or death during sex Shortness of breath	Encourage counseling on realistic restrictions that may be necessary Instruct patient and spouse on alternative positions to avoid strain Suggest that patient avoid large meals several hours before sex Advise patient to relax; plan medications for effectiveness during sex
Cerebrovascular accident (stroke)	Depression May or may not have sexual activity changes Often erectile disorders occur; decrease in frequency of intercourse and sexual relations Possible problems: Change in role and function of partners Decreased physical endurance, fatigue Mobility and sensory deficits Perceptual and visual deficits Communication deficit Cognitive and behavioral deficits Fear of relapse or sudden death	Encourage counseling Instruct patient to use alternative positions Suggest use of a vibrator if massage ability is limited Suggest use of pillows for positioning and support Suggest use of water-soluble jelly for lubrication Instruct patient to use alternative forms of sexual expression

therapy. Evidence from this study did suggest that HRT was most useful in treating menopausal symptoms such as hot flashes. Each woman must consider evidence of her own needs and make her own decisions regarding HRT therapy.

Regaining Sexual Function. After heart attacks, strokes, and abdominal surgery, the aged need not be categorically condemned to abstinence from coitus for the remainder of their lives. Recuperative time is usually 4 to 6 weeks or several months before sexual intercourse can be resumed. After a myocardial infarction, intercourse can be initiated when scar tissue has formed (8 to 14 weeks) and no evidence is observed of ventricular arrhythmias or aneurysms. One method used to test if the individual is able to expend the energy necessary for intercourse is to evaluate the effect on the cardiopulmonary status of rapidly walking up two flights of stairs. Individuals with arrhythmias may need reassurance with a treadmill test to allay their anxiety regarding sexual activity.

Manual stimulation (masturbation) may be an alternative that can be used early in the recovery period to maintain sexual function, if the practice is not objectionable to the patient. Studies show that masturbation is less taxing on the heart and makes less of an oxygen demand (Woods, 1983).

Although self-stimulation is steeped in myth and fear, masturbation is a common and healthy practice in late life. Individuals without partners or with spouses who are ill or incapacitated find that masturbation is helpful. As children, today's aged population were stopped from practicing this pleasurable activity with stories of the evils of fondling a person's own genitals. Masturbation provides an avenue for resolution of sexual tensions, keeps sexual desire alive, maintains lubrication and muscle tone of the vagina, provides mild physical exercise, and preserves sexual function in individuals who have no other outlet for sexual activity and gratification of their sexual need (Butler and Lewis, 1990, 2002).

The aged may or may not have difficulty discussing intimate areas with individuals who are comfortable and capable of dealing with the subject. The nurse has the responsibility

Table 17-3 Chronic Illness and Sexual Function: Effects and Interventions—cont'd

Condition	Effects/problems	Interventions
Chronic obstructive pulmonary disease (COPD)	No direct impairment of sexual activity, though affected by coughing, exertional dyspnea, and activity intolerance Medications may lead to erectile difficulties	Encourage patient to plan sexual activity when energy is highest Instruct patient to use alternative positions Advise patient to plan sexual activity at time medications are most effective Suggest use of oxygen before, during, or after sex, depending when it provides the most benefit
Diabetes	Sexual desire and interest unaffected Neuropathy and/or vascular damage may interfere with erectile ability. About 50% to 75% of men have erectile disorders; a small portion have retrograde ejaculation Some men regain function if diagnosis of diabetes is well accepted, if diabetes is well controlled, or both Women have less sexual desire and vaginal lubrication (Katzm, 1991) Decrease in orgasms/absence of orgasm can occur; less frequent sexual activity; local genital infections	Recommend possible candidates for penile prosthesis Instruct patient to use alternative forms of sexual expression Recommend immediate treatment of genital infections
Cancers Breast	No direct physical affect. There is a strong psychologic effect: Loss of sexual desire Body-image change Depression Reaction to partner	Encourage individual or group counseling
Most other cancers	Men and women may lose sexual desire temporarily Men may have erectile dysfunction; dry ejaculation; retrograde ejaculation Women may have vaginal dryness, dyspareunia Both men and women may experience anxiety, depression, pain, nausea from chemotherapy, radiation, pelvic surgery, hormone therapy, nerve damage from pelvic surgery	

to help maintain the sexuality of the aged by offering the opportunity to discuss. Rarely are sex histories elicited from the elderly patient. Physical examinations do not include the reproductive system unless it is directly involved in the present illness. However, when questions about sexual issues are asked, or when the elderly are examined, the nurse needs to be particularly cognizant of the era and culture in which the individual has lived to understand the factors affecting conduct.

To assist and support the aged in their sexual needs, nurses should be aware of their own feelings about sexuality. Nurses must question their attitude toward old people (single, married, and homosexual) who hold hands or caress or fondle each other. Only after confronting the person's own attitudes, values, and beliefs can the nurse provide support without being judgmental.

Sex in the Nursing Home

Approximately 5% of elders live in institutional environments. Expressions of sexuality are considered in many of these settings (nursing homes, long-term care, chronic disease hospitals) to be a disturbing or behavioral management problem. To consider these expressions as such is a measure of the taboo against sex and the elderly and a denial of elders' private and sexual life (Butler and Lewis, 2002). White (1982) interviewed residents in 15 nursing homes and found that 91% were sexually inactive, although 17% said they would like to be active sexually. White's study seems to reinforce the concept that sexual interest in the institutionalized is related to prior levels of activity and interest. If sexual activity has been an important method of coping, it is likely to remain so. Sexual education and discussion groups should be provided for staff and residents to decrease the overreactions that are commonly seen and to determine policies that allow consenting individuals to engage in sexual activity in private.

Federal nursing home regulations for intermediate care facilities mandate that a married resident must be given privacy during spousal visits. If both husband and wife are residents, they must be permitted to share a room, if they desire. Skilled nursing facilities are under similar mandates unless medically contraindicated. However, what about individuals in intimate relationships when they are not married?

This question has not been addressed. Unmarried elders in care facilities do not have the choice of intimacy of any kind. Although few cases of sexual privacy invasion have reached the courts, they are likely to increase as people become more aware of their rights. The institutionalized aged have the same rights as noninstitutionalized elders have to engage in or abstain from sexual activity.

NURSING ROLES AND FUNCTIONS

Nurses have multiple roles in the area of sexuality and the aged. The nurse is a facilitator of a conducive milieu in which questions can be asked and in which the aged person's sexuality can be expressed. *Most important is providing privacy and allowing the aged control over their sex lives.* The nurse should be an educator and provide information, as well as guidance, to the aged who need it. The aged should be asked about their sexual satisfaction, because they may not mention it voluntarily. Anticipation of problems in aged individuals' sexual experiences can ward off anxiety, misconceptions, and an arbitrary cessation of sexual pleasure. Validation of the normalcy of sexual activity, or a discussion of the physiologic changes that occur with age, or the effect of illness and treatment that may interfere with sexual activity by altering the routine or interfering with physical performance may be needed. Counseling may also be needed for the aged to adapt to natural physiologic changes and image-altering surgical procedures. The nurse may find that he or she is a consultant and counselor to others who give care to the aged.

Assessment

Discussion of sexuality and sexuality problems may be uncomfortable for both nurse and elder. Nonetheless, learning the significance of sexual function to the elder and the perception of sexual function the elder has without bringing the nurse's own biases into the interaction is important. Box 17-5 provides guidelines for data collection.

Interventions

Interventions will vary depending on the needs identified from the assessment data. A variety of suggested interventions for maintaining sexual function for the aged with chronic conditions has been presented in Table 17-3, and ED has been discussed with available options of treatment. Perhaps one of the most important interventions is education regarding normal age changes related to sexual function and the dimensions of sexuality that provide pleasure.

Counseling and Advocacy. Although old people do seek counseling on sexuality and sexual concerns, we do not always hear them, and many of us are not well enough prepared to help them. Successful and continuing sexual activity is but one sign of healthy aging (see Box 17-5). Some nurses have extensive education in sexuality and are in a position to provide intensive therapy for people with sexual problems.

Although the nurse in the acute or long-term care facility may not be well prepared to engage in sex therapy, providing information about sexual issues in anticipation of questions or in response to questions asked and to treat expressions of sexuality as normal and deserving of respect is possible.

The nurse is also an advocate for the aged. An important goal is to look for ways to provide more home care to maintain the option of privacy and control over a person's sexual life and to investigate possible directions to provide comfort without nursing homes and acute care hospitals exerting their authority over sexual expression.

Last, the nurse may become involved in considering issues that might enable the aged to remain in their own homes rather than be subjected to institutionalization.

Evaluation

Elders whose sexuality needs are fulfilled will consider their sexual life with satisfaction. This attitude will be apparent through verbal and nonverbal expression, the individual's self-image, and involvement and concern about others.

In summary, the nurse has a variety of roles in ensuring the sexuality of the aged: facilitator, educator, consultant, counselor, and advocate. Sexuality is an amalgamation of biologic, psychologic, and social moral elements that affect pleasure, adaptation, and a general feeling of well being in the aged.

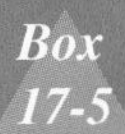

Guidelines for Obtaining Data about Sexual Needs and Concerns

General

What do you think about romance at this stage of your life?
When you were growing up, did people you knew discuss sex and romance?
What were you told about sex when you were a child?
How do you feel about discussing it now?
Do you think it is a very important part of life satisfaction for people of all ages?
What does sexuality mean to you?
How important has sexual activity been in your life?
What were you told about masturbation?
What values and morals influence your feelings about sex now?
How are your needs of intimacy being met now?

Sexual Satisfaction

Have you experienced any changes in your sexual relationships lately?
To what do you attribute this change?
What type of sexual activities have you usually enjoyed the most including such things as hugging, kissing, sleeping together, intercourse, and so on?
Do you or your partner take any prescription medications? What are they? How often do you take them? Have you experienced any changes in your level of energy since starting them? What about feelings of overall well-being? Any changes in sexual desire or activity?

Alterations in Self-Perception

How has growing old changed your lifestyle or things you enjoy doing?
How has the change in your health or the health of your partner altered your lifestyle or your goals?
How do you rate your general health?
On a scale of 1 to 10, how would you describe your satisfaction with your life?
On a scale of 1 to 10, how would you describe your satisfaction with your sexual relationships?

Relationships with Others

Have you ever discussed sexual topics with your spouse, friends, family, or health care professional?
Who do you talk to when you have problems of any kind or just want someone to talk to?

Environment

With whom do you live?
Does your present living situation foster opportunities to express your sexuality?

For men

Have you noticed any change in intensity of your ejaculation, orgasm, or ability to attain or maintain an erection?
Have you ever had an orgasm without ejaculation?
Has your level of enjoyment with sexual relations altered as a result of these changes?
Have you had any problems with urethral discharge or urination?

For women

Have you experienced any vaginal soreness or irritation after sexual intercourse? How long does it last? Any problems with urgency or with burning in urination after intercourse? Have you experienced abdominal contractions or back pain after intercourse?
Have you any problems with vaginal discharge or itching?
Have any of these problems interfered with your sexual pleasure?
Have you or your partner experienced any changes in your health status recently? How have these changes affected your sexual relationship?

From Burke MM, Walsh MB: *Gerontologic nursing: wholistic care of the older adult*, ed 2, St Louis, 1997, Mosby.

Human Needs and Wellness Diagnoses

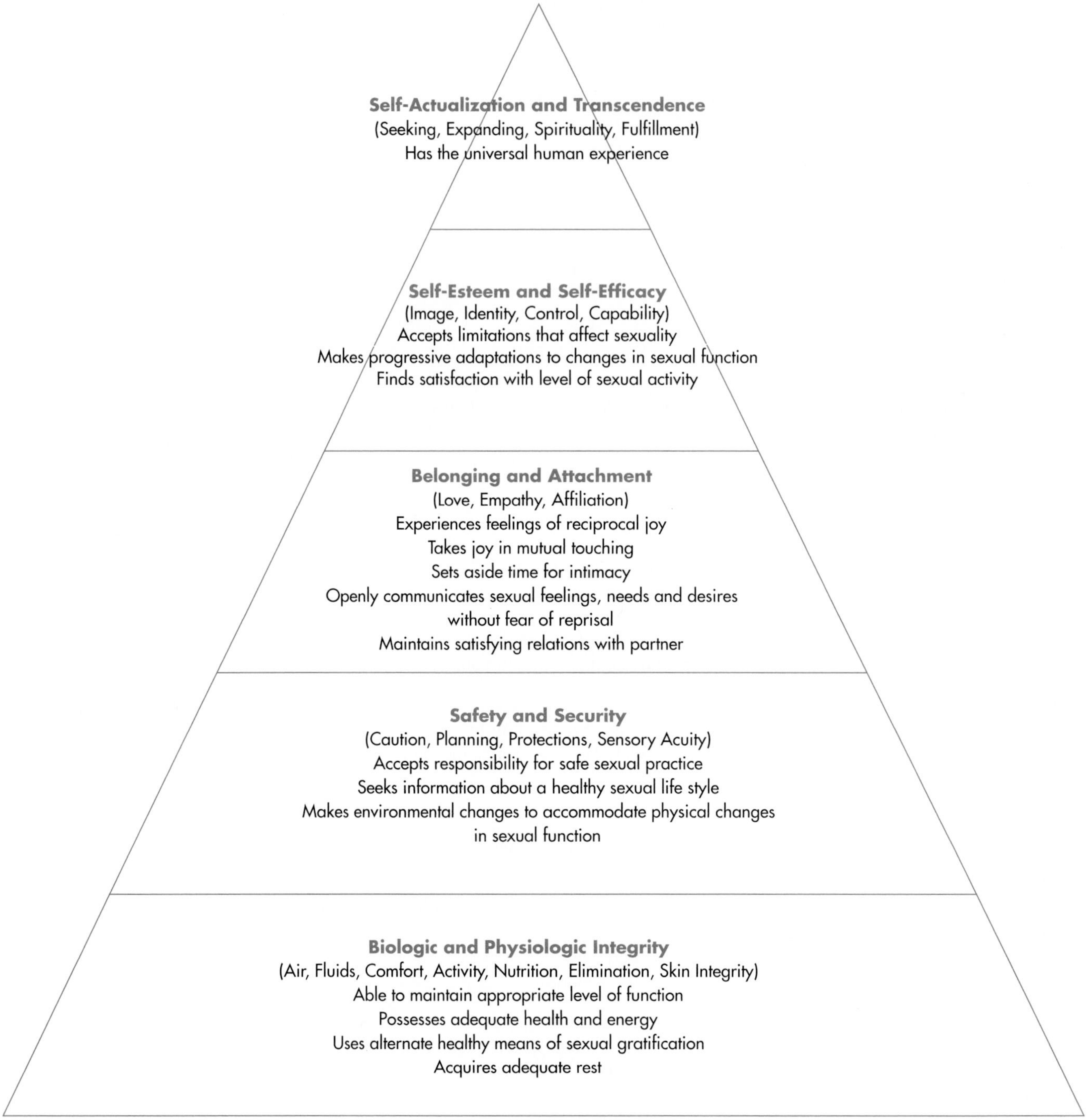

Self-Actualization and Transcendence
(Seeking, Expanding, Spirituality, Fulfillment)
Has the universal human experience

Self-Esteem and Self-Efficacy
(Image, Identity, Control, Capability)
Accepts limitations that affect sexuality
Makes progressive adaptations to changes in sexual function
Finds satisfaction with level of sexual activity

Belonging and Attachment
(Love, Empathy, Affiliation)
Experiences feelings of reciprocal joy
Takes joy in mutual touching
Sets aside time for intimacy
Openly communicates sexual feelings, needs and desires without fear of reprisal
Maintains satisfying relations with partner

Safety and Security
(Caution, Planning, Protections, Sensory Acuity)
Accepts responsibility for safe sexual practice
Seeks information about a healthy sexual life style
Makes environmental changes to accommodate physical changes in sexual function

Biologic and Physiologic Integrity
(Air, Fluids, Comfort, Activity, Nutrition, Elimination, Skin Integrity)
Able to maintain appropriate level of function
Possesses adequate health and energy
Uses alternate healthy means of sexual gratification
Acquires adequate rest

These are not all the possible wellness diagnoses that may be identified. The above are examples of nursing diagnoses that should be considered when planning care for the older adult.

KEY CONCEPTS

- Touch provides sensory stimulation, reduces anxiety, facilitates reality orientation, and provides pain relief, comfort, and sexual expression.
- The absence of touch, a powerful sense, threatens survival.
- Sexuality is love, sharing, trust, and warmth, as well as physical acts. Sexuality provides an individual with self-identity and affirmation of life.
- Sexual activity continues in old age, though adaptations are needed for the age-related changes of the male and female genital systems.
- Generally speaking, medications, ill health, and lack of a willing partner affect sexual activity.
- Older adults with alternative lifestyles, such as gay men, lesbians, bisexual, and transgender, are disenfranchised by govermental laws and rules that do not bestow the same economic, emotional, and physical security enjoyed by heterosexual couples.
- AIDS awareness and the practice of safe sex among older adults are still lacking. Health professionals, too, do not consider older adults at risk for AIDS, even though the incidence of AIDS in the older population is rapidly increasing. Finding appropriate services for the older adult with AIDS may prove difficult.
- The major role of the nurse in older adult sexuality in the community or long-term care settings is education and counseling about sexual function, adaptations for age-related changes, chronic conditions, and the maintenance of sexuality for the older adult's health and pleasure.

▲ CASE STUDY

George was a 70-year-old man who had been widowed for 6 years. He lived alone in a lovely home in the hills of San Francisco. His many friends tried to introduce him to a lady that would be attractive to him, but they were unaware of his real concerns. Although George was attracted to young, energetic women, often barely older than his daughters, he was justifiably cautious regarding their sincere attraction to him because he had a considerable estate. In addition, his sexual desire was waning, and his capacity for sexual performance was unpredictable. One thing George expressed fairly frequently was, "I don't like demands made on me." To further complicate the picture, George had begun to take finasteride to reduce his benign prostatic hypertrophy (BPH) that had become increasingly troublesome. The medication further reduced his sexual desire. In addition, George's sleep pattern was disturbed by the need to arise three or four times each night to void. George came to the clinic for follow-up evaluation of his BPH, and while talking with the nurse, he began crying uncontrollably, much to his embarrassment and the nurse's surprise because George had always seemed a rather stolid and stoic fellow, reluctant to discuss feelings.

Based on the case study, develop a nursing care plan using the following procedure*:

List comments of client that provide subjective data.

List information that provides objective data.

From these data, identify and state, using accepted format, two nursing diagnoses you determine are most significant to this client at this time. List two client strengths that you have identified from the data.

Determine and state outcome criteria for each diagnosis. These criteria must reflect some alleviation of the problem identified in the nursing diagnosis and must be stated in concrete and measurable terms.

Plan and state one or more interventions for each diagnosed problem. Provide specific documentation of sources used to determine appropriate intervention. Plan at least one intervention that incorporates the patient's existing strengths.

Evaluate success of intervention. Interventions must correlate directly with the stated outcome criteria so as to measure the outcome success.

STUDY QUESTIONS/ACTIVITIES

How would you begin discussing sexuality with George?

What are the factors that may be underlying George's sexual distress?

Discuss BPH and its prevalence and usual effects.

With a partner, role play and demonstrate your interpersonal interaction with George in this situation.

What resources or recommendations would you suggest for George?

RESEARCH QUESTIONS

What do women find are the most troubling changes in their sexuality as they grow older?

What do men find are the most troubling changes in their sexuality as they grow older?

What are the differences in sexual feelings and expression in the 60-year-old, the 70-year-old, the 80-year-old, and the 90-year-old individual?

What are the chronic disorders that most affect sexual performance of men and women, and how are they affected?

How many individuals over 60 have ever been given the opportunity to provide a thorough sexual history?

What community and health resources are available to meet the needs of older gay men and lesbians?

REFERENCES

Ackerman D: *A natural history of the senses,* New York, 1995, Vantage Books.

---

*Students are advised to refer to their nursing diagnosis text and identify possible or potential problems.

Adelman M: Stigma, gay lifestyles and adjustment to aging: a study of late-life gay men and lesbians, *J Homosex* 20:3, 1990.

Anderson CJ, Newton K: *Geriatric nursing,* St Louis, 1966, Mosby.

Baker B, Crowley S: AIDS crisis reaches those 50 plus, *AARP Bull* 35(2):5, 1994.

Barnes MM: Female genital disorders. In Beers MH, Berkow R, editors: *The Merck manual of geriatrics,* ed 3, Whitehouse Station, NJ, 2000, Merck Research Laboratories.

Barnett K: A survey of the current utilization of touch by health team personnel with hospitalized patient, *Int J Nurs Stud* 9:195, 1972a.

Barnett K: A theoretical construct of the concepts of touch as they relate to nursing, *Nurs Res* 21:102, 1972b.

Beers MH: Male hypogonadism and impotence. In Abrams WB, Beers MH, Berkow R, editors: *The Merck manual of geriatrics,* ed 2, Whitehouse Station, NJ, 1995, Merck Research Laboratories.

Benary-Isbert M: *The vintage years,* New York, 1968, Abingdon Press.

Beresford JM, Barrett CJ: The widow's sexual self: a review and new findings. Paper presented at the meeting of the Gerontological Society of America, Boston, November 22, 1982.

Berger R: *Gay and gray: the older homosexual man,* Binghamton, NY, 1995, Hawthorn Press.

Berlin H: Your doctor discusses: sexuality in mature/late life, *Planning for Health* 21:2, 1978.

Billhorn DR: Sexuality and the chronically ill older adult, *Geriatr Nurs* 15(2):106, 1994.

Boyarsky RE: Sexuality and the aged. In Steinberg FU, editor: *Cowdry's care of the geriatric patient,* ed 6, St Louis, 1983, Mosby.

Brier J, Rubenstein D: Sex for the elderly? Why not? *Perspect Aging* 2:7, 1977.

Buczny B: Impotence in older men: a newly recognized problem, *J Gerontol Nurs* 18(5):25, 1992.

Burke MA, Knowlton CN: Sexuality. In Burke MM, Walsh MB, editors: *Gerontological nursing,* St Louis, 1992, Mosby.

Butler R, Lewis M: Sexuality. In Abrams WB, Berkow R, editors: *Merck manual of geriatrics,* Rahway, NJ, 1990, Merck Sharpe and Dohme Research Laboratories.

Butler R, Lewis M: Sexuality. In Beers MH, Berkow R, editors: *The Merck manual of geriatrics,* ed 3, Whitehouse Station, NJ, 2000, Merck Research Laboratories.

Butler R, Lewis M: *The new love and sex after 60,* New York, 2002, Ballantine Books.

Butler R, Lewis M, Hoffman E, Whitehead ED: Love and sex after 60: how to evaluate and treat the impotent man, *Geriatrics* 49(10):27, 1994.

Colton H: *The gift of touch,* New York, 1983, Seaview/Putnam.

Cosgray R, Davidhizar R: *Touch among the elderly*. Report of unpublished research, Cincinnati, 1988, Jewish Hospital Third Annual Nursing Research Conference.

Deevey S: Older lesbian women: an invisible minority, *J Gerontol Nurs* 16(5):35, 1990.

DeNigola P, Peruzza M: Sex in the aged, *J Am Geriatr Soc* 22:380, 1974.

Denny NW, Quadango D: *Human sexuality,* St Louis, 1992, Mosby.

Diokno AC, Brown MB, Herzog AR: Sexual function in the elderly, *Arch Intern Med* 150:197, 1990.

Erikson E, Erikson JM, Kivnick HQ: *Vital involvement in old age: the experience of old age in our time,* New York, 1986, Norton.

Flaxman N: Personal conversation, June 13, 1996.

Fletcher JW: Sexually transmitted viral diseases in the elderly. In Cooper JW, editor: *Antivirals in the elderly,* New York, 1995, Pharmaceutical Products Press.

Fletes M: Human immunodeficiency virus infection. In Abrams WB, Beers MH, Berkow R, editors: *Merck manual of geriatrics,* ed 2, Whitehouse Station, NJ, 1995, Merck Research Laboratories.

Fordham F: *An introduction to Jung's psychology,* Baltimore, 1970, Penguin.

Freedman M: Diversity with a difference: gay and lesbian aging, *Aging Today* 16(5):7, 1995.

Gerchafsky M: Impotence: the problem men don't talk about, *Ad Nurse Pract* 3(3):13, 1995.

Goldblatt R: Factors influencing sexual behavior, *J Am Geriatr Soc* 20:49, Feb 1972.

Goodroad BK: HIV and AIDS in people older than 50, *J Gerontol Nurs* 29(4):18, 2003.

Hall ET: *The hidden dimensions,* Garden City, NY, 1969, Doubleday.

Ham RJ: Sexuality. In Ham RJ, Sloane PD, editors: *Primary care geriatrics,* ed 3, St Louis, 1997, Mosby.

Hite S: *The Hite report,* New York, 1977, Dell.

Hooyman N, Kiyak HA: *Social gerontology: a multidisciplinary perspective,* ed 4, Needham, MA, 1996, Allyn & Bacon.

Huss AJ: Touch with care or a caring touch, *Am J Occup Ther* 31:12, 1977.

Jacobi J: *The psychology of CJ Jung,* New Haven, CN, 1973, Yale University.

Jarvik L, Small G: *Parent care,* New York, 1988, Crown.

Jourard S: *The transparent self,* New York, 1964, Van Nostrand.

Kaiser FE: Sexual dysfunction in men; sexual dysfunction in women. In Beers MH, Berkow R, editors: *The Merck manual of geriatrics,* ed 3, Whitehouse Station, NJ, 2000, Merck Research Laboratories.

Kass MJ: Sexual expression of the elderly in nursing homes, *Gerontologist* 18:372, 1979.

Katzm L: Chronic illness and sexuality, *Am J Nurs* 9(1):56, 1991.

Kehoe M: Have you ever seen a lesbian over 60? *The Aging Connection* 4(4):4, 1988.

Kelly J: The aging male homosexual: myth and reality, *Gerontologist* 17:328, 1977.

Kelly J: Homosexuality and aging. In Marmor J, editor: *Homosexual behavior: a modern reappraisal,* New York, 1980, Basic Books.

Kolata G: Hormone replacement study abruptly halted, *San Francisco Chronicle*, July 9, 2002, reprinted from the New York Times.

Kreiger D: Therapeutic touch: the imprimatur of nursing, *Am J Nurs* 75:784, 1975.

Lewis MI: Sexuality. In Abrams WB, Beers MH, Berkow R, editors: *Merck manual of geriatrics*, ed 2, Whitehouse Station, NJ, 1995, Merck Research Laboratories.

Maddocks J: Sexual health and health care, *Postgrad Med* 58:52, 1975.

Miller CA: *Nursing care of older adults,* Glenview, IL, 1990, Scott Foresman/Little Brown Higher Education.

Miller J: The first language, *UCSF Magazine* 13(3):31, 1992.

Money J, Tucker P: *Sexual signatures: being a man or woman,* Boston, 1975, Little, Brown & Co.

Montagu A: *Touching: the human significance of the skin,* ed 2, New York, 1978, Harper & Row.

Montagu A: *Touching: the human significance of the skin,* ed 3, New York, 1986, Harper & Row.

Moon TD: Male genital disorders. In Beers MH, Berkow R, editors: *The Merck manual of geriatrics,* ed 3, Whitehouse Station, NJ, 2000, Merck Research Laboratories.

Nay R: Sexuality and the aged women in nursing homes, *Geriatr Nurs* 13(6):312, 1992.

Quam JK, Whitford GS: Adaptation and age related expectations of older gay and lesbian adults, *Gerontologis*t 32(3):367, 1992.

Raphael S, Robertson M: Lesbians and gay men in later life, *Generations* 6:16, 1980.

Robertson M: The older lesbian, master's thesis, Carson, CA, 1979, California State University, Dominguez Hills.

Sakauye KM, McDonald WM: The impact of caring touch on quality of life in a nursing home (abstract), Chicago. Proceedings of the Third Congress of the International Psychogeriatric Association 3:131, 1987.

Saxon SV, Etten MJ: *Physical changes and aging,* ed 3, New York, 1994, Tiresias Press.

Schiff I: Menopause and ovarian hormone therapy. In Abrams WB, Beers MH, Berleow R, editors: *Merck manual of geriatrics,* Whitehouse Station, NJ, 1995, Merck Research Laboratories.

Schuerman DA: Clinical concerns: AIDS in the elderly, J *Gerontol Nurs* 20(7):11, 1994.

Sherman D: Effects of medications on sexual function, *Contemp Long Term Care* 15(7):64, 1992.

Shippee-Rice R: Sexuality and aging. In Fogel C, Lavver D, editors: *Sexual health promotion,* Philadelphia, 1990, WB Saunders.

Slusher MP, Mayer CJ, Dunkle RE: Gay and Lesbians Older and Wiser (GLOW): a support group for older gay people, *Gerontologis*t 36(1):118, 1996.

Some older Americans not practicing safe sex, *UCSF Health Lett* 19(2):4, 1993.

Starr BD: Sexuality and aging. In Eisdorfer C, editor: *Annual review of gerontology and geriatrics,* vol 5, New York, 1985, Springer.

Stevenson RT, Courtenay BC: Old people, orgasms, and God: a replication determining the relationship between religiosity and attitudes of nurses' aides toward sexual expression among older adults in nursing homes (abstract), *Gerontologist* 22:261, 1982.

Thayer S: Social touching. In Schiff W, Foulke E, editors: *Tactile perception: a source book,* Cambridge, 1982, Cambridge University Press.

Torassa U: Chronicle Medical Writer, UCSF study says hormone therapy not for heart patients, *San Francisco Chronicle*, July 3, 2002, Health section, p. A4.

Walz T, Blum N: *Sexual health in later life,* Lexington, MA, 1987, DC Heath Co.

Whipple B, Scura KW: The overlooked epidemic: HIV in older adults, *Am J Nurs* 96(2):23, 1996.

White C: Sexual interest, attitudes, knowledge, and sexual history in relation to sexual behavior in the institutionalized aged, *Arch Sex Behav* 11:11, 1982.

Wiley D, Bortz II WM: Sexuality and aging: usual and successful, *J Gerontol: Med Sci* 51a(3):M142, 1996.

Woods NF: *Human sexuality in health and illness,* ed 3, St Louis, 1983, Mosby.

Woods NF: Sexuality and aging. In Reinhardt AN, Quinn MD, editors: *Current practice in gerontological nursing,* vol 1, St Louis, 1979, Mosby.

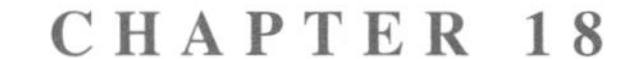

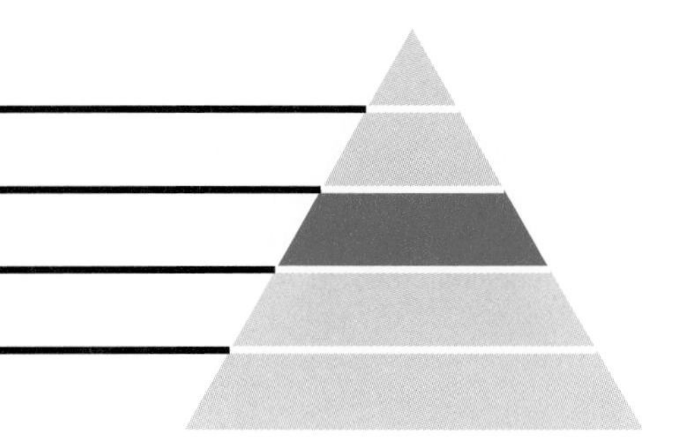

CHAPTER 18

Relationships, Roles, and Transitions

Priscilla Ebersole

A youth speaks

I'm really worried about retirement! That is ridiculous at my age, but I keep reading and hearing about Social Security and Medicare running out of money for the baby boom generation. Those are my parents! What about me?

Joseph, age 30

An elder speaks

I thought when my children left home that my most important job was done. But they came home again and again, and then my mother-in-law came to live with us. Finally, the kids were really on their own and married, so now I take care of the grandchildren while they both work to make ends meet. I just pray daily that my husband will remain healthy. I don't think I could deal with one more thing.

Esther, age 64

LEARNING OBJECTIVES

On completion of this chapter, the reader will be able to:

1. Identify several important roles that elder members of society usually fulfill.
2. Discuss changes in family structure and functions that are occurring.
3. Describe the various functions of grandparents.
4. Enumerate several caregiver concerns and current societal supports.
5. Relate some of the factors that must be considered in the decision to retire.
6. Explain the issues in adapting to a major role change such as retirement or widowhood.
7. Discuss the development of a volunteer role in late life.

This chapter examines the various relationships, roles, and transitions that are characteristic in later life. Important relationships include that of spouse, partner, parent, grandparent, great grandparent, sibling, and friend. The role functions of these relationships shift as societal norms and economics change. Biomedical technology, political agendas, social expectations, and worldwide economic fluctuations are continually changing the face of aging. Even more changes are expected among singles, families, and retirees in the next 10 years as the first wave of "baby boomers" enters young-old age. The population from 45 to 54 years of age has increased by 4.3% since 1999 (U.S. Administration on Aging, 2000). The major concerns of this group are adequate health care coverage, the preservation of social security, and caregiving demands (American Association of Retired Persons [AARP] Public Policy Institute, 2002a, 2002b). This major change in the aging landscape is only one of many massive social changes that have altered the patterns of work, family, and kinship structures in recent decades. In this chapter, we are chiefly concerned with the impact of these numerous changes on the quality of life and range of possibilities for elders in their most important affiliations. Individuals live longer, families are smaller, more women work, and caregiving becomes an expectable concern. Thus social change and individual need continue to change the nature of the life course and affiliative inclinations.

Role transitions likely to occur in later life include working to retirement and volunteering, grandparenthood, widowhood, divorce, and becoming a caregiver and service recipient. These transitions may occur predictably or by unanticipated events. Retirement is an example of a predictable event that can, and should, be planned for long in advance. Divorce, widowhood, and widowerhood may occur unexpectedly and create emotional chaos in the transitional phase. Transitions that are signaled by experiences of family and friends or anticipatory events alert a person to the impending shift and sometimes define the passage through ritualized activities. Most difficult are the transitions that incorporate losses rather than gains in status, influence, and opportunity. The move from independence to dependency and becoming a care recipient is particularly difficult. Conditions that influence the outcome of transitions include personal meanings, expectations, level of knowledge, preplanning, and emotional and physical reserves. The ideal outcome is when gains in satisfaction and new roles offset losses.

RELATIONSHIPS

The classic study of Lowenthal and Haven (1968) has been studied and elaborated many times since its inception. The importance of caring relationships as a buffer against "age-linked social losses" is demonstrated in the study. Maintaining a stable intimate relationship was more closely associated with good mental health and high morale than it was a high level of activity or elevated role status. Individuals seem able to manage stresses if some relationships are close and sustaining. Increasingly evident is that a caring person may be a significant survival resource. Social bonding increases health status through as yet undetermined physiologic pathways, though studies in psychoneuroimmunology are giving us clues (see Chapter 22).

This segment of the chapter will familiarize the reader with relationships as experienced in old age within generations and between generations. A network of kin, friends, and acquaintances can sustain the older adult and give life meaning. We might use the analogy of a tree that withstands storms and drought through an extensive root system, which provides stability and nourishment that may be helpful; such is old age. The ground around the tree must be tended to keep it thriving. We may find ourselves best caring for the aged by caring for those who are important to the aged.

Primary relationships are intimate associations that provide a strong sense of sharing and belonging; these are the deep roots of our tree analogy. Relationships that are more formal, impersonal, superficial, and circumstantial are often time limited, sometimes intense but with a tendency to dissipate. These relationships are the surface network of roots that extend outward in many directions and are sustained by their profusion but wither with neglect or insignificance. Thus the primary network may need professional strengthening to bear the increasing demands.

Friendships

Friendships are individually defined because they manifest certain degrees of intimacy not generally available and are often marked by the length of an enduring relationship. Friendships are very special because they are selected rather than obligatory. Bleiszner (2001) found that 88% of individuals between 65 and 85 years of age maintain contact with friends and neighbors, and these contacts, in many cases, were as meaningful as those with family. Trust, demonstrations of caring, and mutual problem solving were important aspects of the friendships. Bleiszner (2001) suggests that "because of the high value placed on shared activities, frequent contact, and good communication, professionals should be sure to provide settings where elders can interact with others who have similar interests and can talk privately about what is important to them" (p. 51). Because close friendships have such influence on the sense of well being of elders, anything done to sustain them will be helpful. Nurses may include in their assessment questions about older individuals' friendships and their importance and availability.

Mentoring Relationships

Professionals and, in some other situations, older adults may develop intense reciprocal relationships with younger adults, and vice versa. These relationships often have an intimacy that is similar to that of parent and offspring (Fingerman, 2001). In the case of the elder, a relationship may fill a need for offspring that were never produced. In some cases, these relationships may be more satisfactory because the inherent generational expectations are attenuated by the absence of obligation. Elder retired academics often become involved with young, neophyte students and professionals, the elder benefiting from fresh ideas and the younger from the wisdom of the elder. When the relationship is not one of mentoring, it may be a replacement of the idealized parent or grandparent that is no longer or was never available. "Catherine was the great grandmother I never knew." "Rose was a model of gracious aging." "Mary Opal was a mentor and a surrogate mother."

FAMILIES

Family evokes strong impressions of whatever an individual believes the typical family should be. Because everyone comes from a family, these impressions have powerful symbolic meanings. However, family structures are rapidly changing and diverging from these idealized notions. Approximately 42% of today's families are married couples without children. Single-parent families, blended families, childless families, and fewer families altogether are common. Four- and five-generation families are also becoming common (Kutza, 2001). The U.S. Census (2001) defines a family as "a householder and one or more people living in the same household who are related to the householder by birth, marriage or adoption"

(p. 6). This very restricted definition of family is used for purposes of census tabulation.

Family members form the nucleus of relationships for the majority of the old and the back-up system when they become dependent. Most older adults possess a large intergenerational web of significant people, including sons, daughters, stepchildren, in-laws, nieces, nephews, grandchildren, and great grandchildren, as well as partners and former partners of their offspring. All of these people may play an important part in maintaining later life satisfactions. A concern is that the changes in family structure, frequent marital dissolution, and alternative lifestyles with no clear line of responsibility from adults to elders may result in baby boomers having few if any individuals willing to take on the caretaking responsibilities when they become old (Kutza, 2001).

Blended Families and the Elderly

Jane: "Last Thanksgiving we felt the full impact of blended families: our young family of four children had in 40 years grown to the point that with every manipulation we could construct, we could barely accommodate the 24 people who sat down to give thanks. These included the parents of both daughters-in-law, the stepchildren of both sons and daughters, as well as their mutual children, the daughter of one of the stepdaughters, and one ex-son-in-law, as well as our own sons and daughters." It is doubtful that this situation is unusual for an elderly matriarch.

In later life, extended family may be composed of several sets of in-laws, children-in-laws, and stepchildren, as well as direct descendants. The love and loyalty a person feels toward parents of ex-mates may be strong. Shared aspects of grandparenting the children in the family and vital relationships have often developed regardless of the divorces and remarriages of offspring.

Couple Relationships

The most significant and binding relationship is usually that of the couple. However, the chance of a couple going through old age together is exceedingly slim. Approximately 40% of men and 80% of women over age 75 have no spouse (U.S. Administration on Aging, 2000). Men who survive their spouse into old age ordinarily have multiple opportunities to remarry if they wish. A woman is less likely to have an opportunity for remarriage in late life.

Couple relationships are becoming more diverse, involving varying degrees of habit, culture, intimacy, shared backgrounds, and instrumental and emotional support. In late marriages or remarriage, developing an intimate, sharing relationship between individuals who have had 75 or 80 years of separate experiences, often bringing conflicting ideologies into the new relationship, is an enormous challenge.

Couples in late life have needs, tasks, and expectations that differ from those in their earlier postparental years. Some couples have been married over 60 years. People married 50 years or more may describe a happy marriage as related to congruence of perception. This view does not necessarily mean that couples agree, but rather that they know what to expect from each other. However, people who stay together for one half century or more may not have been happy doing so.

Many of the following issues may put a severe strain on couples in the last phase of life:

- Deteriorating health of one partner
- Unequal efficacy in task accomplishment
- Economics
- Previous marriages
- Relationships with children
- Incongruent sexual needs
- Mismatching of personal needs for activity or disengagement
- Inability to support each other through crises
- Negative attitudes about aging

Nurses may learn a great deal, in addition to assisting couples in defining the value of the relationship, by discussing with the couple the strengths in their relationship, as well as the difficulties. Couples may seldom have tried to articulate these difficulties or their thoughts about spousal caregiving clearly.

Lesbians, Gays, Bisexual and Transgender Couples. There are many nontraditional ways of viewing family, although these views are less common among the old than the young. Nevertheless, we are increasingly aware of the varied family styles of the aged and those that have developed among lesbians, gays, bisexual, and transgender (LGBT) couples. Although the issue of same-gender couples marrying is before the courts, it is not legal in most states to do so. However, many of these people enter into marriage contracts and are legally registered as domestic partners. The extent to which older people are involved in such relationships is unknown. Much more knowledge of cohort and generational differences between age groups is needed to understand the recent, dramatic changes in the lives of lesbians and gays in family lifestyles. Cahill and South (2002) contend that the limited research that exists on the topic indicates that the decades of discrimination have led to a "crisis competence" in these individuals, which tends to make aging issues actually less traumatic for them.

Lesbian women and gay men in long-term committed relationships often share homes, resources, and professional interests. In cases in which the relationship was not clearly defined, the grief surrounding the loss of the partner becomes difficult because the loss may be unrecognized by others and pass without ritual or social sanctions. This type of grief has been defined as "disenfranchised grief," which can be particularly difficult to resolve (Doka, 2002).

Issues that are currently of concern to society and the LGBT that need further investigation are the impact of homophobia on late life health, retirement and leisure issues, and the hidden incidence of abuse and neglect (Claes, Moore, 2000).

In terms of elderly parents and relationships with adult gay offspring, Allen and Wilcox (1996) found that coming to terms with the disclosure of the adult child involved several transitions. These issues were denial, acceptance, complacency, and in the majority of cases, the move toward political activism and advocacy for the civil rights of gays, as well as other groups suffering discrimination. These elders became stimulated to work for social change.

Parental Relationship

The relationship with parents in which an understanding human exchange can occur is the hallmark of maturation of both parties and the high-water mark of the parent-child relationship. In adulthood, relationships between the generations become increasingly important for most people. Older parents enjoy being told about the various activities and successes of their offspring, and these adult children begin to see aspects of themselves that are and have developed from their parents. At times, the relationships may become strained because the younger adults are more concerned with their own spouses, partners, and children. The parents are no longer central to their lives, though offspring may be central to the lives of their parents (Fingerman, 2001). The most difficult situations occur when the elder parents are openly critical or judgmental about the lives of their offspring. In the best of situations, adult children shift to the role of friend, companion, and confidant to the elder.

Some of the most important and often problematic relationships in late life are those between mother and daughters. Sons seem more likely to idolize mothers. History and position in the family must be considered. Issues of maternal expectations and degree of control during youth will emerge later to be resolved again and again. These issues are ever in flux, as in many other long and intense relationships. The major dimensions in all such intimate role relationships are the way in which differing expectations were resolved and communication patterns. The major difference in the female generations is the increasingly open opportunities to daughters that were closed to the mothers.

Studies of the special experience of older mothers of adult children often focus on the adults as they relate to their mothers needs. However, from personal experience, I can speculate that many older mothers are the keepers of secrets. Adult children and often grandchildren have some aspects of their lives they have shared only with the trusted mother or grandmother who can be trusted to never divulge their secrets. Mothers are the listeners to the fears, events, and anxieties that cannot comfortably be told to anyone else. We know that although this relationship is not the privilege of all mothers, it is a treasured aspect of the mothering role, perhaps more treasured as the person ages and knows that these secrets will quietly be carried with them as they leave this existence.

Studies of the fathering relationship of adult children have been neglected. Anecdotally, some people find praise or time alone with the father during youth to have lasting impact on later self-esteem and performance (Waldren, 1995; Lindgren, 2001).

The father's secrets may involve the negotiations and manipulations that he had found that were necessary to "launch" his children in the best way possible. One example that we can consider would be that of Joseph Kennedy. Traditionally, the father has assisted the sons or daughters, most particularly the sons, into the world in which they may best achieve success, often following in the father's shadow. As a man ages, he will likely see the adult child surpassing him in accomplishment. Fathers with a generous nature are able to revel in the increasing capabilities of the following generation without exacting obeisance from them. These ideas are speculative, but they might be fruitful areas for research.

Grandparenting

About 72% of elders over age 65 have three or more grandchildren. About 13% of adults over age 65 have no grandchildren (National Council on the Aging [NCOA], 2002). We tend to read and hear most about the ever-increasing number of grandparents that are assuming primary parental roles and responsibilities. We do know that, for many, parenting is a great joy but has delayed their own plans for travel and retirement. Moreover, for elders who are ill, parenting can be an exhausting burden. However, grandparenting involves so much more. As the term implies, the "grands" are a step beyond parents in their concerns, exposure, and responsibility. The age, vitality, and proximity of both grandchild and grandparent produce a kaleidoscope of possible activities and interactions as *both* progress through their aging processes. Historically, the emphasis has been on the progressive aging of the grandparent as it affects the affinity, but little is said about the effects of the growth and maturation of the grandchild as these affect the relationship. The most that can be said with assurance is that these relationships must be addressed individually.

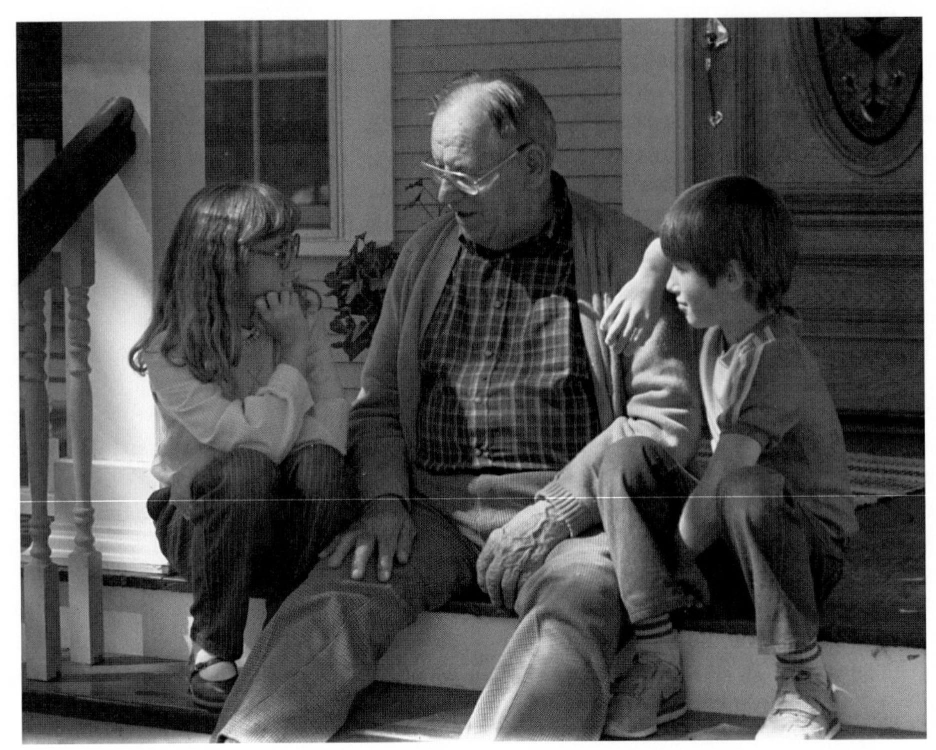

A grandparent listens. (Courtesy Rod Schmall.)

- What are the satisfactions the grandparent experiences?
- What are the problems they encounter in grandparenting?
- What in their biopsychosocial and geographic situation impedes their desired interactions with the grandchild?
- To what ages of the grandchildren have they felt most attuned?
- What special times or interactions have given them the most pleasure?

Similarly, both the grandchild and the grandparent must be addressed to understand what this dyadic relationship means to each (Box 18-1).

Example: Although grandchildren are most affectionate and involved with grandparents from ages 3 until 13, with many stages and activities in between, the relationship matures as the grandchild does and becomes more affiliative and appreciative. With a grandparent, the adolescent can be both childish and playful or discuss adult issues but does not need to swing wildly between dependence and independence as they do with parents. As adolescents approach adulthood and become absorbed with their own lives, the grandparental relationship is less intense or involved, other than with those that are primary caregivers in the child's daily life. Young adults are often given economic assistance as their material needs grow and those of the grandparents diminish. In addition, mileposts of achievement are particularly important to recognize. "My older grandchildren are as proud of me and my accomplishments as I am of theirs."

The most meaningful time has been taking a planned vacation to someplace of the grandchild's choice on the child's

Box 18-1 Grandparenting

Don't give advice about child rearing.
Rules of behavior should relate only to your own home.
Give the child undivided attention during projects, games, and reading.
Be a link with the past; tell grandchildren about their parents and about you when you were a child.
Support the parents in their decisions; never undermine.
Create memories and traditions.
Offer the gift of your time: nature walks, baking cookies, and so on.

Long-Distance Grandparenting

Brief and frequent cards and letters are useful; send clippings, cartoons, and riddles; use colorful stickers and stamps.
Audiotapes and videotapes that you produce are appreciated; storytelling, reading, or singing.
Celebrate special days and firsts (lost tooth, day of school, mastery of a new situation).
Telephone frequently.
Visit as often as you can.

From Good grandparenting, *Mayo Clinic Health Letter* 11(1):6, 1993.

ninth birthday; just one grandchild and I having exclusive time together. I have been fortunate enough to be able both energetically and economically to do this with each of the eight grandchildren. A latecomer, 12 years younger than the others, has been an unexpected great joy.

An Internet site (seniors-site.com/grandparenting) provides an excellent set of guidelines for grandparents:

- Rule-making is not a grandparent's task.
- Grandchildren need your attention and interest in their activities.
- Grandchildren need to hear of their parents' childhood and youth.
- Celebrating special times creates memories and continues traditions.
- Grandchildren need help exploring their world while they are young.
- Offering assistance without interference is recommended.

Sex and lineage are greatly influential in the meaning of grandparenthood (Somary and Stricker, 1998). Chan and Elder (2000) note a great matrilineal advantage in grandparenting relationships. The majority of grandchildren "perceive their grandparents as having active and influential roles in their lives" (Roberto and Skoglund, 1996, p. 107).

Great Grandparenting

Great grandparenthood has been rarely studied, although 40% to 50% of older people in the United States will live long enough to become great grandparents (U.S. Administration on Aging, 2000). Stereotypically, great grandparents have been consigned to a rocking chair and shawl. Today, for a man or woman of 65 years of age, still young and vital, being a great grandparent is not unusual; there are also numerous great-great grandparents.

In most cases, the great grandparental role is modeled after the role as grandparent. The middle generation's attitudes and involvement with their parents and grandparents largely determine the quality of the relationship. For most people, the intensity of the relationship is diminished compared with that of grandparenting. Many identified the great grandchildren only as the children of their grandchild. These great grandparents sent obligatory gifts and wanted to be loved and respected, but few had as close relationships as they did with their grandchildren. Great grandchildren seemed to validate the vitality and success of the family, and the great grandparents enjoyed tracing the patterns of inheritance and personality traits (Wentowski, 1985).

Wentowski (1985) suggests that a study of age-matched grandparents and great grandparents might better sort out the difference in grandparenting and great grandparenting. The author explored the perceptions that great grandparents have of their kinship role and found three significant trends: (1) It is not perceived as a primary kinship role but linked only in the generational context. (2) It is important emotionally, but there is little involvement in the daily lives of great-grandchildren. (3) A diluted sense of obligation exists toward the great grandchildren. Doka and Mertz (1988) found three main aspects of the great grandparenting role: diversion, renewal, and appreciation of longevity. Most studies have focused on young great grandchildren. Not surprisingly, little is known about adult great grandchildren because this requires super-survival. Roberto and Skoglund (1996) found that although the adult grandchildren reported "respect" for the great grandparent, they held no specific role in their lives.

In advanced age, the family role may be supplanted by a symbolic social role as representatives of living history. In some cases, a great grandparent outlives the grandparent and may assume some aspects of a grandparental role. Nurses may explore the meaning of being a great grandparent with these clients, who rarely have role models appropriate to current times and may be defining their function in a unique manner. Age, physical health, living arrangements, and family relationships surely influence the status and roles of great grandparents, but these factors are poorly studied. As more and more older adults become great grandparents, we will doubtlessly learn more about the significance of the role. An area ripe for investigation is that of the increasing number of grandparents who have virtually raised a grandchild and then see the progeny of that child more as a grandchild than they do a great grandchild.

Siblings

As individuals age, they often have more contact with siblings than they did in the years when family and work demands were more pressing. Widowed, divorced, and never-married siblings may share a home and travel together. These relationships became increasingly important because they have a long history of memories and are of the same generation, similar backgrounds, and often ambivalent early relationships (Bedford, Avioli, 2001). The strongest of sibling bonds is thought to be the relationship between sisters. When blessed with survival, these relationships remain important into late old age (Scott, 1996). In some remarkable cases, such as the Delaney sisters, the two personalities complement each other and function well together in coping with the demands of independent living at great old age. Bessie, age 101, was feisty and abrupt, whereas Sadie (age 103) proceeded to do what was needed with quiet determination (Delaney, Delaney, 1993). Of course, much has to do with age differences, place in the family, and personality. Service providers should inquire about sibling relationships of past and present significance.

I remember the days when I detested Buddy, especially in our adolescence, but he is the only one still alive who has been a part of my entire life. Now, when we reflect on our divergent paths it is with a mixture of pleasure and poignancy. When our parents, other siblings and mates died we held each other together. Others call him Joe, but he will always be my Buddy.

Other Kin

Interaction with collateral kin (cousins, aunts, uncles, nieces, and nephews) generally depends on proximity, preference, and the general availability of primary kin. Maternal kin are often emotionally closer than those in one's paternal line. These relatives may provide a reservoir of kin from which to find replacements for missing or lost intimate relationships for singles or childless people as they grow older. These elders often seem to be attached to a favorite niece or nephew on whom they rely to maintain some family connection and, in some ways, serve as a surrogate for the child they never had.

Marge had been scrimping to remain in the deluxe life-care community where she had resided for 20 years. Inflation and taxes caught up with her investment returns. She often did not have her evening meal to reduce her expenses but passed it off by saying, "I can do without those calories." Marge had no children, but her favorite nephew kept in touch. When he called to request money for his graduate school tuition, Marge felt guilty that she couldn't provide it. Her nephew was 40 years old. This is not an aberrant situation. We have heard many similar stories. The transfer of assets and funds to the younger generations is a frequent economic trend in families of today and seems to have especially important psychologic value for elders without direct heirs. It is one way in which some elders seek to establish their place in the kin network and generational flow.

Surrogate Family Forms: Fictive Kin. For many older people without families, an effort might be made by the individual or service providers to develop a cadre of fictive kin. Fictive kin are nonblood kin who serve as "genuine fake families," as expressed by Virginia Satir. These nonrelatives become surrogate family and take on some of the instrumental and affectional attributes of family. Some elders who are alone adopt television families and speak of them as if they were related. Primary care providers or case managers often become fictive kin. Professionals must be aware of the tendency for elders to develop close ties of affection and dependency with fictive kin and must be sure to keep the boundaries that are necessary in each of these situations.

CAREGIVING ROLES

The face of caregiving has changed and may include family, friends, and paid and unpaid workers, as well as volunteers in the home. Some middle-aged adults may also be involved in caring for the elderly parents of previous mates. Even though generally considered a women's issue, in more and more cases, male caregivers are providing various kinds of care from the most intimate to the most instrumental (Houde, 2001). These men are less often the primary caregivers. Caregivers are considered by professionals to be "the hidden patient" (Schulz and Beach, 1999, p. 2216). These caregivers frequently experience depression and physical and emotional exhaustion (Yates et al, 1999). The common problems that create difficulties include race and ethnicity, advanced age of the caregiver, high-intensity caregiving needs, insufficient resources, and dementia of the care recipient (Navaie-Waliser et al, 2002). Not all caregivers experience consequential stress. Factors that seem to make the experience most physically and emotionally difficult are:

- Excessive demands from the care recipient (Zarit and Zarit, 1998)
- Competing role responsibilities
- Caregiver values and beliefs (Noonan and Tennestedt, 1997)
- Quality of previous relationship between caregiver and care recipient (Whitlack and Noelker, 1996).

In this segment of the chapter, caregiving will be considered in some depth because it is one of the most crucial phenomenon of current times (Box 18-2).

Family Caregiving

It has been a cliché: "If she took care of her seven children, why cannot they among them take care of her?" In reality, the family members are heavily involved in the care of their elders and frequently neglect their own needs in deference to the care of other family members. Recently, the U.S. Administration on Aging (AOA) in conjunction with the National

Box 18-2 Family Support System Assessment

Size	Number in extended family that are accessible
	Number of daughters that are accessible
	Number of sons that are accessible
	Number of grandchildren, nephews, nieces, confidants, siblings
Ability	Economic status of each
	Poverty
	Lower middle
	Middle
	Upper middle
	Wealthy
Willingness	Frequency of involvement
	Monthly
	Weekly
	Daily
	Constant
Functions	Contributions to aged member
	Money
	Chores
	Transportation
	Listening and psychologic support
	Functional assistance
Deterrents	Other demands
	Work
	Travel
	Adolescent children
Recent stresses	Poor health
	Job change
	Moves
	Deaths

The strengths of the family or possible dysfunctional aspects can be assessed in a superficial but helpful manner by using the Family APGAR (Smilkstein et al., 1982).

Family Givers Support Projects has given serious attention to the needs of these families. The AOA has developed the *Resource Guide and Survival Tips.* Sources are available on the Internet at www.aoa.gov/carenetwork/nfcsp-resource-guide.html and www.aoadhhs.govcarenetwirj/survival.pdf (Family Caregiver Alliance, National Center on Caregiving, 2002). Literally hundreds of studies have been conducted involving the caregiving role of midlife people with parents, parents-in-law, and sometimes grandparents, as well as children and grandchildren. Shirley Chater (personal communication, 1998), a previous director of the Social Security Administration, dubbed this the "double whopper."

Caring for Parents

The role of elders with adult children is most often studied as a caregiving issue. Adult children are sometimes said to reverse roles with parents when the parents become old and dependent. This scenario has a demeaning connotation, as if the elder becomes a child again. In illness and deterioration of the elder, the adult child may at times feel parental, but the inner child always remains in need of the protective and guiding parent. No matter how mature a person becomes, the parent symbolizes security and acceptance, regardless of the reality or facts. These dynamics often make the caregiving role very complex and difficult.

Filial obligation toward the parents is different than filial affection and seems to be somewhat related to proximity. The sense of obligation toward mothers tends to override role conflicts and even attenuated affections. Daughters involved in other roles seemed to feel less obligation toward fathers and in-laws, and the sense of obligation is somewhat related to affectional ties. The dynamics of filial obligation in this study were related to sex, proximity, education, income, culture, and multiplicity of role demands (Welsh and Stewart, 1995). These factors need considerably more study before an understanding can occur involving the complexity of issues that affect feelings about the significance and variables in close and superficial caregiving relationships. Fingerman (2001) reminds us that the parent's reaction to the offspring's caregiving has not been well investigated. In a small study in Ireland, McCann and Evans (2002) found that most of these people who were receiving extensive assistance with basic activities of daily living were satisfied with the care received but thought that their caregivers showed signs of anger and frustration. The major concerns of the care recipients involved what would happen if the caregiver were not available, worries about the cost of care, and the fact that the caregiver's health was suffering (Box 18-3).

Grandparents Raising Grandchildren

Grandparenting requires a revival of remnants of a previous role and may or may not involve any personal developmental changes or significant life pattern shifts. Some grandparents confront major situational transitions and role adaptations as they take on the function of parents. In cases in which grandparents, and most especially a single grandparent, take on the

Box 18-3 Planning to Add an Aged Member to the Household

Questions you need to ask:

- What are the needs of the new member and of the family?
- Where will space be allotted for the new member?
- How will this new member be included in existing family patterns?
- How will responsibilities be shared?
- What resources in the community will assist in the adjustment phase?
- Is the environment safe for this new member?
- How will family life change with the added member, and how does the family feel about it?
- What are the differences in socialization and sleeping patterns?
- What are the aged person's strong needs and expectations?
- What are the aged person's skills and talents?

Modifications you need to make:

- Arrange semiprivate living quarters if possible.
- Regularly schedule visits to other relatives to give each family times of respite and privacy.
- Arrange day-care and senior activities for the older person to help keep contact with members of his or her own generation.

Discuss potential areas of conflict:

- *Space:* especially if someone has given up his or her space to the aged relative.
- *Possessions:* old person may want to move possessions into house; others may not find them attractive or may insist on replacing them with new things.
- *Entertaining:* times when old and young feel the need or desire to exclude the other from social events.
- *Responsibilities and chores:* old may feel useless if they do nothing and in the way if they do something; young may feel that their position is usurped or may be angry if they wait on parent.
- *Expenses:* increased cost of home maintenance, food, clothing, and recreation may not be shared appropriately.
- *Vacations:* whether to go together or alone, the young may feel uneasy not taking older person out and resentful if they must.
- *Child rearing:* disagreement over child rearing policies.
- *Child care:* grandparental babysitting may be welcomed by family and resented by older person or if not allowed, older person feels lack of trust in capability (McGreehan and Warburton, 1978).

Decrease areas of conflict by:

- Respecting privacy.
- Discussing space allocations.
- Discussing elderly person's furnishings before move.
- Making it clear ahead of time when social events include everyone or exclude someone.
- Clearing decisions about household tasks—-all should have responsibility geared to ability.
- Paying a share of expenses and maintaining a separate phone reduces strain and increases feelings of independence.

full parenting role out of a sense of obligation, duty, or guilt, these transitions and adaptations are especially difficult. Some grandparents believe, correctly or incorrectly, that their deficiencies in parenting are the cause of their adult children's inability to parent. In these cases, grandparenting is not only a transition requiring reorganization of lifestyle, relationships, and patterns of behavior, but also one in which therapeutic support groups can be of enormous value. The wide range of involvement with grandchildren must be examined individually to determine the effects of the role.

Certain lifestyle factors of a child's parents that have greatly increased the need for grandparents to act as primary caregivers include substance abuse, child abuse and abandonment, mental illness, parental death, parental incarceration, teen pregnancy, unemployment, and poverty. As would be expected, although many of these children are deeply disturbed and need mental health services, the grandparents will also need family counseling (Brown-Standridge and Floyd, 2000). Ghuman and colleagues (1999) found that 51 youths among a group of 233 youths being treated at a community mental health center were living with grandparents.

Grandparents who provide 30 hours per week are *extensive* caregivers but not considered *primary* caregivers. Custodial grandparents are those that have primary responsibility for raising a grandchild for 6 months or more (Fuller-Thomson and Minkler, 2001). Estimates suggest that grandparents or other relatives are raising over 2 million children with no parents present. This number has increased by more than 50% since 1990. Approximately one third of these children are within the formal foster care system. Another 2.5 million children are living with grandparents or other relatives, but one or both parents resided with them. Twenty percent of these grandparents were over 65 years of age, and 50% of the children were under 6 years of age (Troope, 2000). Although this situation cuts across all socioeconomic and ethnic strata, these families are more likely to live in poverty and have inadequate health and insurance coverage. Temporary Assistance to Needy Families (TANF) can be helpful to grandparent-headed households (Mullen and Einhorn, 2000). These programs vary tremendously from one state to another and can be awarded as "child only" benefits, regardless of the income and assets of the grandparent. However, frequently, these services offer only short-term assistance benefits rather than long-term aid. Many complexities may be found in the administration of these funds. People interested in such programs should contact their state social services department.

Grandparents also frequently experience problems with legal issues, housing, and within the educational system. Nonetheless, Roe and Minkler (1999) note that in terms of health and school adjustment, children raised solely by grandparents fared better than those in single-parent families. Generations United *(www.gu.org)* is committed to address the legislative, administrative, and community policies that are needed to improve the lives of children and adults in these special caregiving situations (2000).

Although grandparents raising grandchildren is not a new phenomenon, in many ways, it may be harder now, largely because of three reasons: (1) Most young-old women are in the workforce outside the home. (2) Current "welfare reform" sends many single mothers out of the home to work. (3) and Parental divorce complicates the visitation and caregiving expectations. Children of divorce present particular problems for grandparents. Some are cut off from contact with a loved child and must seek legal visitation rights. Although national laws allow grandparents to seek visitation rights, the decision is up to the particular court and judge hearing the appeal. The most difficult cases tend to emerge when a son or daughter has divorced and the children are in custody of the daughter-in-law or son-in-law who then remarries (Hushbeck, 2002). When grandparents are not given the right to see the grandchildren, these children must be helped to recognize and express their grief (Drew and Smith, 1999). A comprehensive book by Hayslip and Goldberg-Glen (2002) provides extensive information regarding the custodial care of grandchildren, including cultural variations and clinical, legal, and service-related policies involved in surrogate parenting. Supportive interventions presently in place include numerous formal and informal groups that provide education, resource guides, help with homework, and nutrition and local experts who discuss legalities and financial concerns. Many Internet resources and chat rooms are also available.

Speculations about the effects and frequency of grandmothers raising grandchildren in culturally diverse families are numerous. A recent study of the preferences for custodial care or co-parenting of grandchildren revealed some differences that may reflect cultural expectations. The study of 1000 grandmothers in Los Angeles, conducted by Goodman and Silverstein (2002), showed differences in the experiences and well being of white, Latino, and African American grandmothers. African Americans were satisfied with co-parenting or total custodial care, Latinos preferred the co-parenting situation, and whites expressed no difference. Although myths and clichés abound, little is actually known about cultural variations because much depends on immigration patterns, socioeconomic situation, and availability of family members.

A study of Asian immigrant women and their ability to find community resources to help with caregiving showed that if family and friends were already established, connections were easily made, although community outreach programs are not routinely extending information to these people in any systematized manner (Neufeld, 2002). Many grandmothers emigrate from the Pacific Rim countries to the United States for the specific purpose of caring for grandchildren while the parents are getting established.

Spousal Caregiving

The most demanding and hazardous of caregiving roles are those of one aged spouse to another when the care recipient suffers dementia. Because of the intensity and constancy of demands, caregivers of people with dementia have given up most other aspects of their lives and even contact with other family members (Ory et al, 2000). In many ways, this type of care becomes similar to caring for an 18-month-old child that needs constant protection and assistance. The greatest tragedy is that the elderly demented person is not learning, growing, and exploring and often reaches the point at which the caregiver is not even recognized. The caregiving spouse finds this situation extremely stressful because long established patterns of intimacy are no longer possible, and evidence of appreciation are not seen. One man said, "Caring for my wife is difficult now because she no longer recognizes me as her husband. I have become a stranger to her and she treats me as such. Because I am no longer viewed as her husband, she will not let me touch her or share the same bed. And, I have been told more than once to 'get out of the house because it's not your home'" (American Society on Aging, 2002, p. 6). In such cases, the nurse must talk about the grief for the lost partner.

Role Reversal in Spousal Caregiving

A rather domineering husband was head of the household, made decisions, and managed the money. A sudden stroke left him unable to walk without assistance. Memory and speech were also affected. The husband became increasingly dependent on his wife, who was overwhelmed with trying to be the "stronger" of the two. She was physically healthy but was unable to see well. She became profoundly depressed and found that her husband needed more care than she was able to provide. She agreed to nursing home placement two or three times but was very critical of nursing home care and took him home prematurely, without adequate supportive services.

Assuming an unfamiliar role is difficult for both parties. The nurse should be alert to situations in which health care personnel may be able to provide supports and resources that make it possible for an individual to assume new responsibilities without being totally overwhelmed. When a spouse is ill and the mate needs to take over functions for both, someone must be available to give reinforcement, encouragement, and relief. A day-care program, routine visits from a community health nurse, or periodic assistance from a home health aide or a housekeeper may make it possible for the couple to continue to live together. One important consideration is counseling the couple to maintain as much independent function as possible for both people.

Long-Distance Caregiving

Long-distance caregiving is increasing in importance as families find their elders either unable or unwilling to be moved to a place convenient for the family. In addition, the downsizing of many industries has forced working families to transfer to places remote from older family members. Numerous independent providers are available to mobilize resources in the area in which the elder lives. Although these services may be expensive, they are far less expensive than alternative living arrangements or institutional placement. The most likely source of assistance can be found by checking the telephone book's list of community services in the place in which the elder resides. It is usually wise for a family member to make a visit to the elder to assess the total situation because the elder may not admit to increasing dependency and may be reluctant to discuss particular problems. A personal encounter with any care planners is essential to evaluate their competence.

Role of Nonfamily Caregivers

Close relationships often develop between older adults and their nonfamily caregivers. Over 50% of family caregivers use nurses, homemakers, and other personal care providers to assist in the care of their elder dependents (Piercy, 2001). These providers may include friends and hired or volunteer caregivers from a church or agency. Piercy found that only 40% of the care recipients actually had living relatives. The caregivers not only provide substantial physical care, but they are also often involved with the elder, when possible, in social activities such as dining, concerts, and church events. Conditions that foster closeness include continuity of caregiver, social isolation of the elder, homogeneity of the client-caregiver, and the caregiver performing extra tasks and small personal attentions. The client will sometimes describe a paid caregiver as "my family." Piercy says, "Practitioners who work with older adults need to acknowledge and support the efforts of friends, neighbors and other nonkin who assist dependent older adults" (p. 43). A caveat should be added that is explained in Chapter 16. Dependent and lonely elders with assets may be victimized by apparently doting caregivers who may exert undue influence.

Role of Nursing Professionals in Providing Support for Caregivers

Nurses are often the primary care providers and case managers for elders and their family caregivers in the home and community. The nurse monitors progress and manages chronic disorders of the elder while continually remaining aware that the total family configuration is the client. A comprehensive assessment of the family system must be conducted, and professional and lay resources must be made available to the family as needed. Ideally, a team of professionals, including the nurse, social worker, mental health counselor, and occupational therapist, should make the initial comprehensive assessment. This assessment should include the Caregiver Strain Index developed by Robinson (1983; Sullivan, 2002). This source is available through the John A. Hartford Foundation Institute for Geriatric Nursing, which has blanket permission to use professionally (2002) (Figure 18-1).

The elder's and family's well being depends on the ability and motivation of the family to obtain and provide direct care and supportive services. Thus the nurse's role is to teach, monitor, and strengthen the family system so as to maintain health and wellness of the entire family structure. The New

I am going to read a list of things that other people have found to be difficult. Would you tell me if any of these apply to you? (Give examples.)

	Yes = 1	No = 0
Sleep is disturbed (e.g., because is in and out of bed; wanders around at night)		
It is inconvenient (e.g., because helping takes so much time; it's a long drive over to help)		
It is a physical strain (e.g., because of lifting in and out of a chair; effort or concentration is required)		
It is confining (e.g., helping restricts free time; cannot go visiting)		
There have been family adjustments (e.g., because helping has disrupted routine; there has been no privacy)		
There have been changes in personal plans (e.g., had to turn down a job; could not go on vacation)		
There have been other demands on my time (e.g., from other family members)		
There have been emotional adjustments (e.g., because of severe arguments)		
Some behavior is upsetting (e.g., because of incontinence; has trouble remembering things; accuses people of taking things)		
It is upsetting to find has changed so much from his/her former self (e.g., he/she is a different person than he/she used to be)		
There have been work adjustments (e.g., because of having to take time off)		
It is a financial strain		
Feeling completely overwhelmed (e.g., because of worry about __________; concerns abourt how to manage)		
TOTAL SCORE (Count yes responses. Any positive answer may indicate a need for intervention in that area. A score of 7 or higher indicates a high level of stress.)		

Figure 18-1. Caregiver strain index. (From Robinson B: Validation of a Caregiver Strain Index, *J Gerontol* 38:344, 1983. Copyright: The Gerontological Society of America.)

York University (NYU) Spouse Caregiver Intervention Study reported by Mittleman (2002) found the most useful of the interventions studied included a few sessions of counseling to the caregiver and other involved family members and a support group for primary caregivers, as well as ongoing telephone support. These interventions, when available, can alleviate much of the stress of caregiving (Box 18-4 and Table 18-1).

The overlapping activities of the various professionals must be organized in a way that is not overwhelming to the caregivers. Coordinating the resource allotment, monitoring functional status, and providing for health needs of the family unit are important activities of the registered nurses and advanced practice nurses working with caregivers. These nurses also assess and supervise the effectiveness of any lay workers and family members that may be needed in the home to sustain the elder. A major expectation of nurses is that they will teach, demonstrate, and evaluate the ability of caregivers to provide necessary interventions with the elder in their care. Given the "sicker-quicker" status of hospital stays, initial evaluation of the families caregiving abilities must begin immediately and continue through recovery and rehabilitation (Figure 18-2).

To reduce caregiver stress, nurses are advised to use all means and resources at their disposal to:

- Restore a sense of control and effectiveness in the situation.

Table 18-1 Positive Outcomes Reported by the Clients and Caregivers

Outcomes	Caregivers' comments	Clients' comments
Social enjoyment	—	It was an outing. An excuse to go out and talk to people!
Increased knowledge	I am more aware now. I know what things to look for.	I enjoyed the assessment. I learned from it.
Reduced stress	The support was very good. There was tremendous amount of guilt going on. . . . Assessment helped us to deal with these things.	I was reassured that this was part of an illness. I had an explanation why this was happening.
Enhanced skills and feelings of competence	It proved very useful for our learning process in terms of her management (referring to client) and my own coping.	I learned how to cope better with my disability. I'm more positive as a result of it.
Better family communication and collaboration	They helped with communication with family. Our children now better understand how to support me.	—
Improved decision-making	I don't know what we would have done without the geriatric services . . . It helped us to make decisions.	—
Greater access to services	Everything came out of that assessment: The diagnosis, home services, day program.	—
Positive health outcomes	If it wasn't for the assessment she wouldn't be here today. She may have died in her apartment.	—

From Aminzadeh F et al: Comprehensive geriatric assessment: exploring clients' and caregivers' perceptions of the assessment process and outcomes, *J Gerontol Nurs* 28(6):9, 2002.

Box 18-4 Goals of Family Support Groups

Learn to accept the elder as he or she is now; let go of the past.
Learn the balance between protectiveness and smothering.
Recognize one's own needs as fundamental to caring for others.
Learn to share and cope with disappointment.
Discuss resurgence of feelings of loss during holidays and anniversaries.
Share knowledge of how to deal with family and community.
Develop a caring and sharing network within the group.
Deal with feelings of guilt, helplessness, and hopelessness.
Identify realistic ways to assist in the care of the elder.

Modified from Richards M: Family support groups, *Generations* 10(4):68, Summer 1986.

- Reinforce any social supports that are available to the caregiver.
- Find opportunities for group participation with other caregivers.
- Advise routine times of respite and assist caregiver in finding respite sources.

The rewards for some people in caregiving depend most on the extent to which the following are present in the relationship (Cohen, Colantonio, and Vernich, 2002):

- Companionship
- A sense of fulfillment
- Feeling of meeting an obligation
- Ability to provide a quality life
- Increased knowledge about self and aging
- Improvement in relationship with the care recipient
- Increased sense of self-worth
- Sufficient financial resources
- Feelings of capability

These items provide guidelines for health care providers' discussion with caregivers and, when appropriate, with care recipients. The stresses, expectations of future needs and problems, and the positive aspects of the caregiving situation should be explored. Schmall, Cleland, and Sturdevant (2000) suggest the following:

- Tailor programs and services to the unique situation of caregiver and care recipient.
- Urge the caregiver to take care of self.
- Encourage caregiver to maintain activities important to his or her well being.
- Allow the caregiver to express negative and angry feelings toward the care recipient.
- Encourage the caregiver's efforts to use all available resources and assistance.

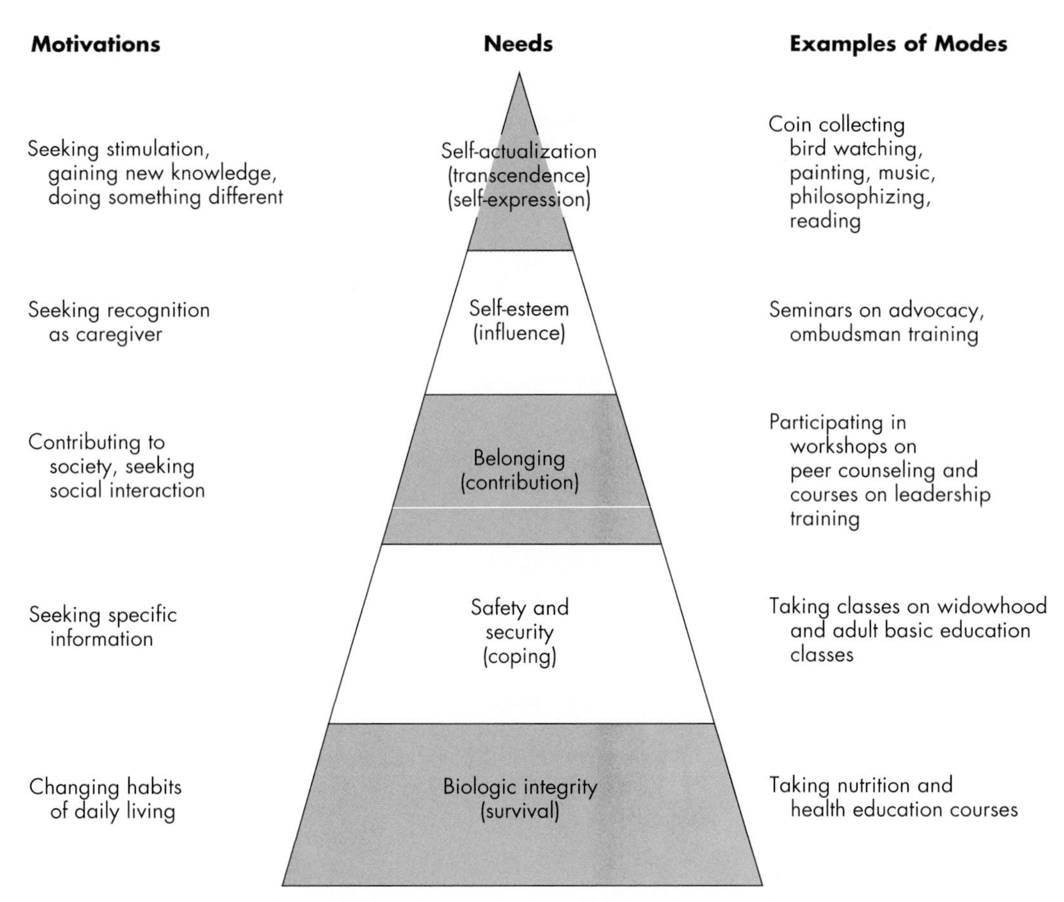

Figure 18-2. Family support problems and interventions.

- Include all directly involved parties in decisions about care.
- Praise whatever is being done well and encourage letting go of things that have not gone well.

TRANSITIONS

Transitions require letting go of certain habits and structures and developing new ones. Some feeling of loss and bewilderment is nearly always present, and anticipation of new roles and opportunities often occur. In aging, many of the transitions incorporate more losses than gains in lifestyle. Friends and family experiencing similar events may make the transition somewhat easier. A rehearsal of an anticipated event may often take place in the setting in which it is likely to occur. This rehearsal may be planned or subliminal, as when an elderly lady accompanies her friend to the funeral parlor to make funeral arrangements. Although probably not consciously identifying the possibility in her own life, she is nevertheless preparing in advance and vicariously experiencing the event. Transitions that make use of past skills and adaptations are less stressful than those that are entirely unfamiliar. Some shifts, such as from functional independence to functional dependence, cut across many aspects of life and require major changes in lifestyle.

In cases of role accumulation, such as that of grandparent or caregiver, some previous life experiences will be useful. The shifts in family and filial relationships are often gradual and do not require abrupt role deletion or role reversal. Some shifts, however, are abrupt and undesired.

Although cohort effects and appropriate role models are critically important in how one develops in a new role, increasingly, rapid changes in sociopolitical climates have made historic roles incongruent with the times. The few role models displayed in the media are often inappropriate to an individual. The ease of major role transitions will depend on the following factors:

- Relevance of proposed models
- Supportive milieu
- Presence of sustained roles not affected by particular role transition
- Age appropriateness of change
- Geographic and cultural milieu
- Personality and motivation in regard to constancy or change

The potential for developing new, fulfilling life patterns is ever present and is enhanced during periods of role transition. Influential dimensions promoting growth rather than stagnation during transitions are anticipatory planning, awareness of problems, positive or negative attitudes, and a sense of control (by far the most important).

Gender Considerations in Role Transitions

Cohort and gender differences are inherent in all of life's major transitions. Many of the present generation of very old women likely retained much of their homemaking role throughout their adult years. Therefore work, caregiving, and grandparental roles may not have varied significantly. However, most women of the young-old group have had work roles outside the home and may find the transitional periods require more adaptation.

Men may have major role disruptions and sometimes experience severe loss of status with the departure from the work role, which tends to be a major transition in their lives that requires important shifts in life patterns. Some years ago, Antonovsky and Sagy (1990) identified four central tasks of men in the transition to retirement: (1) active planning, (2) reevaluation of sources of satisfaction, (3) reexamining one's worldview, and (4) attending to health maintenance. These tasks must be evaluated again as many women are highly involved in careers and may find retirement a wrenching departure. In terms of adapting to divorce or loss of spouse, men are far more likely than old women to find another mate and return to similar relationship patterns.

RETIREMENT

Retirement is no longer just a few years of rest from the rigors of work before death. Retirement is a developmental stage that may occupy 30, even 40 years of a person's life and may involve many stages. The transitions are blurring because numerous pursuits and opportunities may occur after one has "retired." Tafford (2002) is addressing this relatively new segment of adult life. She examines the unprecedented aging in the life cycle and contends that people know as little about it as they did about adolescence at the turn of the century (Age Beat on Line, 2002). Undoubtedly, the numerous patterns and styles of retiring have produced more varied experiences in retirement.

Nursing concern must focus on the group of retirees who did not expect retirement at the time when they left the workforce. These individuals are likely to suffer detrimental effects and be in need of counseling and assistance through the transition. These individuals are also likely to experience job separation as a crisis and have a traumatic role transition triggered by an unplanned job termination resulting from illness or company *downsizing,* a euphemistic term for cutting out jobs (Box 18-5).

Labor Force Participation

Just as Social Security was initially seen as a mechanism for resolving unemployment, early retirement is a means of regulating the labor supply. Employers encourage early retirement of older, more expensive workers by offering attractive incentives. Early retirement programs may be so attractive that individuals retire earlier than they had planned or expected and without sufficient preparatory time.

Box 18-5 Issues in Retirement Potential

1. Financial need versus resources
2. Employability
3. Rewards derived from employment
   - Wages sufficient for needs and morale
   - Satisfaction level, possibility for resolution of job frustrations
   - Meaning of job, contact with friends, source of prestige
4. Psychosocial characteristics—-attitudes toward retirement
   - Attitudes of significant others (advising? directing?)
   - Strength of work ethic
   - Effect of retirement on prestige
5. Personality factors
   - Time orientation (past, present, future)
   - Active versus passive in planning
   - Rationalism versus fatalism as life stance
   - Type-A versus type-B personality (hard-driving, easy-going)
   - Inner directed versus other directed (enjoyment of self or need for high level of external motivation)
6. Level of information about retirement
   - Planning programs on job, adult education, or community programs
   - Awareness of friends and family who have retired and how influenced by them
7. Pressures to retire
   - Compulsory, age discriminatory
   - Unemployment (how long?)
   - Job retrogression (being moved down the ladder)
   - Skill obsolescence (opportunities for developing other skills?)
   - Peer pressure (organized or informal)
   - Employer pressure (reduced incentives to continue work, increased incentives to retire)
   - Family pressure (spouse's working status)
   - Health, discomfort, or disability interfering with job performance and dependability

Clearly, the goals of government and industry are in conflict related to the older work force. Government cannot afford a large body of nonworking individuals, and industry cannot afford to keep these individuals in top salaried positions. With recent events that have seriously threatened pension security and portability, more workers are remaining in the workforce. "The long term trend toward ever-earlier retirement has halted" (Ekerdt and Dennis, 2002, p. 1). The work scene continually changes and becomes more complex as government policies, technology, and world economics continually destroy jobs and create new ones. The balance between downsizing and creating new jobs is quite askew in some regions and industries (Figures 18-3 and 18-4).

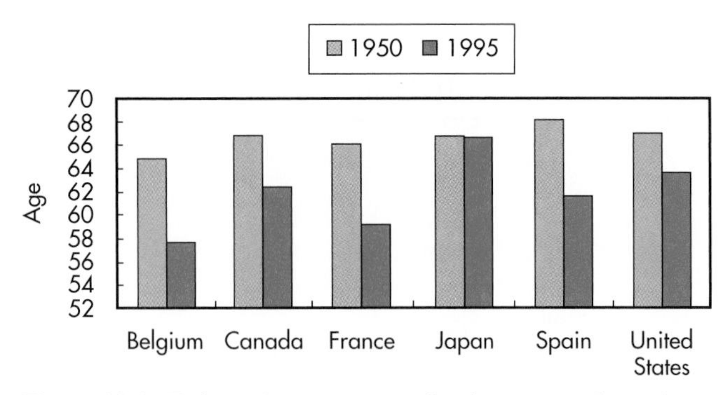

Figure 18-3. Estimated average age of retirement: male workers, selected countries, 1950 and 1995. (Source: Organization for Economic Cooperation and Development, 1998.)

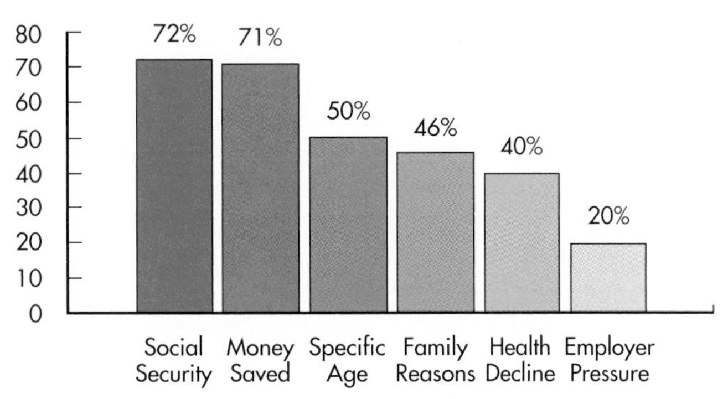

Figure 18-4. Reasons for retiring. (From National Council on the Aging [NCOA]: *American perceptions of aging in the 21st century,* Washington, DC, 2002, www.ncoa.org.)

Retirement and the Work Role Transition

Decisions to retire are often based on attitude toward work, chronologic age, health, and self-perceptions of ability to adjust to retirement (Taylor and Shore, 1995). Retirement intentions are variable and include four types of "retirement": to retire from work, to change jobs, to partially retire, or to work for self (Ekerdt et al, 1996). When a person speaks of retirement or analyzes research, knowing exactly what the individual means by retirement is important because of the many issues that must be considered (Box 18-5).

Part-time work during retirement is viewed by the working public of all ages as a desirable option. Temporary work agencies are now actively recruiting older workers who may wish to keep up their skills and decide when and where they want to work. Employers seek these older workers because they are often more reliable and dependable. Seniors over age 65 can now earn up to any amount without endangering Social Security benefits. Older adults who wish to go into business for themselves have a few advantages over younger people, such as more financial independence, established credit, knowledge, and a wide circle of contacts. "Bridge jobs" that provide part-time work in the move toward self-employment or nonemployment have proved to ease the retirement transition (Quinn and Kozy, 1996).

These alternatives seem to be the wave of the future with increasing numbers of agencies, institutions, and corporations offering retirement incentive programs to workers with extensive seniority. These programs frequently involve gradual reductions in work. Retirement must be examined from several angles: a "post-career" job, exit from long-term job and return again, partial retirement, *ad hoc* arrangements with long-term employers to meet changing work needs and capacities, retire to self-employment, and numerous variations. Retirement patterns are becoming more complex, and many individuals of retirement age are now working out of their home office with numerous electronic supports. Corporations and older workers find this situation ideal. The concern is often around the continuation of benefits, which, at this point, may constitute 35% to 40% of the total employee compensation (O'Brien, 2002).

Some researchers are now focusing on the differences between "crisp" and "blurred" transitions from the labor force (Mutchler et al, 1997). Individuals in partial retirement are thought of as blurred, and those with abrupt stoppage of work life, crisp. The crisp transition is unidirectional and complete, whereas blurred transitions are characterized by repeated exits, entrances, and unemployment spells. These transitions are likely related to economic status. The crisp retirement occurs when a long-term employee leaves the work world completely.

Blue collar–white collar–pink collar differentiations are inadequate to explain the meaning of any work role. Academics, nutritionists, rocket scientists, and auto mechanics may be equally bored or stimulated by their work. One man very succinctly stated the heart of the issue of work: "An orthopedic surgeon and a carpenter are basically doing many of the same things but using different materials." An artist or a plodder can do either job. The results and the level of satisfaction will differ. Work must be examined from a life and personality perspective rather than simply by job identification, though some jobs inherently carry more status and thus may be harder to give up. The person's identity is sometimes greatly defined by the company or institution of one's life commitment. Is retirement more difficult for an individual who has been with one company for most of his or her adult life? These situations are becoming increasingly rare as people move up and out in companies, just as they do in home ownership.

Retirement Planning

Retirement planning is advisable during middle age and essential in late middle age. However, people differ in their focus on the past, present, and future, as well as their realistic ability to "put away something" for future needs. Retirement preparation programs are usually aimed at employees with high levels of education and occupational status, those with private pension coverage, and government employees. Thus the people most in need of planning assistance may be least likely to have any available or the resources for an adequate retirement. Individuals who are retiring in poor health or are disadvantaged and in lower socioeconomic levels need specialized counseling. These groups are neglected in retirement planning programs. Dennis (2002), president of the International Society of Retirement planners, said, "There is a tremendous need to reach low-income individuals regarding these matters."

Retirement decisions are based on a large number of personal questions, including:

1. What do I want to do?
2. Who needs me, and what are my best opportunities?
3. What am I best able to do?
4. What is the meaning of my life?
5. What should my life accomplish or contribute?
6. Am I financially independent for the rest of my life if I live 30 more years?
7. What is the condition of my health?
8. Do I enjoy spending a great deal of time with my spouse?
9. Can I afford to completely retire from paid work?

Retirement education plans are supplied through group lectures, individual counseling, booklets, videocassettes, and computerized modules. However, at this juncture, and in light of the many hazards recently experienced by preretirees, planning is often insufficient. Dennis (2002) notes that many individuals currently have very high expectations for the final third of their lives. Although federal laws encourage increased participation in company-sponsored 401(k) plans, these plans are proving to be shaky in many instances. When considering retirement, Dennis notes the following areas that are essential to consider: How adequate are (1) company-provided retirement benefits, (2) Social Security and Medicare benefits, (3) company-provided postretirement health care, and (4) financial planning. Thoughtful financial planning must include distribution options and tax consequences (LaRock, 2001). The adequacy of retirement income is dependent not only on work history, but also on marital history. The poverty rates of divorced older women are excessively high. Couples that have had previous marriages and divorces have significantly lower available economic resources than those in first marriages. Child support, divorce settlements, and pension apportionment to ex-spouses may have diminished retirement income. This problem is an ever-increasing impediment to retirement because, among couples presently approaching retirement age, less than one half are in a first marriage (U.S. Divorce Statistics, 2002). Policies have been based on the traditional lifelong marriage, and this is no longer appropriate.

Dennis (2002) notes that retirement planning is really life planning and that the process is best accomplished when, early on, individuals determine their goals, values, and motivations in life. This assessment requires personal reflection and thought about the choices in everyday life that provide satisfaction and that the individual will wish to continue in later life (Shagrin, 2002). Retirement planning has become a highly specialized professional field. For people who can afford it, engaging a retirement planner in early adulthood is wise. Nurses need to be familiar with these sources of information and discuss the need for retirement planning with their clients (see Resources).

Couples and Retirement Planning. Husbands' retirement plans tend to be made around pension wealth, health, and the characteristics of the work environment, whereas wives appear to be more concerned about husband's health than their own when formulating retirement expectations (Pienta and Hayward, 2002). Increasingly, however, professional women are retiring much after their husbands, particularly if the husband is older and has benefits from several retirement systems.

A pattern that has been common to the retirement decision is that of the wife adapting to the husband's needs. Older women are now becoming more assertive about their own retirement plans because many more women are engaged in professions and positions of status than they were in previous decades.

Atchley's seminal studies (1979) identified variables affecting couple adjustment to retirement: (1) effectiveness of communication; (2) decision-making patterns relating to money, space, and use of time; (3) role orientation (traditional or shared); and (4) level of affection and intimacy. These variables are likely not new issues but only those previously submerged by the obligations of work and family. Released from these demands, the problems already within the relationship fulminate.

Gender Considerations in Retirement Planning. Inadequate coverage for women in retirement is frequent because their work histories have been spasmodic and diverse. Women are often called on to retire earlier than anticipated because of family needs. A recent study from Cornell University, reported by Family Caregiver Alliance, National Center on Caregiving (2002), found that late midlife women are five times more likely to retire early to care for an ill or disabled husband than those who are not caregivers. The study also found that male caregivers who are caring for their wives retire earlier than those who are caring for a person other than a spouse.

Whereas most men have always worked outside the home, it has been only within the last 30 years that this has been the expectation of women. Therefore large cohort differences exist.

Traditionally, the variability of women's work histories, interrupted careers, the residuals of sexist pension polices, Social Security inequities, and low-paying jobs created hazards for adequacy of income in retirement. The scene is gradually changing in many respects, but the gender bias remains. Basing retirement calculations on gender and projected survival statistics is now illegal, though until the early 1980s, women were allotted less pension income based purely on their expected longevity in comparison to men. Although this is no longer true, women who retired 20 or 25 years ago remain penalized because of gender.

Older women are very likely to have several years of no earnings calculated in the averages that determine the amount of their Social Security benefits. Some women find that they will receive more if their Social Security benefits are calculated on their husband's earnings; this may be true even though widowed or divorced. The Social Security Administration must be contacted regarding these issues because many variables may be used.

The complexity of the issues includes differences between retirement patterns of single and married women and men. Single and married women differ in the degree of dependency on their own benefits and in work history. Pension coverage and health are useful predictors of retirement for men but not as much so for women. For single women, recent income is an important factor in the decision to retire. For women and men, the most significant factors in adaptation to retirement are health, income, and social involvement.

Retirement Planning for LGBT Couples. Barriers to equal treatment in retirement for LGBT couples include job discrimination, unequal treatment under Social Security, pension plans, and 401(k) plans (Cahill and South, 2002). LGBT couples are not eligible for Social Security survivor benefits, and unmarried partners cannot claim pension plan rights after the death of the pension plan participant. These policies definitely put LGBT elders at a disadvantage in retirement planning.

Early Retirement

Early retirement may be a consequence of job dissatisfaction or boredom, unemployment, weeding out top wage and salary personnel, making room for advancement of younger personnel, moving operations to a foreign country, outmoded skills, cost-effectiveness factors, poor health, or personal choice. Although some people of late middle age choose to retire from the labor market, many are being forced out by unemployment. Regional, occupational, and personal variables account for unemployment in late middle age. Many people in early retirement made the decision because of some of the factors cited previously. For many people, job reshuffling and subtle, or not-so-subtle, pressures have forced them out.

The Regional Coordinating Council for Older Workers (RCC) has been established in all nine federal regions to develop older worker programs. One of these agencies, Operation ABLE (in several regions), offers seminars to assist the older professional in a job search. Other similar programs include Second Careers, Forty Plus, Experience Unlimited Job Club, The Los Angeles Council on Careers for Older Americans, and AARP Works.

Career transition programs have appeared in several universities across the United States. Senior Corp of Retired Executives (SCORE) has proved to be a dynamic organization using the talents of retired individuals. Many groups and communities have established job banks to match employers and older workers.

Despite legislation, many subtle pressures, such as the high unemployment rate among youth, may force individuals to retire when they wish to continue working. Many corporations would rather employ two young workers at much lower rates of pay than retain the experienced older worker who commands a high salary.

Before taking a complaint to a lawyer, the following questions should be asked: Are you in the right age group? Were you doing your job to the satisfaction of management? Were you dismissed without cause? Were you replaced by someone younger? An older worker who believes his or her employer is discriminating on the basis of age should contact the nearest Equal Employment Opportunity Commission office.

Problems in adjustment to retirement usually are short lived and focus on impingement on time or unrealistic expectations of the spouse. However, when either spouse is impaired, negative consequences can result for both partners. People who have saved and planned for retirement activities and then find their companion unable to participate are particularly unhappy.

Nurse's Role in Assisting in Retirement Preparation

1. What are the chief work-related satisfactions, and what might compensate for the loss of those?
2. Are friendship networks tied to the job?
3. How do spouse and family enter into the decision-making process?
4. Is there an opportunity to test partial work status or nonworking status before actual retirement?
5. Has sufficient information been available regarding retirement planning?
6. Is the work situation more stressful than it is satisfying?
7. How much of self is defined by job status?
8. Is competitive activity an important source of satisfaction?

Successful retirement adjustment depends on socialization needs, energy levels, health, variety of interests, amount of self-esteem derived from work, presence of intimate relationships, and general adaptability.

1. Talk to clients over 50 years of age about any retirement plans they may have.
2. Make clients aware that the transition to retirement is experienced as a crisis with manifestations of grief in many people.
3. Work with couples whenever retirement may be a possible stressor in their relationship.
4. Institute nursing research regarding the effects of retirement.

The inequities inherent in various work roles compound over time, and thus cumulative progress or cumulative disadvantages result in major differences in retirement compensation and comfort. To our dismay, the service industries that employ caregiving professionals are among the least likely to provide health care and adequate retirement for their employees (Hirshorn et al, 1996). The increasing number of nurses working in long-term care at various levels and at numerous sites must band together and give retirement planning a high priority for themselves. The American Nurses' Association and other nursing organizations must expand their efforts beyond the "hospital" nurse. We as members must institute action. Nurses need to think of and plan for their own retirement needs. Just as we often say, "Physician, heal thyself," we would admonish, "Nurse, take care of thyself."

Satisfaction in Retirement

The most powerful factors in retirement satisfaction are health status, sufficient income, and the option to continue working. Adequate income is often tied to the ability to continue some type of remunerative activity. Health conditions are the least subject to control by the retiree and apparently the most critical to perceived quality of life (Dorfman, 2002).

Preretirement programs are often helpful in terms of ultimate satisfaction in postretirement, but few programs actually have any plan for follow-up assessment. Nurses can consider postretirement assessment as significant as the preretirement planning. Postretirement counseling may be needed. Anticipating psychologic reactions to such a major event is difficult. Support groups for retirees might be particularly beneficial in the first year following retirement.

In the best of situations, retirement offers couples, both of whom have been working, an opportunity for more relaxed interactions and pursuit of mutual interests that may have been neglected while fulfilling obligations. Although household division of labor tends to remain much the same, satisfaction in the roles is increased when time pressure is decreased (Dorfman, 2002). Increasingly, the timing of retirement is not synchronous. A pattern of men retiring earlier than their wives is emerging because women may have entered the work force later and are just reaching their potential when the husband is ready to retire. Dorfman also points out that in the best situations, with more time and resources, retirees have the opportunity to develop special relationships with their grandchildren (Box 18-6).

Gender and Life Satisfaction in Retirement. Levels of preretirement commitment to the job, satisfaction with the spouse, and intrinsic self-esteem continue to influence postretirement self-esteem (Reitzes et al, 1996). Overall, positive preretirement expectations are apparently the greatest predictor of satisfaction in retirement, regardless of race, gender, or ethnicity (Honig, 1996).

Opportunities for New Development

Retirement is often thought of as a time to develop secondary interests and challenges. Our present elders are perhaps the only ones who have, in large numbers, the health, the vitality, education, affluence, and the opportunity to make retirement the most creatively productive and gratifying stage of life. Retirement can be the time when the individual is free to pursue a lifelong avid interest. Sara worked in a chemistry lab until retirement . . . then she began teaching creative writing and published her first book at age 80 (Ruffner, 1991). After spending much of his life as a prison officer, Joe built a trimaran and, with arduous study, became a certified celestial navigator through the U.S. Power Squadron. At age 63, Joe and his eager wife were ready to sail the seven seas (Pierre, 1992). Now, at age 67, Joe and his wife have settled into a comfortable routine with their Web pages, which occupy much of their waking time. The Bennetts left the utopia of Sun City, Arizona to work on medical mission ships serving the South Pacific Islands (Bennett, 1993). Apparently, for the fortunate individuals, retirement years can indeed be the best years of their lives and the most gratifying.

Box 18-6 Phases of Retirement

Remote: Future anticipation with little real planning
Near: Preparation and fantasizing regarding retirement
Honeymoon: Euphoria and testing of the fantasies
Disenchantment: Letdown, boredom, sometimes depression
Reorientation: Developing a realistic and satisfactory lifestyle
Stability: Personal investment in meaningful activities
Termination: Loss of role resulting from illness or return to work

VOLUNTEERISM

Volunteer service provides an attractive role for many aged who have previously not had the luxury of investing time without monetary return. Interestingly, although women have traditionally volunteered, men have experienced the greatest increase in volunteerism among the elderly. Most people involved in volunteer work believe that they are contributing to the community and filling gaps in services that might otherwise be unmet. Thus self-esteem and a sense of usefulness prevail. Successful programs expect a lot from their volunteers and invest considerable time in training and sustaining their interest. Clear guidelines, periodic review, and feedback are critical to the success of any volunteer program.

Some of the programs that include or require senior volunteers are National Network on Aging (Nursing Home Ombudsman Program, National Nutrition Program), ACTION (Foster Grandparents [FGP], Retired Senior Volunteer Program [RSVP], Volunteers in Service to America [VISTA], Senior Companion, Peace Corps), Legal Service Corporation, SCORE (Small Business Administration), Department of Veterans Affairs, and National Volunteer School Program (teacher aides). Many of these volunteers are paid or are given other inducements to supplement low incomes. Though considered volunteer activity, all ACTION programs provide some minimal income or sustenance. Ms. Lillian Carter is an excellent example of a volunteer devoted to public service through the Peace Corps. Another, of personal acquaintance, is Cynthia Kelly, first editor of the Geriatric Nursing Journal. At approximately the age of 70, Kelly went with the backing of the Peace Corps to Micronesia to teach children.

One of the predominant reasons for joining volunteer groups is the social contact with other volunteers. Many volunteer activities involve working with people who are in need of special attention. These situations provide opportunities for expressing altruistic motives. Investment of self and contact with others seems to result in an enriching experience.

Health Care Volunteers

Elderly volunteers serve in hospitals and nursing homes. Some of the myriad of activities includes acting as foster grandparents, tutoring ill children, rocking infants, and writing letters for or visiting with ailing elders. Johns Hopkins Hospital has had such a volunteer program for 60 years and finds the services of elders invaluable.

Older volunteers have been used extensively in nursing homes without pay. One concern is the tendency for older adults to become depressed when constantly exposed to the limitations of their age peers. Counselor availability will be critical to the success of a program. This activity can be in the form of group discussions led by a consistent coordinating individual. An ACTION program that was designed specifically to train and pay older people who may wish to work in nursing homes would be desirable, and during this time of nursing shortage, it is probably essential.

A newsletter from a long-term care facility posted in settings in which senior citizens gather or reside, explaining various volunteer activities (such as entertaining, office work, transportation aide, cafeteria attendants, activity assistants, workshop assistants, boutique salespeople, gardeners, and friendly visitors) would be a useful method of recruiting volunteers.

Peer Counseling

Several institutions have peer counseling training programs in which older volunteers learn interviewing skills and develop their ability to deal with patients who are lonely, depressed, or dying. These volunteer roles have potential for maintaining or elevating self-esteem of volunteers and patients and hold great potential for meeting the needs of many elders. The older generation, often skeptical of professional counseling, will more readily accept the help of peers, especially if identified as volunteers rather than counselors. Based on their understanding of the painful experiences of old age, older adults can add a dimension of friendship and empathy to the counseling function. Nurses can assist in identifying clients most likely to benefit from peer counseling.

A growing number of peer counseling programs are appearing across the United States. These programs train elders to help other elders deal with the major transitions of life: relocation, death of a spouse, retirement, or other crises that occur in the process of aging. Some counselors provide telephone counsel, and others go to the home or visit people who are institutionalized. The proviso is that the elder request help and the response be prompt. Some programs are based in churches, in suicide prevention services, retirement centers, senior centers, and institutions. (For further information regarding development of peer counseling services, see Resources at the end of the chapter.)

Box 18-7 **Steps in Development of Volunteer Role**

1. Volunteer role uses skills from previous work or community experience. A gain in status, prestige, and community sanction is experienced.
2. Volunteer role improves interest in self and others. Dependence is reduced, and interdependence is created.
3. Feedback is gained from recipients of services. Self-view is improved, and resourcefulness is recognized.
4. Social and psychologic stimulation is found in volunteer settings. Personal growth and development occur as skills are refined.
5. Community rewards and recognition are awarded. New roles of social significance are internalized.

Volunteer Training and Roles

Training programs, supervision, and ongoing support are critical to the success of volunteer programs (Musson et al, 1997). The following considerations guide the development of successful volunteer programs:

Administrative support of volunteers
Clearly determined goals for the program
A specific orientation program with printed support materials to give volunteers
Buddy systems to orient and reinforce volunteer role and expectations
Periodic evaluations and modifications as needs indicated by volunteer participants
Determination of specific awards and rewards to sustain interest and involvement

Individuals should be encouraged to begin minimal participation in volunteer programs before work role discontinuation. This type of activity can serve as a bridge of continuity. Certain identifiable steps exist in the full development of a role as a volunteer (Box 18-7). Group involvement and group meetings will solidify and strengthen the identification with the volunteer role.

An important point to remember is that altruism never dies. In some way, elders invariably wish to be contributing members of society as long as they live. Nurses may explore the possibilities with elders and discuss latent interests they may wish to develop and ways they can contribute to others from their vast store of life experience and creative endeavors.

WIDOWS AND WIDOWERS

Losing a partner, when a close and satisfying relationship has lasted a long time, is a psychic amputation. The mourning is as much for self as it is for the dead individual. Part of oneself has been destroyed, and even with satisfactory grief resolution, that previous self will never return. People who reorganize their lives and invest in family, friends, and activities will find later that they will still miss their "other half" profoundly. The loss of spouse is a stage in the life course that can be anticipated but seldom is. Many studies have found widowers often marry quickly but subvert their grief and may never fully adapt to the loss. Widows often experience conflicts with children and family over their decision to remarry. This conflict is frequently related to inheritance and relationship complications.

The transitional phase of grief, if handled appropriately, leads to the confirmation of a new identity, the end of one stage of life and the beginning of another. Seldom in life is there such an abrupt and distinct breach that creates intense pain but offers the opportunity for the emergence of a new identity.

Widowhood

About 35% of elders will be widowed at 65 years of age (NCOA, 2002); most of these elders will be women. The gender gap continues until at age 85 when the ratio reaches 41 men for every 100 women (NCOA, 2002). Older women are three times more likely than men are to be widowed (Kutza, 2001). For people who have been married for many years, widowhood is the most difficult adjustment a person can face, aside from the loss of a child, and exemplifies some of the principles of transitions. Older spouses are somewhat prepared for and expect that one must die before the other, but the loss of a child is not expected.

The Swedish twin study, which has followed over 2000 twins since 1984 (Lichtenstein et al, 1996), describes the recently widowed (less than 3 years) and the long-term widowed (more than 5 years). This study gives some guidelines for expectations of the process of transition from bereaved widow to adjustment. In addition, these studies found that the young-old were more stressed than the oldest-old during the adaptational process, although both groups ultimately achieved a satisfactory adaptation.

A pattern of working outside the home in a gratifying position may provide women with confidence, independence, and autonomy that can act as a buffer during the stress of grieving. Because widowhood and poverty often go hand in hand, working women probably have more resources to provide a healthier lifestyle.

Transitions in Widowhood

Acute reactions usually subside by the second year, and making the past a part of a person's personal history becomes possible. Maintaining an intact role in work or the community may attenuate the confrontation with the emptiness at home.

Patterns of adjustment can be seen in Box 18-8. These stages of the transition to a new role as a widow or widower are proposed as guides to intervention rather than as predictive or prognostic indicators. Each individual grieves in his or her own time and manner. Great cultural variations play a part in the experience of widowhood that have not been sufficiently addressed.

Box 18-8 Patterns of Adjustment to Widowhood

Stage One: Reactionary (First Few Weeks)
Early responses of disbelief, anger, indecision, detachment, and inability to communicate in a logical, sustained manner are common. Searching for the mate, visions, hallucinations, and depersonalization may be experienced.
INTERVENTION: Support, validate, be available, listen to talk about mate, reduce expectations.

Stage Two: Withdrawal (First Few Months)
Depression, apathy, physiologic vulnerability occur; movement and cognition are slowed; insomnia, unpredictable waves of grief, sighing, and anorexia occur.
INTERVENTION: Protect against suicide and involve in support groups.

Stage Three: Recuperation (Second 6 Months)
Periods of depression are interspersed with characteristic capability. Feelings of personal control begin to return.
INTERVENTION: Support accustomed lifestyle patterns that sustain and assist person to explore new possibilities.

Stage Four: Exploration (Second Year)
Individual begins new ventures, testing suitability of new roles; anniversaries or holidays, birthdays, and date of death may be especially difficult.
INTERVENTION: Prepare individual for unexpected reactions during anniversaries. Encourage and support new trial roles.

Stage Five: Integration (Fifth Year)
Individual will feel fully integrated into new and satisfying roles if grief has been resolved in a healthy manner.
INTERVENTION: Assist individual to recognize and share own pattern of growth through the trauma of loss.

Personal interests and attributes, if long suppressed in the role of wife, sometimes spring forth as a plant sprouting in the springtime. The self, previously embedded in the identity of another, tries to emerge from the cocoon, not always successfully. Nonetheless, individuals who do emerge gain a new identity.

The diversity in lifestyles of widows is extreme. However, a new breed of older widow is emerging: the career-minded cosmopolitan who is active in family, religious, recreational, and political groups and not geographically restricted. Better educated and financially sound, these widows are better able to reorganize their lives after the heavy grief is over; they are self-sufficient and manage their homes and lives with a sense of well being (Figure 18-5).

Sophie had a long time to deal with her husband's gradual loss of the battle with a virulent cancer. As a nurse, she comprehended that he would not win, but she nevertheless maintained the hope that recovery was possible. Her weekly reports of their painful but poignant saga via e-mail to her large network of friends and professional acquaintances served to maintain an enormous support system. This

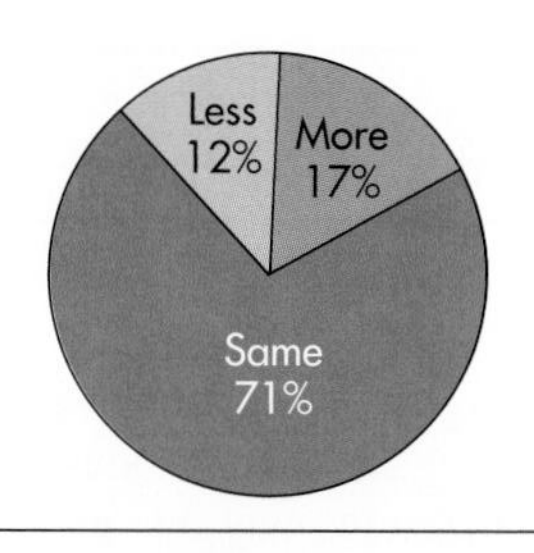

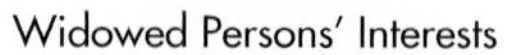

Survey Question: Compared to when your spouse was alive, do YOU have more interest, less interest, or about the same amount of interest in having contact with relatives and friends?

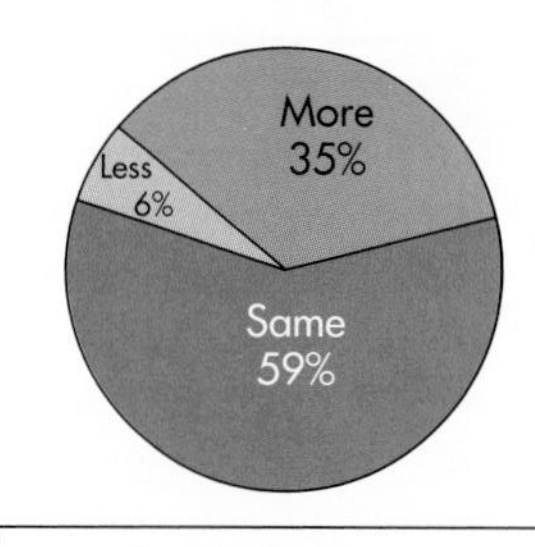

Friends' & Relatives' Interests

Survey Question: Do your relatives and friends show more interest, less interest, or about the same amount of interest in having contact with you?

Figure 18-5. Effect of widowhood on social participation. (From Utz RL et al: The effect of widowhood on older adults' social participation: an evaluation of activity, disengagement, and continuity theories, *The Gerontologist* 42[4]:522, 2002.)

network also allowed her to journal her thoughts as she and Ben progressed together in their pilgrimage. Now, 2 years later, she has rebuilt a productive and rewarding life for herself though remaining actively responsive to her need for ritual and spontaneous expressions of her grief.

The long-term effects of spousal loss pervasively influence the lives of many in terms of health and life satisfaction. Widowhood significantly increases the likelihood of being placed in a nursing home as the individual becomes dependent.

Widowers

Widowers are an elusive group, their grief often hidden in a facade of "manliness." Although sometimes found in grief support groups, widowers usually carry their pain alone. Historically, when maternal death rates were high, a man often had three or four wives and as many as 30 children. The old man, when widowed, remained the patriarch of the family with his needs attended by daughters, unmarried sisters, and other women within the family. Now, with the extended family dispersed, the widower is usually left to his own devices, as long as he is functional.

Hogstel (1985) found that although the experience of widowers is, in many ways, similar to that of widows, some distinct differences do exist. Widowers who must, for whatever reasons, reside with a son or daughter find the adjustment difficult and threatening. These men also report receiving fewer manifestations of affection; hugs and holdings are much less frequent than those given to widows. Although many men remarry precipitously, they often fear impotence and frequently experience it in the second marriage. This condition can most often be remedied but may, too often, simply be accepted fatalistically. The following suggestions from Hogstel (1985) for working with widowers will be useful to nurses:

- Sponsor self-help groups in the community for widows and widowers.
- Discuss sexuality and recommend therapy when needed.
- Watch for signs of severe depression and make immediate contact with family, referral for mental health, or both.
- Arrange classes for cooking and other homemaking skills.
- Provide information about homemaking services.
- Provide information about resources such as Senior Centers, AARP, and RSVP.
- Encourage involvement in volunteer programs, such as SCORE.
- Encourage churches to sponsor programs, groups, and outings for older widowers.

Wives have traditionally been the "kin-keepers" (Troll et al, 1979). Ties with relatives and friends are maintained, and wives are usually the organizers of social and recreational activities. Even when the husband's career has been the central socializing force, the wife has been the social agent. When the wife dies, the husband is set adrift without his rudder. Single women will immediately see the widower as a potential candidate; and the widow who is marriage minded may, in his grief, make precipitous decisions. In grief support groups, if he can find a group not devoted only to widows, the widower is grossly outnumbered and less able to openly express grief, as well as being vulnerable to "women bearing pies."

Even though middle- and upper-class Caucasian men are seen as occupying the power base in society, they are among those most deprived of supports when grieving. To the extent that they have occupied the role of provider, they are further deprived by having no one left to provide for.

In search of patterns of adaptation among widowers, we have gathered experiential and anecdotal data from friends, acquaintances, and colleagues. We are aware that this data has limited application, but it may enhance awareness and stimulate much-needed research on this subject.

Andrew was widowed at 60 years of age after he had cared for his wife through a long and painful illness. His monogamous marriage of 40 years to a professional woman who had commandeered his life as she did her career left him with few internal or external resources. His career in the Army and the pattern of depending on his wife resulted in his having made few decisions about his own life. Andrew was content to have others tell him what to do. His wife designed his social life, and his commanding officers dictated his work life. Andrew had given some thought to what he would do when his wife died and immediately began searching for a female companion. His female companion was a professional woman, similar to his wife in many ways. A disinterested observer would have immediately seen his attempt as an object replacement. Andrew's friends and family misunderstood his lack of open grief and apparent disregard of a "decent period of mourning." They withdrew from him at the time he most needed their support. Unfortunately, Andrew's new companion did not like his dependency, which, exacerbated by grief, overwhelmed her. She also began to withdraw. Within 6 months after the death of his wife, Andrew was searching the "singles" advertisements and had joined several singles clubs. The saga of the search continued for years, always ending with the woman leaving, often because he was unable to really give himself to the relationship. He was unable to find his wife. Andrew is now a lonely man of 70 years, still searching but with even less interest. He talks a lot about feeling old and wonders if he will live much longer. Materially he is well off, but socially he is poverty stricken.

Chester's wife died of a virulent and invasive cancer 6 weeks after it was diagnosed. This marriage, Chester's second, had been one of mutual respect, love, and companionship. Both people were writers and had lived in the rarefied atmosphere of writers and publishers in New York City; they had dozens of friends and acquaintances but few intimates because they had lived for each other and their careers. Chester's psyche, frail at best, was grievously wounded. He was unable to function and eventually lost his job. He returned to his previous hometown on the West Coast and attempted to reestablish a bond with his first wife and his two children, who had become physically and emotionally distant over the years. Failing in that attempt was another blow to his ego. Chester found a nongratifying job and even managed to keep it, although he spent his evenings isolated in a small apartment, drinking, crying, and sleeping. His neglect of his physical needs and lack of emotional support eroded his health. Chester was hospitalized several times. His grief consumed him for 3 years. Finally, Chester met a woman he thought he loved, a writer, somewhat like his wife, but his physical deterioration had left him impotent, and the relationship was short lived. Chester returned to New York City and found a job as an editor that demanded all his time and thought. His work has become his obsession, and he has become even more demanding of himself and others.

George was a traditional man, a successful lawyer and a courtly gentleman. His family life had been as circumscribed and well planned as were all the other elements of his existence. George nursed his wife through a long illness with the assistance of his daughters. He was dutiful and loving. When his wife died, he had many helpful friends and assistance from his family. After 2 years, George's grief subsided, and he began to think of another relationship. Friends were helpful and introduced George to various women, but he found that women had changed in their expectations and relations with men. These women were too liberated for him to understand. After the failure of two attempts to court women, George began to develop self-doubts that were uncharacteristic of him. He attempted to meet other women, but his diffident approach was mistaken as lack of interest and was not successful. He is still trying to find a woman who will appreciate him, and he will with the help of his friends.

Abe was more fortunate than most widowers. His wife openly planned with him for his survival after her death. She found a grief therapist for him and a financial manager. Abe's wife not only gave him permission to find new female relationships, but also recommended it. In addition, Abe and his wife had a large network of friends and family among the Jewish community. Abe grieved openly after her death and sought solace with her sister's family. He was included in all of their activities and encouraged to make their home his emotional shelter. Abe saw his grief therapist weekly and more often when needed, and he left the management of his financial affairs to his advisor. He was thus able to work through his grief without other impediments. He found it very difficult to be at home alone and scheduled activities every evening of the week to avoid it. Finally realizing that the home held too many memories for him, Abe moved. After several brief relationships with women, he found one who was right for him. With the passage of 5 years and consistent support, Abe has achieved a new life for himself in which he appreciates his new companion for herself.

Although these vignettes are limited in their application, the following themes can be identified:

- The search for the lost mate
- The neglect of self
- The inability to share grief
- The loss of social contacts
- The struggle to view women as other than wife
- The erosion of self-confidence and sexuality
- The protracted grief period

Nurses can be instrumental in resolving some of these issues by encouraging the individual to share thoughts and feelings with friends and family, to emphasize the need for maintaining male friendships, to provide resources such as groups or grief therapists, to encourage delay in making female attachments, and to discuss the effects of depression on sexuality. Nurses who are empathetic and responsive may find that the grieving man misunderstands their intentions. The point must be made clear, sometimes repeatedly, that the individual during grief is vulnerable to inappropriate alliances with women and must recover before the energy to make a real investment is possible.

Nurse's Role with Widows and Widowers

Nurses working with the bereaved will need to review Lindemann's classic grief studies to understand the initial somatic responses of the bereaved (Lindemann, 1944). Supporting the grieving person requires an extension of self to reconnect the severed person with a world of warmth and caring. Each gesture crosses the void to bring the lost back to the land of the living. No one nurse or one family member can accomplish this task alone. Hundreds of small, caring gestures build strength and confidence in grieving person's ability and willingness to survive.

Feelings of the bereaved are not orderly or progressive; they are conflicted, ambivalent, suicidal, full of rage, and often suspicious. Widows and widowers may exhibit personality disorganization that would be considered mentally aberrant or frankly psychotic under other circumstances.

Admittedly, some people handle grief with less apparent decompensation. The reason for emphasizing extreme reactions is to avert mislabeling and focusing on pathologic conditions. Grief reactions must be accepted as personally valid and useful evidences of healing.

How then does a nurse recognize an aberrant, mentally unhealthy grief reaction? Immediately assessment is difficult, because grief reactions are so individual. People with few familial or social supports are very likely to need professional help to get through the early months of grief in a way that will facilitate recovery. Therefore the nurse will need to assess the support network rather than focus on unusual symptoms. If adequate support is available, reintegration can be expected in 2 to 5 years.

Additional information about dying, death, and grief can be found in Chapter 24.

Divorce

In the past, divorce was considered a stigmatizing event, though today it is so common that a person is inclined to forget the ostracizing effects of divorce from 60 years ago. One couple, recently celebrated their fiftieth anniversary. The offspring of the couple said, "What kind of freaks are you? No one stays married that long!" Nonetheless, Some elders are firmly tied to the adage, "until death do us part."

At age 65 and beyond, 11.5% of women and 9.2% of men are divorced (U.S. Bureau of the Census, 2001). People who divorce in late life have been largely neglected in research and support services. The number of people who seek divorce after that age is unknown, but divorce, as well as marriage and remarriage, must often be considered within the context of economics. In the last few years, the number of divorced elders has increased much more rapidly than the increase in the elderly population. This statistic may largely be a cohort effect. As divorces increase in couples of all ages, many more enter the ranks of the aged. At present, 50% of all first marriages and 60% of remarriages end in divorce (U.S. Divorce Statistics, 2002). Although generational and individual differences in expectations exist from marriage, older couples are becoming less likely to stay in an unsatisfactory marriage. Health care professionals need to avoid assumptions and be alert to the possibility of marriage dissatisfaction in old age. Nurses need to ask, "How would you describe your marriage?"

Long-term relationships are varied and complex, with many factors forming the glue that holds them together.

John's arthritis, vision, and hearing deficits prevent him or his wife Jennie from enjoying the camping, skiing, and outdoor activities they shared most of their adult lives. Both John and Jennie love good food and have pleasant times together, though Jennie often feels hampered by John's disabilities. She has never believed a wife should pursue her own interests regardless of those of the husband. Jennie's children say, "Come mother, go with us to the mountains." Her reply, "I can't leave Dad here alone." Jennie does not necessarily expect life to be the way she would like it. She remembers the struggles, the losses, and the pain she and John have shared throughout their lives. These memories bind her more strongly to him than the happy moments. Jennie will not likely divorce her husband of 40 years, though they share few interests and abilities.

Margaret, her sister, says, "Why don't you get out and do something?" Margaret talks about divorcing her husband of 50 years. She has not told him yet because she feels as though she is a traitor. However, Margaret says, "We really never shared anything. He was always pursuing his interests but thought I should be there waiting whenever he wanted me. I felt like a widow most of my married life, so I have decided to make a real break. I am concerned about finances, though. I might not have enough if I go out on my own." She may, in fact, not leave but remain in the situation because of guilt and fear.

Lanza (1996) studied the divorces of older women and found them attributed to their husbands' infidelity, retirement, or simply growing apart. Wives often tended to blame themselves, believing that they were in some way deficient, otherwise the divorce would not have occurred. Lanza concluded that marital breakdown is more devastating in old age because it is often unanticipated and may occur concurrent with other significant losses.

Health care workers must be concerned with supporting a client's decision to seek a divorce and with assisting him or her in seeking counseling in the transition. A nurse should alert the client that a divorce will bring on a grieving process similar to that of the death of a spouse and that a severe disruption in coping capacity may occur until an adjustment to a new life is made. The grief may be more difficult with which to cope because no socially sanctioned patterns have been established, as is the case in widowhood. In addition, tax and fiscal policies favor married couples, and many a divorced elderly lady is at a serious economic disadvantage in retirement.

Transition from Health to Illness

Recognition of and adaptation to a chronic disorders and disabilities (see Chapter 8) is likely to incur many transitions during remissions and exacerbations, such as arthritic conditions. Other, more stable and progressive chronic disorders require ongoing adaptations. For example, the move from being a "healthy" elder to that of an elderly "diabetic" requires changes in lifestyle, self-concept, and relationships.

John was a highly sexual person. He adapted fairly well to the dietary changes and was able to tolerate his propensity to develop infections. However, as John became increasingly aware of his impotence, his whole self-image was threatened. He no longer felt "manly" and became quite suicidal. Early affiliation with a group confronting similar issues assisted John in the adaptation to the altered role requirements necessitated by his chronic illness. In all transitions, adequate preparation and support during the progression can mean the difference between success and failure in satisfactory adjustment.

Roles of Client and Nurses

During the transition from familiar roles to new ones, an individual needs the freedom to try various possibilities in an accepting atmosphere that encourages success, tolerates failure, and recognizes that progress is not accomplished by slow, even steps. In real life, progress follows a more wayward, uneven course. The individual is easily distracted and often falls back to the familiar. A nurse is most helpful in providing an accepting milieu that encourages independence and exploration and the realization of the uncertainty inherent in transitions.

Human Needs and Wellness Diagnoses

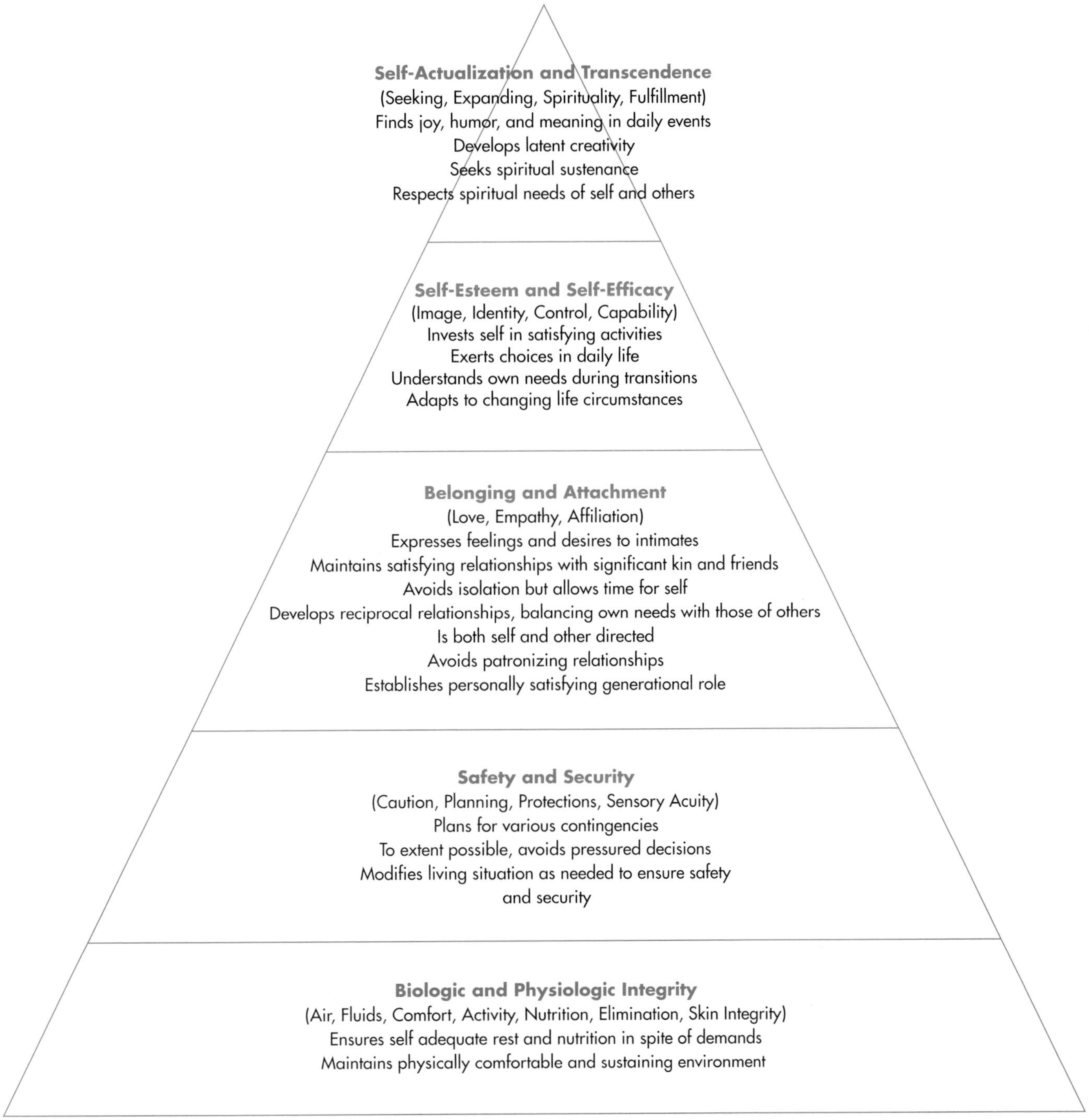

Self-Actualization and Transcendence
(Seeking, Expanding, Spirituality, Fulfillment)
Finds joy, humor, and meaning in daily events
Develops latent creativity
Seeks spiritual sustenance
Respects spiritual needs of self and others

Self-Esteem and Self-Efficacy
(Image, Identity, Control, Capability)
Invests self in satisfying activities
Exerts choices in daily life
Understands own needs during transitions
Adapts to changing life circumstances

Belonging and Attachment
(Love, Empathy, Affiliation)
Expresses feelings and desires to intimates
Maintains satisfying relationships with significant kin and friends
Avoids isolation but allows time for self
Develops reciprocal relationships, balancing own needs with those of others
Is both self and other directed
Avoids patronizing relationships
Establishes personally satisfying generational role

Safety and Security
(Caution, Planning, Protections, Sensory Acuity)
Plans for various contingencies
To extent possible, avoids pressured decisions
Modifies living situation as needed to ensure safety and security

Biologic and Physiologic Integrity
(Air, Fluids, Comfort, Activity, Nutrition, Elimination, Skin Integrity)
Ensures self adequate rest and nutrition in spite of demands
Maintains physically comfortable and sustaining environment

These are not all the possible wellness diagnoses that may be identified. The above are examples of nursing diagnoses that should be considered when planning care for the older adult.

KEY CONCEPTS

- Roles define individual and societal expectations of function.
- In a rapidly changing society, roles quickly become anachronistic.
- Transitions are akin to shedding of skin as a new one is generated.
- Ability to successfully negotiate transitions and develop new and gratifying roles depends on personal and environmental supports, timing, clarity of expectations, personality, and degree of change required.
- Elders may perceive more losses than gains in the transitions of aging.
- Caring family or pseudo-family relationships are critical to an elder's adaptation to the transition in aging.
- Caregiving activities occupy much of an elder's time, either as the caregiver or the recipient of care.
- Spousal caregiving is most onerous when involving dementias and lack of resources.
- Grandparents are increasingly assuming primary caregiving roles with grandchildren.
- Mid-life individuals are often caring for individuals from generations before and after them.
- A major transitional issue for an elder is moving from health to illness and redefining the individual in terms of a chronic disorder. Nurses must ensure that this new definition does not become the identity of the individual.
- The work role transition is the major change for men and is increasingly becoming so for women, though women often continue their homemaker-caregiver role without interruption.
- Numerous patterns of retirement exist at present, and therefore retirement per se cannot be viewed categorically.
- Preretirement planning and postretirement follow-up significantly affect positive adaptation to the transition.
- Definite gender differences exist in the roles and transitions common to the aging process.
- Volunteerism is becoming increasingly attractive to elders who feel the need to express their altruistic motives; some opportunities also supplement retirement income.
- Loss of spouse is the role change that has the greatest potential for maladaptation, and nursing support can make a significant positive difference in the transition.
- Widowers are a neglected group in the literature and in the service arena. These men are particularly vulnerable to maladaptive behaviors and deterioration.
- The role reversal from provider to dependent can be difficult and must be recognized and explored with the individual.

▲ CASE STUDY

Sandy was a professor at a small, private college in a metropolitan area. Although she had taught nursing for 25 years and thoroughly loved her work, it had been a demanding year and she was very tired. A rumor had recently circulated that the college was in trouble financially. Some of the most affluent alumni were no longer able to be trusted for gifts and endowments because the football coach had not produced a winning team for several years. Because the tuition was becoming exorbitant, the college had recently lost some students to one of the three state college campuses within driving distance of the city. The trustees of the college, in a move to cut expenses, offered an incentive to professors who were willing to retire early; an extra year of service credit was presented for every 6 years worked. Sandy was only 55 years of age but thought that the 4 years of extra credit would bring her near the minimum retirement age for Social Security (an error, of course, because her age did not change with her service credit). Rather impulsively, Sandy decided to accept the offer, after telling colleagues, "Well, you know how I love to travel. Why wait until I'm too old to enjoy retirement? Why don't you think about the offer, too? This is a once-in-a-lifetime opportunity." Near the end of the academic year, the celebrations began: recognition, plaques, expressions of gratitude from students, and envy from her associates. The send-off was wonderful. In the summer, Sandy withdrew her savings and booked a cruise to the Greek islands. The journey was lovely, and she enjoyed every moment. Sandy began to feel depressed when she got off the ship but knew it was only because the elegant cruise was over. However, as fall came around, Sandy began to feel more depressed. Most of her friends were teachers, and they were all back at work. Sandy briefly thought of going to Pittsburgh to visit her sister but decided against the idea because she and her sister had really never been very compatible. Then, Sandy was hit with some of the realities of early retirement: she was unable to withdraw any of her considerable tax-deferred savings before she was 59½ years of age without significant penalty, her health insurance coverage was considerably less comprehensive after retirement, her colleagues were all busy, and she was very bored. Then, the real blow fell. The college, in desperation, had dipped into the retirement funds to remain solvent, and the retirees' pensions were now at risk. Sandy's sister, who was a nurse, called to announce that she wanted to come and stay a few days while she attended a conference in the city. When she arrived, Sandy overwhelmed her with the litany of woes. If you were Sandy's sister, what would you do?

Based on the case study, develop a nursing care plan using the following procedure:*

List the client's comments that provide subjective data.

List information that provides objective data.

From these data, identify and state, using accepted format, two nursing diagnoses you determine are most significant to this client at this time. List two client strengths that you have identified from the data.

*Students are advised to refer to their nursing diagnosis text and identify possible or potential problems.

Determine and state outcome criteria for each diagnosis. These criteria must reflect some alleviation of the problem identified in the nursing diagnosis and must be stated in concrete and measurable terms.

Plan and state one or more interventions for each diagnosed problem.

Provide specific documentation of sources used to determine appropriate intervention. Plan at least one intervention that incorporates the client's existing strengths.

Evaluate the success of intervention. Interventions must correlate directly with the stated outcome criteria to measure the outcome success.

STUDY QUESTIONS/ACTIVITIES

Identify several important family and social roles that elder members of your family fulfill. Discuss how their roles differ from those of their parents.

What are the factors to consider in role transitions, and how can transitions be made smoother?

What factors must be considered in the decision to retire?

Discuss the differences you would expect in adaptation to retirement between an individual who retired because of ill health and one who retired because he or she desired to do so.

How do you think retirement differs for men and women?

Describe what you think would be an ideal retirement.

Plan specific ways in which you would present a retirement seminar to workers in a computer microchip factory.

Explain the major issues in adaptation to a major role change such as retirement and widowhood.

Discuss how you think an individual can prepare in advance for widowhood.

Discuss the meanings and the thoughts triggered by the students' and elders' viewpoints expressed at the beginning of the chapter. How do these vary from your own experience?

RESEARCH QUESTIONS

Who and how many couples over age 55 are in the LGBT category?

What are the significant factors in relationships between fathers and adult children?

What are the roles and activities of great grandparents with great grandchildren?

What are the differences between grandparenting and great grandparenting?

What are the reactions of elders to the care given by their offspring?

How many elders had been with one company for the majority of their working life?

How does retirement affect these individuals?

What are the patterns of adaptation of widowers? How different for young-old and old-old?

Who divorces in late life and for what reasons?

REFERENCES

Age Beat on Line: *The Newsletter of the Journalists Exchange on Aging,* 2(15): July 2002. Available at *paul@asaging.org*

Allen KR, Wilcox KL: Becoming an activist: older parents of adult gay children. Paper presented at the meeting of the Gerontological Society of America, Washington, DC, November 19, 1996.

American Association of Retired Persons Public Policy Institute: *Characteristics of uninsured 50-64 year-olds in 2000,* Washington DC, 2002a, AARP. Available at *www.aarp.org/ppi*

American Association of Retired Persons Public Policy Institute: *Health care coverage among 50-64 year-olds in 2000,* Washington DC, 2002b, AARP. Available at *www.aarp.org/ppi*

American Society on Aging: CARE Pro-Module 3: June 2002. Available at *www.asaging.org*

Antonovsky A, Sagy S: Confronting developmental tasks in the retirement transition, *Gerontologist* 30:362, 1990.

Atchley RC: Issues in retirement research, *Gerontologist* 19:44, 1979.

Bedford VH, Avioli PS: Variations on sibling intimacy in old age, *Generations* 25(2):34, 2001.

Bennett: Mercy on the main, *Modern Maturity* 36(1):6, 1993.

Bleiszner R: "She'll be on my heart": intimacy among friends, *Generations* 25(2):48, 2001.

Brown-Standridge MD, Floyd CW: Healing bittersweet legacies: revisiting contextual family therapy for grandparents raising grandchildren in crisis, *J Marital Fam Ther* 26(2):185, 2000.

Cahill S, South K: Policy issues affecting lesbian, gay, bisexual, and transgender people in retirement, *Generations: J Am Soc Aging* 26(11):49, 2002.

Chan CG, Elder GH: Matrilineal advantage in grandchild-grandparent relations, *Gerontologist* 40(2):189, 2000.

Chater S: Speech at Hartford Geriatric Nursing Center, New York, 1998.

Claes JA, Moore W: *J HHS Admin* 23(2):181, Fall 2000.

Cohen A, Colantonio A, Vernich L: Positive aspects of caregiving: rounding out the caregiver experience, *Int J Geriatr Psychiatr* 18:184, 2002.

Delaney S & E: *Having our say: the Delaney sisters' first 100 years,* New York, 1993, Kodansha International.

Dennis H: The current state of retirement planning, *Generations* 13(2):38, 2002.

Doka KJ: Disenfranchised grief: lessons for those serving older clients, *Aging Today* 23(4):13, 2002.

Doka KJ, Mertz ME: The meaning and significance of great-grandparenthood, *Gerontologist* 28(3):192, 1988.

Dorfman LT: Health conditions and perceived quality of life in retirement, *Health Soc Work* 20(3):192, 2002.

Drew LA, Smith PK: The impact of parental separation on grandparent-grandchild relationships, *Int J Aging Human Dev* 48(3):191, 1999.

Ekerdt D, Dennis H: Introduction to retirement: new chapters in American Life, entire issue of *Generations* 26(11), 2002.

Ekerdt DJ, DeViney S, Kosloski K: Profiling plans for retirement, *J Gerontol* 51(3):S140, 1996.

Family Caregiver Alliance, National Center on Caregiving: *Caregiving Policy Digest* 11(11):3, 2002.

Fingerman KL: A distant closeness: intimacy between parents and their children in later life, *Generations* 25(2):26, 2001.

Fischer LR: Respect—the key to valuing today's older volunteers, *Aging Today* 17(6):11, 1996.

Fuller-Thomson E, Minkler M: American grandparents providing extensive child care to their grandchildren: prevalence and profile, *Gerontologist* 41(2):201, 2001.

Generations United P 11. Available at *www.gu.org*

Ghuman HS, Weist MD, Shafer ME: Demographic and clinical characteristics of emotionally disturbed children being raised by grandparents, *Psychiatr Serv* 50(11):1075, 1999.

Goodman C, Silverstein M: Grandmothers raising grandchildren: family structure and well-being in culturally diverse families, *Gerontologist* 42(5):676-689, 2002.

Hayslip B, Goldberg-Glen RS: *Grandparent raising grandchildren: theoretical, empirical, and clinical perspectives*, New York, 2002, Springer.

Hirshorn BA, Tetrick LE, Sinclair RR: Understanding the provision of postretirement health care and pension benefits: which firm characteristics are most explanatory? *Gerontologist* 36(5):637, 1996.

Hogstel M: Older widowers: a small group with special needs, *Geriatr Nurs* 6(1):24, 1985.

Honig M: Retirement expectations: differences by race, ethnicity, and gender, *Gerontologist* 36(3):373, 1996.

Houde SC et al: Men providing care to older adults in the home, *J Geron Nurs* 27(8):13, 2001.

Hushbeck C: Grandparents' visitation rights, *Aging Today* 23(5):11, 2002.

Kleyman P: Age beat online, *Journalists Exchange on Aging and the American Society on Aging* 2(25), 2002.

Kutza EA: Living longer, living better: policy presumptions and new family structures, *Pub Pol Aging Rep* 11(3):12, 2001.

Lanza ML: Divorce experienced as an older woman, *Geriatr Nurs* 17(4):166, 1996.

LaRock S: Key components, topics of successful preretirement counseling program, Employee Benefit Plan Review, November 2001.

Lichtenstein P et al: A co-twin control study of response to widowhood, *J Gerontol B: Psychol Soc Sci* 51(5):279, 1996.

Lindemann E: Symptomalology and management of acute grief, *Am J Psychiatr* 101(2):141-148, 1944.

Lindgren HC: Personal communication, San Francisco, 2001.

Lowenthal MF, Haven C: Interaction and adaptation: intimacy as a critical variable, *Am Sociol Rev* 33:20, 1968.

LTC-Alert: Dramatic growth of aging boomers in one year, from George Sherman, 2001. Available at *gsherman@ris.net*

McCann S, Evans DS: Informal care: the views of people receiving care, *Health Soc Care Comm* 10(4):221, 2002.

Mittleman MS: Family caregiving for people with Alzheimer's disease: results of the NYU spouse caregiver intervention study, *Generations* 26(1):104, 2002.

Mullen F, Einhorn M: The effect of state TANF choices on grandparent-headed households, AARP Public Policy Institute Paper #2000 (October 2000).

Musson ND, Frye GD, Nash M: Silver spoons: supervised volunteers provide feeding of patients, *Geriatr Nurs* 18(1):17, 1997.

Mutchler JE et al: Pathways to labor force exit: work transitions and work stability, *J Gerontol* 52B(1):S4, 1997.

National Council on the Aging (NCOA): American perceptions of aging in the 21st century, Washington DC, 2002, NCOA. Available at *www.ncoa.org*

Navaie-Waliser M et al: When the caregiver needs care: the plight of vulnerable caregivers, *Am J Pub Health* 92(3):409, 2002.

Neabel B, Fothergill-Bourbbonnais F, Dunning J: Issues in family care family assessment tools: a review of the literature from 1978-1997, *Heart Lung* 29(3):196, 2000.

Neufeld A et al: Immigrant women: making connections to community resources for support in family caregiving, *Qual Health Res* 12(6):751, 2002.

Noonan AE, Tennestedt SL: Meaning in caregiving and its contribution to caregiving well-being, *Gerontologist* 37:785, 1997.

O'Brien LR: *Office manager,* Pacifica, CA, 2002, Van Go Painting Company.

Ory M et al: The extent and impact of dementia care: unique challenges perceived by family caregivers. In Schulz R, editor: *Handbook on dementia caregiving,* New York, 2000, Springer.

Pienta AM, Hayward MD: Who expect to continue working after age 62? The retirement plans of couples, *J Gerontol* 57B(4):S199, 2002.

Piercy KW: We couldn't do without them: the value of close relationships between older adults and their nonfamily caregivers, *Generations* 25(2):41, 2001.

Pierre JH: Personal communication, Salem, OR, 1992.

Quinn JF, Kozy M: The role of bridge jobs in the retirement transition: gender, race, and ethnicity, *Gerontologist* 36(3):363, 1996.

Reitzes DC, Mutran EJ, Fernandez ME: Does retirement hurt well-being? Factors influencing self-esteem and depression among retirees and workers, *Gerontologist* 36(5):649, 1996.

Roberto KA, Skoglund RR: Interactions with grandparents and great-grandparent: a comparison of activities, influences, and relationships, *Int J Aging Human Devel* 43(2):107, 1996.

Robinson B: Validation of a caregiver strain index, *J Gerontology* 38:344, 1983.

Roe KM, Minkler M: Grandparents raising grandchildren: challenges and responses, *Generations* 22(4):25, 1998-1999.

Ruffner SS: *A liberal education,* Santa Barbara, CA, 1991, Fithian Press.

Schmall V, Cleland M, Sturdevant M: *The caregiver help book: powerful tools for caregiving,* Portland, 2000, Legacy Health Systems.

Schulz R, Beach SR: Caregiving as a risk factor for mortality: the caregiver health effects study, *JAMA* 262:2215, 1999.

Scott JP: Sisters in later life: changes in contact and availability. In Roberto K, editor: *Relationships between women in later life,* New York, 1996, Haworth Press.

Shagrin SS: Retirement saving and financial planning, *Generations* 26(11):40, 2002.

Smilkstein G, Ashworth C, Montano D: Validity and reliability of the family APGAR as a test of family function, *J Fam Pract* 15(2):303-311, 1982.

Somary K, Stricker G: Becoming a grandparent: a longitudinal study of expectations and early experiences as a function of sex and lineage, *Generations* 38(1):53, 1998.

Sullivan MT: *Caregiver strain index, from Robinson,* New York, 2002, John A Hartford Foundation Institute for Geriatric Nursing.

Tafford A: *The bonus decades,* New York, 2002, Basic Books.

Taylor MA, Shore LM: Predictors of planned retirement age: an application of Beehr's model, *Psychol Aging* 10(1):76, 1995.

Troll L, Miller S, Atchley R: *Families in later life,* Belmont, CA, 1979, Wadsworth.

Troope M: *Grandparents and other relatives raising children,* Washington, DC, 2000, Generations United.

U.S. Administration on Aging: *Facts about older Americans,* 2000. Available at *www.aoa.gov*

U.S. Bureau of the Census: *Statistical abstract of the United States: 2002,* ed 122, Washington, DC, 2001, U.S. Government Printing Office.

U.S. Divorce Statistics: DivorceMagazine.com, December 2002. Available at *www.divorcemag.com/statistics/statsUS.shtml*

Waldren RK: Dad made night special, reminisce, *Psychol Rep* 76(2):482, 1995.

Welsh WM, Stewart AJ: Relationships between women and their parents: implications for midlife well-being, *Psychol Aging* 10(2):181, 2003.

Wentowski G: Older women's perceptions of great-grandmotherhood: a research note, Gerontologist 25(6):593, 1985.

Whitlack CJ, Noelker LS: Caregiving and caring. In Birren JE, editor: *Encyclopedia of gerontology: age, aging and the aged,* San Diego, 1996, Academic Press.

Yates ME, Tennestedty S, Chang BH: Contributors to and mediators of psychological well-being for informal caregivers, *J Gerontol: Psychol Sci* 54B(1):12, 1999.

Zarit SH, Zarit JM: *Mental disorders in older adults,* New York, 1998, Guilford Press.

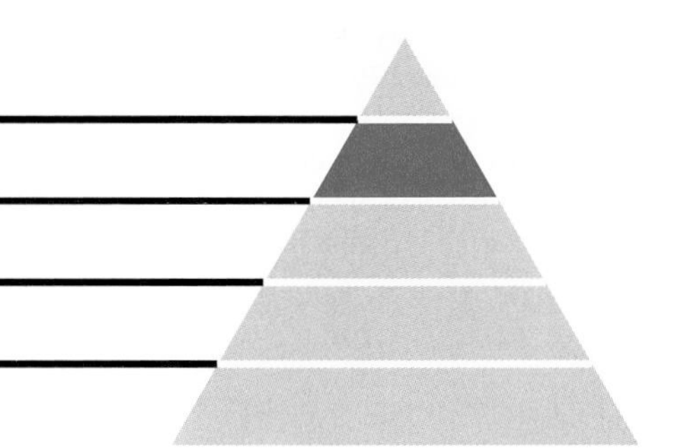

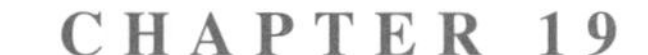

CHAPTER 19

Gender and Culture

Patricia Hess

A youth speaks

The old ones, in their seventies or eighties, with long memories of hardships faced and perhaps only partially (if at all) surmounted, deprived of education, made to feel hopelessly inarticulate, and obviously out of "the American mainstream," they are nevertheless men and women who seem to have held stubbornly to a peculiar notion: that they are eminently valuable and important human beings, utterly worth the respect, even admiration, not to mention the love, of their children and grandchildren.

Description of the Chicanos of New Mexico in Coles R: *The old ones,* Albuquerque, 1973, University of New Mexico Press.

LEARNING OBJECTIVES

On completion of this chapter, the reader will be able to:

1. Identify personal factors contributing to ethnic and cultural sensitivity.
2. Relate major historical events that have affected each cohort of elders.
3. Compare several different ethnically based approaches to health care.
4. Specify some gender characteristics that have been identified in recent studies.
5. Explain various ways in which ethnic groups may be incorporated into the larger culture.
6. Discuss approaches that facilitate an appreciation of diverse cultural and ethnic experiences.
7. Formulate a care plan incorporating ethnically sensitive interventions.

Differences Related To Birth Circumstance

Geographic origin, historical events, cohort position, and gender create significant individual differences within any culture. As our aged become more diverse and heterogeneous we are constantly challenged to understand their needs and help them obtain access to appropriate resources.

Competent role enactment requires a bio-psycho-socio-political-spiritual-cultural perspective. The increasing specificity and accumulation of knowledge on any of these topics make this charge appear not only impossible but one of sheer grandiosity. If we hope to approach this commitment to persons of various cultures, cohorts, and social strata we must learn to be expert listeners—to fact and innuendo, to nonverbal messages, to the subjects that are avoided, to messages acted out, to group statements as well as those of individuals. *We must become skilled in deciphering the unstated agenda in political and economic communication.* And we must certainly try to understand the messages some of our minority citizens receive through the structure of our health care system.

In this chapter we consider old people from other cultures and subcultures; those whose childhoods were marked by distant social and world events; youth of another time and place; and the marked gender differences that existed. We suggest ways that nurses may help the elderly preserve their individuality.

Cohorts

A *cohort* (in geographic circles) is a group of people born within the same time span, most often a decade. Thus a cohort would contain all the people born in the United States between 1900 and 1909. These rigid boundaries fit nicely with statistical and actuarial tables but not so well with people. However, it is useful to consider the "cohort effects" of major national and world events. How would a child of 7 be affected by the Great Depression? A youth of 17? A man of 27? Each would be influenced to a different degree by the same event. Usually political ideology and wars affect adolescents and young adults profoundly; health patterns and educational changes significantly affect children's lives. Mature adults are affected most by relocation and financial and natural disasters. They have accumulated more, have established extensive personal networks, and have much to lose. Wars, economic disasters, great discoveries, shifts in moral values, and progress in health care will alter how one experiences life.

Birth cohort effects have been recognized as significant, but few intensive/extensive, qualitative longitudinal studies exist to elucidate the impact on one's life of his or her cohort. Even more difficult is to account for the effects of geography on cohort. Seigler and colleagues (1992) briefly discuss this phenomenon as it has affected centenarians of Georgia. Segregation, population composition, religious predominance, differences in opportunity for formal education, and numerous other factors interrelate with cohort, raising far more questions than answers.

Elders are the embodiment of living history. They tell it like it was from their vantage point, and in the process, if we listen, they tell us about themselves; they tell us how and why they grew up as they did. Reminiscing has been one of the most entertaining means elders have for sharing their life story and enriching the young. Each cohort has a different view, and each individual within the cohort carries innumerable variations of the story. Older persons will vary greatly in how they view the world, and part of this variance results from the impact of historical eras and beliefs surrounding them.

The study of the aged is anthropologic. Our aged citizens and immigrants form a mosaic of multicultural backgrounds and decade differences. Each decade closes the door on a vanishing breed. *A civilization disappears with the death of each cohort.* The urgency of meeting their needs and preserving the heritage they carry becomes more pressing as technologic advances propel us forward with ever-increasing speed. To properly serve them and learn from them, we must stop to listen.

In the United States today there are the rural aged in communities; the rural aged on farms; the urban aged in ghettos; the urban aged in exclusive penthouses; the suburban aged living with families, spouse, or alone; the retired aged who have sought warm climates; the migrant aged; the settled aged; the immigrant aged; the native-born aged; and the first-, second-, and third-generation aged from countries around the world. The aged can also be described by their state of health or illness, by their marital and family status, by cohort, and by gender.

Many studies focus on generational differences and the conflicts or alliances between generations. We suggest that each generation has a unique perspective of life based on its historic spot in time, and although the individual's view may shift and change, some remnant of the cohort effect will always remain. Cohort and gender differences, in addition to the discussion here, are addressed throughout the text.

Gender

Gender, which refers to the personal, cultural meaning of biologic differences, is fundamental to personal identity and is the primary way in which experiences are organized. There are some definite gender variations in demographics (Table 19-1). Gender incorporates those and other less measurable characteristics that are the result of a coalescence of cohort, culture, and genetics. Environmental influences, social expectations, and early training, as well as innate capacities, all seem to fall within the purview of these three categories. Interestingly, in the previous editions of this textbook we did not have a category related to gender alone because there was so little to be found that identified gender characteristics in the old.

We are now finding more studies related to gender. In 1990 an entire issue of *Generations* (the journal of the American Society on Aging) was devoted to gender and aging (American Society on Aging, 1990). Gender-focused research centers have also been created. The goals of a gender-focused research center include such aims as the following:

- Basic and clinical research related to gender-specific needs and characteristics
- Developing and testing gender-specific therapeutic strategies
- Providing gender-appropriate health recommendations
- Disseminating research findings that promote understanding of gender-specific issues

To identify the relevance of gender is exceedingly difficult and requires a breadth of perspective and objectivity not easily achieved by either sex. In the last two decades we have moved

Table 19-1 Gender-significant Statistics (Not Including Ethnic Variations)

At age 65 and over	Male	Female
Population	14.4 million	20.8 million
Life expectancy at birth	72.2 years	79.8 years
Life expectancy at 65	16 years	19.2 years
Married	77%	43%
Widowed	13%	47%
Live in family	81%	58%
Live alone	16%	40%
Median income	$19,168	$10,899
Below poverty level	7.5%	12.2%
Employed	17%	10%
Need help with ADLs	18%	26%
Need help with IADLs	19%	35%
Annual days of restricted activity	30	36
Suicide/100,000	152.6	19.2
Alzheimer's disease per 100,000 (age adjusted)	30.8	28.1
Heart disease–related deaths per 100,000	2058.5	1712.0

Data from US Census Bureau: Gender 2000: census 2000 brief, *www.census.gov*; Administration on Aging: Profile of older Americans: 2000, *www.AOA.gov/aoa/Stats/profile*; Administration on Aging: Highlights 2001, *www.AOA.gov/aoaprofile2001/highlights.html*.

from simply describing biologic differences to an emphasis on the shaping of gender roles by socialization patterns, and we are now in a phase of describing gender in terms of social structure and cultural patterns (Hendricks, 1990; Hooyman and Kiyak, 1996).

Gender-specific information, although accruing, remains limited. The important message is that one must not make presumptions about the aged and their needs. Be cognizant that culture, cohort, and gender have all influenced the client's values, perceptions, and needs. Discuss these issues.

Survival and the Gender Gap. At every age, beginning in embryo, females outlast males. In later life it was thought that female hormones protect against hypercholesterolemia and heart disease. They also tend to enhance the immune system. However, women have a higher incidence of autoimmune diseases and nonfatal conditions that contribute to frailty and functional decline. Although women have fewer suicides in old age, they are more likely to suffer from anxiety and depression. These data are confounded by the fact that women seek help for physical and emotional disorders more frequently than do men. It has been thought that men tend to be more stoic and less likely to express feelings and, in the work setting, are subject to stressors that have particularly devastating effects on their survival. Clearly, many of these assumptions were cohort based and were never backed by solid evidence. Speculations regarding the contributions of the Y and the X chromosome to sex/gender differences abound. So far, nothing conclusive can be shown, although obviously these account for some inherent differences.

Gender Issues. One of the major issues in late life is that of caretaking. Numerous studies have shown caretaking as primarily a woman's role. Many frail old women take care of a frail old spouse to the detriment of their own health. And after years of subverting their own needs, they become so intermingled with those of the spouse that on the death of the spouse, they are at a loss for filling the empty time and heart (Ebersole, 1996). Interestingly, a study done by Kaye and Applegate (1995) provided strong support for the unwavering devotion and direct caregiving capacity of old men, most often caring for a spouse with a disabling chronic illness. Because of our gender stereotypes, we may not have looked closely enough at the actual caregiving situation with old couples.

Another gender statistic that has been widely accepted must be examined; that is, that a significantly greater number of older women are afflicted with Alzheimer's disease. The incidence of Alzheimer's disease increases exponentially with age so that the extended survival of women skews the statistics.

Women. "In neither the women's movement nor the old age movement have concerns of older women been centrally featured" (Hudson and Gonyea, 1990). Women, in numbers sufficient to influence policy, have never been a part of our governing bodies. For older women, cohort socialization and socioeconomic status have played a large part in subduing activism. Older women are becoming more active politically, but considering that they were the first generation given the right to vote, there is much yet to be done.

The Older Women's League (OWL) grew out of the White House Mini-Conference in Des Moines in 1980. The organization continues to be a strong political advocate for the needs and concerns of older women. The major goals of the organization are to improve the status and image of older women while achieving economic and social equity and building a mutually supportive network.

Woods and Shaver (1992) describe the launching of the Center for Women's Health Research at the University of Washington, under the aegis of the National Center for Nursing Research.

Cardiac care given to women is usually not as intense or as immediate as that given to men. Older women with a heart disorder can expect to be treated less energetically than men. More women than men die of heart attacks each year. There are several possible reasons: hormonal protection before menopause may give a false sense of security to women, as well as their physicians; heart drugs have not as yet been tested on older women, so the normal reactions and side effects are unknown. The risk of death for women who have coronary artery angioplasty is five times that of men of the same age with similar medical histories, and women are two to three times less likely to survive coronary artery bypass (FDA Consumer, 1996). A study of "clot-busting" drugs found that the drugs worked just as well with both men and women except that 1 month later 13% of the women, compared with 5% of the men, died. It was thought that this occurred because the women in the study were at least 10 years older than the men of the sample and had more cardiac risks factors such as high blood pressure and diabetes, yet the gender differences in mortality rate could not be fully explained (Christensen, 1997). Throughout adult life, before age 65, men are much more at risk for heart disorders. Legato (2002), in her book *Eve's Rib,* wrote that research protocols and public health policies reflect intellectual mistakes of astounding proportions and undoubtedly affect the health and lives of many women over the years, and Legato notes that physiologic details are only beginning to emerge.

Many topics related to concerns unique to women have been identified. Those most related to older women include breast self-examination and female aging experiences in various ethnic groups. Journals and newsletters devoted to women's health issues tend to focus on few topics relevant to older women except breast cancer, menopause, and osteoporosis. Some medical centers have now developed special health history forms for women that include, in addition to basic health history and physical examination, detailed information about reproductive organs, sexual history, lifestyle factors, psychologic well-being, and special health support services that are desired. In reality, aside from the specificity of questions regarding reproductive organs, these special histories should be useful for men as well. Little is actually known about the characteristics of very old women.

We often hear about unequal distribution of economic resources between men and women. Yet there are numbers of old women who inherit vast estates on the death of their husbands. It is possible that the maldistribution of resources within the gender is a critical problem that gets little attention. However, it is clear that very old women who have not worked outside the home and did not have wealthy husbands are likely to be poverty stricken if they survive to outlive their limited savings. The vast majority of women across cultures in the United States who worked earned less than their male conterparts or are first-, second-, or third-generation immigrants and did not work.

Studies specific to women have been appearing in recent years. Wagnild and Young (1990), in an attempt to describe the characteristics of resilient older women, found five underlying themes through using a grounded theoretical research approach. Equanimity, self-reliance, existential aloneness, perseverance, and meaningfulness all seemed to constitute resilience and gave evidence of successful psychosocial adjustment. Grounded theory must be rigorously replicated if it is to be relevant.

A longitudinal study of over 500 remarkable women born between 1900 and 1910 was conducted by Day (1992). She has identified three characteristics common to all: a strong sense of independence, dedication to interests outside of self, and gratifying social relationships.

The women's issues that are prominent and will continue to make inroads in the twenty-first century include the following:

- An aging society that consists primarily of women because they are the fastest growing segment of society
- Inadequate health and long-term care
- Economic jeopardy with the threat to Social Security, as well as insufficient pensions

Men. It is difficult to find studies devoted to describing any abiding characteristics of aged men. A largely male veteran sample has formed the basis for a mass of research on "the aged." These data formed the basis for conclusions about aging that, when presented, often lacked gender specificity but were applied as if they were appropriate. A case in point is the oft-repeated statistic that the aged are more highly suicidal than any other group. This is untrue. Aged men, particularly white men, have the highest suicide rates. Women do not. Gender-significant variations are presented in Tables 19-1 and 19-2.

A number of questions arise when discussing gender issues. Some questions to ponder include the following:

- Why, if older women have so many disadvantages, do they survive longer and seemingly maintain morale, in spite of being old, poor, and alone?
- Why is it so difficult for men to seek medical help before serious, life-threatening conditions occur?
- What effect will the baby boomers have on gender parity or disparity?

Table 19-2 Gender Differences

	Male	Female
Mental disorders	Addiction Personality disorders	Neuroses Depression
Cognitive function (specific capacities)	Spatial ability Accuracy Mathematics	Processing information Verbal skills
Personality	Both sexes are thought to become more androgenous—"gender free"	
Role behavior (most likely troublesome)	Work transition	Poverty
Living situation		
With spouse	73%	41%
With relatives	7%	17%
Alone or with nonrelative(s)	20%	42%

Population Diversity

The United States continues to experience a "gerontologic explosion" of ethnically diverse adults 65 years of age and older that will persist for at least the next 30 years (Administration on Aging, 2001). Approximately 14% of the population was age 65 and older in 1995. The year 2000 saw a decrease to 12% in the aged population as those born during and following the depression reach age 65. By 2010 the baby boomers will again increase the older population to 14%. By 2025 older adults will make up about 20% of the population (U.S. Bureau of the Census, 2000; Administration on Aging, 2001). In approximately 30 years, minority elders will represent 25% of the total aged population.

The U.S. Bureau of the Census (2000) projects that Hispanics will represent 13%; African Americans 17%; Asian and Pacific Islanders 12%; and Native Americans, Eskimos, and Aleuts 11% of the elder population. White elders will constitute only 47% of the older population.

The present and expected growth and diversity of the elderly population means that nurses will be caring for a significant number of minority elders, both new immigrants and citizens, immediately and in the future. Standard care approaches will not necessarily be appropriate for the emerging group of elders and the subgroups who are ethnically and culturally diverse in needs, abilities, and resources. Figure 19-1 illustrates the expected population growth and distribution by ethnicity of the aged, 65 years of age and over, by 2050.

Minority Elders. The number of minority elders in the United States has increased faster than white elders (Figure 19-2). There are now more than 2.9 million African Americans over 65 years old, 2.5 million Hispanics, 9.6 million Asian/Pacific Islanders, and approximately 180,000 Native Americans (U.S. Bureau of the Census, 2000). Each has special social and cultural needs.

The status of minority elders in the United States reflects the social, economic, and discrimination barriers. In 1994 one fifth (19%) of the older population was poor or near poor (American Association of Retired Persons, 1995); In 2000 10.2% of adults 65 and older were at or below the poverty level (U.S. Bureau of the Census, 2000). Figures 19-3 and 19-4 graphically show the poverty rates over a 41-year period for those 65 and older and for minorities in general. The percentage of elderly Hispanics living in poverty is the highest of all the minority groups at 38.8%.

Sharing a home with an adult child is more common among the ethnic elderly than among whites. African American elderly persons commonly live with family members or family members live with them, and only 3% over 65 and 12% age 85 and older are institutionalized.

Hispanic elderly persons often (72%) live with a family member; 3% over age 65 and 10% age 85 or older are institutionalized.

Among the Asian/Pacific Islander elderly, 96% live in the community, 77% live with someone, and 2% over age 65 and 10% over age 85 live in institutions. One fourth of the Native American elderly live on reservations, 66% live with family members, some live alone, and 13% were institutionalized after age 85 (Hooyman and Kiyak, 1996). The question arises as to whether this is due to cultural factors or economic necessity.

The sex ratio is approximately 141 women for every 100 men. As age increases, the sex ratio for the 65 to 69 age-group increases from 118 women per 100 men to 237 women per 100 men for the 85 and older age-group (Administration on Aging, 2000).

Immigration in Late Life. There was a great wave of European immigration in the early part of the twentieth century. The influx of aged Asians, Filipinos, and other individuals from the Pacific Rim to the western states has been significant in the past 20 years.

European immigration consisted of many youths and families, but the immigration from Asia and the Pacific Islands

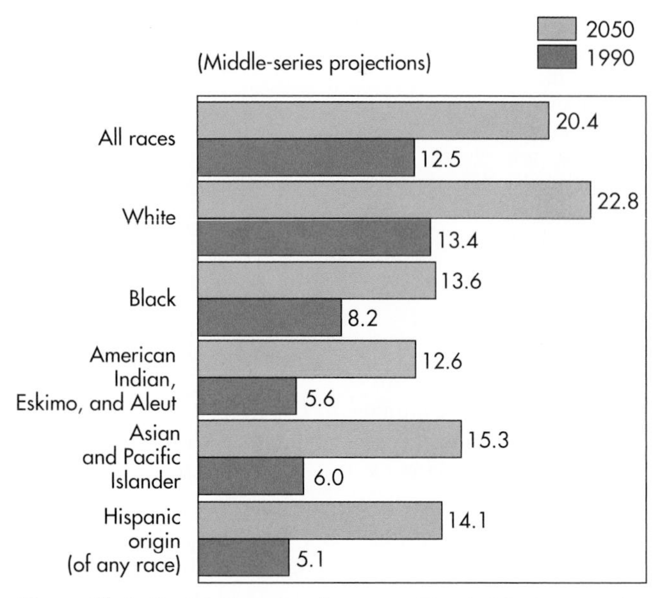

Figure 19-1. Racial diversity of persons 65 and older in percent, 1990 versus 2050. (Source: Hobbs FB: The elderly population, U.S. Census Bureau. Available at *www.census.gov/population/www/pop-profile/elderpop.html*)

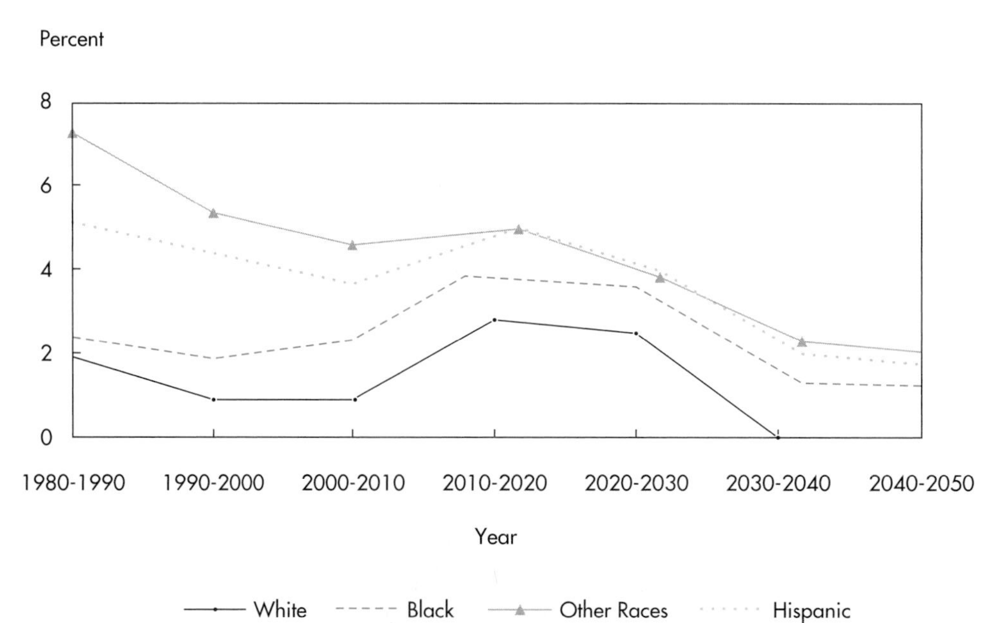

Figure 19-2. Annual rate of increase in elderly population by race and ethnicity: 1980-2050. (Modified from Angel JL, Hogan DP: The demography of minority aging populations. In *Minority aging,* Washington, DC, 1994, Gerontological Society of America.)

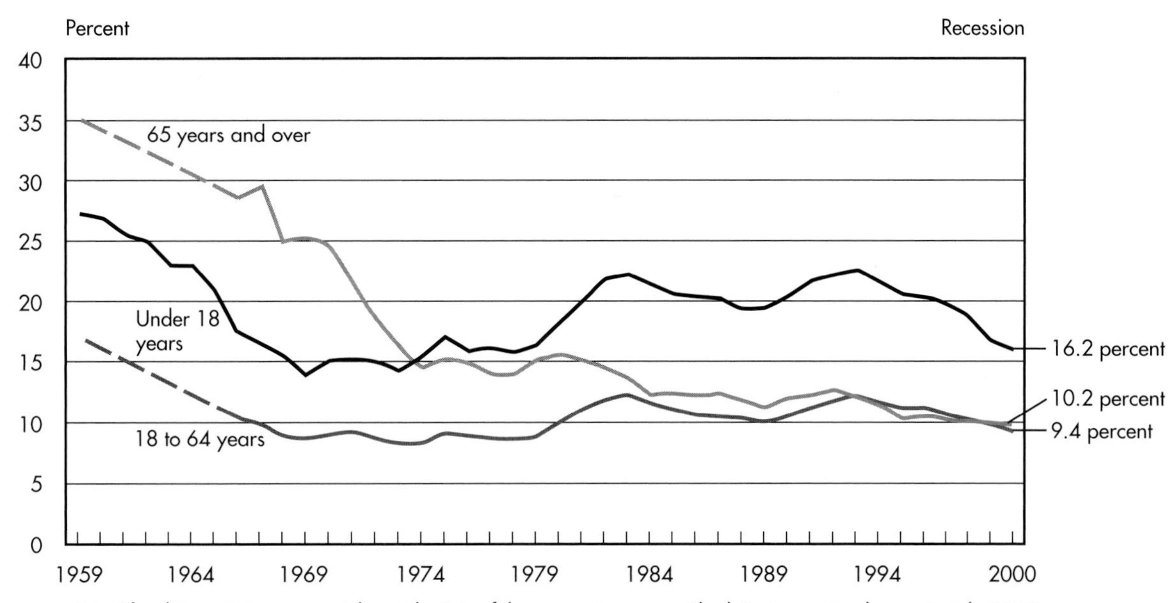

Figure 19-3. Poverty rates by age: 1959-2000. (Source: U.S. Bureau of the Census: Current population survey, March 1960–2001.)

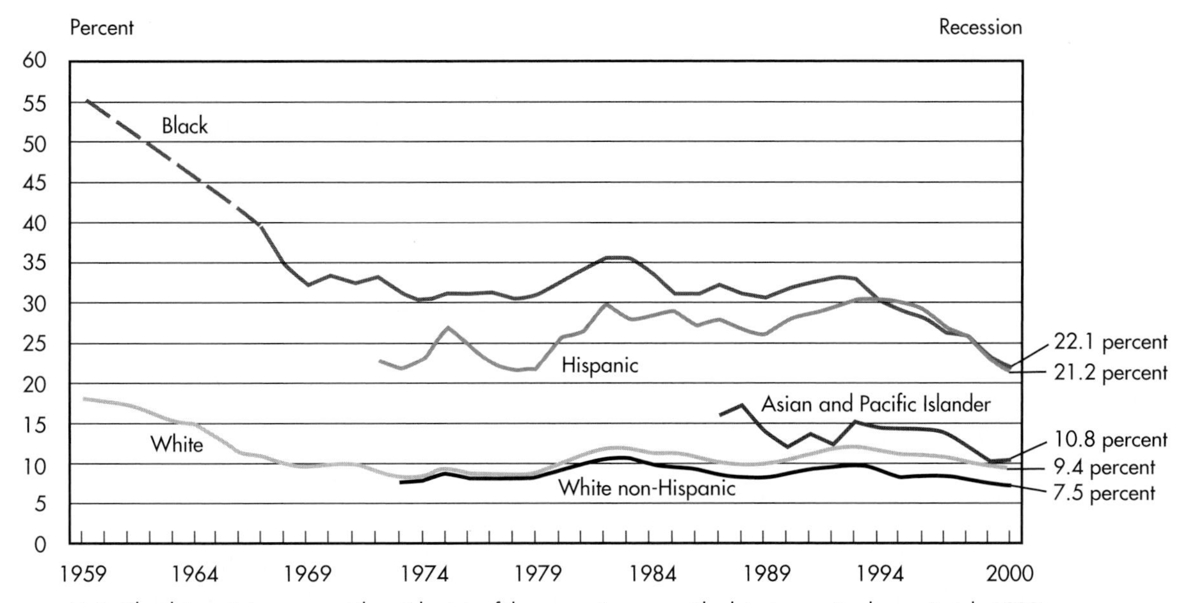

Figure 19-4. Poverty rates by race and Hispanic origin: 1959-2000. (Source: U.S. Bureau of the Census: Current population survey, March 1960-2001.)

is often of elders who have come to the United States to join their children. They mourn the "old country" and wish to return, but their children want to watch over and care for them. Relocation to a new culture and language in late life has not been thoughtfully examined in the literature, but from anecdotal information the relocation seems to impinge on the sense of personal continuity and security. Resources that are available are underused, and the transplanted individual may lack the social and cultural nourishment necessary for satisfaction even though survival needs may be met at a higher level than in the mother country. Table 19-3 documents foreign-born population age 65 and older (naturalized citizens and noncitizens who have immigrated to the United States).

Sarina came to the United States in 1986 at the urging of her oldest son. He provided home, security, and love, but she missed the farm in the Philippines, and she worried about her son and grandchildren

Table 19-3 Naturalized and Noncitizen Foreign-Born Population Ages 65 and Older (from 1990-2000)

	Ages 65-74	Ages 75-84	Ages 85+
Total (%)	1778 (14%)	965 (10%)	373 (7%)
Male (N = 1347) (12%)	102 (7%)	54 (4%)	5 (0.03%)
Female (N = 1769) (11%)	141 (7%)	40 (2%)	19 (1%)

From Foreign-born population age 55 years and over by sex, citizenship, year of entry, and age: March 2000. In U.S. Census Bureau: *Current population survey, March 2000,* Special Populations Branch, Population Division. Internet release date: June 1, 2001.

who remained in the Philippines and pleaded to return. She was alone during the day while her family all worked or went to school. She consciously avoided learning English because her Tagalog was her last link with the past and her roots. Her isolation and depression were clearly related to the discontinuity of lifestyle and relationships.

Language. We seldom think of language as the foundation of self-concept, but the self is continuously constructed and inextricably bound up with the linguistic categories available in a given culture (Berman, 1991). We can only conceive of ourselves within the language we know.

To make each contact with the elderly fully meaningful, shared communication is essential. Communication with persons of a different culture, ethnic group, or geographic region is an issue not only of language but also of idiom, style, jargon, voice tone, and inflection.

Even if it were possible for a nurse to learn all these vagaries, it would likely not be useful. It would be similar to entering a family and using all the pet names and phrases treasured by the family. In most cases the artificiality and intrusive nature of such an action would be irritating.

Asking the individual about a phrase can be illuminating. In turn, we must remember that as health professionals our jargon and idiomatic expressions may be perceived as frightening or threatening. They will most certainly increase the social distance between the provider and the client.

Never assume you know what an aged person means. Ask him or her. If the primary language of the person is not English or is different from that of the care provider, every effort should be made to find an interpreter (one who processes oral language, which preserves meaning and tone and registers the original language without adding or deleting anything) rather than a translator (who only restates words from one language to another) (Purnell and Paulanka, 1998; Enslein et al, 2002). In old age people find comfort in their mother tongue. However, when family members are used as interpreters, they may be unable to aid a care provider because of role conflicts or inability to use medical terms appropriately. Often messages to the client and the provider are based on the interpreter's perception of the situation, and vital information may be withheld or omitted to shield the client from family embarrassment. Whenever possible, health care personnel should use the services of a professional interpretor who is available to or assigned to the setting in which the care provider works.

In working with these elders, nurses must recognize the importance of their identification with past patterns and relationships. They are often living on the edge of anonymity. The most significant intervention is to find someone who speaks their language and can discuss their previous lifestyle. (See Box 19-1 regarding the use of interpreters.) They may also enjoy senior centers designed specifically for their cultural needs. Churches may be another important source of other elders of the same ethnic background. Families need to understand that no matter how pleasant the surroundings, displaced individuals long for the old ways and are experiencing a grief process. If they can be encouraged to talk about the losses,

Box 19-1 Hints to Working with Interpreters

- Use a trained and professional interpreter.
- Before an interview with a client, try to meet with the interpreter to explain the purpose of the session.
- Try to get an interpreter of the same sex, age range, and social status as the client, particularly if sensitive subject information is needed or given.
- Encourage the interpreter to meet with the client before the session to identify the educational level, attitudes toward health and health care, and the depth and type of information and explanation needed.
- Look and speak directly to the client, not the interpreter.
- Be patient. Interpreted interviews take more time because longer explanatory phrases are often needed.
- Use short units of speech. Long, involved sentences or complex discussions create confusion.
- Use simple language. Avoid technical terms, professional jargon, slang, abbreviations, abstractions, metaphors, and idiomatic expressions.
- Encourage the interpreter to avoid inserting his or her own ideas or interpretations or omitting information.
- Listen to the client, and watch nonverbal communication (facial expression, voice intonation, body movement) to learn about emotions related to a specific topic.
- Clarify the client's understanding and the accuracy of the interpretation by asking the client to tell you in his or her own words what the client understands, facilitated by the interpreter.
- Avoid using family members unless client preference. Children, especially young ones, should strongly be discouraged to interpret because of cultural barriers, hierarchy, and lack of language proficiency.

Modified from Lipson JG, Dibble SL, Minarik PA, editors: *Culture and nursing care: a pocket guide,* San Francisco, 1996, UCSF School of Nursing Press; Purnell LD, Paulanka BJ: Transcultural diversity and health care. In Purnell LD, Paulanka BJ, editors: *Transcultural health care,* Philadelphia, 1998, FA Davis.

they may experience the relief that comes with ventilation in the presence of a concerned listener. These individuals often neglect health care because they may not know what is available to them; language is a barrier to information and expression of health needs. In addition, they may be frightened by the health care system and, in some instances, in the country illegally, thus creating additional fears.

Ethnicity. The terms *ethnicity* and *culture* are frequently used interchangeably. In reality, a distinct difference exists in meanings. Ethnicity is a complex phenomenon. It is a social differentiation based on cultural criteria (Giger and Davidhizar, 1991; Gunter, 1991; Spector, 1996). Most important, there is a shared identity.

An ethnic group may share common geographic origins, migratory status, race, language, and dialect. Religious factors (ties that transcend kinship, neighborhoods, and community boundaries) are also important in ethnicity. Traditions, values, symbols, literature, folklore, and diverse food preferences also should be considered a part of ethnicity. Settlement and employment patterns, special interests or politics in the homeland and in the United States, and an internal sense of distinctiveness or perception of external distinctiveness are additional facets of ethnicity that must be considered (Giger and Davidhizer, 1991; Gunter, 1991; Spector, 2000).

Thus ethnicity involves three components: culture, social status, and support systems. These components influence the way people feel about themselves and how they interact with their environment (Hooyman and Kiyak, 1996). Moore (1971) cites five characteristics that constitute an ethnic minority:

- Each group has a specific history.
- The history has been accompanied by discrimination.
- A subculture develops.
- Coping structures develop.
- Rapid change occurs.

Our obligation is not to seek out minutiae of rituals and folkways or differences in habits of living, but to respect those important to the individual. When we insist on regimented care, we infringe on an individual's ability to maintain his or her own cultural orientation.

Writers create a recipe book that often focuses on nutritional patterns, folk medicine, death rituals, and specific cultural beliefs of ethnic groups. *These generalities may not meet individual needs and may serve only to stereotype a person into artificial boundaries.* It is therefore difficult to write about or do justice to the Mexican American (also referred to as Chicano), Raza Latina (Latin American), black American (African American), Native American (American Indian), or Asian and other groups because of the internal heterogeneity that exists within each ethnic community.

For example, it is estimated that there are 2.2 million American Indians who speak 250 different languages besides English. Each of the more than 500 federally recognized tribes, nations, bands, and native villages or groups have different customs, mores, and needs (Kramer, 1996; Spector, 1996; U.S. Bureau of the Census, 2000). Spanish-speaking persons are often lumped together as if a homogeneous group, but there are Mexican Americans, Puerto Ricans, Cubans, Central and South Americans, and Spaniards. All these people may be labeled Hispanic, which tells little about individual and group differences. Yet each major category shares certain distinctive cultural aspects. For this reason, general information is presented, which may help the caregiver develop an elemental and broad understanding basic to various cultural groups.

Ethnic elders prefer programs and services where the staff reflect the ethnic background and speak the language of the elderly clientele.

Adequate and quality health care for the minority elders of today and tomorrow revolves around the issues of appropriate programs for them and cultural relativism. One of the most pervasive barriers to improving services has been the failure of caregivers to recognize race as a critical factor in the provision of such services. Others have noted that effective service delivery to ethnic elders requires a conscious effort to be responsive to the cultural uniqueness of these elderly populations. An example of just what cultural relativism in a senior center can do is described by Ochoco and Shimamoto (1987). They found that by introducing ethnic-related activities at a senior center in Hawaii they were able to increase patient self-esteem, independence, and satisfaction. Many of the participants had been passive, dependent, and depressed.

Two thirds were widowed women who had originally emigrated from Japan. Because a language barrier existed, some of the widows lived with children and deferred to their wishes to the neglect of their own self-esteem and self-concept. The community health nurse who activated the group wished to strengthen the sense of self in group members through a focus on cultural heritage. In addition to health teaching sessions and education about the aging process, the nurse used reminiscence and construction of a collective oral history to stimulate interaction and the sense of accomplishment. This model is adaptable to many community and institutional settings.

Culture

Rousseau, an eighteenth-century romantic, believed human nature to be noble and essentially scarred and distorted by civilization and culture. However, when Victor, the Wild Boy of Aveyron, was found at the end of the century, sociologists and anthropologists were confronted with the reality that the "noble savage" does not exist apart from a culture and an organizing experience represented by symbols. The capacity to develop these and the degree to which they are developed is the essence of human nature. Geertz (1973) says that we are incomplete or unfinished animals who finish ourselves through culture. Culture is, in its simplest concept, bonding with a group through collective interests or concerns, and thus the capacity for communicating these concerns becomes the root of culture. It then becomes easier to understand the origins and development of a culture that in vanished ages was at the mercy of certain geographic formations and natural resource availability (Geertz, 1973).

Culture, on the other hand, is an integrated pattern of behavior, a learned way of acting, communicating (language), and thinking of a particular group that is transmitted to others (Giger and Davidhizar, 1991; Gunter, 1991; Purnell and Paulanka, 1998). Culture guides thinking, decision making, and actions (Leininger, 1978; Purnell and Paulanka, 1998).

Fejos (1959) defines culture as "the sum total of socially inherited characteristics of a human group that comprises everything which one generation can tell, convey, or hand down to the next; in other words, the non-physically inherited traits we possess." Culture is something each of us carries around for a lifetime.

Habayeb (1995) suggests that culture is a complex concept of interrelationships among beliefs, values, language, social relationships, and other factors. Habayeb goes on to state that culture is usually narrowly defined in terms of "color, religion, and geographic location" and "when cultural diversity is discussed in nursing, it is only in terms of minority or ethnic clients."

The nature of culture provides personhood and social relationships. It is the means of creating and limiting human choices and is expressed and identified by interlaced symbols; culture is an extension of biologic capabilities and can be two places at once—in the person's mind and also in the environment as artifacts or spoken word.

Any one definition of culture is too circumscribed, omitting salient aspects of culture and becoming too global to have any substantive meaning (Spector, 1996). For the purpose of having some definition, culture is the social process that is learned, changed, and taught. It is the matrix that influences (both consciously and unconsciously) successive generations. Particular aspects of culture such as knowledge, beliefs, art, law, morals, and customs are retained and passed on unaltered from one generation to the next, or fall by the wayside depending on the social, political, and economic forces in our lives (Bohannan, 1992).

The cultural matrix influences the self-concept and interactions of the individual in coping with and adjusting to life circumstances. It is the sum of intellectual, behavioral, and emotional expressions of living formed by a group of persons and transmitted to succeeding generations. Culture is the substratum that nourishes ethnic expressions. For example, the aged Jewish (culture) immigrants clustered together in Venice, California, form a subculture based on their ethnicity and expressed characteristically by certain ceremonies and language idiosyncrasies that convey their collective generational, geographic, and cultural identity. Variations exist in all cultures in all groups; some hold strong traditional values, and others are more contemporary.

Many of the differences in the elderly attributed to cultural variation may in reality be indications of educational differences, socioeconomic status, language limitations, misunderstanding or unawareness of potential resources, and wariness of the white middle-class professional agency personnel.

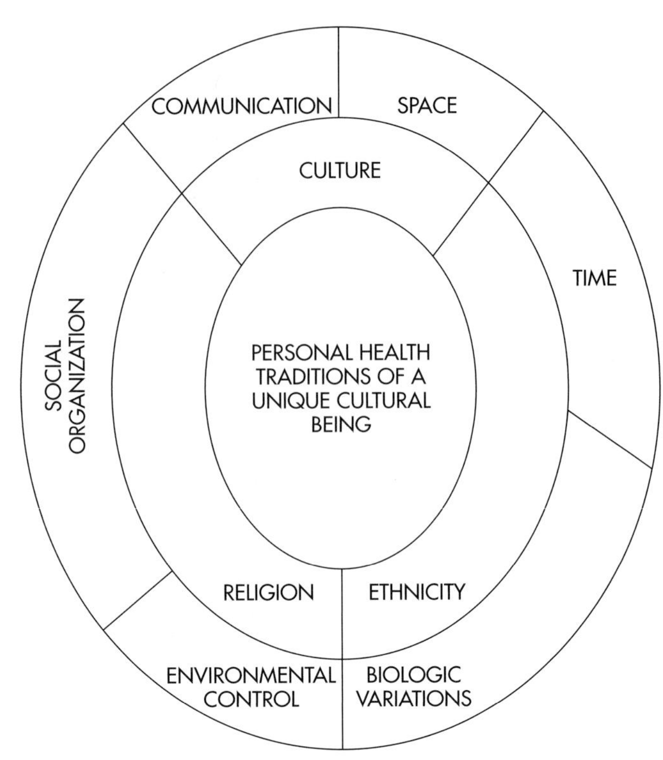

Figure 19-5. Personal health traditions of a unique cultural being. (From Spector RE: *Cultural diversity in health and illness,* ed 5, Upper Saddle River, NJ, 2000, Pearson Education, Inc., p 89.)

To fully understand another culture, one must enter into an unknown conceptual world in which time, space, religion, tradition, and wellness are expressed through a unique language that conveys these formulations about the nature of the world and humanity. Heritage consistency is a component of many features: communications, space, time, socialization, environment, and biology. These in turn affect culture, religion, and ethnicity. Collectively, the personal uniqueness is established. With regard to health, Figure 19-5 illustrates the relationship of these components. Terms that are associated with cultural consistency, such as assimilation, acculturation, socialization, ethnicity, ethnocentrism, and xenophobe, are important to understanding cultural diversity and acquiring cultural sensitivity (Box 19-2).

Assimilation and Adaptation

Four forms of assimilation occur, according to Spector (2000). These are culture, marital, primary structural, and secondary structural assimilation.

Culture assimilation is reflected in the ability to speak excellent English. *Marital assimilation* is recognized through the intermarriage of persons of different groups. *Primary assimilation* and *secondary structural assimilation* are determined by the extent of social mingling and friendship between groups. Primary assimilation reflects relationships that are warm and friendly in all settings (home, social groups, church),

Box 19-2 Definition of Terms Associated with Culture

Heritage consistency: The degree to which a person's lifestyle reflects his or her traditional culture; determination of one's cultural, ethnic, and religious background

Socialization: The process of being raised within a culture and acquiring the characteristics of that group

Acculturation: Becoming a competent participant in the dominant culture, even though one will always be identified as a member of a minority culture

Assimilation: The process of giving up or rejecting one's current cultural identity to develop a new cultural identity

Ethnicity: Belonging to a particular ethnic group within a cultural and social system based on such traits as religion, linguistics, and ancestral or physical characteristics

Ethnocentrism: The belief in the superiority of one's own ethnic group

Xenophobe: One who is unduly fearful or contemptuous of strangers or foreigners, especially as reflected in his or her political and cultural views

whereas in secondary structural assimilation, there is a nondiscriminatory sharing, but it is cold and impersonal in nature.

There has been much concern about aged immigrants and how culture facilitates or hinders their adjustment to old age. Pierce and colleagues (1978-1979) and Spector (1985) believed that various kinds of acculturation were more critical to functional adaptation than others. For example, outward adaptation to the Anglo culture that incorporates language, dress, and behavior was seen as superficially important. On a deeper level, traditional personal value orientations, including concepts of time, man to nature, and relationships, were more likely to remain in the original cultural context. Individually, it was found that most people had unique patterns of acculturation, each incorporating certain aspects of the Anglo culture and retaining some from the original homeland. This study demonstrated the difficulty in making conclusive statements related to one culture or another, and we should hesitate to make assumptions. Nurses need to spend time finding out those aspects of culture that remain significant to the individual (cultural relativism). If a language barrier exists, it is imperative to find an interpreter. In most universities and some high schools there are students of language who may be flattered to assist. (Refer to Box 19-1 regarding the use of interpreters.)

Cultural Competence and Sensitivity

Nurses must avoid an *ethnocentric* stance, that is, the belief that the values and practices of one's own culture are the best ones (Spector, 1996; Estes, 2002).

Cultural competence and sensitivity is being aware of the issues related to culture, race, gender, sexual orientation, social class, economic situations, and many other factors (Meleis et al, 1995; Pender et al, 2002) through knowledge and the ability to intervene appropriately and effectively. In sum, cultural competence encompasses a complex combination of knowledge, attitudes, mutual respect, skill, and negotiation (Chrisman, 1992). Attitudes are affected by experience, flexibility, empathy, and language facility. Skill includes cross-cultural communications, cultural interpretation, assessment, cultural interpretation of the assessment, and intervention (Lipson, 1996; Spector, 2000; Estes, 2002).

Knowledge is what the nurse learns and knows about the client, family, and community and their behaviors. Essential is knowledge of the person's way of life, ways of thinking, believing, and acting—knowledge obtained through personal experiences. Over time, the nurse builds up a reservoir of information about the beliefs of his or her clients and how they behave. An additional reservoir of knowledge comes from the clients and their families. Often nurses turn to these sources for information about ways they cope with chronic conditions and past health problems. Members of the health community who come from specific cultural backgrounds can also afford valuable data. A final source of knowledge comes from the literature. Books, pamphlets, articles, and journals can be significant sources of information about cultures different from that of the nurse. This knowledge needs to be taken and related to professional principles of nursing care. A common example of this is when a client adheres to his or her food customs, which are contrary to the client's therapeutic regimen. The nurse must weigh the nutritional value of the customs in order to recommend a reasonable substitute that will conform to the client's health state.

Mutual respect is closely allied with knowledge. It is working "with" the client rather than "on" the client. Knowledge allows the nurse to recognize and react more positively to seemingly strange and even bizarre health beliefs and practices. A nonjudgmental reaction due to knowledge about the ethnic group can signal to a client that the nurse trusts and respects the individual. Mutual respect is fundamental to culture-sensitive care because it opens opportunities for innovative planning of care that depends on trust between client and nurse (Chrisman, 1992; Abbot et al, 2002; Pender, 2002).

Negotiation should attempt to preserve helpful beliefs and practices, accommodate beliefs that are neither helpful nor harmful from the viewpoint of Western medicine, and repattern harmful beliefs or practices (Jackson, 1993). When repatterning is necessary, it is important to try to make the change without compromising underlying belief systems. When there is an impasse between client and nurse with each person perceiving the issue as nonnegotiable, the foundation of knowledge and trust or mutual respect that has been achieved will be helpful in seeking a goal that will optimize health outcomes beneficial to the client and still support the nurse's technical and ethical concerns.

In summary, the following steps are suggested to attaining cultural sensitivity and competence (Grossman, 1994; Spector, 1996, 2000):

- Know yourself: examine your own values, attitudes, beliefs, and prejudices and your cultural heritage and identity.
- Confront biases and stereotypes.
- Don't judge: don't measure others' behavior against your beliefs and values.
- Keep an open mind: attempt to look at the world through other cultures' perspectives.
- Respect differences among people: each group has strengths and weaknesses. Appreciate inherent worth of diverse cultures, value them equally, and do not consider them inferior to one's own.
- Listen! Develop the ability to hear things that transcend language, and foster understanding of the client and his or her cultural heritage and the resilience that supports family and community that comes from within the culture.
- Be willing to learn: this requires interest in people's beliefs, values, and practices. Travel, read, and attend events in the local ethnic or cultural events in the community.
- Become skilled in cultural assesment as a basis for designing culturally appropriate interventions.
- Develop an awareness and understanding of the complexities of the health care delivery system—its philosophy, problems, biases, and stereotypes—and become keenly aware of the socialization process that brings the care provider into this complex system.
- Be resourceful and creative: there are many ways to accomplish the same thing. Adapt your nursing interventions to suit different cultures and individuals.

Cultural Groups

Demographic and descriptive data about various cultural groups are useful in helping nurses to understand how and where they appear in the host culture. In many instances now there are printed and audiovisual materials available to assist the ethnic elder.

Asian/Pacific Island Americans. There are at least 30 different languages and cultures subsumed under Asian/Pacific Islanders. Statistical data lump the Chinese, Japanese, Asian Indians, Cambodians, Filipinos, Guamanians, Hawaiians, Samoans, Vietnamese, and others under the category of Asian/Pacific Islanders. This extremely diverse group contains elders who immigrated to the United States during the turn of the century, children born to these immigrants, and elderly refugees, primarily from Southeast Asia, who entered the United States in the 1970s and 1980s. Approximately 820,000 (7.7%) Asian/Pacific Islanders are 65 years of age and older. Of these, 64,000 (7.8%) are 85 years or over. As of the 2000 census, 49% of Asian/Pacific Islanders were concentrated in the Pacific Northwest and Pacific states. California has the largest single concentration of Asian/Pacific Islanders in that region (4.2 million). Smaller enclaves reside in other states, mainly in metropolitan areas, with only 10% or less living in rural areas (U.S. Bureau of the Census, 2000).

Although Asians vary immensely, they share certain characteristics that include a cyclic view of time, careful and orderly management of space, religious views that reinforce the importance of ancestry and tradition, languages written in imagery and expressed in subtleties, health practices that focus on vital balances within the organism, and, traditionally, a greater concern for collective goals than for individual pursuits, though this is changing among the young. Table 19-4 lists health problems, risk factors, and areas for health education for Asian/Pacific Island elderly.

Chinese. The aged Chinese who emigrated to the United States have special needs, and it is suggested that to serve them best the health care providers should communicate through the youth in the family, who are often within the U.S. educational system and conversant with the ways of the elders as well as those of the dominant culture (Lin, 1988). One of the frequent errors whites have made in attempting to respond to cultural needs is to assume that all members of a cultural or ethnic group share the same characteristics—a kind of benign stereotyping. We are becoming more discriminating now and are beginning to understand the vast differences within racial and cultural groups of the same generation but of different geographic roots. Lin (1988), a Chinese nursing student from Taiwan, refused to speculate about the needs of elderly Chinese who were not from Taiwan because she felt they were so distinctly different.

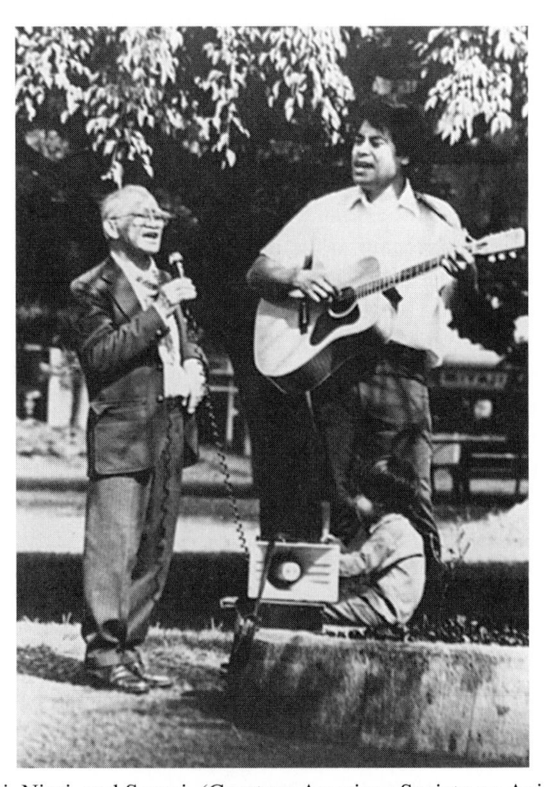

Issei, Nisei, and Sansei. (Courtesy American Society on Aging.)

Table 19-4 Leading Health Problems of Asian/Pacific Island Americans, Modifiable Risk Factors, and Education Areas

Diseases	Modifiable factors	Education areas
Filipinos, Japanese, Native Hawaiians, Chinese		
High blood pressure	Lack of exercise, smoking, obesity, diet (high sodium)	Proper use of medications Nutrition: sodium, cholesterol recipe modification
Japanese, Native Hawaiians		
Coronary heart disease	High blood pressure, high cholesterol levels, smoking, diabetes, alcohol	Exercise Preventive services/screening for hypertension and diabetes
Japanese, Chinese, Native Hawaiians		
Cancer	Smoking, diet, alcohol	
Japanese, Filipinos, Chinese, Koreans, Native Hawaiians		
Diabetes	Diet, obesity, lack of exercise, alcohol	

From American Association of Retired Persons: *Healthy aging: Making health promotion work for minority elders,* Washington, DC, 1990, The Association; Brangman SA: Minorities. In Ham RJ and Sloan PD, editors: *Primary care geriatrics,* ed 3, St Louis, 1997, Mosby; Cultural assessment. In Estes MEZ: *Health assessment and physical examination,* ed 2, Pacific Grove, CA, 2002, Delmar.

The Chinese are often known as quiet and noncomplaining patients. Caregivers interpret this as ideal behavior, but it may indicate conflict over modern treatment practices versus the traditional therapies and their tendency to hide feelings. Medical care may not be sought, or it may be rejected because of lack of funds, location of services, and lack of culturally sensitive health care services and personnel. The absence of bilingual staff creates a language barrier, often preventing adequate expression of these concerns. The strong belief in maintaining harmony may also be a factor in compliant behavior.

The traditional Chinese believe that health is physical and spiritual harmony, which originates from ancient Taoist religion and philosophy. The individual must seek harmony within the environment. Wood, fire, earth, metal, and water are the guiding principles for human beings.

Yin, the female negative energy (symbolized by cold, dark, and emptiness), and yang, the male positive energy (symbolized by light, warmth, and fullness), must be in balance for health to prevail. Yin protects vital strength of life, and Yang protects the body from outside forces. The body is viewed as a gift of the parents and forebears, which should be well cared for and maintained. Any procedure that is intrusive detracts from body harmony. Any disruption of harmony is regarded as the sole cause of disease.

Traditionally diagnosis was made by inspecting, listening, smelling, asking questions, and palpating for pulses. Male physicians were not allowed to touch women; diagnosis was made by using a figurine on which the woman indicated the malady. From this background, diagnostic studies performed in modern medical practice are not understood. Painful procedures may create confusion. The Chinese, however, accept immunization and x-ray examinations willingly.

Treatments by moxibustion, acupuncture, and herbal medicine to restore the balance of yin and yang are used by those Chinese who refuse modern medical assistance or are used in conjunction with today's medical practices. Health-seeking behavior is based on "whatever works." Western medicine is used for acute conditions, whereas Eastern medicine and cultural healers are used for chronic problems.

There are few left of the Chinese elderly who as young men immigrated to the United States early in the twentieth century with intentions of bringing the family later but, because of restrictive immigration laws, could not. When immigration laws relaxed after World War II, the Chinese were again thwarted by China's restrictive laws; people could not return to or leave China. However, by 1965, large numbers of refugees who had relatives in the United States were able to come to this country (Spector, 1996).

Japanese. Although increasingly acculturated to the United States, the feelings and attitudes of the older Japanese are strongly rooted in the cultural values and norms of their homeland. The Japanese Nisei (first American-born children of Japanese immigrants) were routinely sent to Japan by their parents (Issei) to be educated and socialized and as a means of cultural perpetuation. The Japanese immigrants did not expect much in terms of assimilation, equality, or expanded job opportunities; instead of demanding change, patience prevailed until opportunities arose.

Most Issei live in areas designated "Little Tokyo" or Nihonmachi, which remain relatively safe havens for the Japanese elderly. Traditional filial piety *(koko),* keeping problems to themselves, face-saving behaviors, limited fluency in the English language, and unfamiliarity with the social service bureaucracies are reasons for not using the larger community's resources. Discriminatory and hostile behaviors of health care providers are further barriers.

The Nisei adopted values and expected behaviors of American culture, but they were slow to be accepted and included in personal or social relationships with whites. The worst discrimination suffered by this group occurred during World War II, when over 70,000 American-born Japanese were confined to "relocation camps." Simultaneously, many of the young male Nisei were serving in the U.S. Army and stationed in Europe. There is probably a residue of bitterness, even among the Sansei (third generation) and Yonsei (fourth generation), although their devotion to politeness may cover these feelings. In the early 1990s the U.S. government acknowledged the inequities and disruption to the lives of the

Japanese Americans and made monetary restitution to those who had been interned in the relocation camps.

As part of cultural behavior, the elder may refuse an offer or offered object out of a sense of overpoliteness before accepting the offer. In the hospital, the Japanese patient may not turn on the call light until in dire need so as to not bother the staff. One perceives his or her own needs as less important than others (Morioka-Douglas and Yeo, 1990). The elders who speak only Japanese are more responsive to caregivers, friends, and family who speak their language.

Most important, the Japanese elder expects respect and tact when interacting with caregivers. Giving a command to a Japanese elder is an insult. The aged person needs only respect and understanding of expectations to comply. Attention to the specific manifestations of these cultural values will lead to better assessments, interpretations, and conclusions.

African (Black) Americans. Approximately 6.6% of the 34.5 million African Americans are 65 years or over. About 9% (313,289) of African American elders are 85 years of age or older (U.S. Bureau of the Census, 2000). The work history of African American elders has seldom produced Social Security and pension benefits adequate to meet their needs in late life. Elderly black women in rural areas are triply disadvantaged, and about 65% of them live in poverty. Within the black population, ethnic diversity is complex. Immigrant blacks come from African countries, the West Indies, Dominican Republic, Haiti, and Jamaica and bring with them the varied beliefs and customs of these regions, as well as their commonalties.

Health in black cultures is generally viewed as harmony with nature, and illness is viewed as disharmony. The mind, body, and spirit are not viewed separately. The black health belief system is an amalgam of ethnic origins, remnants of folk and formal medicine practiced over 100 years ago and influenced by Christianity, nativistic religions, sympathetic magic (Snow, 1974), and selected beliefs from modern scientific medicine. Many black elderly continue to use folk medicine practices when orthodox medicine and procedures do not work. Urban blacks are known to occasionally visit black cultural or religious healers.

Caregivers who do not understand beliefs and practices or have their own fears, insecurity, or misinformation may approach the black client with a demeaning action or tone of voice. The client may be told about problems in medical jargon, which produces fear of manipulation, feelings of alienation, and a sense of being talked down to and subjugation.

Elderly blacks usually react with patience, perseverance, and fatalistic acceptance of their fate. Time orientation differs between blacks and whites, with blacks functioning on a more flexible time orientation. Awareness of this difference in perspective dictates greater flexibility when providing care to the black elder. Another issue requiring some insight is the use of black English, which evolved from West Africa during the period of slavery. A combination of English words and West African language patterns creates a highly oral, stylized, rhythmic, and spontaneous language. Meaningful interaction is conveyed by the intonations and inflections of speech. Caregivers may gain some understanding of the specific health beliefs and practices important to a particular black client simply by careful observation and discussion with the individual.

We frequently hear of disadvantaged African Americans and their shorter life expectancy when compared with whites. A study by Manton and colleagues (1979; Gibson, 1994) demonstrates the hardiness of very old blacks. Those who live past 75 years of age are likely to outlive their white cohorts. This is called the *mortality crossover* (Manton et al, 1979; Markides and Mindel, 1987; Hooyman and Kiyak, 1996). After age 85, both African American men and women have a lower incidence of heart disease, arteriosclerosis, and cancer. Blacks who survive to 85 years of age are considered "old-old." They are sturdier than whites, have a lower mortality rate, and often appear much younger. According to Stokes (1979), the black elderly seem to accept old age better and maintain higher morale than the white elderly.

It is estimated that one third of the African American community has no form of health care reimbursement, and the large majority of that group do not receive attention to health problems until they become critical. During the Reagan administration, a task force to study the health status of black Americans was established (Pinkleton, 1988). The six major problems identified were (1) cancer; (2) heart disease and stroke; (3) infant mortality rate; (4) diabetes; (5) homicide, suicide, and unintentional accidents; and (6) chemical dependency. Hooyman and Kiyak (1996) indicate that the leading causes of morbidity and mortality among elderly African Americans are heart disease, cancer, and cerebrovascular accidents (stroke). Obesity, which can lead to diabetes, hypertension, and end-stage renal disease, is prevalent among African American women. Table 19-5 lists the health problems, risk factors, and areas for health education for the elderly. The report of the task force indicated an excess of deaths in the African American population, a disparity between the number of deaths in this minority population compared with a similar group in a nonminority population. A large number of African Americans are dying because of their life histories, current economic situation, and impaired access to health care. The task force identified the following social characteristics that particularly influence health status of minorities: (1) demographic profiles, (2) nutritional status and dietary practices, (3) environmental and occupational exposures, and (4) stress and other coping patterns. It is thought that some coping patterns engendered by substandard housing, education, and employment have put elders at risk or have been singularly etiologic to the identified major health problems. It is known that the life expectancy of African Americans is 5.6 years less than that for whites. In 1988, Pinkleton, a black professor at Hampton University, made a plea for increased numbers of competent, autonomous, African American nurses to provide comprehensive health

Table 19-5 Leading Health Problems of Black Americans, Modifiable Risk Factors, and Education Areas

Diseases	Modifiable factors	Education areas
Heart disease, cardiovascular disease	High blood pressure, high cholesterol levels, smoking, diabetes, diet, obesity, lack of exercise	Nutrition (salt, cholesterol levels), (weight loss and control), exercise
Stroke		
Cancer	Smoking, diet, alcohol	Smoking cessation, nutrition, referral for alcohol abuse counseling
Diabetes	Diet, obesity, alcohol, lack of exercise	Exercise, preventive services/screening for hypertension and diabetes
Cirrhosis of the liver	Alcohol	Referral for alcohol abuse counseling

From American Association of Retired Persons: *Healthy aging: Making health promotion work for minority elders,* Washington, DC, 1990, The Association; Brangman SA: Minorities. In Ham RJ and Sloan PD, editors: *Primary care geriatrics,* ed 3, St Louis, 1997, Mosby; Cultural assessment. In Estes MEZ: *Health assessment and physical examination,* ed 2, Pacific Grove, CA, 2002, Delmar.

services for the increasing numbers of black elders. African American nurses are likely to "speak their language" and in so doing increase their comfort and responsiveness.

Black elders have unique histories and adaptive patterns that are often neglected because their cultural and social needs are not recognized. Recognizing typical patterns of behavior, while not to be used as stereotypes, will help nurses work more sensitively. Compared with the majority of individuals, the education of African American elders has been neglected, and these elders are poorer, have less adequate housing, and have a shorter life span. They experience more chronic health problems, illnesses, and injuries than similar groups of whites. All of these factors must be given special consideration.

Church members are an important source of support to elderly African Americans. They develop a hierarchy of assistance, from family to friends and then neighbors and church members, before they seek help from formal organizations. Findings from the extensive National Survey of Black Americans (NSBA) show that over 80% of blacks receive support from church members (Dilworth-Anderson, 1992; Walls, 1992). This study found that elderly African Americans have an extensive support network of family, friends, and church. Belgrave and colleagues (1993) suggest that the multigenerational households may be a function of age, mental and socioeconomic status, and health. In addition, the African American is less likely to be in a nursing home, with only 3% after age 65 and 12% age 85 and older (Hooyman and Kiyak, 1996).

A young black nursing student chose, for her community elder assignment, to work with "Auntie Grace"—not a relative, but a member of the church community. Auntie Grace was old, poor, and obese, lived alone in a deteriorating home, and had great difficulty ambulating. The student's major assignment was to learn about aging and adaptation from Auntie Grace. Auntie Grace gave art lessons to several young children, and when the student realized how much she loved them, the talk turned to children. She was astonished to find that Auntie Grace never had children because she had inherited her father's dark color rather than her mother's lighter complexion, and she was afraid the same would happen to her children. The student and I discussed the impact of the previous generational perspective and the great sacrifice the old woman had made to protect unborn children from segregation and injustice. Auntie Grace did not regret her decision but took pleasure in enriching the lives of others' children. This old black woman, with a family history of slavery, enriched our lives as well.

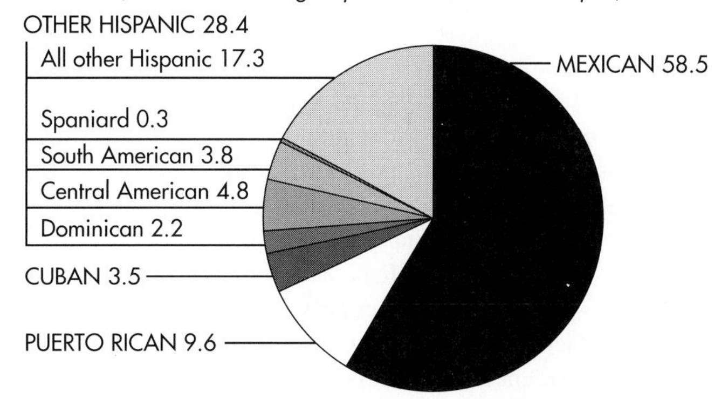

Figure 19-6. Diversity within the Hispanic population: 2000. (Source: U.S. Bureau of the Census: Census 2000 summary file 1.)

Hispanic Americans. Hispanics are culturally diverse with unique cultural heritage, histories, and dialects. Hispanics come from Mexico, Central and South America, Cuba, Spain, and Puerto Rico (Figure 19-6); many of these groups prefer to be identified by descriptors more appropriate to their specific cultural heritage, such as Chicano, Latino, or Latina. As a broad ethnic group, the term *la gente de la raza* (people of the race) is a genetic determination to which all Spanish-speaking people belong regardless of class differences or country of origin (Monrroy, 1983). Mexican Americans are the largest group of Hispanic people in the United States. This highly diverse population includes native born, legal immigrants, and undocumented immigrants. Over 1.7 million (4.9%) are 65 years old or older. Of this group, 9%, or approximately 140,000 Hispanic elders, are 85 years of age or over (U.S. Bureau of the Census, 2000).

Though Hispanic Americans live in every state in the nation, most live in the west or south. The vast majority (73%)

of these elders live in barrios and groups of 100,000 to 300,000 in four states. California (31.3%) and Texas (18.9%) attract Hispanic groups from Central America and Mexico; Florida (7.2%) seems to attract Cubans; and New York (8.8%) attracts Hispanics from the Caribbean Islands and Puerto Rico (U.S. Bureau of the Census, 2000).

Many Hispanics, particularly Mexican Americans, believe that health and illness are "God's will," and they are expected to maintain their own equilibrium in balance with the universe by proper behavior, proper nutrition, and work. Illness may be prevented by praying, adorning oneself with religious medals and amulets, and maintaining religious symbols in the home. Illness, when it occurs, is the result of imbalance or is a punishment for an evil deed. Illness occurs because of (1) imbalance of cold, hot, wet, or dry humors; (2) dislocation of body parts, the "evil eye" (magic or supernatural); (3) fright or envy; or (4) wrongdoing. Illness is seen as punishment. When illness is serious, magic or religious practices are used.

Caregivers often become annoyed with Mexican Americans because they do not respond to time the way Anglos do. Time orientation for the Mexican American is relative, and time is measured by day and night and by need (Monrroy, 1983; de Paula et al, 1996; Spector, 2000; Estes, 2002).

A Mexican American nurse, Carmen Altamirano Wilson (1988), wrote of elderly Hispanic people as a unique and culturally special group particularly sensitive to evidence of respect or lack of it. They are intensely proud. She shares the following evidence: "Pobres pero orgullosos. El orgullo si podemos tener porque eso no se compra en las boticas!" Her translation is, "Poor but proud. Pride is something we can possess because it is something we don't have to buy." Respect is evidence to the aged Hispanic of his or her worth and merit. When not treated respectfully, the elder assumes he or she is in some way undeserving of respect. Health providers must address elderly Hispanics formally and avoid familiarity until (if ever) the elder indicates differently. Elders have a strong sense of privacy and feel they are able to handle their own problems within the family with the help of church and faith. Many believe that God will not give them a cross too heavy to bear and that if they follow His will He will take care of them. Daily prayer sustains them, and their faith provides comfort and peace. They are cautious, nonaggressive, and humble when giving and receiving. They give as a thanksgiving to God and expect nothing but His blessing in return (Wilson, 1988).

A Hispanic's evaluation for health care may be influenced by these attitudes. For example, outright criticism is seldom given because the individual may feel he or she is somehow getting what is deserved and is unworthy of anything better (Wilson, 1988). Keeping in mind that the profile given by Wilson cannot be applied to all aged Hispanics, it can do no harm to anyone to give respect, consider privacy, and proceed with formality until the client indicates otherwise.

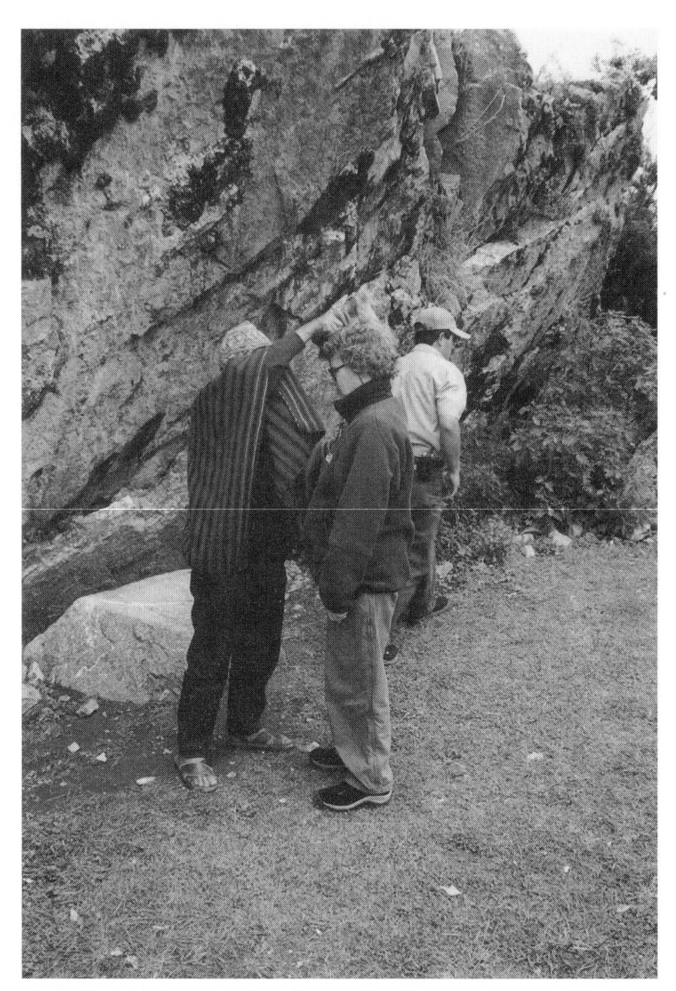

Curandero a Paca performing a healing ceremony. (Courtesy Patricia Hess.)

Many old persons of all cultures value their faith and tend to feel fatalistic about "the burdens God has given me to bear." It will rarely be possible or useful to convince them otherwise. If you suspect that this may be true of your client, ask him or her about the story of Job and thoughts about it.

It would be helpful if caregivers demonstrate interest in the Hispanic subgroup with which the elder is affiliated, and it would be a beginning of respect, understanding, and sensitivity. The Hispanic usually prefers to be addressed by his or her last name. Ask what is preferred. Respect and courtesy toward elders are important in the Hispanic culture, as are privacy and modesty.

Hispanics do not want to hurt anyone's feelings, so they will not readily express dissatisfaction. Even when the individual does not understand what is said, he or she will usually respond with a polite affirmative reply. It is important for the caregiver to be aware of this and be sure that the individual truly understands.

Respect for life, family structure, hard work, and involvement in the care and education of the children are expectations in Hispanic culture (de Paula et al, 1996; Hooyman and Kiyak,

Table 19-6 Leading Health Problems of Hispanic Americans, Modifiable Risk Factors, and Education Areas

Diseases	Modifiable factors	Education areas
High blood pressure	Lack of exercise, obesity, eating habits	Nutrition (balanced diet, salt, sugar, cholesterol), weight loss and control
Diabetes	Lack of exercise, obesity, eating habits, alcohol	Preventive services/screening for hypertension and diabetes
Cancer	Eating habits, smoking, alcohol	Referral for alcohol abuse counseling, smoking cessation

From American Association of Retired Persons: *Healthy aging: Making health promotion work for minority elders,* Washington, DC, 1990, The Association; Brangman SA: Minorities. In Ham RJ and Sloan PD, editors: *Primary care geriatrics,* ed 3, St Louis, 1997, Mosby; Cultural assessment. In Estes MEZ: *Health assessment and physical examination,* ed 2, Pacific Grove, CA, 2002, Delmar.

1996; Spector, 1996). Aged Hispanics are increasingly without a role. Their children have increased social status and educational levels, whereas their own status and respect have decreased. Their children do not seem to need their knowledge and wisdom to survive today. The aged live either in small towns far away from their children or in cities surrounded by a system that does not need their skills. The role they had envisioned in their old age has not materialized.

Table 19-6 provides insight into the leading health problems of Hispanic Americans, the risk factors, and areas of health education. It appears that some of these factors relate directly to the degree of enculturation rather than to ethnicity or poverty (Espino and Maldonado, 1990). Hooyman and Kiyak (1996) point to social and cultural barriers that interfere with care. Mistrust of white medical providers, stigma associated with mental health services, reliance on folk medicine, religious healing, and less health insurance coverage are seen as significant issues.

Native Americans. The Native American elders include the American Indians and the Alaskan Natives (Eskimos and the Aleuts). This combined group has the fastest growing elderly population. It is expanding at about twice the rate of white and black elders. The number of elders over 75 years of age has doubled, and by 2050 this population will have reached 38% of the Native American population. The 2000 census determined that 3.5% of Native Americans are 65 years of age or older, and 2.1% are 75 years of age or older. One quarter of the Native American elders live on American Indian reservations or in Alaskan Native villages. Over half of the Native American elders reside in California, Arizona, New Mexico, Texas, and Oklahoma, with the remainder living throughout the other states (U.S. Bureau of the Census, 2000). Native Americans are the largest group of elders to reside in rural areas.

Health means living in harmony with nature and the ability to survive under exceedingly difficult circumstances for the approximately 500 recognized tribal groups and recognized nations with 200 native languages (Hooyman and Kiyak, 1996; Spector, 2000). The earth and the self are tied; what affects one affects the other. The body is treated with respect and is viewed as having two parts, a positive and a negative energy.

Every sickness or pain that occurs results from something that happened in the past or will in the future, representing a cause-and-effect relationship. Some tribes, however, relate illness to evil spirits.

A Native American converses in low tones and expects to be listened to with attentiveness. To ask the person to repeat or to say "huh" is inappropriate. Notes should not be taken; they are taboo. The nurse must develop acute mental processes for retaining information such as assessment data. Questions are not well received. Instead, declarative statements such as, "You have a pain that keeps you awake" are seen as evidence of respect. The American Indian elderly expect the caregiver to deduce the problem by intuition rather than by questioning (Wilson, 1988; personal experience, Hess, 2000). In addition, one must be aware of the strong importance of nonverbal communication (Cuellar, 1990; Kramer, 1996; Spector, 1996).

Self-esteem is based on the ability to help others by giving advice to younger members of the tribe and being regarded as a source of wisdom. Cooperation is a source of pride, and competition is discouraged (Martin, 1977).

Table 19-7 lists the leading health problems with the risk factors and areas of health education for Native American elders.

Various tribes may have specific rituals that are performed at death, such as burying certain personal possessions with the individual. Consulting with members of the specific tribe to gain insight into special rituals during sickness and at death would be advantageous for nurses working with Native American patients.

MULTICULTURAL NURSING PERSPECTIVES

Most universities now have an international division or section or ethnic study programs to represent and attend to the needs of students of foreign backgrounds. Nursing schools and nursing students may find valuable ideas and assistance toward providing appropriate care through cultivating ties with persons of a particular culture or country or through collaboration with representatives of university ethnic study programs. In addition, cross-cultural research that is conducted

Table 19-7 Leading Health Problems of Native Americans and Alaskan Americans, Modifiable Risk Factors, and Education Areas

Diseases	Modifiable factors	Education areas*
Heart disease	High blood pressure, smoking, high cholesterol levels, diabetes, obesity, diet, lack of exercise	Preventive services/screening/inoculations, support groups or referral for alcohol abuse counseling, smoking cessation, nutrition (fats, fiber), weight loss and control, exercise
Cancer	Smoking; alcohol; high-animal-fat, low-fiber diet	See above
Accidents	Alcohol	See above
Chronic liver disease and cirrhosis	Alcohol	See above
Diabetes	Diet, obesity, lack of exercise, alcohol	See above
Pneumonia/influenza	Malnutrition, alcoholism, smoking, diabetes	See above

From American Association of Retired Persons: *Healthy aging: Making health promotion work for minority elders,* Washington, DC, 1990, The Association; Brangman SA: Minorities. In Ham RJ and Sloan PD, editors: *Primary care geriatrics,* ed 3, St Louis, 1997, Mosby; Cultural assessment. In Estes MEZ: *Health assessment and physical examination,* ed 2, Pacific Grove, CA, 2002, Delmar.
*All the education areas noted are interrelated.

by investigators representing both cultures continues to be desperately needed.

As Lin noted (1988), professionals visiting a country for short periods rarely discover the real needs and problematic issues. It is interesting to note how few studies of ethnic or foreign elders have been conducted by persons indigenous to the group.

If nurses are unfamiliar with a particular ethnic group, churches or associations (e.g., Polish American Alliance, Celtic League, Jewish Family and Children's Society, Slovak League of America) can be helpful in identifying interpreters or persons who can serve as a cultural resource. Consulates for various countries may provide a list of organizations specific to a cultural group. Schools of nursing have begun addressing cultural aspects in their curriculum. Nurses who graduated before this time and who are working may need to individually seek these experiences. Suggestions for upgrading knowledge about the minority aged include the following:

1. Develop interest in and commitment to the needs of minority groups.
2. Become involved in experiences with diverse ethnic and cultural groups.
3. Learn about historical and cultural roots of ethnic variations.
4. Respond to the diverse needs within your community.

Cultural and Health Belief Systems

There are a number of health belief systems that fall into three categories and are actively practiced today as they have been in the past. These are the biomedical or Western system, the personalistic or magicoreligious system, and the naturalistic or holistic system. The diversity of the population has brought the strong potential for a clash of health belief systems, language, and attitudes about health and illness between the care provider and the client. Many of the beliefs and practices do not fit into the traditional format of health care as most care providers know it.

The *biomedical,* scientific, or Western medical belief system espouses that disease is the result of abnormalities in structure and function of body organs and systems. It is still a dominant belief that permeates the thinking of those educated in Western health care. The objective term *disease* is used by care providers, and *illness* is a subjective term to describe symptoms of discomfort or sickness. A personal state of illness has distinct social dimensions. Assessment and diagnosis are directed at identifying the pathogen or process causing the abnormality and removing or destroying the cause or at least repairing or modifying the problem through treatment. Highly skilled clinicians use the scientific method, and sophisticated laboratory and other procedures, to stem the disease or disease process. Prevention in this belief system is to avoid pathogens, chemicals, activities, and dietary agents known to cause malfunction.

Personalistic or *magicoreligious* beliefs may have originated in groups that were relatively small, isolated, and illiterate and lacked contact with ancient high civilizations (Jackson, 1993). Those who follow the beliefs of the personalistic or magicoreligious system believe that illness is caused by active purposeful intervention of agents of the supernatural, such as gods, spirits, and other nonhuman beings. Ghosts, ancestors, evil spirits, or humans in the form of witches or sorcerers are believed to be responsible for sickness. The individual is considered a victim, an object of aggression or punishment. A person may be put under a spell by a disgruntled neighbor so that the person cannot eat or sleep. A dead relative may be angry that his or her wishes were not followed and send an animal to bite the person, cause a growth, or cause a woman to be infertile.

Identification of the agent behind these events and rendering it harmless, lifting a spell, or reversing the method used by the agent is the aim of treatment. Once the agent is known, the "curer" or person can take steps to resolve the situation. Physical symptoms are secondary to finding the initial cause of the dilemma. Making sure that social networks with one's fellow humans are in good working order is the essence of prevention in this health belief system. Therefore avoiding angering family, friends, neighbors, ancestors, gods, and so on and adherence to and the correct performance of rituals are very important. Etiologies of the personalistic beliefs may be intertwined with religious beliefs. Entities that cause illness may be expanded to explain that the deities, ghosts, or spirits are the cause of crop failures, accidents, financial reversals, and so on.

Naturalistic or *holistic* health beliefs consider *sickness* to be an impersonal systemic term. Health is due to equilibrium of the elements of the body such as hot and cold. These must be in balance or harmony. When this is not so, illness is present. The current naturalistic beliefs stem from the ancient civilizations of China, India, and Greece (Jackson, 1993).

Traditional Chinese medicine is the basis for the health belief system and practices today of such countries as Japan, Vietnam, Korea, Taiwan, Singapore, Hong Kong, and China. In India and some of its neighboring countries, Ayurvedic medicine, which arose in ancient India, is still practiced. Humoral pathology, practiced by the ancient Greeks, was disseminated both east and west and was embraced by the Muslim culture and by Spanish and Italian explorers. Variations of humoral pathology can be found in the medical systems of rural and some urban people in Latin America, in the Philippines, and in some low-income blacks and whites in the southern United States. These beliefs are also found in sophisticated and unsophisticated populations in Iran, Pakistan, Malaysia, and Java (Jackson, 1993). In the United States and other countries that are steeped in the biomedical system, the aforementioned beliefs are considered "folk medicine."

Though the origins of naturalistic beliefs are different, they all consider illness the result of an excess of heat or cold that enters the body and causes an imbalance. Hot and cold is generally metaphoric, although at times temperature is an aspect. Various foods, medicines, environmental conditions, emotions, and bodily conditions (menstruation, pregnancy, etc.) may posses the characteristics of either hot or cold (Jackson, 1993; Spector, 1996, 2000).

Diagnosis is concerned with identifying the cause of the disease as either hot or cold in origin. Remedies are divided into hot and cold. Treatment then is focused on using the opposite element; if the disease is the result of excess hot, treatment will be with something that has cold properties, and vice versa. The treatments may take the form of herbs, food, dietary restrictions, medications from Western medicine that have hot and cold properties such as antibiotics, massage, poultices, and other therapies. Naturalistic curers are physicians or herbalists who specialize in symptomatic treatment and know which medicines will restore the body's equilibrium. Prevention is directed at protecting oneself from extremes of heat and cold in both the literal and metaphoric senses.

One may recognize a melding of the various health system beliefs in oneself and others. Therefore it behooves care providers to become sensitive to and versed in these systems to better understand, not necessarily agree with, persons for whom they are providing care, while recognizing their own ethnocentric tendencies. Table 19-8 illustrates variations in illness beliefs between the biomedical and other ethnically based models.

Culture and Health Practices

Attempts to discover and assess health practices and preferences within various groups often yield fascinating results. Elders who grew up in remote areas of any country, including the United States, where traditional health services were scarce or unavailable, developed a number of unusual health practices. Some are physiologically sound, and others may have been beneficial because of the placebo effect. It is important to include this type of information in a health assessment. Even though the client may not admit to presently using any historical folk remedies or unusual practices, awareness of the possibility is important. Encourage and incorporate these practices unless the practice is clearly detrimental. We know that belief and hope have therapeutic benefits. Alternative healers must also be discussed and encouraged if the client believes they are important. Some of the barriers ethnic elders experience can be seen in Figure 19-7.

Many questions have been raised about the advisability of using indigenous health care providers and agency personnel to serve the elderly of ethnic minorities. We believe this is ideal but not always possible. A sensitive nurse needs to become aware of her or his own cultural roots, embrace them, and enjoy them, but keep them in proper perspective in the nurse-client relationship. As with clients of all backgrounds, one nursing function of great importance is to support the ties with family or reference group that maintain the aged person's sense of solidarity.

Encourage family members to prepare specially enjoyed foods and perform significant rituals. Locate priests, monks, rabbis, or ministers who may comfort the aged person. When alternative healing methods are used, respect them as judiciously as the traditional. A sense of caring is conveyed in these gestures of personal recognition. Caring can surmount cultural differences.

Assessment. A cultural history is one way to understand where the aged adult's health beliefs lie. There are few tools or instruments that assist the nurse to elicit health care beliefs and at the same time identify to the nurse his or her own perceptions of the beliefs. Given the necessary data, the nurse is able to use this information to negotiate a clear understanding of problems and solutions with the client or the individual who is the appropriate support figure in the client's life. One must keep in mind that there may be great generational cohort and cultural differences between practitioner and client.

Table 19-8 Explanations of Illness: Biomedical and Behavioral

	Biomedical model	Behaviorally ethnic model
Etiologic beliefs		
Social causes of illness	Usually limited to the stress model or attributed to paranoia.	Many social indiscretions can cause illness. Blaming oneself or others for symptoms is common.
Environmental causes of illness	Exposure to known pathogens, toxins, and social stress may cause symptoms.	Dietary indiscretion can cause hot-cold imbalance in the body. Drafts may cause symptoms.
Blood conditions as causes of illness	Limited to specific hematologic disorders or hypertension.	Many conditions of the blood (too thick, thin, high, low, or stagnant) can cause illness.
Symptom presentation and interpretation		
Altered states of consciousness (trance, visions)	Likely to be considered abnormal.	Often considered to be normal or desirable.
Attitudes toward pain	Stoicism expected unless complaints are congruent with clear organic pathology.	Either total stoicism or emotional expression of pain is healthy and expected.
Focus on physical symptoms	May be considered a psychiatric syndrome.	Expected, proper way of showing distress.
Treatment expectations		
Who is the patient?	Individual is focus of decision making and care.	The family must be involved in decision making.
Beliefs about self-medication and alternative practitioners	Considered potentially dangerous or undesirable.	Self-medication and consulting with traditional healers are common.

Modified with permission from Johnson TH, Hardt EJ, Kleinman A: Cultural factors in the medical interview. In Lipkin M Jr, Putnam SM, Lazare A, editors: *The medical interview,* New York, 1994, Springer-Verlag.

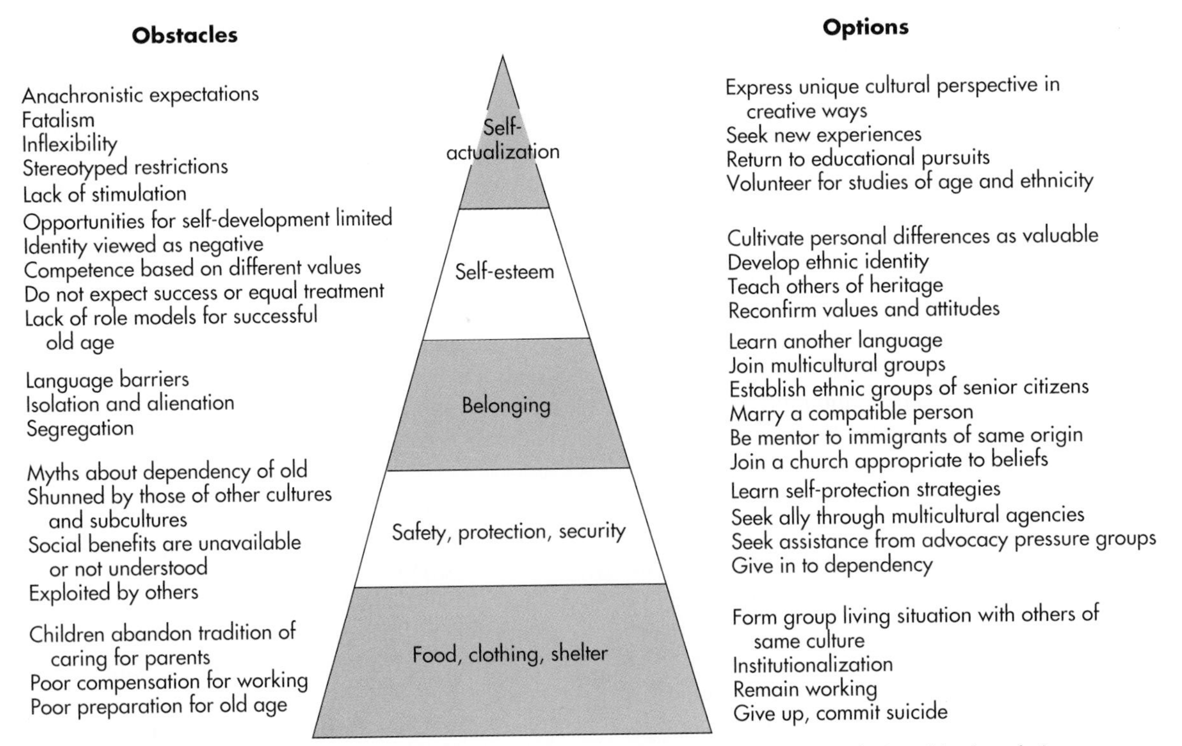

Figure 19-7. Cultural barriers to meeting needs. (Modified from Smith D et al: *A multicultural view of drug abuse,* Boston, 1978, GK Hall & Co.)

To provide quality care to ethnic elders, a comprehensive cultural assessment is important. This type of assessment takes time. It is clear that not all situations allow for this, but even if it must be done bit by bit over time, it will be valuable to the caregiver in better understanding how to work with and within the culture of the client. The exploratory models developed by Kleinman (1980) and Pfeifferling (1981) have helped caregivers obtain needed information in a culturally sensitive manner (see Appendix 19-A). Box 19-3 offers an adaptation of these models for use in a cultural health assessment. Evans and Cunningham (1996) offer specific assessment topics and items to be assessed in Table 19-9.

Usually information gleaned about minority elders concerns the type of practitioners, rituals, and medications, but little attention is given to the activities of daily living that are so vital to care of the aged (Gunter, 1991). To plan for immediate and long-term care, Gunter (1991) offers an assessment of personal care practices of minority aged. These are

Table 19-9 Nursing Care for the Ethnic Elder

	Assessment	Interventions
Ethnicity	Number of years living in United States. Age at immigration (immigrant vs refugee). Degree of affiliation with ethnic group or assimilation to U.S. culture.	Be sensitive to historical events that influence elders' perception of self and authority of health care providers. Demonstrate respect for elder by using surname and providing care in a manner sensitive to cultural norms.
Communication	English as primary or secondary language. Level of fluency. Barriers to communication such as sensory deficits, lack of privacy, distractions. Meaning of nonverbal gestures.	Use of translator for exchange of health information. Document system for communicating basic needs between patient and staff. Provide patient access to sensory aids (glasses, hearing aids, pocket talkers). Eliminate background noise and provide optimum lighting. Smile, offer gestures of assistance with basic needs (warm blanket, glass of water).
Health perception	Perception of health problem, causes, and prognosis. Response to pain, illness and death.	Educate patient/family about disease process and medical treatments. Identify and document reasons for behavior. Develop system for identifying and rating pain.
Folk practices	Use of cultural healers, herbal medicines, alternative health practices and beliefs.	Obtain order for use of folk remedies as indicated. Educate patient regarding contraindications for folk remedy and discourage use if dangerous.
Health care system	Previous hospitalization experiences. Current hospitalization planned or emergency?	Encourage patient to express fears regarding hospitalization and treatments. Keep patient/family informed of patient's progress.
Religion	Spiritual practices and beliefs. Level of incorporation of spiritual practices into healing/dying process.	Allow privacy and space for religious articles and practices. Arrange for visit from spiritual leader. Refer patients to hospital chaplain. Document beliefs about death and burial.
Food	Beliefs regarding food and healing. Use of hot/cold system. Specific food preferences.	Obtain consultation with dietitian. Incorporate food preferences into menu selection. Ask family to supply familiar foods. Document use of hot/cold practices as they relate to nursing care.
Social support	Current living situation. Support of family or community (or both).	Encourage family participation in care. Encourage visits or phone calls with peers.
Decision making	Primary decision maker for health care. How does the patient make decisions? Who is needed for decisions?	Involve family when providing patient with health care information. Arrange for family conference if disparity exists between goals of patient, family, or health care team.
Discharge planning	Expectations for care after hospitalization and during future years of aging. Financial status that affects discharge planning and long-term health status. Ability of patient/family to support discharge needs.	Involve family in discharge planning. Obtain consult for social services. Refer patient to community resources for legal advice, transportation, meals, shopping, and emotional support.

From Evans CA, Cunningham BA: Caring for the ethnic elder, *Geriatr Nurs* 17(3):105, 1996.

Box 19-3 Cultural Assessment Related to Client's Health Problem

The clinician may need to identify others who can facilitate the discussion of the client's problem(s).

1. How would you describe the problem that has brought you here? (What do you call your problem; does it have a name?)
   A. Who in the community and your family helps you with your problem?
2. How long have you had this problem?
   A. When do you think it started?
   B. What do you think started it?
   C. Do you know anyone else with it?
   D. Tell me what happened to them when dealing with this problem.
3. What do you think is wrong with you?
   A. What does your sickness do to you?
   B. How severe is it?
   C. What might other people think is wrong with you?
   D. Tell me about people who don't get this problem.
4. Why do you think this happened to you and why?
   A. Why has it happened to the involved part?
   B. Why do you get sick and not someone else?
   C. Will it have a long or short course?
   D. What do you fear most about your sickness?
5. What are the chief problems your sickness has caused you?
6. What do you think will help clear up this problem? (What treatment should you receive; what are the most important results you hope to receive?)
   A. If specific tests, medications are listed, ask what they are and do.
7. Apart from me, who else do you think can make you feel better?
   A. Are there therapies that make you feel better that I don't know? (May be in another discipline.)

Adapted from Kleinman A: *Patient and healers in the context of culture: an exploration of the borderland between anthropology, medicine, and psychiatry,* Berkeley, 1980, University of California Press; Pfeifferling JH: A cultural prescription for mediocentrism. In Eisenberg L, Kleinman A, editors: *The relevance of social science for medicine*, Boston, 1981, Reidel.

depicted in Table 19-10. Some of these orientations literally cannot be expressed in another language and cannot be fully understood outside the culture. As stated earlier, nurses must avoid an ethnocentric stance, that is, the belief that the values and practices of one's own culture are the best ones (Gunter, 1991). Ethnocentrism will be discussed again later in this chapter.

Brislin and Pederson (1982) approach this dilemma by taking a "culture-general" approach. Rather than focus on eating habits, religious customs, interpersonal etiquette, and decision-making styles, they train the caregiver in self-awareness and sensitivity. This is a wise approach for health care providers who daily encounter clients from extremely different cultural backgrounds with varied levels of assimilation into the host culture. Gaining insight into one's own values and assumptions encourages a perspective that respects the validity and tenacity of others' values and assumptions. For example, a missionary in Japan experienced a severe identity crisis when she realized that her religious myths and traditions were no more rational than those of Shintoism or Buddhism.

This segment of the chapter combines both "culture-general" and "culture-specific" approaches to assist the caregiver in recognizing adaptations that influence responses to care, while simultaneously hoping the student will remain aware of self and avoid stereotypic expectations.

Nursing concerns must focus on overall health care for minority elders by assisting them to gain access to needed services through ascertaining affordability, efficacy, accessibility and availability of information, client satisfaction, respect for clients' health beliefs, illness perspective, and informal support systems.

Caring for the Minority Elderly

The consumers of health care are increasingly being cared for in the home, and providers must adapt strategies to the beliefs and culture of the individual if we hope to be useful. Folk remedies abound among the various ethnic elders and among the dominant culture. We, the dominant cultural group, also embrace many of the beliefs brought in from other shores and welcome the relief from the mechanistic approaches of our

Table 19-10 Areas of Assessment of Personal Care Practices of Minority Elderly

Activities of daily living	Coping strategies	Environment	Family or significant support	Attitudes toward caregivers/professionals
Eating	Problem solving	Home	Availability	Preferences
Feeding		Housekeeping		
Nutrition				
Bathing	Stress	Safety and support/reassurance	Acceptance	Rejections
Dressing	Pain/discomfort	Institution arrangements		
Toileting	Loneliness	Artifacts		
Continence	Religion, prayer, meditation			
Mobility/disability				

This form may be used as a comparative assessment of minority elders. From Gunter LM: Cultural diversity among older Americans. In Baines EM, editor: *Perspectives on gerontological nursing,* Newbury Park, CA, 1991, Sage.

Western, technology-dominated culture. We listen with interest to the efficacy of mind control over body ailments and aches. We embrace acupressure, acupuncture, and other modes of relief that would have been anathema to our thinking as we entered the age of human mechanical efficiency. We may have matured to the awareness of the human mind and meanings as a counterbalance to our extreme efficiency. This small world, in the expanding universe, has not yet lost its anthropomorphic orientations. We have much to learn from those ancient and enduring civilizations that bring from their history another cognitive mode of existence.

The nurse and the health care system have strong ethnocentric tendencies; that is, the individual's or the group's (the health care system) beliefs and ways of providing care are considered the most desirable when dealing with illness or health care. In essence, Western medicine and nursing care are considered superior to others. This latter statement is ethnocentrism (Leininger, 1978; Gunter, 1991; Grossman, 1994; Spector, 1996; Estes, 2002). To combat this and provide sensitively designed care, many components of the individual's life system must be considered (Box 19-4; see Table 19-9).

We must also become acutely aware of the influence of our own values, beliefs, and prejudices before we can hope to understand another's. If we do not become sensitive to the influence of values and beliefs on health we will be unable to provide effective care. Scientific problem solving, the foundation of nursing care planning, is necessary but not inclusive.

Box 19-4 Guidelines to Nursing Interventions for Ethnic Elders

Respect the cultural preferences in food, music, and religion.
Design teaching to the vocabulary and attitude of the individual.
Listen attentively to complaints because these may be the clues to health problems.
In people of color, the signs of some disorders (pallor, cyanosis, ecchymosis) may be masked by color; buccal cavity coloration is significant.
For base physical assessment on norms for the ethnic group, keep in mind that adequate light is especially important in skin assessment for turgor, blemishes, and cyanosis; eye lenses, nail beds, palms of the hands, and soles of the feet can be revealing.
Listen for signs of depression, often in the form of hypochondriasis and apathy.
Inquire about losses and the individual's adaptation to them.
Gather information about lifestyle preferences and incorporate it into the care plan.
Inquire about health practices the individual finds effective.
Identify spiritual resources and incorporate into the care plan; contact the minister and church friends.

Intuition, superstition, belief, faith, and hope are necessarily woven into effective care packages. Jackson (1993), Grossman (1994), and Spector (1996) believe provider self-awareness is fundamental to this process. The nurse must also be cognizant that standard assessment tools, which attempt to identify aspects of an elder's ability to be independent physically and cognitively, may not be sensitive to changes in meaning not intended by developers of the tests when applied to ethnic minorities (Mouton and Esparza, 2000).

In caring for the aged a knowledge of history and culture is necessary. The nature of diseases is changing, and new health problems have emerged. Fads and fashion in health care have changed significantly, as has the delivery of care. Many elders remember when the family physician would advise an ocean voyage to combat illness, would accept eggs in payment for services, would taste or smell urine as a diagnostic test, and would remain with a laboring woman for several hours before delivering the infant at home.

A particularly sensitive physician recently asked if one of my Chinese students could act as interpreter for an elderly Chinese woman who had just been admitted to the hospital. The student, having been in the United States only 2 years, was delighted to speak in her mother tongue, and the elderly woman became noticeably calm as they talked. The physician was grateful and praised the student for her assistance. It was only later I learned that the student's mother had died a few months before and her last days were spent in physical and psychologic misery because she was unable to understand what was being done to her in the hospital. This became the student's motivation for entering nursing.

In schools such as ours where varied ethnic groups abound, it is wise to make students' language skills known to the professionals in the clinical settings in which they practice. A nursing administrator might keep a computerized list of the various language skills of all personnel and have this service as readily available as the technologic services in the health care system.

A number of measures suggested by Spector (1996, 2000) have already been addressed earlier in this chapter that will assist nurses to deal sensitively with people from other cultures (Box 19-5).

Ethnogeriatric Health Care. The term *ethnogeriatrics* has entered the vernacular of health care professionals; it is a specialty in which we hope to work sensitively with ethnic elders. The prediction of a significant increase in ethnic elders suggests that they will have considerable impact on service needs and delivery. It is expected that the minority elder population will increase by 219% by 2030. California is expected to be 58% non-Anglo by 2030. Other states will also experience this upsurge in non-Anglo elders. In light of this, it will be impossible to think of ethnic elders as incidental to the elderly population as a whole.

When we speak of *traditional* versus *nontraditional* medicine we must clarify these terms. Mitchell (1989) believed that *popular* versus *professional* is more accurate. In most parts of the world there is a formal system of health care and

Box 19-5

Culturally Sensitive Health Care

Ethnic studies are essential in the curricula required of health care providers. Students may be required to interview aged individuals of other cultures. Guest speakers from representative cultures may be invited to classes.
Health care providers must be sensitized to their own perceptions and practices related to health and illness. Consciousness-raising exercises include interviewing family about health beliefs and health practices that have been or are part of the family heritage.
Health care providers should become aware of the complex issues of health care from the client's viewpoint: cost, religious beliefs, interpretation of services, inequality of treatment, and many others of which even the client may be unaware.
More minority persons must be recruited into health care professions. Support services for students entering professional education programs must be made readily available to compensate for deficits experienced in early education and language differences.
Health services must be accessible to ethnic minorities and delivered with respect to cultural beliefs and practices. Neighborhood health centers with indigenous providers are most effective for entry into the health care system and appropriate guidance and referral.

Summarized from Spector RE: *Cultural diversity in health and illness*, East Norwalk, CT, 1985, Appleton-Century-Crofts.

the informal system of "folk medicine" or "popular medicine." Anglos are no exception. We quickly adopt one fad after another that we think may preserve health. The difference between our "popular medicine" and that of many ethnic elders is that theirs is steeped in tradition and ritual. Theirs is truly traditional, and ours is not. In all of health care, from whatever culture, we must recognize the power of the mind in healing and incorporate the significant beliefs and rituals in the pattern of health care if we hope to be successful. And we often discover scientifically that the folk remedies were indeed beneficial.

The basis for much folk medicine was purely making the most of whatever was available. We speak in the past tense because most ethnic elders have now incorporated Western medicine into their care and rarely rely totally on their traditional cures. However, they do often cling to some of these and supplement their professional care as they see fit. Separation of cultural beliefs from economic resources and educational background is exceedingly difficult, and additional "education" related to health care rarely changes individual habits and rituals (Chavira, 1989).

Some guidelines for dealing with ethnic elders who are using a mixture of Western and traditional methods to cure their ills are offered by Mitchell (1989):

- Realize that many ethnic elders do not have a concept of chronic illness that cannot be cured and will continually search for a method to alleviate the problem experienced.
- Determine what the problem is from the client's perspective. What does he or she think is wrong?
- What does the client think caused the problem?
- Does the client understand the treatment plan and how it relates to symptoms?
- Try to find out if the elder is supplementing prescriptions and what the expected result is.
- Alert the individual to signs of adverse reactions to treatment.
- Always try to discover the underlying logic of the client's belief.
- Incorporate folk medicine beliefs if they are not harmful.

Scott and Polacca (1995-1996) also note that a definition of *pathologic condition* and *diagnosis* in one culture may be different in another culture. For example, mental illness may be seen as dysfunctional in one culture but normal or a spiritual phenomenon in another culture. In addition, some cultures do not have concepts equivalent to Western conditions, such as depression (Mouton and Esparza, 2000).

We live in a medicalized society where it is not uncommon to "ask the doctor" what to eat, how and when to have sex, how to discipline children, when to go on a diet, if it is safe to travel, and many other issues of living. This is a rather recent phenomenon. In many other societies and eras a physician was sought only for serious problems, and although we have thought that seeing a physician routinely somehow prevents serious problems from developing, we have found that this is not true. It is becoming evident that the daily decisions one makes and the attitudes one has about life are more important than a yearly visit to a physician.

For many ethnic elders, in particular the Hispanic and Asian elder, life is viewed as a balance of energy and forces; intrusion into body systems and drawing off vital fluids are viewed with alarm. Also, the family and environment are intrinsic to the energy systems and must not be excluded from consideration. Thus we can understand how hospitals, diagnostic procedures, and other unfamiliar elements that disturb the peace can be interpreted as producing more harm than good.

Interestingly, there are some racial differences identified in drug metabolism (Zhou et al, 1989). For example, African Americans with hypertension do not respond as well to beta-blockers, and Chinese men are twice as sensitive to them as are whites. Studies have focused on hypertension because it is easy to measure and is now so prevalent in our society. Isoniazid rapidly inactivates in Native Americans, Asians, and African Americans but can be slowed to some degree with the taking of pyridoxine. It has been suggested that there are many other metabolic differences in ethnic groups that are not as easily identified (Goldstein, 1989; Giger and Davidhizer, 1991).

Mexicans are prone to diabetes and blacks to hypertension. We usually think of these as fundamentally dietary problems, but they may not be. In other words, there is much we have discovered and are still discovering, such as the affect of genetics and lifestyle on different populations. As we work with ethnic elders we are learning with them and about them. We are not the experts with all the answers.

Nurses should not attempt to change the client's beliefs. It is difficult if not impossible and usually is counterproductive. What is helpful is negotiating options with the client. This can be done with knowledge and mutual respect. The nurse should attempt to preserve helpful beliefs and practices, accommodate beliefs that are neither helpful nor harmful from the viewpoint of Western medicine, and repattern harmful beliefs or practices. If the nurse has little or no knowledge of a belief or practice, the nurse should study and evaluate it to determine its helpfulness or its potential harm. The nurse should also keep an open mind, learn about practices, encourage their use, and be flexible, creative, and persistent. In this way preservation of beliefs and practices can be achieved. Respectfully explaining concern about harmful client practices with the offer of possible alternatives may show the client that the nurse is taking the client's beliefs and practices into consideration. It is less likely that the client will be dissatisfied and not return for future care (Chrisman, 1992; Grossman, 1994).

Self-Care. Coulton (1988) presented preliminary evidence regarding the use of medical care among blacks, Hispanics, and Eastern European immigrants. Osteoarthritis is present in 85% of individuals between 75 and 79 years of age and thus becomes a focus of self-care practices for many. Ethnic groups differ in their preferential methods of self-care and the extent to which they use medical care versus traditional healing methods and alternative health practices. Coulton found that Hispanics, although poorest and least educated, were most likely to use medical care and prescription drugs for joint symptoms. They also had more chronic health conditions and generally rated their health poorer than blacks or Eastern Europeans. Crisis/health advice lines to serve specific ethnic populations have proved effective when publicized well within the select group.

Implications of Ethnicity in Long-Term Care. Jones and van Amelsvoort Jones (1986) studied the interactions of nursing staff with groups of elderly persons in a long-term care facility to determine the nature of verbal interactions. Immigrants, Canadian-born elders, and American-born elders were included in the study. Although the study was done in only one small nursing home and the sample was of only 41 elders, it is significant to alert us that we may unwittingly be influenced by subliminal stereotypes and discriminatory feelings. Tape recorders were discreetly placed to determine the nature of verbal content: commands, words, statements, and questions. Most of the verbalization (42%) was in the form of commands. The Canadian group was communicated with most frequently, the ethnic Europeans the least, and the American-born elders in between. Men were spoken to less frequently than women and were more frequently given commands. Relating to ethnic elders in long-term care may be more difficult than has been thought. The most important finding of this study was that during the entire 72 hours in which it was conducted, only 850 words were spoken in all to the entire group of subjects—20 words per person! It appears that elders in this long-term care facility, of whatever ethnic background, were severely deprived of communication. Box 19-6 gives Jones and van Amelsvoort Jones' suggestions (1986) for more meaningful care and communication.

Ethnicity may be one of the major elements of self-concept, and when age and institutionalization make one vulnerable, ethnic heritage becomes even more important. To the Chinese, achieving old age is a blessing, and the elderly are held in high esteem. The old are respected and sought for advice. The family unit is expected to take care of its elder members, and thus there may be a reluctance to use long-term care even when badly needed.

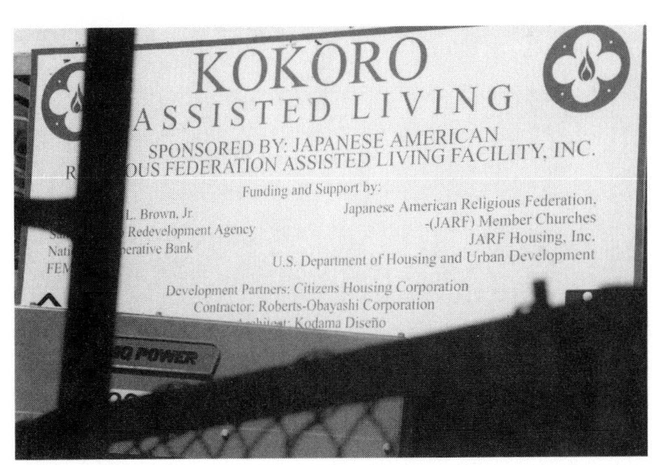

Ethnic-sensitive facility under construction. (Courtesy Patricia Hess.)

Box 19-6 Approaches to Caring for the Ethnic Aged in Long-Term Care Facilities

- Construct monocultural facilities where population demographics warrant.
- Develop transcultural programs in facilities by the incorporation of existing community culture-specific activities, groups, and clubs.
- Establish hiring policies whereby the ethnic roots of the staff reflect the ethnic population as closely as possible.
- Increase cross-cultural long-term care content in nursing school curricula.
- Select roommates with careful consideration of individual needs and preferences.

Originally, nursing home placement for elderly parents was not considered by the Japanese, but the modern Nisei and Sansei (third generation) face the same dilemmas as others when caring for their elderly parents, despite Issei expectations of *oya koko,* or "care for parents." Thus nursing home placement is becoming more common. Nursing homes specifically for the aged Japanese are rare. One does exist near Los Angeles in which familiar traditions are maintained by Japanese staff. There are signs that a few ethnically friendly assisted living and nursing homes are beginning to appear that cater to a specific ethnic group. In these facilities staff are of the same ethnic background or are extremely well versed in the ethnic culture of the residents (KRON TV, news brief, 2001).

There is an increasing cultural diversity in physicians and nurses who are choosing geriatrics and long-term care. These providers of geriatric care are an increasingly heterogeneous cultural group. The countries from which these providers come vary from one part of the United States to another. Some large groups have come from the Philippines, Haiti, and India (Yeo, 1996-1997). There are positive aspects to this trend: (1) they may bring respect for the elder, found in other cultures and less in the youth-driven society of the United States, and (2) they may have the language skills and understanding to better care for the elders and families of their own cultural background. There are concerns as well: (1) the complexities of cross-cultural communications and decision making when second languages are used, and (2) the use of cultural norms not well understood by each other.

Human Need Hierarchy

Maslow's hierarchy may not be relevant to all cultures. As it stands, the hierarchy is applied to all without regard for cultural diversity. Brooks and Nisberg (1974) looked at the hierarchic framework from the black business world perspective and developed the Brooks/Nisberg Need Hierarchy. The import of this approach might serve as a basis for a broader look at human need hierarchies in cultures other than European American.

The Brooks/Nisberg framework presents these levels: (1) staying alive, (2) enjoying life, (3) praising God, (4) getting ahead, and (5) upgrading the race or ethnic group (Figure 19-8). Staying alive; seeking better conditions; basic life necessities of food, clothing, and health care; and recreation are at the first level of human need in the Brooks/Nisberg hierarchy. Economic factors in many ethnic communities interfere with the ability to obtain these survival basics. Interethnic differences exist in eligibility for Social Security and public assistance benefits. Few ethnic groups had survival rates equal to white Americans, so benefit eligibility was not sufficiently considered. Although adjustments have been made and future generations of aged will fare better, the present elderly must cope with this economic inequity.

Enjoyment of life and security within one's own group is the second level of the Brooks/Nisberg hierarchy. The inner community provides an escape from tensions experienced with white society. Major cities tend to have their Nihonmachi, Chinatown, and barrio in which the elderly remain. Traditional ties and cultural identity support the familiar, which has brought pleasure in the past. Here the language, common interests, and interpersonal relationships can remain relatively unchanged.

The third level of which Brooks and Nisberg speak is praising God. Some groups are steeped in deep religious beliefs. At times it is difficult to distinguish that which is culture from that which is religion. Hispanic, Native American, and black cultures look at life as harmony of self with environment sustained through religious practice or following specific tenets. White Americans do not clearly understand the significance of this intense religious foundation in culture. For the

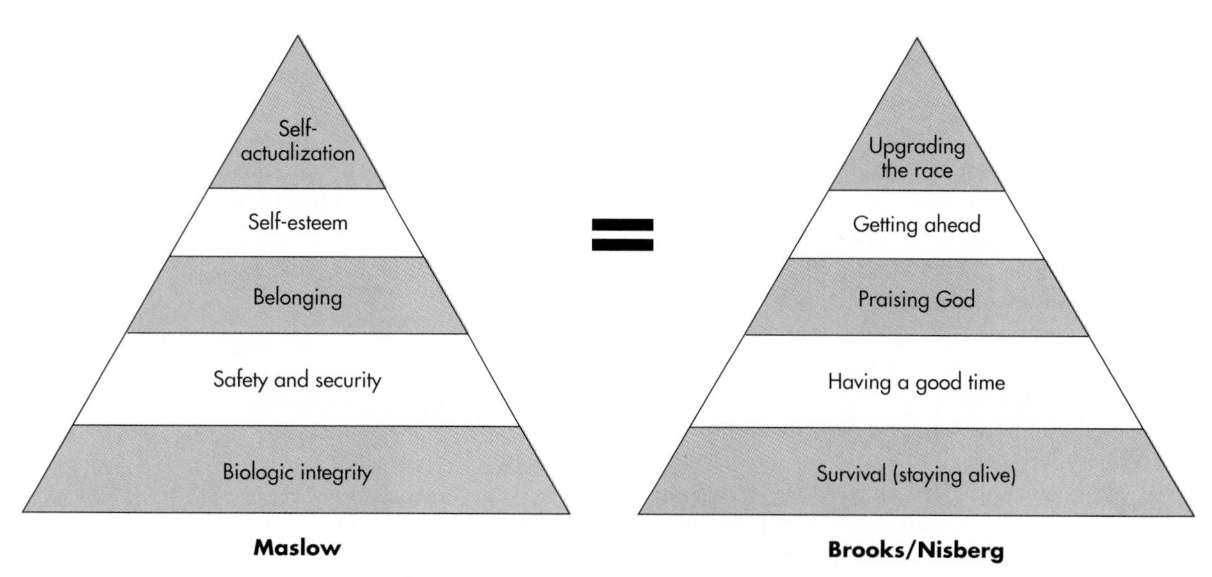

Figure 19-8. Needs hierarchies compared.

average Anglo American, the religious affiliation seems to surface at times of births, weddings, and deaths.

Getting ahead and upgrading the race or ethnic group occupy levels four and five, respectively. This may not be as significant for the aged of today as for the younger representatives of the particular ethnic community, who will be the aged of tomorrow. The potential and desire for self-actualization may not be the highest attainment for persons of certain cultures. In fact, the greatest goal may be to subjugate the needs of the self to others; for example, the Navajo elderly do all they can to help the young "make it" in the new society. Self-esteem may be intricately tied to belonging and contingent on the success of the group rather than on productivity or independent identity.

The ethnic-cultural systemic framework of Orque and colleagues (1983) uses the concepts of Maslow and also seems to incorporate the Brooks/Nisberg hierarchy. Orque's system is holistic and comprehensive in scope and can be used to understand elders in any culture (Figure 19-9). The core of the system contains the basic human needs, which are cyclic in nature because people are continually adapting to their environment. The extent to which each aspect of culture is reflected in meeting these needs depends on the individual's ethnic-cultural system.

Although all the components are universal, the nuances of the components indicate the diversity that exists between groups or individuals.

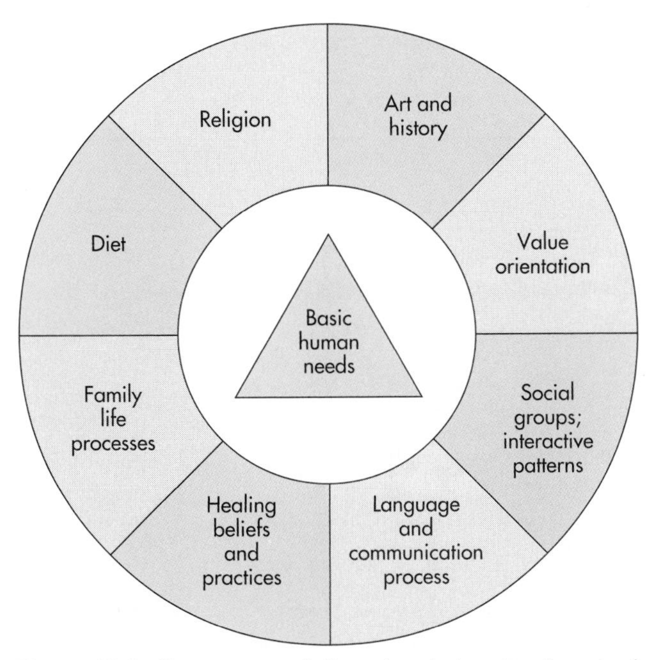

Figure 19-9. Components of Orque's ethnic-cultural systemic framework. (Modified from Orque M, Bloch B, Monrroy L: *Ethnic nursing care: a multicultural approach,* St Louis, 1983, Mosby.)

INTEGRATING CONCEPTS

Family, religion, community, and history are important reference points for self-worth and identity for any individual or ethnic group. Familial supports are variable between groups, social classes, and subcultures, yet the nuclear or extended family is the chief avenue of transmitting cultural values, beliefs, customs, and practices. The family provides orientation, stability, and sanctuary. In a simplistic sense we may say that Asians value familial piety; Hispanics, the extended family (*compadres* translates to *co-parents*); blacks, extended or fictive kin supports; and Native Americans, a system of kinship and line of descent.

Church or religiosity plays a major role in defining many cultures. Religion may function as a consistent experience that affords psychic support in the individual's life. In the black community, religion is a pervasive force and the place to instill self-determination toward change (Moriwaki and Kobata, 1983; Walls, 1992; Hooyman and Kiyak, 1996). The Issei seek religious tradition in the face of aging and death (Kitano, 1969). Padilla and Ruiz (1976) note that Hispanics tend to seek Spanish-speaking clergy rather than mental health professionals when they have emotional problems.

The ethnic community (barrios, nihonmachi, and Chinatown) serves as a buffer and a means of strengthening cohesiveness for elders and others of various cultural groups. Within the community, members are protected from discrimination and the strange language and customs of the dominant society.

Changes are threatening the historical role of the aged and the traditional family. Economic independence and mobility of the younger members of the family are chipping away at the insulation afforded by the community. Intergenerational discontinuities of assimilation create a communication gap between the young and the old. Often the elderly are not proficient in the language of the dominant culture, and the younger members tend not to retain the language of their parents. This may cause isolation and estrangement between the oldest and youngest generations. Members of ethnic minorities are extremely vulnerable in old age. They experience double jeopardy as they may be devalued because of age and ethnicity. Attitudes and economic inequality also contribute to their problems.

Throughout this chapter the aged have been viewed, individually and collectively, as they have been defined and developed by the influence of their time and place in history, their gender, and distinctive group practices and beliefs that have served as the foundation for the self system.

The study of the uniqueness and individuality of each surviving elder is one of the most complex and intriguing opportunities of our day. Realistically it will almost be impossible to become familiar with the whole range of clinically relevant cultural differences of older adults one may encounter, but to attempt to serve them holistically and sensitively is the most challenging opportunity.

Human Needs and Wellness Diagnoses

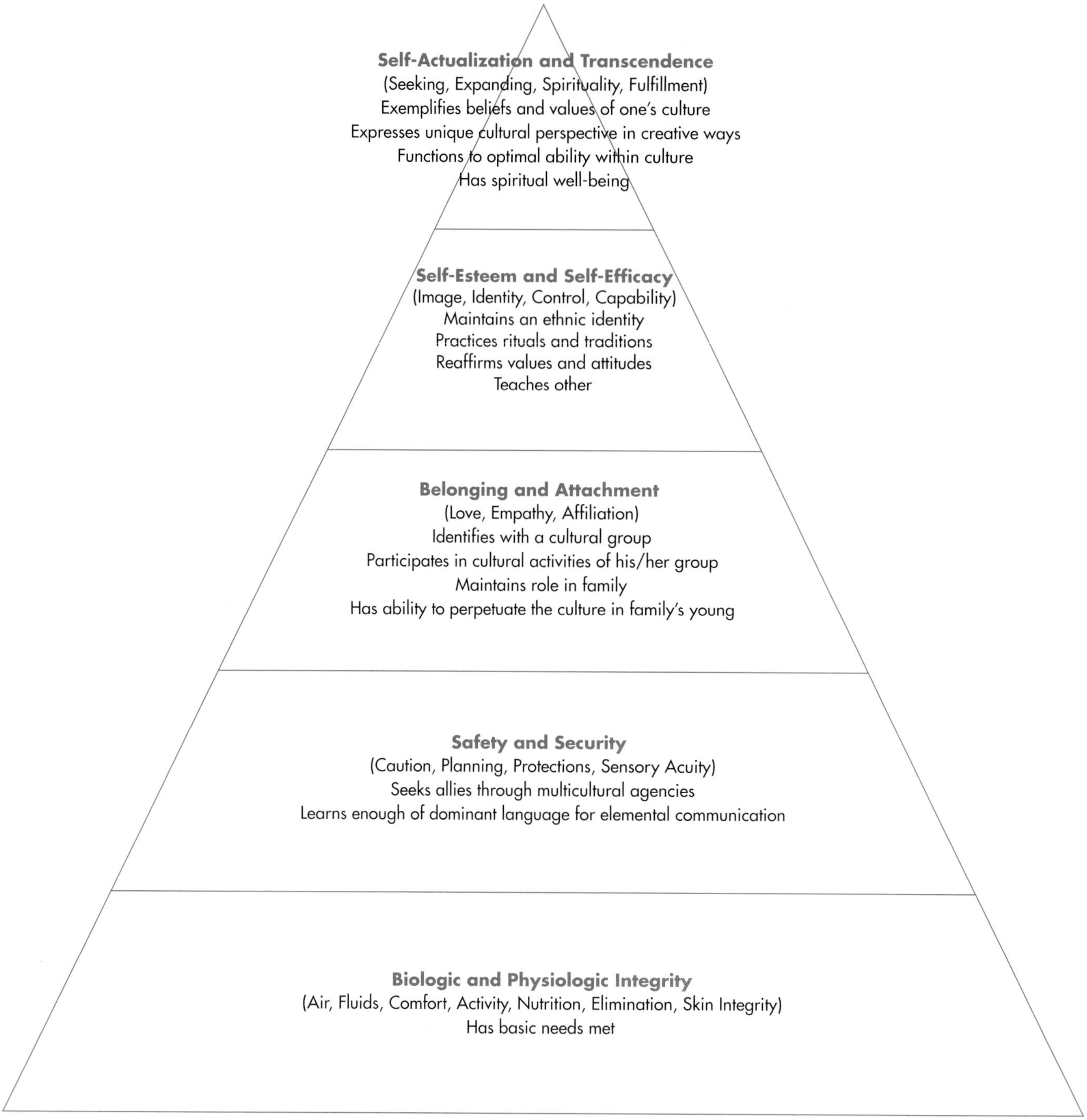

Self-Actualization and Transcendence
(Seeking, Expanding, Spirituality, Fulfillment)
Exemplifies beliefs and values of one's culture
Expresses unique cultural perspective in creative ways
Functions to optimal ability within culture
Has spiritual well-being

Self-Esteem and Self-Efficacy
(Image, Identity, Control, Capability)
Maintains an ethnic identity
Practices rituals and traditions
Reaffirms values and attitudes
Teaches other

Belonging and Attachment
(Love, Empathy, Affiliation)
Identifies with a cultural group
Participates in cultural activities of his/her group
Maintains role in family
Has ability to perpetuate the culture in family's young

Safety and Security
(Caution, Planning, Protections, Sensory Acuity)
Seeks allies through multicultural agencies
Learns enough of dominant language for elemental communication

Biologic and Physiologic Integrity
(Air, Fluids, Comfort, Activity, Nutrition, Elimination, Skin Integrity)
Has basic needs met

These are not all the possible wellness diagnoses that may be identified. The above are examples of nursing diagnoses that should be considered when planning care for the older adult

KEY CONCEPTS

- Cohort groups are convenient for statistical analysis, but such factors as geography, composition, and religion reflect the heterogeneity within groups.
- Gender affects values, perceptions, and the approach to health care assessment and treatment.
- Population diversity is rapidly increasing and will continue to do so for many years. This suggests that nurses will be caring for a greater number of minority elders than they have in the past.
- Ethnicity is a complex phenomenon encompassing geography, language, traditions, symbols, and folklore.
- Culture, social status, and support systems are three components of ethnicity.
- Programs staffed by persons who reflect ethnic elders' background and speak their language are preferred by the elders.
- Culture is a complex concept reflecting the interrelationship of many components.
- Cultural competency and sensitivity require awareness of issues related to culture, race, gender, sexual orientation, social class, and economic situations.
- Stereotyping negates the fact that there is significant heterogeneity within cultural groups.
- Health beliefs of various groups emerge from three general belief systems: biomedical, magicoreligious, and naturalistic. Elders may adhere to one or more of these systems.
- Nurses caring for minority elders must let go of their ethnocentrism before effective caring can occur.
- Family, history, religion, and community are the core of the ethnic elder's self-worth and identity.

▲ CASE STUDY

Georgia was a misfit. She had always been a misfit. She felt that she was born in the wrong time and most of the time was in the wrong place. She was born in China in 1920, the child of missionary parents. Her parents had built and managed a school for orphaned children in Shanghai. There were many problems and uprisings in China, and when she was 15 the political situation and threat of war were so intense that her parents were asked to leave the school and return to the United States. They were then sent to an Appalachian mining village to manage a small school and clinic. Having grown to adolescence in China, she felt more Chinese than Anglo. She had a difficult adjustment in the poverty-stricken rural mining village in Appalachia, so unlike where she had been. In a few years her parents sent her to a private religious college, mainly attended by the children of the affluent elders of the church. She married a young Army officer, and they were immediately sent to France. Her life from then on seemed to consist of nothing but moves as she followed her husband about. She was grateful that she had never had children; as she said, "My life has always seemed so unsettled, I don't think I could have provided any stability for children." As she aged she developed crippling arthritis, and her husband provided much of her care. When she was widowed at 80, she almost immediately entered a nursing home. There she found that most of the staff were Filipino and talked among themselves in Tagalog. Again, she felt out of step with the prevailing culture she found herself in. She became very difficult to get along with, and the staff were at their wits end trying to please her. You recently went to work as director of nursing in the facility Georgia is in. How will you help her and the staff maximize their life satisfactions?

Based on the case study, develop a nursing care plan using the following procedure:*

List comments of client that provide subjective data.

List information that provides objective data.

From these data identify and state, using accepted format, two nursing diagnoses you determine are most significant to this client at this time.

Determine and state outcome criteria for each diagnosis. These must reflect some alleviation of the problem identified in the nursing diagnosis and must be stated in concrete and measurable terms.

Plan and state one or more culturally relevant interventions for each diagnosed problem. Provide specific documentation of source used to determine appropriate intervention. Plan at least one intervention that incorporates the client's existing strengths.

Evaluate success of intervention. Interventions must correlate directly with the stated outcome criteria in order to measure the outcome success.

STUDY QUESTIONS/ACTIVITIES

Define the terms *culture, ethnicity, ethnocentricity, cultural sensitivity,* and *cultural competence.*

Identify several personal values or beliefs that are derived from your ethnic and cultural roots.

Relate major historical events that have affected your birth cohort and explain in what way your cohort has been affected.

Discuss several different ethnically based approaches to health care.

Describe characteristics that you believe are specific to your gender.

Construct a cultural genogram and discuss your roots.

Discuss ways in which you have learned to appreciate cultural and ethnic differences.

Privately list your stereotypes and "ethnocentrisms" for various ethnic groups and explore the basis of these beliefs

---

*Students are advised to refer to their nursing diagnosis text and identify possible or potential problems.

(taught, fear, experience, lack of knowledge). Then consider what can be done to be more culturally sensitive and competent.

Select a food or particular behavior and examine differences in custom that arise from ethnic/cultural interpretations.

Describe the advocacy role of nurses who care for ethnic elderly.

Formulate a care plan incorporating ethnically sensitive interventions.

Plan strategies to provide care that is culturally sensitive and acceptable without losing a focus on the individual's own aging experience.

RESEARCH QUESTIONS

What are the chief difficulties in providing nursing care for individuals from an entirely different background from one's own?

Which personality types thrive best in a homogeneous environment, and which thrive best in a heterogeneous environment?

What are the factors that identify a group as an ethnic minority?

What are the enduring cohort differences that are unlikely to change throughout life?

How is cultural sensitivity incorporated into a curriculum?

What are the outcomes of an integrated cultural approach versus a separate-course approach in a curriculum?

All aspects of differences in the aging man and the aging woman need to be more clearly understood. No comprehensive comparative studies exist that factor in cohort, culture, and gender.

REFERENCES

Abbott PD et al: Improving your cultural awareness with cultural clues, *Nurse Pract* 27(2):44, 2002.

Administration on Aging: Profile of older Americans 2000. Available at *www.AOA.gov/aoa/stats/profile*

Administration on Aging: Highlights 2001. Available at *www.AOA.gov/aoa/stats/profile/2001/highlights.html*

American Association of Retired Persons: *Healthy aging: making health promotion work for minority elders,* Washington, DC, 1990, The Association.

American Association of Retired Persons: *A profile of older Americans 1995,* Washington, DC, 1995, The Association.

American Society on Aging: Gender and aging, *Generations* 14(3), 1990 (entire issue).

Belgrave LL, Wykle ML, Chio JM: Multigenerational households: more a function of aging, mental and socioeconomic status and health, *Gerontologist* 33(3):379, 1993.

Berman HJ: From the pages of my life, *Generations* 15(2):33, 1991.

Bohannon P: *We, the alien: an introduction to cultural anthropology,* Prospect Heights, IL, 1992, Waverly Press.

Brangman SA: Minorities. In Ham RJ, Sloan PD, editors: *Primary care geriatrics,* ed 3, St Louis, 1997, Mosby.

Brislin RS, Pederson P: *Cross-cultural orientation programs,* New York, 1982, Cardier Press.

Brooks WC, Nisberg JN: Effects of cultural differences on motivation, *Personnel Administrator* 51:28, Oct 1974.

Chavira J: *Common remedies used by Mexican American elders: Their source and use: Traditional and nontraditional medication use among ethnic elders.* Conference sponsored by The Stanford Geriatric Education Center, San Jose, CA, April 28, 1989.

Chrisman NJ: Culture-sensitive nursing care. In Patrick M et al: *Medical-surgical nursing,* Philadelphia, 1992, JB Lippincott.

Christensen D: Heart attack shows gender bias, study finds, *J Am Coll Cardiol* 29:35, 1997.

Coulton C: *Ethnicity, self care and use of medical care among the elderly with joint symptoms.* Paper presented at the Veterans Hospital and Medical Center Gerontology Resource and Educational Center, Cleveland, OH, October 1988.

Cuellar J: *Aging and health: American Indian/Alaska Native, Stanford Geriatric Education Center Working Paper Series,* no 6, *Ethnogeriatric Reviews,* Stanford, CA, 1990.

Day AT: Remarkable survivors: insights into successful aging among women, *Aging Today* 13(6):10, 1992.

dePaula T, Lagana K, Gonzalez-Ramirez L: Mexican Americans. In Lipson JG, Dibble SL, Minarik PA, editors: *Culture and nursing: a pocket guide,* San Francisco, 1996, UCSF Nursing Press.

Dilworth-Anderson P: Extended kin networks in black families, *Generations* 17(3):29, 1992.

Ebersole P: Editorial, *Geriatr Nurs* 17(4):149, July/Aug 1996.

Enslein J et al: Evidence-based protocol: interpreter facilitation for individuals with limited English proficiency, *J Gerontol Nurs* 28(7):5, 2002.

Espino DV, Maldonado D: Hypertension and acculturation in elderly Mexican Americans: results from 1982-84 Hispanic males, *J Gerontol* 45(6):M209, 1990.

Estes MEZ: *Health assessment and physical examination,* ed 2, Pacific Grove, CA, 2002, Delmar.

Evans CA, Cunningham BA: Caring for the ethnic elder, *Geriatr Nurs* 17(3):105, 1996.

FDA Consumer 29(9):4, 1996.

Fejos P: Man, magic, and medicine. In Goldstone I, editor: *Medicine and anthropology,* New York, 1959, International University Press.

Geertz C: *The interpretation of cultures,* New York, 1973, Basic Books.

Gibson R: The age-by-race gap in health and mortality in the older population: a social science research agenda, *Gerontologist* 34:454, 1994.

Giger JN, Davidhizar RE: *Transcultural nursing,* St Louis, 1991, Mosby.

Goldstein M: Overview of geriatrics and medications. Traditional and nontraditional medication use among ethnic elders. Conference sponsored by the Stanford Geriatric Education Center, San Jose, CA, April 28, 1989.

Grossman D: Enhancing your cultural competence, *Am J Nurs* 94(7):58, 1994.

Gunter LM: Cultural diversity among older Americans. In Bains EM, editor: *Perspectives on gerontological nursing,* Newbury Park, CA, 1991, Sage.

Habayeb GL: Cultural diversity: a nursing concept not yet reliably defined, *Nurs Outlook* 43:224, 1995.

Hendricks J: Gender and aging: Making something of our chromosomes, *Generations* 14(3):5, 1990.

Hess P: Various seminars, Exploring Health Care in the Southwest: The Navajo Perspective, Navajo Nation Reservation, Arizone, June 10-17, 2000.

Hobbs FB: The elderly population, U.S. Census Bureau. Available at *www.census.gov/population/www/pop-profile/elderpop.html*

Hooyman N, Kiyak HA: *Social gerontology,* ed 4, Boston, 1996, Allyn & Bacon.

Hudson RB, Gonyea JG: A perspective on women in politics: political mobilization and older women, *Generations* 14(3):67, 1990.

Jackson LE: Understanding, eliciting, and negotiating clients' multicultural health beliefs, *Nurse Pract* 18(4):30, 1993.

Jones D, van Amelsvoort Jones G: Communication patterns between nursing staff and the ethnic elderly in long-term care facility, *J Adv Nurs* 11:265, 1986.

Kaye LW, Applegate J: Men's style of nurturing elders. In Sabo D, Gordon D, editors: *Men's health and illness,* Thousand Oaks, CA, 1995, Sage.

Kitano H: *Japanese Americans,* Englewood Cliffs, NJ, 1969, Prentice-Hall.

Kleinman A: *Patients and healers in the context of culture: an exploration of the borderland between anthropology, medicine, and psychiatry,* Berkeley, 1980, University of California Press.

Kramer J: American Indians. In Lipson JG, Dibble SL, Minarik PA, editors: *Culture and nursing care: a pocket guide,* San Francisco, 1996, UCSF School of Nursing Press.

KRON TV: News brief, 2001.

Legato MJ: *Eve's rib,* New York, 2002, Harmony Book, Crown Publishing Group, a division of Random House.

Leininger M: *Transcultural nursing concepts, theories, and practices,* New York, 1978, Wiley.

Lin H: Personal communication. Case Western Reserve University, Cleveland, 1988.

Lipson JG: Culturally competent nursing care. In Lipson JG, Dibble SL, Minarik PA, editors: *Culture and nursing care: a pocket guide,* San Francisco, 1996, UCSF School of Nursing Press.

Manton K, Poss SS, Wiing S: The black/white mortality crossover: investigation from the perspective of the components of aging, *Gerontologist* 19:291, 1979.

Markides KS, Mindel CH: *Aging and ethnicity,* Sage Library of Social Research, vol 163, Newbury Park, Calif, 1987, Sage.

Martin K: Native American customs bear on service delivery, *Generations* 1(2):24, summer 1977.

Meleis A et al: *Diversity, marginalization and culturally competent health care: issues in knowledge development,* Washington, DC, 1995, Academy of Nursing.

Mitchell F: Folk beliefs and health practices of ethnic elders. Traditional and non-traditional medication use among ethnic elders. Conference sponsored by the Stanford Geriatric Education Center, San Jose, CA, April 28, 1989.

Monrroy LA: Nursing care of Raza/Latina patients. In Orque MS, Block B, Monrroy LSA: *Ethnic nursing care: a multicultural approach,* St Louis, 1983, Mosby.

Moore JW: Situational factors affecting minority aging, *Gerontologist* 11:88, 1971.

Morioka-Douglas N, Yeo G: *Aging and health: Asian/Pacific Island American elders, Stanford Geriatric Education Center Working Paper Series,* no 3, *Ethnogeriatric Reviews,* Stanford, CA, 1990.

Moriwaki S, Kobata F: Ethnic minority aging. In Woodruff R, Birren J, editors: *Aging,* ed 2, Monterey, CA, 1983, Brooks/Cole.

Mouton CP, Esparza YB: Ethnicity and geriatric assessment. In Gallo JJ et al, editors: *Handbook of geriatric assessment,* ed 3, Gaithersburg, MD, 2000, Aspen.

Ochoco L, Shimamoto Y: Group work with the frail ethnic elderly, *Geriatr Nurs* 8:185, 1987.

Orque MS, Block B, Monrroy LSA: *Ethnic nursing care: a multicultural approach,* St Louis, 1983, Mosby.

Padilla A, Ruiz R: Prejudice and discrimination. In Hernandez CA, Haug MJ, Wagner NN, editors: *Chicanos: social and psychological perspectives,* ed 2, St Louis, 1976, Mosby.

Pender NJ, Murdaugh CL, Parsons MA: Health promotion in vulnerable populations. In Pender NJ, Murdaugh CL, Parsons A, editors: *Health promotion in nursing practice,* ed 4, Upper Saddle River, NJ, 2002, Pearson Education, Prentice-Hall.

Pfeifferling JH: A cultural prescription for mediocentrism. In Eisenberg L, Kleinman A, editors: *The relevance of social science for medicine,* Boston, 1981, Reidel.

Pierce R, Clark M, Kaufman S: Generation and ethnic identity: a typological analysis, *Int J Aging Hum Dev* 9:19, 1978-1979.

Pinkleton N: The status of black health care, 1988: implications for the health management of the elderly, *GNP Newsletter* 21:2, summer 1988.

Purnell LD, Paulanka BJ: *Transcultural health care,* Philadelphia, 1998, FA Davis.

Scott RW, Polacca M: Staying in balance on the fourth hill of life: mental health and elderly Native Americans, *Dimensions* 2(4):1, 1995-1996.

Siegler IC, Longino CF, Johnson K: The Georgia centenarian study: comments from friends. In Poon LW, editor: *The Georgia centenarian study,* Amityville, NY, 1992, Baywood.

Snow LF: Folk medicine beliefs and their implications for patient care: a review based on studies among black Americans, *Ann Intern Med* 81:82, 1974.

Spector RE: *Cultural diversity in health and illness,* East Norwalk, CT, 1985, Appleton-Century-Crofts.

Spector RE: *Cultural diversity in health and illness,* ed 4, East Norwalk, CT, 1996, Appleton-Century-Crofts.

Spector RE: *Cultural diversity in health and illness,* ed 5, Upper Saddle River, NJ, 2000, Prentice-Hall.

Stokes LG: Growing old in the black community. In Reinhardt AM, Quinn MD, editors: *Current practice in gerontological nursing,* St Louis, 1979, Mosby.

U.S. Bureau of the Census: *Statistical abstract of the United States: 1995,* ed 115, Washington, DC, 1995, U.S. Government Printing Office.

U.S. Bureau of the Census: The 65 yrs and over population: 2000. Census brief. Available at *www.census.gov*

U.S. Bureau of the Census: Gender 2000. Census brief, summary file 1. Available at *www.census.gov*

U.S. Bureau of the Census: The white population: 2000. Census brief, issued Aug 2001. Available at *www.census.gov*

U.S. Bureau of the Census: The Hispanic population. Census 2000 brief, issued May 2001. Available at *www.census.gov* (click on "Minority Links").

U.S. Bureau of the Census: The Native Hawaiian and other Pacific Islander Population: 2000. Census 2000 brief, issued Dec 2001. Available at *www.census.gov* (click on "Minority Links").

U.S. Bureau of the Census: The Asian Population: 2000. Census 2000 brief, issued Feb 2001. Available at *www.census.gov* (click on "Minority Links").

U.S. Bureau of the Census: The American Indian and Alaska Native: 2000. Census brief, issued Feb 2002. Available at *www.census.gov* (click on "Minority Links").

U.S. Bureau of the Census: The black population: 2000. Census 2000 brief, issued Aug 2001. Available at *www.census.gov* (click on "Minority Links").

U.S. Bureau of the Census: American FactFinder census 2000 summary file 1 (SF 1) PCT12: Sex by age [209]-universe: total population. Available at *factfinder.census.gov/home/en/datanotes/expsf1u.htm*

U.S. Bureau of the Census: American FactFinder, DP-1 profile of general demographic characteristics: 2000. Census 2000 summary file 1 (SF 1). Available at *factfinder.census.gov/home/en/datanotes/expsf1u.htm*

U.S. Bureau of the Census: Table 3. Black or African American population by age and sex for the United States: 2000. Internet release date: Feb 25, 2000, summary file 1. Available at *www.census.gov*

U.S. Bureau of the Census: Poverty in the United States: 2000. Available at *www.census.gov*

Wagnild G, Young HM: Resilience among older women, *Image J Nurs Sch* 22(4):252, 1990.

Walls CT: The role of church and family support in the lives of older African Americans, *Generations* 17(3):33, 1992.

Wilson C: Health care and the Hispanic elderly: dehumanization or what, *GNP Newsletter* 21:3, summer 1988.

Woods NF, Shaver JF: The evolutionary spiral of a specialized center for women's health research, *Image J Nurs Sch* 24(3):223, 1992.

Yeo G: Ethnogeriatrics: cross-cultural care of the older adult. In *Geriatrics: a clinical care update, Generations* 20(4):72, 1996-1997.

Zhou HH et al: Racial differences in drug response: altered sensitivity to and clearance of propranolol in men of Chinese descent as compared with American whites, *N Engl J Med* 320:565, 1989.

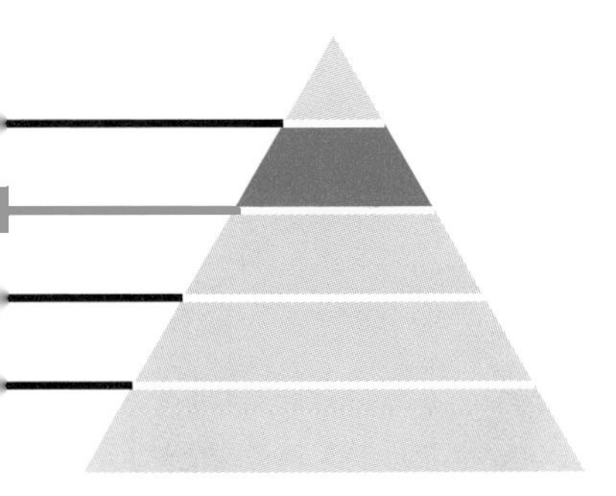

APPENDIX 19-A

Cultural Status Examinations

PFEIFFERLING MODEL*

1. How would you describe the problem that has brought you here?
   NOTE: The clinician may need to identify others who can facilitate the discussion of the client's/patient's problem.
   a. Who in the community and your family helps you with your problem?
2. How long have you had this problem?
   a. Do you know anyone else with it?
   b. Tell me what happened to them when dealing with this problem.
3. What do you think is wrong with you?
   a. What might other people think is wrong with you?
   b. Tell me about people who don't get this problem.
4. Why has it happened to you and why now?
   a. Why has it happened to the involved part?
   b. Why do you get sick and not someone else?
5. What do you think will help clear up this problem?
   a. If specific tests or medications are listed, ask what they are and what they do.
6. Apart from me, who else do you think can make you feel better?
   a. Are there therapies that make you feel better (some discipline) that I don't know about?

KLEINMAN EXPLANATORY MODEL†

1. What do you call your problem? What name does it have?
2. What do you think caused it?
3. When do you think it started?
4. What does your sickness do to you?
5. How severe is it? Will it have a long or short course?
6. What do you fear most about your sickness?
7. What are the chief problems your sickness has caused for you?
8. What treatment should you receive? What are the most important results you hope to receive?

---

*Modified from Pfeifferling JH: *In service provider briefings.* Material prepared by Gutierrez-Mayka M, Henderson JN, Poiley EF, editors; University of South Florida Geriatric Education Center, Suncoast Gerontology Center, funded by Bureau of Health Professions, Health Resources and Services Administration (#DHHS AH64019-04), 1981.

†From Kleinman A: *In service provider briefings: ethnic minority elderly—better understanding for better care.* Material prepared by Gutierrez-Mayka M, Henderson JN, Poiley EF, editors, University of South Florida Geriatric Education Center, Suncoast Gerontology Center, funded by Bureau of Health Professions, Health Resources and Services Administration (#DHHS AH64019-04), 1981.

CHAPTER 20

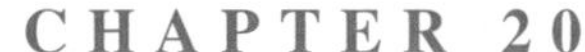

Rural Aging

JoAnn G. Congdon

An elder speaks

The way I look at it, I think you are better off in a nursing home. That is how I maintain my independence. I would hate being dependent on my children.

Anna, age 82

LEARNING OBJECTIVES

On completion of this chapter, the reader will be able to:

1. Develop a broad sensitivity to the multiple, complex issues facing rural older adults.
2. Acknowledge the wide variations among rural communities.
3. Describe personal characteristics of rural older adults historically.
4. Discuss cultural features of rural populations.
5. Identify rural challenges to accessing and receiving health care.
6. Discuss effective strategies to facilitate nursing care in rural settings.
7. Compare features of rural versus urban nursing practice.
8. Be cognizant of organizations that are resources for rural older adults.

The purpose of this chapter is to give the reader an awareness of the life ways and culture of older rural Americans and what it is like to practice nursing in a rural community. The information was taken from the gerontology, nursing, rural, sociology, and research literature. Relevant historical perspectives are highlighted, along with rural concepts, characteristics, health status, and health care features. An attempt was made to present some of the unique features about aging and nursing in rural environments. Rural older adults are different from their urban counterparts, and these differences have both advantages and disadvantages. It is important for the reader to understand the difficulty in generalizing research information across rural settings because great regional diversity exists in the social, cultural, ethnic, and economic structures of rural communities across the United States.

Additionally, the roles of rural nurses are distinct from those of their urban peers. Rural nurses provide care to sparse populations living in large, often isolated geographic areas that have limited resources. They are challenged to become expert generalists, to be nonjudgmental, and to develop the characteristics of resiliency, creativity, and resourcefulness. They often have little or no separation between their professional and personal lives. On the other hand, they are respected, hold public visibility, and have a great deal of autonomy and flexibility in delivering nursing care (Bushy, 2000). See Table 20-1 for a comparison of rural and urban nursing practice.

AGING IN RURAL AMERICA

Older rural persons are often portrayed in a romanticized stereotype of leading peaceful, healthy, independent existences with strong families and environments to support them in their aging years. As more data become available on rural older persons, this stereotype is disappearing and more dependable information is emerging about the day-to-day realities of older rural men and women and their families. The intent of this chapter is to present the current state of knowledge on rural older adults and to introduce nurses to the critical dimensions, issues, and trends in rural health care and unique aspects of nursing practice with rural older adults.

Krout and Coward (1998) explained the recent increase in interest in rural older adults within the field of gerontology as being attributed to a number of factors, including the following:

- A growing exposure of the aging population in research journals and scholarly publications

Table 20-1 Comparison of Rural and Urban Nursing Practice on Select Characteristics*

Feature	Rural	Urban
Clients	Of all ages and across the life span Personally acquainted with many of them Sense of connectedness to the community despite geographic distances	More likely to focus on one or two age-groups Usually not personally acquainted
Scope of practice	Expected to wear many hats Interface with other disciplines Greater opportunity for expanded roles	More precise job description for each discipline
Roles	Generalist role Role overlaps with other disciplines	More opportunities to specialize Disciplines have more clearly delineated roles
Resources (materials, other professionals, technology, fiscal, and other)	Sometimes fewer formal services Greater flexibility in planning and delivering nursing care Informal networking facilitates continuum of caregiving	Usually have more (there always are some limitations) Greater structure in planning and delivering nursing care within an institution
Patient/client health conditions and diagnosis	Exposure to clients with wide range of health conditions and diagnoses Opportunities to become an "expert generalist"	Specialize; work with fewer types of conditions and diagnoses
Degree of autonomy	Greater Fewer peers with whom to consult	More limited Better access to peers and other professionals
Pace	Generally slower	Usually more intense; hurried
Public visibility	High public visibility—known by many locals Difficult to remain anonymous	Less visibility Easier to maintain anonymity
Discharge planning and client follow-up	Formal processes as mandated by regulatory agencies within health care facility Familiarity with clients means increased opportunities for nurse-client interaction outside of facility; continues informally after discharge (in community settings) Creativity encouraged to prevent fragmentation of care	Formal process as mandated by regulatory agencies, usually limited to within facility (hospital, clinic, agency) Formal referrals to other agencies and providers
Coordination of a continuum of care for clients	Extended family and familiarity among residents facilitate integration of informal services with formal services Flexibility in planning continuum of care with family system	Reduced access to informal networks Greater reliance on formal services
Status in community	Nursing viewed as an occupation of status, usually highly esteemed Few nurses means high public visibility Acknowledged as a community health resource Well thought of by community (individual variations)	Denser population means less public visibility More nurses and other health professionals—recognition is dispersed among them
Community involvement (informal health education; local policy development)	Multiple roles in home and community social systems (church, school, civic groups, etc.) Plays many roles in health care facility that extend into community roles Little differentiation (less clear boundaries between work, home, and community)	Community activities/roles shared by more people having a particular interest in that activity
Confidentiality	Can be problematic due to familiarity among residents and the visibility of their actions to others	Less problematic because of less familiarity and public visibility but must always be a concern
Quality-of-life issues	Small-town atmosphere Family, recreation, and lifestyle opportunities differ from those of highly populated settings Regional variations—vary from community to community	Regional variations—vary from community to community

From Bushy A: *Orientation to nursing in the rural community,* Thousand Oaks, CA, 2000, Sage.
*Note: There are wide variations among and between rural and urban communities and individuals. Therefore these characteristics are experienced in varying degrees by individual residents in both settings.

- An increase of federal and foundation funding for research related to the aging population
- The farm crisis of the early 1980s, which heightened national and academic awareness of rural issues
- The national awareness of the changing demographics of Americans, particularly the rapid aging of our population
- The growing interest of gerontologists to better understand the diversity of older Americans, and in particular rural older adults, and the importance that residence plays as a variable that adds to this diversity
- The fact that approximately 25% of all older adults in this country reside in rural areas, consistent with rural populations in many other developed countries

RURAL CONCEPTS

Definitions

Rural areas have several prominent features, including low population size and density, small communities, physical remoteness, distance from urban resources, and relative dominance of natural ecology. However, great diversity and lack of consensus exist in attempts to define the seemingly simple term *rural,* and this has created problems for researchers, clinicians, and policy makers. Inconsistent definitions exist among and within individual agencies. For example, the U.S. Bureau of the Census classifies residence of people based on population size and residential population density. The Census Bureau defines *rural* as a "territory outside places of 2,500 or more inhabitants, or outside an urbanized area. An urbanized area comprises one or more places and the adjacent densely settled surrounding territory that together have a minimum of 50,000 persons" (Special Committee on Aging, 1992, p. 1; Rural Information Center Health Service, 2001). The Office of Management and Budget (OMB) classifies areas as either metropolitan or nonmetropolitan based on whether the area has a large city and suburbs (Johnson-Web et al, 1997). The OMB defines *nonmetropolitan areas* as those outside a metropolitan statistical area (MSA). MSAs are areas that include a city of 50,000 or more, or an urbanized area with at least 50,000 inhabitants and a total MSA population of 100,000 or more (Rural Information Center Health Service, 2001). The use of these national definitions for rural does not accurately describe the differences among rural regions, farms, nonfarms, villages, towns, and urban satellite areas. A well-known prominent characteristic of rural America is its diversity. Rural America varies not only by region, community size, and type, but, most distinctly, by its social and economic diversity (Special Committee on Aging, 1992; Havens et al, 2001).

For the purposes of this chapter, it is not essential to enter into a discussion of the complexities of the finer distinctions between urban and rural differences; therefore *rural* is defined as "a generic term referring to the end of the residential continuum that includes towns and open country with small or widely dispersed populations remote from large metropolitan cities" (National Institute of Nursing Research, 1995, p. 26). Approximately one in four persons age 65 and older in the United States lives in a rural community. Even though rural residence is sometimes equated with farming, only about 6% of rural Americans actually reside on farms (McLaughlin and Jensen, 1998). Most rural older adults live in or near small towns.

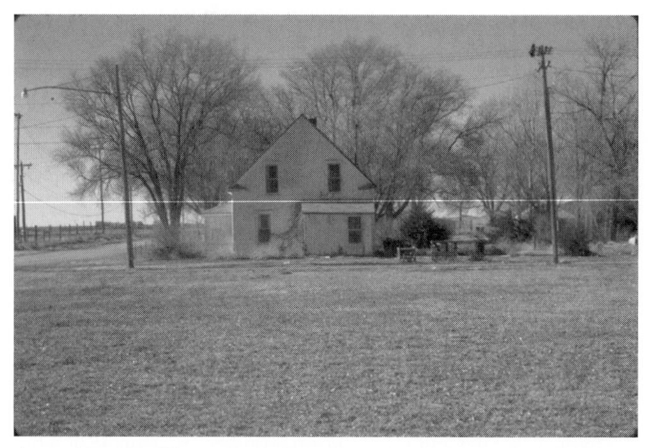

A rural home. (Courtesy JoAnn Congdon and Joan K. Magilvy.)

Characteristics of Rural Older Adults

Age, Gender, and Race Composition. In rural areas, as compared with urban, there is a lower percentage of individuals ages 19 to 54 and a higher percentage of those above 55. An interesting phenomenon accompanying this rural-urban age difference is the high age-dependency ratio. This ratio is calculated by the number of elders and children (those over 64 and under 18 years of age) divided by the number of working-age persons (19 to 64 years of age). The result indicates the extent to which there are working-age persons available to support those who are more dependent—mainly children and elderly persons. The rural age distributions indicate that the nonmetropolitan areas have the smallest number of working-age persons and thus a potentially smaller base of support for the very young and the elderly population (Coward et al, 1994). Many rural areas have been aging through the loss of young adults who move to more urban areas for economic and job-related purposes and from an influx of retirees. Older persons who remain in the rural areas and retirees become an ever-increasing proportion of the total population (Reeder, 1998).

Approximately 60% of all persons age 65 and older are women. In the age-group of 65 to 84 there are about 70 men for every 100 women. In the oldest-old (above 85 years of age) there are about 38 men for every 100 women. In rural or nonmetropolitan areas the imbalance among elderly men and women is not as great. In the age-group of 65 to 84, the number of men living on rural farms exceeds the number of women. The difficulty of living alone on a farm and the trend of older farm widows to move into small towns may account for these figures. Among those age 85 and older the sex ratios are lower, but the pattern is similar (McLaughlin and Jensen, 1998).

The older rural population is less racially and ethnically diverse than those under 65 years of age, but this population is becoming more diverse with the increases in the number of older persons. The extent of racial and ethnic diversity varies from region to region of the country. For example, rural African American elders have greater concentrations in the southern states, American Indians are concentrated more in the southwest and northern plains, and Hispanics and Asians are the smallest groups of rural older adults. Asians, Pacific Islanders, and Hispanics (of any race or ethnic group) are particularly concentrated in metropolitan areas, whereas over half of American Indians, Eskimos, and Aleuts live in nonmetropolitan areas (Special Committee on Aging, 1992). Overall, there is a predominance of whites in both rural and urban areas, but in nonmetropolitan areas approximately 92% of persons over age 65 are white compared with 88% of metropolitan older adults (McLaughlin and Jensen, 1998).

Marital Status, Housing, and Family Conditions. Marital status and living arrangements of older persons have significant influence on overall well-being, social support, poverty status, and health. Older adults who live alone are much more likely to lack social support and are more likely to experience health problems, poverty, and a lower quality of life. Older adults in rural areas are slightly more likely to be married than are urban elders. Approximately 53.6% of nonmetropolitan elders are married and living with spouses compared with 50.5% of metropolitan elders (McLaughlin and Jensen, 1998). Even though marriage is more prevalent in rural areas, it is important to note the decline in marriage with advancing age. For example, Coward and colleagues (1994) reported that for those age 65 to 74, about 68% of rural elderly are married; from age 75 to 84 the marriage rate declines to 48%, and for those over 85 years of age, marriage drops to 28%. These declines in marriage are due to widowhood rather than divorce or separation. They report no differences across residence areas in percentages of older persons never married.

Home ownership can be a valuable asset, and most older persons in all areas own their own homes. However, rural elders are more likely to own their own homes and to be free of mortgage payments than their urban counterparts. In 1998 approximately 87% of rural elders age 60 years and older owned their own homes as compared with 81% of urban older adults (Rogers, 1999). The advantage seems to stop there because rural elders tend to have older homes that are lower in value, substandard, and in need of more repairs, as measured by incomplete plumbing, deficient kitchen facilities, electrical defects, and insufficient heating and maintenance (Rogers, 1999).

Rural households are larger than those in urban areas and often contain multigenerations because of economic needs (Bushy, 1998). An exodus of younger generation from rural communities to urban areas has depopulated many rural communities. Younger persons and professionals are attracted to metropolitan areas for better economic and more lucrative opportunities. The availability of skilled, high-paying jobs is low in rural America. This out-migration pattern of rural young generations has also contributed to some erosion of traditional family structures and networks. On the one hand, as this migration pattern continues, healthy older persons have the potential of becoming an important source of human capital for rural communities (Dorfman, 1998). On the other hand, as the remaining and growing older population becomes an increasing proportion of the rural population, there is a concomitant demand for more health and social services and long-term care in these rural communities. There is some evidence to suggest that declining health, reduced income, and widowhood contribute to migration of the oldest-old to more urban areas where there are more health and social services and where their children live (Siegel, 1993).

Education, Income, and Poverty. Gains in education attainment of older persons have been rising remarkably and are most notably reflected in the young-old. Along with these gains in education has come modest improvement in economic conditions. Young-old rural adults are better educated than the oldest-old. Rogers (1999) reported that about 61% of rural elderly age 85 and older have not completed high school whereas only 28% of those 60 to 64 had not done so. This low educational level has contributed to lifelong limited employment opportunities, lesser incomes, lower retirement incomes, higher poverty rates, and decreased health status. Higher-educated older persons will be better informed and have the skills to take advantage of community programs and services designed to benefit them. Analogous with the higher educational levels will come higher expectations and demands for an increase in the quality and number of health care services for older rural persons (Rogers, 1999).

As a group, rural older women are more economically vulnerable and disadvantaged than urban older women. When compared with their urban counterparts, they are worse off and spend more time in poverty than women in urban or metropolitan areas (McLaughlin, 1998). McCulloch (1998) attributed several explanations for this representation of rural older women: lower levels of education, lower earnings, scarce employment opportunities, competition for jobs that fall within a narrower range of occupations, less prospects for promotion, more part-time employment or employment without benefits, lower pensions, and the high likelihood that rural older women will be living alone as they age.

Although the rural older population in America fares less well economically than their urban counterparts, there have been some slight gains. Bushy (2000) reported that persistent poverty counties have decreased over the last three decades. The United States Department of Agriculture defines *persistent poverty counties* as counties in which 20% or more of the population lived below the poverty line in each of the decades from 1960 to 1990. Jobs grew in these persistent poverty counties, but low-skill jobs, low incomes, and high unemployment rates continue. The persistent poverty counties are most heavily concentrated in the Southeast, in Appalachia, in the Southwest, and on Native American reservations. In addition to the problem of poverty, it is estimated that about 40% of all rural families fall into a category that is described as near poor or working poor (Bushy, 1998). These are families that have members who are employed, but they cannot afford to buy health insurance, nor do they qualify for public assistance because their income level is above the poverty line. The families that do have some coverage struggle with copayments and deductibles.

Transportation. Transportation and access to local services has been a continuing problem in rural America. Most rural older persons rely on private vehicles and equate mobility with the automobile (Kihl, 1993). There are limited public or nonprofit transport systems available in rural America, and, if available, many times they have low levels of utilization. Krout (1994) reported that research shows that rural elders have lower levels of service awareness and tend to distrust the service bureaucracy. He concluded that this combination of availability problems with transportation along with low levels of service awareness and rural cultural attitudes may result in low utilization of the services that are available. Additional transportation barriers include long distances to health care services, poor and inadequate road conditions, and lack of dependable vehicles (Bushy, 1998).

If rural residents are to maintain access to goods and services and any quality of life, they must typically rely on their own private vehicles. It is not uncommon for older rural residents to continue to drive despite considerable problems with vision, hearing, reflexes, and mobility (Kihl, 1993; Magilvy and Congdon, 1994). Researchers report hearing numerous stories from rural health care providers and family members about even the oldest-old making incredible efforts and taking risks in order to drive despite their tremendous physical and mental handicaps. For many rural elders, the loss of driving privileges is synonymous with the loss of independence.

Elderly Migration to Rural Communities. Retirement migration to rural parts of the country is a growing but not easily understood phenomenon in the United States. As a whole, elderly persons are less likely to migrate than are younger persons. Older persons who do migrate tend to be younger, in good health, married, white, and relatively well off economically (Longino and Smith, 1998). They frequently have preestablished links with the rural community through vacationing, visiting relatives or friends, or following associates who migrated earlier (Cuba, 1991). The reasons for rural migration vary greatly, ranging from a yearning to return to rural roots, tiredness of crowded and hurried conditions in the cities, desire for tranquility and beauty of the country, and the belief that life is simpler, less stressful, and less costly in rural areas.

In 1990 the U.S. Department of Agriculture designated 478 nonmetropolitan counties as retirement destinations based on a 15% or more of net elderly in-migration (Reeder and Glasgow, 1990). These retirement counties tend to have a more recreational environment, with many lakes, national parks, and forests, and they tend to be in close proximity to cities. They are located in clusters in areas such as rural California, Oregon, Arizona, New Mexico, the Ozarks, the panhandle of Florida, and the upper Great Lakes (Longino and Smith, 1998).

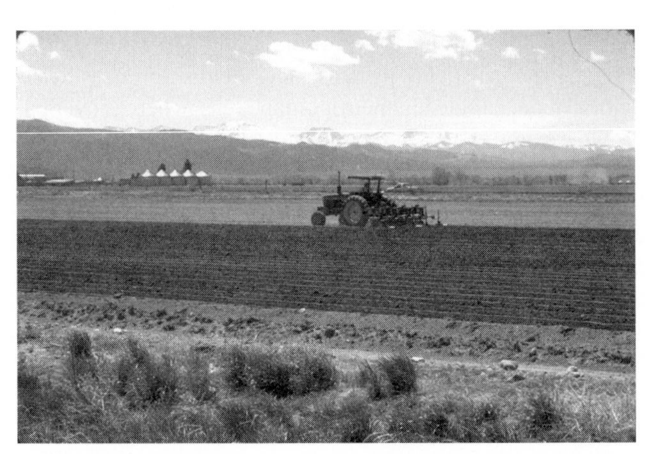

A rural farmer. (Courtesy JoAnn Congdon and Joan K. Magilvy.)

Longino and Smith (1998) described two patterns of retirement movement that they contend have stood for many decades. The first type is lifestyle or amenity motivated, such as urban retirees moving to a rural area to meet their expectations of retirement and to increase their quality of life. The second pattern of movement occurs after a decline in health, a decline in functional ability, or death of a spouse, and is usually in the direction of an urban area. Overall, this second type of move involves a higher number of migrants than the first.

Significant and uneven rural population shifts occurred throughout the 1990s, with much of the rural population growth concentrated in about 40% of rural counties (Health and Human Services Rural Task Force, 2002). The inward migration dynamics of elderly persons, along with a substantial continued out-migration of young people from rural areas, tends to complicate the age, social, economic, and net migration structures of some rural counties. In the short run, this migration pattern appears to benefit the rural areas economically, but more research is needed to fill the gaps in our knowledge about the long-term impact of elderly migration on rural communities (Longino and Smith, 1998).

Health Status

Rural-dwelling older adults are a population at risk for disease and disability because of their multiple, complex health problems, lower socioeconomic status, and barriers to accessible health services (Congdon and Magilvy, 1996). Recent studies have begun to dispel the myth that life in rural America is healthy, care free, and low stress (Wallace and Wallace, 1998). The reality is that rural older adults face vast health challenges. In addition to coping with the problems of aging, rural elders face some vulnerability just by living in rural America. There is a dimension called "triple jeopardy" related to older persons that results from a combination of growing older, residing in a sparsely populated and remote rural setting, and contending with a greater prevalence of certain demographic conditions that negatively affect health (Coward et al, 1996). The data reveal that older rural persons experience a great number of health risks and chronic health problems and that older rural populations generally report poorer perceptions of health status than the urban populations (Special Committee on Aging, 1992). In the 1997 *Current Population Survey,* the rural elderly reported their health status as fair/poor more often than their urban counterparts. Elderly rural residents with fair/poor health status reportings were consistently about 6% higher than urban residents for all groups 60 years of age and older (Rural Information Center Health Service, 2001). In the aggregate, rural U.S. populations experience greater morbidity and higher crude rates of mortality than nonrural populations (Yawn et al, 1994).

Bushy (2000) reported that morbidity and mortality information suggest that rural residents experience high incidences of depression, alcohol abuse, domestic violence, incest, and child neglect. Poor economic conditions and stress-producing rural occupations such as farming, fishing, mining, and forestry may exacerbate these conditions. Isolated farmers are particularly vulnerable to depression and stress-related illnesses.

Acute Conditions. Although there are several important methodologic issues in assessing rural-urban differences in health status of older persons that contribute to inconsistencies and narrowness in study findings, some rural population trends and patterns are worth noting. Older rural residents experience a greater number of acute conditions such as infections, parasitic diseases, acute bronchitis, pneumonia, digestive system conditions, total injuries, sprains and strains, open wounds, lacerations, nonmigraine headaches, and number of persons injured per year than their urban counterparts (Wallace and Wallace, 1998; National Center for Health Statistics, 1994). Many of the injuries encountered in rural areas are due to farm-related occupations along with operating dangerous machinery and working in risky weather conditions.

Chronic Conditions. As persons age, regardless of residential, economic, environmental, or social variables, their number of major chronic health conditions increases. Chronic diseases are the major causes of morbidity and mortality among people age 65 and over in the United States (Hennessy et al, 2001). However, there are some overall variations in urban/rural rates of chronic health conditions. Rural residents have higher rates of the following: arthritis and associated functional limitations and disability, cataracts, hearing impairments, loss of extremities, deformities or orthopedic impairments, ulcers, diabetes, bladder and kidney problems, hypertension, heart disease, and emphysema (National Center for Health Statistics, 1994; Jordon et al, 1995; Wallace and Wallace, 1998).

Health Risks. Health risk factors of rural older adults include obesity, physical inactivity, smoking, moderate drinking, poverty, lack of health insurance, chronic diseases (e.g., heart disease, diabetes, and hypertension), functional impairments, poor dental health, hazardous occupations, higher death rates and serious injuries from motor vehicle accidents, water impurity, and variable weather conditions (Shreffler, 1996; Kumar, 2001; Gamson et al, 2002). These factors are all relevant and important when assessing determinants, emergence, and burden of chronic disease, functional limitations, dependence, and risk of mortality (Hennessy et al, 2001). At the same time researchers caution that the epidemiologic findings in one geographic region do not necessarily generalize to others because of the heterogeneity of rural populations and regions (Wallace and Wallace, 1998).

Coward and colleagues (1994) reviewed the evidence that exists about residential differences in the health status of rural older adults. When interpreting the literature they recommend caution because the data are not always easy to interpret, and further research is needed to clarify the issues. With these concerns in mind, they list several patterns that emerge from their review of the literature:

1. The health of rural elders does differ from that of their urban counterparts, but the differences are not universal across all indicators of health, and they do not always place the rural elderly at a disadvantage.
2. There are significant differences with the rural population along a number of specific health dimensions, especially between farm and nonfarm elders. Rural elders who are still engaged in a farming enterprise are among the healthiest of all elders, whereas rural nonfarm elders have the worst health profiles, compared with the inhabitants of any other residential category.
3. Compared with elders living in all other residential categories, rural nonfarm elders report a higher number of medical conditions, more functional limitations, and difficulty performing a greater number of activities of daily living (ADLs) and instrumental activities of daily living (IADLs). Moreover, both rural farm and rural nonfarm elders perceive their health to be poorer than that of their urban counterparts.

Coward and colleagues (1994) continue to remind us that the rural nonfarm elders represent a much larger segment of the rural population than rural persons still engaged in farming, and that the better health of rural farmers does not make up for the poorer health status of the larger group of nonfarm elders. They also note that although farm elders may be the healthiest of all older adults, they often perceive their health as poor. They give two possible explanations for this seemingly paradoxic finding: (1) because life on a farm is so physically demanding, even small amounts of disability can be perceived as onerous and limiting by older persons living in these settings, and (2) because farm elders may still be actively working, they perceive any health impairment as a great impediment to their ability to perform ADLs.

CULTURAL CHARACTERISTICS

The concept of culture is most often used with reference to different societies or national origins, but it can also mean the differences by geographic regions or other subgroups within a nation (Bureau of Health Professions, Health Resources, and Services Administration, 1995). *Culture* is variously defined as the way of life of a population or part of a population; knowledge; the accumulation of information; a constructed reality; systems of norms; and a learned system of meaning (D'Andrade, 1984). Incorporating these definitions, rural life is a culture. And rural lifestyles and culture predispose older adults to have certain characteristics. These characteristics include a propensity to be self-reliant and independent, use a high level of self-care activities, seek health assistance through an informal health care system, value privacy, and demonstrate a need for reciprocity (Craig, 1994; Magilvy et al, 1994; Stoller and Lee, 1994; Congdon and Magilvy, 1996). Others have described rural residents as having a "greater suspicion of governmental and agency assistance, and greater investment in the maintenance of self and family independence" (McCulloch, 1995, p. 331). In fact, independence may be valued so strongly in rural culture that it may be the impetus that allows an older person to accept assistance for the sake of maintaining independence (Weinert and Long, 1990; Winstead-Fry et al, 1992), or it may lead to a pattern of resisting, neither seeking nor accepting assistance (Longino and Smith, 1994). Longino and Smith (1994) state that "dependence, even on medical authority, is not considered a virtue among many rural elders" (p. 237). Magilvy and colleagues (1994) reported that some elderly persons refused home care services because they viewed the government paperwork to qualify for these services as infringing on their privacy.

Rabiner and colleagues (1997) studied the relationship between metropolitan and nonmetropolitan residential location and self-reported ability to perform basic, mobility, and instrumental activities of daily living, as well as to assess the degree to which the levels and types of functional limitations affect metropolitan versus nonmetropolitan older adults' performance of self-care activities. They found many insignificant differences between the rural and urban participants in their abilities to perform functional tasks, but older adults from nonmetropolitan areas were more likely to report performing self-care activities both in the presence and absence of disability. The researchers concluded that nonmetropolitan older adults may discount the significance of declining functional status, thus normalizing the trajectory of aging in a different way than do their metropolitan counterparts. They give four possible explanations that some of their findings may be due to rural-urban cultural differences. These explanations may help us to further understand the unique cultural characteristics of the rural elderly (Rabiner et al, 1997).

Their first explanation is that rural older adults may have a tendency to report fewer health problems because of their strongly held values of independence and self-sufficiency, similar to those reported earlier. These rural elderly are more likely to perform independent self-care activities in the presence or absence of functional limitations, so the limitations do not get reported. A second reason is that "rural older adults may be more likely to express a sense of contentment in the face of seemingly objective deprivations" (Rabiner et al, 1997, p. 27). Other researchers have reported similar explanations. Magilvy and Congdon (1994) described rural older persons who tolerated significant health problems to remain in their own homes. They further explained that financial, social, and geographic constraints may lead some rural older adults to lowered health expectations and constrain them from seeking advanced health care services (Congdon and Magilvy, 1998b). Still others have suggested that older people who grew up in rural environments are more likely to have limited expectations and a more developed sense of fatalism (Foner, 1986). Rabiner and colleagues' (1997) third explanation is that rural older adults may compare their current situation with that of their peers and consider their health to be better than the health of those in their peer group. Stoller and Forster (1992) further explained this phenomenon by stating that some older rural adults have accepted negative stereotypes of aging but consider themselves exceptions to these stereotypes. Another explanation may be that some may normalize these limitations as a natural part of the aging process. Their fourth explanation of why rural older adults may be less likely to report functional limitations is that they are fearful that these limitations may lead them into a nursing home. This latter explanation is found often in the rural literature.

Spirituality and Faith

In a series of ethnographic studies on the health of rural older adults, Congdon and Magilvy (1998a; Magilvy and Congdon, 2000) reported that churches and religions were vital forces in the communities they studied and that many family and social activities were centered in the rural churches. The faith community assumed a responsibility to minister to the body as well as to the spirit and soul. Older adults, their families, caregivers, and ministers of faith believed that health care and faith were important in achieving healing and positive health outcomes. A strong integration of faith, spirituality, and health existed in the lives of rural older adults. Many rural residents believed that the church held the community together, and that religion and spirituality were important for physical and mental well-being.

Martinez's (1999) work in southern Colorado supports the notion that spirituality is integral to rural life and health; she found that as rural older adults aged, their spiritual health intensified. Older residents often described health as a balance with the spiritual, emotional, and physical aspects of the self. Health was achieved and maintained when one's actions were in harmony with one's values of faith, spirituality, and religion. For the rural Hispanic elders in her study, life's joys and sufferings provided opportunities to serve God, family, and community in the spirit of their faith.

In a discussion of rural health promotion programs, Mochenhaupt and Muchow (1994) confirmed that rural churches are appropriate and available sites for the delivery of health promotion and disease prevention services. Churches are trusted in rural areas whereas outsiders, or persons outside the community, may be viewed with suspicion and doubt. Rural church-based health promotion was most successful when it occurred within congregations and was incorporated into the healing mission and leadership of the church.

Care delivery approaches in rural settings that are culturally congruent and compatible with people's values are the most likely to succeed. Parish nursing has been suggested as an example of a health delivery program that is highly likely to succeed in rural locations (Brown et al, 1996). The concept of parish nursing is culturally well suited to many rural settings in that it places care in a trusted community institution and can provide improved access to and comprehensiveness of care.

HEALTH SERVICES

Although a variety of health care facilities serve the health needs of people living in rural America, a number of rural scholars agree that fewer and a narrower range of services are generally available to and used by rural older adults. Krout (1998, p. 247) summarized these service disadvantages as being variously attributed to a lack of financial and human capital, urban biases in government funding and reimbursement mechanisms, a lack of economic development because of small population size and low population densities, a shortage of adequately trained health care providers, and a rural culture of individual self-reliance that promotes the use of the informal care system.

Rural Hospitals

America's rural hospitals are commonly an integral and major component of the rural community. They have long-standing relationships with their communities and are interwoven into rural life. They are sources of community identity, worth, self-respect, and pride, as well as a major employer and purchaser in the local economy (Duncan, 1994; Schlenker and Shaughnessy, 1996).

Most rural hospitals are nonprofit, but there are also those owned by state and local governments and corporations. In 1996 there were 2226 rural hospitals in the United States. Most of these are small, under 100 beds, and are heavily dependent on Medicare revenues (Rural Information Center Health Service, 2001). Compared with urban settings, rural hospitals are modest institutions in terms of beds, employees, and revenues; are usually housed in older physical plants; and provide a narrower range of medical services (Duncan, 1994). In the 1980s the United States experienced a crisis in health care costs, and dramatic national cost containment efforts took place. Rural hospitals did not fare well from the increased external regulations and cost-cutting changes; consequently, closures accelerated. From 1980 to 1991 a total of 363 rural hospitals were closed, an average of about 30 per year. Although the decline stabilized in the remainder of the 1990s, rural hospitals continue to close. From 1991 to 1999, approximately 116 rural hospitals closed (Rural Information Center Health Service, 2001).

In some rural communities where full-service hospitals have been closed, limited-service hospitals are being used as a means of maintaining health care services. These hospitals provide emergency and low-intensity services (services that do not require intensive or critical care units) and are allowed flexibility in staffing and licensing requirements (Shreffler et al, 1999). Evaluation studies have indicated that these limited-service institutions are a cost-effective solution for maintaining access to acute care services for sparsely populated, remote rural communities that cannot maintain a fully licensed hospital (Shreffler et al, 1999).

Duncan (1994) suggested that rural hospitals, like rural residents, experience a kind of multiple jeopardy. He explained that elderly patients who have the greatest need for local hospital services may also be the least economically desirable, because Medicare reimbursement rates are below costs for rural hospitals. Survival of rural hospitals depends, in part, on providing services for patients who pay at rates that provide a reasonable margin of revenue. These patients are the privately insured or Medicare patients with generous Medigap coverage. Schlenker and Shaughnessy (1996) attributed some rural hospital survival to increased diversification of services, such as swing beds and long-term care. The long-term care services include home health and skilled nursing care. Rural hospitals are presently more involved in long-term care than their urban counterparts, and this pattern of involvement is increasing over time.

A unique example of long-term care use by rural hospitals was the advent of swing beds. Swing beds are acute care hospital beds that are used to provide nursing home care. The term *swing bed* refers to a change in the level of nursing care without the patient being moved from the facility or, frequently, even the bed (Palumbo, 1992). The Omnibus Budget

Reconciliation Act of 1980 allowed eligible rural hospitals with under 50 beds to be certified by Medicare and Medicaid to provide swing bed care. The assumption was that it would be more cost effective to provide long-term care in low-occupancy hospitals in rural areas then to build new nursing homes (Schlenker and Shaughnessy, 1996). Swing beds allow rural hospitals to fill beds, provide postacute care for patients, provide a bed for a patient until one becomes available in a nursing home, or provide beds for patients who would have to travel long distances to obtain skilled nursing care (Rowles, 1996). This swing bed program may make the difference between survival and closure for some rural hospitals. In addition to the swing bed program, in recent years many rural hospitals have added their own long-term care units, which are part of or adjacent to the hospital.

Home Care

Home care has been shown to enhance quality of life and promote a holistic, family-centered approach to the care of rural older adults with acute, postacute, rehabilitative, chronic, and end-of-life conditions (Magilvy, 1996; Congdon and Magilvy, 1998b). Home care focuses on a variety of needs and services that include both medical services and social services. Medical services include skilled nursing care, rehabilitative and restorative therapies, and hospice care and may require the services of providers such as registered nurses, certified nursing assistants, and physical, occupational, speech, and other therapists. Social services focus on providing home-delivered meals, personal care, and assistance with ADLs and IADLs, including preparing meals, shopping, paying bills, using the telephone, doing housework, and providing respite care. The medical services are generally funded by Medicare or Medicaid, and the social service monies usually come from the Older Americans Act (OAA) and Social Service Block Grants (SSBGs) (Krout, 1998).

In rural America the types of services and availability may differ by region. The number and availability of providers and agencies are inconsistent across the country. Magilvy (1996) reported that geographic conditions, economic variables such as funding and reimbursement mechanisms, and local adaptations in the provision of home care that are consistent with local preferences and culture all contribute to the diverse patterns of care. Home care is delivered in a number of settings and by an array of professionals, paraprofessionals, and agencies. It can be delivered in the person's own home, in the home of a relative, in assisted living facilities, or in foster care. The majority of long-term rural home care is provided by informal sources such as family caregivers or friends in the community or by free-standing clinics or agencies affiliated with hospitals (Magilvy, 1996; Krout, 1998).

Congdon and Magilvy (1998b) observed that home care as an integral part of long-term care can be both a socially and culturally acceptable form of holistic health care for an older rural population that fiercely values independence and freedom from institutional restraints. In a series of ethnographic studies, they reported that care at home facilitates independence, self-care activities, and the management of complex health needs over time (Congdon and Magilvy, 1998b; Magilvy and Congdon, 2000; Congdon and Magilvy, 2001). Rural lifestyles and culture challenged persons to use their informal resources and to live with and tolerate significant health problems. Combined with the informal support of family and neighbors, home care surfaced as a major strength in health care delivery and transitions for rural older adults and their families. The commitment and resourceful strategizing of rural nurses was central to accessing both informal and formal home care services for older persons and to the successful delivery of the services.

Nursing Homes

Rural nursing homes have evolved into an important health care resource because often they are the only long-term care option available. Because of this, rural nursing homes have developed in a different way than their urban counterparts (Rowles, 1996). Glover (2001) pointed out that moving to a local nursing home enables long-time rural residents to continue to be part of the community. The residents are well known by the nursing home staff and vice versa.

There is evidence to suggest that rural nursing homes are different from urban nursing homes in the following ways: elderly nursing home residents tend to be younger at the time of entry and less impaired functionally (Green, 1984); rural nursing homes tend to treat chronic care residents rather than those with strong rehabilitation potential (Shaughnessy, 1994); and rural nursing homes have assumed the role of assisted living or other alternative housing options for some of their residents who might have had other options if they resided in urban areas (Rowles, 1996; Congdon and Magilvy, 1998a).

In a series of ethnographic studies conducted in rural Colorado, Magilvy and colleagues found that nursing homes were viewed with mixed feelings by rural older adults and their family members (Magilvy et al, 2000). Caring for one's aging parents was a tradition in the rural communities studied, but frequently health care providers believed that families kept their older members in the home beyond a reasonable period of time. Hispanic family members especially struggled to meet family obligations of "caring for our own." A religious leader in the Hispanic community supported the view that some families waited too long to seek assistance with caregiving, because caregivers became exhausted and care deteriorated. Although family remains an important and treasured aspect of the Hispanic culture, societal, economic, and family changes have altered the ability of families to provide support to Hispanic elders. Responsibilities for caregiving are beginning to fall to nonfamily care providers such as home care nurses, case managers, personal care providers, homemakers, and nursing home staff.

On the other hand, many older adults and their family caregivers were relieved and thankful for the available nursing homes because they would not have been able to provide care without the facilities. The nursing homes contributed to the wholeness of the community and to the health and well-being of the residents. They served as an extension of the home and were considered a rich part of the community. Some older adults felt relieved that they were not burdening their families, and for some, making the decision to move to a nursing home enabled them to maintain their independence and autonomy within the family system (Magilvy et al, 2000).

However, transitions to nursing home were often problematic and of a crisis nature. Most admissions occurred following hospitalizations, and decisions were made quickly with little or no planning (Magilvy et al, 2000; Congdon and Magilvy, 2001). Families had often not considered care beyond the hospital. For some older persons and their families, accessing any type of assistance was intimidating, and they dreaded dealing with institutional bureaucracy, filling out endless forms, and gaining certification of eligibility for services. The presence of an ill or frail spouse or limited family resources could also complicate the transition. After hospitalization for an acute illness or during a period of extreme family or individual stress, the nursing home was sometimes the only choice.

Informal Care

Family members and circles of informal care are primary sources of assistance for both healthy and frail older adults living in rural community settings (Magilvy et al, 1994; Stoller, 1996). Spouses, adult children, extended relatives, friends, and neighbors provide unpaid services that include assistance with meals, household tasks, shopping, personal care, health-related care, errands, transportation, and companionship. Congruent with rural culture, health care providers such as nurses and health care aides are also integral parts of the formal as well as the informal system. Nurses and other health care providers live, shop, work, and worship in the rural communities and are neighbors and friends of elders needing care. For example, a public health nurse's brief trip to the grocery store might entail an extended conversation with a neighbor about a health problem or a commitment to drop off health care supplies to a homebound person on her way home from work (Magilvy et al, 1994).

One of the persistent differences between rural and urban older persons is that rural elders are more likely to be married and tend to be younger, and thus they are less likely to have experienced widowhood (Stoller and Lee, 1994; Stoller, 1996). Higher rates of married status among rural older adults also reflect lower rates of divorce, particularly among farmers (Coward et al, 1994). Rural elders also are less likely to be childless and tend to have more children than urban dwellers. However, they are no more likely than urban dwellers to have access to their children as they age (Stoller, 1996).

Community churches, religious organizations, caring ministries, senior centers, home-delivered meals, and local meal sites are also part of the informal but essential network that assists frail older adults to remain independent in their own homes. Some senior centers have posted lists of programs that offer volunteers who are willing to clean, cook, chop wood, or do other chores to assist elderly persons in need (Magilvy et al, 1994).

The informal care systems are strong and highly developed in rural settings. Weinert and Long (1990) contended that these informal systems are the core of rural health care and that the formal health services and providers frequently support the informal system. To understand this strong informal care system, it helps to place it in the context of rural culture and life. Important characteristics such as dignity, independence, a need for privacy, the importance of reciprocity, and hardiness are embedded in rural culture. For example, Craig (1994) described the significance of reciprocal relationships that emerged between older residents and their community members. The need to reciprocate for the help one received was critical for the older adults in her study. This reciprocity was not only beneficial for the integrity of the older adults, but it also enhanced the health of the entire community. Magilvy and colleagues (1994) summarized their findings of the informal care system by extending a word of caution. Although research supports the view that the informal circle of care is a substantial strength of the rural health care system, "policy makers and health care providers cannot relinquish responsibility for care to the informal network. Critical examination of whose needs are being met at whose expense must be constantly assessed if meaningful and ethical services are to be provided" (p. 32).

RURAL NURSING

Rural nursing is defined as "the provision of health care by professional nurses to persons living in sparsely populated areas" (Long and Weinert, 1998, p. 4). Organized efforts for rural nursing service were initiated early in the twentieth century by frontier nurses such as Lillian Wald and Mary Breckinridge. In 1912 Lillian Wald was instrumental in establishing the Rural Nursing Service, which was renamed a year later as the Town and Country Nursing Service. Mary Breckinridge began the Frontier Nursing Service in 1925 in rural Appalachia and greatly expanded the nursing role in primary health care (Weinert and Long, 1991). High standards for nurses were strictly maintained in the early education and experience of rural nurses. Because Wald believed that rural work was diverse, demanding, and independent, she recruited only the most capable and dedicated women for rural nursing. Breckenridge, disturbed with the limited preparation and education of the lay midwives who were practicing in rural regions of the Appalachians, replaced them with frontier nurses who were prepared in general nursing, public health, and midwifery. The context and framework for nursing in rural environments that was established by Wald and Breckenridge is still relevant in today's nursing world (Bushy, 2000).

Scharff (1998, p. 21) described rural nursing practice as follows:

> Being rural means being a long way from anywhere and pretty close to nowhere. Being rural means being independent or perhaps being alone. Being a rural nurse means that when a nurse saves a life, everyone in town recognizes that she or he was there, and when a nurse loses a life, everyone in town recognizes that she or he was there. Being rural means turning inward for answers, because there may be nobody to turn to outward. Being rural means that when a nurse walks into the emergency room, it may be her or his spouse or child who needs a nurse and at that moment, being a nurse takes priority over being anyone else. Being a rural nurse means being able to deal with what she or he has got, where she or he is, and being able to live with the consequences.

Key Concepts of Rural Nursing

In their ongoing work to develop a theory base for rural nursing, Long and Weinert (1998) noted a pattern of certain concepts and relational statements appearing repeatedly in their data collected in rural Montana. These concepts and perceptions include the following:

- Rural dwellers define health primarily as the ability to perform their work, to be productive, and to do their usual everyday tasks. The ability to carry on one's daily activities takes precedence over comfort, cosmetic, and life-prolonging aspects of health. The researchers noted that rural residents tolerated pain, even for extended periods, as long as it did not interfere with their ability to function.
- Rural dwellers are self-reliant and resist accepting help from those seen as "outsiders" or from agencies seen as national or regional "welfare" programs.
- Rural health care providers, such as nurses, must cope with a certain amount of professional isolation, a lack of anonymity, and a sense of role diffusion. Rural nurses feel a sense of isolation from their peers, have a lack of privacy about their personal lives, have difficultly separating their roles in the community from their roles of professional caregiver, and are expected to perform a variety of diverse and unrelated tasks while working. On a single shift a nurse may work in the delivery room, in the emergency room, and on a medical-surgical unit. During the weekend or an evening shift, the nurse may be expected to carry out the tasks reserved for a pharmacist or dietitian. The lack of anonymity also extends to rural clients and their families. Persons living in a rural setting understand that there are very few secrets in a rural community. Everyone seems to know everything (Glover, 2001). For example, rural persons may be reluctant accessing mental health services with the knowledge that others may recognize their car outside the clinic and know they are there. This lack of anonymity leads to the reduced use of rural mental health services.

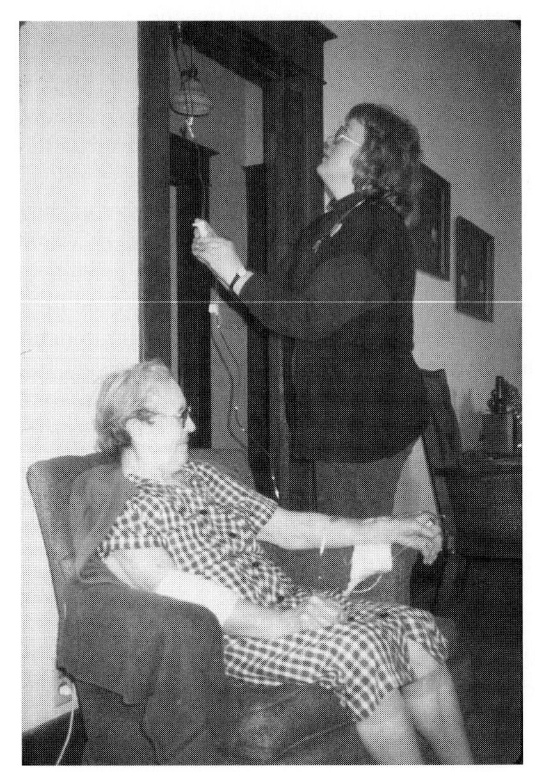

Rural home care nurse treating an older adult. (Courtesy JoAnn Congdon and Joan K. Magilvy.)

Based on their research in Montana, Long and Weinert (1998) offer several implications for rural nursing practice. Because work is of major importance to rural residents, health care clinics, programs, and appointments must fit with rural work schedules. Health promotion education and programs should be related to work issues and the prevention of long-term disabilities that may prevent someone from carrying out his or her work or usual activities. These features will be more meaningful to rural residents rather than preventive measures that emphasize a more comfortable way of living. Glover (2001) added that rural health care providers must learn to be aware of the unspoken community rules, or else they risk being considered untrustworthy or outsiders.

The characteristic of rural people to be self-reliant may influence rural persons to delay seeking health care until they are seriously ill or debilitated. Nurses must learn to be nonjudgmental about this feature and to stress appropriate preventive health strategies or behaviors. With appropriately delivered information, rural residents can learn to make satisfactory decisions regarding the delicate balance of when to rely solely on self-care behaviors and when to seek professional care.

Because of the common practice for rural nurses to work in several speciality areas each week or even within a day, it is helpful for rural nurses to have a strong background in leadership and generalist skills. Scharff (1998), in her study of rural nurses in western Montana, northern Idaho, and eastern Washington, described the *newcomer* and the *old-timer,* terms that are commonly used in rural areas in relation to nursing staff tenure and group acceptance. Nurses who move to rural communities to work should not expect to be accepted immediately. It generally takes time to make the transition from a new-comer to an old-timer. There is no particular time limit identified when a nurse finally makes this transition, nor any clear way to arrive at a level of acceptance. Scharff estimated that it generally takes 3 to 5 years in combination with a certain amount of competence and common sense to be fully accepted. Scharff summarized her thoughts on rural nursing by stating that "the newcomer practices nursing in a rural setting, unlike the old-timer who practices *rural* nursing" (p. 38). Long and Weinert (1998) suggested that involvement in community activities may facilitate being known in the community and thus assist with acceptance. They caution that nurses who choose to maintain a separate professional and personal life may have a more difficult time adjusting to rural culture and environment. Glover (2001, p. 333) added that "health care providers who separate themselves and don't identify with the community may be viewed with suspicion and their judgments challenged."

Current Changes in Rural Nursing

Workforce Differences. Rural nurses are older than their urban counterparts, partly due to their longevity in the rural communities and rural health care institutions. As rural communities lose population and rural hospitals close, the percentage of nurses working in rural hospitals also declines. With the aging of the rural population and the increasing numbers of older persons, rural nurses are needed to provide acute, chronic, and long-term care to growing numbers of elderly persons. The increasing use of biotechnology such as telemetry and telehealth systems allows rural health care providers to consult quickly and efficiently with urban-based experts. Because of these changes, hospital and home care nurses need acute care skills to manage the increased complexity of care in rural areas (Bushy, 2000).

Workforce estimates project that the demand for rural nurses with baccalaureate degrees will increase with the extension of managed care organizations in rural communities (Bushy, 2000). As in urban areas, there is a shift from hospital acute care to community-based care. The greatest nursing needs will be in public health, home care facilities, ambulatory care, and nursing education programs. The question is whether rural facilities will be able to compete economically for nurses with higher educational levels. Rural registered nurses with baccalaureate degrees make lower salaries than their urban counterparts, have lower raises as experience and longevity on the job increase, and receive lower bonuses for earning advanced practice preparation (Bushy, 2000). On the other hand, some authors argue that the cost of living is lower and the quality of life higher in rural settings; thus nurses must assess all the variables when considering the advantages and disadvantages of rural nursing. In any case, if rural providers do not reward productivity and invest solidly in their rural nurses, they will continue to lose them to more urban-based centers (Bushy, 2000).

Strategies to educate, recruit, and retain nurses and other health care providers to rural areas of this country are underway across the country. Innovative educational programs using computer and interactive technologies are being delivered to rural outreach sites. Many schools of nursing are offering and encouraging clinical rotations in rural sites, using local providers in collaboration with academic faculty as preceptors. Introduction of rural high school students to the profession of nursing, exposure of nursing students to rural environments, recruiting students with rural backgrounds to nursing schools, and the increased use of advanced practice nurses in underserved rural areas are examples of the wide variety of strategies nationwide to recruit and retain nurses in rural areas.

Changes in the Nature of Nursing. Historically, through a variety of practices, rural nurses have been committed to providing care to those most in need and to improving the health of their communities. Rural nurses are noted for their resilience, flexibility, ingenuity, and adaptability and for their connectedness to their communities. They are part of the rural system that values taking care of one's own. However, the past two decades of national health care turbulence and economic challenges have directly affected the roles of rural nurses. Congdon and Magilvy (1995), in an ethnographic study employed to enhance the understanding of rural culture and aging as the context in which home care services are provided, studied home care nursing in eight rural Colorado counties. One of their key findings was the theme of the changing spirit of rural nursing. Rural nurses perceived overwhelming documentation requirements as impeding rural practice, decreasing the quality of nursing care, and changing the spirit of rural community nursing from an emphasis on caring and community service to a focus on reimbursement. One nurse, in a comment that was heard repeatedly throughout the study, said, "The back of public health nursing is being broken because of the priority on generating revenue. Preventive care that emphasizes teaching and self care is being replaced by a system obsessed with only cost-containment" (Congdon and Magilvy, 1995, p. 20).

The enormous volume of home care admission paperwork, tedious and complex documentation requirements for reimbursement for services, lower rural reimbursement rates, barriers to providing culturally congruent care, and limited educational preparation for interpreting complex health policy regulations were perceived as factors contributing to the practice changes. The documentation burden led to fewer home visits per nurse per day, decreased job satisfaction, and increased nursing staff turnover. The rural nurses in the study perceived that the traditional system that affirmed the provision of nursing care as the most important value was being threatened with a preoccupation with health care regulations. Customarily, rural nurses will spend extra time and effort in the provision of care because they feel linked to the community with strong ties and relationships. Most of their patients are not strangers. Rural nurses take pride in their self-directedness and independence in practice, and they are not unlike their rural patients in their dislike for too many government regulations and policies. Care is usually not refused just because a person cannot afford it. "Freebies," or free care, was observed, but nurses said the practice is not as prevalent as in the past.

The majority of the nurses who provided direct care in the home were prepared at less than the baccalaureate level and had little or no formal education for public health or home care roles. Some of them discussed openly their desire for skills to better work within the changing health care system. However, one of the successful strategies that the rural nurses used to deal with the frustrating and seemingly ever changing reimbursement regulations was to collaborate and network with other nurses in adjacent counties. The nurses creatively pooled their resources, worked to ensure that home care staff kept current with the changes, and learned coping and management techniques from each other. Taking this opportunity to optimize their collective strength and working together to problem solve led to increased job satisfaction for the home care nurses and helped to rekindle the spirit of rural nursing.

Human Needs and Wellness Diagnoses

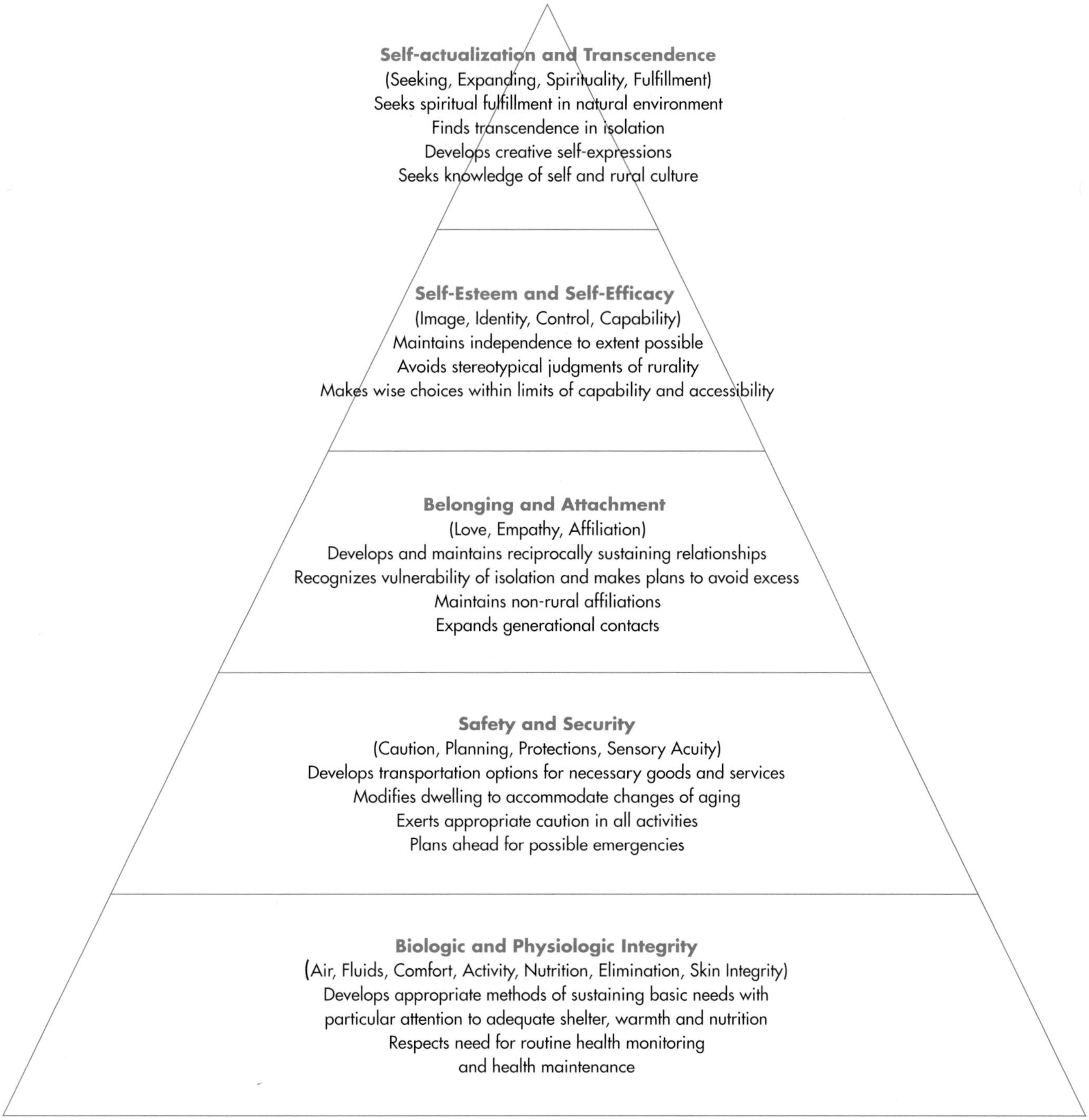

Self-actualization and Transcendence
(Seeking, Expanding, Spirituality, Fulfillment)
Seeks spiritual fulfillment in natural environment
Finds transcendence in isolation
Develops creative self-expressions
Seeks knowledge of self and rural culture

Self-Esteem and Self-Efficacy
(Image, Identity, Control, Capability)
Maintains independence to extent possible
Avoids stereotypical judgments of rurality
Makes wise choices within limits of capability and accessibility

Belonging and Attachment
(Love, Empathy, Affiliation)
Develops and maintains reciprocally sustaining relationships
Recognizes vulnerability of isolation and makes plans to avoid excess
Maintains non-rural affiliations
Expands generational contacts

Safety and Security
(Caution, Planning, Protections, Sensory Acuity)
Develops transportation options for necessary goods and services
Modifies dwelling to accommodate changes of aging
Exerts appropriate caution in all activities
Plans ahead for possible emergencies

Biologic and Physiologic Integrity
(Air, Fluids, Comfort, Activity, Nutrition, Elimination, Skin Integrity)
Develops appropriate methods of sustaining basic needs with particular attention to adequate shelter, warmth and nutrition
Respects need for routine health monitoring and health maintenance

These are not all the possible wellness diagnoses that may be identified. The above are examples of nursing diagnoses that should be considered when planning care for the older adult.

KEY CONCEPTS

- Great regional diversity exists in the social, cultural, ethnic, and economic structures of rural communities across the United States.
- There is lack of national consensus on the meaning of the term *rural.*
- Approximately 25% of persons age 65 and older live in rural communities.
- The older rural population is less racially and ethnically diverse than those under 65 years of age.
- Younger persons and professionals are leaving rural areas for increased economic opportunities in urban areas.
- Retirees are leaving urban areas for rural retreats.
- Rural older adults are at risk for disease and disability because of their multiple, complex health problems, low socioeconomic status, and barriers to appropriate health care services.
- Health risk factors of rural older adults include obesity, physical inactivity, smoking, moderate drinking, poverty, inadequate or lack of health insurance, chronic diseases, poor dental health, higher death rates, and serious injuries from motor vehicle accidents.
- Rural older adults who are still engaged in farming are among the healthiest of all elders, whereas rural nonfarm older adults have the worst health profiles.
- Rural older adults have a propensity to be self-reliant, are independent, use a high level of self-care activities, seek health assistance through an informal system of care, value "insider care," and demonstrate a need for reciprocity.
- Older rural persons have a tendency to underreport health problems and to tolerate significant health problems to remain independent in their own homes.
- Financial, social, geographic, and cultural constraints may lead some older rural persons to lowered health expectations and constrain them from seeking advanced health care services.
- A strong integration of faith, spirituality, and health exists in the lives of rural older adults.
- Family members and the informal system of care are the primary sources of assistance for community-dwelling rural older adults.
- Rural older adults define health in terms of being able to work or carry out their usual daily activities.
- Rural health care providers must cope with a certain amount of professional isolation, a lack of anonymity, and a sense of role diffusion.
- Rural nurses are not unlike their rural patients in their dislike for too many government regulations and policies.
- Successful rural nurses are expert generalists.

▲ CASE STUDY

Maude, an 85-year-old widow and retired schoolteacher, developed breast cancer with metastases. She lived alone and was active in her community. She developed pain and swelling of her right leg and was hospitalized. She was diagnosed with deep venous thrombophlebitis. Maude was discharged to home with treatment, but she soon realized that she could not live independently, even with substantial help from her church and friends. She chose to move into a nursing home that was right down the street, where her friends could continue to visit. Many of the staff at the nursing home had been friends of her daughter, and she had watched many of them grow up. At the time of admission to the nursing home, Maude was of sound mind. She completed a medical power of attorney form and named her only child, Sarah, as her medical power of attorney representative. Sarah had moved away years ago and the two were not close. Maude was always trying to find ways to improve their relationship. Over a period of time, Maude became confused and forgetful. The doctors said that she had less than 6 months to live and recommended a comfort care plan. Maude had continuous problems with pain in her right leg. She began to vomit blood. Sarah was contacted, and she insisted that her mother be hospitalized to get the bleeding stopped. She did not want her mother to bleed to death. She disagreed with the doctor about the comfort care plan and demanded that everything be done for her mother, including hospitalization for tests and cardiopulmonary resuscitation (CPR) if necessary. The staff in the nursing home was upset with the decisions of the daughter. Sarah had never come to visit her mother, and she had never asked Maude what her wishes were regarding end-of-life care. The staff, by contrast, had a rich sense of what Maude would want, based on numerous conversations with her as she faced her own illness and death, and through conversations with her about other friends and family members. They had watched her gradual decline and they wanted to make sure that she remained comfortable. They believed Sarah's decisions were based on guilt and not based on any actual knowledge of her mother's wishes or experience of her mother's care. (Modified from *Journal of Rural Health* 17(4):333, 2001.)

Based on the case study, develop a nursing care plan using the following procedure:*

List comments of the client that provide subjective data.

List information that provides objective data.

From these data identify and state, using accepted format, two nursing diagnoses you determine are the most significant to the client at this time.

Determine and state outcome criteria for each diagnosis. These must reflect some alleviation of the problem identified in the nursing diagnosis and must be stated in concrete and measurable terms.

Plan and state one or more interventions for each diagnosed problem. Provide specific documentation of source used to determine appropriate intervention. Plan at least one

*Students are advised to refer to their nursing diagnosis text and identify possible or potential problems.

intervention that incorporates the client's existing strengths.

Evaluate success of intervention. Intervention must correlate directly with the stated outcome criteria in order to measure the outcome success.

STUDY QUESTIONS/ACTIVITIES

Although this case could also happen in an urban setting ("the daughter from out of town" is a familiar scenario), what specific features of the case are characteristic of a rural setting?

Why do you think Maude chose to move into this particular nursing home?

Why do you think the nursing home staff feels a strong ethical responsibility to intervene in Maude's behalf? Taking into account what you have learned about the rural health care system, what is at stake for the nursing home staff?

What are your thoughts on confidentiality? Do you think it is an issue in this rural case study?

RESEARCH QUESTIONS

What are the ways that rural older adults and their families are coping with increasing chronic illnesses and frailty?

How do informal systems operate in rural communities?

What are the critical aspects that facilitate continuity between the informal and formal health care systems in a rural community?

What is the relationship between spirituality and rural health behaviors, quality of life, and the management of chronic illness?

What is the impact of a community-based parish-nursing program on the health and quality of life of rural older adults?

How can rural nurses facilitate smooth transitions among levels of health care for rural older adults and their families?

How do rural bioethical issues of the older adult differ from urban ones?

How can health care providers balance the ethical obligation of confidentiality and maintain the trust of the rural community?

REFERENCES

Brown NJ, Congdon JG, Magilvy JK: An approach to care management for rural older adults: parish nursing, *New Horizons* 5:7, 1996.

Bureau of Health Professions, Health Resources, and Services Administration: *A national agenda for geriatric education: white papers,* Washington, DC, 1995.

Bushy A: Health issues of women in rural environments, *J Am Med Wom Assoc* 53(2):53, 1998.

Bushy A: *Orientation to nursing in the rural community,* Thousand Oaks, CA, 2000, Sage.

Congdon JG, Magilvy JK: The changing spirit of rural community nursing: documentation burden, *Public Health Nurs* 12(1):18, 1995.

Congdon JG, Magilvy JK: Health status of rural older adults, *New Horizons* 5(24):4, 1996.

Congdon JG, Magilvy JK: Rural nursing homes: a housing option for older adults, *Geriatr Nurs* 19(3):157, 1998a.

Congdon JG, Magilvy JK: Home health care: supporting vitality for rural elders, *J Long-Term Home Health Care* 17(4):9, 1998b.

Congdon JG, Magilvy JK: Themes of rural health and aging: a program of research, *Geriatr Nurs* 22(5):234, 2001.

Coward RT et al: An overview of health and aging in rural America. In Coward RT et al, editors: *Health services for rural elders,* New York, 1994, Springer.

Coward RT, Netzer JK, Peek CW: Obstacles to creating high quality long-term care services for rural elders. In Rowles G, Beaulieu J, Myers W, editors: *Long-term care for the rural elderly,* New York, 1996, Springer.

Craig C: Community determinants of health for rural elderly, *Public Health Nurs* 11(4):242, 1994.

Cuba LJ: Models of migration decision making reexamined: the destination search of older migrants to Cape Cod, *Gerontologist* 31:4, 1991.

D'Andrade RG: Culture meaning systems. In Shweder RA, Levine RA, editors: *Cultural theory: essays on mind, self, and emotion,* Cambridge, MA, 1984, Cambridge University Press.

Dorfman LT: Economic status, work, and retirement among the rural elderly. In Coward RT, Krout JA, editors: *Aging in rural settings,* New York, 1998, Springer.

Duncan RP: Rural hospitals and rural elders. In Coward RT et al, editors: *Health services for rural elders,* New York, 1994, Springer.

Foner A: *Aging and old age: new perspectives,* Englewood Cliffs, NJ, 1986, Prentice Hall.

Gamson L et al: Identifying rural health priorities and models for practice, *Journal of Rural Health* 18(1):9, 2002.

Glover JJ: Rural bioethical issues of the elderly: how do they differ from urban ones? *Journal of Rural Health* 18(1):332, 2001.

Green VL: Premature institutionalization among the rural elderly in Arizona, *Public Health Rep* 99(1):58, 1984.

Havens B et al: Finding and using rural aging data: an international perspective, *Journal of Rural Health* 17(4):350, 2001.

Health and Human Services Rural Task Force Report to the Secretary: *One department serving rural America,* 2002, U.S. Department of Health and Human Services.

Hennessy CH et al: The public health perspective in health promotion and disability prevention for older adults: the role of the Centers for Disease Control and Prevention, *Journal of Rural Health* 17(4):364, 2001.

Johnson-Webb KD, Baer LD, Gesler WM: What is rural? Issues and considerations, *Journal of Rural Health* 13(3):253, 1997.

Jordon JM et al: The impact of arthritis in rural populations, *Arthritis Care Res* 8:242, 1995.

Kihl MR: The need for transportation alternatives for the rural elderly. In Bull CN, editor: *Aging in rural America,* Newbury Park, CA, 1993, Sage.

Krout JA: Rural aging and community-based services. In Coward CN et al, editors: *Health services for rural elders,* New York, 1994, Springer.

Krout JA: Services and service delivery in rural environments. In Coward RT, Krout JA, editors: *Aging in rural settings,* New York, 1998, Springer.

Krout JA, Coward RT: Aging in rural environments. In Coward RT, Krout JA, editors: *Aging in rural settings,* New York, 1998, Springer.

Kumar V et al: Health status of the rural elderly, *Journal of Rural Health* 17(4):328, 2001.

Long KA, Weinert C: Rural nursing: developing the theory base. In Lee HJ, editor: *Conceptual basis for rural nursing,* New York, 1998, Springer.

Longino CF, Smith MH: Epilogue: reflections on health services for rural elders. In Coward CN et al, editors: *Health services for rural elders,* New York, 1994, Springer.

Longino CF Jr, Smith MH: The impact of elderly migration on rural communities. In Coward RT, Krout JA, editors: *Aging in rural settings,* New York, 1998, Springer.

Magilvy JK: The role of rural home and community based services. In Rowles GD, Beaulieu JE, Myers WW, editors: *Long-term care for the rural elderly,* New York, 1996, Springer.

Magilvy JK, Congdon JG: Circles of care: rural home care for older adults, *Rural Clinician Quarterly* 4(2):3, 1994.

Magilvy JK, Congdon JG: The crisis nature of health care transitions for rural older adults, *Public Health Nurs* 17(5):336, 2000.

Magilvy JK, Congdon JG, Martinez RJ: Circles of care: home and community support for rural older adults, *Adv Nurs Sci* 16(3):22, 1994.

Magilvy JK et al: Caring for our own: health care experiences of rural Hispanic elders, *Journal of Aging Studies* 14(2):17, 2000.

Martinez RJ: Close friends of God: an ethnographic study of health of older Hispanic adults, *Journal of Multicultural Nursing and Health* 5(1):40, 1999.

McCulloch BJ: Aging and kinship in rural context. In Blieszner R, Bedfor VH, editors: *Handbook of aging and the family,* Westport, CT, 1995, Greenwood Press.

McCulloch BJ: *Old, female, and rural,* New York, 1998, Haworth Press.

McLaughlin DK: Rural women's economic realities. In McCulloch BJ, editor: *Old, female, and rural,* New York, 1998, Haworth Press.

McLaughlin DK, Jensen L: The rural elderly: a demographic portrait. In Coward RT, Krout JA, editors: *Aging in rural settings,* New York, 1998, Springer.

Mochenhaupt RE, Muchow JA: Disease and disability prevention and health promotion for rural elders. In Krout JA, editor: *Providing community-based services to the rural elderly,* Newbury Park, CA, 1994, Sage.

National Center for Health Statistics: Current estimates from the National Health Interview Survey, 1994, *Vital Health Stat* 10:189, 1994.

National Institute of Nursing Research (NINR): *Community-based health care: nursing strategies, report of the NINR Priority Expert Panel,* NIH pub 95, Bethesda, MD, 1995, National Institutes of Health.

Palumbo MV: Swing beds: providing extended care in rural acute-care hospitals. In Winstead-Fry P, Tiffany JC, Shippee-Rice RV, editors: *Rural health nursing,* New York, 1992, National League for Nursing Press.

Rabiner DJ et al: Metropolitan versus nonmetropolitan differences in functional status and self-care practice: findings from a national sample of community dwelling older adults, *Journal of Rural Health* 13(1):14, 1997.

Reeder R: *Retiree-attraction policies for rural development,* AIB-741, Economic Research Service, Washington, DC, 1998, U.S. Department of Agriculture.

Reeder RJ, Glasgow NL: Non-metro retirement counties' strengths and weaknesses, *Rural Development Perspectives* 6:12, 1990.

Rogers CC: *Changes in the older population and implications for rural areas. Rural development research report number 90,* Food and Rural Economics Division, Economic Research Service, Washington, DC, 1999, US Department of Agriculture.

Rowles GD: Nursing homes in the rural long-term care continuum. In Rowles GD, Beaulieu JE, Myers WW, editors: *Long-term care for the rural elderly,* New York, 1996, Springer.

Rural Information Center Health Service (RICHS): Rural health statistics, Beltsville, MD, 2001. Available at *www.nal.usda.gov/ric/richs/stats.htm*

Scharff JE: The distinctive nature and scope of rural nursing practice: philosophical bases. In Lee HJ, editor: *Conceptual basis for rural nursing,* New York, 1998, Springer.

Schlenker RE, Shaughnessy PW: The role of the rural hospital in long-term care. In Rowles GD, Beaulieu JE, Myers WW, editors: *Long-term care for the rural elderly,* New York, 1996, Springer.

Shaughnessy PW: Changing institutional long-term care to improve rural health care. In Coward CN et al, editors: *Health services for rural elders,* New York, 1994, Springer.

Shreffler MJ: An ecological view of the rural environment: levels of influence on access to health care, *Adv Nurs Sci* 18(4):48, 1996.

Shreffler MJ et al: Community decision-making about critical access hospitals: lessons learned from Montana's medical assistance facility program, *Journal of Rural Health* 15(2):180, 1999.

Siegel JS: *A generation of change: a profile of America's older population,* New York, 1993, Russell Sage Foundation.

Special Committee on Aging, United States Senate: *Common beliefs about the rural elderly: myth or fact?* Serial no 102-N, Washington, DC, 1992, U.S. Government Printing Office.

Stoller EP: The role of family in rural long term care. In Rowles GD, Beaulieu JE, Myers WW, editors: *Long-term care for the rural elderly,* New York, 1996, Springer.

Stoller EP, Forster LE: Patterns of illness behavior among rural elderly: preliminary results of a health diary study, *Journal of Rural Health* 8(1):13, 1992.

Stoller EP, Lee GR: Informal care of rural older adults. In Coward CN et al, editors: *Health services for rural older adults,* New York, 1994, Springer.

Wallace RE, Wallace RB: Rural-urban contrasts in elder health status: methodologic issues and findings. In Coward RT, Krout JA, editors: *Aging in rural settings,* New York, 1998, Springer.

Weinert C, Long KA: Rural families and health care: refining the knowledge base, *Journal of Marriage and Family Review* 15(1/2):57, 1990.

Weinert C, Long KA: The theory and research base for rural nursing practice. In Bushy A, editor: *Rural nursing,* vol 1, Newbury Park, CA, 1991, Sage.

Winstead-Fry P, Tiffany JC, Shippee-Rice RV: *Rural health nursing,* New York, 1992, National League for Nursing Press.

Yawn BP, Bushy A, Yawn RA: *Exploring rural medicine,* Thousand Oaks, CA, 1994, Sage.

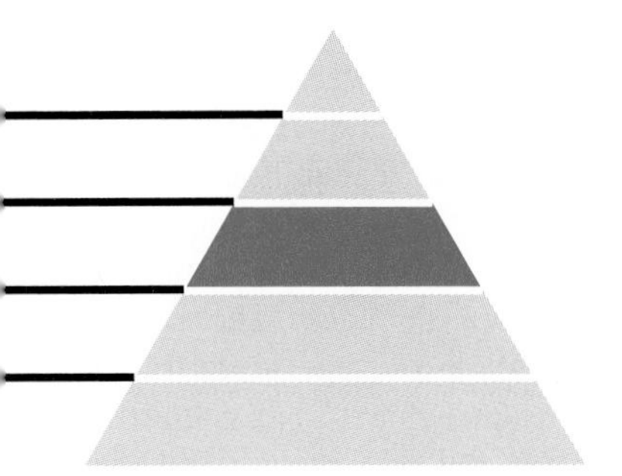

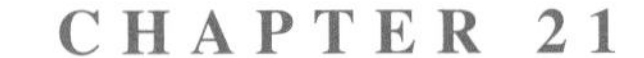

CHAPTER 21

Cognition

Ann Schmidt Luggen

A student speculates

I imagine I am in my late eighties and my husband and I live with our daughter. I am experiencing an unpleasant physical change; I am losing my memory. I can sharply remember all details about events that happened a long time ago, but often fail to recall what happened 2 hours ago. Although this situation scares me and I wonder what will happen if my family gets tired of my forgetfulness, I remind myself that I live with the people who love and care for me very much and will not desert me at the time when I need them the most.

Tatyana, age 30

An elder speaks

It has been quite a relief to be in this retirement home ... everyone here forgets names and words, and I don't feel alone when I'm forgetful.

Liz, age 78

LEARNING OBJECTIVES

On completion of this chapter, the reader will be able to:

1. List five purposes of a cognitive assessment.
2. Explain reasons nurses may provide an accurate assessment of cognitive status.
3. Describe similarities and differences between dementia and delirium.
4. Relate six ways in which cognitive impairment is measured.
5. Describe the parameters and methods used in a comprehensive assessment of cognitive function.
6. Develop a nursing care plan for an individual with irreversible dementia.
7. Develop a nursing care plan for an individual with reversible dementia.

COGNITIVE FUNCTION

This chapter addresses normal cognition of the aged and the various situations, disorders, and diseases that influence cognitive processes and at times produce temporary or permanent cognitive decline. We remain oriented to the healthy aging model while we examine each of the states of mentation in old age as having the potential for comfort and pleasures. All elders are deserving of active nursing intervention to maintain the highest practicable level of function and satisfaction.

We have artificially separated cognitive function from mental health, though they are in most ways interdependent. The mind is in some ways limited by the capacities of the brain, yet just as in medicine, there is a danger of evaluating the person by the measured and tested efficiency of cells and organs. Nowhere is this more important than in examining the cognition of the aged. Citing John Morris, professor of neurology at Washington University in St. Louis, Crowley (1996) says that if brain function becomes impaired in old age, it is a result of disease, not aging.

Adult Cognition

Cognition is the process of acquiring, storing, sharing, and using information (Bunton, 2001). Cognitive development of the aged is often measured against the norms of young or middle-aged people, which may not be appropriate to the distinctive characteristics of the aged. More and more theorists are now speculating about the possibility of unique cognitive powers of old age, as did Plato.

In his seventy-third year the great Erik Homburger Erikson, when writing of Freud, noted that in Freud's sixty-eighth year he became aware of a phase of regressive development and the "all-enveloping duality of life and death" (Erikson, 1975, p. 33). This awareness of reflective regression seems to be a stage of cognitive development characteristic of late life. Individuals become absorbed with memories and meanings.

Berry (1974) provides a good example in Old Jack, who sat in a rocking chair on the veranda of the general store, immersed in the span of his years and the meanings of events. He failed to see what was going on around him or recognize people not because of cognitive decline but immersion in memories (Berry, 1974). It is doubtful he would remember, if asked, what he ate for breakfast, or even if he ate breakfast. Various cognitive activities may appear impaired if we are not alert to differences that occur in the process of aging.

The determination of intellectual capacity and performance has been the focus of a major portion of gerontologic research. In general, cognitive functions may remain stable or decline with increasing age (Beers and Berkow, 2000). The cognitive functions that remain stable include attention span, language skills, communication skills, comprehension of discourse, and visual perception. The cognitive skills that decline are verbal fluency, logical analysis, selective attention, object naming, and complex visuospatial skills (Beer and Berkow, 2000). Interrelationships between intelligence quotient (IQ) and mental and physical health are exceptionally strong. However, in general, intellectual abilities appear to plateau in the fifties and sixties and begin to decline in the seventies. Elderly people do maintain their ability to understand situations and learn from new experiences. These findings are significant to satisfaction in old age because the capacity for effective lifestyle management and cognitive resources contribute to adaptation and enjoyment in old age (Figure 21-1).

The Aging Brain

It has been generally assumed that cognitive function declines in old age because of a decreased number of neurons, decreased brain size, and diminished brain weight. Although these losses are features of aging, they are not consistent with deteriorating mental function (Sugarman, 2002), nor do they interfere with everyday routines. Neuron loss occurs mainly in the brain and spinal cord and is most pronounced in the cerebral cortex. The neuronal dendrites atrophy with aging, resulting in impairment of the synapses and changes in transmission of the chemical neurotransmitters dopamine, serotonin, and acetylcholine. This causes a slowing of many neural processes. However, overall cognitive abilities remain intact. We now understand that continued development requires appropriate levels of

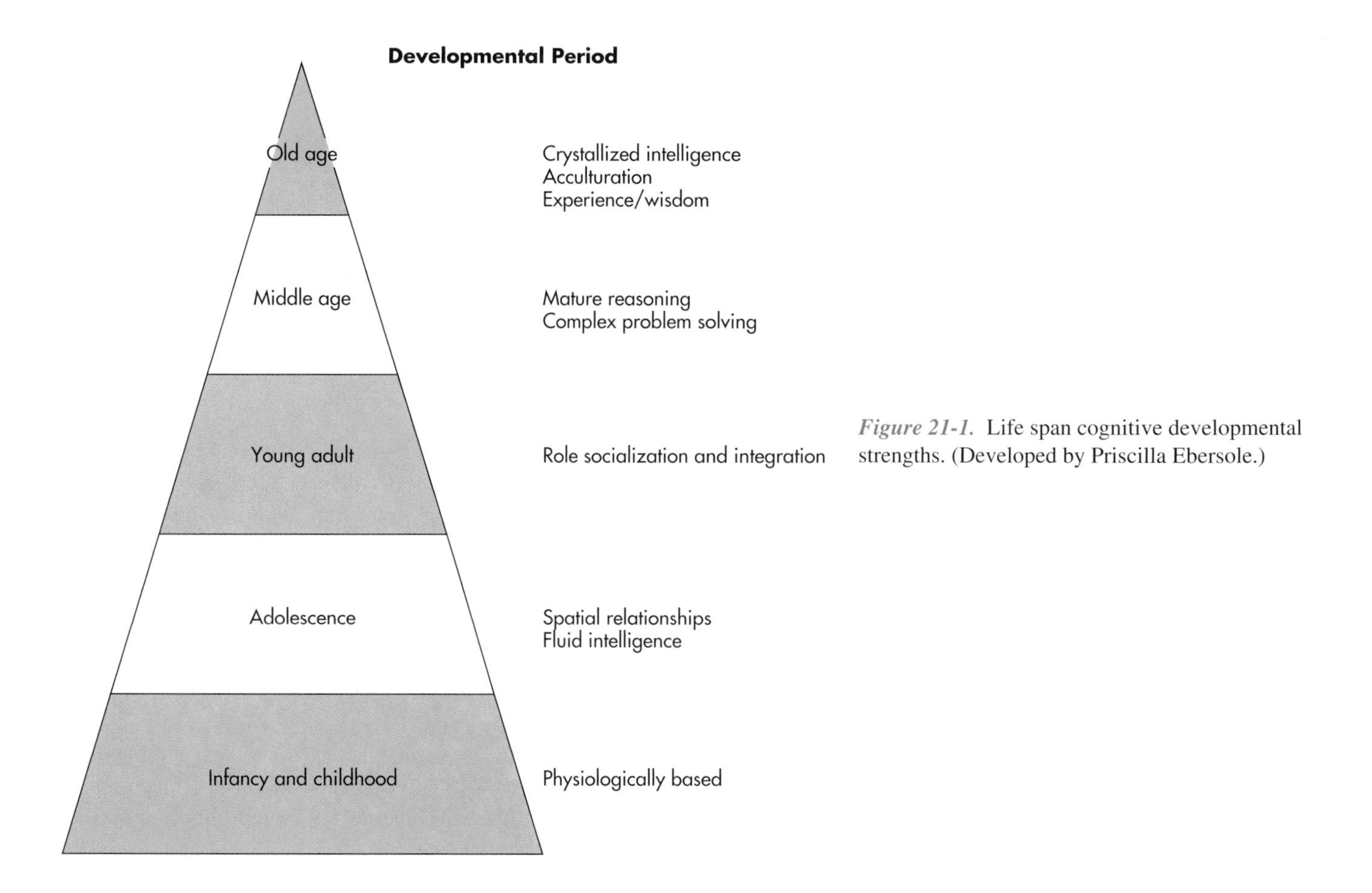

Figure 21-1. Life span cognitive developmental strengths. (Developed by Priscilla Ebersole.)

challenge and stimulation throughout life. There is untapped potential for patterning and learning through stimulating brain cells to expand function. This is shown most remarkably in the retraining of speech and other functions following a stroke.

Memory Retrieval. Memory can be thought of as having three components: immediate recall; short-term memory, which may range over minutes to days; and remote or long-term memory (Gallo et al, 2003). Interestingly, older persons' self-reports of memory loss do not correlate with objective measures of memory function. Normal older adults may complain of memory problems, but their symptoms fit what is called *benign senescent forgetfulness* or *age-associated memory impairment* (AAMI) (Gallo et al, 2003). In this instance, the person may not recall details of a situation but does remember the situation or experience. The memory fluctuates and details not remembered at one time may be remembered later. This type of impairment is not progressive, nor is it disabling (Box 21-1).

Older adults with significant memory loss will often have concomitant intellectual deficits (Gallo et al, 2003). This has been called *malignant memory loss* because these subjects have a higher mortality rate than those who do not have this type of memory loss. Those with malignant memory loss forget the details of situations and even the situation itself. They may confabulate about the forgotten details. The practicality of these distinctions in everyday life is that even though older subjects show some decrements in information processing, reaction time, perception, and attentional tasks, the majority of functioning remains intact and sufficient. Familiarity, previous learning, and life experience compensate for the minor loss of efficiency in the basic neurologic processes. In unfamiliar, stressful, or demanding situations these changes may be more marked.

Scientists are finding that nerve cell regeneration does occur in the hippocampus of the brain, where memory formation occurs (National Institutes of Health, 2002). They have found that stress decreases the capacity for generation of new nerve cells. Present research focuses on the factors linking stress and nerve cell regeneration. There is also evidence that estrogens may enhance memory function in postmenopausal women and may delay memory loss related to Alzheimer's disease (AD). Research at the National Institute on Aging (NIA) has demonstrated that there is greater blood flow to the brain areas involved in memory formation in older women receiving estrogen replacement therapy (ERT) than in postmenopausal women not receiving ERT (Maki and Resnick, 2000). Still other research on the "plasticity" of the brain, the integration of "nature" and "nurture," is based on the physical changes that occur in the brain that result from new memories and the addition of new neurons. This causes a change in hormones and a remodeling of the brain itself. Through this plasticity, experience constantly changes the brain. This is good evidence for us to continue to learn and grow and experience the world around us even into very old age.

Box 21-1 Memory Loss

Memory loss: forgetfulness, amnesia, impaired memory; a result of brain damage or severe emotional trauma. Common causes include the following:

- Aging
- Alzheimer's disease
- Neurodegenerative illness
- Head trauma or injury
- Seizures
- Stroke or TIAs
- Electroconvulsive therapy, especially prolonged
- Alcoholism
- Benzodiazepines and barbiturates

Source: National Institutes of Health: Memory loss, 2002. Available at *www.nlm.nih.gov/medlineplus/ency/article/003257.htm.*

Learning in Later Life

Basic intelligence remains unchanged with increasing years. Spatial awareness and intuitive, creative thought may decline (Batchelor, 2001). Verbal abilities do not change. However, elderly people may have many barriers to learning. These include memory impairment, vision and hearing impairment, fatigue, and delayed cognitive processing (Anderson, 2001). The older adult will demand that there be relevance in any teaching situation; new learning must relate to what the elder already knows. The elder is in control of what and how much is learned and the degree of participation in a learning situation, and the elder will monitor his or her own progress and pace.

Anderson (2001) has described methods to combat memory decline and enhance learning. She lists the following suggestions:

- Promote physical comfort (fluid intake, toileting)
- Eliminate distractors (noise, traffic)
- Ensure that glasses are clean and on, and that hearing aids are in place and working
- Increase the amount of time allowed for the learning situation, especially if it involves psychomotor skills
- Treat the elder with respect and dignity at all times in the learning situation
- Ensure that the information given is at the appropriate educational level
- Use examples that are relevant to the elder's life
- Ensure that visual aids are of a large size; yellow or orange paper is preferable
- Encourage verbal responses and allow time for responses
- Reinforce correct responses immediately, and correct incorrect responses immediately
- Set realistic and achievable mutual goals

Mental Frailty. An interesting concept proposed by Wolanin (1997) has to do with *mental frailty.* The concept is

Table 21-1 Domains Assessed in Mental Status, Cognitive Function, and Dementia

Mental status	Cognitive function	Dementia
	Attention span	Attention span
Affect and mood		
Level of consciousness		Level of consciousness
General speech		
	Learning ability	
Intellectual performance	Intelligence	Intellectual performance
Abstraction		Abstraction
Attention		
Concentration	Concentration	
Insight		
Judgment	Judgment	Impaired judgment
Memory	Memory	Memory impairment
Orientation	Orientation	Disorientation
Thought content		
	Perception	Perceptual disturbances
		Personality changes
	Problem solving	
Physical appearance and behavior		
	Social intactness	
Psychomotor behavior	Psychomotor ability	Psychomotor activity
	Reaction time	
		Sleep-wake cycle disturbances

From McDougall GJ: A review of screening instruments for assessing cognition and mental status in older adults, *Nurs Pract* 15:11, 1990.

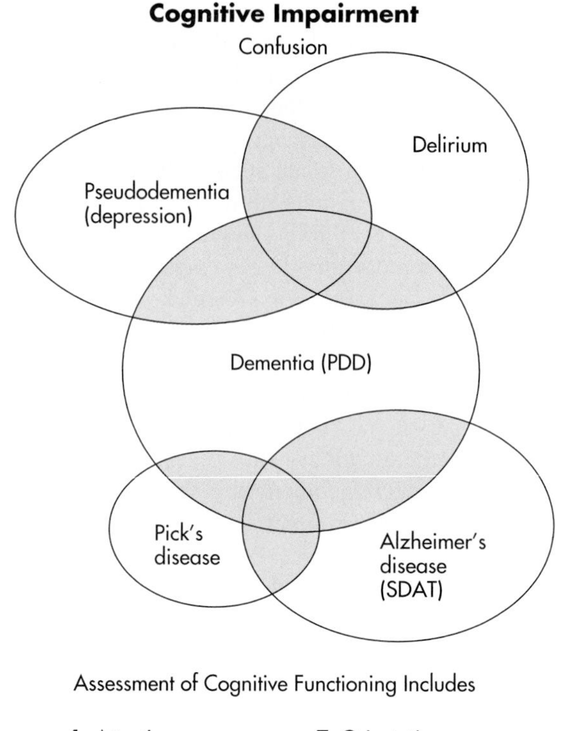

Figure 21-2. Relationship of Alzheimer's disease to other manifestations of cognitive impairment.

rooted in the triad of change, stress, and support. The elder has a sense of continuity of self that persists throughout life and must be maintained to properly filter and integrate events into the persona. When undesired, unexpected, or overwhelming changes occur—sociologically, psychologically, or physiologically—the elder needs stress relief and familiar supports to maintain the disturbed balance of self-perception. When these are not available at the appropriate time and degree to maintain the sense of the continuity of the predictable self, the elder's mentation goes awry and various psychologic and cognitive disturbances emerge. Nurses are in a position to restore the personal continuity of the elder by focusing on the familiar, obtaining the support of those within the individual's comfort zone, and immediately reversing to the extent possible the overwhelming changes and relieving stress. This concept needs considerably more attention.

Cognitive Impairment

Cognitive impairment (CI) is a term that describes a range of disturbances in cognitive functioning, including disturbances in memory, orientation, attention, and concentration (Warner and Butler, 2001). Other disturbances of cognition may affect intelligence, judgment, learning ability, perception, problem solving, psychomotor ability, reaction time, and social intactness (Table 21-1). The CI diagnosis is easily missed in primary care practices. In one study (Holzer and Warshaw, 2000), the researchers reviewed medical records in two geriatric evaluation centers. They found that there is probably a constellation of symptoms that may be associated in diagnosing early AD. This constellation includes missing recall items on the mini-mental state examination (MMSE), difficulty with calculations, repetition, getting lost while driving, forgetting the names of relatives, and poor judgment, especially in the area of hygiene. Recall was the symptom that provided the greatest clue to early diagnosis of AD.

Cognitive Assessment. The evaluation of cognition requires a formal focused assessment (Figure 21-2). Casual informal interviews with those who are socially adept or highly educated may not uncover a cognitive deficit that is present. A thorough medical assessment should be performed to rule out medical causes of CI. The following is a guide to conducting a mental status examination and is useful as a screening tool for cognitive impairment (National Institutes of Health, 2002). See Box 21-2 for an overview of cognitive assessment.

Box 21-2 Overview of Cognitive Assessment

A. Concepts and categories
  1. Definition: cognitive function: the processes by which an individual perceives, registers, stores, retrieves, and uses information
  2. Categories of cognitive change/decline
    a. The dementias (e.g., Alzheimer's, vascular) are chronic, progressive, insidious, and permanent states of cognitive impairment
    b. Delirium/acute confusion: an acute and sudden impairment of cognition that is considered temporary, generally an identifiable, biophysical cause
    c. Impairment in thought processes

B. Assessment
  1. Methods of assessment
    a. Formal—cognitive testing using standardized instruments
      i. Advantages: standardized; enables comparison across individuals and nurses
      ii. Disadvantages: individual performance influenced by pain, education, fatigue, cultural background, and perceptual and physical abilities
    b. Informal—through structured observations of nurse-individual interactions
      i. Advantages: may have greater meaning about individual's actual cognitive ability-performance
      ii. Disadvantages: difficult to make judgments regarding change in individual condition; variability in interpretation
  2. Other considerations for assessment
    a. Characteristics of the environment for assessment
      i. Physical environment
        —Comfortable ambient temperature
        —Adequate lighting but not glaring
        —Free of distractions (e.g., should be conducted in the absence of others and other activities)
        —Position self to maximize individual's sensory abilities
      ii. Interpersonal environment
        —Use individual's self-paced rate for assessment
        —Emotionally nonthreatening
    b. Timing considerations
      i. Timing should reflect the actual cognitive abilities of the individual and not extraneous factors
      ii. Times of the day to generally avoid
        —Immediately on awakening from sleep, wait at least 30 minutes
        —Immediately before or after meals
        —Immediately before or after medical diagnostic or therapeutic procedures
        —When patient has pain or discomfort

From Foreman MD et al: Assessing cognitive function, *Geriatr Nurs* 17(5):228, 1996.

Depression must be ruled out or appreciated before conduct of the cognitive assessment. It can be difficult to differentiate depression from dementia without a formal assessment of the latter. See Chapter 23 for further discussion of depression.

Orientation. Ask some or all of the following questions: time, date, season; the place in which you live; what type of building do you live in, what city and state do you live in; your name, age, and occupation? Nurses need to know that assessment of time, place, and person does not constitute an assessment of cognition.

Attention span. Test the patient's ability to complete a thought. This may be done in casual conversation or by asking the patient to follow a series of directions. Base conclusions on performance.

Recent memory. Ask questions about recent events that have taken place in the patient's life. Ask about family, other people, and places that are part of recent events.

Remote memory. These are questions about people and events that took place early in the older person's life. Ask about childhood, school, and historical events that took place early in the patient's life.

Word comprehension. This tests knowledge of commonly known items such as keys, pens, and flashlights. Point to the items and ask the patient to name them.

Judgment. Ask the patient a question that allows alternative solutions to a certain situation. For example, ask what the patient would do if he or she had a flat tire while driving on the expressway, or ask what he or she would do if a pot of milk began to boil over on the stove.

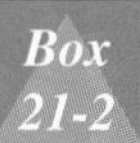

Box 21-2 Overview of Cognitive Assessment—cont'd

3. Parameters of assessment
    a. Alertness/level of consciousness: the most rudimentary cognitive function and level of arousal, or responsiveness to stimuli determined by interaction with individual and determination of level made on the basis of the individual's best eye, verbal, and motor response to stimuli
        i. Alertness—able to interact in a meaningful way with the examiner
        ii. Lethargy or somnolence—not fully alert; individual tends to drift to sleep when not stimulated, diminished spontaneous physical movement, loses train of thought, ideas wander
        iii. Obtundation—transitional stage between lethargy and stupor; difficult to arouse, meaningful testing futile, requires constant stimulation to elicit response
        iv. Stupor or semicoma—individual mumbles/groans in response to persistent and vigorous physical stimulation
        v. Coma—completely unable to be aroused, no behavioral response to stimuli
    b. Attention: ability to attend/concentrate on stimuli: can follow through with directions, especially a three-stage command; is easily distracted
    c. Memory: ability to register, retain, and recall information both new and old; does individual remember your name? Is individual able to learn and remember new information?
    d. Orientation to time, place, and person
    e. Thinking: ability to organize and communicate ideas; thoughts should be organized, coherent, and appropriate perception: presence/absence of illusions, delusions, or visual or auditory hallucinations
    f. Psychomotor behavior: ability to comprehend and perform simple motor skills; relative to execution ability to ask the individual to perform certain ADLs/LADLs, or to perform a three-step command, and to copy a figure
    g. Insight: ability to understand oneself and the situation in which one finds oneself
    h. Judgment: ability to evaluate a situation (real or hypothetical) and determine an appropriate action

C. Outcomes of assessment
1. Individual
    a. Detection of deviations will be prompt and early with appropriate care and treatment instituted in a timely manner
    b. Plans of care will appropriately address corrective and supportive cognitive function
2. Health care provider
    a. Assessment and documentation of cognitive function
    b. Appropriate strategies to address any deviation in cognitive function
    c. Competence in cognitive assessment
    d. Evidence of ability to differentiate among the different types of cognitive change/decline
3. Institution
    a. Documentation of cognitive function will increase
    b. Referral to appropriate advanced practitioners (e.g., geriatrician, geriatric/gerontologic or psychiatric clinical nurse specialist or nurse practitioner, consultation-liaison service) will increase

ADLs, Activities of daily living; *IADLs*, instrumental activities of daily living.

A normal examination is determined when there is orientation to person, place, and time; a normal attention span; and intact recent and remote memory. The patient has normal word comprehension, reading, and writing. The patient's judgment is intact and appropriate.

An abnormal examination will reveal deficits in one or more areas. Orientation to time is usually first lost, then place, then person. Causes may be alcohol overuse, low blood sugar, head trauma, fluid and electrolyte imbalances, or nutritional deficiencies such as vitamin B_{12}, vitamin C, thiamine, and niacin. Fever is also a cause of abnormal examination, as are hypothermia, which causes confusion; hypoxemia from chronic pulmonary problems; and environmental factors such as heavy metal poisoning or heat stroke (National Institutes of Health, 2002).

An abnormal examination of attention span is when the patient is unable to complete a thought or is easily distracted by stimuli. Some causes of this are confusion, negativism, manic-depressive illness, attention deficit disorder (ADD), histrionic personality disorder, and schizophrenia.

An abnormal examination of recent and remote memory is uncommon in the general elderly population. Recent memory loss with intact remote memory indicates an organic syndrome. Remote memory loss occurs when patients have disorders such as AD.

Aphasia is the term for loss of word comprehension, reading, and writing. Causes of aphasia include dementia of AD, stroke, head trauma, and transient ischemic attacks (TIAs).

Loss of judgment is a considerable problem in everyday life because we use this skill during much of each day in

Box 21-3 Mild Cognitive Impairment

Normal memory changes: Momentary lapses, misplaces items, forgets names
Mild cognitive impairment: Persistent, troublesome problems, forgets facts quickly, poor recall of reading or poor recall of details of simple drawings; forgets important events repeatedly; may or may not progress
Dementia: Additional problems of cognition—orientation, language, attention, gradual decline

Box 21-4 Common Causes of Confusion in the Elderly*

- Drug intoxication
- Circulatory disturbances
- Metabolic imbalances
- Fluid imbalance
- Major medical and surgical treatments
- Neurologic disorders
- Infectious processes
- Nutritional deficiencies
- Abrupt loss of significant person
- Multiple losses in short span of time
- Moves to radically different environments

*Shown in rank order of occurrence.

everything we do, and it can be vital in many situations. Impaired judgment may be due to organic brain diseases, dementia of AD, emotional dysfunction, mental retardation, and schizophrenia.

The first population-based study of cognitive impairment in the United States was reported in the journal *Neurology* (Unverzagt and Hendrie, 2001). The authors suggest that this condition may be far more prevalent than previously thought. The study looked at cognitive impairment that falls short of AD or other dementias in community-dwelling African Americans in Indianapolis, Indiana. Nearly one in four had measurable problems. This prevalence increased with age—about 10% every 10 years after age 65. Nearly 38% of those 85 and older had some cognitive impairment, short of dementia. However, looking at the data another way, 45% of elderly subjects at age 85 and older were cognitively normal, and 79% of elders age 65 to 74 were cognitively normal. The authors state that this is consistent with the few studies that have been conducted in other countries. A study conducted by the NIA on elders with mild cognitive impairment is due to be completed late in 2002 (Box 21-3). This study has three groups randomized to receive placebo, vitamin E, or donepezil (Aricept), a drug used to treat AD. This study may assist in early diagnosis and treatment of AD and other dementias to slow decline and prolong function (*www.alzheimers.org/nianews19.html*).

Confusion

Confusion is a broad and imprecise term that conveys little specific meaning; it is a clinical term used to describe a patient's behavior. According to Wolanin (1997), nurses use the nursing diagnosis "confusion" synonymously with the medical diagnosis of "organic brain syndrome." Sometimes, however, *confusion* is used to refer to an acute state, and *organic brain syndrome* is used to refer to a chronic state. Therefore the two terms are used in different contexts based on the acuity of the confusional state. This imprecision of meaning among nurses leads to inconsistent reporting of patients' behavioral manifestations. In addition, the *Diagnostic and Statistical Manual of Mental Disorders* revises acceptable terminology with each edition, which further adds to professionals' confusion with terminology.

Acute confusional state (ACS) is a term used by many health professionals. It is used synonymously with *delirium* to describe severe confusion with hyperactivity (Beers and Berkow, 2000). Still others use the term *delirium* to describe severe confusion and use the term *acute confusional state* to describe a mild disorientation to place and person. See Box 21-4 for common causes of confusion in the elderly.

Delirium is the proper term for the clinical assessment of an ACS. Any alteration in mentation may be loosely labeled *confusion,* and thus comparisons of delirium, dementia, and depression may be helpful in making a cursory judgment. These can be seen in Table 21-2.

Delirium.

Although the official nomenclature of the syndrome is delirium, it has been called many other names: acute confusional state, acute brain syndrome, confusion, intensive care psychosis, metabolic encephalopathy, postcardiotomy delirium, and toxic psychosis. Delirium is a clinical state characterized by an acute or subacute fluctuating change in mental status, with inattention and altered levels of consciousness (Beers and Berkow, 2000).

Delirium is common in older adults (Beers and Berkow, 2000). Hospitalized elderly patients 70 years and older have a delirium incidence of 10% to 25% and postoperatively 15% to 65%, the higher number for emergency surgery such as repair of hip fracture. In our experience, delirium of a prolonged nature occurs not uncommonly in older patients after surgery. It also occurs with some frequency after chemotherapy. Family and other caregivers need to be informed that this can occur but will usually remit. However, long-term cognitive deficits sometimes occur in these instances.

Risk factors for delirium. Old age, dementia, functional impairments, and medical comorbidities are risk factors for delirium (Beers and Berkow, 2000). See Box 21-5 for a definition of the mnemonic DELIRIUM, which identifies factors that often precipitate delirium.

Table 21-2 A Comparison of the Clinical Features of Delirium, Dementia, and Depression

Clinical feature	Delirium	Dementia	Depression
Onset	Acute/subacute, depends on cause, often at twilight or in darkness	Chronic, generally insidious, depends on cause	Coincides with major life changes, often abrupt
Course	Short, diurnal fluctuations in symptoms, worse at night, in darkness, and on awakening	Long, no diurnal effects, symptoms progressive yet relatively stable over time	Diurnal effects, typically worse in the morning, situational fluctuations, but less than with delirium
Progression	Abrupt	Slow but uneven	Variable, rapid or slow but even
Duration	Hours to less than 1 month, seldom longer	Months to years	At least 6 weeks, can be several months to years
Awareness	Reduced	Clear	Clear
Alertness	Fluctuates, lethargic or hypervigilant	Generally normal	Normal
Attention	Impaired, fluctuates	Generally normal	Minimal impairment, but is easily distracted
Orientation	Generally impaired, severity varies	Generally normal	Selective disorientation
Memory	Recent and immediate impaired	Recent and remote impaired	Selective or "patchy" impairment, "islands" of intact memory
Thinking	Disorganized, distorted, fragmented, incoherent speech, either slow or accelerated	Difficulty with abstraction, thoughts impoverished, judgment impaired, words difficult to find	Intact but with themes of hopelessness, helplessness, or self-deprecation
Perception	Distorted, illusions, delusions, and hallucinations, difficulty distinguishing between reality and misperceptions	Misperceptions usually absent	Intact, delusions and hallucinations absent except in severe cases
Psychomotor behavior	Variable, hypokinetic, hyperkinetic, and mixed	Normal, may have apraxia	Variable, psychomotor retardation or agitation
Sleep-wake cycle	Disturbed, cycle reversed	Fragmented	Disturbed, usually early morning awakening
Associated features	Variable affective changes, symptoms of autonomic hyperarousal, exaggeration of personality type, associated with acute physical illness	Affect tends to be superficial, inappropriate and labile, attempts to conceal deficits in intellect, personality changes, aphasia, agnosia may be present, lacks insight	Affect depressed, dysphoric mood, exaggerated and detailed complaints, preoccupied with personal thoughts, insight present, verbal elaboration
Assessment	Distracted from task, numerous errors	Failings highlighted by family, frequent "near miss" answers, struggles with test, great effort to find an appropriate reply, frequent requests for feedback on performance	Failings highlighted by individual, frequently answers "don't know," little effort, frequently gives up, indifferent toward test, does not care or attempt to find answer

From Foreman MD et al: Assessing cognitive function, *Geriatr Nurs* 17(5):228, 1996.

Clinical presentation. The essential features of delirium are "reduced ability to maintain attention to external stimuli and to appropriately shift attention to new external stimuli, and disorganized thinking, as manifested by rambling, irrelevant, or incoherent speech" (American Psychiatric Association, 1994) (Box 21-6). There is difficulty in shifting, focusing, following commands, and processing and sustaining attention to both external and internal stimuli; sensory misperception; and a disordered stream of thought. Irrelevant stimuli can easily distract the delirious individual. Perceptual disturbances are common and may result in misinterpretations, illusions, and hallucinations. Recent memory is lost. In addition, disturbances of the sleep-wake cycle and psychomotor activity are present. The elderly patient may have some awareness of the disturbances and feel that he or she "is losing my mind" (Stanley, 1999). Nurses and other health care professionals may see delirium in younger people and assume it to be transient and reversible. Older people are often labeled "senile," and the precipitant or cause is neither sought nor actively treated to reverse the underlying physiologic or psychologic problems.

Classifications of delirium. Delirium can be classified as *hyperactive,* about 25% of cases, in which agitation and psychomotor activity are present (Beers and Berkow, 2000). In

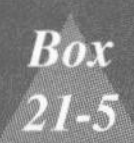

Box 21-5

DELIRIUM

Drug use—especially new drugs or changes in dosage of previously used drugs such as sedatives, antidepressants, anticholinergics, opioids, antipsychotics, antiparkinson agents
Electrolyte abnormalities—hyponatremia, hypoxemia
Lack of drugs such as sudden withdrawal of a previously used drug—may occur at hospitalization
Infection—especially urinary tract infections and respiratory infections
Reduced sensory input—visual disturbances, darkness, deafness, isolation, sudden changes in environment
Intracranial incidents—stroke, meningitis, seizure
Urinary retention and fecal impaction
Myocardial incidents—myocardial infarction, heart failure, arrhythmias

Box 21-6

DSM-IV Criteria for Delirium

1. A disturbance in consciousness, diminished awareness of environment, and decreased ability to focus, concentrate, or shift attention.
2. A change in cognition such as disorientation, loss of recent memory, or lanaguage disturbance or a new perceptual disturbance not accounted for by a preexisting dementia.
3. These disturbances tend to develop over a short period of time (hours to days) and fluctuate during the course of the day.

Delirium due to medical condition. There is evidence from the history and physical examination or laboratory tests that the disturbance is due to direct physiologic consequences of a general medical condition.

Delirium due to substance intoxication. There is evidence from the history or physical examination or laboratory test that either (a) symptoms listed in the first two criteria developed during the substance intoxication, or (b) the drug use is the etiology related to the disturbance.

Delirium due to substance withdrawal. There is evidence from the history, physical examination, or laboratory tests that the symptoms listed in the first two criteria developed during or shortly after the withdrawal of a substance.

Delirium due to multiple causes. There is evidence from the history, physical examination, or laboratory tests that the delirium has more than one etiology—either more than one medical condition, or a medical condition plus an adverse drug effect or substance intoxication.

Adapted from American Psychiatric Association: *Diagnostic and statistical manual of mental disorders,* ed 4, pp 129, 131-133, Washington, DC, 1994, The Association.

hypoactive delirium, 25% of cases, psychomotor activity is decreased and may be misdiagnosed as depression because of apathy and somnolence or not be detected at all. In *mixed* delirium, about 35% of cases, the psychomotor activity may have hyperactive and hypoactive features. Unfortunately, failure to diagnose delirium or misdiagnosing it occurs in nearly 80% of cases. This is less likely to occur with a team approach of nurses, physicians, family members, and others.

Pseudodelirium is a delirium-like state that occurs as a result of psychosocial stressors, depression, mania, severe anxiety, disturbances in the sleep-wake cycle, and physical or psychosocial stress. It usually ends in either full recovery or death, although it may result in some degree of permanent dementia if the causal factors go unattended. An accurate diagnosis of delirium, dementia, depression, and pseudodementia is a challenge because all present symptoms of CI. If the condition is an abrupt confusional onset, it is probably not a dementia but delirium and may be reversible. However, dementia caused by a stroke or anoxia may occur abruptly.

Nursing interventions. Nurses can reduce the discomfort of delirium. In our experience, we have found the most effective intervention to be the continuous presence of one reliable family member or friend who will provide ongoing reassurance that the experience is caused by toxicity and will subside in a few hours or days. We have also used students in this manner and found it effective. In addition to psychologic manifestations of acute cerebral impairment, physical symptoms such as vasomotor instability; elevated pulse and respiration; temperature fluctuations; tremors of fingers, hands, lips, and facial muscles; headache; and generalized weakness are often present. An individual with acute organic brain disorder is physically ill, as well as cognitively impaired. Any condition that compromises the cellular function of the brain will cause an acute organic brain disorder. Delirium is a common psychiatric complication of physical illness and of treatments for physical illness in the elderly. In our experience, it is a more common signal of physical illness of the elderly person than symptoms such as fever, pain, or tachycardia. Elderly individuals with some degree of dementia are particularly likely to develop transient delirium in response to physical illness, drug intoxication, and psychosocial stressors. Delirium is typically of abrupt onset and brief duration.

Prevention and Early Management of Acute Confusional States. Approximately 10% to 20% of all older patients admitted to hospitals exhibit some symptoms of acute confusion, and the same percentage develop delirium after surgery. The onset of delirium during hospitalization depends on the patient's illness and care management while hospitalized. Preventing or minimizing these occurrences is often possible through early and correct diagnosis, treatment of underlying disorders, removing causative factors, avoiding iatrogenic complications, judicious use of short-term medications, maintaining fluid and electrolyte balance, and supporting the patient and family (Beers and Berkow, 2000). Failure to provide this needed care may result in loss of function and life-threatening complications.

A focused workup of the older patient with acute confusion or delirium is usually necessary for a correct diagnosis. Depending on suspicions, one may test for fluid and electrolyte balance, urinalysis and culture (if a urinary tract infection [UTI] is suspected), complete blood count to evaluate for bleeding or anemia, and chest x-ray and oxygen saturation if respiratory infection, pulmonary embolus, or heart failure is suspected. An electrocardiogram may be done if there is suspicion of a cardiac problem or arrhythmia. Serum drug levels may be drawn if toxicity is a possibility. A computed tomography scan or magnetic resonance imaging (MRI) may be done if a stroke is suspected.

Requesting that the family stay with the patient as much as possible, even through the night, can be highly beneficial in preventing or minimizing delirium. The patient should be encouraged to use sensory aids such as glasses and hearing aids to maintain contact with the new environment. Clocks and calendars that are visible from a distance can be beneficial. Patients should be placed in rooms near the nurses' station to ensure early intervention.

Drugs are sometimes used for chemical restraint in the agitated patient, especially in alcohol withdrawal. Benzodiazepines are often used for this purpose. Risperidone may be given in low doses because it is a high-potency antipsychotic. These drugs are used for agitation when there is fear that the patient may hurt himself or herself. Assessing for oversedation is important when these types of drugs are given.

Irreversible Dementia

In contrast to delirium, which is usually a reflection of an acute physiologic disturbance, or severe depression, dementia is an irreversible state that progresses over years in the decline of intellectual function. It is an umbrella term used to describe a number of diseases that impair cognition (usually memory and thinking). In days past, we used terms such as *senility* and *hardening of the arteries* to describe dementia.

Dementia usually progresses gradually over a period of years; however, it can begin abruptly. It affects memory, orientation, language, judgment, visuospatial skills, concentration, and the ability to sequence tasks (Alzheimer's Organization, 2002). It is one of the most serious disorders that affect older adults. The prevalence increases with increasing age, doubling every 5 years after age 60.

Types of Dementia. Alzheimer's disease (AD) is the most common type of dementia. However, there are a number of other common causes. These include vascular dementia (large or small strokes or multiinfarct dementia), dementia of Parkinson's disease (usually Lewy-body dementia), dementia of pernicious anemia, and dementia of hypothyroidism, to name just a few.

Primary dementia is composed of AD, Pick's disease, frontal lobe dementia syndromes, and some mixed dementias that have an AD component (Beers and Berkow, 2000). *Vascular dementias* include multiinfarct dementia, lacunar state, Binswanger's disease, and mixed vascular dementia. *Dementias associated with Lewy-body disease* include Parkinson's dementia, progressive supranuclear palsy, and diffuse Lewy-body disease. *Dementia due to toxic ingestion* includes alcohol-associated dementia and dementia due to heavy metals or toxic exposures. *Dementia due to infection* includes viral infections such as human immunodeficiency virus (HIV)–associated dementia and postencephalitis syndromes. Spirochetal infections are neurosyphilis and Lyme disease. Prions cause Creutzfeldt-Jakob disease. *Dementia due to structural brain abnormalities* includes normal-pressure hydrocephalus, chronic subdural hematomas, and brain tumors. Potentially reversible conditions that are to be considered in the differential diagnosis of dementia include hypothyroidism, depression, and vitamin B_{12} deficiency (Beers and Berkow, 2000). Depression is considered a *pseudodementia,* because it mimics the symptoms of dementia (Gerdner and Hall, 2001).

Reversible dementias or dementias that can become stabilized include drug intoxications, central nervous system (CNS) infections, metabolic disturbances such as vitamin deficiencies, thyroid disorders, liver and pancreas disorders, and chronic renal failure. Brain tumor or brain injury may be reversed or stabilized. Normal-pressure hydrocephalus is uncommon but may be treated with a shunt that diverts cerebrospinal fluid away from the brain (Alzheimer's Organization, 2002). See Box 21-7 for disorders causing or simulating dementia.

Most dementias are not reversible. These include AD, multiinfarct dementia, Parkinson's dementia, Lewy-body disease, Pick's disease, acquired immunodeficiency syndrome (AIDS) dementia, and Creutzfeldt-Jakob disease. There are many more but they are extremely rare.

Symptoms of Dementia. The earliest feature of dementia is impairment in short-term memory. These patients will ask the same questions over and over. Forgetting where belongings are placed can eventually lead to paranoia about theft. Word finding becomes difficult. The elderly person may describe "those things on your feet" in place of the word "shoes." Activities of daily living (ADLs) that were usually a matter of course become difficult, for example, driving. The change in level of functioning eventually becomes obvious despite efforts to hide problems. Other changes in early dementia include mood swings, such as depression, euphoria, irritability, hostility, and agitation. Agitation may occur if the person is confronted with his or her problem (Beers and Berkow, 2000). There may be a more acute decline if the older person is subjected to a sudden change, such as hospitalization. Disorientation and behavioral changes may occur. This decline may not improve after the patient returns to his or her home. See Boxes 21-8 and 21-9 for useful dementia tools.

Intermediate dementia is characterized by the loss of ability to perform ADLs. Learning new information becomes difficult. The usual normal environmental cues and social cues are not functioning, and this increases disorientation. There

Box 21-7 Disorders Causing or Simulating Dementia

Disorders Causing Dementia

Degenerative diseases:
- Alzheimer's disease
- Pick's disease
- Huntington's disease
- Progressive supranuclear palsy
- Parkinson's disease (not all cases)
- Cerebellar degenerations
- Amyotrophic lateral sclerosis (ALS) (not all cases)
- Parkinson-ALS-dementia complex of Guam and other island areas
- Rare genetic and metabolic diseases (Hallervorden-Spatz, Kufs', Wilson's late onset metachromatic leukodystrophy, adrenoleukodystrophy)

Vascular dementia:
- Multiinfarct dementia
- Cortical microinfarcts
- Lacunar dementia (larger infarcts)
- Binswanger disease
- Cerebral embolic disease (fat, air, thrombus fragments)

Anoxic dementia:
- Cardiac arrest
- Cardiac failure (severe)
- Carbon monoxide

Traumatic dementia:
- Dementia pugilistica (boxer's dementia)
- Head injuries (open or closed)

Infectious dementia:
- Acquired immunodeficiency syndrome (AIDS)—dementia and opportunistic infections
- Jakob-Creutzfeldt disease (subacute spongiform encephalopathy)

Disorders That Can Simulate Dementia

Psychiatric disorders:
- Depression
- Anxiety
- Psychosis
- Sensory deprivation

Drugs:
- Sedatives
- Hypnotics
- Antianxiety agents
- Antidepressants
- Antiarrhythmics
- Antihypertensives
- Anticonvulsants
- Antipsychotics
- Digitalis and derivatives
- Drugs with anticholinergic side effects
- Others (mechanism unknown)

Nutritional disorders:
- Pellagra (B_6 deficiency)
- Progressive multifocal leukoencephalopathy
- Postencephalitic dementia
- Behçet's syndrome
- Herpes encephalitis
- Fungal meningitis or encephalitis
- Bacterial meningitis or encephalitis
- Parasitic encephalitis
- Brain abscess
- Neurosyphilis (general paresis)

Normal pressure hydrocephalus (communicating hydrocephalus of adults)

Space-occupying lesions:
- Chronic or acute subdural hematoma
- Primary brain tumor
- Metastatic tumors (carcinoma, leukemia, lymphoma, sarcoma)

Multiple sclerosis (some cases)

Autoimmune disorders:
- Disseminated lupus erythematosus
- Vasculitis

Toxic dementia:
- Alcoholic dementia
- Metallic dementia (e.g., lead, mercury, arsenic, manganese)
- Organic poisons (e.g., solvents, some insecticides)

Other disorders:
- Epilepsy (some cases)
- Posttraumatic stress disorder (concentration camp syndrome—some cases)
- Whipple disease (some cases)
- Heat stroke
- Thiamine deficiency (Wernicke-Korsakoff syndrome)
- Cobalamin deficiency (B_{12}) or pernicious anemia
- Folate deficiency
- Marchiafave-Bignami disease

Metabolic disorders (usually cause delirium, but can be difficult to differentiate from dementia):
- Hyperthyroidism and hypothyroidism (thyroid hormones)
- Hypercalcemia (calcium)
- Hypernatremia and hyponatremia (sodium)
- Hypoglycemia (glucose)
- Hyperlipidemia (lipids)
- Hypercapnia (carbon dioxide)
- Kidney failure
- Liver failure
- Cushing syndrome
- Addison's disease
- Hypopituitarism
- Remote effect of carxinoma

From Office of Technology Assessment: *Losing a million minds: confronting the tragedy of Alzheimer's disease and other dementias*, Washington, DC, 1987, U.S. Government Printing Office.

Box 21-8 Functional Dementia Scale

Circle one rating for each item:
1 None or little of the time
2 Some of the time
3 Good part of the time
4 Most or all of the time

Patient ____________

Observer ____________

Position or relation to patient ____________

Facility ____________

1	2	3	4	(01)	Has difficulty in completing simple tasks on own, e.g., dressing, bathing, doing arithmetic.
1	2	3	4	(02)	Spends time either sitting or in apparently purposeless activity.
1	2	3	4	(03)	Wanders at night or needs to be restrained to prevent wandering.
1	2	3	4	(04)	Hears things that are not there.
1	2	3	4	(05)	Requires supervision or assistance in eating.
1	2	3	4	(06)	Loses things.
1	2	3	4	(07)	Appearance is disorderly if left to own devices.
1	2	3	4	(08)	Moans.
1	2	3	4	(09)	Cannot control bowel function.
1	2	3	4	(10)	Threatens to harm others.
1	2	3	4	(11)	Cannot control bladder function.
1	2	3	4	(12)	Needs to be watched so doesn't injure self, e.g., by careless smoking, leaving the stove on, falling.
1	2	3	4	(13)	Destructive of materials around him, e.g., breaks furniture, throws food trays, tears up magazines.
1	2	3	4	(14)	Shouts or yells.
1	2	3	4	(15)	Accuses others of doing him bodily harm or stealing his possessions—when you are sure the accusations are not true.
1	2	3	4	(16)	Is unaware of limitations imposed by illness.
1	2	3	4	(17)	Becomes confused and does not know where he/she is.
1	2	3	4	(18)	Has trouble remembering.
1	2	3	4	(19)	Has sudden changes of mood, e.g., gets upset, angered, or cries easily.
1	2	3	4	(20)	If left alone, wanders aimlessly during the day or needs to be restrained to prevent wandering.

From Moore JT et al: A functional dementia scale, *J Fam Pract* 16:498, 1983.

is loss of judgement and increasing confusion, which can be a precipitant to falls. Paranoia becomes significant in about 25% of patients (Beers and Berkow, 2000). Wandering becomes problematic as the patient is unable to recognize or find his or her bedroom or other familiar place. In long-term care facilities this can be a significant problem as the resident tries to find a familiar place.

Severe, late-stage dementia is a difficult period for all caregivers as the patient becomes totally dependent and is unable to perform any ADLs, including toileting and feeding. This person no longer recognizes loved family members. Ambulation becomes more and more difficult. Swallowing may become impaired, which increases risk of malnutrition, dehydration, and infection (often the cause of death in AD). The diagnosis is not made if these features are due to clouding of consciousness, as in delirium; however, delirium and dementia may coexist (American Psychiatric Association, 1994). The most common reasons for coexistence of delirium and dementia in elderly patients are multiple medications, fluid and electrolyte imbalance, systemic disease, and malnutrition. There are, of course, numerous other disorders causing or simulating dementia.

Dementia has biopsychosocial components that produce disruption in behavior, cognition, affect, and socialization. The tendency to equate dementia and chronic organic brain disorders with a fatalistic approach to care is unwarranted. Irreversible dementia, by the nature of the label, promotes the belief that nothing can be done. This is rooted in our mechanistic approach to illness. Recovery and growth are not expected, but often careful evaluation of all factors involved, both primary and secondary, will reveal that improvement in function and enjoyment may be facilitated.

Box 21-9 Mini-Mental State Inpatient Consultation Form

Maximum Score	Score	
		Orientation
5	( )	What is the (year) (season) (date) (day) (month)?
5	( )	Where are we (state) (country) (town) (hospital) (floor)?
		Registration
3	( )	Name three objects: 1 second to say each. Then ask the patient all three after you have said them. Give one point for each correct answer. Then repeat them until he learns all three. Count trials and record.
		Attention and Calculation Trial
5	( )	Serial 7s. Give one point for each correct. Stop after five answers. Alternatively spell "world" backwards.
		Recall
3	( )	Ask for three objects repeated above. Give one point for each correct.
		Language Trial
9	( )	Name a pencil and a watch (two points). Repeat the following "No ifs, ands, or buts" (one point). Follow a three stage command: "Take a paper in your right hand, fold it in half, and put it on the floor" (three points). Read and obey the following: "Close your eyes" (one point). "Write a sentence" (one point). "Copy design" (one point). Assess level of consciousness along a continuum.
		Alert — Drowsy — Stupor — Coma
	TOTAL ( )	

From Folstein MF, Folstein S, McHugh PR: Mini-mental state: a practical method for grading the cognitive state of patients for the clinician, *J Psychiatr Res* 12:189, 1975.

Alzheimer's Disease or Senile Dementia of the Alzheimer Type. Alzheimer's disease (AD) was described by Dr. Alois Alzheimer in 1906 and is a cerebral degenerative disorder of unknown origin. The prevalence is greater than 4 million Americans and may be said to include their families, because it is a disease that produces maximum impact on families as well as the patient (Alzheimer's Organization, 2002). It is not just a disease of the old, but the incidence increases with aging. AD was described by Dr. Alzheimer as neurofibrillary tangles and senile plaques. This has been confirmed. The tangles and plaques represent the death of nerve cells, neurons, throughout the brain. The brain shrinks to about one third of its normal weight. The tangles consist of a protein called *tau* that "clogs" the insides of brain cells and their connections. Tangled tau is seen in most people of old age but is less widespread in the brain compared to those with AD. Deposits of beta amyloid also accumulate abnormally in the brains of patients with AD. Researchers have found that there are changes in the ways that glucose disperses in the brain of AD patients (Alzheimer's Organization, 2002). The disease is progressive and is accompanied by increasing forgetfulness, confusion, inability to concentrate, personality deterioration, and impaired judgment. The cause of the disorder is still unknown, although there is a genetic factor in the gene that codes for tau and is associated with dementia that doubles the occurrence within susceptible families to 4% as opposed to 2% of the general population.

Senile dementia of the Alzheimer type (SDAT) was the term used to describe the Alzheimer's disorder as diagnosed by clinical research criteria but not histologically verified. SDAT was the usage suggested by the National Institute of Neurological and Communicative Disorders and the Alzheimer's Disease and Related Disorders Association Work Group. In the more recent publication of the DSM-IV, senile dementia of the Alzheimer type is no longer considered an appropriate category. Rather, it is classified as dementia of the Alzheimer's type (DAT) with subsets of early onset or late onset (Box 21-10). It is further refined into subtypes such as with delirium, with delusions, with depressed mood, with behavioral disturbance, or uncomplicated.

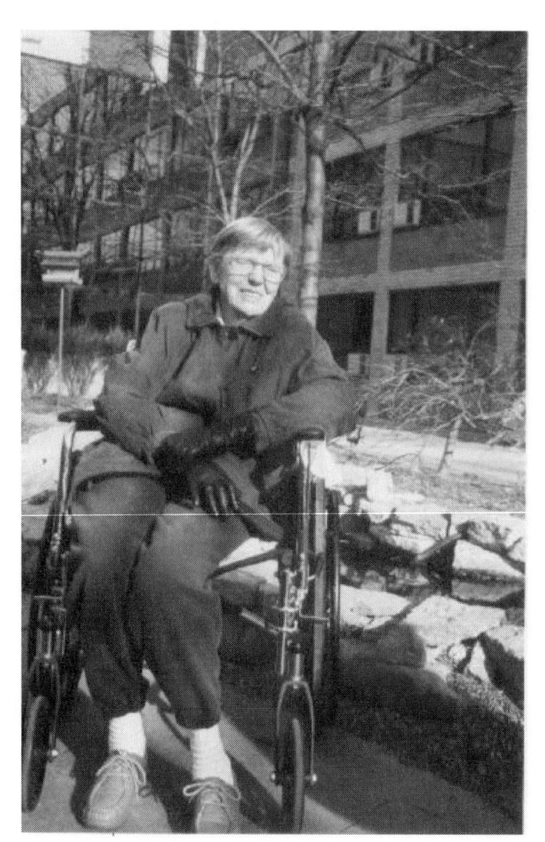

Thelma with end-stage Alzheimer's disease. (Courtesy Ann Luggen.)

Box 21-10 DSM-IV-TR Criteria for Dementia of Alzheimer's Type

1. Multiple cognitive deficits manifested by the following:
   a. memory impairment, and
   b. either aphasia, apraxia, agnosia, or executive function disturbance
2. Significant impairment of social and work-related function caused by deficits in cognition in 1a and 1b and is a decline from previous functioning.
3. There is gradual onset of deficits and progressive cognitive decline.
4. The cognitive deficits in 1a and 1b are not caused by the following:
   a. Central nervous system disturbances that cause progressive memory deficit such as Parkinson's disease, cerebrovascular disorders, subdural hematoma, brain tumor
   b. Conditions known to cause dementia such as hypothyroidism, pernicious anemia, folic acid deficiency, neurosyphilis, hyperparathyoid disease with hypercalcemia
   c. Substances, drugs
5. The deficits are not caused by delirium.
6. The deficits are not accounted for by major depression or schizophrenia.

Adapted from American Psychiatric Association: *Diagnostic and statistical manual of mental disorders,* DSM-IV-TR, Washington, DC, 2000, The Association.

Box 21-11 Criteria for Alzheimer's Diagnosis

- Dementia present, established by clinical and neuropsychologic examination
- Deficits in at least two areas of cognition
- Progressive worsening of memory and other cognitive functions
- No disturbances of consciousness
- Onset between ages of 40 and 90
- Absence of other disorders to account for dementia

Alzheimer's is common with very old age. Only about 3% of elders age 65 to 74 have AD; however, about 20% of those age 75 to 84 and nearly 50% of those age 85 and older have AD (Alzheimer's Organization, 2002). It is extremely rare before age 65. Because more people are living into the seventh, eighth, and ninth decades, the number of diagnosed cases of AD is estimated to nearly triple in 50 years unless we find a method of prevention.

Diagnosis of Alzheimer's disease. The only accurate method of diagnosing AD is to perform a brain biopsy or autopsy, though some promising gene research and structural MRI may enable us to predict or diagnose with a high level of accuracy. At this time, AD is diagnosed by clinical and neuropsychologic examination; it is characterized by deficits in at least two areas of cognition, progressive worsening of memory and other cognitive functions, no disturbances of consciousness, an onset between ages 40 and 90, and the absence of other disorders to account for the dementia (Alzheimer's Organization, 2002). See Box 21-11 for criteria for the diagnosis of Alzheimer's disease.

Researchers at Massachusetts General Hospital and Harvard Medical School examined patients with early signs of AD using MRI to look at specific areas of the brain found to be affected early in AD with significant loss of neurons (Alzheimer's Organization, 2002). The patients were followed over a 3-year period to determine who developed AD, as diagnosed by the standard medical/neuropsychologic examination. The MRIs were 100% accurate in discriminating between patients who were normal and those who had mild AD. The MRIs were 93% accurate in discriminating between patients who were normal and those who initially had memory impairments and ultimately developed AD. The area of the brain the researchers examined was the entorhinal cortex.

Another interesting study developed to diagnose AD involves an odor identification test (National Institute on Aging,

2002). Researchers from Columbia Presbyterian Medical Center in New York studied 90 men and women with minor memory problems and other mild cognitive impairments, subjecting them to a "scratch and sniff" test. They tested 40 distinct smells, for example, peanuts, soap, and menthol. The results, published in the *American Journal of Psychiatry,* revealed that of the 30 older adults who scored well on the smell test, none developed AD in the follow-up period of nearly 2 years. However, 19 of the subjects reported a good sense of smell but scored poorly on the smell test and went on to a diagnosis of AD in the follow-up period. The researchers purport that inability to recognize smells, combined with the lack of awareness that olfactory sense is impaired, may be useful as a predictor for AD.

Risk factors for AD include increasing age, family history and genetics, female gender, and presence of Down syndrome. Down syndrome is a genetic disorder involving chromosome 21, which produces amyloid precursor protein (APP); APP plays a role in the deposition of beta amyloid, the substance involved in the senile plaques of AD. In a 1996 study, researchers with the MIRAGE project tracked lifetime risk of AD of 13,000 people (Alzheimer's Organization, 2002). By age 80, people with AD in both parents had a 54% risk, which is 1.5 times the risk of the disease in people with only one affected parent and 5 times the risk of people with two unaffected parents. Further, with identical twins, if one develops AD, the other's risk is 40% to 50%, arguing for a genetic predisposition.

Possible risk factors for AD have been identified. These include environmental toxins, low formal education and occupational attainment, previous head trauma, and cerebrovascular disease (Alzheimer's Organization, 2002). The environmental toxins are unknown; for many years aluminum was suspect, but it is no longer a major consideration. The well-known Nun Study conducted by Dr. David Snowden at University of Kentucky has brought new speculation about AD. In this study, 675 Catholic sisters joined the study from 1991 to 1993 and donated their brains at death. It was found that the presence of tiny strokes or TIAs in combination with the plaques and tangles significantly increased the clinical manifestations of AD. This study, funded by the NIA and published in the *Journal of the American Medical Association* (*JAMA*) in February 1996, also found that cognitive ability in youth is linked to development of AD in later life. The women who had poor scores on measures of cognitive ability as young adults were found to be at higher risk for AD and low cognitive function in late life.

In other reports, head trauma, even one minor incident in early life, makes one more prone to AD than a person without trauma (Alzheimer's Organization, 2002). The size of the risk is not yet known.

A recent study in England and Wales, described in *The Lancet* (Medical Research Council, 2001), had findings that contradict much of our physiologic findings in AD. In this large study, consent was obtained to examine subjects' brains at autopsy. The mean age of death was 85 for men and 86 for women. Both cerebrovascular (78%) and AD (70%) pathology was present in 48% of subjects, and 64% had features indicating AD. But 33% of nondemented people had equivalent densities of neocortical neuritic plaques and neurofibrillary pathology. The researchers state that additional factors are needed to determine whether or not "moderate burdens of cerebral AD-type pathology and vascular lesions are associated with cognitive failure" (Medical Research Council, 2001, p. 169).

Disease course. The course of this disease ranges from 1 to 15 years; typical life expectancy is 8 to 9 years after symptom onset, with death usually occurring because of pulmonary infections, urinary tract infections, decubitus ulcers, or iatrogenic disorders. Current research focuses on many aspects of AD: anatomy, biochemistry, diagnosis, genetics, language, memory, nutrition, perception, pharmacology, physiology, psychosocial issues, virology, and vitamin therapy. Symptoms of depression may be the first and earliest signs of AD, occurring up to 3 years before the disease is diagnosed. In the past, researchers have questioned whether depression is an early sign of AD or a risk factor for the disease. The belief at this time is that depression is not a risk factor, but an early sign of AD. Further, the belief is that the depression of AD is not mood related, but rather motivation related, indicating lack of interest and energy and difficulty with concentration. The researchers state that this indicates that depression is not related to the patient's feelings about losing cognitive abilities, but actually reflects changes in the brain's areas of attention and energy. See Box 21-12 for stages of Alzheimer's disease.

Theories. In addition to the genetic theories known and proposed, a number of other avenues are being pursued in the effort to find a cause for AD. Atherosclerosis, cerebrovascular disease, and AD have been linked because researchers in

Box 21-12 Stages of Alzheimer's Disease

Mild Stage (2-5 Years)

Symptoms: memory loss and forgetfulness; unable to hold job, complete tasks; trouble recognizing the meaning of numbers; loses initiative, loses interest in hobbies, loses judgment

Moderate Stage (2-8 Years)

Symptoms: forgets how to get dressed, bathe; wanders; does not recognize friends, family; anxious, personality changes; insomnia, anxiety, delusional

Severe Stage (1-3 Years)

Symptoms: memory completely lost, does not recognize family; difficulty swallowing; no control of bowel and bladder; does not understand words; likes music, touch the Netherlands found that individuals with atherosclerosis were three times more likely to have AD (Christensen, 1997). More recent evidence has been provided by the Nun Study. This suggests that changes in blood vessels in the brain may trigger the deterioration that occurs in AD. This is complicated by the fact that the likelihood of developing any kind of dementia increases as atherosclerosis progresses.

The beta amyloid theory hypothesis is that as the brain perceives microscopic beta amyloid as foreign, primitive immune cells (microglia) serve as "biologic garbage collectors" that continuously try to clear them away (Nash, 2000). This results in a state of chronic inflammation that injures nearby neurons. Other scientists believe that the protein COX2, which rises steeply in the brains of patients in the early stages of AD and is a response to cell injury, may induce the inflammatory response and not beta amyloid. Antiinflammatory drugs, such as COX2 inhibitors, have emerged as a possible therapy for AD and clinical trials supported by the NIA have begun. These trials are testing COX2 inhibitors and naproxen (National Institute on Aging, 2001).

The E4 allele of apoE, a protein involved in cholesterol transport, has been genetically linked and is a risk factor of AD. There is an E2 allele that appears to be protective against AD, and there is an E3 allele that is neither protective nor causative for AD. Those people with the E4 allele develop AD at an earlier age than those without E4. At this time, genetic testing for apoE genotypes is not recommended by any government or organizational bodies.

Recent thought is that APP, the beta amyloid precursor, is definitely a susceptibility gene for AD, but there are other precursors as yet undiscovered (Nash, 2000). The newest proposal is a gene called A2M on chromosome 12 that seems to mediate the rate at which neurons produce beta amyloid.

At this time there is great competition among the "TAUist" and "BAPtist" (beta amyloid protein researchers) scientists. Tau, which normally supports the axons carrying signals from one nerve cell to another, "goes bad" and clumps into the tangles (Nash, 2000). In 1998 researchers found a form of dementia with a mutation of the tau gene. In 1999 the BAPtists, in animal studies of mice genetically engineered to develop plaques, developed a vaccine with beta amyloid; to their great surprise, the animals remained plaque free. When the vaccine was given to mice who already had numerous plaques, the plaques "melted away" when vaccinated. There are plans to test this in humans (Nash, 2000). More recently a causative brain enzyme has been found, gamma secretase, and pharmaceutical companies at this time are developing drugs to inhibit it.

A number of scientists believe that cholesterol may be a factor. Just as it contributes to heart disease, it may contribute to AD. In recent studies at New York University, researchers put mice on high-fat diets and observed the increased rate at which beta amyloid accumulated in their brains. When they gave the mice cholesterol-lowering drugs, the rate of accumulation slowed (Nash, 2000).

Recently, clinical research trials have begun looking at homocysteine, which is linked to an increased risk of developing AD over time. This amino acid is known to be linked to an increase in heart disease risk (Aldridge, 2002). A new study reported in the *New England Journal of Medicine* followed 1092 subjects from the Framingham study for 8 years, measuring their homocysteine levels. Of these, 111 developed dementia and 83 cases were AD. They found that the higher the homocysteine level, the greater the risk for AD (Aldridge, 2002). This kind of information from research allows us to consider a preventive stance in nursing toward AD.

The cholinergic theory is based on the understanding that acetylcholine, an important chemical neurotransmitter in the brain, is deficient. AD-affected areas of the brain have cholinergic activity that is reduced by 80% to 90%. New medications, the cholinesterase inhibitors, have been developed based on this theory. The inhibition of cholinesterase allows more acetylcholine to be available for cognitive functioning. Tacrine, a first-generation cholinesterase inhibitor, came out in 1993 (Novartis, 2000). This drug had hepatotoxicity concerns and is little used today. Donepezil, a second-generation drug, came out in 1997 and has become a useful drug in AD management. In 2000 rivastigmine tartrate (Exelon) became available and was a marketing success in the management of mild to moderate AD. Long-term studies are needed to determine how successful these drugs will be.

Other reports of agents that may affect the AD process include studies of estrogen, antioxidants such as vitamin E, and nerve-growth factors (Nash, 2000). A Dutch study states that moderate alcohol consumption may reduce the risk of dementia and suggests that alcohol may affect the AD process (Breteler, 2002). The researchers followed 8000 subjects 55 years of age and older for 6 years, examining the relationship between alcohol consumption and dementia. The researchers concluded that light to moderate alcohol consumption (one to three drinks per day) was associated with a 42% risk reduction for all dementias and a 70% reduction for vascular dementias. This information should not be too surprising to us, because we know from earlier studies that alcohol, especially red wine, is protective for cardiac and cerebrovascular disease due to its ability to reduce platelet aggregation or alter the blood/lipid ratio. Further rationale is that there may be a direct effect on cognition by stimulation of acetylcholine release—acetylcholine is known to facilitate memory and learning processes. It should be noted, however, that high alcohol intake inhibits acetylcholine production.

Recent reports suggest that long-term use of nonsteroidal antiinflammatory drugs (NSAIDs) reduces the risk of AD. A prospective study followed nearly 7000 subjects, 55 years and older, for an average of 6.8 years (Veld, 2001). The researchers found that subjects who used NSAIDs for at least 2 years had a significantly reduced risk for development of AD, though not for vascular dementia. Taking NSAIDs for any length of time reduced risk as well. Doses of NSAIDs had no relationship to risk in the subjects. Interestingly, the use of oral salicylates (aspirin) was associated with an increased risk of vascular dementia and a fivefold increased risk if they took oral salicylates for more than 2 years.

Parkinson's Dementia. Parkinson's disease (PD) results from the progressive loss of dopaminergic cells from the substantia nigra in the brainstem (Moore and Clarke, 2001). Though the etiology of primary parkinsonism is unknown, the death of substantia nigra cells within the basal ganglia results in a marked reduction in dopamine and is the cause of symptoms of tremor, muscular rigidity, akinesia, and loss of postural reflexes. There is an 80% to 90% loss of the dopamine-producing cells by the time the person becomes overtly symptomatic (Burke and Laramie, 2000). There is a young-onset PD that begins before age 40, but the mean age of onset is 65, and PD is common in all older adults, men and women equally (Moore and Clarke, 2001). At least 40,000 new cases are diagnosed every year and 50% are older than 70 (Kovach and Wilson, 1999; Burke and Laramie, 2000). First-degree relatives have twice the risk of developing PD (Moore and Clarke, 2001). Diagnosis has often been one of exclusion; however, more recently, the diagnosis requires two of four cardinal symptoms: resting tremor, bradykinesia, cogwheel rigidity, and postural instability (Boss, 2002).

Recent research suggests that a folic acid deficiency may increase susceptibility to PD (National Institute on Aging, 2002). Mouse studies reveal that low amounts of folic acid result in increased amounts of homocysteine in the brain. Homocysteine causes damage to the DNA of nerve cells in the substantia nigra. When the mice were fed folate, these nerve cells were able to repair damaged DNA. Many people who have PD may suffer from malnutrition, because the drugs they take cause nausea frequently. It is prudent then to give vitamin therapy that includes adequate amounts of folic acid (400 mg qd).

Secondary PD is caused by several medications (see Chapters 8 and 10). Among them are antipsychotics, antiemetics, antihypertensives such as verapamil and captopril, the antiangina drug diltiazem, the drugs valproate and phenytoin, and some of the common anticancer drugs such as vincristine and cytarabine (Burke and Laramie, 2000). Other causes are exposure to carbon monoxide, infarcts of the substantia nigra, brain tumors, and other metabolic and degenerative disorders. Depression and anxiety are common in individuals with primary or secondary parkinsonism and may occur in 80% of these individuals. The most common initial symptom is tremor of one hand and the pill-rolling motion of the fingers.

About 30% of people with PD develop dementia, and dementia is most common in those older than 70 (Boss, 2002). In institutionalized residents with PD, 80% have dementia. The PD patients with associated dementia (Lewy-body dementia) have a loss of cholinergic cells in the basal nucleus of Meynert, neuron loss, senile plaques, neurofibrillary tangles in the neocortex, and amyloid changes in small blood vessels (Boss, 2002). Lewy bodies are diffusely spread in neocortical neurons. Most elderly patients who have had a long course of PD develop dementia (Kovach and Wilson, 1999). The DSM-IV states that the dementia is a direct result of pathophysiologic changes that occur in the presence of PD.

The depression associated with PD is believed to be an endogenous depression, inherent in the pathology of PD (Boss, 2002). It is reasonable to assume that an exogenous depression may also occur with the progressive nature of the disease.

Nurses will best serve the clients by following the medications carefully, because the adverse effects of antiparkinsonian drugs may increase the dementia. The dopaminergic drugs that improve motor disability are associated with symptoms of psychosis (Cummings, 2000). Only early assessment and intervention can bring relief. Medications and individualized treatment plans are critical to the care of the person with PD because no curative therapy is available, and there is no evidence that any drug delays the progression of disease (Moore and Clarke, 2001). The challenge to client, family, and nurse is to maintain the highest possible level of functioning. At times the progress of disease is rapid, but most patients remain functional for many years.

Vascular Brain Disorders. Dementia of vascular disease origin, usually a subcortical dementia, is the second most prevalent dementia and often coexists with AD (Johnson, 2002). There are a number of vascular dementias—multiinfarct dementia, strategic infarct dementia, lacunar state, Binswanger's disease, and mixed vascular dementia (Beers and Berkow, 2000). They are marked by several distinguishing characteristics (American Psychiatric Association, 2000): multiple cognitive deficits manifested by memory impairment and aphasia, apraxia, agnosia, or executive function deficit (Box 21-13). These cognitive deficits cause significant impairment in daily functioning. There are behavioral and memory disturbances that fluctuate considerably and are unpredictable. This causes great difficulty for caregivers. Some of the focal neurologic signs and symptoms that may be observed include increased deep tendon reflexes, positive extensor plantar response, pseudobulbar palsy, gait disturbance, and extremity weaknesses (Figure 21-3). The dementias associated with brain infarction are often lacunar infarcts (Beers and Berkow, 2000). See Box 21-14 to differentiate the vascular dementias.

Intracerebral hemorrhage and the interruption of an adequate supply of blood and nutrients to the brain, resulting in tissue damage, accounts for most strokes in older adults. It is the third leading cause of death in the United States and many other countries (Beers and Berkow, 2000), and the incidence and mortality rate increase with age. It is now thought that immediate treatment, within 3 hours of the first symptoms of a blood clot in the brain, may prevent some of the brain cell death. Treatment begun within 90 minutes of symptomatology doubles the chance of full recovery (Haney, 2002). An intracerebral hemorrhage is not amenable to this treatment. The prevalence of cerebrovascular disease varies with race and gender (higher in blacks and men, but may be higher in white men older than 75) (Beers and Berkow, 2000). Risk factors are prior TIA or stroke, myocardial infarction, rheumatic heart disease, hypertension or diabetes in an adult older than 75, coronary artery disease, congestive heart failure, atrial fibrillation, hyperlipidemia, peripheral arterial disease, smoking, lack of exercise, and obesity.

Box 21-13 Vascular Brain Disease

Vascular brain disease may result from any of the following:
- Arteriosclerotic plaques blocking circulation to cerebral cells.
- Blood dyscrasias interfering with platelet and clot formation.
- Cardiac decompensation, resulting in insufficient perfusion to the brain.
- Cerebrovascular hemorrhage (strokes) of small or large magnitude.
- Diabetic deterioration of blood vessels.
- Primary hypertension causes deterioration of capillary walls because of sustained pressure; cerebral cells dependent on the deteriorated capillaries no longer function. Over time, hypertensive persons show greater decrements in cognitive performance than persons with normal blood pressure.
- Rupture of cerebrovascular or aortic aneurysms.
- Sustained severe anemia.
- Systemic emboli lodging in cerebrovascular pathway.
- Transient ischemic attacks (TIAs) lasting up to 24 hours, resulting from spasms of blood vessels in certain segments of the brain, which produce temporary disturbances in sensation, cognition, and motor activity, and are often a warning of impending stroke.

Treatment of vascular brain disorders begins with risk reduction. In addition, it includes taking aspirin, 75 mg, or anticoagulants to prevent thrombosis. Sadly, one study found that 75% of elderly stroke survivors in nursing homes do not receive medication to prevent further strokes (Agency for Healthcare Research and Quality, 2001). Using a statin to lower cholesterol may be of benefit in stroke prevention. Fit older adults with symptomatic carotid artery stenosis may benefit from endarterectomy. No clinical trials have demonstrated that these treatments slow the progression of vascular dementia (Beers and Berkow, 2000).

Transient ischemic attacks. In addition to major brain attacks, there are transient ischemic attacks (TIAs) caused by impaired circulation that last only a few minutes. The attacks occur suddenly and are usually completely resolved in 1 to 24 hours, and 75% last less than 5 minutes (Beers and Berkow, 2000). One third of people who have a TIA will have a stroke.

Box 21-14 Differentiating the Vascular Dementias

Multiinfarct dementia: major cerebral infarcts in two or more arteries in anterior, middle, or posterior territories; stepwise decline in cognition, each step another ischemic episode

Strategic infarct dementia: single infarct in crucial area of brain such as thalamus; gradual rather than stepwise decline

Lacunar state, Binswanger's: multiple small infarcts, usually in the periventricular white matter; cognitive impairment in some areas, other areas unaffected

Mixed dementia: combination of other vascular dementias and symptoms

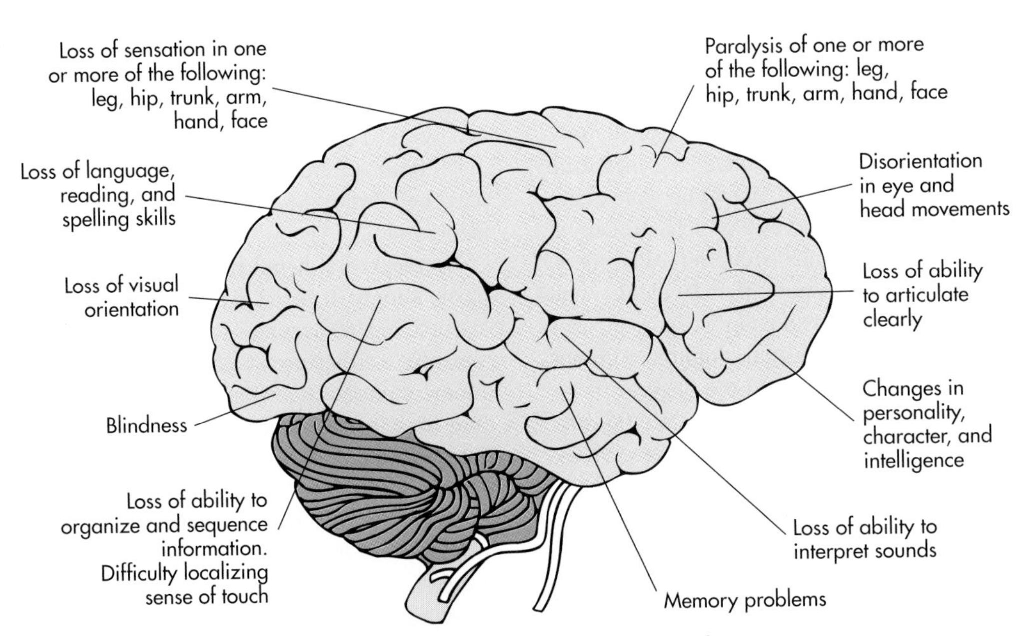

Figure 21-3. Brain areas affected by stroke.

The stroke may occur days to years after the TIA. The TIA is caused by temporary occlusion of an artery in the brain (a thrombus or an embolus). Elders with carotid artery stenosis who have a hypotensive episode may also suffer a TIA. Signs and symptoms include sudden onset of monocular blindness, difficulty seeing in one or both eyes, disturbance in speech, weakness or numbness in one arm or leg, vertigo, ataxia, generalized weakness, confusion, or loss of consciousness (National Institute for Neurological Disorders and Stroke, 2002). Strokes and the chronic symptoms and needs are discussed more fully in Chapter 8.

After a TIA or recovery from a stroke, there is considerable fear of further events. To restore some sense of security to the patient, the following steps should be taken:

1. Install a telephone with a long cord or a portable phone and post emergency numbers on the phone.
2. Instruct the patient to avoid rising rapidly from a lying or sitting position to a standing position.
3. Engage family, friends, or agencies in a daily telephone check to determine the client's status.
4. Subscribe to "Lifeline" or other emergency call method through a community hospital or service.

Pick's Disease. Pick's disease is a rare progressive degenerative brain disorder, a tau disease, involving atrophy of the frontal and temporal lobes of the cerebral cortex. Pick's disease is an uncommon type of dementia with clinical features similar to AD and is often misdiagnosed. It was discovered by a Czechoslovakian physician, Arnold Pick (1851-1924), and has a distinctive histopathology of degenerating neurons that contain globular intracytoplasmic filamentous inclusion bodies. The clinical distinction between AD and Pick's disease is often difficult; however, Pick's disease shows gradual progression, beginning in the fifth or sixth decade of life (Cotter, 2002). Patients exhibit amnesia, aphasia, and loss of socially appropriate behavior and inhibitions (Gerdner and Hall, 2001). There is profound alteration in personality characterized by inertia but with preservation of memory function. Language disorders occur, such as incorrect use of grammatical terms, sound-based errors ("bat" for "cat"), and anomia (inability to find the correct word). Further, the ability to recognize familiar faces and objects is lost (Cotter, 2002).

Huntington's Disease. Huntington's disease (HD) is inherited and can occur in 40- to 50-year-old persons, in whom it progresses rapidly, or in 60- to 70-year-old persons, in whom it progresses slowly. Patients exhibit characteristic choreiform movements, which need to be differentiated from senile chorea that occurs as isolated symptoms in elders older than 60 (Beers and Berkow, 2000). HD exhibits personality changes, cognitive impairments, and psychiatric signs of depression and psychosis. It should not be dismissed from consideration as a cause of dementia in the aged but does remain rather rare, and the chorea makes the diagnosis obvious.

Other Dementias. Other causes of dementia in older adults include a variety of sources. Toxic ingestion of alcohol for longer than 10 years can impair short-term memory and other cognitive domains (Beers and Berkow, 2000). Acute infections may cause delirium, and chronic infections may cause dementia. HIV-associated dementia is probably the most common of these and occurs late in the disease process. Encephalitis may cause an acute-onset dementia that may become chronic with a postencephalitis syndrome. Neurosyphilis and Lyme disease may also cause dementias that, if diagnosed early, may be at least partially reversible.

Developmentally Disabled Elders. The number of developmentally disabled elders (DDEs) is rapidly increasing, primarily because of medical advances and healthier living conditions that maintain them longer than in previous generations. Interestingly, individuals with Down syndrome (trisomy 21) who survive until old age develop the pathogenic hallmarks of AD (Beers and Berkow, 2000). Functional limitations in the biologic, social, and psychologic spheres may be a major cause of frailty in the DDE. Those elders are particularly dependent on their environment for stimulation, and in its absence behaviors suggestive of dementia may emerge.

Many aspects of the aging process apparently are prematurely experienced by the developmentally disabled. Their average age of death is younger than healthy persons—death in women/men is 79/73 in healthy adults but 67/63 in elders who are developmentally disabled (Brown, 2002). Thus they may experience musculoskeletal changes, sensory decline, problems from medication use over long periods of time, and certain disease states earlier. It is important to look for behavioral changes in those who have communication problems because these may indicate an underlying health disorder. Age-related hearing loss and vision loss are two of the problems that affect DDEs just as they affect healthy adults, but these problems may be discovered only by observing and acting on behavioral changes (Bagley, 2002; Flax, 2002). Retirement needs and responses to relocation present special considerations.

INTERVENTIONS: CARING FOR THE PERSON WITH DEMENTIA

Much of dementia care takes place in the home and is provided by an aging spouse or in a nursing home where it is provided by aides. Therefore nurses will be most effective when they assist the caregivers in whatever setting to understand the nature of dementia and the interventions likely to be most effective. Overall, interventions must match expectations with capacities, incorporate earlier life skills and interests, and provide a calm, caring, and structured environment. These are mighty challenges to nurses and direct caregivers wherever they may be.

Determining the strengths of the dementia-afflicted older person requires staff commitment and patience. Too often the obvious deficits create an unwarranted assumption that the individual has nothing left of personality that is valuable. In an atmosphere of acceptance individuals will show their maximum potential. Staff can reinforce independence and prevent shame by helping the patient only with things he or she has tried and is unable to accomplish. This requires patience and hope and providing assistance at the minimum level necessary.

Basic Nutrition

Individuals with dementia exhibit numerous behaviors that interfere with adequate nutritional intake. The nursing challenge is to increase functional behaviors during the process of eating or being fed. Encourage the patient to feed himself or herself; assist when it becomes necessary. Someone very knowledgeable described this as communication and as an art. The caregiver must develop a sensitivity to the subtle cues the patient gives and be responsive to them.

Common problems encountered in the feeding process include the following:

- Refusal to open mouth without extra stimulation such as coaxing it open with a spoon
- Closing mouth inappropriately; extrusion and disturbed tongue movements; hoarding food in mouth
- Inability to swallow
- Coughing when swallowing
- Spitting out food

General interventions should include: establishing a pleasant dining experience; addressing the person by name and touching the person; using a large cloth napkin, rather than a bib; and introducing the resident to others at the table (O'Neill, 2000). Explain the content of each bite, and observe if it is desired or not. Offer sips of fluid between bites, holding spoon ready while talking to and touching resident, hugging resident when successfully taking and swallowing bite. For each resident there are particular behaviors of the nurse that will facilitate the process. The caregiver with sensitivity to the individual's eating patterns, preferences, life history, and present symptoms can respond more effectively to the patient's eating preferences.

A recent study by Simmons and colleagues (2001) described a one-on-one feeding trial. Fifty percent of the participants significantly increased their oral food and fluid intake during mealtime. It cost a great deal in staff time—an average of 38 minutes per resident per meal versus the 9 minutes usually given by nursing home staff.

Dealing with Agitation

Agitation is defined as inappropriate verbal, vocal, or motor activity not explained by apparent needs, confusion, medical condition, or social/environmental disturbances (Valle, 2001). Agitation is pervasive among individuals suffering from AD. It can be verbal, physical, vocal, or sexual. Behaviors commonly seen and heard include pacing, undressing publicly, handling things inappropriately, restlessness, screaming, and repeated vocalizations.

Valle (2001) describes a general approach to those displaying frequent aggression:

- Identify and treat primary medical illnesses that may be the underlying problem (e.g., pain, infection, dehydration, electrolytes, anemia)
- Limit "prn" medicines
- Review the medications
- Specify/quantify target behaviors for the treatment plan
- Develop realistic goals for improvement
- Identify needs that are not being met (pain, hunger, thirst, toileting, fatigue, fear)
- Plan behavior management:
  - A—antecedents
  - B—behaviors
  - C—consequences
- Psychiatric assessment

Pharmacologic Management. According to Valle (2001), "Bactrim is the best antipsychotic in the world." There is no medication that is approved by the Food and Drug Administration for the treatment of behavioral disturbance or agitation and aggression associated with dementia. All the medications that we use to manage aggression are "on trial." Key assumptions are "start low, go slow" and "keep going." Titrate a dose upward until there is benefit or toxicity. Back down from toxicity.

Nonpharmacologic Management. The most important factor is to avoid the overstimulation so common in the environment of an elder with AD. Change the environment so that it is nonthreatening. Limit isolation. Provide soothing sounds, music; give gentle touch; and subdue or brighten the lights depending on the need for relaxation or orientation.

Feelings of helplessness, anger, fatigue, or anxiety may result in abusive, acting-out behavior (Roach, 2001). Patients become agitated easily and frequently, and caregivers often have great difficulty knowing the cause or how to intervene. A systematic and individualized approach is necessary because agitation is often a multidimensional problem. It is often demonstrated in aggressive behaviors such as hitting and biting, spitting, motor restlessness, verbal abuse or yelling and screaming, and resistance to care. Difficult behaviors often occur at bath time.

Causes of agitation may include hypoxia, delirium, urinary tract infection, fatigue, or, often, pain. Even small environmental changes and psychologic stress must also be considered. See Box 21-15 for antecedents of agitation. All of these factors should be explored. Too often the agitation is considered just another demonstration of dementia, although there is considerable evidence today that agitation or a change in behavior is related to pain.

Care must be individualized to preserve dignity. In spite of cognitive deficits and behavioral aberrations, these clients are sensitive to attitudes and seem to know instinctively whom they can trust. Approaching the patient in a gentle, nonthreatening manner sets an emotional climate (O'Neill, 2002); facial expression, eye contact, gestures, and fluidity of movement convey messages. Burke and Laramie (2000, p. 419) describe "touching with love." Moments of pleasure and joy

Box 21-15 Antecedents of Agitation

Cognitive Impairment
Acute and chronic brain syndrome (delirium, dementia)

Psychiatric Disorders
Depression
Manic-depressive illness (bipolar disorder)
Agitated depression
Involutional depression
Schizophrenia
Paraphrenia

Internal and External Stimuli/Situational Anxiety
Unresolved past stressors
Intracerebral or extracerebral stress
Sensory isolation
Invasion of personal space

Sensory Impairment
Impaired hearing
Impaired sight
Communication losses

Physical Disorders
Acute hypoxia
Pain or discomfort
Infectious processes
Parkinsonism
Fatigue
Cardiovascular disorders
Renal disorders
Neurologic disorders
Electrolyte disturbances
Endocrine disturbances

Pharmacologic Effects
Antipsychotic medications
Drug toxicity
Drug withdrawal
Psychotropic drugs

From Gerdner LA, Buckwalter KC: A nursing challenge: assessment and management of agitation in Alzheimer's patients, *J Gerontol Nurs* 20(4):11, 1994.

must not be overlooked as sources of brief satisfaction, distraction, and respite from the underlying anxiety. Affection, appreciation, and touch may provide some moments of meaning.

Coping with Problem Behaviors

Management of common problems such as incontinence, immobility or constant wandering, shouting, spitting, and aggressive actions constitutes a heavy burden for nursing staff.

Nursing responsibilities include the following:

1. Carefully observe and record mood, behavior, and memory. Erratic changes in the last two areas would be less indicative of AD than would a slowly progressive loss of functional abilities. They suggest an infectious process, especially a UTI, or pain.
2. Manage behaviors with the use of as few psychotropic medications as possible. They tend to increase the patient's difficulty negotiating the environment.
3. Try different methods to control the behavior, such as distraction via music or increased or decreased environmental lighting.
4. Avoid changing routines: make surroundings as predictable as possible.
5. Groom the patient carefully; encourage independence in this area, but if he or she is unable, do not leave him or her untidy. Try to find a time when the resident is in a mood to bathe and dress and maintain the schedule.
6. Provide occupational therapy geared to the patient's abilities.
7. Work with the family toward premorbid grief resolution. Support the family and instruct in particular ways to interact in a helpful manner.
8. Provide the patient with consistent reality orientation. However, correcting the patient by, for example, telling the patient that his or her mother died 10 years ago is harmful to a distressed person who has lost capacity (Burke and Laramie, 2000).
9. Avoid using physical or chemical restraints.
10. Provide a mildly stimulating environment.
11. Interact in a caring and supportive manner.
12. Make every effort toward consistency of caregivers.

Improving Communication

Bartol's pioneering studies in the nursing care of individuals with dementia in the late 1970s alerted nurses to the extreme difficulties of communicating with a patient in the advanced stages of AD. Memory loss, aphasia, apraxia, agnosia, and overwhelming disorientation make verbal communication meaningless. Communicating with the cognitively impaired elderly patient requires special skills (Box 21-16). At this late stage of AD, most patients are bed-bound or chair-bound and have lost the ability to talk, walk, and provide any self-care (Burke and Laramie, 2000). Ideas for communication are to continue speaking quietly with eye contact, patting and touching the patient lovingly, smiling, and personalized kinds of comfort care because the patient is no longer aware of what is happening. The nurse's calm concern will do much to alleviate anxiety and cultivate client and family responsiveness. Actions, however, will have more influence than words in such situations. The sound of communication is a humanizing factor, even though words may not be understood. See Box 21-17 for communication guidelines.

Preventing Catastrophic Reactions

In the 1950s Goldstein coined the term *catastrophic reaction* to describe the overreaction toward minor stresses that occurs in demented patients. Usually catastrophic reactions occur when

Box 21-16 Communicating with the Cognitively Impaired

Be patient; the individual may lack comprehension but may respond to repeated and varied attempts to communicate.

Keep routines the same and provide written reminders. Repetition is often necessary.

Introduce one idea and allow time for response. A demented person may require inordinate amounts of time to respond.

Use the active tense when speaking; for example, "Eat this apple."

Demonstrate and give pictures of eating the apple or whatever you wish the person to do.

Additional and specific information may tap some element of comprehension. Use redundant cueing; for example, "Bite the apple with your teeth."

Ask closed, specific questions; for example, "Do you want to eat the apple?" If the individual does not answer, offer another alternative after waiting for a response; for example, "Are you hungry?"

Remember: the patient is likely to become even more frustrated than you when messages are not understood. Intersperse verbal activities with periods of quiet touch or stroking.

Box 21-17 Communication Guidelines: Do's and Don'ts

1. Orient yourself to the individual. Make sure you are at eye level with the person. Look for signs of agitation or withdrawal.
2. Assume the person understands more than he or she is able to express. Watch how the person communicates, and use that knowledge to converse.
3. Recognize the misperceptions and misunderstandings. Avoid complicated issues.
4. Avoid noisy and busy environments. Find out if the person has a hearing or visual disorder and compensate for it.
5. Convey messages through touch, expressions, posture, head movement, eye contact, gesture, and position relative to the person with dementia. Speech should be in a low, audible tone.
6. Be concrete and direct.
7. Use short sentences or questions. Ask questions that require yes/no or either/or answers.
8. Try again and be redundant.

From Proulx G: When someone you know has a memory problem: some of the "do's and don'ts" to help you communicate, *Baycrest Bulletin* 8(1):3, 1996, Baycrest Centre for Geriatric Care, Toronto, Canada.

the person becomes overwhelmed by sensory input and acts out in an aggressive manner (Ham, 2002). This often occurs at the worst time—at a family reunion, for example, or on the family vacation. This can be the first indication of AD. It will be precipitated by fatigue, overstimulation, inability to meet expectations, and misinterpretations. Interventions to avert or minimize this reaction include those proposed by Wolanin and Phillips (1981) in their classic work on confusion (Box 21-18).

Box 21-18 What to Do for Catastrophic Behavior

The patient with Alzheimer's may exhibit a sudden temporary worsening in behavior related to buildup of stress, fatigue, or physical discomforts. Thinking deteriorates (cognitive inaccessibility) and the patient becomes unable to communicate (social inaccessibility). The patient experiencing a catastrophic episode is generally frightened or panicked, feels unsafe, and exhibits strong potential for injuring himself or others.

How to prepare for it: A person's catastrophic episodes are usually the same each time. Ask the caregiver how the patient usually acts when tired or overwhelmed: Does he become fearful? Agitated? Wander? Act more confused? Become combative? Ask what the caregiver does to calm the patient.

Immediate measures: Place the patient in a quiet room, eliminating all extraneous stimuli, including people. Regard the patient as frightened. Focus your interventions on returning the patient's sense of mastery or control over his or her environment.

- Assess for and eliminate all potential stressors, such as full bladder, restraints, catheters, pain.
- Provide a "time out" of at least 30 minutes to 1 hour. If possible, ask the caregiver to sit quietly with the patient. (No TV or talking except quiet, gentle reassurance.)
- If the patient's combative behavior poses an immediate hazard to himself or herself or to others, provide physical or chemical restraints in the least restrictive manner possible. However, if the patient is not combative unless approached, simply supervise while maintaining a safe distance, using the "time out" to defuse the situation.
- Remain calm: this is a time-limited event. Talk in low, calm, reassuring tones to help the patient feel safe and secure. Do not attempt to argue with the patient's belief. ("They are not constructing that building in your yard, you are in the hospital!") Usually the patient will not believe such a comment; instead, it will heighten his or her anxiety.
- Chart the symptoms of the event, time of onset, duration, and successful interventions.
- Prevent further episodes by simplifying the daily schedule, increasing rest periods, evaluating environmental stressors, limiting visitors, controlling pain, and using other interventions.

From Wolanin MO, Phillips LR: *Confusion: prevention and care,* St Louis, 1981, Mosby.

Recognize that the feelings of distress may linger in a patient after he or she has forgotten the precipitant. Time spent with an uninvolved person may help. The nurse present during the reactions may instinctively respond with anger or irritation. It is important for the nurse to express her annoyance or impatience to another staff member. We believe it is futile to talk of caring, patience, and gentleness with patients without learning to handle irritating behaviors.

Even grossly disoriented persons, often seen as helpless and hopeless, may briefly respond with warmth and pleasure when stimulated. For those persons the goal is not orientation but rather human contact. Care should be directed toward fostering good general health and maintaining locomotor skills and functional preservation in all areas of behavior. Reality orientation and environmental awareness may be futile. Listening with respectful attention to any attempts to communicate is most important. This can lead to reminiscing, even though patients may not even remember the names of their spouse or children. See Box 21-19 for orientation guidelines.

The management of ambulatory institutionalized patients with dementia presents many problems to the staff and the institutional milieu. Disorientation, wandering, rummaging, irritability, loss of social inhibition, and combativeness are difficult for other patients and for staff. There are nonpharmacologic ways to deal with this; it will be different for each patient. For example, the catastrophic reactions of certain patients respond readily to distraction, but avoid multiple distractions as in a busy, noisy environment. The infectious nature of agitated behaviors often results in overreactions of caregivers as well. Slow, calm, deliberate action is much more likely to be effective. Other methods of containment include speaking slowly and clearly; using one-step commands when giving direction; being willing to repeat or rephrase; and trying to get the patient's attention in a calm environment (Burke and Laramie, 2000).

It is becoming more common in the care of the patient with AD to design a facilitative environment, a special care unit that supports the remaining functions of the afflicted. Burke and Laramie (2000) identify general principles for day-to-day caregiving: promote function and independence as the patient and situation allow; prevent disability as long as possible; and help, but do not do, as long as possible.

Box 21-19 Orientation Guidelines for Working with Confused Elderly

1. Add as many visual cues to the setting as you can. When patient's vision is impaired, heavy reliance on consistent auditory input is essential. Check patient's hearing aids and eyeglasses for effective function.
2. Make the environment as predictable as possible by using anticipatory planning, printed schedules, and a safe, routine schedule. When changes must be made, introduce them slowly and rehearse expected performance with the individual involved.
3. Insist on a thorough physical and neurologic examination of the patient to rule out organic bases of confusion. Remember that too many intrusive or diagnostic procedures in a short time will increase confusion.
4. Assess the stresses the patient has experienced recently and within the last 2 years.
5. Either a lack of stimulation or an overload of changes can result in confusion. If sensory deprivation or lack of stimulation is the problem, add color, texture, flavor, and noncompetitive activity to the daily schedule. If an overload of new expectations and adaptations has occurred, providing environmental stability, reduced expectations, rest, and continuity of supportive personnel is essential.
6. When confusion is extensive and organically based, reduce expectations to those that can be accomplished and give consistent, immediate praise for any degree of success. This must be done by all personnel, and long-term consistent efforts are essential.
7. No matter what degree of confusion is present, individuals remain sensitive to warm affect and caring gestures. Providing a relationship that conveys the value of each human regardless of functional capacity is of the utmost importance. Achieving the patient's recovery may not be realistic, but caring in the presence of deterioration and decline is high-level nursing.
8. Finally, when working with individuals whose ability to give accurate feedback and warm gratitude is impaired, the nurse may develop a solid personal, peer-support system. Those peers who understand the disappointments and struggles are in the best position to listen to each other. Sharing feelings, anger, exasperation, and humor allows the nurse to continue in a very difficult task.

Reality Orientation

Reality orientation is a term much used and abused. Approximately 30 years ago a specific program of reality orientation (called RO) was begun in Tuscaloosa, Alabama, to stimulate staff members' interest in and hope for the profoundly disoriented patients in their care. This program was useful because it provided caregivers with a specific program and structure that resulted in increased interaction with patients and some hopeful interventions. In the intervening years it has been found that some of the expectations were unrealistic, but the interest in communicating with the individual resident has been sustained. At present the thrust of programs is toward identifying with elements of the individual's past and helping the individual and the staff to appreciate the connections and the feelings. It remains important to retain the following concepts that evolved out of the RO programs:

1. A calm, caring atmosphere
2. Dependable routines and structured expectations
3. Clear communication in simple words; brief and consistent instructions
4. Consistent caregivers

5. An RO board containing information about date and place consistently maintained to give residents an opportunity to remain oriented to dates, times, and important events
6. Connecting present situations with past similar experiences to accentuate strengths and capitalize on the tendency for remote memories to be more intact than retention of recent events

Box 21-19 provides guidelines for working with the confused elderly.

Validation Therapy

Validation therapy was developed by Naomi Feil in the 1980s and involves following the patient's lead and responding to the issues of importance to the patient rather than interrupting to supply factual data. Even the most bizarre misinterpretations and actions carry a message if we will listen. This does not mean that we reinforce the client's action or misinformation; it means that we respond sensitively and reorient the client only when there is legitimate reason for doing so.

Martha, a resident with AD in a nursing home where I worked, used to call out loudly, "Mimi!" to the dismay of the other residents and the staff. We talked to her daughter, who told us that Mimi was Martha's great aunt, who had raised her as a child. The staff worked at finding out what "Mimi" meant to Martha but did not talk about the reality that Mimi was long gone. After time spent with Martha, letting her talk in "fits and starts" about Mimi, it became clear that "Mimi" was a call for love and protection, because she was in pain.

Reality orientation is not useful for those with advanced AD. It is best used for those in early-stage AD, when you want to have large clocks and calendars and the daily weather available. In late-stage AD, those things lose importance and meaningful things are those at the very base of our being—love, warmth, feeling, gentleness, and pain.

Joe was dying of invasive cancer that had metastasized to his brain. He was disoriented, inattentive, and unable to make reasonable judgments about most events that were transpiring; at least, that was the way it appeared to an observer. But was Joe able to meet his needs? The need to die, the need to say goodbye to those he would not see again, and the need to inform those "on the other side" that he was on his way were of overwhelming significance to him. He spoke to people who were not visible to anyone else, he accused a family member of interrupting a Cheyenne death ceremony, and he became irate when told that no one had been there. From his viewpoint, many people had been there. A sensitive nurse need only have said, "Tell me about the ceremony."

Healthy Aging in Dementia: Environmental Alterations

Beyond searching for a cure for AD, we need to develop new care models that emphasize the reduction of symptoms and help the person retain a "sense of self" (Eastman, 2001). Florence Nightingale's environmental therapy of fresh air, sunlight, clean and pleasant surroundings, and good nutrition is as effective today as it was in the nineteenth century. Reducing external triggers of agitation, confusion, and stress is a good starting point in environmental manipulation. Identify the triggers and plan how to lessen them. Provide opportunities for private time.

Support the elder with AD to be as autonomous and independent as possible. Bonnel (2000) describes the challenge of dressing a patient with dementia. Not only is dressing a complex task, but the elder with AD will not like having his or her personal space "invaded." Bonnel gives this advice:

- Approach the elder calmly, slowly, and in a pleasant manner (not the rush we so often see, which causes anxiety).
- Give simple directions.
- Find the balance between helping the elder and encouraging the elder to act for herself or himself (individualizing the care based on the patient's status).
- Do not be overly helpful—this may lead to patient apathy or agitation and aggression.
- Maintain a positive emotional environment by communicating calmly and in a friendly manner.
- Break tasks into components—for example, "Put this arm into the sleeve."
- Keep clothing and dressing simple—loose fit, simple fasteners, fresh clothes out and available, few choices, but choices; lay out clothes in the order that they would best be put on.
- Be flexible—if the client is upset and becoming irritable, come back later and try again.

John Zeisel (Eastman, 2001) describes some ideas for therapeutic environmental designs. Many are for long-term care unit consideration, but some can be created at home in the community.

- Meaningful common space—"the hearth is a hard-wired memory" (Eastman, 2001, p. 18). Elders with AD will relate well to a common space with a fireplace and comfortable chairs.
- Safe outdoor gardens—accessible, provide directional cues, walkways that are clear with places to stop and sit along the way.
- Supports for independence—low-tech supports such as rails in hallways, raised toilets with arms, the word "toilet" outside the door, see-through drawers.
- Sensory comprehension—quiet colors on walls with an occasional accent wall for interest. No glare or stripe patterns on the floors. Familiar odors, such as baking bread and fresh-washed laundry smells, are cues that help orient elders.
- Private spaces—to be alone at will. Having one's own room is the best start on this. Personalize it with beloved objects, photographs, and artwork.

Joseph Weiner, an architect, agrees that environments can provide a therapeutic setting for dementia patients (Eastman, 2001). He suggests getting rid of overhead paging systems, blue fluorescent lights, noxious smells, and clanging noises. This environment fosters overstimulation for the patient and a poor work environment and poor living environment.

For mildly confused people, clocks and calendars and an indoor sign naming the institution would allow people to orient themselves. How often have you seen anything visible in patients' rooms that indicates the name of the hospital they are in? In mental health units it is common to have rooms that appear "homelike" and staff members in street clothes. How could you find out where you were if you awoke in such a setting? Would you believe you were in a hotel (one of the most common misperceptions of place)? We must be more careful in assessing disorientation. Perhaps environmental cues are lacking. When RO is considered necessary, there are several ways it can be facilitated.

Dim lighting can be confusing and make vision difficult for those already impaired. There is new evidence that bright light improves the circadian rhythms of dementia patients in the long-term care setting (American Geriatric Society, 2002). Because fragmented sleep patterns and daytime sleeping are barriers to good geriatric care, this information may enhance care in this setting.

Memory Enhancement

Memory loss is one of the most common complaints of people over 50, and it is often blamed on aging (Mayo Clinic, 2001). The most frequent intervention is to simply tell the individual, "Don't worry, there is nothing wrong with you." This advice is rarely heeded, and the person continues to worry and silently remain concerned. A second approach is for the older adult to practice memory training and memory exercising.

Most people who forget things have many things on their mind—a kind of overload. Paul Takahashi, a geriatrician at Mayo Clinic and an expert on cognitive decline, developed a list of ways to keep the memory "nimble":

- Exercise your mind—challenge it and it will grow
  - Play a musical instrument
  - Do crosswords or puzzles
  - Switch careers
  - Develop a new hobby
  - Learn a foreign language
  - Read
- Stay active—it improves mood
  - Aerobic activity five times per week
  - Strength training two to three times per week
  - Stretching every day
- Eat and drink healthy
  - Fruits and vegetables—enriched diet (antioxidants)
  - Drink eight glasses of water per day—fill a water bottle and keep it with you
  - Skip the soft drinks and coffee at lunch; drink water instead
- Develop a system of reminders/clues
  - Write it down
  - Develop a routine for everything—store things in the same place every time
  - Set up clues—put your car keys on the stove, so you remember to check and see if it is turned off before you leave
  - Repetition—when meeting someone new, say the person's name several times in conversation after being introduced
- Take time to remember
  - We are less efficient in processing new information
  - Experience compensates for this loss
  - Slow down and pay full attention to the task at hand—be attentive

In a nutshell, "use it or lose it" certainly applies to elders and their memory performance.

Support Groups

Most of the intervention strategies suggested can be applied in small groups of three or four individuals. These are particularly useful with those who have mild to moderate dementia. Group techniques and guidelines can be found in Chapters 18 and 23. However, expectations must be geared very thoughtfully to the capacities of the group to avoid agitation and catastrophic reactions.

Caring for the Developmentally Disabled with Mental Retardation

Developmental disabilities are pathologic conditions that start developing before age 18, and most persist throughout life, though some can be effectively treated. Those individuals with developmental disabilities that have produced cognitive deficits have special needs. Caring for those who have been mentally impaired throughout their lives is somewhat different than caring for the elderly person who has developed dementia late in life. Although the individual with AD may not remember what happened yesterday, he or she has a lifetime of experiences and skills that may remain to some degree until the later stages of the disease.

The aged who have developmental disabilities have often spent the majority of their lives in institutions and may have had very limited exposure to the community outside. Moving out of a state institution into a group home and involvement in sheltered workshops are comparatively recent phenomena. Roberts and Davis (1988) provide one of the few studies that report the particulars of success in reintegrating these individuals into community life and activities. They are first assigned an escort, or buddy, to accompany them into each new activity but are soon able to launch into some activities unescorted. They attend senior meals and senior programs in which they are involved in music, art, and other activities that stimulate interest and self-expression. Most important, they have the opportunity to make friends with other seniors.

These community-oriented programs provide a model for other states, and training materials have been developed. We believe this model deserves replication. More attention must be given to delineating the characteristics of this population.

Those experienced in working with them believe the following:

- The profoundly retarded rarely survive to old age because they often have multiple physical incapacities. In general, retarded persons experience greater deficits in vision, hearing, and strength than other aged persons. Accurately assessing and enhancing their sensory capacities as necessary is extremely important.
- The educable (mildly) retarded may not have had the advantage of any education in youth, and their potential has been undeveloped. Most grew up in a time and place in which programs for the developmentally disabled were unavailable. Many were given no formal schooling, remaining sheltered by the family or spending a lifetime inappropriately institutionalized.

The mentally retarded in nursing homes are usually physically and mentally impaired and physically and socially dependent and have an excess of empty time. They readily adapt to the nursing home environment, possibly because their expectations are lower than those of other aged persons and because they were institutionalized before aging. Nurses may effectively use Maslow's hierarchy as a guide to needs assessment. Those patients who are congenitally cerebrally impaired may have limited hopes and expectations, but their human needs remain: comfort, protection, security, acceptance, pride, and self-expression.

Creative nurses will seek to enhance sensual pleasures; promote personal ties; and provide an orderly, predictable environment. One might think of retardation as a condition in which an individual is sensorially ill equipped for the place and time in which he or she lives. For example, imagine a medieval peasant set in the middle of New York City or one transported through time and space to a place where the mode of communication is through thought transference, and intellect depends on tuning in to electromagnetic waves through antennas we do not possess. One might expect fear, anxiety, and attempts to conform to or mimic what others are doing. Anger and mood swings could be expected to accompany such feelings of vulnerability.

Working with the developmentally disabled is somewhat more difficult than working with those who have had social skills and lost them. Retarded older women may wish to play with dolls. Both older men and women may never have developed a sense of modesty. They should be trained to interact in an appropriate manner to promote interpersonal acceptance. Rather than behavioral modification programs depending on tangible rewards, we favor those that provide immediate rewards of warmth and praise for each small success. Both methods are useful.

Some innovative programs have been found that are designed for the retarded elder. One psychologist shared her experience working with retarded adults in a program designed to tap nondominant (nonintellectual) cerebral activity (Murphy, 1979). Arts, music, and movement conducted in an atmosphere of acceptance and noncompetitiveness aroused feelings of pleasure and self-esteem in the program participants.

Another aspect of aging and retardation is encountered frequently. We have known several cases in which an elderly parent has become disabled and unable to continue the care of a retarded adult child. In those cases, the retarded adult has been placed in a long-term care institution, and the aged parent is worried and grief stricken over the inability to continue sheltering and protecting the adult child. Retarded adults living with the frail elderly, in institutions and at home, often assume a helping role if they have such skills. Some are abusive of the aged parent. The Friends of Philadelphia are particularly concerned about assisting the aged parents to deal with developmentally disabled adult children and have developed a booklet of helpful guidelines (Schwartz and Kelly, 1996).

Families of Patients with Dementia

There are special problems with caring for severely demented individuals because they are psychologically absent and physically present. Ambiguity and ambivalence exist in all aspects of care. Some caregivers with the capacity for retrospective reverie can sustain themselves with memories of the individual; others who do not stray into the past but focus entirely on the present often find the burden intolerable.

The recent film *Iris* starred Judi Dench as Iris Murdoch, the brilliant scholar and libertine from Oxford University. Iris had an amazing career and life as a philosopher and novelist to her final days living, and suffering, with Alzheimer's disease. It is an amazing love story of a man who, despite the challenges, frustrations, and pain of caring for Iris, loved her to the end.

Roger Rosenblatt (1998, p. 98) wrote an essay in *Time* about the inner turmoil of living with his 90-year-old mother in her Alzheimer's world for over 14 years. He writes, "In a way, the disease demonstrates the essential incomprehensibility of the human mind by reducing it to pure puzzle. It represents all that is impenetrable about who people are and what they think." He quotes Alexander Pope: "This long disease, my life." Rosenblatt agrees: "That's Alzheimer's, especially in my mother's case." He muses further, "I wonder if my mother is losing all her words one by one, until she eventually will be down to her last word, the only word left her in the world. What word would that be?"

We can feel the pain of caring for a loved one who has AD. The help is derived from encouraging the caregiver to recite incidents from the better times. Seventy years of living leave a legacy of love. What do we say to the tree when ravaged by parasitic mistletoe? You are the bearer of a gift of love. Can we know that the gift the demented elder gives is the endurance of the aberration that terrorizes? Must we be held hostage by this dread threat of old age? Can we remember that life is more than momentary cerebral synapses? It is the total piece that has been woven, and if at the end there are ragged edges, are they fault or fringe? We know full well the strain that loved ones endure when the beloved is out of touch with reality and incapable of behaving in socially acceptable ways. Yet, when in the depths of despair, can we be reminded of the better times?

Caregivers and Coping. Families report that the greatest source of stress is watching the deterioration and being unable to help. The process of caregiving has been studied by numerous individuals. These studies are discussed in Chapter 18, but some reports are particularly relevant to this section.

Belgrave and colleagues (1993) determined that black caregivers have significantly lower levels of knowledge about caregiving than a comparable group of white caregivers. The distress experienced by caregivers includes their perception of burden and is evidenced by depression, anxiety, hostility, and other similar manifestations. Most patients with AD are cared for at home, and this care is particularly demanding. The caregiver must provide more hours of care and suffer more adverse consequences than caregivers of those with chronic illness without dementia (National Academy on an Aging Society, 2000). The coping strategies used by caregivers of Alzheimer's patients have a strong influence on the mental health of the caregiver and the patient.

Too much stress is damaging for the caregiver as well as for the person in care. Learning the signs of caregiver stress is an important intervention for nurses to communicate to caregivers (Figure 21-4). Caregivers will recognize these phrases associated with the signs (Alzheimer's Association, 1999):

- Denial—about the disease and its effect on the person with it: "I know Dad will get better."
- Anger—at the person with AD and with others, that there is no cure, that others do not understand how this affects your life: "If he asks that same question one more time, I'll scream."
- Social withdrawal—no time for friends or social pleasures: "I don't care about being with the neighbors any more."
- Anxiety—about facing one more day and what the future holds: "What happens when he needs more care than I am able to give?"
- Depression—this affects the relationship with the person with dementia and the caregiver's ability to cope: "I don't care anymore."
- Exhaustion—it interferes with completing *necessary* tasks: "I am too tired to do this."
- Sleeplessness—a never-ending list of concerns: "What if he wanders out of the house and falls and hurts himself?"
- Lack of concentration—the caregiver begins losing ability to perform familiar tasks: "I was so busy that I forgot we had an appointment."

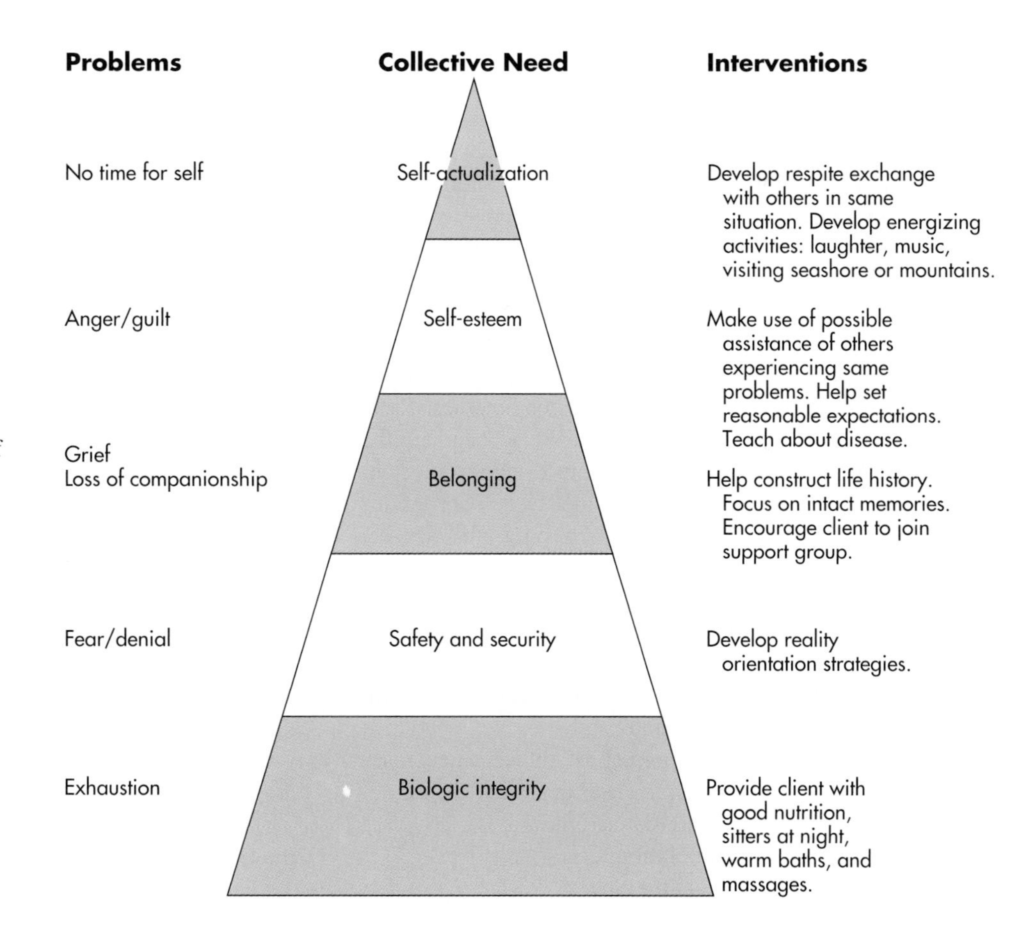

Figure 21-4. Hierarchy of needs of families caring for family members with SDAT.

- Personal health—mentally and physically declines: "I can't remember the last time I felt well."

If the spouse or caregiver is experiencing some of these signs, it may be time for respite care, day care, nursing home placement, or other supportive intervention to help. One study (Lieberman and Fisher, 2001) examined the effects of nursing home placement versus maintaining community placement for patients with AD on changes in family caregiver health and well-being over time (2 years). The family caregiver health and well-being did not improve over time following placement or maintaining the elder at home. Female caregivers and spouses had greater declines in health and well-being compared with other family caregivers regardless of home or long-term care placement.

When families must finally be separated by institutionalization, the maintenance of some mutually shared activities can ease the pain and guilt. Group and recreational activities in which family members and elders participate are useful. Open communication with and accurate information for the family and the elder cultivate an atmosphere of trust. Spouses in particular need special consideration when separated by dementia.

With understanding staff, shame is diminished in the community-residing spouse, and acceptance will gradually emerge. In the ideal nursing home setting the feelings, attitudes, communication, and actions of the staff are the cornerstones of the milieu that tap the wellspring of dignity in each individual, no matter how impaired.

Day Care. The use of adult day care to care for the disabled demented elderly is increasing. Day care provides a safe and supportive environment that can give family members respite while providing a positive emotional atmosphere for the elder. Guiding principles for activities are prevention of harm to the elder (and other patients) and maintaining competence in areas in which the individual is most capable in a pleasant, positive environment. These units require heavy staffing (usually a ratio of 1 : 3) and may not prevent the cognitive decline of the patient, but they do enhance quality of life and reduce psychosocial dysfunction. Restlessness, anxiety, and agitation that often occur in the demented patient are kept to a minimum by the calm, nonthreatening, positive environment provided by these programs and centers. The main goals for such programs are the following:

1. To provide respite and support of caretakers
2. To provide socialization and stimulation appropriate for the demented patient
3. To help family members keep the individual in the community as long as is appropriate
4. To assist family with placement of patient when necessary

Day care units include such features as the following:

- Therapeutic and recreational activities
- Mental and social stimulation
- Exercise and movement therapy
- Music therapy and entertainment
- Nursing and social work consultation
- Caregivers' support group
- Nutritious hot meal
- Transportation

Respite care, foster care, and assisted living settings are other methods that families may use to relieve the pressures of caregiving. These are discussed elsewhere in the book.

LEGAL ISSUES IN GERIATRIC PSYCHIATRY

In 1986 the American Psychiatric Association Task Force on Forensic Issues in Geriatric Psychiatry was organized to develop a guide for the evaluation of the older patient and to review the legal issues that psychiatrists would encounter in their work with geriatric patients. Nurses must be cognizant of these issues to ensure legal protection of self and patient.

Establishing Competence

The evaluation of a patient's cognitive capacity and judgment is at the core of most legal dilemmas that health care personnel face, whether an issue of consent, commitment, or civil or criminal law. *Competency* is a legal term and has precise meaning (Goldstein, 2002). A patient is competent unless the courts have declared him or her incompetent and the patient is not able to understand the consequences of his or her actions (Springhouse, 2002). Legal competence is based on a physician's or other health professional's assessment. When an elder becomes confused alternating with clarity, this should be documented by the health professional at the time of assessment and how a decision about competency was made. Competency is also task specific—the patient must be competent to handle finances and make medical decisions. He or she may be declared competent for one, but not the other. Competency is having the mental capacity for the task at hand (Goldstein, 2002).

It is important that the client not be sedated at the time of evaluation; he or she must be alert. Further, it is important to clarify where the question of competence originated. The family may have ulterior motives, the physician may be distressed by noncompliant behaviors, the health care system may be responding to difficulties in patient management, and the patient may be concerned about proving legal competence. All of these sources have different reasons for wishing competence to be evaluated.

Many schemes and protocols have been proposed to judge competence, but at best there may be ambiguity about the patient's cognitive capacity and judgment. Most important, the patient must be informed that when cognitive capacity is being evaluated for legal purposes, there is no confidentiality.

Data gathering to establish competency will ideally include the following:

1. Thorough neuropsychiatric evaluation
2. Physical functioning

3. Mental status examination
4. Depression assessment
5. Anxiety state assessment

Cautions are needed related to source and accuracy of data. As mentioned earlier, the source of the data; the accuracy of the informant; the observational skills of the appraiser; and the time, place, and pacing of the interview are of critical importance. The presence of depression or anxiety states has a significant influence on the quality of patient response. Criminal issues of the elderly most often involve drunken driving, shoplifting, exhibitionism, and occasionally homicide. In all these situations, competency may be called into question. Additional discussion of competence, guardianship, powers of attorney, and the legal ramifications can be found elsewhere in this book.

End-of-Life Decisions and Physician-Assisted Suicide

At present there is a move, with much controversy, to legally support assisted suicide. This has been condoned in some cases for devastating and painful illnesses when an individual felt unable to endure life any longer. Media reports have kept the public aware of the controversy over assisted suicide for individuals who are incapable of deriving sufficient meaning from continued existence. Ethical opinion is divided (Goldstein, 2002). Most physicians today do not have sufficient knowledge about their patients to make such a profound decision. Euthanasia is even more controversial than assisted suicide; in euthanasia the physician goes beyond providing the patient with the means for suicide, and actually performs some act that causes death.

Attention to advance directives and quality of life is a concern for families of individuals with progressive and unremitting dementia. Usually, it has been assumed that decisions for persons suffering from dementia would be made by a court-appointed conservator or family member, but this has not included any decisions regarding assisted dying. However, at least one study has demonstrated that some individuals with dementia can decide appropriately regarding treatments they wish at the end of their lives. Thirty percent of demented residents at the Frances Schervier Home in the Bronx, New York, were consistent in their decisions about naming a proxy, and 27% were consistent in decisions regarding resuscitation. We expect this may at some time extend to decisions regarding assisted suicide. Further discussion of these issues may be found in Chapter 24.

The numerous ethical and humane issues involved in planning and caring for the mentally impaired individual are not nearly fully addressed in view of individual and societal needs. We can expect ongoing discussion and concern about these devastating situations and hope for some real solutions. The nursing role will always be to support and assist families of these victims and provide all possible means toward comfort and momentary pleasures for the victims.

Human Needs and Wellness Diagnoses

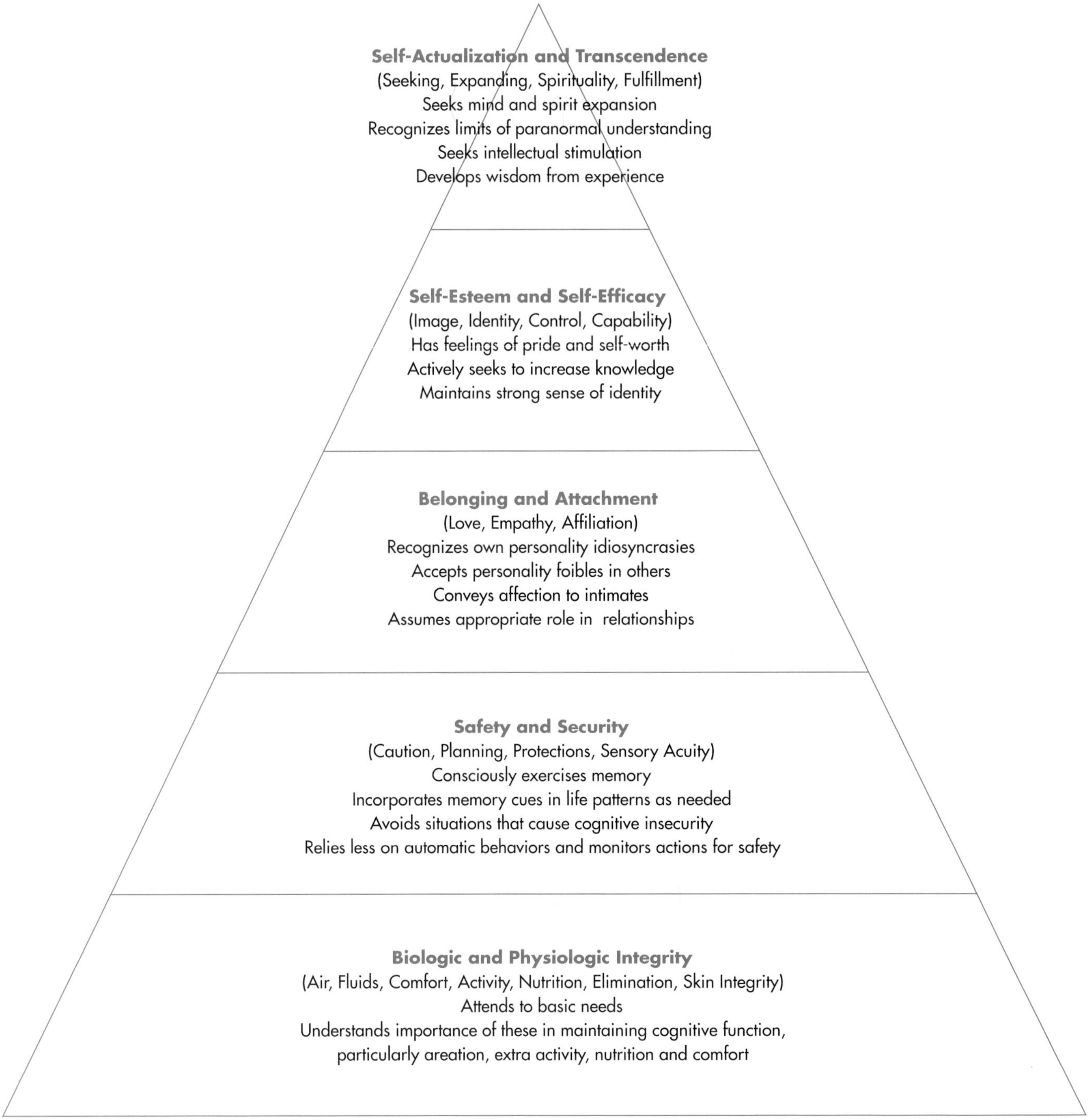

Self-Actualization and Transcendence
(Seeking, Expanding, Spirituality, Fulfillment)
Seeks mind and spirit expansion
Recognizes limits of paranormal understanding
Seeks intellectual stimulation
Develops wisdom from experience

Self-Esteem and Self-Efficacy
(Image, Identity, Control, Capability)
Has feelings of pride and self-worth
Actively seeks to increase knowledge
Maintains strong sense of identity

Belonging and Attachment
(Love, Empathy, Affiliation)
Recognizes own personality idiosyncrasies
Accepts personality foibles in others
Conveys affection to intimates
Assumes appropriate role in relationships

Safety and Security
(Caution, Planning, Protections, Sensory Acuity)
Consciously exercises memory
Incorporates memory cues in life patterns as needed
Avoids situations that cause cognitive insecurity
Relies less on automatic behaviors and monitors actions for safety

Biologic and Physiologic Integrity
(Air, Fluids, Comfort, Activity, Nutrition, Elimination, Skin Integrity)
Attends to basic needs
Understands importance of these in maintaining cognitive function,
particularly areation, extra activity, nutrition and comfort

These are not all the possible wellness diagnoses that may be identified. The above are examples of nursing diagnoses that should be considered when planning care for the older adult.

KEY CONCEPTS

- Cognitive function has been the most studied topic in age-related research.
- It has long been assumed that cognitive decline is a necessary concomitant of aging, but recent studies demonstrate the potential of the aging brain for regeneration.
- The distinctive cognitive capacities of the aged have hardly been investigated and are poorly understood.
- Age-associated memory impairment (AAMI) refers to the common forgetfulness that many elders experience. This is usually attributed to distraction, preoccupation, or performance anxiety. It is poorly understood but must be met with reassurance that this is not an evidence of impending dementia.
- Cognitive impairment that is significant is a disease process and must be regarded as such. Some of the dementias are treatable, and some are not. Nurses need to advocate for thorough assessment of any elder who appears to be experiencing genuine cognitive decline and inability to function in important aspects of life.
- Delirium, sometimes referred to as acute confusional states, is the result of physiologic imbalances and may be caused by a variety of biologic disturbances. Delirium is characterized by fluctuating levels of consciousness, sometimes in a diurnal pattern, and frequent misperceptions and illusions.
- Medications are frequently the cause of delirious states in the aged.
- Irreversible dementias follow a pattern of inevitable decline accompanied by decreased intellectual function, personality changes, and impaired judgment. The most common of these is Alzheimer's disease.
- Alzheimer's disease has been the subject of enormous amounts of research in attempts to understand the causes. Genes, latent viruses, enzyme and neurotransmitter deficiencies, environmental toxins, and psychosocial stressors have all been implicated to some degree. Research is continuing in attempts to discover ways to protect against or halt the progress of the disease. At this time there is no known cure, though some medications being developed seem to slow the progress of the dementia for a time.
- HIV-related dementia is often overlooked in the aged; there is an ageist assumption implicit in this neglect.
- Vascular brain disorders (brain attacks) are caused by interruption of the blood supply to the brain because of clots, hemorrhages, and vascular spasm or occlusion. Many of these situations can be remedied and serious brain damage prevented if treatment is immediate.
- Developmentally disabled elders are a rather new phenomenon because these individuals usually died long before they reached old age. Those who have survived have special needs related to the levels of development they may or may not have achieved. These individuals should not be treated as if demented but given opportunities carefully matched to the level of their abilities.
- Assessment of cognitive impairment is complex. Nurses may do a cursory assessment with any number of brief mental status examinations and need to request more thorough assessment when there is an indication of dementia.
- Individuals who are mentally impaired respond best to calmness, few demands, clear communication, and predictable routines. They are hypersensitive to chaotic situations and may develop catastrophic reactions when demands exceed their ability.

▲ CASE STUDY

William was 69 years old and had been a successful builder until his retirement from business 4 years ago. His wife, Caroline, of 30 years was a high school teacher. Their marriage had been minimally gratifying, but both enjoyed their work and had felt they led a full and satisfying life. They had no children but had developed a large social network over the years; most were friends who were in some way work related. Six months ago William began to seem restless; he was easily angered and embarrassed himself and his wife several times by being verbally abusive during a social function with their friends. William was also less careful about his grooming; because he had always been most meticulous about his appearance, his wife was quite alarmed that he seemed not to notice or care. After returning from one particularly exhausting vacation trip, William became enraged when he thought someone had stolen his wallet. He ignored his wife's efforts to calm him and became even angrier. Later his wife found his wallet in an inner suit jacket pocket. He ordinarily kept his wallet in the back pocket of his trousers. His wife began to feel anxious and frightened of him, though he had never physically abused her. She urged him to see the doctor for a "general checkup" but was not surprised that he refused. She went to the doctor for tranquilizers to quell her anxiety. He gave her a prescription for Prozac and sent her on her way. Her nurse-neighbor dropped by one day and found her in tears saying, "I just can't stand it anymore. William is not like himself. We used to have such fun and now he is angry all the time." As the nurse-neighbor, how would you help Caroline and William?

Based on the case study, develop a nursing care plan using the following procedure:*

List comments of client that provide subjective data.

List information that provides objective data.

From these data identify and state, using accepted format, two nursing diagnoses you determine are most significant to this client at this time.

---

*Students are advised to refer to their nursing diagnosis text and identify possible or potential problems.

Determine and state outcome criteria for each diagnosis. These must reflect some alleviation of the problem identified in the nursing diagnosis and must be stated in concrete and measurable terms.

Plan and state one or more interventions for each diagnosed problem. Provide specific documentation of source used to determine appropriate intervention.

Evaluate success of intervention. Interventions must correlate directly with the stated outcome criteria in order to measure the outcome success.

STUDY QUESTIONS/ACTIVITIES

Discuss ways in which you might help an individual who is complaining of memory loss.

Is there any evidence that cerebral cells may regenerate?

What are some of the differences between delirium and dementia?

Discuss some reasons you might suspect an elder with dementia to have HIV dementia.

Identify several signs of early dementia.

How can Alzheimer's disease be diagnosed accurately?

Develop a nursing care plan for dealing with an individual with agitated dementia.

How could you communicate best with an individual who is perseverating?

What is the essense of validation therapy?

What memory aids might you suggest for a person who is forgetful?

What is the most difficult thing for a family dealing with a demented elder? Why do you think this is so?

Discuss elders you have known who are between 85 and 90 years old and evidences of their intact cognition or signs of dementia.

RESEARCH QUESTIONS

What is the prevalence of dementia in community-dwelling older adults?

What methods of memory enhancement are most effective in the long term?

REFERENCES

Agency for Healthcare Research and Quality: Two-thirds of elderly stroke survivors in nursing homes are not receiving medications to prevent further strokes, *Research Activities* number 253, Sept 2001.

Aldridge S: Homocysteine raises Alzheimer's disease risk. Available at *www.healthandage.com* (accessed Feb 14, 2002).

Alzheimer's Association: *Women and Alzheimer's disease: a major issue for the next millenium* (pamphlet), Chicago, 1999, Alzheimer's Association.

Alzheimer's Organization: Questions and answers on launch of NIA memory impairment study, 2002. Available at *www.alzheimers.org/nianews/nianews19.html*

American Geriatric Society, 2002. Available at *www.americangeriatrics.org/news/dementia*

American Psychiatric Association: *Diagnostic and statistical manual of mental disorders,* ed 4, Washington, DC, 1994, The Association.

American Psychiatric Association: *Diagnostic and statistical manual of mental disorders,* DSM-IV-TR, Washington, DC, 2000, The Association.

Anderson M: Communication process. In Luggen AS, Meiner S, editors: *NGNA core curriculum for gerontological nurses,* ed 2, St Louis, 2001, Mosby.

Arie THD: Acute confusional states. In Abrams WB, Beers MH, Berkow R, editors: *Merck manual of geriatrics,* ed 2, Whitehouse Station, NJ, 1995, Merck Research Laboratories.

Bagley M: Hearing changes in aging people with mental retardation, 2002. Available at *www.thearc.org/faqs/hearinginaging*

Batchelor N: Normal aging changes. In Luggen AS, Meiner S, editors: *NGNA core curriculum for gerontological nurses,* ed 2, St Louis, 2001, Mosby.

Beers MH, Berkow R: *Merck manual of geriatrics,* ed 3, Whitehouse Station, NJ, 2000, Merck Research Laboratories.

Belgrave L, Wykle M, Choi J: Health, double jeopardy and culture: the use of institutionalization by African-Americans, *Gerontologist* 33(3):379, 1993.

Berry W: *Memory of Old Jack,* New York, 1974, Harcourt Brace.

Bonnel W: Dementia patients and challenges with dressing, *NCGNP Newsletter* number 68, p 4, summer 2000.

Boss B: Alterations of neurological function. In McCance K, Huether S, editors: *Pathophysiology: the biologic basis for disease in adults and children,* ed 4, St Louis, 2002, Mosby.

Breteler M: Moderate alcohol consumption may reduce risk of dementia, *Lancet* 359(9303):281, 2002.

Brown A: Aging with developmental disability, *Women's Health Issues,* 2002. Available at *www.thearc.org/faqs/whealth*

Bunton D: Normal changes with aging. In Maas ML et al, editors: *Nursing care of older adults: diagnoses, outcomes, and interventions,* St Louis, 2001, Mosby.

Burke MM, Laramie JA: *Primary care of the older adult: a multidisciplinary approach,* St Louis, 2000, Mosby.

Christensen D: Hardening of the arteries linked to Alzheimer's disease, *Medical Tribune News Service,* Jan 16, 1997.

Cotter VT: Dementia. In Cotter VT, Strumpf N, editors: *Advanced practice nursing with older adults,* Philadelphia, 2002, McGraw-Hill.

Crowley SL: Aging brain's staying power, *AARP Bulletin* 37(4):1, 1996.

Cummings JL: Managing psychosis in patients with Parkinsons' disease [editorial], *N Engl J Med* 340(10), 2000.

Eastman P: Environmental therapy aids Alzheimer's patients, *Caring for the Ages* 2(9):1, 18, 2001.

Erikson E: *Life history and the historical moment,* New York, 1975, WW Norton.

Flax M: Aging with developmental disabilities: changes in vision, 2002. Available at *www.thearc.org/faqs/visfact.*

Folstein MF, Folstein S, McHugh PR: *Mini-mental state: a practical method for grading the cognitive status of patients for the clinician,* 1975, Pergamon.

Gallo JJ, Fulmer T, Paveza G: *Handbook of geriatric assessment,* ed 3, Boston, 2003, Jones & Bartlett.

Gerdner LA, Hall GR: Chronic confusion. In Maas ML et al, editors: *Nursing care of older adults: diagnoses, outcomes, and interventions,* St Louis, 2001, Mosby.

Goldstein MK: Ethics. In Ham RJ, Sloane PD, Warshaw GA, editors: *Primary care geriatrics,* St Louis, 2002, Mosby.

Ham RJ: Dementias [and Delirium]. In Ham RJ, Sloane PD, Warshaw GA, editors: *Primary care geriatrics,* St Louis, 2002, Mosby.

Haney DQ: Study: faster ER care treats strokes better, *Associated Press,* Sunday, Feb 10, 2002.

Holzer C, Warshaw G: Clues to early Alzheimer dementia in the outpatient setting, *Arch Fam Med* 9(10):1066, 2000.

Johnson BP: The elderly. In Frisch NC, Frisch LE, editors: *Psychiatric mental health nursing,* ed 2, Clifton Park, NY, 2002, Delmar.

Kovach CR, Wilson SA: Parkinsons' disease. In Stanley M, Beare P, editors: *Gerontological nursing,* ed 2, Philadelphia, 1999, FA Davis.

Lieberman MA, Fisher L: The effects of nursing home placement on family caregivers of patients with Alzheimer's disease, *Gerontologist* 41:819, 2001.

Maki P, Resnick S: ERT stimulates blood flow to key memory center in the brain, *Neurobiol Aging* 21(2):373, 2000.

Mayo Clinic: Keeping health in mind: 10 tips to keep your memory sharp, 2001. Available at *www.mayoclinic.com/findinformation/healthylivingcenter/invoke.cfm?objectid=8D8*

Medical Research Council: Cognitive function and ageing study, *Lancet* 357:169, 2001.

Moore AP, Clarke C: PD, *BMJ Clinical Evidence,* issue 6, Dec 2001.

Murphy M: Personal communication, 1979. Living Arts Center, Oakland, CA.

Nash JM: The new science of Alzheimer's, *Time* 56(3):51-57, 2000.

National Academy on an Aging Society: *Alzheimer's Disease and Dementia: A Growing Challenge* (newsletter), number 11, p 1, 2000.

National Institute on Aging: *Questions and answers on launch of NIA.* Available at *www.alzheimers.org/nianews/nianews19.html*

National Institute on Aging: Alzheimer's disease anti-inflammatory prevention trial (ADAPT) launched. Jan 30, 2001. Available at *www.alzheimers.org/nianews/nianews37.html*

National Institute on Aging: Folic acid deficiency may increase susceptibility to Parkinson's disease. Jan 14, 2002. Available at *www.alzheimers.org/nianews/nianews42.html*

National Institute for Neurological Disorders and Stroke: *Transient ischemic attack.* Information page, 2002. Available at *www.ninds.nih.gov/health_and_medical/disorders/tia_doc.htm*

National Institutes of Health: Memory loss, 2002. Available at *www.nlm.nih.gov/medlineplus/ency/article/003257.htm*

Novartis: *Emerging therapies in Alzheimer's disease,* East Hanover, NJ, 2000, Novartis Pharmaceutical Corporation.

O'Neill PA: *Caring for the older adult,* Philadelphia, 2002, WB Saunders.

Roach S: *Introductory gerontological nursing,* Philadelphia, 2001, JB Lippincott.

Roberts R, Davis G: Expanding options for seniors with mental retardation, *Aging* 357:17, 1988.

Rosenblatt R: This long disease. Essay, *Time,* Jan 12, 1998, p 98.

Schwartz D, Kelly C: *A guide for hospital staff working with adult patients with developmental disabilities,* Gwynedd, PA, 1996, Elders with Adult Dependents.

Simmons SF, Osterweil D, Schnelle JF: Improving food intake in nursing home residents with feeding assistance, *J Gerontol Series A Biol Sci Med Sci* 56:M790, 2001.

Springhouse: *Better elder care,* Springhouse, PA, 2002, Springhouse.

Stanley M: Acute confusion. In Stanley M, Beare P, editors: *Gerontological nursing,* ed 2, Philadelphia, 1999, FA Davis.

Sugarman RA: Structure and function of the neurologic system. In McCance KL, Huether SE, editors: *Pathophysiology: the biologic basis for disease in adults and children,* ed 4, St Louis, 2002, Mosby.

Ten commandments for caregivers, *Caregiver,* spring 2001, p 8.

Unverzagt F, Hendrie H: Cognitive impairment high among older people. *NIA News,* Alzheimer's disease research update, Nov 12, 2001. Available at *www.alzheimers.org/nianews/nianews41.html*

Valle G: Behavioral issues in elderly patients with dementia: a geriatrician's perspective. Presentation to Greater Cincinnati Gerontological Nursing Association, Cincinnati, Mar 2001.

Veld BA: Long term NSAID use tied to decreased risk of AD, *N Engl J Med* 345:1515, 2001.

Warner J, Butler R: *Alzheimer's disease. Clinical evidence number 6,* London, 2001, BMJ Publishers.

Wolanin M: Mental frailty, *Geriatr Nurs* 18(2), 1997.

Wolanin MO, Phillips LR: *Confusion: prevention and care,* St Louis, 1981, Mosby.

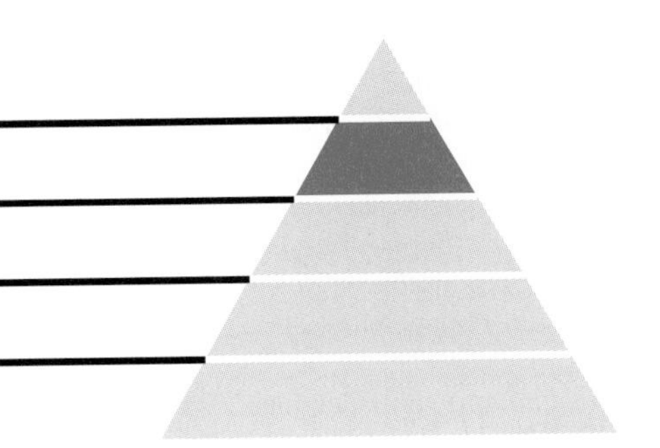

CHAPTER 22

Stress, Crises, and Health in Aging

Priscilla Ebersole

A student learns

My grandmother told me that every day should be an adventure. It isn't enough I have to worry about school, gang fights, gaining weight and everything else. Now I have to worry about something happening to her! She travels all the time.

Ashley, age 15

An elder speaks

You know, I'm 83 years old! I've seen so many changes in my lifetime but the world seems such a dangerous place now. I worry so about my grandchildren and the things they must deal with in the future.

Sarah, age 83

LEARNING OBJECTIVES

On completion of this chapter, the reader will be able to:

1. Identify several aspects of stress.
2. Relate several stressors that are likely to occur in late life.
3. Recognize physiologic responses to stress.
4. Discuss common reactions to crises.
5. Describe posttraumatic stress disorder and other devastating crises.
6. Discuss coping styles and methods of resolving stress and crises.
7. Enumerate several stress-related illnesses.
8. Explain the healthful aspects of resolving stress and crisis.
9. Describe several methods of restoring a sense of control.

STRESS

Stress is a given in any complex society. Stress is any event or situation that brings about bodily or mental tension. Without stress there would likely be little motivation in living other than filling most basic needs. Perhaps many of the stressors we subject ourselves to are unnecessary, but these are highly individual matters. Some people thrive on high levels of stress; others are depleted by it. In this chapter we try to understand the ability of individuals to cope with stress and crises and the mechanisms that translate these into illness or healthy adaptations. Our focus is on stress and crises and the events, likely to occur in the process of growing old, that may create disruptions in daily life that drain one's inner resources or require the development of new and unfamiliar coping strategies. We are now, as a society, experiencing nonspecific stressors that are unpredictable, are uncontrollable, and produce a constant level of anxiety and insecurity that is ever present, although it is more intense for some individuals than others (depending to a large extent on their earlier life experiences). We have not yet measured the emotional "fallout" from the terrorist attacks of September 11, 2001, and their aftermath. Becoming alert to evidences of decompensation and helping individuals regain equilibrium on a healthier level are the goals of this chapter.

Acute Stress

Acute stress is seldom productive in that it is an internal state perceived as a threat to self. A stress response exists whenever there is a discrepancy between what the individual expects and that which requires change or recognition of uncertainty (Eriksen et al, 1999). Healthy stress levels motivate one toward growth, whereas a stress overload diminishes one's ability to cope effectively. Stress may arise from external events and situations or inner dictates. Most people recognize visible manifestations of acute stress such as increased body movement or excessive talking, irritability, sweaty or clammy hands, insomnia, and accelerated heart rate.

Proximal Stressors

Proximal stressors are those that are in the present and that require prompt action and inner resources to avert crises. Proximal stressors are often acutely uncomfortable, are pronounced, and require immediate adaptive energy on an ongoing, daily basis for a brief time. The effects of these are mitigated by personality, available resources, environmental situation, contextual issues, and presence of chronic stressors. The number and frequency of stressors experienced in a given period of time must be considered (Box 22-1).

Distal Stressors

Distal stressors have "gone underground," and the individual may be unaware of their presence. They are more often chronic and sometimes imbedded in personality. These are likely to be attenuated as current demands fluctuate as some taxing situations are resolved.

Box 22-1 Stressors of the Aged

- Incompetency proceedings
- Inheritance conflicts
- Abandonment: fear of dying alone/not being found/painful death
- Hospitalization
- Institutionalization
- Separation from personal physician
- Sensory changes (vision and hearing)
- Housing and home maintenance
- Lack of protection when frail and vulnerable
- Limited mobility and lack of transportation
- Unnamed concerns about the future
- Fears of senility
- Social losses, loss of driver's license
- Acute and chronic pain
- Medications
- Abuse and neglect
- Loss of pet
- Rent increases
- Caregiving of a demented spouse
- Illness
- Relocation
- Loss of children
- Loss of cohorts
- Loss of siblings
- Loss of friends
- Dispersal of significant belonging

Chronic Stressors

Chronic stressors tend to be those categorized as constant or remote events and are contextual, such as a nongratifying marriage, childhood scars, or inability to carry out desired activities. For elders, contextual issues often involve a living situation that produces constant discomfort and dismay, functional disabilities, enduring chronic illnesses and pain, abusive caregivers, generally poor health, and internalized ageism. Inability to manage activities of daily living (ADLs) is a major and ongoing stress factor for older persons. Anxiety responses and chronic disorders may erupt during an increase in events that are stressful or worrisome.

Chronic stress is likely to activate depression, and this creates physiologic changes that can result in illness and further exacerbate stress. This cyclic process may be the source of numerous illnesses. Perhaps some of the aging process itself is a result of a lifetime of numerous stresses and adaptive demands; essentially, the body runs out of energy.

Hassles. Hassles are the small daily events, everyday stressors that are seldom given much thought. Hassles are generally minor harassments. These include everyday irritants in daily life involving home maintenance, transportation, balancing checkbooks, finances, waiting in lines for goods or services, or waiting on hold during phone calls. An overload of daily hassles may adversely affect well-being and health status even more than major life disruptions. Home maintenance and environmental and social hassles are particularly onerous for old people who have depleted energies.

In combination with major stressful life events, hassles create psychologic, and sometimes physiologic, problems. Gerontologists seriously consider the impact of hassles on stress levels, coping energy, and style of coping.

It may be useful to keep a diary of daily events because many individuals are unaware of small hassles; the diary may help to identify irritating problems and patterns that are readily subject to solution. Stetson (1997) uses diaries to assist individuals to identify self-healing activities in which they select one hassle they wish to modify and then develop a concrete plan to accomplish that with weekly, measurable goals.

Worry. A common perception about elderly people is that they worry excessively about the stresses associated with the aging process, such as declining health, limited finances, and decreased opportunities for social involvement. The feeling that the events in one's life are the result of fate, chance, or luck creates worry. Powers and colleagues (1992) developed a worry scale that may assist the elderly to make a more specific appraisal of their worries (Figure 22-1).

Stressors Experienced in the Process of Aging

Some stressors that are common to the aged are listed in Box 22-1. We believe in the holism and integration of the entire organism within its environment. The narrowing range of biopsychosocial homeostatic resilience and changing environmental needs as one ages may produce a stress overload that can occur unexpectedly. This is often signaled by the

Instructions: Below is a list of problems that often concern many Americans. Please read each one carefully. After you have done so, please fill in one of the spaces to the right with a check that describes how much that problem worries you. Make only one check mark for each item.

THINGS THAT WORRY ME. . .

	Never	Rarely (1-2 times per month)	Sometimes (1-2 times per week)	Often (1-2 times a day)	Much of the time (more than 2 times a day)
Finances					
1. that I'll lose my home					
2. that I won't be able to pay for the necessities of life (such as food, clothing, or medicine)					
3. that I won't be able to support myself independently					
4. that I won't be able to enjoy the "good things" in life (such as travel, recreation, entertainment)					
5. that I won't be able to help my children financially					
Health					
6. that my eyesight or hearing will get worse					
7. that I'll lose control of my bladder or kidneys					
8. that I won't be able to remember important things					
9. that I won't be able to get around by myself					
10. that I won't be able to enjoy my food					
11. that I'll have to be taken care of by my family					
12. that I'll have to be taken care of by strangers					
13. that I won't be able to take care of my spouse					
14. that I'll have to go to a nursing home or hospital					
15. that I won't be able to sleep at night					
16. that I may have a serious illness or accident					
17. that my spouse or a close family member may have a serious illness or accident					
18. that I won't be able to enjoy sex					
19. that my reflexes will slow down					
20. that I won't be able to make decisions					
21. that I won't be able to drive a car					
22. that I'll have to use a mechanical aid (such as a hearing aid, bifocals, a cane)					
Social conditions					
23. that I'll look "old"					
24. that people will think of me as unattractive					
25. that no one will want to be around me					
26. that no one will love me anymore					
27. that I'll be a burden to my loved ones					
28. that I won't be able to visit my family and friends					
29. that I may be attacked by muggers or robbers on the streets					
30. that my home may be broken into and vandalized					
31. that no one will come to my aid if I need it					
32. that my friends and family won't visit me					
33. that my friends and family will die					
34. that I'll get depressed					
35. that I'll have serious psychological problems					
Other worries					
36.					
37.					
38.					
39.					
40.					

Figure 22-1. The Worry Scale. (From Powers CB, Wisocki PA, Whitbourne SK: Age differences and correlates of worrying in young and elderly adults, *Gerontologist* 32[1]:82, 1992.)

appearance of cognitive impairment that will be alleviated as the stress is reduced to the parameters of the individual's adaptability.

Stress tolerance is variable and based on current as well as ongoing stressors. For example, if an elder has lost a significant person in the previous year, the grief may be manageable. If he or she has lost a significant person and developed painful, chronic health problems, the consequences may be quite different and can be highly stressful (Box 22-2).

Assessment of Stress Levels

Assessing stress level is a complex issue with many variables, both personal and environmental. The confluence of daily hassles; distal, chronic, and proximal stressors; worries; and functional capacities all create a stress load. Though many life event stress evaluation scales have been developed, none that presently exist can measure age variances as well as these other factors. We favor using any of them as tools to focus discussion of the various events and to suggest other factors that may be creating stress. Adolph Meyer's seminal concept (1951) of evaluating numerous strands in a lifeline perspective is likely to be useful. A discussion of the clustering of events and situations at various times can be very revealing. Figure 22-2 can be used as a model. Smyth and colleagues (1999) found that writing about stressful life experiences tended to be helpful.

Box 22-2 Stressors Identified by Community Elders*

- Sensory changes (vision and hearing)
- Necessity to relocate
- Housing and home maintenance
- Protection when frail and vulnerable
- Limited mobility and lack of transportation
- Fears of senility
- Social losses, loss of driver's license
- Depression/bereavement
- Management of acute and chronic pain
- Medications
- Protection from abuse and neglect
- Retirement of physician
- Loss of pet
- Rent increases
- Prevention of illness

From Ebersole P: Data obtained from nursing students' interviews of community elders, Holistic Nursing Course, San Francisco State University, San Francisco, 1988.
*Items not ranked in order of significance.

One factor that is seldom given sufficient consideration is the stress created by positive events. Pasupathi and colleagues (1996) used a modified Holmes and Rahe stress scale to determine the influence of age and socioeconomic status on the degree of stress in adapting to events ordinarily seen as positive, yet disruptive. Age seemed to make little difference, but individuals of lower socioeconomic status who had experienced a positive event seemed to find it more stressful, perhaps more surprising, and requiring alterations in lifestyle. The researchers suggest that positive events have not been given sufficient attention as adaptive challenges and stress producers.

Selye (1974) notes that stress inventories need to be more cognizant of individual differences. Self-knowledge allows us to judge whether we are running above or below the stress level that suits us best. The elderly are more prone to the adverse effects of stress and anxiety on the heart. Increased heart rate, blood pressure, insomnia, and irritability are some of the signs that an individual has exceeded the optimum stress level. In the frail old, confusion may be the signal of stress overload.

Stress Management

There has been a large body of research in the last 25 years on the effects of stress on aging and adaptation (Hughes et al, 1988; Avison and Gotlib, 1994; Cohen, 1995; Turner and Wheaton, 1995; Ensel et al, 1996; Trilling, 2000). Researchers

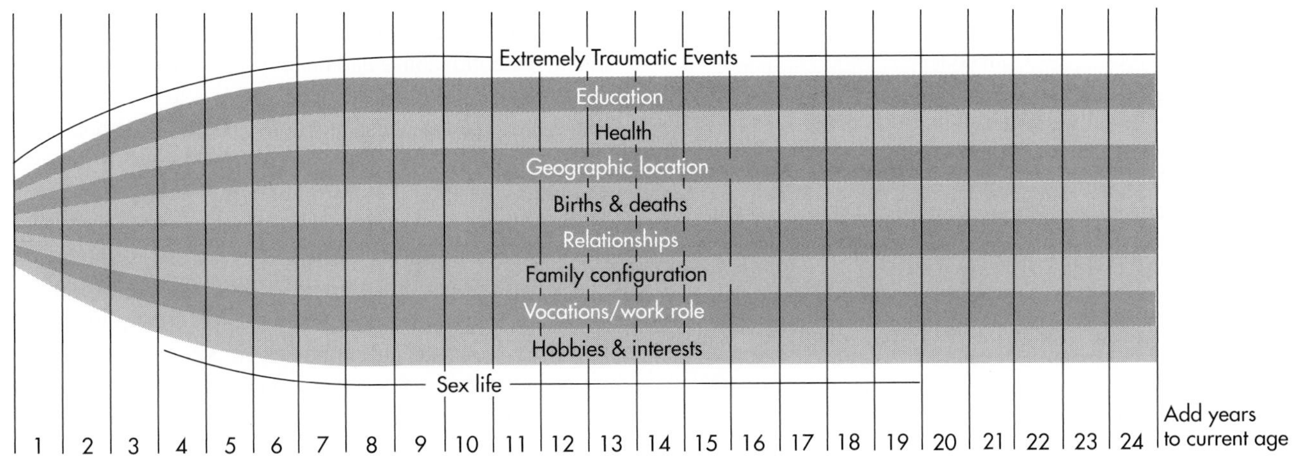

Figure 22-2. Life chart.

concerned with the effects of stress on the lives of elders have examined many moderating variables and have concluded that cognitive style, coping strategies, social skills, personal efficacy, support systems, and personality are all significant to stress management. Humans have two qualities that allow them to make the most or the least of stressful situations: awareness and choice. Stress mediators that are useful include religion, optimism, and hypnosis (Ishler et al, 1995; Koenig, 2000). Factors that influence one's ability to manage stress include the following:

- Health and fitness
- A sense of control over events
- Awareness of self and others
- Patience and tolerance
- Support groups
- Personal stability zones or a strong sense of self
- Beliefs and values

CRISES

Crises constitute a major, temporary disruption in coping capacity, whereas stress involves ineffectual or effectual coping and may be sustained over long periods. The term *crisis* was first introduced by Erich Lindemann (1944) after the Coconut Grove fire. It is defined as the lack of defense or coping mechanisms to deal with sudden and unexpected intrusions into a life situation that was previously experienced as satisfactory. A distinction between crisis and stress is related to time. Crises occur abruptly, are time limited, and are always resolved as an individual initiates some action and reestablishes equilibrium on a higher or lower level of personal organization.

The disequilibrium of crises cannot remain for more than a few weeks, thought to be about 6 weeks, but this is not necessarily true of older persons; this is a fruitful area for investigation. Ultimately crises are expressed in higher levels of coping or deterioration in efficacy and feelings of failure. A crisis event for one person may be perceived only as a stressor by another.

Major crises events for elders have always been the death of children, spouse, and siblings. Now the undercurrent of terrorizing events made boldly evident to the entire population has resulted in amplified reactions to all other crises and sometimes intense reactivation of early traumatic life experiences. Crises common to the aged are listed in Box 22-3.

Box 22-3 Crises Common to the Aged

- Abrupt internal and external body changes and illnesses
- Other-oriented concerns: children, grandchildren, spouse
- Loss of significant people
- Acute discomfort and pain
- Breach in significant relationships
- Fires, thefts
- Injuries, falls
- Translocation
- Aphasia, abrupt loss following stroke
- Abrupt loss of mobility or source of transportation
- Major unexpected drain on economic resources; for example, house repair, illness
- Abrupt changes in housing, especially without warning, to a new location, home, apartment, room, or institution
- Death of roommates in institutions

Posttraumatic Stress Disorder

Posttraumatic stress disorder (PTSD) is a prevalent and disabling disorder that flares into a coping crisis periodically. Psychologic trauma plays a causal role in the disorder and is characterized by specific psychobiologic dysfunctions. The disorder was first recognized following the Vietnam War, and since then many persons previously thought to be maladjusted have been identified and treated for PTSD. Debriefing, group and individual psychotherapy, and medications have been used with varying degrees of success (Stein et al, 2000).

Crisis situations such as experienced by World War II combat veterans and prisoners of war, Jewish holocaust survivors, and those who have been imprisoned and tortured may initially seem intolerable, but the victims often settle into the rarefied routine, not normal but ongoing, until the situation is experienced as a series of ever present, high-level stressors. The influence of disciplined training, group trauma, and support in these situations has, to our knowledge, not been examined, but it seems likely that these factors defer the actual personal chaos and breakdown of coping activities, which then are deferred until a later time and emerge as PTSD.

These breakdowns may erupt later as nightmares, intrusive images, personality disorders, and physiologic disturbances such as arthritis and digestive disorders. These reactions are often activated by the weakened psychic and immunologic defense systems that may accompany the stressors of aging and the loss of loved ones (Buffum and Wolfe, 1995). One 80-year-old man noted that startle reactions, uncontrolled aggression, and alcohol abuse had been ongoing problems following his survival of the Battle of the Bulge over 50 years ago, though he noted that these reactions had diminished somewhat in recent years. These data need considerably more study because the particular cohorts suffering these events are now well into their seventies and eighties, and some are in their nineties. Tom Brokaw (2001) has given us insights as these veterans are now confronting and talking about the horrors they had long suppressed. Port and colleagues (2001) examined longitudinal changes in symptom levels and prevalence among former prisoners of war (POWs) from World War II and found that prevalence rates and symptoms of PTSD increased significantly over the 4-year measurement interval.

Holocaust Survivors

Though the adjustment of most holocaust survivors indicates that they possess effective coping abilities (Schmitt et al, 1999), recent terrorist events have reactivated earlier horrors for many (personal conversations with holocaust survivors, Jewish Home for the Aged, San Francisco, 2002). Some studies indicate that the children of these survivors (now entering the ranks of the young-old) suffer emotional maladjustments related to the parents' denial or repression of the trauma (Kellerman, 2001; Kogan, 2002). Some of these adult-children do not know their true identity and suffer high rates of somatization, depression, and anxiety (Amir and Lev-Wiesel, 2001). Critical to adaptive strengths are the individuals' developmental level and sense of control (Lev-Wiesel and Amir, 2000). The psychologic impact of the terrorist attacks on PTSD sufferers may exacerbate already shaky personality adaptations. To some degree our whole society has been deeply shaken by these events.

Madge was a 92-year-old Jewish woman of great dignity, self-sufficiency, and personality strength. Her adaptability to several moves, bereavement, and the loss of her belongings in a fire were remarkable demonstrations of her fortitude. Shortly after her ninety-second birthday she began telling her daughters she felt anxious and fearful but did not know why. She became immobilized and would not leave her bed and complained of sleeplessness and nightmares. Possibilities to consider are a psychologic overload that created a belated posttraumatic stress reaction. Elements of the aging process that eroded her strong sense of self, strength depletion, residual and chronic stressors, and other unknown factors apparently reactivated psychic trauma experienced in her childhood through the loss of family members in the holocaust.

"Acts of God"

Tornadoes, hurricanes, cyclones, floods, firestorms, and earthquakes, often termed "acts of God," are some of the events that result in the crisis of homelessness. Rotton and Dubitsky (2002) found that following disaster exposure an increase in salivary immunoglobulin A occurs in students. Whether this is applicable to the aged is unknown, but it demonstrates the physiologic reactions to intense, uncontrollable events. Nurses involved in caring for those exposed to natural disasters were greatly concerned about their own family safety, pet care, and personal safety as they were ministering to others. It is suggested that disaster protocols must be clarified and family commitment versus professional obligation must be carefully considered (French et al, 2002).

Benezra (1996) identified individuals who had experienced extremely traumatic events that created intense fear and helplessness. Those who coped successfully without enduring problems seemed to exhibit the following characteristics: secure and supportive relationships, ability to freely express or fully suppress the experience, avoided dwelling on trauma, favorable circumstances immediately following the trauma, productive and active lifestyles, learning from the experience, strong faith/religion/hope, sense of humor, biologic strength, and endurance.

Crisis Assessment

Crisis assessment must take into account the recency of the event, effectual or ineffectual efforts to cope, and the available supports. The following are guidelines for determining the seriousness of a crisis:

Stage 0—No crisis but rather a request for information.

Stage 1—Mild crisis with ability to mobilize own resources after ventilating concern.

Stage 2—Emerging crisis; client insightful but desiring specific help.

Stage 3—Emergent crisis, second grade. Client recognizes need for assistance but uncertain what, where, or how to obtain. Counseling and referral necessary. Future crisis likely but client open and willing to use help when necessary.

Stage 4—Moderate crisis. Decompensation impending, behaviors mostly ineffective, but client making attempts to resolve problem. Assistance can be deferred for a short time.

Stage 5—Moderately severe crisis. Client agitated, disoriented, severely depressed.

Stage 6—Severe crisis. Client presents likelihood of a life-threatening situation; client pleading for help, praying, trying ineffectively to escape the situation.

Stage 7—Very severe crisis. Client in an immediate life-threatening situation; unable to focus on present situation; often engaged in irrelevant activities; for example, looking for makeup or comb when the house is on fire.

The elderly themselves and their families need more education in recognizing the early warnings of an impending crisis. Any of the reactions identified in stages 3 through 7 need immediate attention. Referrals may come from family members, a nonrelative, or a professional. Rarely does the aged person seek crisis assistance. Therefore the first action is to assess the degree of crisis and respond to the appropriate level of disorganization.

Long ago, Robert Butler (1967), the first director of the Institute on Aging, identified four factors that significantly affect individual perception of crisis events in old age:

1. *Extrinsic factors.* The social or personal impact of losses and the degree of lifestyle reorganization required to adapt are significant in crisis resolution.
2. *Intrinsic factors.* Personality bents such as a pessimistic or optimistic outlook on life affect interpretation of events.
3. *Reserve capacity.* Depletion as a result of physical disabilities, chronic illness or stress, and brain damage may predispose one to experience small irritations as crises.
4. *Past history.* Capacity for surviving, adapting, and maintaining a positive self-view throughout life will influence ability to tolerate crises and stress in old age.

We have not found a better way of delineating the various influences on crisis impact for the aged. The important thing to remember is the great individual variability in definition of a crisis event. For some the loss of a pet canary is a crisis;

others accept the loss of a good friend with grief but without personal disorganization.

Once an event has been identified as being of crisis proportions, the following actions must be taken:

- Immediate support of the individual and communication of concern
- Availability of a responsive person at any time the individual needs support
- Identification to the individual of any positive adaptive efforts
- Identify and establish some patterns of coping
- Provide information about available resources
- Follow up after resolution of the crisis to determine level of adaptation

EMOTIONS AND ILLNESS

There is much we do not yet understand about the connection between emotions and health and illness, but it has become obvious that the mind and body are integrated and cannot be approached as separate entities (Kelley, 2001). A common experiment to illustrate this is, "Concentrate on biting into a lemon and notice your salivary reaction." We know some emotions for some people result in physical illness, particularly those that produce negative emotions (Kiecolt-Glaser et al, 2002). Data suggest that persons with low psychosocial resources are vulnerable to illness and mood disturbance when their stress levels increase, even if they generally have few current stressors in their lives. Sustained stress can lead to such physical consequences as heart disease, hypertension, bowel irritation, and skin disorders. These conditions, when identified with stress as a major factor, are called *stress-related diseases.* Raison and Miller (2001) have found a bidirectional relationship between the brain and the immune system. Cannon (1932), Meyer (1951), and Selye (1956), the fathers of stress theories, recognized that responses to life events often resulted in illness. The general adaptation syndrome (GAS) identified by Selye (1956) is composed of the alarm reaction, the stage of resistance, and the stage of exhaustion. The body responds to stress through the GAS (fight or flight). Fight or flight is an inborn response and part of the human character. It is frequently referred to as an "extra squeeze of adrenaline." At times it provides the individual with what seems to be superhuman power to escape from danger or the necessary stamina to complete essential detailed information by a deadline.

The hormonal activity initiated by the alarm reaction triggers the sympathetic nervous system to respond by elevating blood pressure, pulse, and respirations and increasing metabolism and blood flow to the muscles. Biochemical changes begin, and the varied defense mechanisms of the body attempt to organize as a united front. At this point, while the body is mobilizing its forces, the individual's resistance is lowered. Once mobilization of defenses is completed, resistance rises to meet the threat. Adaptive capacity of the body is used to establish the individual at a new level of functioning or return the person to the prestress level; in other words, a return to a balanced state.

Most stressors produce change only in the first two stages; more serious stressors can lead to the exhaustion stage and death. However, exhaustion does not always terminate in death; when only part of the body is involved, the exhaustion stage may be reversible. The fight-or-flight syndrome seems much attenuated in the aged. As one gets older and homeostatic resilience decreases, the exhaustion stage may occur earlier and more frequently.

Some researchers have found that early life events, such as parental loss, continue to exact an emotional price throughout life (Ensel et al, 1996; Johnson and Barrer, 2002). Resurgence of traumatic memories is often triggered by current crises and losses. In addition, the weighting of events at any given time is dependent on concurrence of both positive and negative events; recency of exposure; timing, interval, and duration of the event; number of roles occupied by the individual; and general affective state of the subject.

Psychoneuroimmunology

From the seminal thoughts of Cannon, Meyer, and Selye decades ago, hundreds of studies, and a whole science of psychoneuroimmunology, have emerged, most within the last decade. Earlier studies, from 1939 onward, were chiefly published in *Psychosomatic Medicine.* It is generally accepted now, even by the medical profession, that emotions can wreak havoc with health and may be the source of many illnesses. Diseases thought to be triggered by psychologic factors that influence the immune system include cardiovascular disease, osteoporosis, arthritis, type 2 diabetes, certain cancers, frailty, and functional decline (Kiecolt-Glaser et al, 2002). In recent years there has been a dramatic increase in research related to the psychobehavioral modulation of immune function and attempts to assay the actual stress-related impairment of the immune system (Vedhara et al, 1999). Some studies contend that personality factors and perception of environmental events are also influenced by the individual's genetic makeup (Hickie et al, 1999; Kemeny & Laudenslager, 1999).

The intricate nature of these factors is illustrated by a brief vignette:

An ambitious, successful, optimistic middle-aged woman was abruptly widowed. There was some evidence of genetic familial mood disorders, but these had never been given serious thought by Mrs. K. Six weeks after the violent death of her husband, she developed crippling rheumatoid arthritis in both wrists. She was fully aware that this reaction was directly related to the death of her husband. She was immobilized and unable to work for 6 months. This anecdote illustrates the complexity and uncontrollability of these reactions. The body will dictate its own timing toward health, and individuals should be encouraged to respect this.

Dependency and Loss of Control

Impaired ability to maintain self-care is likely to deteriorate to the point of precipitating a dependency situation. Functional independence is the decisive factor in an old person's capacity to hold out at home and avoid family or institutional care. It is the basis of establishing the limits beyond which assistance and support become indispensable.

The aged person may, as part of a continuing lifestyle or pattern, have a dependent personality. The dependency need originated in early life but may remain dormant until physical, mental, social, or economic resources are threatened or lost. The impact directly affects the individual's capacity for mastery or gratification and activates feelings of helplessness. The aged person then exhibits loss of confidence; anticipates failure; and experiences shame, diminished self-esteem, and a sense of incompetence.

Anger, fear, and fear of retaliation can immobilize the aged person or mobilize him or her to seek help through a display of helplessness, hypochondriasis, or angry manipulation of others. This dependency is sometimes cultivated by caregiving staff who consciously or unconsciously are motivated by the assumed roles of healer, protector, and nurturing mother.

What about those aged who continue in their dependency and are never restored to a state of autonomy? We believe this occurs when supports are inadequate or missing during critical stress periods. Those aged who deteriorate mentally, emotionally, and physically exert a perverse kind of control through their dependency.

The nursing function is to redirect any evidence of control toward preserving the integrity, personality, and self-esteem of that individual. If power is properly redirected, some measure of life control can be restored. Even when people are unable to make decisions regarding their own personal care, they may still be able to participate if given direction and assistance. For example, giving the patient a washcloth and standing by to help if requested, rather than doing for the patient, reinstates an element of control. Nurses must examine their capacity to tolerate untidiness, inefficiency, and delay in the interest of promoting some measure of independence.

Regardless of the cause of the dependency of the aged person, the most constructive role the caregiver or nurse can assume is that of confidant, advocate, counselor, and encouraging supporter. These roles foster independence within the confines of the elderly person's capacity. Stressors often reach crisis proportions when the family with insufficient knowledge is confronted with life, death, and illness situations. The nurse will iterate all of the actions taken by the couple that were helpful and will explain those that are essential and will need to be taken in the future.

Helplessness. Helplessness may be a result of repeated ineffective attempts to deal with stressors or crises. Seligman (1975) introduced the concept of "learned helplessness" into the vernacular of gerontologists. It is based on studies of mice that show they will continue to seek food through a maze even when they receive a predictable electric shock. However, when the shocks become unpredictable, they cease trying. Extrapolated to humans, we believe that actions with unpredictable results over time eventually result in the individual's retreat into helplessness. Powerlessness is defined as "perceived lack of control over a situation and that actions will not significantly affect an outcome." In uncertain and inconsistently demanding situations, helplessness, powerlessness, and perceived lack of control erode the personality of individuals. The loss of health is often the precursor to loss of control and signals fatalistic acceptance of impairment, disability, discomfort, and old age. Uncertainty of illness and outcome is seen as a particularly debilitating situation in which coping may be seriously undermined (Mishel, 1988). Nurses, remembering this, must make special efforts to reinstitute personal control, particularly with the ill aged. Feelings of powerlessness and helplessness can arise from any of the sources identified in Box 22-4.

COPING

Coping strategies are the stabilizing factors that help individuals maintain psychosocial balance during stressful periods. More broadly, coping strategies are any efforts toward stress management; things that people do to avoid being harmed by life strains, or overt and covert behaviors to reduce or eliminate psychologic distress. Two major categories of coping behaviors are those that actively and directly deal with the problem and those that are designed for

Box 22-4 Sources of Feelings of Helplessness

- An unsuccessful illness-related regimen
- The implacable structure of the health care environment
- Interpersonal interactions
- A lifestyle of helplessness
- Repeated attempts to exert control that have failed
- Inability to predict a consistent outcome of certain actions

The pervasiveness of the powerless feeling can be categorized from the most to the least severe in the following manner:

- Verbalization of lack of influence over outcome
- Depression when condition deteriorates in spite of compliance with health regimen
- Apathy
- Nonparticipation in care or decisions when opportunities are provided
- Expressed frustration over limitations
- Expressed doubt regarding role performance
- Passivity
- Disinterest in information regarding care
- Dependency on others with the accompanying feelings of resentment, anger, and guilt
- Reluctance to express true feelings
- Agreeing readily to whatever may be suggested
- Expressed uncertainty about fluctuations in energy and functional ability

avoidance of the problem. Holahan and Moos (1986) found that depressed persons used avoidance coping increasingly as their depression became more profound and that individuals who adapted to stress with little physical or psychologic strain were less inclined to use avoidance coping than were those who showed psychologic dysfunction under stress.

Lazarus and Folkman (1984) distinguish between problem-focused strategies and those that are emotion focused. For example, if one's elderly parent demands to be waited on, a direct method to solve the problem would be to discuss with the elder the assistance that can realistically be given and what is needed. In an effort to avoid the problem and reduce emotional frustration, one might take a Valium and go to bed, hoping that the problem would eventually resolve itself. Some emotion-focused strategies may be healthy, such as centering oneself or meditating, but are still an avoidance of the actual issue (Box 22-5).

The aged are more frequently in a position of decreased ability to cope with daily hassles, cumulative life events, and other stressors because of their waning energy and adaptive capacity. The deficits in adaptability are most evident in neuroendocrine interactions and in the responsiveness of the nervous and endocrine systems. It does not make a difference whether stress is physical or emotional; the aged require more time to recover or return to prestress levels than when they were younger. Various means of stress reduction exist, such as meditation, biofeedback, tai chi, progressive relaxation, and visualization (see Chapter 3). Moderately vigorous exercise is one of the best ways to handle stress (Woods et al, 2002). Other methods include yoga, prayer, deep breathing, imagery, laughter, and massage.

Elders respond positively to most of these interventions. Some individuals use one; others use a combination of holistic methods to achieve inner balance (Maes, 2001). Mind-body therapies that integrate cognitive, sensory, expressive, and physical aspects are most helpful (Eliopoulos, 2000; Bauer-Wu et al, 2002). These data are significant for nurses as we identify and reinforce successful coping mechanisms. Because we often focus exclusively on the problem-solving mode, we may forget that there are many ways to solve a problem besides resolving it.

As elders confront problems that cannot be reversed or logically resolved, they obviously resort to other mechanisms that help them successfully cope with the issue. Encouraging the sharing of early memories is often useful in comprehending the coping style of an elder and helping the elder remember how he or she coped successfully. Application of what one has learned from a previous situation can help dissipate the intensity of stress.

Occasionally getting lost in some creative pursuit is an excellent means of dealing with stress. For some, knitting is helpful, whereas others find that painting a pastoral scene or the side of the house may be satisfying. Stroking a pet, rocking on a porch, or watching fish swim in an aquarium can serve as tranquilizers. Others enjoy fishing, a game of golf, reading a book, or listening to music. Still others find writing poetry a means of releasing frustration and stress. Physical activity is an appropriate means of handling stress for some individuals. These activities provide time to revitalize after a stressful incident, although if used continually as a means of avoiding resolutions they may become less effective (Box 22-6).

Box 22-5 Coping Strategy Items

Active-Cognitive Strategies

Prayed for guidance and strength
Prepared for the worst
Tried to see the positive side of the situation
Considered several alternatives for handling the problem
Drew on my past experiences
Took things a day at a time
Tried to step back from the situation and be more objective
Went over the situation in my mind to try to understand it
Told myself things that helped me feel better
Made a promise to myself that things would be different next time
Accepted it; nothing could be done

Active-Behavioral Strategies

Tried to find out more about the situation
Talked with spouse or other relative about the problem
Talked with friend about the problem
Talked with professional person (e.g., doctor, lawyer, clergy)
Got busy with other things to keep my mind off the problem
Made a plan of action and followed it
Tried not to act too hastily or follow my first hunch
Got away from things for a while
Knew what had to be done and tried harder to make things work
Let my feelings out somehow
Sought help from persons or groups with similar experiences
Bargained or compromised to get something positive from the situation
Tried to reduce tension by exercising more

Avoidance Strategies

Took it out on other people when I felt angry or depressed
Kept my feelings to myself
Avoided being with people in general
Refused to believe that it happened
Tried to reduce tension by drinking more
Tried to reduce tension by eating more
Tried to reduce tension by smoking more
Tried to reduce tension by taking more tranquilizing drugs

From Holahan C, Moos R: Personal and contextual determinants of coping strategies, *J Pers Soc Psychol* 52(5):946, 1987.

Box 22-6 Ways of Coping Checklist Responses

Most Frequent Responses
- Pray
- Remind self that things could be worse
- Maintain pride
- Look for the silver lining
- Turn to work or activity
- Keep feelings from interfering
- Try to analyze the problem

Least Frequently Used Coping Activities
- Talk with someone who can help
- Get professional help
- Apologize
- Take it out on others

Personal and Contextual Determinants of Coping

Factors such as sociodemographics, personal disposition, and contextual issues all affect ability to cope with crises. Contextual issues include such things as education, marriage and economic status, personal flexibility, logical choice, and problem-focused coping strategies.

Most elders, during the aging process, are confronted with loss, threats, and deprivation when their socioeconomic status is likely to be reduced and their health compromised. On the positive side they have developed, over time, numerous survival strategies that have been effective to one degree or another, and they are likely to have developed an internal locus of control. This should be the focus on an interaction with any elder: identify past patterns that have been productive.

Ongoing demands of a situation, up to a point, engender an increase in coping efforts, but just as there are individual pain thresholds there are also stress thresholds. We have not yet tried measuring elders' stress on a coping scale from 1 to 10. This might be a fruitful study.

There is the presumption that the use of certain coping strategies is largely a result of situational or personality variables. In fact, it may be that the coping style itself may result in the emergence of certain previously submerged personality characteristics and situational effects.

Hardiness and Buffers

Hardiness and "buffers" are concepts that attempt to explain the ability of some individuals to withstand enormous stress. *Hardiness* is a term that has captured the imagination of researchers interested in determining the differences in coping capacity of ostensibly similar elders. The cornerstones of hardiness are control, competence, and compassion (Kobasa, 1979). Hardiness, the combination of personality characteristics of vigor, resilience, commitment, and control, apparently buffers the illness-related effects of stress (Felton, 2001; Hagberg et al, 2002). Buffers against decompensation with stress come from social supports and are usually seen as the most important coping resource (see Chapters 17 and 18). Life goals and a sense of purpose or meaning undergird hardiness.

The relevance of hardiness to nursing practice is in assisting individuals to regain a sense of control over their lives, to feel committed or deeply involved with some activity that gives meaning, and to anticipate change as exciting. These may seem lofty goals, but they have been observed under the most extenuating circumstances.

Central to hardiness is the viewpoint that stress is a decision-making challenge and that meaning comes from making decisions. Stressful situations are seen as opportunities for growth. Clients should be apprised of any evidence of hardiness in their actions. This can reinforce their strength and coping abilities. Individuals should be asked the meaning of certain events in their lives and what they are learning from these challenging situations.

The seminal studies of Warheit (1979) to measure stress factors and effective coping strategies revealed that people generally use a progressive pattern of resources in the following order:

1. Own inner resources
2. Assistance from spouse, children, parents, or family members
3. Interpersonal networks, friends
4. Assistance from professionals and agencies
5. Cultural beliefs, values, symbols, and myths

Depending on the effectiveness of these resources, three levels of response to stress were evoked. Transient symptoms of stress were present in most subjects; some developed psychologic or physiologic illness syndromes; and those most severely affected became socially dysfunctional. From this study it seemed that life event stressors are mitigated by various strategies. We suggest that culturally embedded beliefs and expectations may be a major aspect of one's own inner resources and therefore high on the list of coping strategies.

Establishing Control

The previous discussion of crises, stress, and coping has shown the importance of a sense of control in preventing illness, disability, and deterioration. Crises, stress, chronic illness, and depression can erode self-esteem and the sense of mastery and induce feelings of "oldness." In these cases it is not uncommon for aged persons to seek an ally to whom they can temporarily relinquish control. The health care provider must be alert to the need for this short-lived splinting support (Wolanin and Phillips, 1981). The individual, injured and limping psychologically, physically, or both, needs a support person to help him or her regain psychic stability. The immediate availability of such support in a crisis may be the most critical element in achieving higher levels of function.

Symbols of Control. Some people have symbols of control that suffice in the absence of real influence. For example, Catherine's cane conveyed her authority. She kept it near her at all times, slept with it, and threatened to use it to defend herself if necessary. It was lost in transferring to another facility. She said, "Well, I think they've about got me now. I'm lost without my cane."

When dealing with vulnerable patients, be alert to their symbols of control. Some common ones are money, presence of family, pictures of family, hoarding of supplies or food, refusal of meals, demanding small or large amounts of attention, compulsive placement of personal articles, and other ritualistic behaviors. Respond to the latent message of a need for control, and work with the patient to reinstate legitimate control.

In one facility a dying woman was extremely demanding about the details of her morning care. One student nurse was able to comply without resentment because she understood the need to establish some order in the events of the day to compensate for lack of control over impending death. This was a legitimate use of patient power, although sometimes inconvenient for staff members.

Nurses also have power symbols: uniforms, special equipment, records, standing above rather than sitting by a patient, closing and opening doors without permission, medications, and addressing patients in familiar terms. We might consider ways to diminish the overwhelming influence of our power symbols on vulnerable patients.

Specific suggestions for establishing control are provided by Aasen (1987):

1. Identify issues in which residents have control, such as arrangement of personal items and selection of clothing. Loss of some autonomy in a situation is often perceived as a global loss of control. Particular areas of control must be emphasized.
2. Provide realistic opportunities for choice of alternatives in areas of interest. Choices of books, music, newspapers, snacks, and music are always possible.
3. Too many choices may have the negative effect of making decisions difficult and confusing, which will further emphasize the feeling of loss of control.
4. Opportunities to share personal talents, hobbies, and interests can be made available. First efforts may be disappointing, but persistence is advised. Gentle encouragement and lack of pressure for performance are recommended. Singing, reciting poetry, and playing the piano are only a few of the talents some elders may be "hiding under a bushel."
5. Discuss and reinterpret irrational beliefs (cognitive restructuring) that one has no control.
6. Give information and rationale for situations in which resident does not have control.

Choices. Generally, it is thought that beginning with small and valid choices is the most logical approach to reestablish a sense of control. As with all persons who are insecure about their position and uncertain of outcomes, the choices should be limited, be clear, and have visible results. For example, bathing seems to be one of the inflexible expectations in many institutions. Logically we know elders' skin should be protected against drying, and yet we feel so much better if the individual is clean, dry, powdered, and tucked into a neatly made bed. Can we ask patients to identify their bathing habits and adjust our schedule to their expectations? Unfortunately, the Saturday night bath ritual from the childhood of many of our elders is no longer considered adequate.

Meals are most important events in exercising control and personal preferences. Could a buffet cart be available for persons to choose from when they are hungry or feel inclined to eat? There are many healthy and attractive foods that can be always available to be served cold or heated in a microwave oven. Undoubtedly, there would be concern about persons on special diets who might select foods that were banned. John Morley, recent editor of *The Gerontologist* and notable researcher, believes there should be no dietary restrictions in long-term care institutions regardless of physical disorders. He believes that food restrictions, whether imposed by self or others, result in unintended weight loss and have negative results on the overall health of older individuals (Thomas et al, 2000). The Geriatric Center at Johns Hopkins Hospital instituted buffet meal services and found residents very receptive and appreciative (Remsburg, 2000). Robinson and Rosher (2002) began a beverage cart service in their facility. The many choices that were readily available increased residents' fluid consumption and sparked their interest.

Another area of choice that is significant is that of roommates. Unit supervisors may collaborate on ways to better match residents in long-term living situations. Perhaps there could be patient profiles of interests and abilities that could be shared with a new patient, thus involving him or her in selecting a compatible roommate.

All resident/patient choices may require extra effort and planning from staff, and the commitment to the goal of patient initiative and increased independence must be reinforced. Participation is invited in activities in which the client is unlikely to fail, such as making a collage with the assistance of the activity director. If the client adamantly refuses, the activity director will need to discuss reasons and other options. Together they can evaluate the validity of the reasons and try to pinpoint specifics and find something the elder really enjoys.

When some small gains are made in ADLs, the individual can be assisted to begin a daily log of events that produce momentary satisfaction. Each thing that was partially completed or attempted can be logged and discussed. Self-esteem and a sense of effectiveness is engendered because an individual is able to see concrete evidence of moving to a higher level of function.

WELLNESS AND GROWTH

The term *eustress* is defined as good stress engendered by challenging, demanding situations in which an individual feels capable and in control (Selye, 1978). Selye's recipe for good stress is as follows: (1) seek your own stress level, which fits you best; (2) choose your own goals, not ones imposed by others; and (3) develop altruistic egoism—look out for the self by being necessary to others and earning goodwill. Competence and usefulness make this feasible. Selye's recommendations are important to nurses as well as their aged clients.

In this chapter we have tried to present situations that often confront people in the aging process. With some people, events become catastrophic, whereas others seem to handle similar events well. Some events present immediate crises and others result in stress overload and breakdown of coping mechanisms. We have discussed many of these factors. A half century after Selye's seminal observations of the relationship of stress and illness and the numerous studies of psychoneuroimmunology, we still have only a beginning understanding of the mechanisms that create positive adaptations. Stress is a constant in our lives and those of our clients. The geriatric nurse is in a position to assist an individual in seeking meaning from untoward events. The presence of the nurse and his or her sensitivity in attending to the individual's immediate situation in a way that moves an individual toward higher levels of wellness is truly the art and the joy of nursing.

Human Needs and Wellness Diagnoses

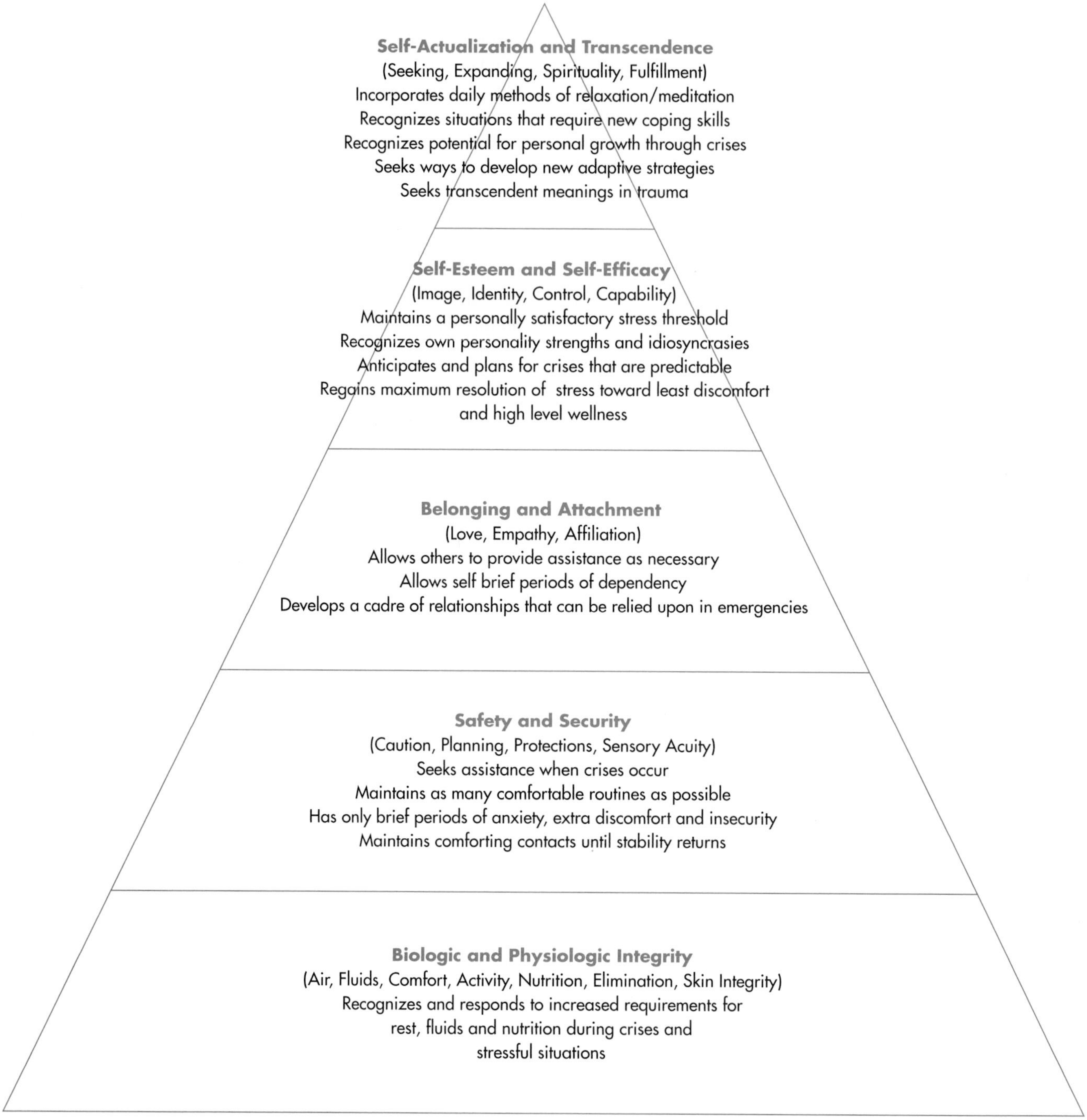

Self-Actualization and Transcendence
(Seeking, Expanding, Spirituality, Fulfillment)
Incorporates daily methods of relaxation/meditation
Recognizes situations that require new coping skills
Recognizes potential for personal growth through crises
Seeks ways to develop new adaptive strategies
Seeks transcendent meanings in trauma

Self-Esteem and Self-Efficacy
(Image, Identity, Control, Capability)
Maintains a personally satisfactory stress threshold
Recognizes own personality strengths and idiosyncrasies
Anticipates and plans for crises that are predictable
Regains maximum resolution of stress toward least discomfort and high level wellness

Belonging and Attachment
(Love, Empathy, Affiliation)
Allows others to provide assistance as necessary
Allows self brief periods of dependency
Develops a cadre of relationships that can be relied upon in emergencies

Safety and Security
(Caution, Planning, Protections, Sensory Acuity)
Seeks assistance when crises occur
Maintains as many comfortable routines as possible
Has only brief periods of anxiety, extra discomfort and insecurity
Maintains comforting contacts until stability returns

Biologic and Physiologic Integrity
(Air, Fluids, Comfort, Activity, Nutrition, Elimination, Skin Integrity)
Recognizes and responds to increased requirements for rest, fluids and nutrition during crises and stressful situations

These are not all the possible wellness diagnoses that may be identified. The above are examples of nursing diagnoses that should be considered when planning care for the older adult.

KEY CONCEPTS

- Disturbing emotions experienced over extended periods may result in depletions of the immune system and resulting illnesses.
- Crises and stressors are experienced by the aged less frequently than among younger adults but often have more devastating consequences.
- Crises have the potential for producing individual growth and higher levels of function as a result of successful mastery of the situation.
- If timely support and appropriate interventions are not activated during a crisis situation, the individual is likely to stabilize at a lower level of function than that before the crisis.
- Methods of assessing the impact of stressful events are inadequate if they do not consider chronic stressors that may exist over long periods of time, the particular population profile of the individuals being assessed, the individual's personality, the recency and frequency of events, and very early traumatic events that erode the individual's sense of security.
- Stress management strategies must be designed to meet individual needs because some methods may in fact be experienced as an additional stressor; for example, a shy, reticent elder would be unlikely to find body massage soothing and relaxing.
- Though helplessness and dependency are often seen as negative qualities, they may be temporarily adaptive and stress reducers in certain situations within the family or institutions.
- Reestablishing feelings of adequacy and control is the sine qua non of crisis resolution and stress management.
- Health care providers must develop ways to manage personal stressors if they are to be effective in helping others through crisis and stressful situations.
- Psychoneuroimmunology is attracting considerable attention as the relationship of emotions and disease and the particular physiologic responses involved are becoming clearer.

▲ CASE STUDY

Mrs. M is an 85-year-old Hispanic woman, recently moved from her home in Guadalajara to the home of her daughter and son-in-law in Los Angeles. She has been sent home from the hospital with draining lower leg ulcerations needing daily dressings, intermittent oxygen required to combat cerebral anoxia, and a gastrostomy tube for feeding. The decision to have her cared for at home was made by the physician, with the assistance of a Hispanic social worker and the patient, with the hesitant approval of her 60-year-old diabetic daughter and 67-year-old retired son-in-law. Mrs. M wanted to go back to her home in Guadalajara where her church and friends were and where she felt confident she could manage. While in the hospital and discussing the plans with the doctor, visiting nurse, social worker, and patient, the daughter and son-in-law thought the plan sounded feasible but not desirable. The husband said, "Where will we put her? Who will take care of her?"

When Mrs. M arrived at their home by ambulance and was settled in her bed, she began to retch, and the gastrostomy tube exuded greenish, clotted fluid. The couple were not prepared sufficiently and had no coping skills for such a situation. Mrs. M and her daughter and son-in-law panicked and called 911. Mrs. M was returned to the hospital, and the immediate crisis was quickly resolved; however, the stress was enormous and though brief will influence the ability of the couple to continue supporting home care for Mrs. M. Their feelings of efficacy have been eroded.

As a home care nurse, what would be your first intervention? What resources would you consider essential to their coping? How could the problems in this case have been averted?

▲ CASE STUDY

Aaron and Anna had a comfortable existence as the managers of a small hotel in upstate New York. They had downgraded from a large and lovely home when they retired but had been able to move most of their treasured possessions to the manager's cottage they occupied adjacent to the hotel. At 75 years old they felt fortunate to remain active, healthy, and generating an income. Their lives had provided much satisfaction, and this was a time to enjoy the rewards for long years of hard work and relative success. Their duties at the hotel were not strenuous because employees took care of the manual duties. They were in the control center—guiding, problem solving, and delegating—their dream retirement! One night while they were at a concert their cottage caught fire, and unfortunately, almost all their possessions were destroyed before the blaze was brought under control. Aaron repeatedly said, "I'm so glad we were not there and that we are safe." Anna wrung her hands constantly and chanted over and over, "My mother's photos are gone; my grandmother's quilts are gone; my Spode china is black." Clearly, for Aaron this was another hazard of living; for Anna it was the loss of the substance of her existence, definitions of her identity. Ordinarily one thinks of rape, traumatic injury, or cataclysmic events before worrying about the need to avert later PTSD. In Anna's case this was truly a cataclysmic event. Fortunately, the firemen recognized the magnitude of Anna's crisis reaction and called for assistance. An alert public servant called a crisis counselor to spend some time with Anna.

Based on these case studies, develop a nursing care plan using the following procedure:*

---

*Students are advised to refer to their nursing diagnosis text and identify possible or potential problems.

List comments of client that provide subjective data.
List information that provides objective data.
From these data identify and state, using accepted format, two nursing diagnoses you determine are most significant to this client at this time. List two client strengths that you have identified from data.
Determine and state outcome criteria for each diagnosis. These must reflect some alleviation of the problem identified in the nursing diagnosis and must be stated in concrete and measurable terms.
Plan and state one or more interventions for each diagnosed problem.
Provide specific documentation of source used to determine appropriate intervention. Plan at least one intervention that incorporates the client's existing strengths.
Evaluate success of intervention. Interventions must correlate directly with the stated outcome criteria in order to measure the outcome success.

STUDY QUESTIONS/ACTIVITIES

Discuss differences between crises and stress, and describe methods to discriminate between the two situations.
Talk to elders in your neighborhood and ask about their crises and stressors within the past 6 months or 1 year. How frequently did they experience the loss of a friend or relative? Interview an elder in a nursing home and ask about the events or situations that are most troubling to him or her. List the crises and stressors you have experienced in the past year and compare the differences and similarities in the three lists.
Discuss your thoughts about the science of psychoneuroimmunology.
Explain methods of restoring a sense of control and averting excessive dependency.
Discuss the meanings and the thoughts triggered by the students' and elders' viewpoints expressed at the beginning of the chapter. How do these vary from your own experience?
As a group project, develop a life events rating scale for an elderly population that includes the following considerations:

- Events and other possible sources of social stress
- Significance of event in relation to age, gender, cohort, and culture
- Desirable and undesirable events
- Comprehensiveness of events listed
- Roles occupied by the individual at the time of the survey
- Affect of the individual at the time of the survey
- Time frame, recency, and duration of event

Construct a life chart for yourself and consider events around times when you were greatly stressed.

RESEARCH QUESTIONS

What items would be important in the development of age-specific tools to determine the nature of anxiety in the old?
What are the events that are particularly malignant crises for elders?
In what areas of life do elders feel they have the least control?
What are the most common or frequent worries of elders?
What is the impact on stress management of various personality gender differences?
Develop a tool for measuring coping capacity of elders on a scale of 1 to 10 (similar to pain assessment tools).

REFERENCES

Aasen N: Interventions to facilitate personal control, *J Gerontol Nurs* 13(6):21, 1987.
Amir M, Lev-Wiesel R: Does everyone have a name? Psychological distress and quality of life among child holocaust survivors with lost identity, *J Trauma Stress* 14(4):859, 2001.
Avison WR, Gotlib IH: Future prospects for stress research. In Avison WR, Gotlib IH, editors: *Stress and mental health: contemporary issues and prospects for the future,* New York, 1994, Plenum.
Bauer-Wu SM: Psychoneuroimmunology: part II. Mind-body interventions, *Clin J Oncol Nurs* 6(4):243, 2002.
Benezra EE: Personality factors of individuals who survive traumatic experiences without professional help, *Int J Stress Management* 3(3):147, 1996.
Brokaw T: *The greatest generation,* New York, 2001, Bantam-Dell.
Buffum MD, Wolfe NS: Posttraumatic stress disorder and the World War II veteran, *Geriatr Nurs* 16(6):264, 1995.
Butler RN: The crises of old age, *RN* 30:47, 1967.
Cannon WB: *The wisdom of the body,* New York, 1932, WW Norton.
Cohen S: Psychological stress and susceptibility to upper respiratory infections, *Am J Respir Crit Care Med* 152(4):S53, 1995.
Eliopoulos C: Using complementary and alternative techniques—boosting immunity, *Director* 8(4):142, 2000.
Ensel WM et al: Stress in the life course: a life history approach, *J Aging Health* 8(3):389, 1996.
Eriksen HR et al: The time dimension in stress response: relevance for survival and health, *Psychiatr Res* 85(1):39, 1999.
Felton BS, Hall JM: Conceptualizing resilience in women older than 85: overcoming adversity from illness and loss, *J Gerontol Nurs* 27(11):46, 2001.
French ED, Sole ML, Byers JF: A comparison of nurses' needs/concerns and hospital disaster plans following Florida's hurricane Floyd, *J Emerg Nurs* 28(2):111, 2002.
Hagberg M, Hagberg B, Saveman BI: The significance of personality factors for various dimensions of life quality among older people, *Aging Ment Health* 6(2):178, 2002.
Hickie I et al: Complex genetic and environmental relationships between psychological distress, fatigue and immune function: a twin study, *Psychol Med* 29(2):268, 1999.
Holahan C, Moos R: Personality, coping and family resources in stress resistance: a longitudinal analysis, *J Pers Soc Psychol* 51:389, 1986.
Holahan C, Moos R: Personal and contextual determinants of coping strategies, *J Pers Soc Psychol* 52(5):946, 1987.

Hughes DC, Blazer D, George L: Age differences in life events: a multivariate controlled analysis, *Int J Aging Hum Dev* 27:207, 1988.

Ishler KJ et al: Religious coping, general coping and controllability: testing the hypothesis of fit. Paper presented at the 48th Annual Meeting of the Gerontological Society of America, Los Angeles, Nov 18, 1995.

Johnson CL, Barrer BM: Life course effects of early parental loss among very old African Americans, *J Gerontol B Psychol Sci Soc Sci*, 57(2):S108, 2002.

Kellerman NP: Psychopathology in children of holocaust survivors: a review of research literature, *Isr J Psychiatry Relat Sci* 38(1):36, 2001.

Kelley KW: It's time for psychoneuroimmunology, *Brain Behav Immun* 15(1):1, 2001.

Kemeny ME, Laudenslager ML: Beyond stress: the role of individual difference factors in psychoneuroimmunology, *Brain Behav Immun* 13:73, 1999.

Kiecolt-Glaser JK et al: Psychoneuroimmunology: psychological influences on immune function and health, *J Consult Clin Psychol* 70(3):537, 2002.

Kiecolt-Glaser JK et al: Psychoneuroimmunology and psychosomatic medicine: back to the future, *Psychosom Med* 64(1):15, 2002.

Kobasa SC: Stressful life events, personality and health: an inquiry into hardiness, *J Pers Soc Psychol* 37(1):1, 1979.

Koenig HG: Psychoneuroimmunology and the faith factor, *J Gender Specific Med* 3(5):37, 2000.

Kogan I: "Enactment" in the lives and treatment of holocaust survivors' offspring, *Psychoanal Q* 71(2):251, 2002.

Lazarus R, Folkman S: *Stress appraisal and coping,* New York, 1984, Springer.

Lev-Wiesel R, Amir M: Posttraumatic stress disorder symptoms, psychological distress, personal resources, and quality of life in four groups of holocaust child survivors, *Fam Process* 39(4):445, 2000.

Lindemann E: Symptomatology and management of acute grief, *Am J Psychiatry* 101:141, 1944.

Maes S: Nurses explore relationships among mind, body, spirit, *ONS News* 16(9):1, 2001.

Meyer A: The life chart and the obligation for specifying positive data in psychopathological diagnosis. In Winters EE, editor: *The collected papers of Adolph Meyer,* vol 3, Baltimore, 1951, Johns Hopkins University Press.

Mishel M: Uncertainty in illness, *Image J Nurs Sch* 20(4):225, 1988.

Pasupathi M, Sjostrom S, Richardson J: Lifespan perspectives on stressful events. Paper presented at the meeting of the Gerontological Society of America, Washington, DC, Nov 20, 1996.

Personal conversations with holocaust survivors, Jewish Home for the Aged, San Francisco, June 6, 2002.

Port C, Engdahl B, Frazier P: A longitudinal and retrospective study of PTSD among older prisoners of war, *Am J Psychiatry* 158(9):1474, 2001.

Powers CB, Wisocki PA, Whitbourne SK: Age differences and correlates of worrying in young and elderly adults, *Gerontologist* 32(1):82, 1992.

Raison CL, Miller AH: The neuroimmunology of stress and depression, *Semin Clin Neuropsychiatry* 6(4):277, 2001.

Remsburg R: *Creating buffet selections in a geriatric unit,* poster session presentation, National Gerontological Association, Washington, DC, October 19, 2000.

Robinson SB, Rosher RB: Can a beverage cart help improve hydration? *Geriatr Nurs* 23(4):208, 2002.

Rotton J, Dubitsky SS: Immune function and affective states following a natural disaster, *Psychol Rep* 90(2):251, 2002.

Schmitt E, Kruse A, Re S: Patterns and influences of coping with traumatic reminiscences in holocaust survivors, *Z Psychosom Med Psychotherapy* 45(3):279, 1999.

Seligman M: *Helplessness: on depression, development and death,* San Francisco, 1975, Freeman.

Selye H: *The stress of life,* New York, 1956, McGraw-Hill.

Selye H: *Stress without distress,* Philadelphia, 1974, JB Lippincott.

Selye H: On the benefits of eustress. In interview by Cherry L, *Psychol Today* 11:60, March 1978.

Smyth MM et al: Effects of writing about stressful experiences on symptom reduction in patients with asthma or rheumatoid arthritis, a randomized trial, *JAMA* 281:1304, 1999.

Stein DJ et al: Psychotherapy for traumatic stress disorder, *Cochrane Database Syst Rev* 4:CD002795, University of Stellenbosch, Tygerberg, South Africa, 2000.

Stetson B: Holistic health stress management program: nursing student and client health outcomes, *J Holistic Nurs* 15(2):143, 1997.

Thomas DR, Ashmen W, Morley JE, Evans WJ: Nutritional management in long term care: development of a clinical guideline, *J Gerontol* 55(12):M725-734, 2000.

Trilling JS: Selections from current literature of psychoneuroimmunology: validation of the biopsychosocial model, *Fam Pract* 17(1): 90, 2000.

Turner RJ, Wheaton B: Checklist measurement of stressful life events. In Cohen S, Kessler RC, Gordon LY, editors: *Measuring stress: a guide for health and social scientists,* New York, 1995, Oxford University Press.

Vedhara K, Fix JD, Wang EC: The measurement of stress-related immune dysfunction in psychoneuroimmunology, *Neuroscientific Biobehavioral Rev* 23(5):699, 1999.

Warheit G: Life events, coping, stress and depressive symptomatology, *Am J Psychiatry* 136:592, 1979.

Wolanin MO, Phillips L: *Confusion: prevention and care,* St Louis, 1981, Mosby.

Woods JA, Lowder TW, Keylock KT: Can exercise training improve immune function in the aged? *Ann N Y Acad Sci* 959:117, 2002.

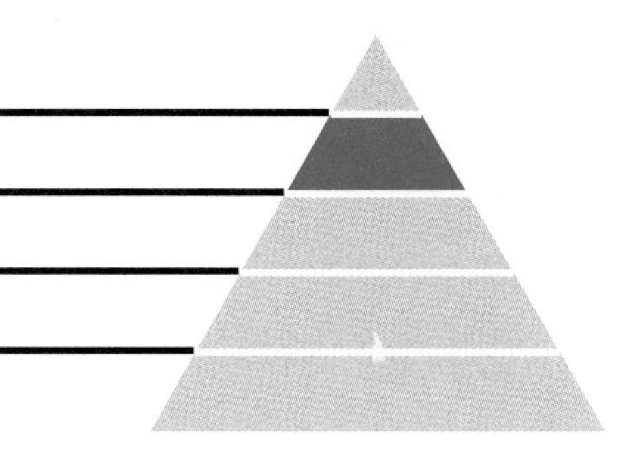

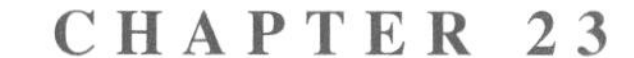

CHAPTER 23

Mental Wellness and Disturbances

Ann Schmidt Luggen

A student speculates

The process of aging scares me. Aging brings up emotions such as low self-esteem, powerlessness, and hopelessness. An old person has to accept the existing gap between the young and the old. I still remember telling my grandmother she was old-fashioned and out of touch. Now, I realize how rude I was to her. By the time I am about 75 years old, I will be just as depressed as some of the elderly I work with.

Rossana, age 28

An elder speaks

I am very irritable and quick to anger, and this is increasing as I age. I think people's strengths increase as they age, and their weaknesses do also.

Madeline, age 78

LEARNING OBJECTIVES

After completing this chapter, the reader will be able to:

1. Differentiate mental health from mental illness in older adults.
2. Name the three most common disturbances of the mental health of elders.
3. Assess the presence of depression in an elder.
4. Recognize elders who are at risk for suicide and conduct a suicide assessment of an elder.
5. Explain therapies that are useful in the care of mentally disturbed elders.
6. Describe methods of communicating with the mentally disturbed elder.
7. Evaluate interventions aimed at promoting mental health in older adults.
8. Relate the nursing concerns in managing a resident with a communication disorder caused by a perceptual disturbance.
9. Develop an individualized nursing care plan for a client with a mental illness.

This chapter presents concepts of mental health wellness and mental illness in old age and provides specific nursing strategies to maintain and promote mental health wellness, self-esteem, and psychologic health of older individuals to the optimum of their capacity. The chapter is divided into three major sections: considerations in mental health of the aged, cognitive disturbances created by psychiatric problems, and therapeutic interventions. Developmental transitions, life events, and situations requiring psychic energy may interfere with the ability to concentrate in many older adults. These factors, though not unique to the old, often influence adaptation. In previous chapters, we examined these challenges in Maslow's hierarchical fashion. We hope that nurses who are caring for the aged will first consider the status of their clients' basic human needs when assessing mental health and illness.

MENTAL HEALTH IN OLD AGE

Mental health of the elderly is difficult to define because the increasing differentiation of personality throughout the life span results in idiosyncratic and sometimes eccentric adaptations in late life. Each individual becomes more uniquely himself or herself the older he or she becomes. The accumulation of life experience, as well as particular situations, emphasizes certain aspects of personality and appearance and diminishes others. Some apparently negative personality characteristics, such as being crusty, disagreeable, grouchy, or grumpy, may be adaptive. Thus a cantankerous old man engaged in coping with a severe illness and stoically protecting others from awareness of his pain might be mentally healthy.

Mental health can be defined as a satisfactory adjustment to one's life stage and situation. We tend to believe certain cultural artifacts such as independence and assertiveness are indices of mental health when they may be maladaptive to certain lifestyles and stages. Using these criteria, it becomes apparent that a contented, but passive, institutionalized older person might be mentally healthy and adapted to the peculiar subculture that demands certain behaviors of those who best manage.

The Diagnostic and Statistical Manual of Mental Disorders, fourth edition, (DSM-IV) (American Psychiatric Association [APA], 1994) provides categorical criteria for diagnosing mental disorders from a medical perspective but is of little help in assessing elders with mental illness because no special characteristics are noted except in age-related cognitive decline. Actual geropsychiatric problems not related to cognitive pathologic conditions are neglected. We contend that some disorders in DSM-IV should be defined more carefully in terms of symptomatologic factors when considering the mental disorders of elders.

We note that mental health in the aged embodies our adaptation to sociocultural roles, cohort differences in expectations, positive relationships, and matured mental well being. In later life, mental health is measured by the capacity to cope effectively with relationships and environment and by the satisfaction experienced in doing so. The individual's response to the environment can be used as a criterion of mental health *only* if the environment provides the potential for mental health. Theoretically, this view is useful. When someone is underrated or "placed in a box," expectations of mental health are reduced, feedback is modified, and a danger of instigating a self-fulfilling prophecy exists. For example, many older people fear that they will lose their intellectual powers as they age and are particularly vulnerable to any implication that confirms their fear. Thus, in a community or society in which ageism is rampant and distribution of mental health resources to the aged has a low priority, as at present, we would expect many mental aberrations in the elderly. The development of holistic, humanistic, interactional, and individualistic models of psychiatric nursing care is critically important in the care of the aged at this time. Using Maslow's hierarchic need model, we might assume that the higher one rises in terms of needs met, the more likely one is to be mentally healthy (Figure 23-1, *A*).

Mental health, as with general health, can be thought of on a fluctuating continuum from wellness to illness. The absence of mental illness does not mean one is mentally healthy, nor does the presence of psychologic symptoms mean one is mentally ill. Individuals move back and forth on the continuum as stressors, supports, health, and resources are ample or scarce (Figure 23-1, *B*).

Freud believed the major determinants of mental health were the capacities to work and love, thus expressing the energies of aggression and Eros. Freud's ideas regarding the centrality of work and love can be expanded in late life to include purposeful living as the work of aging and to include all evidences of altruism as love. In contemporary society, we have added a third capacity, particularly significant to elders, and that is the ability to enjoy leisure.

Erikson thought autonomy, intimacy, integrity, and generativity were all aspects of mentally healthy adult adaptation. These concepts are culture bound and to some extent dependent on semantics. Most importantly, no one is entirely mentally unhealthy, and no one is fully healthy at all times. We can help the elder seek to maximize the healthiest self-attributes.

Mental Health Services for the Elderly

Severe gaps exist in the delivery of mental health services to the elderly who are seeking services. At this time, federal policy and the Community Mental Health Centers Act both exclude the continuing care of individuals with chronic disorders from reimbursement. In addition, a 190-day lifetime limit still remains on treatment in mental hospitals. Psychiatric services may be delivered by a psychiatrist, psychologist, nurse practitioner, or social worker and are reimbursable, and many of the best health maintenance organizations (HMOs) provide mental health and counseling services, as well as programs for special problems, such as addictions. This trend portends somewhat better and more available care.

The elderly patients we have today have endured many situations, including two world wars and the great depression. An unprecedented boom has occurred in medical knowledge and technology, and we are extending human life to ages previously thought improbable (Jarman and Herrera, 2001). Life expectancies will take on a whole new meaning with the "baby boomers" who are accomplishing financial planning, retirement plans, and long-term care insurance, things that were difficult in past generations. We know little how this planning will pan out with this new generation of elders. Interestingly, in this season of our life when we are least able to deal with change, we are exposed to the most dramatic changes. Losing family, friends, loved ones, even children, is a struggle. One must give up one's dog or cat when entering a facility. We lose contact with extended family, status, and position. The most feared loss is the loss of cognitive ability, not remembering simple things—telephone numbers or name of family members or good friends. With whom can we share these concerns? Mental health services is one answer.

Nursing homes, although not licensed as psychiatric facilities and seldom staffed to provide continual mental health assessment or care, are providing the majority of *care* given to elders with psychiatric conditions. Staff cannot treat these elders appropriately because of an insufficient number of

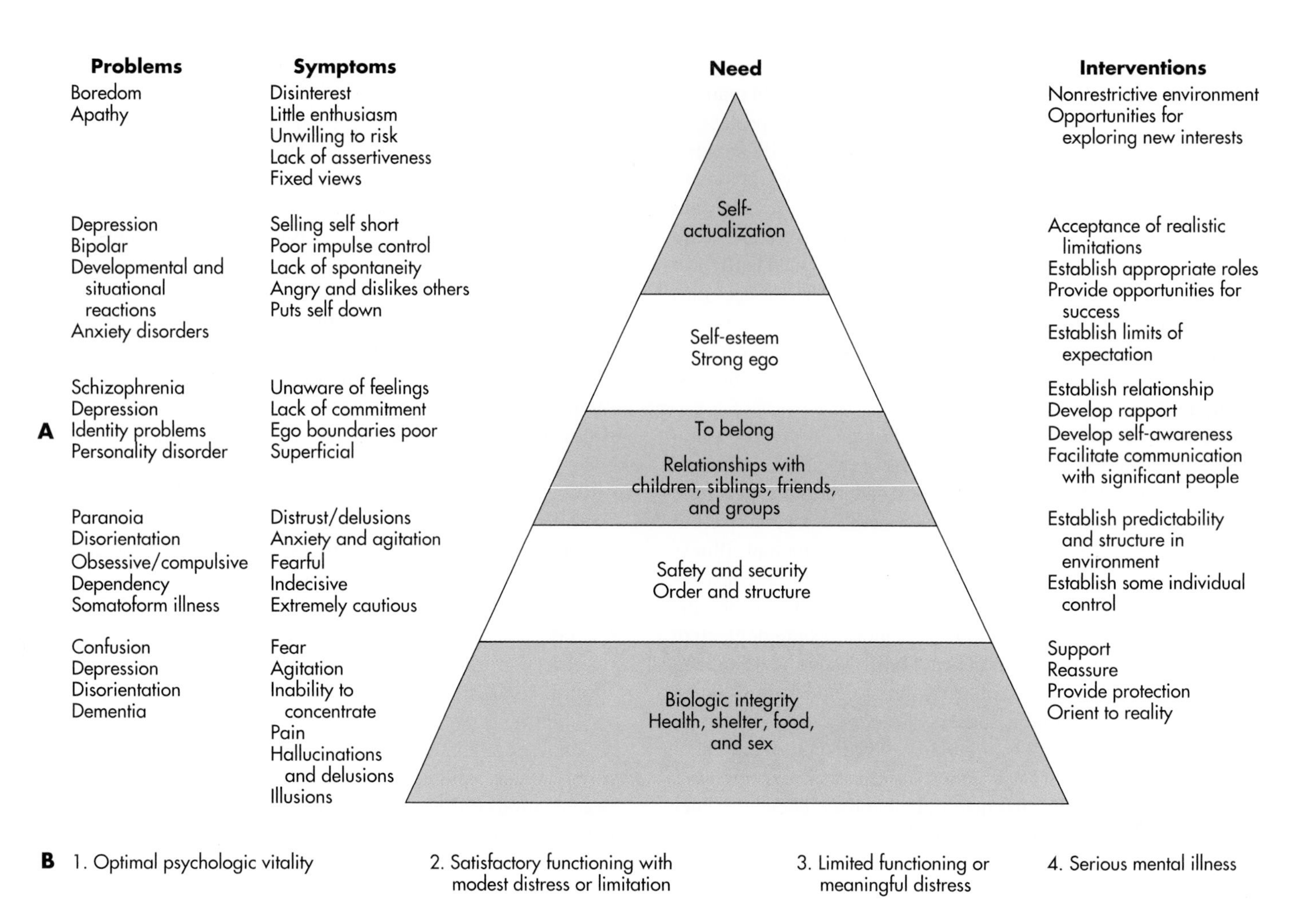

Figure 23-1 **A,** Mental health disorders. **B,** Continuum of mental health and illness.

trained personnel. Some of the obstacles to mental health care in nursing homes are (1) shortage of trained personnel, (2) lack of in-service training in nursing homes related to mental health and illness, and (3) inadequate Medicaid and Medicare reimbursement for mental health services. Recommendations of the U.S. Health Resources and Services Administration (USHRSA) report include additional funding for training, reimbursement, psychiatric and behavioral therapies, and consumer education. This financial support is unlikely to happen given the shift to state fiscal responsibility. However, some progress is being made in nursing homes and long-term care facilities. The various revisions of the Omnibus Budget Reconciliation Act (OBRA) and the implementation of the Minimum Data Set (MDS) have resulted in more resident-oriented and holistic care and the reduction of chemical and physical restraints.

As part of OBRA 1989, Congress recognized nurse practitioners (NPs) as direct providers of services to residents of nursing homes. The reimbursement varies by the type of NP, the health care setting, and the payment level. Medicare directly reimburses the services of NPs in nursing homes and in rural-area settings. Whether these NPs have geropsychiatric specialized training is questionable; probably not. A recent report of the Surgeon General in 2000 spoke to the mental health needs of the elderly population (Jarman and Herrera, 2001). The report verifies the need for therapy services in long-term care settings. Counseling services are now being instituted, which give residents an opportunity to talk with someone and share their struggles. Reminiscent counseling is also beneficial. Feeling pride for one's accomplishments is vital to reaching one's peak.

Geropsychiatric nursing is the specialty care that nurses provide to elders with mental health disorders. Few educational programs focus on this specialty, and all of the professions notoriously neglect the mental health needs of elders. When available, geropsychiatric nursing consultation to facilities is recommended as one method of alleviating some of the lack of specific expertise. However, because this service is not the norm, nurses employed in long-term care must encourage such consultation on an ongoing basis rather than only in occasional provocative situations.

Demographics

America's population grew 74% between 1970 and 1999, from 20 million to 35 million (American Association of Geriatric Psychiatry, [AAGP], 2002). This number will grow remarkably to the extent that in 2030 older adults will make up 20%, rather than 12% of the population that they do now. Nearly 20% of people over 55 years of age experience mental disorders that are not part of normal aging. The most prevalent disorders are anxiety, severe cognitive impairment, and mood disorders. These mental disorders are underreported. The rate of suicide is higher in older adults than it is in any age group, with age 85 and over having the highest suicide rate—twice the national rate.

Less than one half of older adults who acknowledge mental health problems receive any treatment from any provider, and a mental health specialist provides few of the treatments. The rate of utilization is less than that of any other age group.

Medicare provides health insurance, but the coverage is not comprehensive. Only 50% of mental health services are covered, although most recently, it is providing more care to people with Alzheimer's disease. Health insurance does not cover any prescription drugs. Medicare beneficiaries spend nearly 20% of their income for out-of-pocket health care costs. Additionally, people with the lowest income, below poverty level, spent 33% of their income for out-of-pocket expenses (AAGP, 2002).

Psychologic Assessment of Elders

A well-known fact is that depression in the elderly is highly prevalent and treatable but is infrequently recognized or treated. Moorhead and Brighton (2001) report several studies suggesting that a substantial number of elders are suffering anxiety, substance abuse, and somatoform disorders that were also unrecognized and untreated. These findings serve only to confirm the increasing prevalence and neglect of mental disorders in elders. Medical patients with chronic illnesses present with psychiatric disorders such as depression and anxiety in 25% to 33% of cases, though they are unrecognized by primary health practitioners much of the time.

General issues in the psychologic assessment of older adults involve distinguishing among normal, idiosyncratic, and diverse characteristics of aging and pathologic conditions. Baseline data are often lacking from the individual's middle years. Using standardized tools and functional assessment is valuable, but the data will be meaningless if not placed in the context of the patient's early life and hopes and expectations for the future. Distinguishing normal from pathologic aging in a particular individual depends on these factors. Few standardized assessment tools included any old subjects in the development of the tool.

Assessment of mental health includes examination for cognitive function or impairment and the specific conditions of demoralization, depression, paranoia, substance abuse, psychopathologic conditions, and suicidal risk. Assessment of mental health must also focus on social intactness and affectual responses appropriate to the situation. Attention span, concentration, intelligence, judgment, learning ability, memory, orientation, perception, problem solving, psychomotor ability, and reaction time are assessed in relation to cognitive intactness and must be considered when making a psychologic assessment. Assessment includes specific processes that are intact, as well as those that are diminished or compromised.

Obtaining data from elders is best done during short sessions after some rapport has been established. Performing repeated assessments at various times of the day and in different situations will give a more complete psychologic profile. Being sensitive to a patient's anxiety, special needs, and disabilities is important. The interview should be focused so that attention is given to strengths and skills, as well as deficits. A global assessment of functioning is useful (Box 23-1) in assessing the old. Also useful is to take a psychologic inventory of the geriatric client (Box 23-2). See Appendix 23-A for depression rating scales.

Defenses

"Defense mechanisms (or coping styles) are automatic psychological processes that protect the individual against anxiety and from the awareness of internal or external dangers or stressors" (APA, 1994, p. 751). Given the prevalence of anxiety and agitation among the aged, we must question whether the psychologic defensive processes become less efficient in later life, just as do some of the physiologic processes.

In the DSM-IV, the defenses have been grouped in the Defensive Functioning Scale. These hierarchical categories allow the practitioner to categorize coping styles and then indicate the predominant defensive level that the individual exhibits. A glossary of defense mechanisms, somewhat different and healthier than the classic definitions, assists in evaluation. This Defensive Functioning Scale holds promise for evaluating an elder's adaptation. As with all evaluative efforts, micro and macro timing are important, as are fatigue, pain, and stress levels.

Some of the defensive mechanisms of the aged are very healthy and some are inhibitory. We present some of the most predominant.

Denial. Denial of illness, aging, loss, death, or incapacity helps ease one through some of the difficulties of aging. Denial may be difficult to assess because many older people avoid discussion of major concerns and losses, not because they are unaware, but rather because they have a strong enculturation to stoic endurance or have great courage. If denial is present, it is necessary and should be addressed directly only when the elder shows signs that it is weakening.

Al (76 years of age) planned, scheduled, and prepaid for a cruise for himself and his wife the following month. Al's wife was in the process of divorcing him, his cardiac decompensation had nearly immobilized him, he had an unexplained seizure, and his physician told him that he would need to be closely monitored until his

Box 23-1 Global Assessment of Functioning (GAF) Scale

Consider psychological, social, and occupational functioning on a hypothetical continuum of mental health and mental illness. Do not include impairment in functioning caused by physical (or environmental) limitations.

Code	(Note: Use intermediate codes when appropriate [e.g., 45, 68, 72].)
100 91	Superior functioning in a wide range of activities (e.g., life's problems never seem to get out of hand) is sought out by others because of his or her many positive qualities. No symptoms are present.
90 81	Absent or minimal symptoms (e.g., mild anxiety before an examination), good functioning in all areas, interested and involved in a wide range of activities, socially effective, generally satisfied with life, no more than everyday problems or concerns (e.g., an occasional argument with family members).
80 71	If symptoms are present, they are transient and expectable reactions to psychosocial stressors (e.g., difficulty concentrating after family argument), no more than slight impairment in social, occupational, or school functioning (e.g., temporarily falling behind in schoolwork).
70 61	Some mild symptoms (e.g., depressed mood and mild insomnia) OR some difficulty in social, occupational, or school functioning (e.g., occasional truancy, theft within the household), but generally functioning well; has some meaningful interpersonal relationships.
60 51	Moderate symptoms (e.g., flat affect, circumstantial speech, occasional panic attacks) OR moderate difficulty in social, occupational, or school functioning (e.g., few friends, conflicts with peers or co-workers).
50 41	Serious symptoms (e.g., suicidal ideation, severe obsessional rituals, frequent shoplifting) OR any serious impairment in social, occupational, or school functioning (e.g., no friends, unable to keep a job).
40 31	Some impairment in reality testing or communication (e.g., speech is at times illogical, obscure, or irrelevant) OR major impairment in several areas, such as work or school, family relations, judgment, thinking, or mood (e.g., depressed man avoids friends, neglects family, is unable to work, child frequently beats up younger children, is defiant at home, is failing at school).
30 21	Behavior is considerably influenced by delusions or hallucinations OR serious impairment in communication or judgment (e.g., sometimes incoherent, acts grossly inappropriately, suicidal preoccupation) OR inability to function in almost all areas (e.g., stays in bed all day; no job, home, friends).
20 11	Some danger of hurting self or others (e.g., suicide attempts without clear expectation of death, frequently violent, manic excitement) OR occasionally fails to maintain minimal personal hygiene (e.g., smears feces) OR gross impairment in communication (e.g., largely incoherent or mute).
10 1	Persistent danger of severely hurting self or others (e.g., recurrent violence) OR persistent inability to maintain minimal personal hygiene OR serious suicidal act with clear expectation of death.
0	Inadequate information.

From American Psychiatric Association: *Diagnostic and statistical manual of mental disorders,* ed 4, Washington, DC, 1994, The Association.

physical status was stabilized. The clinic nurse believed it would be impossible for Al to surmount all of these problems and take the cruise within the next month.

When Al came to the office to have his blood drawn for liver studies for his Depakote administration, he asked, "I must be well enough to go on my cruise by next month." The nurse saw the opening and began asking astute questions: "What is happening now between you and your wife?" "How far can you comfortably walk now without shortness of breath?" "What will be required of you on the cruise?" "What will you do if you have a problem while cruising?" "Are you worried about another seizure?" Gently helping Al consider the specifics of his situation may help him begin to accept the reality.

Projection. Projection is present when the individual attributes his or her own unacceptable feelings, impulses, or thoughts to another. Fear, anxiety, and anger accompanying uncertainty about one's situation are often not perceived as part of one's repertoire of feelings but rather are projected onto others with whom one comes in contact. The most common projection of elders is rejection of others who are aged or

Box 23-2 Inventory of Psychogeriatric Client: Function and Care Plan

1. **List client's strengths:**
   - Ability to take initiative in caring for self, finances, work project
   - Ability to express feelings
   - Ability to stand up for his or her rights
   - Ability to make decisions
   - Ability to care for self; for example, dressing, going to meals
   - Ability to share with others or show concern for others
   - Enjoyment of music and arts
   - Active participation in organizations
   - Interest in sports
   - Enjoyment of reading
   - Imagination and creativity
   - Special aptitudes; for example, mechanical ability, gardening
2. **Identify predominant defensive coping styles:**
   - Denial
   - Projection
   - Displacement
   - Passive aggression
   - Positive identification
3. **Identify highly adaptive coping styles:**
   - Affiliation
   - Altruism
   - Humor
   - Self-assertion
   - Sublimation
4. **Identify defensive breakdown patterns:**
   - Delusional projection
   - Psychotic suspiciousness
   - Psychotic denial
   - Immobilizing fears
   - Psychotic distortions
   - Apathetic withdrawal
5. **Determine client needs and problems based on:**
   - Reason for seeking assistance by patient, family, and others
   - Medical history and findings (physical, mental, neurologic, and psychologic examinations and tests)
   - Drug use profile (use of prescribed and nonprescribed drugs)
   - Laboratory and diagnostic tests
   - Psychiatric history
   - Social history
   - Mental status
   - Other background information provided by patient, family, and each staff person who has interviewed the patient
6. **Develop a nursing care plan considering:**
   - Patient's problems, needs, and strengths
   - Mutually identified short-term goals
   - Mutually identified long-term goals
7. **State expected outcome of care in terms that can be measured. The following are examples of goals stated in measurable terms:**
   - Socializes more
   - Dresses appropriately—puts on coat or jacket when going outside in cold weather
   - Improves personal hygiene—brushes teeth daily without being reminded
   - Shows improvement in problem areas
   - Improves attitude—discusses problems or concerns instead of hitting or resisting
   - Increases functional independence
   - Reduces hostility—responds when spoken to in a friendly manner
   - Improves self-esteem—goes 1 day without self-criticism
   - Reduces depression—expresses interest in one outside activity
   - States increased enjoyment of activities
   - Reduces suspiciousness—eats a meal without expressing fear of poisoning
8. **Review progress periodically and revise goals as necessary and appropriate.**

disabled, for example, "You won't catch me at the senior center with all those old fogeys. All they do is complain about their illnesses—an organ recital I call it."

Altruism. Altruism is a highly valuable defense against meaninglessness. Elders often become involved in helping others or dedicating their efforts to a good cause. The individual is gratified by the appreciation of others and by personal satisfaction. Laura volunteers to take school children on nature walks. The clear observations and unique views of these children restore her youth as she teaches them and as they all commune with nature. We find this attribute one of the transcendent mechanisms and prefer to categorize it as quite beyond a defense mechanism.

Displacement. Displacement of feelings onto the intentions of others is quite common. The aged often become suspicious of others' intentions toward them because the older person may be quite vulnerable. Rather than feeling the vulnerability or precariousness of their existence, elders may be wary and untrusting of others. This suspicion may progress to a pathologic paranoia and feelings that specific people are biased against them. The initial perceptions are often reality based. For example, one old man would not allow his wife to go anywhere without him because he feared other men would seduce her. He had no realization that this fear is related to his own impotence.

Passive Aggression. Passive aggression is used when outright aggression would be dangerous or unacceptable to self-concept or others' opinions. Elders who are feeling unable or unwilling to carry out expectations of others commonly use passive aggression. Compliance is often a mask for resentment and hostility.

Mary, widowed last year, is expected to move into the cottage her son is having built for her on his property. She does not want to leave the community where her long-time friends are, and she does not like her son's wife. Mary continues to agree with his proposal but quietly resists sorting out the things in her home, always feels ill, and refuses to be available when the real estate agent wants to show her home. In addition, Mary never calls back when her daughter-in-law leaves telephone messages regarding the plans they need to make.

Positive Identification. Positive identification is not listed among the defensive mechanisms in the DSM-IV, but it appears to be a healthy coping activity. Some aged individuals in poor health identify with others who are more physically and psychologically intact, and because of this identification, these elders appraise themselves as more able. Positive identification seems to be a process embodying both hope and affiliation. If Bob Hope or George Burns could be clever, rich, and functional at their ages, then the elder can claim their success through cohort affiliation. These successful people were contemporaries and make the elder feel more effective because of affiliation with the respect they generated.

All of us use defensive strategies, some quite conscious and others that are far beyond our awareness. The more vulnerable we become, the more these defenses are needed. If the individual is maintaining sufficient supports and life satisfactions in the situation he or she is in, let us not disturb the balance, no matter how precarious. Shore up the foundations of strength.

PSYCHIATRIC DISORDERS OF AGING

The incidence of psychiatric disorders in old age has been studied since the 1950s and has shown a rather consistent prevalence rate of 15% to 25% in people over 65 years of age. These data reflect a conglomerate of disorders. Cognitive changes and psychiatric disturbances often go hand-in-hand in aging, but because they are so frequently considered synonymous, we have separated them for more accurate and precise understanding.

Adjustment Disorders

Adjustment disorders are diagnosed when one develops significant emotional or behavioral responses to an identifiable psychosocial stress or stressors (APA, 1994). Clinical significance is noted when the distress that the elder exhibits is in excess of that expected by the nature of the stressor (Box 23-3). The stressors may be single or multiple, recurrent or continuous, and some are more prominent than others in certain developmental periods, such as a move into a dependent situation, which is many elders must confront.

Assessing excessive emotional reactions to certain adjustments required of the aged may be difficult because personality, gender, and cultural factors must be considered, as well as the availability of supportive relationships. Adjustment disorders may be exhibited by profound depression, with or without anxiety, and behavioral disturbances.

Nursing interventions should include anticipatory rehearsal of the event and instigation of a reliable and ongoing support system available to the individual before and after the occurrence. In addition, options and alternatives related to the particular adjustment should be thoroughly discussed and considered, which will reduce the sense of helplessness and irreversibility.

George had all of his teeth removed and both upper and lower dentures put in place in one day. The analgesics made him nauseated, pain kept him awake, and he lost interest in food. These not unusual occurrences continued to be a focus of attention and complaint for him for several months. Whenever anyone said, "How are you?" George would go into a litany about his teeth. Insomnia and weight

Box 23-3 Diagnostic Criteria for Adjustment Disorders

A. The development of emotional or behavioral symptoms in response to an identifiable stressor(s) occurring within 3 months of the onset of the stressor(s).
B. These symptoms or behaviors are clinically significant as evidenced by either of the following:
   (1) Marked distress that is in excess of what would be expected from exposure to the stressor
   (2) Significant impairment in social or occupational (academic) functioning
C. The stress-related disturbance does not meet the criteria for another specific axis I disorder and is not merely an exacerbation of a preexisting axis I or axis II disorder.
D. The symptoms do not represent bereavement.
E. Once the stressor (or its consequences) has terminated, the symptoms do not persist for more than an additional 6 months.

Specify if:
Acute: if the disturbance lasts less than 6 months
Chronic: if the disturbance lasts for 6 months or longer

Source: American Psychiatric Association: *Diagnostic and statistical manual of mental disorders,* ed 4, Washington, DC, 1994, The Association.

loss became serious problems, and he became increasingly nonfunctional.

When the complaints persisted for several months, and after many visits to the dentist because the teeth "didn't fit properly," the prosthodontist recognized an extreme adjustment reaction and referred George for a psychiatric consult. The geriatric NP who saw George convinced him to accompany her to the senior center, which he had previously avoided because of "all the old folks there." The NP introduced him to some of the elders in her caseload who attended the center's meals and activities. Fortunately, the NP was able to establish a tentative relationship between George and a lady who had experienced similar difficulties adjusting to dentures. Much later, George told the NP that she had literally saved his life. He found others who had been as distressed as he was about adjusting to dentures, and he established a friendship with the lady to whom he had first been introduced. To avoid such an intense adjustment, there should have been much preparatory work and discussion of options by George and his dentist and sufficient time elapsed to incorporate the idea of this major change in appearance, self-perception, and sensual pleasure.

Anxiety Reactions

A general definition for anxiety is unpleasant and unwarranted feelings of apprehension, which may be accompanied by physical symptoms (Frohberg and Herting, 1999). Anxiety itself is a normal human reaction and part of a fear response; it is rational, within reason. Anxiety becomes problematic when it is prolonged, exaggerated, and begins to interfere with function. Anxiety states are not as common in elders as they are in younger adults (Reuben et al, 2002). When new onset of anxiety occurs, it is usually related to a physical illness, depression, side effects of medications, or a withdrawal of a medication.

The DSM-IV recognizes many anxiety disorders; the most common one in elderly people is anxiety disorder resulting from a general medical condition (GAD) (Reuben et al, 2002). This type of anxiety occurs in almost 5% of community-living elders (Beers and Berkow, 2000). The criteria for GAD are listed in Box 23-4. Anxiety disorders that occur in older people include phobic disorder, obsessive-compulsive disorder, and panic disorders. Some of the medical disorders that cause anxiety responses include cardiac arrhythmias, delirium, depression, dementia (probably the most common cause of anxiety), hyperthyroidism, hypoglycemia, postural hypotension, pulmonary edema, and pulmonary emboli. Drugs that cause anxiety reactions are anticholinergics, caffeine, beta-blockers, corticosteroids, and over-the-counter drugs such as appetite suppressants, ephedrine, nicotine, and pseudoephedrine. Withdrawal from alcohol, sedatives, and hypnotics will cause symptoms of anxiety. In other cases, precipitants of anxiety reactions may be obscure and difficult to identify. Disturbances in daily routine or ritual that form the basis of security and control may be trigger events for anxiety reactions. One elderly man said with agitation, "If I can just have my newspaper in the morning and find out what's going on in the world, then I can get moving."

Box 23-4 Criteria for GAD

- Excess worry and anxiety about many things more often than not for more than 6 months.
- Inability or difficulty controlling the worry and anxiety
- Worry and anxiety associated with 3 or more of the following:
  - Muscle tension
  - Irritability
  - Difficulty concentrating; mind going blank
  - Sleep disturbances
  - Easily fatigued
  - Restless, on edge
- Worry and anxiety focus about routine life situations, circumstances that may shift from one concern to another
- Worry and anxiety not due to physical effects of drug abuse or medication, or to a medical condition and does not occur during a mood disorder or psychotic disorder

Support Efforts. When dealing with anxiety reactions, look for daily disturbances such as staff or caregiver changes, room changes, and other events over which the individual feels a lack of control or influence. By themselves, these circumstances seldom provoke an anxiety reaction, but they may be the "straw that breaks the camel's back." Anxiety embodies an overwhelming sense of being out of control of one's life and destiny. Restoring the individual's sense of influence as quickly as possible is critical. Discuss feelings and actions that can be taken. In a room change, for instance, how can the individual be alerted in sufficient time to incorporate the idea? How can the new room be personalized? Is there a choice of rooms? We can assist by focusing attention away from the body and onto feelings and problem solving.

A good relationship should exist between the patient and the care provider. An accurate diagnosis needs to be made. Clinical signs that suggest an anxiety reaction include restlessness, edginess, fatigue, difficulty concentrating, irritability, tension, and sleep disturbances. Anxiety is often concomitant with depression. When comorbid conditions are present, they both (or all) need to be treated. A review of medications is in order, thus the medications that cause anxiety may be eliminated. Providing a structured environment may alleviate anxiety in a mildly demented patient. In a cognitively alert patient, cognitive-behavioral therapy is effective, usually in conjunction with medication. Drugs that have been found to be especially useful in elderly anxious patients are paroxetine and venlafaxine (Reuben et al, 2002). Intermediate half-life benzodiazepines are also used; lorazepam and oxazepam are recommended for short-term therapy.

Posttraumatic Stress Disorder

Posttraumatic stress disorder (PTSD) has become a part of our national vocabulary and reminds us of the deep and lasting toll that national disasters take. PTSD was early recognized as an outcome of overwhelmingly stressful experiences of individuals in the war in Vietnam. Only recently realized is that many World War II veterans have lived the majority of their lives under the shadow of PTSD without it being recognized. Seniors under our care now have also experienced the Great Depression, the holocaust, racism, and the Korea conflict (Kennedy, 2001). Now, we know from community surveys that PTSD is fairly common, occurs increasingly in women, and has a lifetime prevalence of 7% to 12% (Culpepper, 2000). The likelihood that a specific trauma will result in long-lived PTSD in women is capped with rape, then child abuse, then being threatened with a weapon, molested, neglected as a child, and physical violence. For men, the greatest trauma is also rape, followed by abuse as a child, neglect as a child, combat, and being molested. The major traumas that occur by frequency in the elderly population are listed in Box 23-5.

According to the DSM-IV, PTSD (recognized by the DSM over 20 years ago) is a syndrome characterized by the development of symptoms following an extremely traumatic event, which involves experiencing, witnessing, or unexpectedly hearing about an actual or threatened death or serious injury to oneself or another closely affiliated person. Individuals often reexperience the traumatic event in episodes of fear and experience symptoms such as helplessness, flashbacks, intrusive thoughts, memories, images, emotional numbing, loss of interest, avoidance of any place that reminds of the traumatic event, startle reactions, poor concentration, irritability, jumpiness, and hypervigilance (Culpepper, 2000). These episodes may occur periodically for years, though they frequently remain submerged until activated by the losses of aging. These individuals may have ongoing sleep problems, somatic disturbances, anxiety, depression, and restlessness. Over the long term, these people are typically impaired in work, have maladaptive lifestyles, and do not develop close relationships.

Ernie may have had PTSD, though it was only speculative following his suicide. On his eighteenth birthday, Ernie joined the U.S. Army Air Corps (precedent to our present U.S. Air Force) in 1941. He was quickly trained and sent to Burma to "fly the hump," the Himalayan mountains in Burma, China, and India. During his 3-year stint, Ernie survived two airplane crashes, saw several of his companions mutilated in crashes, watched the torture of captured Japanese, and witnessed the capture of some of his friends. When Ernie returned to the United States, his hair had turned from deep auburn to pure white. He retired from the service after 20 years but was never really able to work after his retirement. Ernie's life was filled with episodes of alcoholic binges, outbursts of anger, and episodes of abusing others, all seemingly quite out of his control. One friend remained from his "service" days and visited him periodically until his death in 1996. Other relationships seemed to have been superficial and to have had little meaning for Ernie. On his seventy-eighth birthday, which he spent alone, Ernie shot himself. One must wonder how many of the aged veterans of World War II, the most highly suicidal group in the United States, are suffering from PTSD.

Box 23-5 Major Traumas and Injuries Causing Death in Elderly People

- Motor vehicle crashes
- Firearms
- Suffocation
- Falls

CDC: *Aging Trends*, March 2001, Available at *www.cdc.gov/nchs/agingact.htm*.

Support Efforts. PTSD prevention and treatment is only now getting the research attention that other illnesses have received over the years (Culpepper, 2000). The care of the individual with PTSD involves awareness that certain events may trigger inappropriate reactions, and the pattern of these reactions should be identified when possible. The terrorist attacks of September 11, 2001 resurrected memories of past losses for many older adults (Kennedy, 2001), and they relived their grief. These individuals may have experienced fear and sadness and not realized it. Emotions may have been expressed with rage that was irrationally directed at loved ones or caregivers. Fear and unwarranted suspicions may have caused elders to avoid contact with others and become secluded, with a false sense of protection. Gary Kennedy, then president elect of the American Association for Geriatric Psychiatry, offers suggestions for supporting the elder (Box 23-6). Although many elders may be crippled by new traumatic events, others will "rise to the occasion" and perform chance acts of kindness and resilience (Kennedy, 2001). Cognitive-behavioral therapy with pharmacologic therapy will be useful for supporting the patient through PTSD (Culpepper, 2000). Sertraline is the only medication that the U.S. Food and Drug Administration (FDA) has approved to treat PTSD. Trials have been conducted with low-dose fluoxetine that demonstrate improvement in symptoms and function (Culpepper, 2000). Nursing supports also include humor distraction, teaching relaxation techniques, back massage, support groups with guided imagery, therapeutic touch, and information provided to family members (Moorhead and Brighton, 2001).

Obsessive-Compulsive Disorders

Obsessive-compulsive disorder (OCD) is characterized by recurrent and persistent thoughts, impulses, or images (obsessions) that are repetitive, purposeful, and intentional urge or ritualistic behaviors (compulsions) that improve comfort level but are recognized as excessive and unreasonable. These behaviors may seem weird or nasty or horrible (Beers and Berkow, 2000). OCD is an anxiety disorder that significantly impairs function and consumes more than 1 hour each day

Box 23-6 Guidelines for Nursing Care of Suspicious Patients

Remember that anger is pervasive and is not meant for the nurse per se.
Anger is a legitimate expression of feeling.
Suspicious patients will look for flaws or indications of injustice.
Attempt to accept criticism without resentment or defensiveness.
Arguing only increases the struggle for control.
The quality of nursing care may not be measurable by patient progress, particularly if the goals are unrealistic or not relevant to the patient. In other words, paranoia may lift slowly or not at all.
Nursing care should provide for the following needs:

1. Suspicious patients need to learn to trust themselves. Allow the patient to function independently in areas in which success can be achieved and identified.
2. Suspicious patients need to be able to trust others. Nurses should state what they are willing and able to do. Vague promises such as, "I'll be around whenever you need me," only increase opportunities for distrust and disappointment.
3. Suspicious patients need to test reality. When the larger reality is distorted, focus on smaller aspects of reality, for example:
   Mrs. J: The whole world is against me.
   Nurse: What in this room gives you that feeling? Are there certain times when you feel that most strongly?
   Contact with the nurse and her accepting responses reassure the person and decrease the need for a protective delusion.
4. Suspicious persons need outlets for their anger.

(APA, 1994). OCD is common among elderly people, seems to have a genetic component, and occurs mainly in women. The identifying symptom of compulsive hand washing is not common in older adults. These disorders are exaggerated manifestations of a need for control and order and a way of warding off anxiety. Often in elderly people, symptoms are not sufficient to seriously disrupt function and thus may not truly be considered a disorder but rather a coping strategy. If symptoms progress to a point at which they disrupt lifestyle, the elder will need clinical attention.

In the aged, these disorders are often displayed as obsessions about body functions and morbid fears. The compulsive rituals that accompany these thoughts are an effort to ward off anxiety and discharge tension. In the process of carrying out these tension-relief behaviors, the individual may ignore important aspects of life.

Interestingly, the one most consuming compulsive disorder I have observed was related to the control of clocks. One lady had numerous clocks with alarms set for different times of day and night. In dealing with her, staff members considered the symbolic significance of clocks and time and death from an existential perspective. The elder was gradually weaned, one clock at a time, and other gratifying activities were introduced into her schedule, one at a time, and on a precise timetable that staff assured her would not vary. She was also shown her chart to show that she was checked each half hour at night to be sure she was all right.

Another common OCD issue, with both obsessive and compulsive components, is that of bowel management. Jim moved in with his daughter's family and distressed the household with his endless talk about his bowel function and continual preoccupation with the rituals of medications, laxatives, and prune juice. If his prune juice was not available, Jim became extremely upset. His concern about bowel function literally dominated his life and obscured the pleasure that might be encountered living within his daughter's family. Discussing the annoyance that an obsessive-compulsive individual produces or attempting to interrupt the behavior is seldom helpful. In this case, nurses may be most helpful in assisting the family and Jim to talk about the stresses for Jim and the family, related to the move, and to develop a plan that will allow the family and Jim certain privileges and areas of control within the household. As all parties involved feel more secure in the new relationship, the obsessive-compulsive coping style should diminish in intensity.

Support. As in other anxiety disorders, cognitive-behavioral therapy has been shown to be effective in managing OCD along with pharmacologic therapy. Sertraline, paroxetine, fluoxetine, and fluvoxamine are recommended (Reuben et al, 2002). Antipsychotic drugs are not prescribed unless symptoms progress to delusions or other signs of psychosis (Beers and Berkow, 2000).

Substance Abuse and Addictions

Alcohol. Substance abuse often arises in old age as a coping mechanism to deal with loss, anxiety, depression, or boredom. Although alcohol alleviates the distress temporarily in some situations, it may create more problems in carrying out social roles. Alcohol-related problems in the elderly often go unrecognized, though the residual effects of alcohol abuse complicate the presentation and treatment of many chronic disorders of the aged. In the general population, abuse of alcohol is readily recognized because of social and work problems; however, elders may not come under observation as frequently and may essentially "hide out" when they are drinking. Estimates suggest that between 2% and 17% of elders over age 60 have alcohol abuse and dependence (Beers and Berkow, 2000; Brown, Bedford, and White, 1999). Box 23-7 shows the *Healthy People 2010* objectives related to alcohol abuse (U.S. Department Health and Human Services, 2000).

A common belief is that the prevalence of alcohol abuse will increase in elders; more middle-aged adults are at risk because alcohol, in this cohort, has been used throughout their

Box 23-7 Healthy People 2010 Objectives Related to Alcohol Abuse

- Reduce deaths and injury caused by alcohol- or drug-related motor vehicle crashes.
- Reduce number of cirrhosis deaths.
- Reduce alcohol-related hospital emergency department visits.
- Reduce intentional injuries resulting from alcohol-related violence.
- Reduce number of people engaging in binge drinking of alcohol.
- Reduce average annual alcohol consumption.
- Reduce number of adults who exceed guidelines for low-risk drinking.
- Reduce the treatment gap for alcohol problems.
- Increase number of people referred for followup care for alcohol problems.

From U.S. Department of Health and Human Services: *Healthy people 2010,* Washington, DC, 2000, USDHHS. Also available at *www.health.gov/healthypeople.*

lives (Kennedy-Malone, Fletcher, and Plank, 2000). In the present cohort, the prevalence of drinking declines after age 65 (Beers and Berkow, 2000). Reasons include lower lifetime drinking habits than predecessors; female-to-male ratio increases with age, and women drink less; declining health and functional impairments lead to decreased alcohol intake; and alcohol-related illnesses and injuries prevent many from surviving to old age. Men are four times more likely to abuse alcohol than women. Easterners are more likely to abuse alcohol than mid-westerners. In Boston, 70% of elders report drinking in the previous year, and in Iowa, 46% reported drinking alcohol (Beers and Berkow, 2000). Further, the prevalence of elders with alcohol dependence is high in the health care setting—10% to 21% of hospitalized elders and 3% to 49% of nursing home residents. The rate of alcohol-related hospitalizations is higher than it is for myocardial infarction. Elders who are chronically ill are less likely to drink excessively than those who are independent and more socially active.

Physiology. Older people develop higher blood alcohol levels because of age-related changes (increased body fat, decreased lean body mass, and total body water content) that alter absorption and distribution of alcohol (Beers and Berkow, 2000). The liver's ability to metabolize alcohol diminishes with age, and susceptibility to psychomotor effects of alcohol may increase with age. A known fact is that light to moderate drinking is associated with better health, especially in decreased cardiovascular disease. However, more than two drinks a day increases the risk of adverse effects. Elderly who drink to excess are susceptible to cognitive decline, physical decline, functional decline, and increased risk for injury.

Drug Effects. Many drugs that elders use for chronic illnesses cause adverse effects when combined with alcohol. Some drugs can increase alcohol levels by 30% to 40%; cimetidine is one commonly used drug that produces this increase, as are sedatives (Kennedy-Malone, Fletcher, and Plank, 2000). Some drugs suppress central nervous system function, especially benzodiazepines (Beers and Berkow, 2000), and may impair balance, precipitating falls. Acetaminophen taken on a regular basis, when combined with alcohol, may lead to liver failure. Alcohol diminishes the effects of oral hypoglycemics, anticoagulants, and anticonvulsants (Kennedy-Malone, Fletcher, and Plank, 2000). Other effects of alcohol in older people include urinary incontinence, which results from rapid bladder filling, and diminished neuromuscular control of the bladder (Beers and Berkow, 2000). Other effects include gait disturbances from alcohol-caused cerebellar degeneration and peripheral neuropathy, depression and suicide, sleep disturbances and insomnia, and dementia or delirium.

Assessment. Most primary care providers do not diagnose alcohol abuse. A psychosocial assessment should include a mental status examination, the CAGE questionnaire, consisting of four questions, commonly used and thought to be reliable, but seems a bit judgmental. The basic ideas have been incorporated in Box 23-8 in what we believe is a more acceptable form. A geriatric depression scale should be performed, as well as a cultural assessment. Diagnostic tests should include a complete blood count (CBC), liver function tests, chemistries, and an electrocardiogram.

Support. The goal should be abstinence or sobriety; if the patient is in need of withdrawal, hospitalization should be considered. Alcoholics Anonymous should be consulted because it is the most successful group in bringing about sobriety. Antabuse, a drug to help maintain abstinence in healthy patients, is a consideration. Multivitamins and folic acid, magnesium, and thiamine should be strongly considered. The patient should be seen on a regular basis to support continuity and the goals of therapy. The caregiver should watch for gastrointestinal bleeding, malnutrition, cognitive decline, and withdrawal symptoms. Cirrhosis is a problem if the addiction is continued.

Elderly individuals who are abusers of one drug are more likely to be addicted to others. However, using illegal drugs is uncommon among older adults (Beers and Berkow, 2000). Prescribed anxiolytics or other psychoactive drugs may be misused. Nicotine, more common than alcohol abuse, and caffeine may also be misused by the elderly person. Unexplained gastrointestinal, psychologic, or metabolic problems may be signs of the abuse of over-the-counter products.

Many of the traditional ways of dealing with alcoholism have a punitive sound, for example, "Have you ever thought you were drinking too much?" A far more productive approach is to discuss the issue factually. For example, "Many elders find that the stresses, loneliness, and losses of aging are very hard to bear. Some retreat into alcohol use as a way of

Box 23-8 Questions Regarding Abuse of Alcohol

Are you upset when people criticize your drinking? How do you handle that?
Do you believe that you sometimes drink too much? Are there particular occasions when that occurs?
Do you feel disturbed about your alcohol consumption?
Do you drink when you are feeling lonely?
Have you identified a pattern regarding your drinking?
Would you like to stop drinking?

coping. There are treatments and groups that assist individuals in these difficult adjustments. If this is a problem for you or if it becomes a problem, please let us know so we may provide resources or referrals for you." Elders are likely to feel excessively guilty and regretful about alcohol misuse, and reaching out to them with understanding is important. The notion that alcoholism is a genetic or metabolic disorder that can be cured only by a return to God may be useful to some, but we find elders are also responsive to activity enrichment and group support. Several pharmacologic choices are available for dealing with alcohol abuse in addition to cognitive-behavioral therapy and inpatient therapy. Disulfiram is one medication that has been used for a long time, though it is not very effective and has many side effects. Naltrexone is another medication that has been useful as an adjunct to psychosocial therapies (Reuben et al, 2002).

Risks of alcohol and medication mixtures have not been sufficiently emphasized with most elders. A primary goal of geriatric nurse practitioners should be prevention through the education of the provider community, families, and elders about these risks.

Suspicion and Paranoia

Many older people without a history of mental disturbance develop a suspicious or paranoid viewpoint. Various estimates of the prevalence of paranoia range from 5% to 10% of the aged population. Alcoholism or medications, particularly male hormones in combination with antidepressants, can induce these reactions. Paranoia is an early symptom of Alzheimer's disease, appearing approximately 20 months before diagnosis, usually after social withdrawal, depression, and suicide ideation, but before anxiety. Memory loss and forgetfulness may result in an elder being convinced that items are being stolen or that medications are not the correct ones. Fear and a lack of trust originating from a reality base may become magnified, especially when one is isolated from others and from reality feedback. The dynamics seem to be loss of control, inability to evaluate the social milieu appropriately, with the feeling of external forces controlling one's life, which in many instances is true. In addition to these dynamics, an unknown number of elders has a paranoid personality disorder that has simply grown old and more pronounced. These individuals have had a pervasive distrust and suspiciousness of others' motives all of their adult life, assuming that others will harm, exploit, or even deceive them, though they have no basis to support these beliefs (APA, 1994).

Drug intoxication, physical illness, and postoperative psychosis in the intensive care unit are usually transient and different from delirium (Beers and Berkow, 2000) in that they are more organized and elaborate. Although the acute situation must be managed, the treatment is usually resolution of the medical problem or environment or situation.

Paranoia is characterized by suspiciousness and insecurity. Deafness or hearing impairment may accentuate these feelings. Delusions often begin outside the home but move inside the home such that creaking noises in the attic can take on suspicious meaning. Many cases have been encountered in which plots against an older person were real. In the case of simple paranoia, the delusions appear to serve an adaptive function. When an individual becomes incapable of obtaining life's satisfactions or of maintaining function or adequate supplies, the delusions may allow the individual to avoid depression and self-blame and maintain self-esteem by projecting blame onto others or society.

Assessment and Treatment. Direct confrontation is likely to increase agitation, a sense of vulnerability, and the need for the delusion; it may also disrupt the relationship. A more useful approach is to establish a trusting, supportive relationship that is nondemanding and to identify the client's strengths and build on them (see Box 23-6). The nurse should demonstrate respect for the patient and be willing to listen to complaints and fears (Beers and Berkow, 2000). The nurse should not pretend to agree with the paranoid beliefs, but rather ask to understand what is troubling to the patient. Clear information should be given, and clear choices should always be presented to the patient. When offering food, medication, treatments, or resources, relevant information should be given. When patients refuse *necessary* treatments, their decision must be respected. Focusing on decision-making power is most likely to be beneficial. For example, "Mrs. S., it seems you are reluctant to take these medications. I respect the fact that you are cautious about such things. I will get you more information about these drugs. Are there particular reactions you are concerned about? Let me know if you decide to take them"; or "Mrs. J., many people feel angry or afraid when they are ill. Is there anything I can do to make you more comfortable?" Other strategies include not arguing with the patient about disappearing items or trying to rationally explain them. The nurse should try reducing the number of hiding places available and checking wastebaskets before emptying. Whispering in the presence of the patient will increase suspiciousness and should be avoided. Keep an extra pair of glasses and hearing aid batteries available outside the patient's possessions (Brown, Bedford, and White, 1999).

Antipsychotic drugs are often needed for effective management (Beers and Berkow, 2000). The newest atypical antipsychotics (risperidone, olanzapine) are preferred for the suspicious or agitated elder because these drugs have few side effects.

Delusions

A delusional disorder is one in which conceivable ideas, without foundation in fact, persist for more than 1 month. These beliefs are not always bizarre and do not originate in psychotic processes (APA, 1994). Common delusions are of being poisoned, being followed, of their children taking their assets, being held prisoner, or being deceived by a spouse or lover. Delusional disorders in the absence of psychoses usually begin at age 25, with an average at age 40, but continue on into old age. Delusions are intellectual mechanisms for maintaining a sense of control when security is threatened. Delusions are beliefs that guide the individual's interpretation of events and help make sense out of disorder. The delusions may be comforting or threatening but always form a structure for understanding situations that might otherwise seem unmanageable. One old lady persistently held onto the delusion that her son was coming to pick her up and take her home, although her son had been dead for 10 years. The events of her day, her hopes, and her status were all organized around this belief. Clearly, without her delusion, she would have felt forlorn, lost, and abandoned. I have encountered many delusions related to family members and their actions or intentions among the institutionalized aged. As the population ages, encounters with elders with delusions will increase. One study found that 21% of 125 new nursing home residents had delusions (Grossberg, 2000).

The assessment dilemma is often one of determining the truth of the delusional belief and avoiding assumptions. Concluding that someone is delusional is never safe, unless you have thoroughly investigated his or her claims. In one case, an elderly man insisted that he must go and visit his mother. His thoughts seemed clear in other respects (as is often the case with people who are delusional), and I suspected that he had some unresolved conflicts about his dead mother or felt the need of comforting and caring. I did not argue with him about his dead mother, because arguing is never a useful approach to people with delusions. Rather, I used the best techniques I was able to recall to assure him that I was interested in him as a person and recognized that he must feel very lonely sometimes. He continued to say he must leave and go to his mother. When I was unable to delay his leaving no longer, I walked with him to the nurses' station and found that his 103-year-old mother did indeed live in another wing of the institution, and he visited her every day.

Frightening delusions such as those that the world is coming to an end or that one is being poisoned are usually in response to anxiety-provoking situations and are best handled by reducing situational stress, being available to the client, and attending to the fears more than the content of the delusion. Other suggestions are to avoid television, which can be confusing, especially if the patient awakens and finds it on. Additionally, reduce clutter in the patient's room, eliminate large mirrors, and eliminate shadows that can appear threatening (Brown, Bedford, and White, 1999).

Hallucinations

Hallucinations are best described as sensory perceptions of a nonexistent object stimulus and may be spurred by the internal stimulation of any of the five senses. Although not attributable to environmental stimuli, hallucinations may well occur because of the total environmental impact. Hallucinations arising out of psychologic conflicts tend to be less predominant in old age, and those that are generated as security measures tend to increase as the person ages. These hallucinations are thought to germinate in situations in which one is feeling alone, abandoned, isolated, or alienated. To compensate for insecurity, a hallucinatory experience, often a companion, is imagined. Imagined companions may fill the intense void and provide some security, but they may become accusing and disturbing.

The character and stages of hallucinatory experiences have not been adequately defined in terms of the aged. Many hallucinations are in response to physical disorders, such as dementias, Parkinson's disease, physiologic and sensory disorders, and medications. Hallucinations of the aged most often seem mixed with disorientation, illusions, intense grief, and immersion in retrospection, the origins being difficult to separate. Most psychotic states arising in late life are associated predominately with cognitive decline. One elderly lady I know, Florence, fell down her basement stairs, and when I visited her to check on her well being, I found her sitting in a chair in the basement, where she had been for more than 2 days. She was terrified, incontinent, dehydrated, and had a fractured pelvis. She was completely unaware of any physical discomfort, despite what we found to be a severe fracture. She believed a man was watching her from the basement shadows, thus she was afraid to move. This hallucination completely resolved after she was well again, and she has not had a hallucination in the years since this incident.

Determining whether the hallucinations are the result of dementia, psychoses, deprivation, or overload is important for nurses because the treatment will vary. An isolated old person who is admitted to the hospital in a hallucinatory state must be carefully and thoroughly assessed physically and then gradually brought into socializing experiences. He or she should be allowed peripheral participation and retreat when necessary. Individuals in the community who develop hallucinations must be assessed in terms of threats to security, severe physical or psychologic disruptions, withdrawal symptoms, medications, and overload of stimuli. These individuals will need a subdued environment with staff continuity and availability, and comprehensive assessment and care. Psychotropic medications are a significant aspect of management for most hallucinations, although in cases such as that with Florence, managing the physical illness and changing the environment will eliminate the hallucinations without pharmacologic management.

Schizophrenia

Approximately 1% to 2% of people in the United States have schizophrenia. However, although we are unable to find data on the number of elders with this disease, apparently, it almost never occurs *de novo* in elderly people (Heaton et al, 2001). Nonetheless, a sizeable minority of people first show signs of schizophrenia in middle age or old age (Omnicare Formulary, 2002). Schizophrenia may be categorized as late onset (over age 40) or very late onset (over age 60). Furthermore, the rate of suicide in younger patients (middle age) with schizophrenia is nearly three times the rate in comparable people without the illness (Brown, 2001) and do not reach old age. Symptoms of schizophrenia are categorized into positive and negative symptoms. Elders with schizophrenia seem to exhibit primarily positive symptoms, such as memory and speech disturbances, blunted affect, impaired impulse control, combativeness, agitation, hallucinations, and delusions of persecution (Antai-Otong, 2000). Patients with positive symptoms usually have a better treatment outcome compared with those with negative symptoms, such as lack of motivation and spontaneity, impoverished speech, and loss of initiative. Diagnosing psychotic disorders is important to differentiate them from other behavioral disorders because the management is different (Beers and Berkow, 2000). Approximately 10% of demented patients with behavior disorder, and even a higher percentage in nursing homes, show signs of psychosis. Grossberg (2000) found that between 33% and 50% of elderly patients with Alzheimer's disease or dementia develop psychotic symptoms, and 63% to 67% develop delusions or hallucinations.

Theories suggest that many elderly people who are homeless may have chronic schizophrenia; discharged from state hospitals years ago after spending their young adulthood institutionalized, they were simply unable to develop satisfactory living situations. Other elderly people who have schizophrenia and take medication can maintain an adequate lifestyle in the community. When an individual's condition deteriorates and medication reevaluation is needed, hospitalization may be required.

Assessment. Every patient presenting with psychosis should be evaluated for depression, suicidal and homicidal risk, extrapyramidal effects (if they have been taking antipsychotic drugs), and for irreversible movement disorders such as tardive dyskinesia (TD) (Antai-Otong, 2000). The abnormal involuntary movement scale (AIMS) is useful for evaluating early symptoms of TD.

Support. Environmental intervention is the most successful, least expensive, and safest form of treatment (Beers, Berkow, 2000). Behaviors that are appropriate should be supported, maintaining the safety of the patient. Doors should have alarms and locks, floors should be marked (with stripes) to indicate areas to avoid, and signs that the patient can see should direct him or her to the dining room or toilet. Sexual activity is being allowed and even supported in many long-term care facilities today. However, protection must be in place for residents, as well as staff members, who do not wish to participate. Couples can be given rooms together, even double beds, if desired.

Physical activity is important to help avoid emotional or physical outbursts and to promote sleep without drugs (Beers and Berkow, 2000). Getting to know patients well helps the nursing staff know what kinds of cues the patient gives before a burst of agitation; sometimes pacing the floor is a precipitant to an outburst. Drugs are used when the environmental changes are not enough to maintain a safe and tolerable milieu. Sedatives-hypnotics are often used to help the resident sleep. Antidepressants may be given if signs of depression are exhibited. Antipsychotics are given for problem behaviors. Lorazepam and risperidone are given intramuscularly for an acute behavioral problem (Antai-Otong, 2000). Some evidence suggests that beta-blockers, such as propranolol and the drug, carbamazepine, an anticonvulsant, are useful in treating elders with problem behaviors (Beers and Berkow, 2000). More recently, the addition of a mood-stabilizing agent, divalproex (Depakote), is valued as adjunctive therapy (Casey, 2001). At least 40% of elders who take antipsychotics long term will develop extrapyramidal symptoms (Beers and Berkow, 2000). TD occurs in as many as 31% after 43 weeks of neuroleptic (haloperidol, risperidone) therapy (Antai-Otong, 2000). Some new evidence indicates that vitamin B6 alleviates symptoms of TD without adverse effects (Lerner, 2001). However, in this study, when the vitamin was discontinued, the symptoms returned. The newer atypical antipsychotics (clozapine, olanzapine, quetiapine, ziprasidone, and risperidone) given in very low doses, are less likely to cause the irreversible effects of TD and seem to be more effective in very-late-onset schizophrenia (Omnicare Formulary, 2002). The drugs of choice for treatment of schizophrenia in elders as determined by an expert panel from the American Geriatric Society (AGS) are olanzapine and risperidone, and the unacceptable agents are chlorpromazine, mesoridazine, and thioridazine (Omnicare Formulary, 2002).

Bipolar Disorders

The essential features of bipolar I disorder are characterized by the experience of one or more manic episodes with or without an episode of depression (Beers, Berkow, 2000). Mania does occur in old age and may be an exacerbation of a previous disorder, a result of drug therapy (L-dopa, steroids), illness (encephalitic influenza), or head trauma. Bipolar II is characterized by clear-cut episodes of depression without episodes of mania. In many instances, dysfunction is not recognized because the periods of depression may not interfere with function. Bipolar disorders tend to decrease in the intensity of the extremes of depression and elation in the later years (National Institutes of Mental Health [NIMH], 2002) and the individual sinks more frequently into the depressive mode (NIMH, 2002). However, mania does occur in older adults and is a distinct period lasting at least 1 week during which an abnormally and persistent elevated, expansive, or irritable mood is exhibited (Beers and Berkow, 2000). Mania may resemble an agitated depression and be difficult to diagnose. The Geriatric Depression Scale and the Hamilton Depression Scale are useful tools for screening elders. However, a thorough history and physical examination is imperative in making a diagnosis. Thyroid dysfunction should always be part of the differential diagnosis.

Support. The standard treatment has been with lithium, though this medication may not be tolerated well, particularly in the elderly person. Irritable and aggressive people with diagnosed mania are least responsive to lithium treatment. Some of the symptoms that show in the manic stage of bipolar disorders include cognitive impairment, depressed symptoms, irritability and anger, mild confusional states, and paranoid delusions (Grossberg, 2000). Patients who have depressive disorders should be managed with concomitant antidepressants and antipsychotic therapy. Psychotic symptoms in a manic episode will need a mood-stabilizing agent such as lithium, carbamazepine, or valproic acid, either alone or with another antipsychotic drug. Delusions may respond to low-dose antipsychotic agents (Grossberg, 2000).

Commitment by the patient to the treatment regimen may be minimal because of insufficient understanding of the medications and inability to tolerate symptoms of the disease and side effects of the drugs. The patient needs relief from the most troublesome side effects of medication and can be encouraged to discuss these effects rather than simply accepting them. Medication management of an elder with manic episodes is often difficult, and individualizing medication dosages and monitoring lithium levels regularly is necessary. When lithium is ineffective or poorly tolerated, the anticonvulsant agents previously mentioned and calcium channel blockers may be better choices. Medications for the elderly with mania must be carefully prescribed, monitored, and adjusted.

Patient and family education is essential. The family must understand that the individual is not able to control mania and irritating behaviors because of a chemical imbalance in the brain. Family members also need a great deal of support and information (Tables 23-1 and 23-2).

Depression

Depression is one of the psychiatric illnesses appearing most frequently among the aged population, and it is still underdiagnosed. Estimates of prevalence vary radically depending on the qualitative variables being considered and the definition being used. Although estimates suggest that 6% of the population over age 65 meet the DSM-IV criteria for a major depressive disorder (NIMH, 2002), depression conditions of varying degrees in elderly patients is common. Although these patients do not fully meet the DSM-IV criteria for depression, many individuals who are considered depressed are equally severely distressed and often progress to major depression. Dysthymic disorder may be chronic, persistent, and moder-

Table 23-1 Factors in the Self-Management Process

	Self-management efforts		
Motivators	**Successful**	**Unsuccessful**	**Self-assessment parameters**
Wanting to live	Follow professional advice	Deny there is a problem	How you feel
Wanting mental wellness	Talk with people	Overextend self	Intervention frequency
	Take medication	Expect too much from misinformed	Common sense
Wanting to get along with others	Set goals	Stay to oneself	How people treat you
Wanting love	Follow schedule	Be open with family*	How you treat people
To become productive	Be prepared	Do street drugs	Positive results
To feel better about self	Stay active	Rely on others for information	Decreased hospital stay
To avoid problems in family	Seek information	Self-start and stop medication	Behavior
Self-love	Read	Let problems overwhelm	Able to manage daily activities
Because of barriers	Groups	Get angry	
Receiving help	Therapy	Watch TV all the time	
Finally knew what was wrong	Selective disclosure	Not coping with stress	
Costs (e.g., relationships, jobs)	Do not let things get to you	Not seeking help	
Duration of illness	Hospitalization	(A particular hospitalization)	
Symptoms		(A prison group)	
Being hospitalized			
Self-management not an option			

From Pollack LE: Inpatient self-management of bipolar disorder, *Appl Nurs Res* 9(2):71, 1996.
*An unsuccessful intervention for one person may be helpful for another in differing circumstances.

Table 23-2 Self-Management Information Needed for Bipolar Group Patients

Area of concern	Information needed
Understanding bipolar disorder	Education for self and others
	Importance of medication
	Importance of groups
	Importance of therapy
	How to deal with the disorder
	How to manage yourself
	Follow medical advice
	The need to get help
Managing daily life	Set goals
	Schedule self
	Seek support
	Manage stress
	Daily functioning
	Enjoy life
	Importance of exercise
Living in society	Stress management
	Money management
	Society reentry
Relating to others	Anger management
	Need for support
	Be self-aware and independent
Relating to self	Need for good self-esteem
	Avoid substances
	Think positively
	Take responsibility for your life
	Assess self
	Solve problems
	Help self
	Attend groups
	Seek spiritual strength
	Deal with situations
	Seek support
	Meditate
	Exercise mind and body

From Pollack LE: Inpatient self-management of bipolar disorder, *Appl Nurs Res* 9(2):71, 1996.

ately severe, with no clear onset, defined by DSM-IV as depressed mood with two more additional symptoms. These signs may be a sense of hopelessness, sleep problems, lethargy, and diminished appetite (Beers, Berkow, 2000). In older adults, these signs progress to long-term sadness without signs of psychosis (Sahr, 1999).

The presence of clinically significant depression in the community is from 8% to 15% and approximately 30% of institutionalized elderly residents. A significant morbidity and mortality goes hand-in-hand with depression in elders. People with depression will report increased levels of pain, diminished physical functioning, and increased number of days spent in bed (Sahr, 1999) compared with elders without depression but with arthritis, diabetes, or hypertension, which are risk factors for depression.

Etiologic Factors of Depression. Depression in the aged differs in several ways from that of younger adults. One of the major differences is the insidious manner in which depression develops and the concurrency with other events, which results in depression, frequently going unrecognized and untreated. Some researchers even attribute symptoms of depression to *aging*. In fact, the cause of depression in elders is biopsychosocial (Beers, Berkow, 2000). Some of the medical disorders that cause depression are cancers; cardiovascular disorders; endocrine disorders, such as thyroid problems; neurologic disorders, such as Alzheimer's disease, stroke, and Parkinson's disease; metabolic and nutritional disorders, such as vitamin-B_{12} deficiency and malnutrition; viral infections, such as herpes zoster and hepatitis; and elders with advanced macular degeneration, who have twice the prevalence of depression compared with the general population of older adults (Brown, 2001). Most of these conditions are primarily diseases of the aged. Some recent evidence demonstrates that low blood pressure is linked to depression (International Health News Database, 2001). In a study of 2700 elderly Mexicans, 55% had low diastolic blood pressure, or systolic blood pressure, or both. The subjects with hypotension were most likely to be depressed. The researchers believe that overtreatment of hypertension may result in depression. Other important factors of depression are alcohol abuse, some antihypertensive agents, guilt, negative though patterns, cognitive dysfunction, loss of a spouse or partner, loss of social supports, lower income level, and gender (depression occurs more often in women). Heredity is also a factor, especially in late life onset of depression (Beers and Berkow, 2000). In some instances, changes that are displayed on magnetic resonance images are thought to be related to vascular insufficiency. These depressions are called vascular depression.

Major depressive disorders in elderly people have been divided into subgroups. Psychotic subgroups seem to run in families (Sahr, 1999) and are likely to become bipolar. The melancholic subgroup can often be diagnosed as dementia and occurs with higher frequency in older adults. Seasonal onset depressions often occurs with the onset of the fall season, with improved depression in spring. Women who have had postpartum depression when young or middle aged may develop a bipolar disorder with age.

Age, Gender, and Ethnicity. Age and gender differences in incidence and expression of depression in very old age are important to consider. We do not yet know why women survive the ravages of aging better than men. In the young and middle adult years, women seek help for depression twice as frequently as men. By age 65, the gender gap of depression closes somewhat, though women still seek relief more quickly than men and may abuse medications more frequently so as to seek relief. Suicide statistics (discussed later in the chapter) indicate that significant age differences also exist in the frequency of depression among the very old, especially in older men in their 80s. Native Americans have very high rates of depression (Kennedy-Malone, Fletcher, and Plank, 2000). Elderly white men in the United States have the highest rates of suicide, although Asian Americans also have high rates.

Box 23-9 Most Frequent Problems in Late Life Caused by Depression

1. Social isolation, loss of important social support systems
2. Loss of autonomy (psychiatric and physical illness, physical disability)
3. Inactivity (retirement)
4. Loss of reputation, financial problems
5. Relocation of residence
6. Severe insomnia

From Müller-Spahn F, Hock C: Clinical presentation of depression in the elderly, *Gerontology* 40(suppl 1):10, 1994.

Social and Cultural Factors. Social and cultural factors influence the appearance and course of depression. In spite of deep and profound misery, some older individuals may not seek treatment for depression because they, as so many people do, believe that depression is a character weakness to which the person must not surrender and that they should be able to pull themselves out of the *doldrums* by their own efforts. Some families and professionals share this view. Some of the problems most frequently causing reactive depressions are enumerated in Box 23-9. Single or widowed women have a high prevalence of depression especially if chronic illnesses lead to losses in daily activities, lack of social supports, and stressful life events (Sahr, 1999).

Pathologic Factors. Function of the neurotransmitter, serotonin, a chemical messenger of the brain, is altered during depression. Additionally, the number of serotonin receptor sites, which regulate the amount of serotonin, is diminished; changes in cerebrospinal fluid and platelets also occur (NIMH, 2001a).

Diagnosis. The Geriatric Depression Scale, the Hamilton Depression Rating Scale, and the Beck Depression Inventory are often used to screen for depression. Both physicians and patients have difficulty identifying the signs of depression (NIMH, 2001b). We encourage staff nurses to use the simple and reliable tools provided in Appendix 23-A and to alert geriatric nurse practitioners and physicians when evidence of depression exists. The Zung Self-Rating Depression Scale was developed specifically for use in elders with depression. A key to depression management is early identification, diagnosis, and management (Beers and Berkow, 2000). Family members should be alert to subtle changes in personality, especially spontaneity, loss of sense of humor, new onset of forgetfulness, loss of appetite, and new sleep disturbance. Other signs may include wringing the hands, hypersomnia, recurrent thoughts of death, inattention to personal cleanliness or dress, persistent sadness, anxiety, and irritability (Kennedy-Malone, Fletcher, and Plank, 2000). Certain laboratory tests should be considered, mainly thyroid tests, B_{12}, calcium, liver function studies, renal function, electrolytes, CBC, and urinalysis (Reuben et al, 2002).

Hypochondriasis. Hypochondriasis is preoccupation with the idea or fear that the elderly patient has a serious disease (Beers and Berkow, 2000). This belief is a misperception of the body's normal function and processes. These patients may actually have some medical disorders but will not explain the patient's concerns nor the nature and severity of the symptoms reported. These concerns last for approximately 6 months. Elderly people tend to express depression through somatic symptoms. Thus the hypochondriacal preoccupation of the elderly may be a signal of the presence of depression, as are frequent visits to general practitioners. The patients are far less likely to view problems as psychologic, interpersonal, or situational; chief complaints are usually of various physical discomforts (e.g., constipation, gas pain, heartburn). Complaints such as these are too readily dismissed as hypochondriacal when a more holistic approach to the patient would reveal the extent and complexity of problems. Malingering is not uncommon. The patient is rewarded with external gain: he or she may receive financial compensation or relief from obligations and duties (Beers and Berkow, 2000).

Grief. Grief is a normal process that very often occurs or begins before an anticipated death or change, or loss. Dynamics include loss of control, preparation for loss, fear of separation, an uncertain future, and suffering (Beers and Berkow, 2000). Chronic grief and multiple losses may result in profound depression, apathy, and withdrawal from life. Approximately 50% of women older than age 65 are widows, and 13% of men are widowers (Kennedy-Malone, Fletcher, and Plank, 2000). Farberow and colleagues (1992) studied the grief process in people over age 55 through comparisons of spouses of suicides and spouses who lost their mate through illness. This longitudinal study (2.5 years) challenges some previous ideas about the grief process in elders and confirms some concepts already in the literature. Rather than specific, identifiable stages of resolution, the authors found a gradual adaptation to the loss, which was facilitated by a supportive network and prior good coping skills. People in an environmental setting that was stressful and those with other concurrent losses had a more difficult adaptation. The biggest problems were loneliness and managing the tasks of daily living. At the completion of the 2.5-year study, results indicated that both groups were significantly more composed, enthusiastic about life, and relaxed. Adjustment to bereavement is an ongoing life process with no precise point when grieving is over and mourning ends. The pain of loss may remain for a lifetime, felt in a different manner as time passes.

Mark had lived an ordinary life with few demands and few adventures. As he was dying, Mark invented, in his delirium, adventures that he might have had. It was as if Mark's psyche were expressing that element of his nature that had lain dormant for so long.

Fred, who had seemed so superficial and lacking in the capacity for inner exploration, became visibly changed following his seventieth birthday. He began to speak of his past experiences with some insight and to express his uncertainties. He, who had appeared so blasé, expressed tender feelings. Tears would fill Fred's eyes as he speculated about the future of his grandchildren: Would they remember him? Would they care? Would they wonder about him?

This distinct type of depression is born of the existential loneliness each person feels when confronted with the ultimate relinquishment of self. The great drama is ending, and no sequel will ensue. Even people who believe firmly in an afterlife or reincarnation must let go of this particularly unique life and personality.

Institutions. Institutions cause depression, as well as harbor those who are depressed. Commerford and Reznikoff (1996) found that neither religiosity nor social support were significant in reducing depression in nursing home residents. In other words, depression is apparently a result of the impact of the environment, regardless of the quality of external and internal supportive resources. Issues of control may be at the crux of these depressions. Elderly males, without a history of mental illness or cognitive impairment, seem to develop depression and learned helplessness after entering a nursing home. This tendency suggests that immediately after admission to long-term care, strategic patient care planning must include ways in which the individual will be given control of the situation.

Biorhythmicity. Biorhythmicity and the emotional effects of disruptions in light must be considered. Temporal patterns of exposure refers to the length of exposure to solar radiation that maintains health and avoids overexposure. Seasonal affective disorders (SADs) have been given attention by psychologists and others as the source of annual depressive episodes in some individuals. Growing evidence indicates that light-dark cycles are critical to these individuals.

Evidence also suggests some individuals have strong psychophysiologic responses to artificial light. Bright, artificial light has been shown to increase calcium absorption in healthy elderly men and to enhance synthesis of vitamin D, while simultaneously lowering plasma bilirubin. In addition, bright light administered 2 hours each morning for two 10-day periods has reduced agitated behaviors in demented subjects living in a skilled nursing home. The NIMH follow-up studies of individuals suffering winter SAD found that light treatment was safe and effective for most people, but severely affected individuals were nonresponsive to light therapy. Morning walks in natural light may be more effective than treatment with low-dose artificial lighting. Assisting residents of institutions to get outdoors or to use solariums should be a part of the daily care plan because of the apparent physiologic and psychologic needs that respond to appropriate amounts of sunlight. Nurses are largely responsible for the contact a resident has with environmental and natural lighting.

Goals of Treatment. The goals of treatment for depression include (1) decreasing symptoms, (2) reducing risk of relapse and recurrence, (3) increasing quality of life, (4) improving medical health status, and (5) decreasing health care costs and mortality. The changes in the health care delivery system, the emphasis on cost savings, and the increasing number of frail elderly make these goals even more pertinent today than when they were formulated almost a decade ago. Again, early identification and intervention are key (Beers and Berkow, 2000).

Interventions. Interventions are individual and are based on history, what has previously been effective, concurrent illnesses, and severity of illness (Reuben et al, 2002). Psychotherapy is effective in elderly patients with mild recent onset of depression. Psychotherapy is less effective in melancholia (Beers and Berkow, 2000). The addition of pharmaceuticals seems to have the most beneficial effect, though 80% of elders will improve on appropriate medication, psychotherapy, or the combination (NIMH, 2001b). Other considerations are electroconvulsive therapy (ECT) for severe depression; social (family and social support), grief management, cognitive-behavioral therapy; interpersonal therapy; and problem-solving therapy (Reuben et al, 2002).

A strategy we developed fully in one of our earlier editions was the use of dreams for self-expression, understanding, and reestablishing control. We have found this strategy useful because many very depressed people seem to live more in their dream time than they do while awake. We have not corroborated this finding with studies. Reminiscing serves somewhat the same functions, though a very depressed elder may not reminisce spontaneously. Always, in all interventions with depressed elders, the goal is to stimulate them to take control and make the decisions, explain what they want and what they enjoy or appreciate.

Medications. Drug therapies are very effective in managing depression. Most elderly depressed patients will continue on antidepressant therapy for the rest of their lives (Reuben et al, 2002). Older antidepressants include the tricyclic antidepressants (TCAs) and monoamine oxidase inhibitors (MAOIs), which will manage depression but also have important side effects and are thus poor selections for the elderly patient, unless other therapies have failed. TCAs fall into the category of class I antiarrhythmic drugs, which have been responsible for increased cardiac disorders and deaths in people with ischemic heart disease. The newer selective serotonin reuptake inhibitors (SSRIs) are the drugs of choice for most elders with depression and especially for those with conduction defects, ischemic heart disease, glaucoma, and prostate disease (Reuben et al, 2002). The patient's participation in the treatment plan and compliance with medication dosage must be encouraged because clients' motivation may be very low.

Electroconvulsive therapy. ECT is safe and effective (Reuben et al, 2002). ECT is useful in severe depression when obtaining a rapid response via therapy is essential or when the depression is resistant to pharmacotherapy. Patients with psychotic depression, catatonia, and Parkinson's disease with depression appear to respond well to ECT.

Cognitive-behavioral therapy. Cognitive-behavioral group therapy, focused visual imagery group therapy, and education and discussion groups on cognition, depression, and hopelessness have been used with moderate improvement in cognitive function in people with mild depression. These approaches are more effective than analytic therapy or nondirective therapies (Beers and Berkow, 2000). Cognitive-behavioral therapy focuses on negating cognitive errors that are common to mildly depressed elderly: (1) overgeneralizing; (2) "awfulizing"; (3) exaggerating own importance; (4) demanding of others; (5) expecting mind reading; (6) self-blame; and (7) unrealistic expectations.

Social supports. Family interventions may consist primarily of shoring up the person's tolerance, knowledge, and understanding. The following is a summary of interventions that have been found effective with depressed elders:

- Structured, noncompetitive activities
- Opportunities for decisions and to exercise control
- Focus on spiritual renewal and rediscovery of meanings
- Guided autobiography
- Self-analysis through journals and dreams
- Reactivation of latent interests
- Validation of depressed feelings as aiding recovery, not trying to bolster patient's mood or deny his or her despair
- An accepting atmosphere and an empathic nursing response

Professional supports. Encourage the individual to recognize depression as a treatable illness and to seek help. Discussing the nature of the depression with the client is most helpful. Help the client become aware of the presence of depression, the nature of the symptoms, and the time limitation of depression. For example, do not talk him or her out of being depressed; do not console with "life is worth living" or other clichés that only confirm the nurse's inability to comprehend the pain. Present depression as a dynamic process of choosing to experience the depression rather than avoiding it by overactivity, suicide, psychosomatic illness, or substance dependence, all of which can be seen as less healthy options than dealing directly with depression.

Encourage and validate feelings of family, friends, and professionals as clients deal with anger, hostility, and rejection. These feelings intensify the sense of loss and rejection the client is experiencing, further increasing self-deprecation. To the extent possible, the feelings should be defused before approaching the depressed elder. Reminiscence is believed to have particular diagnostic and therapeutic potential for elderly patients. Reminiscence can be used as a means to resolve old conflicts, guilts, and disappointments; for socialization experiences; and as a way to capitalize on the preserved memories of those who may have lost some cognitive capacity. Maintenance of self-esteem and self-continuity are some of the benefits of reminiscence therapy. Reminiscence as a therapeutic strategy is summarized in Box 23-10. Additional discussion of reminiscence is presented later in the chapter.

Box 23-10 Reminiscence as a Developmental and Therapeutic Strategy

Maintain continuity
Extract meaning
Define and develop personal philosophy
Identify cycles and themes
Recapitulate learning and growth
Evolve identity
Provide insight and growth
Integrate and accept regrets and disappointments
Perceive universality

Nurses may help themselves and the client by being present, accepting the client's limited amount of interaction, and continually giving the client choices and clear feedback. When certain expectations of the client exist, state them in the form of options, for example, "It is important for you to get up and get dressed. Movement will increase your circulation and your energy levels. Do you want to get up before breakfast or after breakfast?" The client may respond that he does not want to get up. In that case, the nurse might reply, "You do have the right not to participate. I will return in 30 minutes, after you have given it more thought." On returning, the nurse may ask, "What is your decision?" Use humor: "Do I understand you intend to remain in bed? Remaining in bed ensures that you won't get up on the wrong side!"

Getting into a power struggle over involvement in activities only ensures that the nurse will lose. If this event occurs inadvertently, stop as soon as you recognize it and bring it to the attention of the client, "You will win this game; you can choose to remain in bed and there is little I can do about that."

To be successful, treating depression must include considerations of the individual's premorbid personality, determination of reactive or endogenous origins, symptom relief, social support manipulation, and the importance of a positive relationship with health care providers. The ability to tolerate depression enhances the person's coping capacity in later years. All aged people will be depressed at some time and may better survive these episodes if they can develop a perspective that allows depression to be viewed as a valid and healing life process. A depressive episode is time needed for psychologic wound repair, cleansing tears, protection of the wounded psyche by withdrawal, and the facilitation of repair and restoration of vitality, enthusiasm, and spontaneity. Nurses can facilitate this process by validation. Ronsman (1987) developed an extensive nursing care plan based on Maslow's hierarchy of needs to be used in the care of a depressed patient (Table 23-3).

Suicide

Lying dormant within all of us is an extremely personal equation that determines the point at which the quality of our lives

Table 23-3 Dealing with Depression: The Nursing Process and Maslow's Hierarchy of Needs

Needs	Assessment	Identifying problems	Establishing goals	Intervention	Evaluation
Physiologic needs					
Food and fluid Shelter and warmth Air Rest and sleep Avoidance of pain Sex	Usual and present nutritional, elimination, sleep, and sexuality patterns Physical activity—exercise pattern Emotional pain and discomfort Suicide potential Physical health Medications	Nutritional deficit Dehydration Constipation Sleep pattern disturbance Sexual dysfunction Self-destructive behavior Medications or physical illnesses that may cause depression	Establishing and maintaining adequate biologic functioning in areas of sleep, nutrition, and elimination Relief from emotional pain and discomfort Elimination of drug or disease-induced depression	Assist with ADLs Support of self-care abilities Encouragement to start a physical activity regimen Teach side effects of antidepressants Treat medical problems under poor control Change medications that may cause depression	Feelings of physical satiation Homeostasis Optimal physical health
Safety and security needs					
Feel free from danger Need for a predictable, lawful, orderly world Need to feel in control	Home environment assessment Mental status examination Assessment of visual acuity and hearing Knowledge of disease process Physical mobility	Perceived inability to control feelings or behavior Perceived powerlessness Translocation syndrome Cognitive impairment Alteration in sensory perceptions Impaired physical mobility	Establish predictability and structure in environment Maintenance of a safe environment Realistic understanding of disease course and expected outcome Reversal of treatable confusion	ECT, hospitalization, antidepressive medications for the severely depressed Avoid relocations when possible Correct environmental hazards Encourage a structured daily routine Instruct about disease course and prognosis	Feeling in control of one's disease and optimistic about the future Confidence in the future Feelings of safety, peace, security, protection, lack of danger, and threat
Need for love, belonging, and affection					
Need for contact and intimacy Need for friends Need for a feeling of having a place, "belonging" Need for interactions with others	Family relationships and members Friends that are supportive Recent losses Present and past social interactions	Disruption in significant relationships Social isolation Lack of contact with or absence of significant others Alterations in socialization with reduced social interactions	Maintenance of significant relationships with family and friends Establish community support system Resumption of previous level of social activity	Encourage social interactions that have been enjoyed in the past Encourage interactions with family members, friends, and health caregivers Provide reassuring, supportive atmosphere	Feelings of loving and being loved, of being one of a group, of acceptance
Need for esteem and self-respect					
Need for achievement, mastery, and competence Need for reputation or prestige, appreciation, and dignity Need for love of self	Amount of pleasurable pursuits Emotional or mood assessment Role patterns Coping—stress tolerance pattern Attitude about self, the world, the future	Negative feelings or conception of self Loss of significant roles Unrealistic self-expectations Anxiety Lifestyle change Dependency on others	Acceptance of realistic limitations Establish appropriate roles Achieve self-acceptance Accept ownership of consequences of one's own behavior	Teach problem-solving skills Cognitive therapy Promote self-care Counseling Behavior therapy Relaxation techniques	Feelings of self-confidence, worth, strength, capability, adequacy, and of being useful and necessary in the world

Continued

Table 23-3 Dealing with Depression: The Nursing Process and Maslow's Hierarchy of Needs—cont'd

Needs	Assessment	Identifying problems	Establishing goals	Intervention	Evaluation
Need for self-actualization					
Need for beauty Need for self-expression Need for new situations and stimulation	Occupation, job history Value-belief patterns	Distress of human spirit Loss of zest for life	Expression of self through meaningful recreational activities Exploring new interests	Encourage a nonrestrictive environment Provide beauty in environment Read to the sick or hard of hearing Music	Autonomy Freshness of appreciation Creativeness Spontaneity Feelings of self-fulfillment

From Ronsman K: Therapy for depression, *J Gerontol Nurs* 13(12):21, 1987.
ADLs, Activities of daily living; *ECT,* electroconvulsive therapy.

would be so pathetically poor we would no longer wish to live. This "line of unbearability," as it might be called, usually exists only subconsciously, and we are therefore not normally cognizant of it. However, when we actually find ourselves in an intolerable situation, even for the first time in our lives, we become conscious of our line of unbearability. Once the line of unbearability is crossed, a crisis is triggered. Individuals who still maintain hope cry out for help; those who do not are likely to kill themselves (Miller, 1979).

Although elders make up 13% of the population, they commit 20% of suicides (McAndrews, 2001). White men over 85 years of age commit suicide at an annual rate of 67 per 100,000, approximately six times the national rate (NIMH, 2001b). In contrast, white women of the same age category commit suicide at an annual rate of 6 per 100,000. Women are most suicidal between ages 45 and 54, with an incidence of 8 per 100,000. Suicide rates for white men and white women over age 75 have slightly but steadily increased since 1980. Old blacks have much lower suicide rates (men, 18 per 100,000, and women, less than 1 per 100,000); however, suicide rates of elderly black males have almost doubled since 1980 (U.S. Bureau of the Census, 1995). One of the significant differences in suicidal behaviors in the old and young is the lethality. Eight of ten suicides of males over age 65 were with firearms, and most were successful.

We have stated that health care professionals do not diagnose or manage depression very well in elderly people. Interestingly, in one study of physicians presented with a case study of a depressed man who was alternately presented as young or elderly, physicians treated the young suicidal man but did not treat the elderly man (Uncapher, Arean, 2000). The physicians all correctly diagnosed the situation but treated them differently, with a bias toward the younger male patient. Further, elders who are planning to commit suicide apparently visit their primary care physician very close to the time that they commit the suicide (NIMH, 2001b). Twenty percent of the elders visited the physician on the same day of the suicide, 40% within 1 week and 70% within 1 month. This statistic suggests to us that opportunities for intervening are present but not seen as urgent or not being diagnosed at all.

In primitive societies, the old were expected to commit suicide when their existence was considered a burden to the community. Stories of assisted suicide and mutual suicides are being reported more frequently, and society generally condones the suicide of an aged person who is ill and in pain. In fact, in the current climate of increasing interest in *assisted suicide,* a time may come when we regress to the primitive mode. In the past, the distribution of food was at stake; now, money is the crucial element.

Aged white men in America suffer the most status loss because American white male society is almost wholly devoted to occupational success, often to the neglect of other social roles. Women in all countries have much lower suicide rates. As more women identify themselves with the work role and abstain from having children, statistics may shift.

Common precipitants of suicide include physical or mental illness, death of spouse, substance abuse, and pathologic relationships. Contrary to general opinion, the majority of elderly people who committed suicide were not physically ill. Most of these individuals were depressed (65%) or had other mental health problems. Depression was a potential underlying cause in 53% of cases studied by Haring and colleagues (1987). Twelve percent of the suicides investigated were patients of long-term care.

Suicide of widows and widowers has been attributed by Durkheim (1951) to "domestic anomie," that is, a deregulation of behavior by the loss of spouse that results in a vague and unstructured state of being that lacks guidelines, status, and clear expectations. Widowers are most vulnerable because they are unfamiliar with domestic chores and have often depended on the wife to maintain the comforts of home and the social network of relatives and friends.

Assessing the Suicidal Risk of an Elder. The lethality potential of an elder must always be assessed when elements of depression, disease, and spousal loss are evident.

Delusional and hypochondriacal thinking are risk factors (Lester and Tallmer, 1994). Many studies have shown that, with few exceptions, a suicidal individual has seen a physician within a month before the suicide attempt (American Association of Retired Persons, 1994). Unfortunately, few physicians make a suicide assessment.

Nurses are often in a position to assume responsibility for assessing lethality potential. The clues that are common signals of suicidal intent may be absent, disguised, or misinterpreted in the elderly. However, any direct, indirect, or enigmatic references to the ending of life must be taken seriously and discussed with the elder. Many older people, having grown up in the era when suicide bore stigma and even criminal implications, may not discuss their feelings in this respect. Depersonalizing the subject and discussing it on a more philosophic basis is often helpful, using questions such as the following:

"Under what conditions do you think a person has a right to take his life?"

"What are your opinions about the present interest in active euthanasia and assisted suicide?"

"Do you think suicide is a sign of weakness or strength?"

"Suicide is a taboo subject that many people are uncomfortable discussing, but as a health professional I think it is very important. Have you ever believed that you would be better off dead?"

Typical behavioral clues such as putting personal affairs in order, giving away possessions, and making wills and funeral plans are indications of maturity and good judgment in late life and cannot be construed as indicative of suicidal intent. Other factors such as self-neglect, erratic behavior, suspiciousness, hoarding pills, and personality change are more likely the side effects of illness or progressive dementia than they are of suicidal intent. Even statements such as "I won't be around long" may be only a realistic appraisal of the situation in old age. Requests to die and statements that life has no meaning may indicate despair and hopelessness but often lack the conviction of planned suicide.

In evaluating lethality potential, the informed nurse will recognize the high-risk patient: male, old, widowed or divorced, white, in poor health, retired, alcoholic, with a family history of unsatisfactory relationships and mental illness. A cluster of these factors should be a red flag of distress to all health professionals. Recent traumatic changes, mild dementia, depression, or cerebrovascular disease also increase the danger. Present relationships that are unsatisfactory, critical, or rejecting greatly enhance the potential for suicide.

The straightforward aspects of a suicide assessment include the following:

- Frequency of suicidal ideations
- A formulated plan for suicide
- Availability of means to complete the plan
- Specificity regarding details (e.g., time, place)
- Lethality of the method chosen

Three other factors must be considered in assessing lethality potential:

- Internal resources (personality factors and coping strategies)
- External resources (money, family, friends, and services)
- Communication skills (ability to ask for help and express feelings)

Suicide is a taboo topic for most of us, and a lingering suspicion exists that the introduction of the topic will be suggestive to the patient and may incite suicidal action. Precisely the opposite is true. By introducing the topic we demonstrate interest in the individual and open the door to honest human interaction and connection on the deep levels of psychic need. Superficial interest and mechanical questioning will not, of course, be meaningful. The nature of our concern and ability is to connect with the alienation and desperation of the individual that will make a difference. No matter how much empathy and concern are conveyed, many old people will quietly and methodically kill themselves with never a clue to their intent.

Interventions with a Suicidal Elder. Community health nurses, visiting nurses, and other professionals have a case-finding role in the community that extends beyond traditional boundaries: (1) awareness and use of resources within the high-risk populations and (2) providing depression screening clinics at nutrition sites, senior centers, industrial health sites, churches, and community clubs.

Establishing lifesaving connections with individuals and groups that can be available on demand and that can provide ongoing, long-term counseling, emotional support, and reassurance is the approach to the suicidal elder (Arbore, 1995). Arbore established a 24-hour "Friendship Line" designed especially for elders under the umbrella of suicide prevention. Phone call-in counseling is always available by specially trained volunteers, as well as telephone outreach reassurance and a visiting service. The goal is to intervene before suicide becomes a seriously considered option. Suicide risk and recovery factors are listed in Box 23-11.

Aged suicidal clients are encountered in many settings. Our professional obligation is to prevent whenever possible an impulsive destruction of life that may be a response to a crisis or a disintegrative reaction. In other words, we must be concerned about immediate protection for the highly lethal individual while respecting the individual's right to make the most significant remaining decision open to him or her, namely, whether to live or to die. For some people, our well-planned interventions may restore a sense of self and purpose such that the suicidal individual will deem preservation worthwhile. For other individuals, their final statement of dignity will be in the control of their death.

Actions to deal with the suicidal elderly include:

- Build trust and rapport.
- Overcome fear of responsibility for client suicide.

Box 23-11 Suicide Risk and Recovery Factors

Risk Factors

Depression
Paranoia or a paranoid attitude
Rejection of help; a suspicious and hostile attitude toward helpers and society
Major loss, such as the death of a spouse
History of major losses
Recent suicide attempt
History of suicide attempts
Major mental, physical, or neurologic illness
Major crises or transitions, such as retirement or imminent entry into a nursing home
Major crises or changes in others, especially among family members
Typical age-related blows to self-esteem, such as loss of income or loss of meaningful activities
Loss of independence, when dependency is unacceptable
Expressions of feeling unnecessary, useless, and devalued
Increased irritability and poor judgment, especially after a loss or some other crisis
Alcoholism or increased drinking
Social isolation: living alone; having few friends (The social isolation of the couple is also associated with suicide.)
Expression of the belief that one is in the way, a burden harmful to others
Expression of the belief that one is in an insoluble and hopeless situation
Communication of suicidal intent: direct or indirect expression of suicidal ideation or impulses and symptomatic acts, such as giving away valued possessions, storing up medications or buying a gun
Intractable, unremitting pain—mental, or physical—that is not responding to treatment
Feelings of hopelessness and helplessness in the family and social network
Feelings of hopelessness in the therapist or other helpers; desire to be rid of the patient
Expression of a belief in ageism, especially that the aged should not be
Acceptance of suicide as a solution

Recovery Factors

A capacity for:
Understanding
Relating
Benefitting from experience
Benefitting from knowledge
Accepting help
Being loving
Expressing wisdom
Displaying a sense or humor
Having a social interest
Accepting a caring and available family
Accepting a caring and available social network
Accepting a caring, available, and kowledgable professional and health network

From Richman J: A rational approach to rational suicide. In Leenars AA et al, editors: *Suicide and the older adult,* New York, 1992, The Guilford Press.

- Come to terms with your own suicidal impulses and feelings.
- Recognize and handle resentment of the client who wants to die.
- Listen intently and empathically.
- Focus on the individual's perception of problem.
- Begin to help establish or restore a supportive network.

If suicidal intent has been established, the following interventions, arranged in order of immediacy, are necessary:

1. Reduce immediate danger by removing hazardous articles.
2. Evaluate the need for constant attendance, and arrange for family, friend, or professional to be present during the period of imminent danger.
3. Evaluate the need for medication.
4. Focus on the current hazard or crisis that gives the client the most present distress.
5. Extract a promise from the client not to attempt suicide before your next meeting.
6. Mobilize internal and external resources by getting the individual reinvolved with external supports and reconnected with internal capacities. The caregiver may have to find activities, support systems, transportation, and other resources for the individual.
7. Implement a specific plan of action with an ongoing structured program to obviate long periods that the client may spend alone. Develop a "lifeline" of individuals who can be called at any hour of distress, and plan regular calls to the individual.

In many cases, interventions with depressed elders can be extrapolated to suicidal elders, given that they are often depressed (see discussion earlier in the chapter). Suicide is often a distorted method of regaining control of a person's life. Prevention of suicidal behavior is related to alleviation of depression and restoration of a sense of control in life. Working with isolated, depressed, and suicidal elders continually challenges the depths of nurses' ingenuity, patience, and self-knowledge.

THERAPEUTIC STRATEGIES TO PROMOTE MENTAL HEALTH

Mental health promotion and treatment strategies for the elderly are based primarily in the community and nursing homes, though some geropsychiatric units and some mental health units provide excellent care for elders with mental disorders. Individual integration into the relevant community and family activities with sufficient supports to remain vital and esteemed are the overriding goals of all therapeutic efforts.

Most articles about the mental health of older adults focus on the presence of organic brain disorders as a primary issue. Extensive psychotherapy is rarely reported, and most treatment is somatic. Problems labeled psychotic or neurotic in the young are most often labeled senile in the old. Although many psychologic problems of aging may be accompanied by a cerebral deficit, active therapeutic psychodynamic interventions can be expected to produce some improvement in most cases because dementia seldom exists without some overlay of mental health problems that are potentially reversible or that can be ameliorated. Effective treatment modes include psychoanalysis, psychotherapeutic reminiscence, brief psychotherapy and crisis intervention, somatotherapy, behavioral therapy, family therapy, reality orientation, resocialization, and remotivation. The choice of therapy depends on the needs of the client and method of reimbursement.

Community-Based Psychiatric Care

Elderly psychiatric patients have been treated with Band-Aids and then misplaced and all too frequently forgotten. Now, with the trend of all health care to move the majority of care provision to the community, the mental health providers are creating new comprehensive community psychogeriatric care systems. Canadians in Ontario have found this method most satisfactory. Case finding may be from several sources, and initial screening is often in response to a crisis call from a client, family member, or professional in the community or based in an institution.

When completed, an assessment provides the base for a holistic plan of care. The client and care planning team determine what is both desired and feasible. The range of options is thoroughly examined. Only then is the decision made as to what level of support is needed and whether a move may be necessary. Wherever the site in which the care plan is activated, the client is still provided access to the community-based services that have been identified in the care plan. Periodic assessment of progress toward goals involves all team members, the client, and the family. This community case-managed model can be effectively implemented in any community. As the program becomes more fully developed, an increasing number of caregivers and local resources can be involved. Overall, these programs have proved economically and humanistically effective. Institutions and community groups have worked together to maintain continuity of efforts and consistency of service. The programs appear to be more cost-effective than institutionalization.

Psychotherapy

Goldfarb and Turner (1953, 1955), pioneers in psychogeriatric care, first reported serious attempts at psychotherapy with the aged. These researchers carried out brief (15-minute) semi-weekly therapeutic sessions aimed at increasing self-esteem and reinforcing a therapeutic alliance between psychiatrist and client. In an average of six to eight sessions, 78% of the participants improved their social adaptation and psychologic functions. Interestingly, two thirds of the sample had some cerebral impairment, yet all but 22% of them improved or stabilized. Of the subjects who were psychotic in the absence of organic mental disorders, only one in five improved. Of the subjects with psychoneuroses or personality disorders in the absence of organic mental disorders, all either stabilized or improved. Goldfarb and Turner emphasized the point, made by so many others since their pioneer studies, that treatment is helpful even in cases in which severe dementia is present. These authors found repeatedly that emotional disorganization often exaggerates the picture of dementia. In addition, Goldfarb and Turner advocate warm interactions, focusing on positive transference as helpful to most elderly. In contrast to traditional psychotherapy, the therapist often interjects thoughts, opinions, and personal experiences when relevant (Nowak and Wandel, 1998).

Brief Psychotherapy and Crisis Intervention. These modalities are often surprisingly successful because the elderly are acutely aware that their time is limited and their problems are often clearly apparent. Crisis intervention is discussed thoroughly in another chapter. Brief psychotherapy is often the treatment of choice for the elderly who need to resolve interpersonal problems and develop more effective coping strategies. Issues of transference and resistance, which are the essence of a long-term therapeutic alliance, are not developed in brief psychotherapy. Generally, brief psychotherapy is limited to less than 15 weeks. The emphasis is on important problems in the person's life; goals are limited. The therapist is active in providing direction, guidance, and environmental manipulation. Some therapists recommend a philosophic approach to psychotherapy with older adults.

Brief psychotherapy with the elderly can be successful when conducted by experienced psychotherapists who use brief psychodynamically oriented psychotherapy, psychologic testing, and diagnostic interviews. Psychotherapists are advised to focus on issues of major concern or on ones that will restore a sense of mastery and self-esteem. Nurses, acting as client advocates, are often in the position of encouraging both physician and client to include psychotherapeutic support in the treatment regimen.

Benefits from verbal psychotherapy for aged individuals cannot be predicted from current tests. Individual long-term psychotherapy for the aged in the community is theoretically beneficial but is seldom seen in actual practice. The distance between therapists and potential aged clients is mutually maintained for many reasons. Despite these impediments, several modes of psychotherapy with the aged have been effectively demonstrated.

Psychodrama. Psychodrama has been infrequently used with aged individuals because they have been considered as poor candidates for developing insight and personality change. Nonetheless, the approach can be used effectively. Residents of nursing homes can participate in expressive groups for the purpose of dramatizing physical limitations, death of self and loved ones, and dependencies. These topics, frequently avoided when working with the aged, are potent issues that need to be handled openly and in depth. The participants confront conflictual issues and develop insight into anxieties. Dramatic role-playing not only resolves past issues, but also brings about reinvestment in the present relationships in a group.

Psychodrama and life review have been used successfully to enhance adaptation and life satisfaction. Psychodrama emphasizes the reenactment of troublesome memories that are consuming psychic energy and producing incongruence in an individual's self-concept. The life review and reminiscence activity can be effectively implemented using the techniques of psychodrama. Although used with adolescents, dreams have also been incorporated into psychodrama for further understanding. Imagery-based cognitive training techniques have also been used successfully with elders. The particular techniques used include visual imagery elaboration, verbal judgment, and relaxation. Elders who are intuitive seem to benefit most from psychodrama, life review, and imagery.

Institutionally Based Care. Typically, as mentioned earlier, nursing homes have, by default, been given the task of caring for the mentally disturbed elder. Many facilities have done quite an excellent job in implementing reality orientation (RO), remotivation, and resocialization using group therapy strategies. RO is used primarily for individuals who have some cognitive impairment. Remotivation and resocialization can be adapted to clients with dementias or psychologic disturbances (Table 23-4).

Remotivation Technique. This approach was designed for long-term, chronic psychiatric residents and for use in extended care facilities and nursing homes. Avoidance of emotionally laden issues and a focus on extending opportunities for varied successful experiences are characteristic of remotivation techniques. Butler and colleagues (1991) emphasized five steps in the remotivation technique:

1. Climate of acceptance—establishing a warm friendly relationship in the group
2. Bridge to reality—reading of simple poetry, current events, and so on
3. Sharing the world—developing the topic (introduced earlier) through planned objective questions, using props, and so on
4. Appreciation of the work of the world—designed to stimulate the residents to think about work in relation to themselves
5. Climate of appreciation—expression of enjoyment at getting together and so on

Individuals with little training may successfully use remotivation for the aged in long-term care situations. Student projects in applying remotivation techniques are useful and often result in the youth forming relationships with the aged. The students learn to appreciate the aged, and the elders, in turn, become more interested in life, less irritable, better groomed, and motivated toward interpersonal contacts. The therapeutic value of contact between young students and the psychiatrically disabled aged is thought to be important. Table 23-4 provides some guidelines and comparisons of RO, remotivation, and resocialization.

Pet therapy in nursing homes is generally used to bridge the gap between the resident and the therapist. The dog or cat helps the resident break through apathy and depression. The resident is then better able to respond to caregivers and interact with other residents. Pet therapy consists of a brief session each month in which well-behaved cats and dogs are brought to nursing homes for residents to play with and hold. Animals are selected based on their good temperament and ability to withstand the confusion and the number of people who will hold and play with them. Volunteers from the animal shelter usually accompany pets to ensure the safety of both animals and residents. Nursing homes sometimes adopt an animal that becomes the mascot, and various residents take responsibility for caring for the animal. The Humane Society of the United States offers the following points that should be considered before initiating pet therapy in a nursing home (Wright and Dribben-Gutman, 1981):

1. What does the staff think about the project?
2. Will the facilities lend themselves to such a program?
3. Is space available where the animal can retreat and also be kept out of the way of residents who have no interest in pets or are afraid of them?
4. Can a program schedule be set up to include an animal on a routine basis?
5. Is the local humane society or animal shelter willing to become involved in such a project?
6. If adopting a resident mascot, is adequate food, shelter, and water available for the mascot at all times, and will there be people consistently responsible for the care of the animal?

Reminiscing and Life Review. Reminiscing has been viewed as a particularly adaptive function at the last stage of life. Reminiscence is an activity that can allow clients a sense of security through rehearsal of comforting memories, belonging through sharing, and self-esteem through confirmation of uniqueness. Box 23-12 lists several ways memories and reminiscences can be used effectively for enriching the aging process. For the nurse, reminiscences is a tool of assessment and understanding.

The concept of reminiscence fits well with mechanisms of crisis and grief resolution and seems to be a fitting tool to accomplish some of the work in these situations.

Table 23-4 Differences in Reality Orientation, Resocialization, and Remotivation

Reality orientation	Resocialization	Remotivation
1. Correct position or relation with the existing situation in a community; maximum use of assets	1. Continuation of reality living situation in a community	1. Orientation to reality for community living; present oriented
2. Called reality orientation, and classroom reality orientation program	2. Called discussion group or resocialization to differentiate a social function from a therapeutic need	2. Called remotivation
3. Structured	3. Unstructured	3. Definite structure
4. Refreshments, food, or both may be served for identification	4. Refreshments served	4. Refreshments not served
5. Appreciation of the work of the world; constantly reminded of who he is, where he is, why he is here, and what is expected of him or her	5. Appreciation of the work of the world; reliving happy experiences; encourages participation in home activities relating to subject	5. Appreciation of the work of the group stimulates the desire to return to function in society
6. Class range from 3-5, depending on degree or level of confusion or disorientation from any cause	6. Group range from 5-17, depending on mental and physical capabilities	6. Group size: 5-12 patients
7. Meeting ½ hour daily at same time in same place	7. Meetings three times weekly for ½ to 1 hour	7. Meeting once to twice weekly for an hour
8. Planned procedures: reality-centered objects	8. No planned topic; group-centered feelings	8. Preselected and reality-centered objects
9. Consistency of approach or response of resident responsibility of teacher	9. Clarification and interpretation in responsibility of leader	9. No exploration of feelings
10. Periodic reality orientation test pertaining to residents' level of confusion or disorientation	10. Periodic progress notes pertaining to residents' enjoyment and improvements	10. Progress ratings
11. Emphasis on time, place, person orientation	11. Any topic freely discussed	11. Topic: no discussion of religion, politics, or death
12. Use of portion and mind function still intact	12. Vast stockpile of memories and experiences	12. Untouched area of the mind
13. Resident greeted by name, thanked for coming, and extended handshake or physical contact according to attitude approach in group	13. Resident greeted on arrival, thanked him, and extended handshake upon leaving	13. No physical contact permitted; acceptance and acknowledgment of everyone's contribution
14. Conducted by trained aides and activity assistants	14. Conducted by RN, LPN/LVN, aides, and program assistants	14. Conducted by trained psychiatric aides

From Barns E, Sack A, Shore H: Guidelines to treatment approaches, *Gerontologist* 13:513, 1973.
LPN/LVN, Licensed practical nurse/licensed vocational nurse; *RN,* registered nurse.

Reminiscence is versatile because it is ubiquitous, natural, and embodies the whole of the individual's conscious life experience. Goals of reminiscing are related to enhancing the person's identity, socialization skills, sense of continuity, and coping. The tendency to reminisce can be applied therapeutically in many ways: socialization, remotivation, integration, assessment, and as part of RO. Webster (1993) has tested a reminiscence functions scale that can be used to assess some of these ways. Although used with all ages, the scale demonstrated a significant increase in death preparation functions in people 80 years of age and beyond. Interestingly, the function of teaching and informing remained steady through the forties and beyond.

Life review. Psychotherapeutic reminiscence is akin to psychoanalysis and forms the conceptual base for life review. The life-review concept is only one aspect of reminiscence that may decrease depression with some resolution of disappointments, ventilation, or closure. The exercise involves reviewing remote memories (self-revelation), expressing related feelings (catharsis), recognizing conflicts (insight), and relinquishing viewpoints that are self-inhibiting (decathexis).

Life review occurs frequently as an internal review of memories, an intensely private soul-searching activity, while reminiscing is for pleasure. Sharing and self-expression occurs most in an interpersonal context, often occurring sporadically in a long-term trusted relationship. During periods of crisis and transition, life review occurs quite naturally for many people. This approach is appropriate for any aged person, and Butler has called this process life review. Butler and Lewis

Box 23-12 Suggested Applications of Memories

Legacy identification
- Products
- Contributions
- Qualities of character
- Talents

Scrapbooks
Photo albums
Establish rituals of security and comfort
Work history
Life's turning points—can be mapped out as a road map
Fantasy trips—follow the alternate road
Grief resolution
History of homes
Map life geographically
Historic events—cohort identification
Life history of significant persons—why significant
Sensory stimulation
Develop memory chains
Inventory significant items—why significant
- To whom would he or she like to give them?

Dietary history—significant foods of the past may stimulate appetite
Resolve disappointment
Entertainment

(1983) provide the following guidelines for using life-review therapy:

1. Mastery of the past is the basis for adaptation to the present.
2. Encourage spontaneous life review.
3. Support the search for meaning, problem solving, and emotional gratification.
4. Use an eclectic approach.
5. Confront conflicts and anxieties regarding death, guilt, and dependency.
6. The therapist's stance is that of a dependable confidant.

The psychologically disturbed elderly person may be reluctant or unable to reminisce fluently in dyadic or group situations. Self-view is often distorted, distressed, or suppressed. Group sharing may be useful because it is less intense than dyadic communication and tends to provide balance to extreme feelings. Some nurses are reluctant to stir the memories of older individuals who seem psychologically vulnerable. We would not advocate confrontation or interpretation but rather exploration of all the meanings and feelings relevant to the situation being shared. If anxiety or agitation seems to become an inhibition factor, we would verbally validate the discomfort and move the focus to another group member. Crying, guilt, or regret expressed by group members can be reinforced as an evidence of self-affirmation. We believe the full range of human emotions and experiences are acceptable, and group validation may allow each member to move toward expression and resolution of psychologic pain.

A memory is a gift to the nurse, a sharing of a part of oneself when one may have little else to give. The more personal memories are saved for people who will patiently wait for their unveiling and who will treasure them. Of course, a recitation of life history may be a boring affair. When a nurse finds boredom setting in, it may be helpful to confirm the feeling; "It sounds like life became pretty monotonous for you at that time," or "The small details of life may keep one from thinking of larger problems."

Depressed individuals may ruminate about past inadequacies or illnesses. An unspoken message is often present: "See how sad and helpless I feel. Please take care of me." Nurses fear depression because we begin to feel helpless too. Fromholt and colleagues (1995) found that depressed individuals tended to recall negative memories, but after successful treatment and the recovery from depression, the memories recalled were more positive.

Restoring adequacy and a sense of being cared for requires patience and tolerance of depression. One nurse listened attentively to a long recitation of painful events and then interrupted the flow with "Who helped you get through these difficult times?" Another comment might also be helpful: "You must have a tremendous tolerance for discomfort. How did you survive such trauma?" A nurse must also occasionally restore perspective with a comment such as, "When you are depressed, everything you remember seems to have been miserable. As you recover, you will begin to remember happier times in your life." Nurses demonstrate caring by the willingness to listen to sad and disappointing memories, as well as the joyful, entertaining ones.

A most effective life review would resolve (at least partially) some past conflicts in a manner that would hold significance for the present and future. For instance, a group of elders might indicate some regret about insufficient planning for retirement. Ideally, the group would assess the supremacy of other needs that prevented them from making such plans and arrive at an acceptance of their needs and motives then and now. When working with the elderly in a life-review process, having a clear understanding of goals is important:

1. Is the person reviewing the life course preparatory to letting go? If so, the main goal is acceptance of what has been.
2. Is the individual facing a major crisis in self-esteem or need? The goal will be to identify past coping strategies and gather from them strategies that will be currently effective. Evaluating times when one was effective will sustain confidence in future effectiveness.
3. Is the individual bound in a morass of regret? The goal will be to reenergize the person for present and future function by developing alternative views of past failures.
4. Is the individual suffering the effects of institutionalization? The goal will be to stimulate clear memories of who the person has been and what the person has accomplished to reaffirm uniqueness and individuality.

5. Has the person held long-standing grievances against significant others? The goal will be to explore the complexity of these relationships and provide opportunities for interpersonal resolution with the individuals involved.

Life review occurs periodically throughout the life span. Often used to achieve resolution and identify potential for new directions, in the very old, life review is most likely used to alter views of what has been rather than what will be. The uses of reminiscence, in addition to cognitive stimulation, reduction of depression, and psychologic restitution, are numerous. The nurse can learn much about a resident's history, communication style, relationships, coping mechanisms, strengths, fears, affect, and adaptive capacity by thoughtful listening.

Caring nurses will want to protect themselves and others from boredom. The resident must learn how to relate in a manner that does not drive people away. On occasion, the garrulous chatter is a warm-up for a life review. In these cases, the nurse can facilitate meaning by directing the resident toward critical life passages, for example, "Mrs. J., tell me what it was like for you when you began school." "Mrs. J., do you remember your first date?" "Mrs. J., who was with you when your first child was born?"

Other questions that may guide away from perseveration and circumstantiality are as follows:

"What was your most fearful experience?"
"In your life, when did you feel most proud of yourself?"
"Are there any events in your life you would like to have handled differently?"
"If you could change anything about your past, what would it be?"
"What is the greatest lesson life has taught you?"
"Who was most influential in your life?"
"If you could choose a time and place to live your life, when and where would it be?"
"Did you have any major disappointments in your life?"

These and many other exploratory statements will facilitate the life review. Usually helpful is to begin with descriptions of events, because these are less threatening than sharing fears, failures, and feelings. During any interview, an important aspect is to comment on increasing evidence of anxiety and tension and ask if the interviewee wishes to continue, to sit quietly, or to be left alone. The cathartic release experienced in life-review therapy may be less intensely experienced in old age but is nonetheless therapeutic. Guidelines for life-review therapy are provided in Box 23-13.

An old person is a living history book. However, unlike written history, the story remains flexible and changeable, similar to a kaleidoscope—each shift, however minor, in the person's self-esteem displays another pattern and colorful image. The most exciting aspect of working with the aged is being a part of the full emergence of the life story. Impatience with the early garrulous or tentative process may reduce the possibility of resolution in the resident and inspiration in the nurse.

Box 23-13 Guidelines for Life Review

1. Alert aged individuals to the characteristics and normality of the life-review process.
2. Provide opportunities for aged persons to recapitulate events in their lives (e.g., "What has most influenced the course of your life?" "Who has most influenced the course of your life?").
3. Assist aged individuals to view their life experiences in a broader or different context (e.g., "As you explain your regrets, can you think of other factors that contributed to those events?" "How would you have changed your life then?" "What factors influenced your course of action?" "What would you do differently now?").
4. Facilitate connections between past hopes, present events, and future expectations.
5. Be aware that the process may be carried out sporadically over several months. Live-review is a painful examination of the past and is sometimes avoided.

Group Psychotherapy. This approach may be more practical and acceptable than individual psychotherapy for people with limited incomes and psychologic distress resulting from the aging process. Cohort groups sharing common problems reduce feelings of alienation and ineffectiveness. Intergenerational groups are also successful in promoting understanding of common human needs and conflicts. The importance of group affiliations for the aged is discussed in an earlier chapter. Some guidelines for conducting group therapies are provided in Table 23-5.

Goals of group therapy with the aged are as follows:

1. Reduction in stress-related anxiety
2. Short-term treatment of specific disorders
3. Acceptance of the aging process
4. Resolution of conflicts

Grief Support Therapy. The most common problem of aging, grief resolution, is seldom addressed in the care of the institutionalized elderly. Staff avoidance, lack of skill, ignorance, and lack of concern are a few of the reasons this breakdown may occur. Worley (1996), an experienced grief therapist, has contracted with several long-term care facilities in California to provide grief counseling and has found the response encouraging. With continuation of these efforts and measurement of efficacy, we hope greater interest will develop in implementing grief counseling in nursing homes on a national level. In addition, similar group sessions are conducted on a weekly basis for community residents recovering from losses. Hospitals provide these opportunities as part of community outreach efforts. These "drop-in" groups are open to all community residents and are focused on warm acceptance, immediate support, sharing of feelings, provision of specific information, guidance, and resources in written

Table 23-5 Guidelines for Group Therapies

	Cognitively impaired	Psychologically disturbed	Depressed
Patient selection	No more than five members Age cohorts Both sexes	10 members Varied ages Both sexes	8-10 members Patients with similar problems, for example, grieving, retired Both sexes
Structure	Consistent place and time Frequent 30-minute meetings Co-leaders	Consistent place and time Biweekly 1-hour meetings One leader consistently	Varied meeting places Weekly 1-hour meeting Variable leadership
Process	Connect specific events, things, and places common to group	Members connected through shared feelings and survival strategies	Members focused on successful coping during life span; mutuality encouraged
Goals	Stimulate memory Enhance identity Raise self-esteem Increase socialization skills	Recognize feelings and meaning of suppressed conflicts Enlarge coping strategies Integrate self-view Promote universality	Reduce feelings of hopelessness Restore personal control Increase affectual responsiveness Develop a sense of integrity and acceptance of life as lived Promote caring between members
Nurse's function	1. Provide a comfortable, mildly stimulating environment 2. Select props that will stimulate memories 3. Assist members by giving specific information, reminders, and clues 4. Give praise and recognition for any participation	1. Establish a private meeting and a closed group 2. Plan to focus on specific developmental stages or critical life events 3. Accept and validate all expressions of feeling 4. Clarify multiple meanings of events 5. Reduce anxiety	1. Provide a comfortable, stimulating environment 2. Appeal to sensory memories 3. Focus members' attention on evidence of caring and sharing 4. Demonstrate a caring attitude 5. Allow time to complain

form, and referral for individual therapy when needed. Although these groups are not limited to the aged, the great majority of participants are over 60 years of age. Some participants attend weekly for several years, and some attend a few times or drop in sporadically as they feel the need. The individual is not *"expected"* to follow any particular pattern.

Somatotherapies. Promoting health, nutrition, activity, and rest is crucial to the success of any psychotherapeutic venture. These activities are discussed in many ways throughout this text. We would emphasize the importance of a balance of sleep and activity in maintaining mental health. Sleep is not only essential to daily restoration of function, it is also the domain of the psyche. Interference with sleep delays the integration and resolution of daily events. Psychologic work is accomplished during dream or rapid-eye-movement (REM) sleep, and this work may not proceed efficiently during drugged sleep. The dilemma for nurses is to support the need for rest and dream sleep. At times, individuals may need a hypnotic, but the continued reliance on such substances is physically and psychologically ill advised. Activity during the day and anxiety reduction exercises before sleep may have beneficial results in promoting the natural healing tendencies of the psyche during sleep.

Activity is useful in discharging anxiety and reducing agitated movement. In addition, exercise improves physical reserves, increases bone density, and reduces serum cholesterol. Nurses might consider providing some opportunity for exercise before verbal therapies.

Somatic therapies are often heavily reliant on drugs. Drugs must be used judiciously in the care of the aged. Major and minor tranquilizers often create more problems than they resolve.

ECT may be recommended for middle-aged and elderly individuals who are severely depressed. ECT can be effective and alters the entire affectual response of a severely depressed patient. Clinical experience clearly demonstrates that judicious use of ECT lifts depression and reduces the guilty ruminations that often accompany involutional depressive disorders. The problem is that no one understands exactly what all the cerebral consequences are. ECT has generally fallen out of favor as a treatment mode as more effective antidepressants have been developed. Many authors consider the prudence of discontinuing the use of ECT entirely until mechanisms of the brain are more fully understood and the potential recipients can truly make an informed choice.

Nursing Home Consultation. Monthly psychiatric consultation in nursing homes is another method of attempting to serve the mental health needs of residents. The consultations are primarily useful in increasing staff understanding and acceptance of the emotional problems of residents. Better understanding will also encourage staff members to increase the number of therapeutic programs offered.

Obtaining immediate psychologic evaluation of residents in long-term care settings facilitates rapid and successful adjustment. The information obtained may assist caregivers in structuring care and activities to enhance the resident's strengths and to reduce anxiety.

Information from the resident's family is integral to accurate assessment. The family can be asked about personality characteristics, cognitive abilities, patterns of response to stress and anxiety, history of psychopathologic conditions, and pervasive emotional tone. The resident's perspective and mental status must also be assessed.

Providing continuity of care for geropsychiatric patients across a variety of institutional and community-based settings has not been given adequate attention. Relocation stress and trauma can be reduced significantly by prior preparation, preservation of autonomy, and follow-up by people from the prior setting to assist in problem solving and adjusting to the new setting. Providing programs for information and preparation of individuals and their families when a move is necessary may facilitate the adaptation. Introduction to a "patient pal" from the new unit can ease the way and may increase the self-esteem of both residents.

In dealing with individuals who are experiencing their first admission to a psychogeriatric ward, assessing their life stresses and functional capacity is particularly important before the emergence of the current problems. Most commonly, a major loss precedes the first admission. Although most of these residents have lived independently, they are often discharged to nursing homes. Symptomatology or diagnosis alone is not sufficient to determine the need for a protected setting. This determination should be made with great caution and sensitivity to the self-concept implications, and every effort should be made to restore the residents to the setting of their choice.

NONTRADITIONAL THERAPY AND COUNSELING

Nontraditional therapies are nonthreatening and designed to enhance coping, self-esteem, and respect for individuality. Developing an individualized nursing care plan is essential. Motivating the aged to use traditional counseling and psychotherapy has always been a factor in underuse of mental health facilities. Nontraditional programs and approaches that are therapeutic may be more acceptable to older people than those that have the mental illness stigma.

Peer Counseling

In peer counseling, people without professional training but of similar age and experience help other people. The approach is appealing to both the helper and the helpee and is nonthreatening. The peer concept can facilitate the development of a genuinely supportive relationship and a special rapport. The older person providing service enhances his or her own mental health through the opportunity to engage in productive, other-directed activities. Some ways elders have been used to provide services for other elders include the following:

- Counseling people in retirement transition about benefits, income tax, insurance and investment, and retirement adjustment
- Counseling elders about legal issues and social and personal problems
- Providing for developmentally disabled adults
- Providing senior companions, visitation, and support to residents in nursing homes and to the homebound
- Providing aged advocacy by indigenous elders for minorities

Volunteers in peer support programs need special training in the following:

- Empathic interviewing and listening skills
- Aspects of normal aging
- Special problems of the elderly
- Self-awareness
- Problem-solving methods
- Information and resources available to the aged

Particular topics that may be introduced in peer counselor training sessions include the following:

- Assertiveness training
- Management of depression
- Death and dying, grief
- Evaluation of institutional care
- Working with the disabled
- Use of reminiscence
- Human sexuality

Self-Help Programs

Self-help programs have flourished in the last two decades, as has the use of peer counselors and volunteers. Self-help programs usually follow a "train the trainer" model and recruit from churches, community colleges, and universities in which vital and engaged older individuals can be found. Community and news announcements are also effective in recruiting trainees.

Screening of volunteers is a sensitive issue and must not in any way erode the self-esteem of the individual volunteer. Throughout the process of selection and training, the emphasis must be on the strengths that the volunteer brings. If the qualities necessary for counseling are not present, the person must be routed early to an activity fitting his or her skills.

Providing scheduled supervision and support is necessary, as are providing tokens and awards of appreciation and planning activities in which the peer counselors have opportunities to share and learn from each other. The failure to plan for these needs of the peer counselor or volunteers is likely to result in less than satisfactory results from them as counselors.

Mobile Clinics

A psychogeriatric clinic may become a vital addition to the elder services. The clinic offers multidisciplinary assessment and treatment services. Home assessments, follow-up visits, and psychosocial, nursing, medication, and occupational therapy consultation are included in the comprehensive care plans. Referrals are accepted from anyone in the community. The clinic also provides consultation to nursing homes and ongoing support groups for elders at risk, including such foci as relaxation, memory strengthening, and peer counseling.

Roy and colleagues (1987) reported on services provided in Middletown, New York, through a mobile geriatric treatment team. The team has been able to avert inpatient psychiatric hospitalization for 77% of cases. Comparable efforts have been made in communities throughout the nation and should certainly be given consideration.

Within the home, providing such services is not only cost-effective, but also more attendant to the holistic perspective of an individual's needs. Older people account for only 5% of visits made to mental health clinics and less than 2% of visits to private psychotherapists (Nesbit, 1987). Given that most elders consult their internist when encountering an emotional problem, it is imperative that acceptable and comprehensive methods of meeting their needs are used. The mobile mental health clinics seem to be a step in the right direction.

Additionally, identifying high-risk individuals such as those who are living alone, homebound, recently bereaved, or suffering from repeated falls or hospitalizations and mental deterioration and providing preventive supports might best be accomplished by mobile mental health units.

A similar model uses the services of a psychologist, nurse, geriatric NP, and psychiatrist provide individuals with comprehensive physical and mental health assessments and problem management.

Multidisciplinary community mental health teams will continue to grow because of the multiple health and social needs of the older population and the limited availability of appropriate psychogeriatric institutional care. The geropsychiatric nurse's role is becoming a critical component of human services.

Human Needs and Wellness Diagnoses

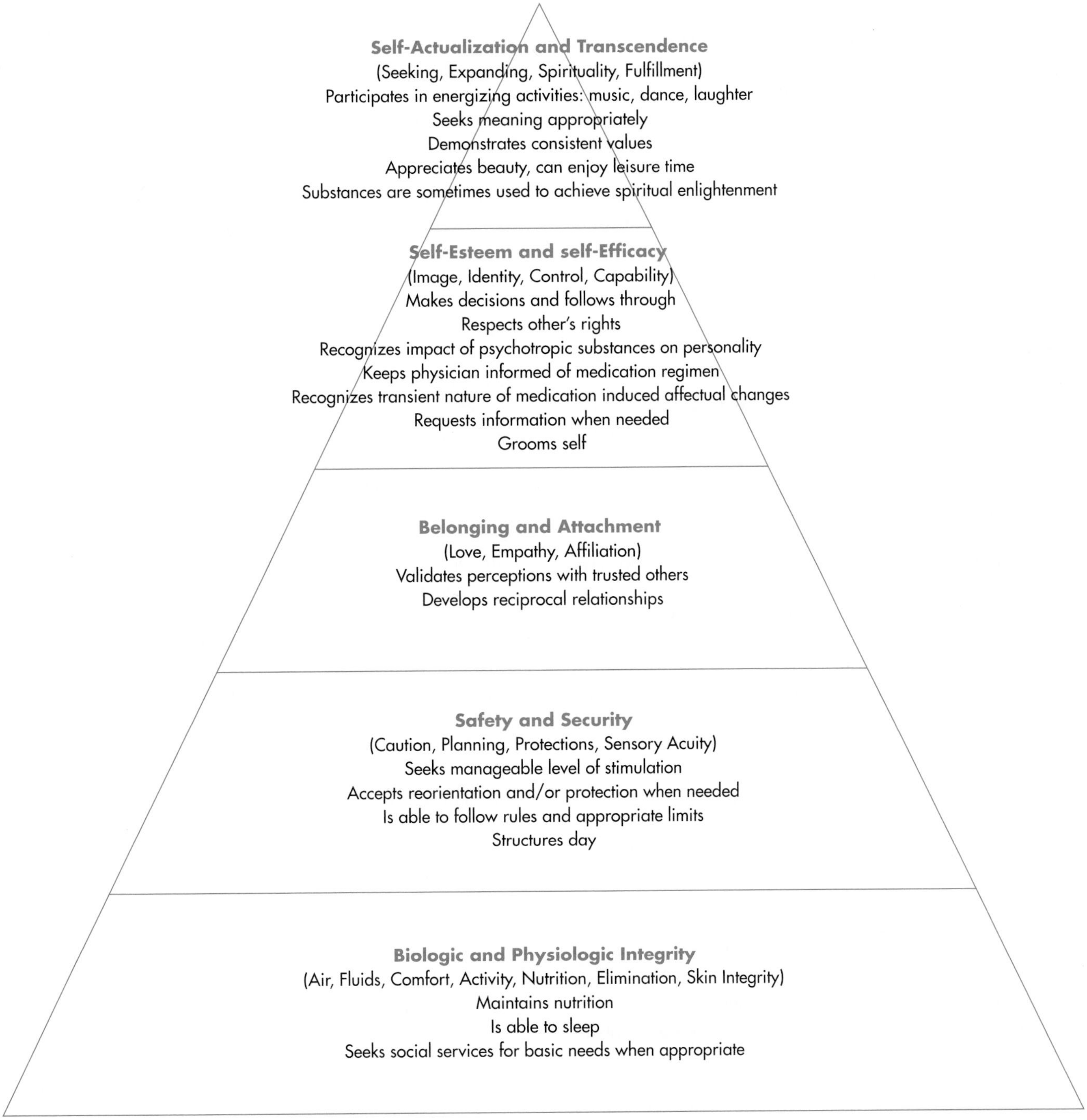

Self-Actualization and Transcendence
(Seeking, Expanding, Spirituality, Fulfillment)
Participates in energizing activities: music, dance, laughter
Seeks meaning appropriately
Demonstrates consistent values
Appreciates beauty, can enjoy leisure time
Substances are sometimes used to achieve spiritual enlightenment

Self-Esteem and self-Efficacy
(Image, Identity, Control, Capability)
Makes decisions and follows through
Respects other's rights
Recognizes impact of psychotropic substances on personality
Keeps physician informed of medication regimen
Recognizes transient nature of medication induced affectual changes
Requests information when needed
Grooms self

Belonging and Attachment
(Love, Empathy, Affiliation)
Validates perceptions with trusted others
Develops reciprocal relationships

Safety and Security
(Caution, Planning, Protections, Sensory Acuity)
Seeks manageable level of stimulation
Accepts reorientation and/or protection when needed
Is able to follow rules and appropriate limits
Structures day

Biologic and Physiologic Integrity
(Air, Fluids, Comfort, Activity, Nutrition, Elimination, Skin Integrity)
Maintains nutrition
Is able to sleep
Seeks social services for basic needs when appropriate

These are not all the possible wellness diagnoses that may be identified. The above are examples of nursing diagnoses that should be considered when planning care for the older adult.

KEY CONCEPTS

- Mental health in old age is difficult to determine because the accrual of life experiences makes for great variations. Mental health must be determined by the gratification or satisfaction that individuals feel within their particular situation.
- Mental health is a fluctuating situation for most individuals, with peaks and valleys of happiness and pain.
- Elders are not well served within the mental health system as it exists today. Neither practitioners nor reimbursement mechanisms are adapted to their needs.
- Psychologic assessment of elders that is based on the common psychometric instruments will usually show deficits because these instruments, with few exceptions, have been designed to test the mental health of young adults.
- Classic defense mechanisms, such as denial, displacement and identification, when used by the elderly, are often life enhancing and necessary to their function.
- Anxiety disorders are common in late life and are best managed by restoring some sense of control to the situation that the individual perceives as out of control.
- PTSD is finally being recognized in the aged who have been subjected to extremely traumatic events. Programs are now available to provide support and insight for these individuals.
- Substance abuse and addictions may be distorted adaptational methods used by some aged to cope with losses and end-of-life concerns. These individuals have been successfully treated by providing supportive groups and relationships.
- Depression is the most common emotional disorder of aging and similarly the most treatable. Unfortunately, depression is often neglected or assumed to be a condition one must "learn to live with." Nurses may be instrumental in ensuring that elders are assessed properly and treated for depression.
- Grief is a component of aging for most individuals as they confront various losses. Grief is not a mental illness, but it often requires grief counseling and support for resolution.
- Suicide is not prevalent among the aged. Women vastly outnumber men in late life, and women are rarely suicidal. Very old white men are highly suicidal and must be assessed for suicidal intent whenever they confront a trauma or catastrophe.

▲ CASE STUDY

Depressive Disorder with Suicidal Thoughts

Jake had cared for his wife, Emma, during a long and painful illness until she died 4 years ago. He found that alcohol provided a way to cope with the stress. Within a year after her death, Jake met a lady to whom he was very attracted, and a few months later, she moved in with him. Jake managed to move his things around until some space was made for her personal items, but neither of them were very comfortable with this, he because he really did not like to move his things from their usual place and she because her allotted space was so small she felt like an intruder. He collected guns, and she shuddered when she saw them. He was an avid fan of John Wayne movies, and she preferred going to the symphony. He liked meat and potatoes, and she was a vegetarian. She also disapproved of his increasing reliance on alcohol. The blending of two such different lifestyles proved difficult. In a few months she moved out, and Jake blamed himself. He said over and over, "I should have done more for her. I'm not good for anything anymore." His friends began to pull away from him, just when he needed them most, because he seemed to talk of nothing but his various aches, pains, and pills and his general discouragement with life. Jake's consumption of alcohol increased markedly. He had some health problems: a mild congestive heart, a lack of exercise, dairy products gave him diarrhea, he was somewhat obese, and his knees were painful most of the time. He routinely visited his allergist, his internist, his orthopedist, and his cardiologist. However, it seemed the more he went to these specialists, the worse he felt. He was taking several medications, and each time he saw one of his clinicians, he came away with another prescription. No one asked about his drinking, and he never mentioned it. He awoke one morning feeling very dizzy, and so he went to his internist later in the day. He began to share the litany of his discomforts, and the physician reminded him that at 76 years of age he could not expect to always feel in top shape.

When he returned from seeing the physician, Jake called his daughter and surprised her by saying he had just decided he would take a week off and go to Hawaii to see if the sun and sand would revive him. Jake was not usually impulsive. His daughter, fortunately, was a psychiatric nurse and was concerned about the change in his behavior.

Based on the case study, develop a nursing care plan using the following procedure:*

List the client's comments that provide subjective data.

List information that provides objective data.

From these data, identify and state, using accepted format, two nursing diagnoses you determine are most significant to this client at this time. List two client strengths that you have identified from the data.

Determine and state outcome criteria for each diagnosis. These criteria must reflect some alleviation of the problem identified in the nursing diagnosis and must be stated in concrete and measurable terms.

Plan and state one or more interventions for each diagnosed problem.

Provide specific documentation of sources used to determine appropriate intervention. Plan at least one intervention that incorporates the client's existing strengths.

---

*Students are advised to refer to their nursing diagnosis text and identify possible or potential problems.

Evaluate the success of intervention. Interventions must correlate directly with the stated outcome criteria to measure the outcome success.

STUDY QUESTIONS/ACTIVITIES

Discuss the variations in symptoms of depression in the old and the young.
Describe some of the reasons we believe that elders are more vulnerable to depression than younger people.
Describe a time when you were depressed and the feelings you had. What did you do about it?
Given the situation in this case, discuss what your thoughts would be if you were his daughter.
Given his daughter's background, what are her responsibilities in this case?
What is the responsibility of a student nurse in the case of suspected suicidal thoughts?
Would you address the possibility of suicidal thoughts if you were the nurse in the physician's office? When and how would you take on this task?
What action should be taken for Jake's protection?
Would you expect that Jake is still grieving over the death of his wife? What are your thoughts about this situation?
What are the clues or indications that an elder is thinking of committing suicide?
What are some of the signs of suicidal intent in young adults? How are these signs different from those of elders?
Under what conditions do you think a person has a right to take his or her life?
What are your thoughts about Jake's use of alcohol?
Do you think suicide is a sign of weakness or strength?

1. Normally older people feel depressed much of the time.
2. Older people are more likely than young people to admit to depression.
3. Most older people talk about suicide but rarely try to kill themselves.
4. Depression of the elderly is helped by medications.
5. Depression may be the cause of forgetfulness.
6. Depression in the elderly is often linked with disease and alcoholism.

▲ CASE STUDY

Bipolar Disorder

Myra is a 71-year-old white woman who was admitted to the geropsychiatry inpatient unit for alcohol abuse and noncompliance with her lithium, which had been prescribed for a diagnosed bipolar disorder. Myra's primary mode of coping with her depression and mood swings has been to drink alcohol, meet abusive men, and play bingo. However, when she stops taking her dose of lithium, she begins to have flights of ideas, argues with her daughters, and tries to pick up men in her apartment complex. After seeing her at home, you discover that she has a long history of being physically abused by her husband, now deceased for 8 years, and has been living with one daughter who has also emotionally and physically abused her, causing her to be hospitalized. Myra's ability to test reality is compromised because of years of denial and low self-esteem. She says, "I used to have lots of times when I felt really good in between the depressions. Now I feel depressed most of the time." She tells you that her daughters harass her and interfere in her life. Your goals as a community-based nurse are to facilitate her independence, that is, being able to live in her own apartment, to assist her with medication compliance, and to intervene with Myra to improve relationships with her daughters. Home visits are approved through Medicare for 2 months after hospital discharge.

Based on the case study, develop a nursing care plan using the following procedure:*

List the client's comments that provide subjective data.
List information that provides objective data.
From these data, identify and state, using accepted format, two nursing diagnoses you determine are most significant to this client at this time. List two client strengths that you have identified from the data.
Determine and state outcome criteria for each diagnosis. These must reflect some alleviation of the problem identified in the nursing diagnosis and must be stated in concrete and measurable terms.
Plan and state one or more interventions for each diagnosed problem. Provide specific documentation of sources used to determine appropriate intervention. Plan at least one intervention that incorporates the client's existing strengths.
Evaluate success of intervention. Interventions must correlate directly with the stated outcome criteria to measure the outcome success.

STUDY QUESTIONS/ACTIVITIES

How will you evaluate Myra's ability to live independently?
What particular strategies are necessary to meet the goals of the nursing care plan?
Given that Myra's primary coping strategy is drinking alcohol, how will you facilitate her sobriety and help her deal with stress?
How much involvement with Myra's daughters do you believe is necessary to assist with her transition back into her own apartment?
Given the short number of visits covered by Medicare, what information does Myra need so as to provide self-care? In other words, the nurse must be teaching Myra how to live independently after discharge from home health care. What does Myra need to know?

*Students are advised to refer to their nursing diagnosis text and identify possible or potential problems.

Discuss the meanings and the thoughts triggered by the students' and elders' viewpoints expressed at the beginning of the chapter. How do these vary from your own experience?

RESEARCH QUESTIONS

What is the prevalence of mental disorders in community-dwelling older adults? What mental health care is nursing able to provide in the home?

How common is alcohol abuse a strategy of self-care used by the mentally ill elderly?

What types of assessment instruments best determine an individual's ability to provide self-care?

Is psychiatric home care a more cost-effective alternative than institutional care?

Discriminate more clearly the types of geriatric depression and develop specificity of treatment based on these findings.

Clarify cause-and-effect relationship between various illnesses and depression.

Identify risk factors, prodromal signs, and their relationship to depressive symptomatology.

Determine in what circumstances antidepressants are useful in grief reactions.

What are the cardinal symptoms of depression in the oldest-old?

To what extent can depression be identified as a major precipitant to suicide?

Although the general status of aged white males is thought to be the best it has been from a socioeconomic perspective, inexplicably, suicide has begun to increase since 1981. What factors may be contributing to this increase?

Do degenerative neurosensory changes predispose a person to depression?

What are some factors that explain the great age difference in peak suicidal behaviors in men and women?

How many physicians consider or evaluate for the presence of depression in elders who see them for physical complaints?

What is the most reliable tool for identifying depression in the elderly?

In what present cultures are the aged most comfortable and honored?

What is the earliest sign of depression that an elder experiences?

REFERENCES

American Association of Geriatric Psychiatry (AAGP): *Geriatrics and mental health—the facts,* 2002. Available at *www.aagpgpa.org/prof/facts_mh.asp*

American Association of Retired Persons: *Suicide by the elderly,* Washington, DC, 1994, AARP.

American Psychiatric Association: *Diagnostic and statistical manual of mental disorders (DSM-IV),* ed 4, Washington, DC, 1994, The Association.

Antai-Otong D: Schizophrenia in the elderly, *Adv NP* 8(3):39, 2000.

Arbore P: *Suicide in the elderly.* Presented at the 48th Annual Scientific Meeting of the Gerontological Society of America, Los Angeles, November 20, 1995.

Beers MH, Berkow R: *Merck manual of geriatrics,* ed 3, Whitehouse Station, NJ, 2000, Merck Research Laboratories.

Brown JB, Bedford NK, White SJ: *Gerontological protocols for nurse practitioners,* Philadelphia, 1999, JB Lippincott.

Brown SI: Depression common among adults with advanced macular degeneration, *Ophthalmology* 108:1893, 2001.

Butler RN, Lewis MI: *Aging and mental health: positive psychosocial approaches,* ed 3, St Louis, 1983, Mosby.

Butler RN, Lewis MI, Sunderland T: *Aging and mental health: positive psychosocial, and biomedical approaches,* ed 4, New York, 1991, Macmillan.

Casey DE: *Improved antipsychotic effect of divalproex combined with risperidone or olanzapine for schizophrenia.* Presented at World Assembly of Mental Health, 26th Biennial Congress of the World Federation for Mental Health, Vancouver, BC, July 22-27, 2001.

Commerford MC, Reznikoff M: Relationship of religion and perceived social support to self esteem and depression in nursing home residents, *J Psychol* 130(1):35, 1996.

Covinsky K: Depressive symptoms and disability progression, *Pepper Rev* 3(3):4, 1996.

Culpepper L: Recognizing and treating post-traumatic stress disorder, *Hippocrates* 14(6), June 2000.

Durkheim E: *Suicide,* Glencoe, IL, 1951 (reprint of 1897 work), Free Press.

Farberow NL et al: Changes in grief and mental health of bereaved spouses of older suicides, *J Gerontol* 47(6):357, 1992.

Frohberg NR, Herting RL: Psychiatry: anxiety disorders. In *University of Iowa family practice handbook,* ed 3, 1999, Virtual Hospital. Available at *www.vh.org/Providers/ClinRef/FPHandbook/Chapter 15/02-15.html*

Fromholt P, Larsen P, Larsen S: Effects of late-onset depression and recovery on autobiographical memory, *J Gerontol* 50(2):P74, 1995.

Goldfarb A, Turner H: Psychotherapy of aged persons. II. Utilization and effectiveness of "brief" therapy, *Am J Psychiatr* 109:916, 1953.

Goldfarb A, Turner H: Psychotherapy of aged persons, *Psychoanal Rev* 42:916, 1955.

Grossberg GT: Diagnosis and treatment of late-life psychosis in the elderly, *Long-term Care Forum* 1(3):7, 2000.

Haring C et al: *Suicide in the elderly,* abstract. Proceedings of the 3rd Congress of the International Psychogeriatric Association, Chicago, March 17, 1987.

Heaton RK et al: The stability and course of neuropsychological deficits in schizophrenia, *Arch Gen Psychiatr* 58(1):24, 2001.

International Health News Database: *Low blood pressure linked to depression,* 2001. Available at *www.yourhealthbase.com*

Jarman RW, Herrera RM: Recognizing and meeting the mental health needs of the elderly in the new century, *The Director* 9(2):49, 2001.

Kennedy GJ: *Helping older Americans cope with crisis.* AAGP press release, September 18, 2001. Available at *www.aagponline.org/new/pressreleases*

Kennedy-Malone L, Fletcher KR, Plank LM: *Management guidelines for gerontological nurse practitioners,* Philadelphia, 2000, FA Davis.

Lerner V: New hope in treating tardive dyskinesia, *AJN* 102(1):23, 2001.

Lester D, Tallmer M: Now I lay me down to sleep, *Contemp Gerontol* 1(3):91, 1994.

McAndrews MM: Lighting the darkness, *Advance for Providers of Post-Acute Care* 73:40, Sept/Oct 2001.

Miller M: *Suicide after 60: the final alternative,* New York, 1979, Springer.

Moorhead SA, Brighton VA: Anxiety and fear. In Maas ML et al, editors: *Nursing care of older adults: diagnoses, outcomes, and interventions,* St Louis, 2001, Mosby.

Müller-Spahn F, Hock C: Clinical presentation of depression in the elderly, *Gerontology* 40(suppl 1):10, 1994.

National Institutes of Mental Health: *A story of bipolar disorder,* 2002. Available at *www.nimh.nih.gov/pub licat/bipolstory08.cfm*

National Institutes of Mental Health: *The neurobiology of depression and suicide,* 2001a. Available at *www.nimh.nih.gov/sciadvances/0011.cfm*

National Institutes of Mental Health: *Older adults: depression and suicide facts,* 2001b. Available at *www.nimh.nih.gov/publicat/elderlydepsuicide.cfm*

Nesbit D: *Attitudinal barriers to delivery of mental health services to the elderly* (abstract). Proceedings of the Third Congress of the International Psychogeriatric Association, Chicago, March 16, 1987.

Nowak KB, Wandel JC: The sharing of self in geriatric clinical practice: case report and analysis, *Geriatr Nurs* 19(1):34-7, 1998.

Omnicare Formulary: *Geriatric pharmaceutical care guidelines,* Covington, KY, 2002, Omnicare.

Reuben DB et al: *Geriatrics at your fingertips, 2002 edition,* Malden, MA, 2002, American Geriatric Society–Blackwell.

Reuben DB et al: *Geriatrics at your fingertips, 2003 edition,* Malden, MA, 2002, American Geriatric Society–Blackwell.

Ronsman K: Therapy for depression, *J Gerontol Nurs* 13(12):21, 1987.

Roy B, Obaid M, Rudick S: Patterns of psychiatric illness in elderly and the role of a mobile geriatric treatment team-management outcome and cost effectiveness (abstract). Proceedings of the Third Congress of the International Psychogeriatric Association, Chicago, March 9, 1987.

Sahr N: Assessment and diagnosis of elderly depression, *Clin Excellence for NPs* 3(3):158, 1999.

Uncapher H, Arean P: Doctors less inclined to treat suicidal elderly, *J Am Geriatr Soc* 48:188, 2000.

U.S. Bureau of the Census: *Statistical abstract of the United States: 1995,* ed 115, Washington, DC, 1995, U.S. Government Printing Office.

U.S. Department of Health and Human Services: *Healthy people 2010,* Washington DC, 2000, USDHHS. Also available at *www.health.gov/healthypeople*

Webster JD: Construction and validation of the reminiscence functions scale, *J Gerontol* 48(5):P256, 1993.

Worley A: *Grief group counseling in nursing homes and community "drop-in" grief support groups,* unpublished manuscript, 1996.

Wright P, Dribben-Gutman B: Animal facilitated therapy in nursing homes, *Nurs Homes* 30:2, 1981.

Yesavage J et al: Development and validation of a geriatric depression screening scale: a preliminary report, *J Psychiatr* 12:63, 1983.

Zung W: A self-rating depression scale, *Arch Gen Psychiatr* 12:63, 1965.

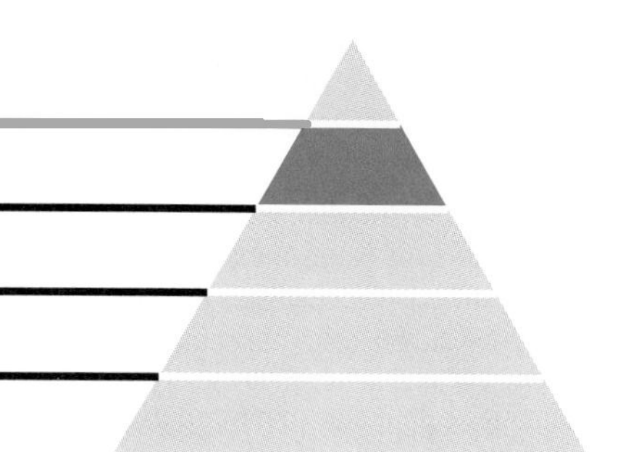

APPENDIX 23-A

Depression Rating Scales

The Zung Self-Rating Depression Scale (SDS) is probably the most widely used test of depression in the elderly. The SDS is a self-administered questionnaire consisting of 20 items that measure areas associated with depression such as mood, well being, optimism, and somatic symptoms (Zung, 1965). The scale incorporates both positive and negative responses. The items are scored on a 4-point scale, ranging from "a little of the time," "some of the time," "a good part of the time," to "most of the time." The responses are given a score of 1 to 4, arranged such that the higher the score, the greater the depression: the statements designated with (1) are given "1" for response "most of the time," and those with (2) are given a "4" for "most of the time." The score is derived by dividing the sum of the 20 items (which are rated from 1 to 4) by the maximum score of 80 to arrive at a number expressed as a decimal. Scores above 0.38 (or a raw score of 50 and over) were associated with depression requiring hospital treatment (Zung, 1965).

The Center for Epidemiologic Studies Depression Scale (CES-D) was developed by the Center for Epidemiologic Studies at the National Institutes of Mental Health for use in studies of depression in community samples. The CES-D contains 20 items. Respondents are asked to report the amount of time they have experienced symptoms during the past week. Typically, a threshold of 17 and above is taken as defining "caseness," although higher cutoff points (e.g., 24 and above) have been suggested.

The General Health Questionnaire (GHQ) is a 60-item self-administered instrument, the purpose of which is to detect the presence of psychiatric distress. A scaled version has been devised and consists of 28 items that test four general categories (seven questions each): somatic symptoms, anxiety and insomnia, social dysfunction, and depression. The GHQ is unusual in that it was developed specifically for use in the primary care setting.

Using the GHQ, respondents rate the presence of anxious and depressive symptoms "over the past few weeks" into one of four categories: "not at all" (coded 1), "no more than usual" (coded 2), "more than usual" (coded 3), or "much more" (coded 4). Each question has four responses: score 1 for either of the two answers consistent with depression and 0 for the other two.

Zung Self-Rating Depression Scale

1. (−) I feel down-hearted and blue.
2. (+) Morning is when I feel the best.
3. (−) I have crying spells or feel like it.
4. (−) I have trouble sleeping at night.
5. (+) I eat as much as I used to.
6. (+) I still enjoy sex.
7. (−) I notice that I am losing weight.
8. (−) I have trouble with constipation.
9. (−) My heart beats faster than usual.
10. (−) I get tired for no reason.
11. (+) My mind is as clear as it used to be.
12. (+) I find it easy to do the things I used to.
13. (−) I am restless and can't keep still.
14. (+) I feel hopeful about the future.
15. (−) I am more irritable than usual.
16. (+) I find it easy to make decisions.
17. (+) I feel that I am useful and needed.
18. (+) My life is pretty full.
19. (−) I feel that others would be better off if I were dead.
20. (+) I still enjoy the things I used to do.

From Zung WK: A self-rating depression scale, *Arch Gen Psychiatr* 12:65, 1965, Copyright © 1965, American Medical Association, with permission. All depression checklists from Gallo JJ, Reichel W, Andersen LM: *Handbook of geriatric assessment,* ed 2, Gaithersburg, Md, 1995, Aspen Publishers.

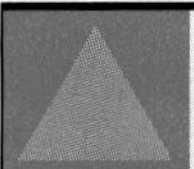

Center for Epidemiologic Studies Depression Scale

INSTRUCTIONS FOR QUESTIONS: Below is a list of the ways you might have felt or behaved. Please tell me how often you have felt this way during the past week.

Rarely or none of the time (Less than 1 day)
Some or a little of the time (1-2 days)
Occasionally or a moderate amount of time (3-4 days)
Most or all of the time (5-7 days)

During the past week:

1. I was bothered by things that usually don't bother me.
2. I did not feel like eating; my appetite was poor.
3. I felt that I could not shake off the blues even with help from my family or friends.
4. I felt that I was just as good as other people.
5. I had trouble keeping my mind on what I was doing.
6. I felt depressed.
7. I felt that everything I did was an effort.
8. I felt hopeful about the future.
9. I thought my life had been a failure.
10. I felt fearful.
11. My sleep was restless.
12. I was happy.
13. I talked less than usual.
14. I felt lonely.
15. People were unfriendly.
16. I enjoyed life.
17. I had crying spells.
18. I felt sad.
19. I felt that people dislike me.
20. I could not get "going."

From Center for Epidemiologic Studies, National Institutes of Mental Health.

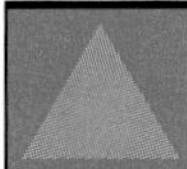

Items from the Scaled U.S. Version of the General Health Questionnaire

A. Somatic symptoms
- A1. Been feeling in need of some medicine to pick you up?
- A2. Been feeling in need of a good tonic?
- A3. Been feeling run down and out of sorts?
- A4. Felt that you are ill?
- A5. Been getting any pains in your head?
- A6. Been getting a feeling of tightness or pressure in your head?
- A7. Been having hot or cold spells?

B. Anxiety and insomnia
- B1. Lost much sleep over worry?
- B2. Had difficulty staying asleep?
- B3. Felt constantly under strain?
- B4. Been getting edgy and bad-tempered?
- B5. Been getting scared or panicky for no reason?
- B6. Found everything getting on top of you?
- B7. Been feeling nervous and uptight all the time?

C. Social dysfunction
- C1. Been managing to keep yourself busy and occupied?
- C2. Been taking longer over the things you do?
- C3. Felt on the whole you were doing things well?
- C4. Been satisfied with the way you have carried out your tasks?
- C5. Felt that you are playing a useful part in things?
- C6. Felt capable of making decisions about things?
- C7. Been able to enjoy your normal day to day activities?

D. Depression
- D1. Been thinking of yourself as a worthless person?
- D2. Felt that life is entirely hopeless?
- D3. Felt that life isn't worth living?
- D4. Thought of the possibility that you might do away with yourself?
- D5. Found at times you couldn't do anything because your nerves were too bad?
- D6. Found yourself wishing you were dead and away from it all?
- D7. Found that the idea of taking your own life kept coming into your mind?

In scoring the Social Dysfunction Rating Scale, the rater assigns a score based on the following six gradations: not present (score 1), very mild (score 2), mild (score 3), moderate (score 4), severe (score 5), and very severe (score 6). This instrument, although not designed to measure degrees of depression, is very useful when assessing the impact of depression on quality of life. The Geriatric Depression Scale (GDS) exists in both short and long forms (Yesavage et al, 1983). The original 30-item form of the GDS has been shown to be an effective screening test for depression in a variety of settings. The short, 15-item version of the GDS was developed primarily for brevity and, in particular, for use in populations such as the medically ill or those with dementia, where the longer form might be burdensome. How well this short form works in these populations, however, is largely undetermined.

The short version of the GDS, similar to its longer predecessor, is an effective screening tool in the cognitively intact. However, in a population of subjects with mild dementias of the Alzheimer's type (DAT), the short form does not appear to retain its validity.

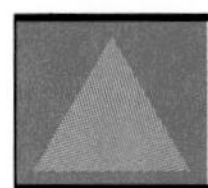

The Short Form of the Geriatric Depression Scale

1. Are you basically satisfied with your life?
2. Have you dropped many of your activities and interests?
3. Do you feel that your life is empty?
4. Do you often get bored?
5. Are you in good spirits most of the time?
6. Are you afraid that something bad is going to happen to you?
7. Do you feel happy most of the time?
8. Do you often feel helpless?
9. Do you prefer to stay at home, rather than going out and doing new things?
10. Do you feel you have more problems with memory than most?
11. Do you think it is wonderful to be alive?
12. Do you feel pretty worthless the way you are now?
13. Do you feel full of energy?
14. Do you feel that your situation is hopeless?
15. Do you think that most people are better off than you?

From Yesavage J et al: Development and validation of a geriatric depression screening scale: a preliminary report, *J Psychiatr Res* 17(1):37, 1982-1983.

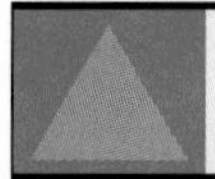

Social Dysfunction Rating Scale

Self-Esteem

1. Low self-concept (feelings of inadequacy, not measuring up to self-ideal)
2. Goallessness (lack of inner motivation and sense of future orientation)
3. Lack of a satisfying philosophy or meaning of life (a conceptual framework for integrating past and present experiences)
4. Self-health concern (preoccupation with physical health, somatic concerns)

Interpersonal System

5. Emotional withdrawal (degree of deficiency in relating to others)
6. Hostility (degree of aggression toward others)
7. Manipulation (exploiting of environment, controlling at other's expense)
8. Overdependency (degree of parasitic attachment to others)
9. Anxiety (degree of feeling of uneasiness, impending doom)
10. Suspiciousness (degree of distrust or paranoid ideation)

Performance System

11. Lack of satisfying relationships with significant persons (spouse, children, kin, significant persons serving in a family role)
12. Lack of friends, social contacts
13. Expressed need for more friends, social contacts
14. Lack of work (remunerative or nonremunerative, productive work activities that normally give a sense of usefulness, status, confidence)
15. Lack of satisfaction from work
16. Lack of leisure time activities
17. Expressed need for more leisure, self-enhancing, and satisfying activities
18. Lack of participation in community activities
19. Lack of interest in community affairs and activities that influence others
20. Financial insecurity
21. Adaptive rigidity (lack of complex coping patterns to stress)

From Linn MW et al: A Social Dysfunction Rating Scale, *J Psychiatr Res* 6:300, 1969.

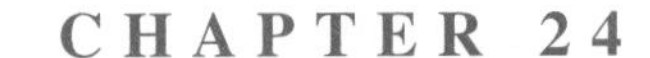

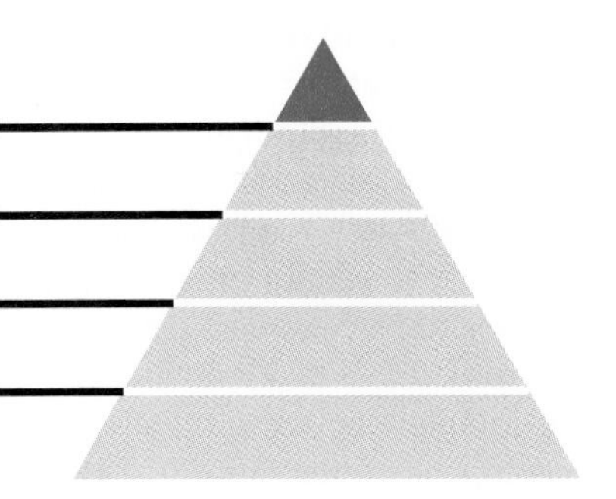

CHAPTER 24

End-of-Life Issues

Patricia Hess

An elder speaks

Losses are the hardest of all experiences. Losing parents is expected; deaths of children hurt. If one lives as long as I have, increasingly, others my age and younger are expiring; and then there is the experience of real loneliness. I sometimes feel like the proverbial last leaf clinging to the tree. By the time I was 50, numerous uncles, aunts, cousins had died; in the last 5 years, my only brother; last week his daughter-in-law. Since living at the Meadows, I have made and lost many friends; we are constantly reminded of the proximity of death.

Lyn, age 85

LEARNING OBJECTIVES

After completing this chapter, the reader will be able to:

1. Differentiate between loss and grief.
2. Explain the different types of grief and the dynamics of the grieving process.
3. Explain the attributes that are required of the nurse to be able to intervene effectively in grief and mourning.
4. List interventions that are helpful to the newly bereaved and those whose grief is established.
5. Discuss the process of dying and the pros and cons of the various theories and frameworks for the dying process.
6. Identify and discuss the needs of the dying and appropriate interventions.
7. Differentiate between the types of advance directives, and explain the role and responsibilities of the nurse as they relate to each of them.
8. Develop an understanding of end-of-life issues.
9. Describe palliative nursing care and the competencies it requires.

LOSS, GRIEF, AND BEREAVEMENT

Loss, dying, and death are universal incontestable events of the human experience that one is unable to stop or control. The numerous physical, psychologic, and behavioral responses that are exhibited are known as grief, mourning, or bereavement.

Loss, similar to death, is an event, whereas dying and grief and mourning are dynamic processes. Loss for elders generally relates to loss of relationships through death (of spouse, friends, and at times adult children), and life transitions (retirement, role change, and relocation from home to a nursing care facility) (Box 24-1).

Dying may be the elder's own or that of a significant other. Regardless, grief and grief work or mourning are intrinsic. Grief and mourning (bereavement) are usually used synonymously. However, in its purest form, grief refers to the individual's response to the event of loss. Mourning incorporates the loss into his or her ongoing life. Mourning is an active process rather than one that is reactive. The behaviors associated with mourning are determined by social and cultural norms that prescribe the appropriate ways of coping with loss in a given society.

The approach in this chapter leans toward a modernistic perspective because of the amount of research that has been disseminated during the twentieth century. *However, an*

Box 24-1 Losses of the Aged

Loss of Relationships
Significant others
Social contacts through:
- Illness
- Death
- Distance
- Decreased mobility

Life Transitions
Significant roles
Financial security
Independence
Physical health
Mental stability
Life-death

important point to emphasize is that no single way to grieve or respond to loss exists. Responses will vary widely among individuals and across cultures.

The experience of death (age, place, and manner of death) has been profoundly altered during the twentieth century. Seventy three percent of deaths each year are of the aged (U.S. Bureau of the Census, 2001). The mean age of death has increased throughout the century. The elderly are the only group of individuals to whom death is considered culturally acceptable (Godow, 1987). This view is a form of ageist discrimination, a subtle denigration of aging. The number of elders surviving into very old age has influenced the experience of death and bereavement.

CONCEPTUAL UNDERPINNINGS OF GRIEF

The majority of grief theories have evolved between the early 1900s and early 1990s and have served as the foundation of what caregivers and society in general have been taught about grieving. Theorists suggested that grief work or mourning occurred in varying number of stages (Bowlby, 1961; Engel, 1967; Parks, 1972; Worden, 1991; Raphael, 1983). Regardless of the theorist, clearly, grief has a beginning (with physical and psychologic manifestations), a middle (considered the work of grieving or mourning) during which time the individual is breaking the bonds that tied him or her to the deceased, and an end (with the individual emerging refocused) having relinquished the ties to the dead person.

These models or theories are based on the Euro-American perspective of breaking the emotional ties between the bereaved and the dead (DeSpelder and Strickland, 1995). Bowlby (1961), known for his attachment and bonding theory, describes a distinct sequence of grieving after loss: numbness, anger, and distress; yearning and searching for the lost figure; disorganization and despair; and reorganization.

Recently, the stages or phases of grief have been examined again with a critical eye. The implication of stages or phases is that young and old griever alike go through grief or mourning in a linear pattern. This view suggests that each stage must be achieved sequentially if one is to grieve well. These models imply that all who grieve should experience each stage or phase, that all the reactions contained therein must occur in a neat chronologic order, and that individuals will progress toward an ending, completion, or resolution of the grief. If this goal is not accomplished, the individual is thought to have grieved poorly or has not adjusted to the loss.

Current concepts about grief recognize that it is not rigidly structured and is without a predictable pattern of responses. The accepted theories do not consider cultural and gender differences. The trend today is to consider grief work as a process. Rando's (1984) theory is a process of seven *R*s: *recognize* the loss, *react* to the separation, *recollect* and *reexperience* the relationship, *relinquish* old attachments, *readjust* to move adaptively in a new world, and *reinvest.* Although Rando was process oriented, the model continued to reflect the linear pattern of other theorists. Stroebe and Schut (1999) proposed a dual process model, which uses aspects of previous theories but suggests a dynamic and interactive process that goes back and forth (oscillation) between loss-oriented and restoration-oriented bereavement. The model does not focus on outcomes, but rather on coping with primary and secondary losses and sources of stress.

The interrelated processes of loss orientation and restoration orientation affect many aspects of daily life to which previous theories did allude or address. For example, loss-oriented coping involves not only dealing with the loss per se, but also coping with ties or bonds to the deceased person, inclusive of ruminations about life together, circumstances and events surrounding the death, and painful memories, as well as yearning for the loss. Restoration-oriented coping includes doing new things, distraction from grief, avoidance or denial of grief, and new role relationships. All of these factors are stressors and issues that require coping. The person in grief alternates between loss-oriented and restoration-oriented coping, which is comparable to confrontation and avoidance of the stressors associated with bereavement. The individual will avoid memories and seek relief by focusing on other things. As stated by Stroebe and Schut (1999), "sometimes there may simply be no alternative but to attend to additional stressors (e.g., managing household chores, or earning a living" (p. 216). Oscillation and mental and physical health are necessary for optimal adjustment over time: the person may take *time off,* be distracted, or need to attend to new things; or confronting some aspect may be too painful at times, thus it is voluntarily or involuntarily repressed. Over time, repeated exposure and confrontation may lead to the reaction response weakening, and the individual no longer thinks about specific aspects of the loss. This model seems to allow for culture and gender differences and emphasizes coping with bereavement rather than outcomes (Figure 24-1). *Coping and bereavement may*

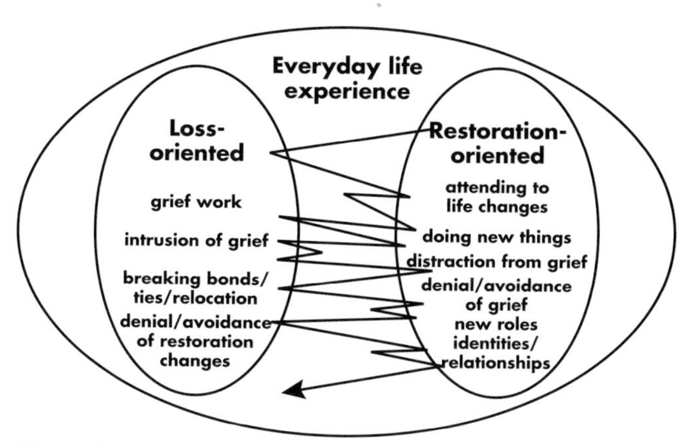

Figure 24-1. A dual process model of coping with bereavement. (From Stroebe M, Schut H: The dual process model of coping with bereavement: rationale and description, *Death Stud* 23:197, 1999.)

differ from one culture to another, one individual to another, and one moment to another.

Rubin (1999) proposes a Two-Track Model of Bereavement, which is described as a multidimensional view. Each track has specific features. Track 1 addresses the way in which people function affectively, interpersonally, somatically, and psychologically in a classical psychiatric sense in response to a major event such as loss or death. Track 2 is concerned with the relationship to the deceased: the way in which the individual is involved in maintaining and changing the relationship with the deceased. This model is also a process model but seems more intricate than that offered by Stroebe and Schut.

Modernistic or Romantistic Approaches

The modernistic and romantistic approaches to grief have been offered by Stroebe and colleagues (1992), suggesting that romantistic and modernistic approaches to grief exist. The modernistic approach proposes specific stages or steps to the grieving process that everyone must experience to become whole again. The focus of life in Western society is to be direct, efficient, and rational. In short, functionality is the key essential in Western society. Therefore, when grief occurs, people are expected to recover from their intense feelings (grief) and return to normal function and effectiveness as quickly as possible. The theories of Lindeman (1944), Engel (1967), Bowlby (1961), and others suggest this approach and the relinquishing of the ties that bind one to the dead. Grief is seen as debilitating and an interference with daily routine.

The romantistic perspective of the grief response facilitates the maintenance of bonds with the dead; it represents fidelity of memories and the essence of the relationship. Ties are deeper than death. To grieve shows everyone the significance of the relationship and the depth of one's spirit. To dissolve the bonds indicates the superficiality of the relationship and denies the self-worth of the survivor and suggests the relationship was a sham. Followers of the modernistic point of view question the normalcy or emotional adequacy of the grieving process of the person who exhibits romantistic beliefs. These modernist believers suggest aberrant, inadequate, or pathologic grieving, thus making an unusual response to grief problematic. Modernistic thought does not seem to facilitate cultural differences in the grief process.

Contemporary studies show grief resolution to be more complex than simply letting go and moving on with life. Examples of ongoing attachments, which to some would be labeled as unhealthy or problematic, are pilgrimages to the Vietnam War Memorial, the Wailing Wall, and to family gravesites. Each year, individuals visit the Vietnam War Memorial in Washington, DC, to remember and leave items that connect them to the their deceased. Similarly, individuals make pilgrimages to the Wailing Wall in Jerusalem, praying and placing little prayer papers in the crevices of the wall. People in other cultures visit the graves of their family members at least once a year to clean the grave, leave food, and commune with their dead relatives.

Postmodern Era

Today, we live in what is being called a postmodern era (DeSpelder and Strickland, 1995). Awareness of the entire experience of the human race heretofore was not available to previous generations. This postmodern influence is reflected in social, political, lifestyle, and art expression; it opens the possibilities to select ideas from all historical periods and cultures. In light of the opposite thoughts on the approaches to grieving, considering the appropriate therapies is also important. Rather than strict adherence to modernistic or romantistic dictums, the expression of grief needs to move toward growth, flexibility, and appropriateness within the cultural context.

An important point to remember is that theories are attempts to address the grieving process; they are helpful to our understanding of grief. Similarities and differences exist, behavior may be the same or different, and the process of grief has been approached differently by those who have developed models, but they should not be imposed on the survivor. Nurses need to know the process of grief to be helpful to the older adult, as well as understanding the dynamics of their own grief.

Types of Grief

Several types of grief need to be addressed briefly, which include acute grief, chronic grief, anticipatory grief, and disenfranchised grief.

Acute grief is similar to a crisis, lasting approximately 4 to 6 weeks. Acute grief has a definite syndrome of somatic symptoms of distress that occur in waves lasting varying lengths of time, usually 20 minutes to1 hour. These symptoms occur every time the loss is acknowledged. Preoccupation with the image of the deceased, as well as a loss of body function or loss by relocation, is a phenomenon similar to daydreaming and is accompanied by a sense of unreality. Feelings of self-blame or guilt are often present. These feelings of guilt may remain unstated, or a verbalized attempt is made to seek validation. Hostility or anger toward usual friendships may occur as a result of the griever's inner struggle. The lack of warmth toward others is another internal struggle that also occurs. Outward behavior may be stiff or formal in interactions with individuals with whom the griever was previously relaxed socially. People usually have typical ways of accomplishing activities of daily living, tasks, and responsibilities. The distraction and restlessness created by acute grief causes feelings of being at *loose ends*. Motivation and zest disappear; tasks and activities take considerable effort to accomplish. Activities such as dressing that normally took 30 minutes now may take hours, and every moment may seem exhausting. The griever becomes overwhelmed with ordinary decisions and activities that have to be performed. These feelings and behaviors are considered loss of patterns of conduct.

Anticipatory grief is the response to an event that has not yet happened or not yet moved from expectation to reality. One can experience this type of grief in preparation for potential loss of belongings, friends moving away, and knowing that a body part or function is going to change. Anticipatory grief is also evident when a person anticipates the loss of a spouse through death. In a sense, the feeling is insulation against that which will be, a dress rehearsal for the actual event that is destined to occur. Healthy anticipatory grief minimizes unfinished business, premature separation, poor communications, and interaction with a dying loved one. Some individuals feel more in control of the situation because anticipatory grief facilitates planning and preparation for death by saying goodbyes in special ways (Zilberfein, 1999). Behaviors similar to acute grief are experienced, including preoccupation with the particular loss and anticipation of the mode of adjustment that might be necessary. Futterman and colleagues (1970) conceptualized anticipatory grief as having five functionally related aspects: (1) acknowledgment—convinced the inevitable will occur; (2) grieving—experiencing and expressing the emotional impact of the anticipated loss and the physical, psychologic, and interpersonal turmoil associated with it; (3) reconciliation of the situation; (4) detachment—withdrawal of the emotional investment from the situation; and (5) memorialization—developing a relatively fixed conscious mental representation of that which will be lost. One frequently sees the struggle of anticipatory grief in families with elders who have been diagnosed with Alzheimer's disease.

Anticipatory grief possesses negative, as well as positive, aspects. If the loss does not occur when or as expected, individuals awaiting the actual loss or death may become hostile and impatient. In the event of a relocation, individuals may become angry or hostile toward the agency, institution, or others who are responsible for the delay. Anticipatory grief can result in premature detachment from an individual who is dying. If premature detachment occurs, family members or others are prevented from reinvesting in the dying individual. This phenomenon is known as the Lazarus syndrome. Premature detachment may deprive family and friends of a final close relationship and prevent resolution of unfinished business. Researchers have found in some instances that grief after anticipatory grief is no less painful than unanticipated loss, but it does allow for less of an assault on the mourner's adaptive capacity (Parks and Weiss, 1983). Some theories suggest that anticipatory grief work among widows helped them adjust to bereavement when the spouse died. Studies by Dessonville and colleagues (1983) revealed that expectancy of death was not related to adjustment to bereavement. Further, rehearsal for the role of widowhood was not related to better adjustment and, in some cases, was actually associated with a poor adjustment. Anticipatory grief, then, can be helpful or harmful to the griever but is recognized as a legitimate phenomenon.

Disenfranchised grief is a grief that a person experiences when the loss cannot be openly acknowledged, publicly mourned, or is not socially supported (Doka, 1989). The person does not have a right to be perceived or function as a bereaved person. In other words, a relationship is not recognized; the loss is not sanctioned or the griever is not recognized. The grief is socially disallowed or unsupported. Disenfranchised grief has frequently been associated with domestic partnerships in which the family of the deceased does not acknowledge the partner of the dead person or in secret liaisons in which the involved party cannot tell others of the strong relationship. Disenfranchised grief can also occur in situations of family discord in which a member of the family is considered the "black sheep" because of unapproved behavior or shirking expected family responsibility. The aged can experience this disenfranchisement when individuals associated and close to them do not understand the full meaning of a retiree's retirement, the impact of the death of a pet, or when gradual losses occur that are caused by chronic conditions that have great impact on the elder but are not seen as important to others. Families coping with a member who has Alzheimer's disease may also experience disenfranchised grief, particularly when others perceive death of the elder as a blessing but fail to support the griever or caregiver who has struggled for years with anticipatory grief and now must cope with the actual death.

Chronic grief has often been called impaired, pathologic, abnormal, or maladaptive grief. Traditional thinking asserts that chronic grief begins with normal grief responses, but obstacles occur that interfere with the normal grieving process. Normal responses are replaced by exaggerated responses. This type of grief may be fostered by the lack of social involvement with others. Individuals who live alone, socialize little, and have few close friends or have an ineffective support network will be more at risk for chronic grief. Issues of guilt, anger, and ambivalence toward the individual who has died are factors that will impede the grieving process until these issues are resolved. Behaviors such as irrational anger, social outbursts, and insomnia that lingers for an extended time or surfaces months or years later, or the appearance of mental or physical ailment, should be suspected as a potential inability to grieve in a healthy, constructive manner. Other behaviors describe maladaptive grief, depending on the interpretation applied to them. The Stroebe and Schut model consider this

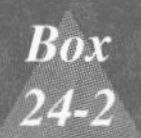

Box 24-2 Guidelines for Psychotherapy for the Bereaved Older Adult

Permit and help the patient put into words and nonverbal expression the pain, sorrow, and finality of bereavement.
Review the relationship of the patient with the deceased (i.e., a life history approach).
Encourage the patient to discuss feelings of love, guilt, and hostility toward the deceased.
Help the patient recognize the alterations in cognition, affect, and behavior secondary to bereavement.
Work with the patient to find an acceptable balance for the future incorporated memory of the deceased.
Avoid interpretations of long-dormant, highly charged intrapsychic conflicts.
Support existing coping mechanisms.
Reassure the patient that the intense suffering and pain are transient.
Allow a positive, even parental, transference to evolve.
Facilitate the transfer of dependency from the deceased to other sources of gratification when necessary.
Decrease sessions with the patient on improvement, but avoid abrupt termination.

grief *complicated grief* in which a disturbance in oscillation occurs whereby the disturbance to the process is in the area of confrontation-avoidance that is necessary for adjustment. This type of grief requires professional intervention of a clinical nurse specialist, a hospice nurse, or a psychologist or psychiatrist with specific training. Guidelines for psychotherapy for bereaved older adults appear in Box 24-2.

Grief Work

The process or experience of mourning takes time, much longer than anyone anticipates. The pangs of grief continue for years, even though the intensity and the resurgence of the grief may become less frequent. In loss by death, grief that remains with us is not unusual. Lund and colleagues (1986) and Arbuckle and deVries (1995) demonstrated that older widows' and widowers' grief is not completed or ended in a prescribed time period. Horacek (1991) referred to this type of grief as *shadow grief.* Shadow grief may inhibit some normal activity but may be a common response that is not considered abnormal. The pain of grief is often exacerbated on anniversary dates (birthdays, holidays, and wedding anniversaries).

Grieving or mourning is often viewed as a *weakness,* a self-indulgence, or a reprehensible habit rather than a psychologic necessity (Parks, 1972). Grief work takes enormous amounts of physical and emotional energy. Grief work is the hardest work anyone can do. Although every culture seems to observe a certain set of behaviors after death, apparently no set of behaviors exists when the loss is of another type. For example, an individual who is seriously ill, who is moved from his or her home (or loses the home), or who retires willingly (or is forced to retire) may not realize that feelings being experienced and behaviors displayed in the weeks that follow are natural and normal responses to loss. In most instances, the individual is labeled *depressed* rather than grieving. The essential point is that after any significant loss or change, some degree of grief and grief work will occur. Influences and manifestations of grief and grief work are depicted in Box 24-3 and Box 24-4.

Grief for the older adult may be longer than others might expect or understand. Confusion, depression, preoccupation with thoughts of the deceased may be mistaken for other conditions such as dementia, deterioration, or depression. Initially, positive feelings about the ability to cope may be evident, but over time the grief response may be exhibited. An attempt to get the older person into routine activities too soon after a significant loss may complicate the grieving process rather than help it. As Stroebe and Schut suggest, oscillation between loss and restoration orientation often includes avoidance or attention to other necessary everyday life experiences that are misinterpreted by others as not dealing with the loss. Multiple loss experiences through acute and chronic illness may be superimposed on relocation, a shrinking support network, economic changes, and role change. This phenomenon can lead to a continual state of grieving, known as *bereavement overload.* No sooner has the individual begun to grieve for one loss than another occurs, and so forth. An individual must grieve one loss before he or she can go on to grieve the next. Multiple loss experiences occur frequently with elders.

Grief Assessment

Mortality of the bereaved during the first year of mourning is greater than it is for those who have not experienced a loss through death. Rees and Lukin (1967) found the mortality rate of the aged surviving spouse to be seven times greater than the average population. As early as 1972, Parks noted a higher mortality rate for widowed males after the age of 75. Exacerbation of dormant conditions such as ulcerative colitis, asthma, congestive heart failure, leukemia, and diabetes may develop during this time (Carr et al, 1970). Mittleman (1996) found that heart attack risk was five times higher than normal 2 days after the death of a significant person and remained elevated for approximately 1 month following the death. Pietruszka (1992) notes that bereaved elders may present clinical symptoms that mimic the signs and symptoms of serious medical and psychologic conditions of the deceased person, which presents a diagnostic challenge to primary care providers. Therefore performing a grief assessment is important to anticipate the problems that grief may precipitate.

Assessment is based on knowledge of the grieving processes and the subsequent mourning. Data are obtained through observation of behavior of the individual elder, keeping in mind the cultural and gender context. Questions should include losses and gains that have occurred within the last year (gains also bring with them some losses), strengths the aged person brings to the situation, what the person values in life, and how grief

Box 24-3 Factors Influencing the Grieving Process

Physical

Illness involves numerous losses.
Each loss must be identified.
Each loss prompts and requires its own grief response.
Importance of the loss varies according to meaning by individual.
Sedatives deprive experience of reality of loss that must be faced.
Nutritional state, if inadequate, leads to the inability to cope or meet demands of daily living and numerous symptoms that grief can cause.
Inadequate rest leads to mental and physical exhaustion, disease, and unresolved grief.
Exercise, if inadequate, limits emotional outlet; increases aggressive feelings, tension, and anxiety; and leads to depression.

Psychologic

Unique nature and meaning of loss
Individual qualities of the relationship
Role body part, self-image, aspect of self was to the individual, family, or both
Individual coping behavior, personality, and mental health
Individual level of maturity and intelligence
Previous experience with loss or death
Social, cultural, ethnic, religious or philosophic background
Sex-role conditioning
Immediate circumstances surrounding loss
Timeliness of the loss
Perception of preventability (sudden versus expected)
Number, type, and quality of secondary losses
Presence of concurrent stresses or crises

Specific to Dying and Death (in Addition to the above)

Role that the deceased occupied in family or social system
Amount of unfinished business
Perception of deceased's fulfillment in life
Immediate circumstances surrounding death
Length of illness before death
Anticipatory grief and involvement with dying patient

Social

Individual support systems and the acceptance of assistance of its members
Individual sociocultural, ethnic, religious or philosophic background
Educational, economic, and occupational status
Ritual

From Beare PG, Myers JL: *Adult health nursing,* ed 3, St Louis, 1998, Mosby.

Box 24-4 Manifestations of Grief

Emotional (Feelings)

Sadness
Anger
Guilt

Physical Sensations

Hollowness in stomach
Lump in throat
Chest pain
Lack of energy
Weakness

Cognitive

Disbelief
Confusion
Hallucinations
- Auditory
- Olfactory
- Visual

Behavior

Sleep disturbance
Appetite disturbance
Absentmindedness
Social withdrawal

Social

Difficulty with interpersonal search for meaning relationships
Dysfunction in work setting

Spiritual

Hostility toward God
Value framework inadequate to cope

is unique to the individual. These questions will help the nurse develop a plan with the older person that will facilitate physiologic and psychologic manifestations of grieving, regardless of whether they are transient or continuing. Inherent in developing intervention strategies is knowledge about the elder's coping mechanisms (effective and ineffective) and support systems on which he or she can rely. (See Box 24-3 to review the physical, psychologic, and social factors that influence grieving; Figure 24-1 puts some of these influences in context of oscillation in the Stroebe and Schut bereavement process.)

A risk factor profile for bereaved spouses was developed by Steele (1992) to identify individuals whose behaviors are suggestive of risk for physical or emotional disturbances. For example, a 70-year-old, middle class, female widow exhibiting despair or optimism, loss of vigor, depersonalization, physical and somatic symptoms, anger, and social isolation may be at risk (Table 24-1).

Table 24-1 Risk Factor Profile of Bereaved Spouses

Demographic category	High-risk bereavement behavior and feelings
Age	
66-85	Despair
76-85	Denial Loss of vigor
Sex	
Female	Depersonalization (shock, numbness, hopelessness) Somatization Physical symptoms Loss of vigor Optimism or despair (loss of meaning or hopelessness) Anger and hostility
Male	Guilt Social isolation Rumination Social desirability
Socioeconomic status	
Upper-middle class	Anger and hostility
Lower class	Guilt Rumination Depersonalization (shock, numbness, confusion) Physical symptoms, loss of vigor
Middle class	Optimism or despair
Quality of relationship	
Extremely close to deceased	Guilt Rumination Depersonalization Physical symptoms, loss of vigor, somatic complaints
Somewhat close to deceased	Anger and hostility Social isolation Optimism or despair

Modified from Steele L: Risk factor profile for bereaved spouses, *Death Stud* 16(5):387, 1992.

Interventions

One of the goals of intervention is to help the individual (or family) attain a healthy adjustment to the loss experience. Actions that can meet this goal are basic and simple; however, the emotional overlay of providers may make the simple difficult. The nurse who is confronted with a person's grief for the first time may feel intense discomfort, fear, and insecurity. The tendency is to be sympathetic rather than empathetic. Confrontation with one's own mortality complicates the interactions. Questions arise in one's mind: What do I say? Should I be cheerful or serious? Should I talk about or even mention the dead person's name?

The nurse requires four strengths to help someone cope with grief. First, the nurse must have spiritual strength, or strength from within. This requirement does not mean that the nurse must have a specific religious orientation or affiliation but must have a positive belief in self. Second, the nurse must find meaning in life. One needs a philosophy to sustain oneself during difficult times. With age, life experiences grow, and a person's philosophy may change or be amended. Nonetheless, at any particular time, the individual should have a philosophy. Third, the nurse must develop emotional maturity. The individual who has always gotten his or her way will most likely have trouble when confronted with deprivation or loss. Fourth, comfort with one's own mortality is essential for working with loss and grief.

The nurse must also be ready to listen. Active listening is an important skill for the nurse who serves as a support person for the griever. Giving advice on how to solve a problem is far easier than allowing a grieving person time and space to express feelings.

When listening, the nurse soon discovers that the actual loss is not of the utmost concern, but rather the fear associated with the loss. If the nurse listens carefully to both the stated and the implied, what will be heard may be phrases such as, " How will I go on?" "What will I do now?" "What will become of me?" "I don't know what to do." "How could he (she) do this to me?" Because the nurse knows resolution occurs with time, such statements may seem exaggerated or melodramatic. Nonetheless, to the one who is grieving, there seems to be no resolution. The griever cannot yet look ahead and know that the despair and other feelings will resolve. Therefore, in the process of active listening, the nurse will clarify what is said to help the person deal with his or her fears about the future.

Listening to the same thing, endlessly repeated, is difficult for the nurse and others. However, reminiscing is important to the griever. Reminiscing allows for the working through of the loss. Reminiscence is a means by which denial can fall by the wayside and allow reality of the loss to filter slowly into the conscious mind. Reminiscence helps the griever acknowledge that the loss is indeed real and that life can go on, even though the future will be difficult and experienced in a different way.

Kelly (1992) talks about re-forming one's life story. By incorporating the loss, and putting the deceased into the life story in a new way (re-forming the story), energy can be invested in all other relationships that exist or may come to be. Drawing out anecdotes and vignettes of the relationship helps the griever keep control over the story and over his or her own life. Encourage the griever to talk and tell the story of the relationship as it had been. Keeping the continuity of the presence of the deceased alive gives permission for the griever to feel the presence of the dead in life. Spirituality (mystical, beyond humans) is linked with specific beliefs or religions. This belief is a basis for faith and religious beliefs. Critical to recovery is the ability of the nurse or caregiver to allow the griever to remain in control. Control is crucial to recovery!

The nurse must not orchestrate the grief process but facilitate the process responses in the cognitive, affective-emotional, behavioral, valuational, and spiritual domains. These responses are incorporated into a three-point approach that the nurse might employ with the grieving person: *talk out, feel out,* and *act out.* The griever initially needs prompt, accurate, and reliable information about what has happened (cognitive).

Talking it out requires active listening when grievers are trying to make sense of the loss and find meaning in it, questioning their values, and constructing new ones to account for the change in their reality (valuation). The expression of and sharing his or her grief and feelings with others, the momentary panics, hysteria, and other sensations accompanying the grief are less frightening when heard by a caring person who can validate their appropriateness (affective, emotional). The belief that individuals who are grieving want to be left alone is incorrect. In actuality, solitude is not the usual desire. The person in grief wants to talk about the loss with people who care.

Feeling it out is a cathartic experience. In many instances, the nurse allows the griever to express hurt, anger, crying, and so forth. The nurse may have to say, "It's okay to [have whatever feelings the griever has]."

Acting out (behavioral) is a natural extension of feelings. Intense physical activity gives one some control over emotions. Ancients used to rend their clothes or tear their hair. Today, the acting out of feelings can be done in many ways, from throwing things, to taking a walk, to busying oneself with tasks, to expressing feelings in creative works. In situations in which acting out predominates, providing a safe means of acting out and a safe environment in which to do so is important to prevent self-harm. Preservation of memories (commemorative activities) is also part of acting out. Planting a tree (rebirth), creating a scrapbook of memories, the wake, and the funeral are all part of acting out.

The nurse's role is also as an advocate who displays the behavioral qualities of responsiveness, authenticity, commitment, and competence (Krohn, 1998). Table 24-2 correlates caring behaviors with caring actions or interventions.

Outliving people one loves may create an emptiness that can never be fully assuaged. Table 24-3 provides a nursing care plan for survivors, whether the survivor is a spouse, domestic partner, friend, companion, or confidant, with suggested interventions. The nurse must be prepared for this most difficult task.

Table 24-2 Caring Behaviors

Behavior	Caring action
Advocacy	Extend oneself to find proper help
	Work to grant reasonable requests
Authenticity	Sharing feelings appropriately
	Honesty
	Use of healing
	Touch
Responsiveness	Be available
	Interact verbally
	Provide comfort
	Provide privacy
	Be nonjudgmental
Commitment and presence	Provide the little extras
	Grooming
	Quiet for talking
	Time
	Presence
Competence	Perform tasks consistently
	Radiate self-assurance in care giving
	Teach simply and completely
Give positive meaning to another's life	Listen
	Touch
	Point out reactions to family
	Praise when appropriate
	Help them gain a sense of control

From Krohn B: When death is near, *Geriatr Nurs* 19(5):276, 1998.

Evaluation

As the mourning proceeds toward an integration of the loss, and a new beginning or re-forming of the life story occurs, the language that the bereaved uses often changes, which is suggestive of progress and growth (Table 24-4).

What is actually helpful to bereaved older persons? Attitudes and actions that have been found to be helpful in coping with grief in widows include the following:

- Keep busy; accept and extend social invitations.
- Help someone else.
- Learn to enjoy some solitary activities.
- Accept your own grief process as unique and individual.
- Talk to others and express feelings.
- Have faith in recovery and maintain beliefs.
- Take one day at a time, and do not expect to follow a timetable of recovery (Rigdon, Clayton, and Dimond, 1987).

In many instances, help given is crisis oriented and soon dissipates. Rigdon and colleagues suggest help over time is much needed. Rather than asking, "What can I do?" a person should simply do something. Accompany the bereaved in a new activity or a new situation, and by action invite them toward the building of a new life.

Newly Bereaved. Nurses commonly provide crisis intervention with the newly bereaved, largely because the majority of deaths occur in the institutional setting, and most of these deaths are of the aged. Nursing actions said to be most helpful during the death or immediately thereafter include the following:

- Kept me informed
- Asked how I was doing and offered support
- Put an arm around me when I cried
- Brought me food
- Knew my name
- Cried with me

Table 24-3 Nursing Care Plan for Survivors

Nursing diagnosis	Expected outcomes	Interventions
Depression, loneliness, social isolation related to loss of spouse, sexual partner, friend, companion, or confidant		
Manifestations: Teariness, crying, sleep disturbance, weight gain, compulsive eating, weight loss, anorexia, fatigue, confusion, forgetfulness, withdrawal, disinterest, indecisiveness, inability to concentrate, guilt feelings; displays feelings of detachment, inferiority, rejection, alienation, emptiness, isolation; unable to initiate social contacts; seeks attention	Short-term and intermediate goals: The survivor will: Develop or use immediate support systems. Express feelings of security. Exhibit meaningful social relationships. Show decreasing signs of depression. Long-term goal: The survivor will demonstrate readiness to build a new life as a single person.	Attempt to develop a therapeutic relationship through touch, empathy, and listening. Listen to perceived feelings. Help person realize that grief is a painful but normal transitional process. Encourage use of other women, daughters, widows, men, and friends as support systems. Encourage balance between linking phenomena (mementos, photographs, clothes, furniture) associated with the deceased and the bridging phenomena (new driving skills, evening classes, new job). Establish contact with Widow-to-Widow. Program for counseling if appropriate. Refer to appropriate agencies.
Anxiety related to increased legal, financial, and decision-making responsibilities		
Manifestations: anger, nervousness, palpitations, increased perspiration, face flushing, dyspnea, urinary frequency, nausea, vomiting, restlessness, apprehension, panic, fear, headache	Short-term and intermediate goals: The survivor will demonstrate adequate decision-making skills in financial and legal matters as evidenced by: Seeking legal aid Writing or calling appropriate agencies Formulating a realistic budget Long-term goals: The survivor will: Cope with legal, financial, and decision-making responsibilities with only a moderate degree of anxiety Make rational decisions about single life	Assist in obtaining attorney if necessary. Encourage contact of Social Security and spouse's employer to ensure receipt of all benefits. Encourage contact of insurance agencies if applicable. Discourage immediate decision-making regarding assets (e.g., home, investments). Encourage seeking of advice from individuals who are trusted. Contact proper social agencies if indigent or in need. Assist in seeking employment if health permits and client so desires. Offer alternatives for decision-making. Refer to any other proper community agencies that offer needed assistance.

From Alexander J, Kiely J: Working with the bereaved, *Geriatr Nurs* 7(2):85, 1986.

- Brought a bed and encouraged me to stay in the room with my dying husband
- Told me to hold my husband's hand while he was dying
- Held my hand
- Got the chaplain for me
- Let me take care of my husband
- Stayed with me after their shift was over (Richter, 1987)

These actions may assist nurses in gaining a clearer perspective of comfort interventions.

Although we do not know the impact of action as related to overall grief recovery, these actions are clearly significant for individuals in their immediate grief. Grief survivors report great variance in the recovery process and deeply resent a professional's efforts to hurry them through it. Even other widows can be a source of distress when imposing their timetable on another grieving widow. The lesson for nurses is to accept whatever the individual is experiencing and exert extreme caution in urging the person to *get going*.

Dysfunctional grief can be assessed only holistically. Is the individual able to maintain self-care? Is the person reaching out to others? Does the individual have a hope for recovery? Is the person searching for meaning in the event? Widows using the greatest number of resources were more functional (Gass, 1987). Caserta and Lund (1993) found, among older adults, that one's intrapersonal resources help reduce negative effects of spousal bereavement. Self-help groups also seemed to assist individuals who did not possess the intrapersonal skills by helping them toward gaining self-esteem and an optimistic meaningful outlook.

Effects of Grief on Sexuality. The absence of a sexual partner following the death of a spouse temporarily cancels an important expressive role of feelings of femininity or masculinity. The intimacy and closeness of a mate provide strong self-affirmation. The loss of this important role results in asexuality for many of the old. Seldom are elders considered as full sexual beings, even when married. When widowed, most

Table 24-4 Perceptual Changes as a Function of Growth after Loss

Before	After
Function, cope, survive	Grow, discover, live
Adjust	Center, balance
Control	Flow with
Pain	Hurt
Pain, illness as negative	Hurt, illness as a sign or signal
Enduring	Reliable
Anxiety (diffuse)	Scared (focused)
Guilt as responsible	Guilt as not fulfilling
Loneliness	Solitude, aloneness
Explain, judge	Understand
Expectations	Wants
Hopelessness	Discouraging
Problems	Challenges
Winning	Succeeding
Time as past, now, or future	Time as a continuum, a flow
Losing	Not realizing potential
Mistake, error	Limited awareness
Assume	Question, reformulate
Tragedy	Tragic opportunity
Pathology	Natural healing, restoration
Responsibility	Awareness of consequences
Symptoms	Reminders
Specialized	Balanced
Search for meaningful existence, happiness	Search for wholeness
Peak or *peek* experience	Fulfilling awareness
Awareness of limits and strengths	Awareness of potential
What is probable	What is possible
Helplessness = weakness, incompetence	Helplessness = a sometimes condition of being alive
Positive or negative feelings	Feelings are signs of being alive
Operate *as if* immortal or in mortal fear of death	Operate *as if* death can occur at any time but without fear or without self-fulfilling prophecies
Death as failure, tragedy, termination, the ultimate loss	Death as transition
Self = individual physical being who is sometimes social and sometimes solitary, but clearly separate from other individuals	Self = all things that have significance for the individual

Developed by Sisneros J, San Francisco State University School of Nursing, 1994.

older women are effectively neutered. Men may seek and find new sexual partners but are vulnerable to *widower's impotence,* a result of guilt, depression, long periods of abstinence from sexual activity, and the strangeness of a new sexual partner. All of these factors may hinder an aged man from consummating a new marriage.

Grief and Gender Differences. Three of four women will be widowed at one time or other resulting from women living longer and frequently marrying older men. Theories suggest that widowhood is less difficult for women than retirement is for men because other widows are available with whom to share leisure time and activities. In many instances, a woman's status increases with widowhood, whereas a man's decreases with retirement (DeSpeleder and Strickland, 1996). The abundance of literature on bereavement focuses on women. This emphasis has lead to the use of the feminine model of grief, which most health professionals use with both men and women, not realizing that perhaps differences in the grief response do exist. Loss and mourning models shed little light on the bereavement of men, particularly in spousal loss in which males are the survivors. The assumption is that men are less emotionally involved in the conjugal relationship than women and therefore are less likely to grieve or express their grief. This assumption was found not to be true (Brabant, Forsyth, and Melanon, 1992; Martin and Doka, 1996, 1998). Evidence shows that men hurt and knew they hurt but did not reach out to others for help. The magnitude of the loss was felt in hurt, pain, and anger.

Men suppressed other emotional responses and hid their vulnerability. Men also carried deep lasting attachments to the deceased spouse (Schreck, 1993). Hopmeyer and Werk (1994) found that women placed *sharing feelings and emotions* first in coping with grief. Men, however, were reluctant to share or seek help. Most men wanted to learn how others solved problems that were similar to their own at first, wanted to be self-reliant next, and then immersed themselves in work. The identification of the feminine and masculine grief response does not mean that every man and every woman follows the pattern ascribed to him or her. What has been derived from these responses is that men and women often mix these gender-specific responses or reverse them, with women responding as men do, and vise versa. Gender and grief work remains an area for further research.

Coping with the Death of a Child. Traditional opinion holds that the death of an adult child may be the most difficult grief an elder must bear. A small study of 12 Jewish and 17 non-Jewish elders whose child died seemed to indicate that the Jewish women accepted and went on with their lives (Goodman et al, 1991). Although this interpretation is questionable, the study points out that the manner in which one integrates the death of a child has to do with the centrality of that child to one's existence, the ability to express grief, aspects of generativity in the lifestyle, and general health and well-being.

Grief and Sibling Death. Death of siblings are particularly hard to integrate because the close affiliation and identification threaten one's mortality to a greater degree than most relationships. In addition, the death of each sibling removes one more member from childhood, one who can confirm and remember shared childhood, youth, and energy (Moyers, 1992). On the other hand, the first sibling who dies may teach the others more about death and coping.

Bereavement as a Growth Opportunity. Survivor coping ability improves when the person is aware that death and bereavement can lead to growth. A change in thinking from limits to potential, from coping to growth, and from problems to challenges are perceptual mindsets that help move one toward growth. Resolving loss and working through the grief process provide incentives, enabling possible important life changes. Transformation from intense focus on self-awareness evolves into a new sense of identity. The loss is placed within the context of growth and life cycles: the lost relationship is changed not ended. By turning to the inner resources, creativity arises from the experience of grief.

PROCESS OF DYING

Nature of Dying

Dying is the most challenging of life experiences and a highly individual and private one. Most of all, dying is coming to terms with being alone. The way in which one reacts to extreme stress, bad news, disappointment, loss, or change governs attitudes and coping with dying. An individual's coping patterns and personality are established early in life, thus most people die as they have lived.

The dying of young and middle-aged people is perceived as tragic, loss of a not fully lived life. Dying and death of an aged person is frequently regarded as a blessing, a culmination of a full and rich life. This view, of course, is presumptive! Many aged have not fulfilled their lives, nor are they ready to die. The dying process for one of advanced years can be a period of positive forward movement, a time of fulfillment and growth, and a completion of life orchestrated by the individual with support, understanding, and assistance of those around him or her.

Elders seek to make sense of their lives in the face of impending death. The remaining time may become a time of life-review or a time to repair former failures, such as resolving a parent-child or sibling-sibling conflict or completing a task that has been left undone.

Dying Process

Dying may take weeks, months, or years; it can be anticipated and, in some instances, predicted. For the aged, dying often arises from degenerative diseases typical of mortality in our society. However, the dynamics of experiencing dying vary greatly based on age, experiences, and culture.

The literature on coping with terminal illness and dying spanned a 20-year period from the 1960s to the 1980s, during which time stages and phases associated with dying were identified. As with the grieving process, the descriptions or expectations were linear structured progressions.

The literature is replete with different yet similar variations of the dying process. People often use these frameworks as a panacea for dealing with the dying. These stage-based approaches lead to obstacles, stereotyping the individual when the person is vulnerable and is coping with dying. Health professionals should not force the terminally ill into preestablished stages; rather, they should take into account the experiences of the individual (Lindley, 1991). The previously established works provide a useful vehicle to facilitate sharing of information about dying.

The benchmark work of Kübler-Ross (1969) focused on untimely dying and death. Participants in Kübler-Ross's study were mainly middle-aged who were confronted with an abrupt cessation of their careers, relationships, and tasks that had been planned. The responses described were largely defense mechanisms. The framework continues to suggest a cognitive grid or guideline of possible moods and coping mechanisms. However, the findings do not provide direction for interventions that would be helpful to a caregiver who is trying to support the dying individual. Kübler-Ross and other researchers did not pursue her findings to confirm validity or reliability of her model or provide further evidence to support her work (Corr, Nabe, and Corr, 2000). Also apparent was that most of the research studies on dying during that time were not focused on the aged. Retsinas (1988) points out that model responses such as those of Kübler-Ross might not be appropriate for the aged because the aged have completed many of the developmental tasks ascribed to adulthood and advanced age.

Keleman (1974) incorporated Kübler-Ross's anger, denial, and bargaining into the first of his three phases of the dying process. These phases were the resistive phase, the review phase, which dealt with unfinished business and the reclaiming of a part of the self by becoming more in tune with the present rather than the past, and the unconscious phase, in which the individual talked about his or her dying calmly and which is comparable to acceptance. In recent years, elders last days are beginning to be recognized and addressed with attention on end-of-life or palliative care.

Corr (1993) suggests three concepts that can be gleaned from the previous interpretations of the dying process, especially that of Kübler-Ross: (1) individuals who are coping with dying are still living and often have unfinished needs that must be addressed; (2) one cannot become an effective provider of care without listening actively to individuals who are coping with dying and identifying with them and their needs; and (3) one needs to learn from individuals who are dying and are coping with dying to come to know oneself better. Corr also points out that the ways in which individuals cope with anything as fundamental as dying number far more than five. People cope with living and dying in a spectrum of varied and individualistic ways. One should not assume that the five stages or types of coping are somehow obligatory or prescriptive in how one must or should cope with dying. Insistence on the individual dying in a particular way, considered to be the correct way by others, imposes additional burdens on the one who is dying.

Theories suggest that any approach to coping with dying should consider a basic understanding of all dimensions and all of the individuals involved. The approach should foster empowerment by emphasizing the options available while the person lives on, emphasizing participation or shared aspects of coping with dying (interpersonal network), and providing guidance for care providers and helpers.

Corr (1995) proffers a task-based concept that addresses coping with dying from an individual's own perspective and with coping tasks grounded in situations that are fundamental markers of human living. The dimensions of coping—physical, psychologic, social, and spiritual—each has a specific function and affords development of interventions.

The physical realm addresses satisfying bodily needs and minimizing physical distress in ways that are consistent with other values. These needs include nutrition, hydration, elimination, and shelter. Maslow also considers these needs as fundamental. Pain, nausea, vomiting, and constipation are among the physical distresses that must be managed. The physical dimension is extremely important because inadequate understanding remains of the management of pain and other symptoms, misplaced fear of addiction, overemphasis on cure, fear of failure, concern about one's own mortality (caregiver's), and feelings of frustration and inadequacy in the presence of dying.

The psychologic dimension promotes three features: freedom from anxiety, fear, and apprehension; autonomy (security); and self-governance or control of one's life (often supported by others) and the texture of one's life that makes it satisfying or bountiful, such as serenity, activity, creativity, and risk of danger.

Relationships with others and society as a whole are the two aspects of the social dimension. Relationships with others—individuals or groups—sustain and enhance interpersonal attachments. Significant ties continue; others fall by the wayside as death nears. The sustained relationships are ones that the dying person believes are important, not those that others think are important. No matter how much individuals think that they are alone, they are connected to society as a whole through family, culture, congregations, and governmental entities. The dying individual may need to call on these resources at some point.

The spiritual dimension from which one draws spiritual vigor and vitality is dependent on the individual's fundamental values and moral commitments of acceptance, reconciliation, self-worth, meaning, and purpose in living. The purpose in living is reflective of Erikson's integrity or wholeness (1963). Spirituality may be formal or informal religiosity, or it may be a life-review, or both. Hope is a key element in coping. Hope involves faith and trust, which may or may not have a religious basis. Hope may be related to a cure, a holiday, the birth of a grandchild, or reconciliation. The definition of hope to the dying individual requires listening carefully to what the meaning of life is to him or her.

Based on task analysis, Corr (1993, 1995), Doka (1993), and Coolican and colleagues (1994) focused on living with life-threatening illness and defined the tasks that address the initial diagnosis, the living-dying interval, recovery or death, and the aftermath. These tasks confront general issues of acute, chronic, and terminal phases of the life-death cycle (Table 24-5).

Much of what Corr, Doka, and Coolican and colleagues offer elaborates on the living-dying trajectory of Pattison (1967). The trajectory explains patterns of coping with a diagnosis of a terminal illness that abruptly confronts an individual. Pattison describes this phase as a crisis.

Table 24-5 Tasks in Life-Threatening Illness

General	Acute phase	Chronic phase	Terminal phase
1. Responding to the physical fact of disease 2. Taking steps to cope with the reality of disease 3. Preserving self-concept and relationships with others in the face of disease 4. Dealing with effective and existential or spiritual issues created or reactivated by the disease	1. Understanding the disease 2. Maximizing health and lifestyle 3. Maximizing one's coping strengths and limiting weaknesses 4. Developing strategies to deal with the issues that the disease creates 5. Exploring the effect of the diagnosis on a sense of self and others 6. Ventilating feelings and fears 7. Incorporating the present reality of diagnosis into one's sense of past and future	1. Managing symptoms and side effects 2. Carrying out health regimens 3. Preventing and managing health crisis 4. Managing stress and examining coping 5. Maximizing social support and minimizing isolation 6. Normalizing life in the face of the disease 7. Dealing with financial concerns 8. Preserving self-concept 9. Redefining relationships with others throughout the course of the disease 10. Ventilating feelings and fears 11. Finding meaning in suffering chronicity, uncertainty, and decline	1. Dealing with symptoms, discomfort, pain, and incapacitation 2. Managing health procedures and institutional stress 3. Managing stress and examining coping 4. Dealing effectively with caregivers 5. Preparing for death and saying good-bye 6. Preserving self-concept 7. Preserving appropriate relationships with family and friends 8. Ventilating feelings and fears 9. Finding meaning in life and death

From Coolican MB et al: Education about death, dying, and bereavement in nursing programs, *Nurs Educ* 19(6):38, 1994.

Living while Dying. The time between the diagnosis and the point of death is the living-dying interval, composed of acute, chronic, and terminal phases. Medical science may extend the length of terminal illness for many years, thus lengthening the living-dying interval.

The acute phase is associated with recent diagnosis of the terminal illness and is usually the peak time of crisis because great uncertainty exists. Crisis intervention is most effective here because the individual, family, and caregivers are struggling to come to terms with impending death. Impending death or the chronic living-dying phase, a segment of the trajectory, is a time during which work-activity patterns, entertainment, and relationships should be maintained as normally as lifestyle permits. Martocchio (1982) describes living-dying patterns as peaks and valleys, descending (stepwise) plateaus, and progressive downward slopes. The patterns may be singular or in combination and may or may not be related to the pathologic parameters of the disease. The terminal phase is ushered in by withdrawal or turning away from the outside world in response to internal body signals that tell the dying person to conserve energy.

The dying process affects everyone involved. Glaser and Strauss (1963) observed a process of sequential interactional dynamics between people who are terminally ill and family, friends, and health professionals, which can still be observed as closed awareness, suspicious or suspect awareness, mutual pretense, and open awareness.

Closed awareness is described as *keeping the secret.* Medical personnel and the family know that the patient will die prematurely, but the patient does not know it. Generally, caregivers invent a fictitious future in which the patient can believe, in the hope that the patient's morale can be boosted.

In *suspicious awareness,* the patient suspects that he or she is going to die. Hints are bandied back and forth, and a contest ensues for control of the information. In truth, the patient wants these suspicions to be wrong.

Mutual pretense is basically called "let's pretend." Everyone knows the patient has a terminal illness and will die, but the patient, family, friends, or medical personnel talk about it—real feelings are kept hidden.

Open awareness acknowledges the reality of approaching death. The patient, family, friends, and medical staff openly acknowledge the eventual death of the patient. The patient may ask, "Will I die?" and "How and when will I die?" The patient becomes resigned to dying, and the family grieves *with* the patient rather than *for* the patient.

Nursing the Dying

In reviewing the literature, a major question arises: When is an aged person dying? The consensus is that physical deterioration is the prime indicator of dying. The less visible, subtle, and frequently misinterpreted indications of an aged person's terminal process are based on psychologic clues. The aged individual without perceptible physical changes that indicate dying may have a sudden and abrupt change in thought or behavior. Coded communication such as saying good-bye instead of the usual good night, giving away cherished possessions as gifts, urgently contacting friends and relatives with whom the person has not communicated for a long time, and direct or symbolic premonitions that death is near are indications that the aged individual is approaching death or is experiencing the process of dying. Anxiety, depression, restlessness, and agitation are behaviors that are frequently categorized as manifestations of confusion or dementia but in reality may be responses to the inability to express feelings of foreboding and a sense of life escaping one's grasp.

Speculation regarding terminal drop has been recognized as a 1- to 4-year period before death, during which time an alteration in psychologic or performance ability, vocabulary, or verbal ability occur (Botwinick et al, 1978; White and Cunningham, 1988; Lentzner et al, 1992). However, this theory remains vague, and no conclusive studies have emerged.

The elderly do not have a clearly marked dying trajectory. Elders often harbor multiple illnesses or pathologic conditions; the list may get longer as the person grows older. Elders also become accustomed to chronic disorders and repeatedly make adaptations in their lifestyle to remain active and defy death.

Institutional settings tend to dissect an individual into component parts, dealing with segments rather than with the living whole. Nurses are caught in the biologic and physical aspects of patient care. Relieving physical symptoms associated with dying is easy and nonthreatening. However, permitting oneself to become involved in a meaningful interpersonal relationship to support the dying aged is extremely difficult for most nurses and other caregivers.

Perhaps caring for the aged is difficult because the nurse brings his or her experience with death, perpetuated myths, and values regarding life and death. Also possible is that the philosophy of acute care settings, the goal of which is to effect cure, governs to some extent care outcomes that the nurse expects. Long-term care facilities often transfer a dying elder to an acute facility that is not able to provide a good death.

The individual who is dying is a symbol of every person's fears of aging and mortality. The nurse follows a social code of living but has no similar code that is sufficient for dying. Many nurses are still not educated in state-of-the-art caring for the dying. The negative cultural norms provide little help in facing death. The caregivers' beliefs about dying, as painful, upsetting, indifferent, or a blessing, will influence the treatment that the dying patient will receive. A study of nursing home personnel demonstrated that nursing personnel who had more negative attitudes toward the aged had a higher death anxiety. These nurses were therefore less able to deal with deaths of the elderly (Depaola et al, 1992). The nurse must become aware of the feelings that have been suppressed when ministering to the dying. When the nurse is able to deal with his or her fears, recognize them honestly, acknowledge the behaviors they produce, and begin to act on such behaviors, the nurse will be able to approach the dying aged in a more honest and caring way.

The development of the art of being with the dying necessitates inner strength, a strength that may or may not have its basis in religious teachings but that definitely stems from a positive belief in oneself. Formulating a philosophy and belief about life will help the nurse through difficult times. Emotional maturity and the ability to deal with disappointment and postponement of immediate desires will have a bearing on the nurse's ability to cope with the deprivation that loss brings. Knowledge of the grieving process and the human responses that grief elicits is also essential for the nurse to effectively and empathetically care for the aged, the family, and himself or herself during the patient's death.

Some nurses are unable to care for the dying because of their own unresolved conflicts and should not be expected to function in these situations. It is important, however, that someone more able to deal with the situation be asked to intervene in the care.

Needs of the Dying

The needs of the dying aged are as threads in a piece of cloth. Each thread is individual but necessary to the integrity and completeness of the fabric. If one thread is pulled, it touches the other threads, affecting the material's appearance, the thread placement, and the stability of the piece. Separating the physical and psychologic needs of the dying aged so as to identify specific interventions and approaches is difficult because they are interwoven. Corr, Nabe, and Corr (2000) suggest the tasks that the dying person needs to address: (1) maintaining sense of self; (2) participating in decisions regarding their life; (3) being assured that their life has value; and (4) receiving appropriate and adequate health care. Within these tasks, the need for freedom from pain, freedom from loneliness, conservation of energy, and maintenance of self-esteem can be identified. These needs are most often neglected in dying elders and when unfulfilled needs impede the ability to reconcile the remainder of life. The needs of the terminally ill individual in hierarchic order are shown in Figure 24-2. The needs of the terminally ill are subsumed in Corr's task approach that follows.

Receiving appropriate and adequate health care includes freedom from pain, conservation of energy, and relief from bothersome physical symptoms. Pain can be relieved by administering analgesics given properly (McCaffery and Pasero, 1999), by positioning, and by other physical measures (see Chapter 9). Frequently, pain expands to occupy the patient's whole attention, isolating him or her from the world. Patients with chronic pain do not respond to the usual methods used with acute pain. *Most nurses make no distinction between the two types of pain* (see Chapter 9).

With any dying person, not just the dying aged, the nurse is placed in conflict. Pain requires the nurse to use a double standard. In acute pain situations, during which pain is expected to dissipate, the nurse is concerned that the patient should be weaned from a narcotic analgesic and given a nonnarcotic drug as soon as possible. Chronic pain requires a regimen of narcotic and adjuvant drug therapy administered around the clock and on time, not just as requested by the patient. *Narcotic addiction of a dying patient is not the issue;* relief of pain is paramount (see Chapter 9). Bernabi and colleagues (1998) note that 83% of nursing facility residents and 40% of patients with cancer in these facilities still had pain that was inadequately treated. Patients over the age of 70 were at increased risk of undertreatment of pain because of fears of addiction, hastening death, and incurring legal liability.

Saint Christopher's Hospice, London, demonstrated over the years the effectiveness of a regimen of pain control. Hospices and oncology units in the United States continue this practice today. When physical pain is controlled proactively,

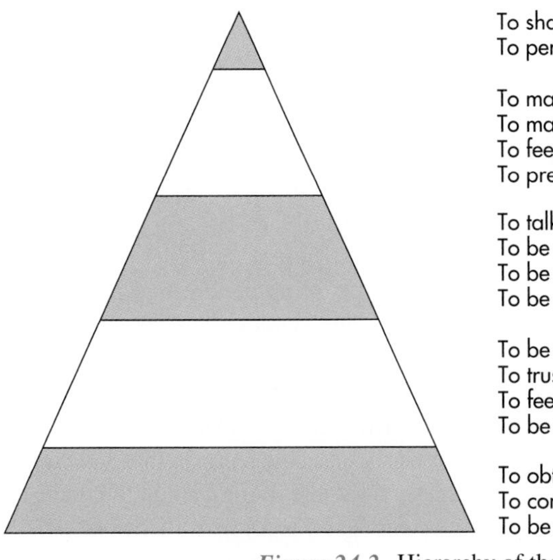

Figure 24-2. Hierarchy of the dying person's needs.

the amount of narcotic medication required by the dying patient does not endlessly increase. *The sooner the nurse realizes that imposing his or her values and fears about addiction on the dying patient is negative care, the sooner physical relief for the dying will be effectively met.* In some sectors of the United States, undertreated pain is beginning to be considered by the legal system as a form of elder abuse. The key to effective care is knowledge of pain control and management. With the methods available today, few patients have pain that cannot be relieved. *One has to remember that pain control does not always mean complete stopping of pain but a level that the person can agree is tolerable and does not interfere with their ability to function* (Fine, 2002).

One tends not to think of *psychologic pain.* However, pain induced by depression, anxiety, fear, and other unresolved emotional concerns of the dying is just as strong and just as real. When emotional needs are not met, the total pain experience, physical and psychosocial, may be exacerbated or intensified. Medication alone cannot relieve this pain. Instead, empathetic listening and allowing the dying person to verbalize what is on his or her mind are important interventions that must be based on the energy level of the one who is dying. If tears and sadness are present, silence and touch are worth more than words might ever convey. Gentleness of touch, closeness, and sitting near the person are appropriate. The acknowledgment and sharing of the nurse's own emotions may be meaningful to the dying person. Diversional activity can sometimes be helpful when pain is present: a backrub to ease tension, a foot massage, or access to a radio or television set. If hearing is impaired, perhaps an amplifier close to the patient's ear would help. If vision is impaired, talking books can be obtained, or a volunteer reader might help. In many instances, all that the dying elder needs to feel safe is someone close by to converse, to listen, and to touch.

The dying aged use great amounts of energy in attempting to cope with the physical assault of illness on the body and with the emotional unrest that dying initiates. Nursing interventions should be directed toward the *conservation of the patient's energy.* How much can the individual do without becoming physically and emotionally taxed? What activities of daily living are most important for the aged person to do independently? Would it be best to bathe the person so he or she could eat alone or feed the patient so he or she could wash him or herself or receive visitors? How much energy does the patient need to talk with visitors or staff members without becoming exhausted? The aged person should be involved in making these decisions. Emotional turmoil and anxiety sap energy. Energy can be spared and anxiety reduced by listening, touching, and providing rest and an environment that permits the patient to make decisions but be dependent as necessary. Conservation of energy is one of the most tangible patient needs the nurse faces. By meeting the needs for freedom from pain, and conservation of energy, the nurse has already begun to intervene on behalf of maintaining self-esteem.

One's sense of integrity or maintenance of self-esteem is the foundation of self-concept. Pride in oneself is a composite of the physical and psychologic attributes of one's years of living. Watching self-image dissolve through loss of independence, loss of the potential for doing (a result of physical disabilities), or loss of body functions such as hearing, seeing, eating, urinating, defecating, or cleaning self is difficult. The person begins to feel ashamed, humiliated, and as a *burden.*

Institutions and caregivers (by their approach and attitude toward the aged) can erode an elder's self-esteem. The number of physicians and others who come to look, prod, and poke in search of diagnoses and learning can invade the aged patient's privacy and dignity. Calling the aged person "Mom," "Pop," or "Dearie" imposes additional insults. Actions such as putting bows in women's hair or applying lipstick on an individual who rarely wears it can be demeaning. The elder may be treated as if he or she has the mentality of a child. Behaviors such as these by caregivers compound the problem for the dying aged.

Withdrawing from the dying aged reinforces the aged person's feeling of worthlessness. When self-esteem is at an ebb, other factors such as psychologic and physical pain, aloneness, and depletion of energy are intensified. Depression aggravates pain and further isolates the individual. The elderly response to dying is influenced by his or her background, past experiences, religious and philosophic orientation, and the prior degree of life involvement. If prior experiences have been negative, the lack of care and attention by caregivers further reduces self-concept.

Self-esteem and dignity complement each other. Dignity involves the individual's ability to maintain a consistent self-concept. Caregivers frequently take control and dignity away from the dying and impose their own expectations on the patient. Essential to the facilitation of self-esteem is the premise that the values of the patient must figure significantly in the decisions that will affect the course of dying.

An important concept for the caregiver to master is that *the dying aged individual is a living person with the same needs for good and natural relationships as the rest of us.* When the caregiver can incorporate this concept, the course of the person's dying process will be significantly improved. Including the person in decisions about care encourages the patient to control the most important event in life.

What can be done to help maintain and bolster self-esteem of the dying aged? Focus on the present and the opportunities that exist in the immediate future. Attention must be paid to the person's hygiene: cleanliness, lack of odors, and personal appearance (without hair ribbons unless requested). Physical comfort is vitally important because with comfort comes security. Caregivers must become good listeners and act as a sounding board to allow the dying aged to express their fears of pain, aloneness, and the struggle with the separation and grief over losses. Caregivers may need to assume the management of necessary body and ego functions for the aged.

This task requires emphasis on respect and helpfulness rather than encouraging dependency, guilt, or conflict. Human contact is vital. One quickly falls into the confusional syndrome of human deprivation: loneliness. As early as 1967, results in sensory deprivation experiments (i.e., touch) revealed a disintegration and loss of ego integrity (dignity) (Pattison, 1967).

Of utmost importance therefore is for the caregiver to use auditory, visual, and tactile stimulation appropriately to nurture and foster self-esteem in the dying aged. Verbal and nonverbal communication is necessary to convey positive messages; hand-holding, placing an arm around the shoulder, or sitting on the edge of the bed conveys to the dying person that the nurse or caregiver is prepared to meet the person on his or her own terms and that the aged person is an individual unique unto self and is appreciated. Providing stimuli such as photographs and mementos, enabling the individual to stay at home, or enabling individuality in the institutional setting engenders self-esteem. Jointly identifying achievable goals through craft work as tangible gifts to others serves as an endearing legacy for the dying aged person.

Loneliness can come from within and from without as well. The dying aged have sustained many losses: loss of friends through death, perhaps loss of spouse, loss of control by institutionalization, loss of meaningful possessions, and loss of physical abilities (sight, hearing, and body functions). Language barriers and cultural differences can also generate loneliness.

In the hospital setting, the nursing staff can easily intensify loneliness by caring for the aged person with detachment, by surrendering to the mechanical technology of the profession, and by avoiding the death situation. In these ways, the nurse truly isolates the old person. Offensive odors emanating from the patient's room or body keep people away. Unrelieved pain, physical or psychologic, intensifies loneliness. Behavior meant to attract attention may in fact distance people. The dying person is frequently placed in a single room or curtained off as signs become more apparent that death is approaching. Care is reduced with decreased tactile and auditory stimulation. Lighting in the room is dim, curtains or shades may be drawn, and people speak in hushed tones or not at all. The dying person perceives these actions as abandonment, the ultimate loneliness. No one wants to die alone; yet, knowingly or unknowingly, nurses foster this loneliness and aloneness. Room location and environment are important considerations to reduce or eliminate loneliness.

Assessing the rationale for isolating the dying person in a single room is critical. For whose benefit is it . . . the patient, the staff, or to protect the uncomfortable visitors to the hospital unit? For some elders, seeing activity when one is confined to bed can be reassuring. Placing the dying older person in a room with several other people can provide the opportunity to share conversation and companionship, as well as security that he or she will not die alone. The patients who remain in the room after a death have the support and solace of each other. When only two people are in a room, the remaining occupant is left alone, a situation that can be frightening and a negative experience. These considerations are highly individual and must be based on patient preference.

If the energy level of the dying elder allows ambulation, he or she should be free to leave the confines of his or her room and associate with other patients, visitors, and staff. When physical tolerance is limited to sitting in a chair, a wheelchair can provide mobility and accessibility to the larger environment with the least energy expenditure. Sitting by the nurses' station or desk is sometimes preferable to sitting alone in one's room. If possible, the patient should be encouraged to wear his or her own clothing.

A pleasant room atmosphere with bright colors and diffuse, high-intensity lighting not only protects the aged from visual discomfort, but also affords a clearer visual contrast of objects. Gray (1976) noted that in the last hours of the dying process, individuals turned toward light. Perhaps this finding supports the value of using bright colors and adjusting lights to keep the patient in touch with life until the end of living.

Live plants and flowers are a way of bringing the outside world in. Memorabilia, pictures, cherished objects, or anything that brings solace should be recognized as important in the care of the dying aged. These tangibles are a means of coping with anxiety and furnish a modicum of security and familiarity in an alien environment. A portable radio (or one with headphones) is easy to reach, conserves energy, staves off loneliness, and provides contact with the outside world. Television, if available, can also be a beneficial outlet for some individuals.

Visitors should be allowed to be with the dying aged any time of the day or night. Night is the most lonely and painful time for the aged. Night is a time of least attention, a time when one thinks and reviews the sorrows and joys of life past and what is to be. Night is also a time of fear of dying alone and no one will know. When a friend or relative cannot stay with the dying person, a mature sitter might be the answer. The sitter's prime responsibility would be psychologic support, not nursing care. If the dying person is part of a hospice program, a volunteer may be available to stay with him or her. Not all elderly dying patients want this attention, but if they do, it should be available.

Some elderly individuals have developed a lifestyle around aloneness. These individuals do indeed prefer solitude. Thrusting any of the nursing care approaches at these people would serve only to aggravate the patient. Being sensitive to the patient's clues and assessing and acting on them accordingly is important. Because of the interactive nature of loneliness and pain (pain may precipitate loneliness, and loneliness can exacerbate pain), the nurse may need to deal with physical and psychologic discomfort separately or together, depending on assessment of the situation.

Assurance that life has value requires maximizing the quality of the dying experience. Many individuals seek reconciliation with God and other people as death approaches. Pain and other disabilities may interfere with this reconciliation. Symptomatic control in a milieu that responds to psychologic, social, and religious needs can facilitate this process of adjustment. *This control requires a multidisciplinary team that includes pastoral care of the dying as a high priority.* Pastoral care seems to facilitate the humanistic approach. Depressed and dying elders often express concerns that have religious overtones. When these concerns are made apparent, pastoral counseling should be available to assist the elder toward spiritual peace.

Participation in decision-making or autonomy is prized and essential to elders in their experience with loss and terminality of life. This need may foster delicate negotiations with the elder, family members, and professional caregivers, regardless of the setting.

Participation in decision-making is a stipulation of the Patient Self-Determination Act of 1991, which refers to the patient being informed of their rights. The Bill of Rights for patients established by the American Hospital Association in 1992 outlined 12 rights of the patient. Before the passage of this Act, a Bill of Rights for Dying Patients was drawn up at a workshop on terminal illness in Lansing, Michigan, in 1975 (Box 24-5). Part of the nurse's responsibility is to ensure that patients' rights are maintained and, if advance directives are not executed, to discuss with patients the value of these rights to ensure their autonomy if and when they cannot speak for themselves.

Communication and control are the borders necessary to complete the fabric of needs of the dying aged. The influence of communication and control is omnipresent in the other needs; without them, the cloth can fray, and attempts to meet the needs will be limited.

Talking helps relieve anxiety; it fills time and fosters the sharing of feelings. The dying aged should never be lied to nor should they be ignored. Lying is betrayal, not listening is interpreted as emotional abandonment, and avoiding the person's room is perceived by the dying as physical abandonment.

Control over one's time of death is a phenomenon that occurs. If care and institutionalization in life are seen as overwhelming negatives by the dying aged person, death can be hastened through the person's own control. The physiologic mechanism is unknown, but theories suggest that hypersensitivity of the sympathetic adrenal system or responses of the parasympathetic nervous system is involved in people who are willing their own death (Watson and Maxwell, 1977). Neglect of the needs of the dying aged encourages the aged person to indeed use this last source of control over life, the willing of death.

Conditions have begun to change as death education for health care personnel has become more available; patients insist on being informed about their illnesses; and the public in general exercises the *right to know* and the *right to die.*

Box 24-5 Bill of Rights for the Dying

I have the right to be treated as a living human until I die.
I have the right to maintain a sense of hopefulness, however changing its focus may be.
I have the right to be cared for by those who can maintain a sense of hopefulness, however changing this may be.
I have the right to express my feelings and emotions about my approaching death in my own way.
I have the right to participate in decisions concerning my care.
I have the right to expect continuing medical and nursing attention, even though *cure* goals must be changed to *comfort* goals.
I have the right not to die alone.
I have the right to be free from pain.
I have the right to have my questions answered honestly.
I have the right to retain my individuality and not be judged for my decisions, which may be contrary to the beliefs of others.
I have the right to expect that the sanctity of the human body will be respected after death.
I have the right to be cared for by caring, sensitive, knowledgeable people who will attempt to understand my needs and will be able to gain some satisfaction in helping me face my death.

From *The terminally ill patient and the helping person workshops,* Lansing, Mich, 1975.

Spirituality and Hope

Spirituality is the basic human quality for hope. Without one's own spiritual nourishment, one cannot meet the same needs in others. A transcendental relationship exists between a person and a higher being. In most instances, spirituality is two-dimensional, that being between God and others. Spirituality may be expressed through religious acts, or through caring human relationships, or both. A person's internal beliefs, personal experiences, and religion are expressions of spirituality. Box 24-6 provides a guide for assessment and intervention of spiritual distress.

Acceptance of death is thought to be easier for individuals with a strong religious faith, regardless of whether they believe in an afterlife (Cartwright, 1991). Siegel and Kuykendall (1990) found corroborating evidence that membership in a church or temple moderated the impact of death. Mickley and colleagues (1992) found that women who were diagnosed with breast cancer and who internally defined religious beliefs contributed significantly to spiritual well being.

Box 24-6 Assessing and Intervening in Spiritual Distress

Assessment

Brief history:
- Losses
- Challenged belief, value system
- Separation from religious and cultural ties
- Death
- Personal and family disasters

Symptoms (defining characteristics) such as the following:
- Unmet needs
- Threats to self
- Change in environment, health status, self-concept, etc.
- Questioning meaning of own existence
- Depression
- Feeling of hopelessness, abandonment, fear

Assessment of cause of spiritual distress
- Depletion anxiety
- Helplessness, hopelessness
- Perceived powerlessness
- Medication reaction
- Hormonal imbalances

Interventions

Create a therapeutic environment.
Assess support system.
Assess past methods of decreasing distress (e.g., prayer, imagery, healing, memories or reminiscence therapy, medication, relaxation).
Determine environmental changes needed to enhance function.
Assess and assist implementation of coping mechanisms.
Refer to clergy.
Evaluate effects of nursing interventions.
Activate and evaluate appropriate community referrals.
Use techniques to assist client and family in reducing spiritual distress.

This belief was characterized by affirmation and satisfaction with life, a relationship with God, and perception that one's life has meaning. Individuals who were extrinsically religious expressed less spiritual well being.

Hope is expectancy of fulfillment, an anticipation, or relief from something. Hope is based on the belief of the possible, support of meaningful others, a sense of well being, overall coping ability, and a purpose in life. Generally speaking, hope is an overall feeling of future good. *Enabling hope* empowers and is an integral thread in one's life. Erickson equates hope with integrity; it is also comparable to Maslow's self-actualization.

The multidimensional nature of hope is expressed through thoughts, feelings, and actions. Hope is activated when a crisis occurs and personal resources are exhausted (Herth, 1990).

Box 24-7 Hope in Aging

Love from others
Interaction with others
Freedom to make choices
Growth through discovery
Future orientation
Active movement toward goals
Life after death

Box 24-8 Eight Attributes of a Good Death (in Priority Order)

Freedom from pain
Being at peace with God
Having family present
Being mentally aware
Having treatment choices followed
Having a sense that life was meaningful
Resolving conflicts
Dying at home

From a study by Steinhauser KE: *JAMA* 284:2476, 2000. Summary by Eastman P: Caring for the ages, *Newsletter of LTC Practitioners* 2(2):1, 2001.

Hope empowers the individual, generates courage, motivates action and achievement, and can strengthen physiologic and psychologic function. Forbes (1994) describes six characteristics of hope that reflect the affective (emotional and sensation), cognitive (imaging, having a future), affiliative (sense of relatedness to others), temporal (time, future, change), and contextual (placing experiences within one's life situation) domains. The characteristics according to Forbes are the following:

- Confidence that change and adaptation is possible
- Relating to others
- Belief in the future
- Spiritual belief
- Active involvement
- Trust

The degree of hope that the dying person possesses depends on caring relationships with others and with caregivers, such as health professionals. Love from others is a message of hope (Box 24-7). In a study headed by Steinhauser (in Easton, 2001) terminally ill patients considered nine attributes for a good death, among them, being at peace with God (Box 24-8).

Dying and the Family

Aged individuals today are most frequently members of a multigenerational family. Although members may be geographically separated, some degree of filial tie exists.

When an elder becomes seriously or terminally ill and cannot uphold his or her role or obligation, the family balance or dynamics are significantly altered. Even the aged person who is single and relies on friends and neighbors finds a change in the relationships. Depending on the role the individual has in the family constellation, problems often begin at the time of diagnosis or shortly thereafter. Roles and traits of the person who is now considered to be dying may create adjustment difficulties in the soon-to-be survivors, whether they are spouse, adult children, or grandchildren. Adult children often begin to see their own mortality through the death of their parent, with the appearance of a new family order.

The idea that family members can remain involved with the dying person can be a constant struggle as they try to withdraw and try to readjust their lives without the dying member. This change requires enormous energy by family members who are already burdened with their own anticipatory grief, daily living, and, in many cases, raising their own children and possibly grandchildren. The conflict is not only grieving for the dying, but also for a part of themselves that will be lost with the death of the parent or significant family member. A number of adaptive tasks are required to facilitate healthy resolution of the loss of a family member.

At times, family members have to separate their own identities from that of the patient's and learn to tolerate the reality that this family member will die while they live on. The ability of the family members to truly support, love, and provide intimacy may lead to exhaustion, impatience, anger, and a sense of futility as the patient's illness drags on and on. Family members may be at different points in grief than the patient, which can hinder communication between the patient and family members. As the illness worsens, physical disability increases, and the patient complains more often, intensifying feelings of helplessness and frustration in family members.

The death may require role changes. For example, an adult child has to grieve the death of one parent while assuming responsibility for the welfare of the remaining parent.

Experiencing the effects of grief requires acknowledgment of current feelings that surface as anticipatory grief. Coming to terms with the reality of the impending loss means that family members must go through many emotional responses in achieving acceptance of the loved one's approaching death. Because people are supposed to die in old age, the grief responses may not be exceptionally intense; but then, too, many filial relationships that seem superficial can result in very deep and acute grief responses.

Family members may feel extremely pressured during the final days of an aged relative's life. These individuals may be caught between experiencing the present and remembering the patient as he or she was, between pushing for more interventions or letting nature take its course, and occasionally wanting to retreat because of a discordant relationship with the patient. Families frequently feel guilt ridden because they are thinking more about their needs rather than those of the dying patient.

Despite the family's grief and pain, the family must give the patient permission to die; let the patient know that it is all right to let go and leave. This gesture is the last act of love and dignity that the family can offer the dying patient. Occasionally, no family is available to say, "It's okay to let go." The task then falls to the nurse who has developed a meaningful relationship with the patient throughout care.

GRIEVING AND THE HEALTH PROFESSIONAL

Whenever an individual invests in something or someone and that something or someone leaves, is gone, or is lost, a need to grieve may exist. By the very nature of the population whom nurses serve, they are forced to confront loss, not only of patients and families, but also of personal loss. Caring for dying patients over time, or watching patients go home and repeatedly return, involves a degree of emotional investment and a feeling of grief that requires resolution.

The nurse's ability to grieve is hampered by the assumption that the role of the caregiver is to be emotionally strong. The nurse has been told that feelings of ambivalence or guilt toward the patient are inappropriate. The nurse attempts to control these feelings by remaining detached, thwarting the acknowledgment or resolution of feelings. The nurse can also experience ambivalence between wanting the dying patient to live and yet to be relieved of suffering in a lingering death. A study of nurses in a rehabilitation center found those affected negatively by patient deaths had been employed at the facility for a longer period or were recently grieving a personal loss (O'Hara et al, 1996). The study also suggested that some nurses are at higher risk for negative impact if they have a strong personal tendency toward immersing themselves in nursing care. This tendency is an example of an earlier discussion of investing oneself without adequate support systems.

Harper (1977) identified a process of adaptation through which health professionals must pass to cope with the stress of caring for the dying. Intellectualization, which focuses on professional knowledge and facts, and occasionally emphasizing philosophic issues, is the first stage of adapting. At this time, conversation with the dying is distant, and a flurry of activity ensues as the caregiver busies himself or herself with physical tasks and reading about the patient's illness in an attempt to allay their own anxieties.

The professional, in the second stage of adapting, is jolted out of this intellectual haven into a confrontation with the realities of the patient's impending death and his or her own personal mortality. Grieving is triggered for oneself and at the same time by genuine compassion for the dying person. Caregivers can feel guilty, frustrated, and hostile. Hostile feelings are not uncommon for caregivers when they attempt to fight their feelings, a phase Harper calls emotional survival. Awareness of depression, pain, mourning, and grief are crucial in this period for the health professional.

The health professional is said to have arrived at self-mastery when he or she is free from identification with the patient's symptoms and is no longer occupied with personal mortality. Self-mastery allows greater sensitivity to the patient without incapacitating effects on the caregiver. This phase is called emotional arrival: moderation, mitigation, and accommodation. The culmination of previous growth and development enables the caregiver to relate compassionately to the patient and fully accept the impending death. The enhanced dignity and self-respect that the caregiver feels allow him or her to give respect and dignity to the dying patient. Through this growth process, the health professional has learned that living can be more painful than dying. Now, concern for the dying can be translated into constructive and appropriate care activities for both the patient and the family. Needless to say, the caregiver must have outside interests and a support network beyond the work setting to maintain a balanced perspective on life. Without this equilibrium, growing and accepting the death of others and oneself will be difficult.

Assessment

Dying Aged. Few, if any, tools are available to assess dying patients. Caregivers, for the most part, have to depend on their understanding of the grieving and dying processes and draw carefully from the literature appropriate behavioral responses. *A danger exists among health professionals of superimposing what they think the patient should feel and do in the dying process.* The purpose of knowing about theories of grief and dying is to recognize emotions and behaviors and to plan interventions accordingly as they appear. An extensive list of items to assess for the dying patient and the illness appear in Box 24-9.

As an individual nears the final days and hours of life, physical, psychologic, and emotional events occur that provide clues to the impending death. Nurses, families, and patients are too often unaware and unprepared for these signs and responses. Tables 24-6 and Table 24-7 provide guidance for these responses.

Family of the Aged. The family, whether biologic or chosen by the aged individual, is often neglected when the aged person is dying. Attention paid to family members revolves around their presence as an obstacle or a nuisance to the caregiving staff. More often than not, animosity toward the family develops, and prejudgments are made about their behavior during this stressful time. As institutions downsize and fewer professional staff becomes available, patients' families may find themselves assuming more care responsibility.

The ability to do a detailed assessment depends on the willingness, availability, and degree of stress of the family, as well as the time constraints of the nurse who will be caring for a group of patients. Using available time, the nurse can acquire information early in the dying patient's illness to help the family cope with the dying process as it progresses. (See Box 24-9 for assessment data that are important to obtain for effective intervention.)

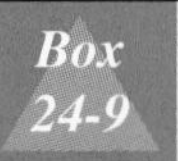

Box 24-9 Assessment of the Dying Patient and Family

Patient

Age
Gender
Coping styles and abilities
Social, cultural, ethnic background
Previous experience with illness, pain, deterioration, loss, grief
Mental health
Intelligence
Lifestyle
Fulfillment of life goals
Amount of unfinished business
The nature of the illness (death trajectory, problems particular to the illness, treatment, amount of pain)
Time passed since diagnosis
Response to illness
Knowledge about the illness or disease
Acceptance or rejection of the sick role
Amount of striving for dependence or independence
Feelings and fears about illness
Comfort in expressing thoughts and feelings and how much is expressed
Location of the patient (home, hospital, nursing home)
Relationship with each member of the family and significant other since diagnosis
Family rules, norms, values, and past experiences that might inhibit grief or interfere with a therapeutic relationship

Family

Family makeup (members of family)
Developmental stage of the family
Existing subsystems
Specific roles of each member

Characteristics of the Family System

How flexible or rigid
Type of communication
Rules, norms, expectations
Values, beliefs
Quality of emotional relationships
Dependence, interdependence, freedom of each member
How close to or disengaged from the dying member
Established extrafamilial interactions
Strengths and vulnerabilities of the family
Style of leadership and decision-making
Unusual methods of problem solving, crisis resolution
Family resources (personal, financial, community)
Current problems identified by the family
Quality of communication with the care givers
Immediate and long-range anticipated needs

From Hess PA: Loss, grief, and dying. In Beare P, Myers J: *Adult health nursing,* ed 3, St Louis, 1998, Mosby.

Table 24-6 Physical Signs and Symptoms Associated with the Final Stages of Dying, Rationale, and Interventions

Physical signs and symptoms	Rationale	Intervention (if any)
Coolness, color, and temperature change in hands, arms, feet, and legs; perspiration may be present	Peripheral circulation diminished to facilitate increased circulation to vital organs	Place socks on feet; cover with light cotton blankets; keep warm blankets on person, but do not use electric blanket.
Increased sleeping	Conservation of energy	Spend time with the patient; hold the hand; speak normally to the patient, even though response may be lacking.
Disorientation, confusion of time, place, person	Metabolic changes	Identify self by name before speaking to patient; speak softly, clearly, and truthfully.
Incontinence of urine, bowel, or both	Increased muscle relaxation and decreased consciousness	Maintain vigilance; change bedding as appropriate; use bed pads; try not to use an indwelling catheter.
Congestion	Poor circulation of body fluids, immobilization, and the inability to expectorate secretions causes gurgling, rattles, bubbling	Elevate the head with pillows, or raise the head of the bed, or both; gently turn the head to the side to drain secretions.
Restlessness	Metabolic changes and decrease in oxygen to the brain	Calm the patient by speech and action; reduce light; gently rub back, stroke arms, or read aloud; play soothing music; do not use restraints.
Decreased intake of food and fluids	Body conservation of energy for function	Do not force patient to eat or drink; give ice chips, soft drinks, juice, popsicles, as possible; apply petrolatum jelly to dry lips; if patient is a mouth breather, apply protective jelly more frequently as necessary.
Decreased urine output	Decreased fluid intake and decreased circulation to kidney	None
Altered breathing pattern	Metabolic and oxygen changes of respiratory system	Elevate the head of bed; hold hand, speak gently to patient *Additional general interventions:* Learn to be *with person* without talking; a moist washcloth on the forehead may be soothing; eye drops may help soothe the eyes.

From Hess PA: Loss, grief, and dying. In Beare P, Myers J: *Adult health nursing,* ed 3, St Louis, 1998, Mosby.

Table 24-7 Emotional or Spiritual Symptoms of Approaching Death, Rationale, and Interventions

Emotional or spiritual symptoms	Rationale	Intervention
Withdrawal	Prepares the patient for release and detachment and letting go of relationships and surroundings	Continue communicating in a normal manner using a normal voice tone; identify self by name; hold hand, say what person wants to hear from you.
Visionlike experiences (dead friends or family, religious vision)	Preparation for transition	Do not contradict or argue regarding whether this is or is not a real experience; if the patient is frightened, reassure them that the feeling is normal.
Restlessness	Tension, fear, unfinished business	Listen to patient express his or her fears, sadness and anger associated with dying; give permission to die.
Decreased socialization	As energy diminishes, the patient begins making his or her transition	Express support; give permission to die.
Unusual communication: out of character statements, gestures, requests	Signals readiness to let go	Say what needs to be said to the dying patient; kiss, hug, cry with him or her.

From Hess PA: Loss, grief, and dying. In Beare P, Myers J: *Adult health nursing,* ed 3, St Louis, 1998, Mosby.

Values, norms, beliefs, and priorities of the family must be recognized and accepted. Rarely do major changes in communication patterns occur just because a family member is dying. Realistic interventions and outcomes that are consistent with the existing family system may foster positive family growth.

Intervention

Interventions have many facets and range from the simple act of hand-holding to dealing with a multitude of emotions. The core of interventions focus on communication, pain and symptom relief, knowledge of available resources, and fostering involvement in and control of decision-making by the patient as long as possible. Many interventions have been mentioned throughout the discussion of the needs of the dying patient. (See Tables 24-6 and 24-7 for interventions that can be taken as death nears.)

Communication includes the verbal and nonverbal exchange among the nurse, the elder, and possibly the family. Although talking with the dying is full of emotional land mines, communication is a vehicle for establishing a trust relationship that can help relieve anxiety. Talking is a way to instruct, explain, divert attention, and amuse. Humor can be highly therapeutic. Nonverbal responses are expressed in facial expressions, touch, and behavior. The dying often experience *touch hunger,* or the lack of human contact through tactile stimulation, such as holding hands or receiving and giving hugs. Procedural touch used in bathing and treatments does not fulfill the touch need.

Knowledge of community resources will help the nurse give direction to the patient and family and help them cope with the physical, emotional, socioeconomic, and religious and spiritual problems that might occur (see Resources).

Loss of health or deterioration resulting from chronic problems, loss of independence, social contacts, finances, and energy threatens control over oneself and the environment.

The nurse's role is that of supporter, facilitator, advocate, and caregiver. Nurses can facilitate meeting patient needs through patient empowerment and control and by providing choices in care such that the patient remains an active participant. Environmental stimulation through social contacts and diversional activities often relieves the sense of isolation and abandonment.

Choosing to be cared for at home is not feasible for all patients, but those who choose to do so should be supported. Ancillary services must be provided that will cooperate with the patient and family. *The patient and family should be aware that if they get into difficulty, they should not consider it a defeat if they have to return to the hospital for care.* The nurse must realize that some emotions and experiences are inexpressible and that the nurse's role is his or her presence, being with the person and the family, and being able to detect feelings of these individuals.

Hospice: An Alternative

The hospice movement, which began in the United States and Canada in 1971, has made *hospice* a familiar word to some health care professionals and the lay public. However, the meaning attached to hospice is still subject to a variety of interpretations. The model for hospice and its concepts was based on way stations, which cared for the sick and tired during the crusades. More than 40 years ago, under the direction of Dr. Cicely Saunders, Saint Christopher's Hospice in London implemented this concept for people who were dying of cancer.

The hospice process or ideology is unique. Hospice is described as the link between the needs of the terminally ill and their families and a staff that employs the medieval concept of hospitality in which a community assists the traveler at dangerous points along his or her journey. The hospice process returns nursing to its roots: humane compassionate care, an ideal that has been the basis of nursing for centuries. The dying are indeed travelers—travelers along the continuum of life—and the community represents friends, family, and specially prepared professionals to care—the hospice team.

The philosophy of hospice care is, "The last stages of life should not be seen as defeat, but rather as life's fulfillment. It is not merely a time of negation, but rather an opportunity for positive achievement . . ." (Ulrich, 1978, p. 20).

The number of hospices has expanded enormously, with over 2000 in the United States, many of which are affiliated with community hospitals. Other hospices are operated by public health agencies, home health agencies, or volunteer groups. The variations in origins and style reflect the particular needs of the community, the style of leadership, funding sources, political forces, available resources for health and social services, and the spiritual care in each community in which hospices are established. Long-term care facilities often have difficulty reconciling the hospice approach to care because of their own rigid interpretation of regulations meant to protect residents from neglect.

Most facilities provide services that incorporate hospice ideals and are developed using the guidelines of the National Hospice Organization (NHO), now called National Hospice and Palliative Care Organization (NHPCO). This organization, formed in 1978, has been in the forefront of promoting standards of hospice care that ensure that the purposes and intent are met. Some facilities offering hospice care may not have appropriately trained staff. Nurses would do well to investigate the quality and staffing of a hospice against the standards of the organization. The NHPCO is committed to developing education in the hospice concept and promoting appropriate legislation, regulation, and reimbursement. A summary of the philosophy and principles that guide hospice are listed in Box 24-10.

Hospice care is usually free to the patient and has been supported by volunteers, public and private funds, and memorial donations. Efforts to incorporate hospice care into health insurance payments and other third-party reimbursement mechanisms resulted in the implementation of hospice benefits under Medicare in November 1983, under the Tax Equity and Fiscal Responsibility Act (TEFRA). In 1986 Congress passed legislation making hospice a permanent Medicare benefit and granted a modest increase in reimbursement rates. Since then, the number of private insurance companies and health maintenance organizations (HMOs) offering a hospice option has increased. The hope is that in this age of accelerating costs, hospice care will save money while making more humane care available to terminally ill patients and their families. The hope is that hospice care will eventually be generally available to all who wish it.

Hospice care is a reorientation in health care for the patient and family. The home usually becomes the primary center of care, and care is provided by family members or friends who

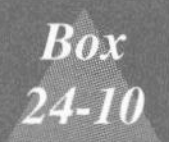

Box 24-10 Summary of Hospice Philosophy and Principles

Hospice is a philosophy, not a facility, one in which the primary focus is on terminal illness.
Hospice affirms life, not death.
Hospice strives to maximize present quality of living.
Hospice offers palliative care to all people and their family members, regardless of age, gender, nationality, race, creed, or sexual orientation, who are coping with a life-threatening illness, dying, death, and bereavement,
The hospice approach offers care to the patient and family as a unit.
Hospice programs make service available on a 24-hour-a-day, 7-day-a-week basis without interruption, even if the patient care setting changes.
Participants in hospice programs give special attention to supporting each other.
Hospice is holistic care.
A highly qualified, specially trained team of hospice professionals and volunteers work together to meet the physiologic, psychologic, social, spiritual, and economic needs of patient and family facing terminal illness and bereavement.
Hospice offers a safe, coordinated program of palliative and supportive care, in a variety of settings, from the time of admission through bereavement, with the focus of keeping the terminally ill patient in his or her home as long as possible.
Hospice offered continuing care and ongoing support to bereaved survivors after the death of someone they love.
Hospice is accountable for the appropriate allocation and utilization of its resources to provide optimum care consistent with patient and family needs.
Hospice has an organized governing body that has complete and ultimate responsibility for the organization. The governing body entrusts the hospice administrator with over-all management responsibility for operating hospice, including planning, organizing, staffing, and evaluating the organization and its services.
Hospice is committed to continuous assessment and improvement of the quality and efficiency of its services.

From The National Hospice Organization: *Standards of a hospice program of care,* Arlington, Va, 1993, The National Hospice Organization; Corr CA, Nabe CM, Corr DM: *Death and dying, life and living,* ed 3, Stamford, CT, 2000, Wadsworth.

are taught basic nursing care, including diet, exercise, and medication needed to care for the dying individual. The person generally wishes to die at home; the family fears this desire because they do not know what to do, and they want the person to die in the hospital. Given the necessary tools and orientation, much of the anxiety is eliminated, and families, with the emotional support of the hospice team, are able to care for the dying at home.

Hospice is available 24 hours every day of the year for its clients, providing, as needed, the services of physicians, nurses, mental health specialists, therapists, social workers, and chaplains. Hospice facilitates a redefinition of relationships. The spouse may not always be the caregiver; it might be a friend or child. For individuals without family, hospice staff and, at times, friends become the patient's family. Someone from hospice is readily available to stay with the patient or family whenever the need occurs. Neither the dying person nor the family is alone during the dying process or during the months of bereavement that follow. A great amount of personal contact, interaction, and sharing takes place between the family and hospice team. Hospice volunteers provide direct or indirect assistance. Chores are performed and friendship and companionship are provided to the patient and family.

The unprecedented contribution of hospice continues to be the reestablishment of control for the dying person. Through polypharmaceutic means, control of distressful symptoms and pain has been accomplished without denying the patient full alertness and the ability to communicate to others. This gift, so to speak, allows normality for the patient. The crux of accomplishing this end is the anticipation of symptoms and intervention by the caregiver before problems occur (see Tables 24-6 and 24-7).

Pain control, the issue that is discussed most frequently when hospice is mentioned, is not exclusively physical pain, but also relief of psychologic, social, and spiritual pain. Heightened physical pain may be the only tangible clue to the existence of the other types of pain. Psychologic pain emerges when loss of control over one's life occurs. The equilibrium is disturbed, and the usual coping mechanisms may not be effective. Social pain can be summed up as "man's inhumanity to man," problems stemming from loss of interpersonal relationships, unfinished business, unsaid good-byes, and non-closure of life. Spiritual pain may be tied to cultural, racial, and religious aspects from which the dying person feels alienated, for example, rituals or participation in group prayers.

Reeducation of the patient and family is another dimension of hospice care. Before teaching is initiated, the hospice team finds out what the patient and family already know, what functional abilities are operant, what unfinished goals remain for the family, and what kind of rehabilitation will facilitate the achievement of the patient's and family's goals.

Pain control and the opportunity to die at home are the key ideas and activities that people associate with hospice. In actuality, hospice represents much more. Hospice supports and guides the family in patient care and ensures that the patient will not die alone and that the family will not be abandoned, regardless of the site of care. Bereavement services for the family extend for a period on an emergency and regular basis after the death of the patient. The hospice staff helps family members learn care techniques, dietary approaches, medication management, and how to handle an assortment of problems that occur in a family in which a member is dying. Life is made as meaningful as possible.

Nurse's Role in Hospice Care. Nursing practice and hospice incorporate the mind-body continuum. Cicely

Saunders refers to nursing as the cornerstone of hospice care. The nurse provides much of the direct care and functions in a variety of roles: as staff nurse giving direct care, as coordinator implementing the plan of the interdisciplinary team or as executive officer responsible for research and educational activities, and as advocate for the patient and hospice in the clinical and political arena.

Thomas (1983) and the *American Nurses' Association's Standards and Scope of Hospice Nursing Practice* (1987) enumerate the special skills, knowledge, and abilities needed by a hospice nurse:

1. Thorough knowledge of anatomy and physiology and considerable familiarity with pathophysiologic causes of numerous diseases
2. Well-grounded skill in physical assessment and in various nursing procedures such as catheterization, colostomy, and traction care
3. Above-average knowledge of pharmacology, especially of analgesics, narcotics, antiemetics, tranquilizers, antibiotics, hormone therapy, steroids, cardiotonic agents, and cancer chemotherapy
4. Skill in using psychologic principles in individual and group situations
5. Great sensitivity in human relationships
6. Personal characteristics such as stamina, emotional stability, flexibility, cooperativeness, and a life philosophy or faith
7. Knowledge of measures to comfort the dying in the last hours

A summary of principles for measuring the quality of care at the end of life are presented in Box 24-11.

Hospice and Palliative Care Nurses Association (*www.hpna.org*) provides guidance in end-of-life care (see Resources). Geriatric theory, nursing concepts, and knowledge of medical management of acute and chronic conditions of elders are brought together to provide the most sensitive and comprehensive care.

Hope. Hope changes as one is dying. Hope for a cure is never abandoned, but the focus of care is on creating an environment that encourages honesty, compassion, and mutual support. The intimacy of everyone working together establishes an environment in which sharing sad and wonderful moments with one another is safe for the patient, family, and hospice personnel.

Box 24-11 Principles for Measuring the Quality of Care at the End of Life

1. **Physical and emotional symptoms**
   Pain, shortness of breath, fatigue, depression, fear, anxiety, nausea, skin breakdown, and other physical and emotional problems often destroy the quality of life at its end. The focus should be on these needs and ensuring that people can count on a comfortable and meaningful end to their lives.
2. **Support of function and autonomy**
   Maintaining a patient's personal dignity and self-respect is extremely important.
3. **Advance care planning**
   Planning ahead allows for decisions to be made that reflect the patient's preferences and circumstances rather than only a response to crises.
4. **Aggressive care near death—site of death, CPR, and hospitalization**
   Although aggressive care is often justified, most patients would prefer to have avoided it when the short-term outcome is death.
5. **Patient and family satisfaction**
   Both patient and family satisfaction should be measured by the following elements: the decision-making process, the care given, and the outcomes achieved.
6. **Global quality of life**
   Overall well being can be good, despite declining physical health. Care systems that achieve this goal should be valued.
7. **Family burden**
   When possible, serious financial and emotional effects from the costs of care and the challenges of direct caregiving should be reduced.
8. **Survival time**
   That death may be too readily accepted is reason to worry. Purchasers and patients need to know that survival times vary across plans and provider systems.
9. **Provider continuity and skill**
   Providers must have relevant skills, including rehabilitation, symptom control, and psychologic support. Care systems must demonstrate competent performance on continuity and provider skill.
10. **Bereavement**
    Survivors may benefit from relatively modest interventions, when immediately available.

Modified from American Geriatrics Society: Measuring quality of care at the end of life, a statement of principles, *AGS Newsletter* 25(3), May/June/July, 1996.
CPR, Cardiopulmonary resuscitation.

CURRENT ISSUES IN DEATH AND DYING

Palliative Care

Palliative care refers to care in the last weeks of life when death is imminent. Nurses are the first-line caregivers at this time. Nonetheless, the number of nursing programs with a specialty in palliative nursing care and little or inconsistent continuing education are few. White, Coyne, and Patel (2001) indicate "A significant gap between scientific knowledge and clinical education regarding palliative and end-of-life care" (p. 147). Palliative care means care at the end of life. Palliative care is all inclusive of the dimensions aforementioned in this chapter and considers the needs and wishes of both the patient and family in an interdisciplinary way. All nurses will encounter end-of-life situations; thus a need exists for incorporation into nursing curriculum and continuing education for professionals who have not had courses in their basic or advanced nursing education. A study by White, Coyne, and Patel (2001) identified core competencies for effective palliative care by nurses (Box 24-12).

Advance Directives

Decision-making on life-prolonging procedures when death is inevitable have become legal, ethical, medical, and professional issues today. The blurring of the lines between living and dying result from technologic advances, the ambivalence of whether death is to be fought or accepted, and the dilemma brought about by medical technologies. Decision-making at the end of life has become increasingly complex because most people die in advanced age from chronic illnesses, dying over a period of years, slowly declining from degenerative conditions, including Alzheimer's disease, Parkinson's disease, and heart failure. Seventy three percent of the deaths each year are elders, making end-of-life decisions a frequent part of this group's needs (Mezey, 1996).

Self-determination is at the core of protecting patients from misuse of the medical system. Many physicians are unaware of or ignore patients' advance directives (ADs). These professionals are inadequately trained to care for the dying and are economically deterred from providing humane compassionate care. *The Patient Self-Determination Act (PSDA),* under which the durable power of attorney (DPA) for health care (DPAHC), the living will (LW), and the directive to physician (DTP) are subsumed, was created by the United States Congress in October 1990 and implemented in all states in December 1991. The intent of the PSDA is based on belief in the preservation of individual rights in decisions related to personal survival. A DPAHC can relate to any medical situation in which the individual becomes unable to communicate his or her own choices. All agencies that receive Medicare and Medicaid funds are mandated to disseminate PDSA information to their client (Mezey, Ramsey, and Mitty, 1994; Mezey, 1996; Berrio and Levesque, 1996). Hospitals and long-term care facilities are responsible for providing written information at the time of admission about the individual's rights under law to refuse medical and surgical care and the right to initiate this refusal in a written AD. HMOs and home health care agencies are required to do the same at the time of membership enrollment or before the patient comes under the care of the agency. Hospices are obliged to inform patients of their self-determination rights on the initial visit (Parkman, 1996; Berrio and Levesque, 1996; Mezey, 1996).

Durable Power of Attorney. A DPA enables an individual to appoint a trusted person as *attorney in fact* and gives this person the power to represent the elder in all legal matters. A DPA should be carefully considered in later life and should be entered into with complete understanding of the risks and benefits. In 1979 the Commissioners on Uniform State Law (a federally appointed commission) adopted the uniform durable power of attorney that will survive a person's incapacity (Cohen, 1987).

Durable Power of Attorney for Health Care. The DPAHC or health care proxy is a legal, notarized or witnessed document by which an individual can express his or her wishes regarding care in acute illness and in dying.

Emanuel and Emanuel (1989) of Harvard developed a medical directive describing hypothetical scenarios to which people creating this directive might respond (Appendix 24-A). Many states have their own forms for the execution of a DPAHC. The forms are available from many agencies, including the state medical association and personal physicians. A resource list of agencies is provided under Resources at the end of this chapter. An example of one state's DPAHC or health care proxy appears in Appendix 24-B.

Autopsy as an Advance Directive. ADs may include the individual's wishes regarding autopsy. For some people, this consideration is insignificant, but for others, it may be very important. Rarely is this topic discussed in nursing literature, and nurses have nearly as many misconceptions as do patients. The informed and sensitive nurse can do a great service to patients by discussing the idea and the procedures, clarifying misconceptions, and advocating for the client's wishes. Importantly, autopsy is a method of quality control that ensures that a misdiagnosis is recognized. Interestingly, even with all the sophisticated diagnostic technologies we now have, autopsy confirms an approximate 10% error rate that has remained constant for over 40 years. The lowest rate of autopsy is among the very old (2.4% at age 90). Common reasons for refusing an autopsy are concern about disfigurement, religious beliefs, cost, and lack of good reason to conduct such a

Box 24-12 Core Competencies for Palliative/End-of-Life Care

The nurse should be able to:

- Talk to patients and families about dying.
- Be knowledgeable about pain control and pain-control techniques (opioid dosing and other pharmacologic interventions).
- Provide comfort-oriented nursing interventions.
- Provide palliative treatments.
- Recognize physical changes that precede eminent death.
- Deal with own feelings.
- Deal with angry patients and families.
- Be knowledgeable and deal with the ethical issues in administering end-of-life palliative therapies.
- Be knowledgeable, and inform patients about ADs.
- Be knowledgeable of the legal issues in administering end-of-life palliative care.
- Be adaptable and sensitive to religious and cultural perspectives.
- Explain the meaning of hospice.

Modified from White KR, Coyne PJ, Patel UB: Are nurses adequately prepared for end-of-life care? *J Nur Sch,* 33(2):147, 2001, Sigma Theta Tau International.
ADs, Advance directives.

procedure. Individuals are rarely approached regarding autopsy, and more than 50% of the time, the autopsy is not mentioned to the family after the death of a loved one. Little is to be gained by the physician in promoting autopsies, and the number of autopsies performed consistently decreases.

Living Will. Introduced in 1970, the LW is a personal statement of how and where one wishes to die. An LW does not acknowledge decisions by a proxy and is activated only when the person is terminally ill and incapacitated. The LW is comparable to the DTP, also known as instructional directives or treatment directives (Appendix 24-C).

Wills Not Related to Health Care. Wills and living trusts are needed to express one's wishes regarding the disposition of assets on death. A will simply states how the estate will be distributed. A revocable trust is more costly and sophisticated but will avoid probate and many management problems. This type of trust ensures ongoing management of the estate without a court-supervised conservatorship because asset preservation and tax planning can be incorporated.

Christian Affirmation of Life. The Catholic Hospital Association approved the Christian Affirmation of Life in 1994, which is similar to the LW but expresses wishes consistent with the religious faith.

Studies by Emanuel and colleagues (1991) showed that approximately 70% of individuals decide against life-sustaining treatments if they become incompetent and have a poor prognosis for survival. Danis and colleagues (1991) found that care followed the AD in 75% of the cases they studied retrospectively. These figures were compiled before the implementation of the PSDA. Three years after the PSDA, Berrio and Levesque (1996) reviewed patient records at their facility and discovered only 17% (N = 551) of the patients had completed an advance directive. Johns Hopkins Hospital found only 31% (N = 526) of patients had completed an AD (Berrio and Levesque, 1996). Other studies have shown rates of completion as low as 4%. The hope is that the completion rate for ADs will be higher in the future.

Gilfix (1987) makes a point that legal planning is essential for protecting victims of Alzheimer's disease and their families. Unless steps are taken well in advance, serious financial and legal repercussions may occur. Because no one can predict future capacities, everyone should consider establishing certain legal protections. For the elderly, this precaution is exceedingly important (Table 24-8).

MacKay (1992) discusses the several methods by which elders may dictate desires regarding control of their medical care and introduces the strengths and limitations of each directive (Table 24-9). Appendix 24-D provides definitions, language, and examples used in advance directives.

Barriers to Completing Advance Directives. Studies have indicated inaccessible documents, level of education, income, age, and race as impediments to executing an AD (Mezey et al, 2000; Havens, 2000; Habel, 2001; Douglas and Brown, 2002). Individuals with high school or lower education, nonwhite, and who exist on a low income tend not to have completed an AD. This tendency is the result in part of the lack of information about ADs and lack of information about subsequent consequences of treatment choices or refusal of treatments. In some groups and cultures, the family is the decision-maker of care issues, not the patient. The fear of putting things in writing, as well as finding someone to serve as proxy, also influences the completion of a directive. Interpreters, used to assist the health care professional with explanations to their non-English speaking patients, may not facilitate a clear translation of an AD (Morrison, 1998; Douglas and Brown, 2002; Havens, 2000; Mezey et al, 2000). The nurse must keep all of these considerations in mind when attempting to ensure that a patient has an AD.

Table 24-8 Advance Directives*

Type	Characteristics
Durable power of attorney (DPA)	Includes specific legal capacities and incapacities that must be specified. Similar to a conservatorship without court-oriented procedures, DPA makes all decisions. Time limits must be specified (Cohen, 1987; Gilfix, 1987).
Durable power of attorney for health care (DPAHC)	Appointment by the individual of a proxy of his or her choosing. DPAHC is authorized by the individual to express his or her wishes regarding care in acute illness and in dying and to make medical decisions when the individual is unable to do so. The proxy may be a relative, friend, or significant other. The DPAHC is a legal document and must be notarized (Delong, 1995; Berrio and Levesque, 1996; Mezey, 1996; Weenolsen, 1996).
Living will (LW) (comparable to directive to physician, instrumental directive, treatment directive)	Personal statement of how one wishes to die. An LW sets forth choices and instructions for personal end-of-life care. Less specific than DPAHC, no provision for proxy is provided (Weenolsen, 1996).
Christian affirmation of life (similar to LW but consistent with Catholic doctrine)	Expresses that the person need not accept extraordinary medical care, but he or she must receive ordinary care, such as food, water, pain relief, and hygiene care (Catholic Hospital Association, 1994; in Weenolsen, 1996).

*Patient Self-Determination Act mandated by Congress in October 1990 preserves an individual's right in decisions related to personal survival.

Table 24-9 Strengths and Limitations of Advance Directives for Nursing Home Use

	Advance directives		
Requirements	**LW**	**DTP**	**DPAHC**
Patient must be competent to initiate this type of advance directive.	Yes	Yes	Yes
Patient must be competent to revoke this type of advance directive.	No	No	Yes
Two witnesses are required.		Yes	Yes
One witness must be a patient advocate or ombudsman designated by the state.		Yes	Yes
Notary public can be substituted for the required witnesses.		No	Yes
Special form is required.	No	Yes	No
Advance directive lasts up to 5 years	Yes	Yes	Yes
Advance directive lasts at least 7 years.	No	No	Yes
Advance directive requires the patient to have an agent or surrogate decision-maker.	No	Yes	Yes
Attending physician is required to be the agent or surrogate decision-maker for the patient.		Yes	No
Patient can select a friend or family member as agent.		No	Yes
Legal liability.		Yes	Yes
Advance directive used only for terminal illness or when death is imminent.	Yes	Yes	No
Agent can become guardian.		No	Yes
Advance directive can go into effect immediately.	No	No	Yes
Advance directive requires 14-day waiting period after terminal illness is determined.	Yes	Yes	No

From MacKay S: Durable power of attorney for health care: is DPAHC the best advance directive for patients residing in long-term care facilities? *Geriatr Nurs* 13(2):105, 1992.
LW, Living will; *DTP,* directive to physician; *DPAHC,* durable power of attorney for health care.

Nurse's Role and Advance Directives. The nurse serves as a resource person who is ready to answer questions openly and honestly about available options. This role requires knowledge and understanding of the PSDA. The nurse is one of the health care professionals who are responsible for ensuring that the individual has the opportunity to learn about and to make an AD. The nurse must also ascertain proper disposition of the AD if it is completed. For the patient who enters a facility with a directive, the nurse needs to ascertain that it is current and contains directives that are reflective of the person's current choices. The document must be easily available to caregivers (placed on the chart where all can see it).

Nursing home residents with cognitive ability have an opportunity to discuss their thoughts regarding life and death decisions with someone. Residents who are perceived to have a lack of cognitive capacity do not get the opportunity to do so nor do residents with communication disorders. All residents should be given the opportunity to execute an AD. Nurses should be aware of the ANA position statement on care and do-not-resuscitate decisions (1992).

In a small study of elder patients who were diagnosed as demented by standard tests, 30% were found to possess the mental ability to understand the nature of a health care proxy and designate a relative as their decision-maker. Twenty seven percent of the participants were able to express their preference for or against a *do not resuscitate* (DNR) option; 21% was able do both a DNR and health care proxy (Schmitt, 1996). Although this study was limited, it suggests that decision-making capacity is not always accurately predicted by screening tests such as the Folstein Mini Mental Status Examination (MMSE) or the Global Deterioration Scale (GDS-2). Further, the question is raised as to who is making the decision of mental capacity. The implication for elders in long-term care facilities is that these elders should not be excluded from consideration in executing an AD.

As a provider of information, the nurse needs to be aware of the types of directives that are legally recognized in the state in which the nurse practices and the terminology associated with directives; for example, surrogate is not recognized as interchangeable with proxy or agent (Weensolen, 1996). The nurse should also be familiar with the AD form or forms used by the organization in which he or she is employed. Forms vary from state to state, institution to institution, and may still be recognized as legal documents (Figure 24-3). Also important is to know is that if one is taken ill in a state other than that in which the directive was executed, reciprocal legislation usually recognizes the original document. The nurse must also be cognizant of the barriers to implementing an AD (Box 24-13). This knowledge will aid in clarifying patient misunderstanding.

The nurse is expected to answer an elder's questions, such as, "Can I just talk about my wishes, or do I have to put it in writing?" or "Does this type of form have to be witnessed?" In addition, the nurse must know how a directive is accomplished. Elders in long-term care facilities usually need two witnesses for their directive, one witness being the

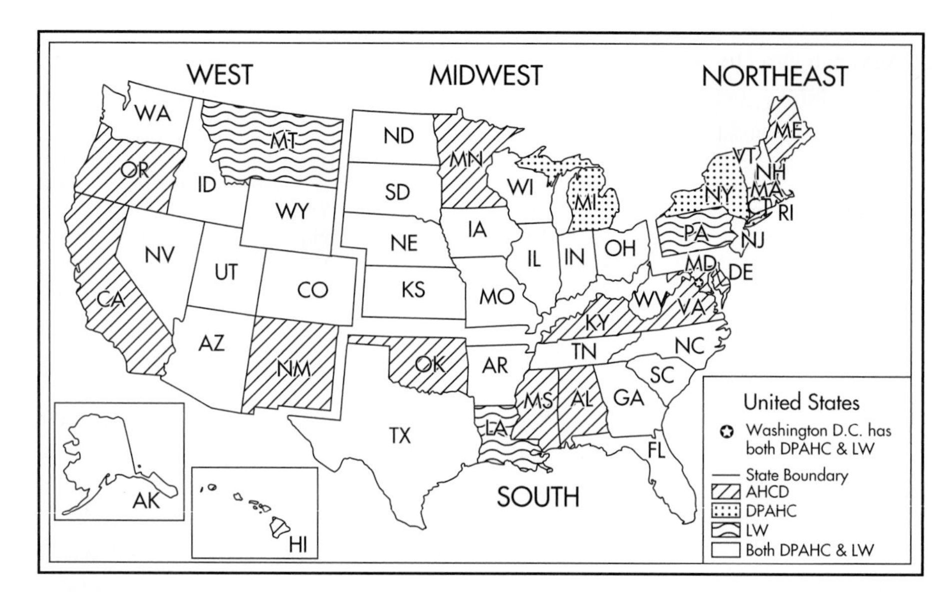

Figure 24-3. Advance Directive documents officially sanctioned by states and Washington, DC. *DPAHC,* Durable power of attorney for health care; *LW,* living will; *AHCD,* advance health care directive. (From Hunt GG, Mahoney JE, Sieger CE: A comparison of state advance directive documents, *Gerontologist* 42[1]:53, 2002.)

Box 24-13 Barriers to Advance Directives Completion

- Inability to speak English
- Need more information
- Religious or ethnic affiliation
- Memory
- Inability to concentrate
- Eyesight
- Hearing
- Print size of document or reading material
- Physician will do what is right
- Waiting for physician to initiate discussion
- Physician waiting for patient to initiate discussion
- Never heard of an advance directive
- Difficult topic to discuss
- Do not want anything such as this in writing; fear of signing life away
- Believe an attorney is needed for completion of forms
- Family structure and support; family makes decisions for ill person
- Procrastination (or wait to do later)
- Fatalism or the acceptance of *will of God*
- Fear of being untreated
- Too fatigued

Modified from Mezey M: Advance directives protocol: nurse's helping to protect patient's rights, *Geriatr Nurs* 17(5): 204, 1996. Berrio MW, Levesque ME: Advance directives: most patients don't have one. Do yours? *Am J Nurs* 96(8):25, 1996; Mezey MD et al: Why hospital patients do or do not execute an advance directive, *Nurs Outlook* 48:165, 2000.

ombudsman from the area office on of aging who serves as a patient advocate.

The nurse may be a patient advocate by bringing family members and the elder together to discuss the difficult issues addressed in making a directive or to simply discuss the elder's wishes. The nurse may be the one who brings the patient and the physician together to ensure that both parties agree on the terms of the directive and whether the physician can honor the patient's wishes. The nurse may also be the one who obtains the appropriate AD form for the elder who is well or ill. Several studies have concluded that counseling by hospital representatives, nurses, and others of hospitalized patients is an effective and generalized way of improving recognition and execution of advance directives (Meier et al, 1996).

As a facilitator, the nurse encourages the elder to think about end-of-life decisions before becoming a patient. However, necessity usually requires this consideration while one is a patient. Elders in long-term care may be vulnerable to loss of control in their life. ADs enable these vulnerable individuals to have some control over care issues at the end of life.

A values assessment, learning what the elder holds important in his or her life and how this relates to his or her desires for health care and quality of life, should be encouraged. Does the elder want measures to be taken to prolong life at all costs, or does he or she wish for a natural death if the alternative may mean prolonged maintenance on machines? Is anyone available with whom the elder feels comfortable who can act as a proxy to ensure that the elder's wishes will be carried out? Answers to these questions are helpful when discussing the elder's wishes. The discussion should include the family, and perhaps the clergy and friends, before a directive is completed so as to identify if those who are to be involved are comfortable with the decisions and will adhere to the directive. For elders without family, the nurse may become a sounding board.

No one can think of all the possible contingencies that might require decisions with serious illness or a current condition. The nurse can help the elder understand treatments that are available to sustain life and the implications of interventions such as resuscitation efforts (cardiopulmonary resuscitation), intubation, and artificial nutrition, as well as the technical terms associated with them.

Suicide. Suicide by the elderly, per se, is mentioned here because it is an alternative way of dying that the aged may choose. Suicide no longer holds the societal stigma it once did. In 1994 the suicide rate was 3.5% in the aged population and is believed to be rising (U.S. Bureau of the Census, 1998). The number of successful suicides increases with age, particularly with aged males, who have a suicide rate twice that of the population as a whole. The motive of the aged who attempt suicide is not to attract attention or to gain sympathy, but rather a genuine desire to end life.

The aged, as mentioned earlier in this chapter, would often rather die than experience the indignities of severe illness, dependency, rejection, and isolation. In their own way, whether in an overt act of suicide or the insidious culmination of excessive or predetermined drug use (such as alcohol or mixing medications), refusal to eat, or the willing of oneself to die, the suicide presents a final statement, an effort to retain control of life and life decisions. Interestingly enough, if the terminally ill aged have needs met in a hospice or other care environment and are kept in the mainstream of life, suicide, although an option, is rarely considered.

Physician-Assisted Death. In May 1992 the *Journal of the American Medical Association* reported that 73% of the general public in a large sample approved of some form of euthanasia. Physician-assisted death, physician-assisted suicide, physician-aid in dying, and active euthanasia are interchangeable terms. Changes in dying in the latter half of the twentieth century have resulted in the patient's right to refuse life-sustaining medical measures and the hospice movement. These changes have also spurred growing debate over physician-assisted suicide and active euthanasia. Reasons for the debate arise from advances in high-tech support systems that maintain cardiac and respiratory function, the increasing aged population, the changing trajectory of illness with large numbers of patients alive for months and years with cancer or other incurable illnesses, limits on health care resources and misconceptions about the rising cost of care of the dying, and greater emphasis on patient autonomy with policy shifts from societal to individual rights (Foley, 1996).

The following definitions are presented to help with understanding key terms used in the discussion of assisted dying. Active euthanasia is "the commission of any act that directly leads to the death of a patient. The intent of the act is to mercifully cause the death of the patient" (Minogue, 1996, p. 64). Physician-assisted suicide occurs "when the physician facilitates a patient's death by providing the necessary means and/or information to enable the patient to end his or her life" (Minogue, 1996, p. 80). An example of physician-assisted suicide might be the physician providing the patient with sleeping pills and instructions about the lethal dose. This form is considered passive euthanasia because the physician has not withheld or withdrawn life-sustaining treatment. The physician who would inject lethal poison into a patient who voluntarily requested to be euthanized would be practicing active euthanasia. At this time, both active and passive euthanasia are considered criminal acts by law.

The Netherlands is held up as the example of the only nation that permits physician-assisted death and active euthanasia. Although physician-assisted death is not legal, it is tolerated (Morrison and Meier, 1994; O'Keefe, 1995; DeSpelder and Strickland, 1996; Hendin, 1996). A comparison between the Netherlands homogeneous population, with almost all possessing medical insurance, and the United States great heterogeneity of races, cultures, religions, languages, lifestyles, and medical access makes arriving at consensus on this issue extremely difficult. Why does one request euthanasia? Indications point to the fear of the loss of dignity, uncontrolled pain, and dependency on others; some are tired of life (Morrison and Meier, 1994). Passage of the Death with Dignity Law by the State of Oregon voters in 1994 and again in 1997 in response to a citizen's ballot initiative became the only state in the nation to have a physician-assisted dying statute. This law enables a terminally ill adult resident of Oregon with fewer than 6 months to live and who is mentally competent to seek the assistance of the physician for the purpose of a dignified death at a time and manner of his or her choosing. Additional criteria of this law include a written and two oral requests at 15-day intervals followed by a 15-day waiting period to certify the person's desire to end his or her life. Two physicians must also certify the diagnosis, prognosis, competency, and voluntary nature of the request. The individual is counseled on alternatives and also receives counseling from a pharmacist. If these criteria are met, the patient's request is granted, and he or she receives the lethal prescription from the physician. The physician is not present when the person decides to take the medication (passive euthanasia). The law prohibits lethal injection (active euthanasia). Since 1997 (to 2001) 141 prescriptions were issued with only 91 terminally ill persons taking full advantage of the opportunity.

Death with Dignity Law. The majority of deaths under this law were terminal cancer. Ninety one terminally ill individuals have taken advantage of the Death with Dignity Law, the majority of whom had terminal cancer (Lee and Brody, 2002; Chronicle News Services, 2002). In 1998 the U.S. Attorney General authorized federal agents to take action against physicians in Oregon who prescribed lethal drugs to patients under the Oregon Law. Prescribing lethal drugs would revoke the physician's license (Verhorvek, 2000). Compassion in Dying Federation challenged this ruling by the Attorney General in U.S. district court. The court upheld the State of Oregon case on every point and issued a permanent injunction, shielding the statute in April 2002 (Chronicle News Services, 2002), and won to block the edict in November 2001.

Table 24-10 Arguments for and against Physician-Assisted Suicide

For	Against
Physicians have a duty to alleviate uncontrollable pain and suffering, including the obligation to provide an assisted death at the competent patient's request.	Society runs the risk of sliding into a practice of involuntary euthanasia and subtle coercion of vulnerable and disenfranchised patients.
Patients have the right to autonomy, which presently includes the right to forego or have withdrawn life-sustaining therapy.	A potential for abuse exists. Involuntary euthanasia has a higher priority in permissive environments in which euthanasia is legal.
Physician-assisted suicide allows the terminally ill to preserve their autonomy and exert final control.	The healing ethos of medical practice may be adversely affected, and public trust in physicians may be eroded.

Data from Morrison S, Meier DE: Physician-assisted dying: fashioning public policy with an absence of data, *Generations* 18(4):48, 1994.

The Attorney General, who insisted on making the law illegal, sought the opinion of the U.S. Supreme Court, which in May 2001 unanimously ruled that no exceptions in federal drug laws existed. The Supreme Court based its decision on California's Proposition 215, which approved medical marijuana use to ease pain of cancer, acquired immunodeficiency syndrome (AIDS), and other illnesses but has been deemed illegal by federal government agencies. The 2002 protective decision by the U.S. district court cited that "the Attorney General misconstrued the court's ruling in the California case, and applied it to Oregon (Chronicle News Services, 2002, p. A3).

Nurses have had strong opinions pro and con on the topic. The American Nurses' Association position statement on assisted suicide was developed to provide nurses with a point of reference for discussion and understanding of the many difficulties involved in the issue of a patient's request to terminate his or her life. The American Nurses' Association advises nurses not to participate in assisted suicide, citing such action a "violation of the Code for Nurses with Interpretive Statements and the ethical traditions of the profession" (American Nurses' Association, 1985; Canavan, 1996, p. 8). The nurse is involved in many end-of-life care situations because she or he is the primary care provider who implements decisions of others around end-of-life care. Such advice should not mean patients who want their life terminated should be abandoned.

Considerable confusion exists regarding terminology and interpretation of what effects the nurse's role may have. Many nurses believe that turning off the ventilator, turning off tube feedings, stopping intravenous fluids, or giving as much pain medication as is needed, even if the side effect is death, constitutes assisted suicide. Nurses must understand that withdrawal of devices such as feeding tubes and ventilators is allowing natural death to occur, which is very different than actively doing something to cause death (Murphy, 1996; Huang and Ahronheim, 2000; Kuebler and McKinnon, 2002).

The general trend in American law is toward greater freedom for the individual to choose when and how to die. Many people believe that patient-assisted suicide might soon be reality based on constitutional grounds of the right to privacy (Messinger, 1993) or the due process clause of the Fourteenth Amendment to the U.S. Constitution (Sedler, 1993; Wilkes, 1996; Carter, 1996).

As a means of stimulating thoughtful discussion on this topic, Table 24-10 includes some pros and cons from Morrison and Meier (1994). Murphy (1996) suggests that now is the time for nurses individually, among themselves, and collectively, in professional organizations, to consider the implications of physician-assisted suicide and what their role will be while it is still a topic of social debate, rather than to be caught unprepared without professional consensus as to their position if it should be legalized, as it might be (Murphy, 1996).

Clearly, continuing discussion and new perspectives are needed to resolve this supremely important question. *California Nurse* (Liaschenko and Drought, 1993) introduced some cogent questions regarding this issue; these are included at the end of the chapter for student discussion.

Planning for the Care of Survivors

As with grief, discussed earlier in this chapter, outliving one's loves may create an emptiness that can never be fully assuaged. Table 24-3 is again cited as an aid to facilitating the needs of survivors. The nurse must be prepared for this most difficult of all tasks.

This chapter has dealt with the apogee and perigee of human experience. The highest levels of nursing function and the deepest feelings are uncovered in the nurse who is privileged to accompany the aged through the processes of fully living the last days before dying.

Human Needs and Wellness Diagnoses

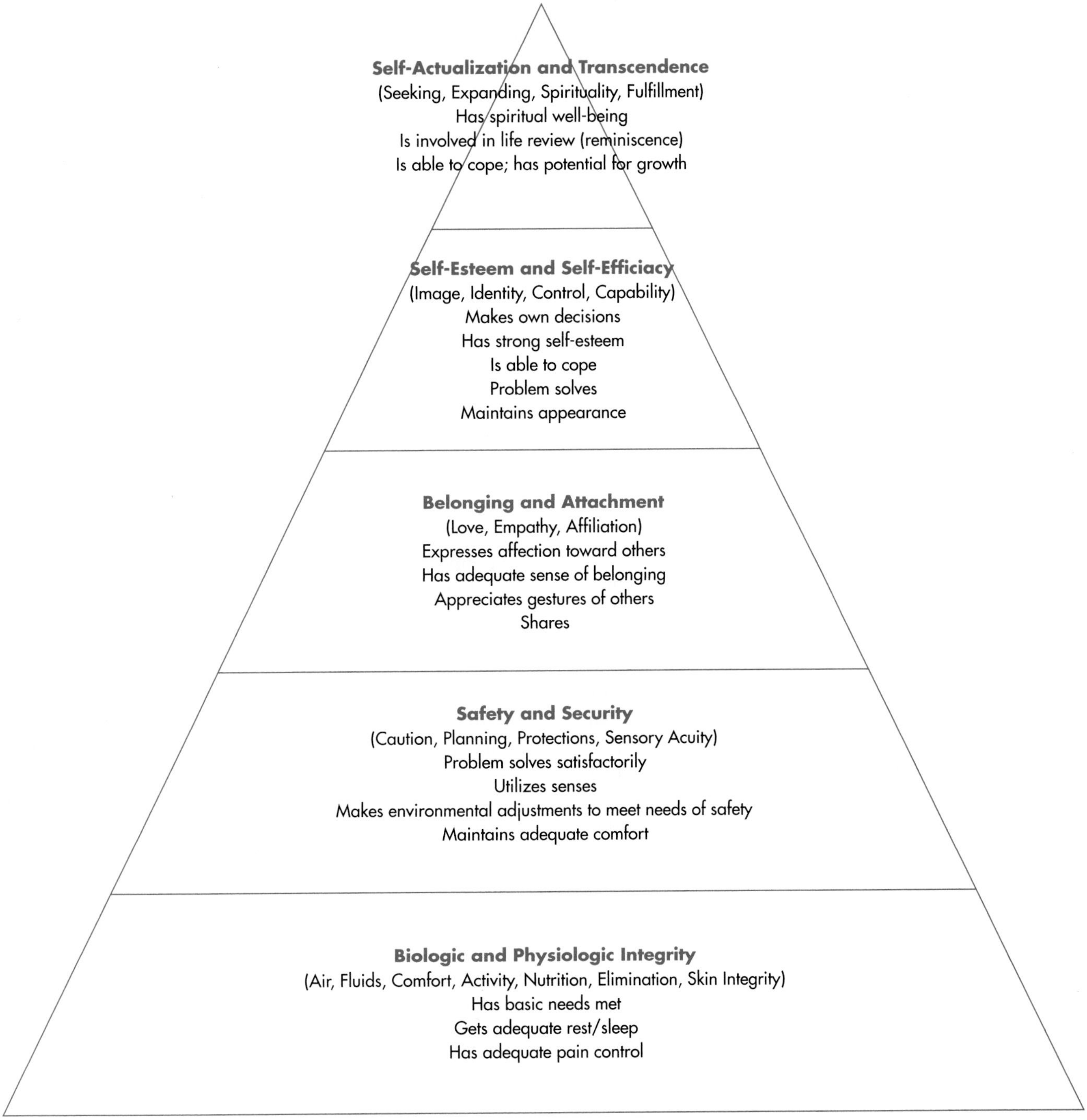

Self-Actualization and Transcendence
(Seeking, Expanding, Spirituality, Fulfillment)
Has spiritual well-being
Is involved in life review (reminiscence)
Is able to cope; has potential for growth

Self-Esteem and Self-Efficiacy
(Image, Identity, Control, Capability)
Makes own decisions
Has strong self-esteem
Is able to cope
Problem solves
Maintains appearance

Belonging and Attachment
(Love, Empathy, Affiliation)
Expresses affection toward others
Has adequate sense of belonging
Appreciates gestures of others
Shares

Safety and Security
(Caution, Planning, Protections, Sensory Acuity)
Problem solves satisfactorily
Utilizes senses
Makes environmental adjustments to meet needs of safety
Maintains adequate comfort

Biologic and Physiologic Integrity
(Air, Fluids, Comfort, Activity, Nutrition, Elimination, Skin Integrity)
Has basic needs met
Gets adequate rest/sleep
Has adequate pain control

These are not all the possible wellness diagnoses that may be identified. The above are examples of nursing diagnoses that should be considered when planning care for the older adult.

KEY CONCEPTS

- Grief is an emotional and behavioral response to loss.
- Many theories or frameworks have been offered that outline grief responses. However, grief responses are individual. One group may consider that which is appropriate for another societal group aberrant.
- One never completely resolves grief. Instead, the individual incorporates the grief as a part of his or her life.
- Dying is a multifaceted active process. Everyone involved is affected: the one who is dying, the family, and the professional caregivers.
- The stages or phases of dying and the type of coping are not obligatory or prescriptive of the way one should die. Such expectations place an added burden on the one who is dying.
- There are tasks that the terminally ill and dying person attempts to resolve in the acute, chronic, and terminal phases of his or her illness.
- An individual is living until he or she has died.
- The dying older adult is a living person, with all the same needs for good and natural relationships with people as are the rest of us.
- Hope is empowering; it generates courage and motivates action and achievement. The degree of hope that a dying individual possesses depends on a caring relationship with others.
- The health professional who cares for the dying must have outside interests and support systems before considering care of the dying.
- Living can be more painful than dying.
- Hospice is a process or unique ideology that links the needs of terminally ill, the family, and staff to fulfill the remainder of a dying individual's life by enabling or returning control to the dying person.
- ADs allow an individual control over life and death decisions by written communication and allows an appointed person (a proxy) to be his or her advocate when he or she is not able to communicate desires personally.
- Most medical and nursing organizations do not support physician aid in dying and suicide. These issues will continue to generate controversy within the health professions for many years to come.

▲ CASE STUDY

Jesse was simply unable to believe that his wife was dying. The physician told Jesse that Jeannette was in the early stages of multiple myeloma, and she might die in less than a year, or she might have remissions and live another decade. Jesse and his wife had worked hard all their lives and raised two sons. Now that they were both retired and financially well fixed, even though they were not yet 65, they had thought the best years of their lives were ahead. However, both Jesse and Jeannette were the type who approached a problem head on, and they gathered all the relevant material they were able to find and assiduously studied all they were able to find about multiple myeloma. Jeannette said that she did not want to mention her problem to others because she thought that she was unable to deal with "their piteous cancer looks." She also stressed that she expected to have long remissions and to live to be 75 years of age, at least. So why trouble friends and family? As a result of her decision, Jesse was unable to share his fear and grief because he had promised to respect Jeannette's wishes in that regard. She began a series of chemotherapeutic drugs, and friends began to notice her lethargy. They began to worry about her, but she insisted, "I'm just fine." Six months passed with a steady downward course in Jeannette's condition. Her sons began to suspect she had a malignancy, and one son, Rob, asked outright, "Are you hiding a serious illness from us?" She denied it, but Rob also noticed that Jesse was withdrawing into himself and frequently retreated into the booze bottle. Rob knew something was wrong but was at a loss. When Rob went to the family physician for his annual checkup, the office nurse said, "Oh, Rob, how is your mother doing now?" At Rob's insistence the nurse told him of his mother's diagnosis.

Discuss your rationale and feelings as the office nurse, and determine a plan of action that seems appropriate at this time. Develop a long-range plan of care for this family.

Based on the case study, develop a nursing care plan using the following procedure:*

List the client's comments that provide subjective data.

List information that provides objective data.

From these data identify and state, using accepted format, two nursing diagnoses you determine are most significant to this client at this time.

Determine and state outcome criteria for each diagnosis. These criteria must reflect some alleviation of the problem identified in the nursing diagnosis and must be stated in concrete and measurable terms.

Plan and state one or more interventions for each diagnosed problem. Provide specific documentation of sources used to determine appropriate intervention.

Evaluate the success of intervention. Interventions must correlate directly with the stated outcome criteria to measure the outcome success.

STUDY QUESTIONS/ACTIVITIES

Explore your responses to being given a terminal diagnosis. What coping mechanisms work for you?

With which awareness approach would you be comfortable?

How would you recognize spiritual distress? Relate particular interventions you think would be helpful to an individual who was feeling spiritually distressed.

*Students are advised to refer to their nursing diagnosis text and identify possible or potential problems.

Discuss what you believe are the significant aspects of "religion" or "spirituality" in your life. Do not think you must do so if the topic is uncomfortable for you to share.
If you believe that you are able, discuss your grief process when you dealt with the loss of someone special in your life.
Practice with a partner several methods that you will use to introduce the topic of dying with a client who is critically ill and is not expected to live.
Describe how you would deal with a dying person and his or her family when these family members are especially protective of each other.
Discuss and strategize how you would bring up the topic of ADs.
What AD is legally recognized in your state?
Explore with family and friends their thoughts on completing an AD.
Complete your own AD.
Student Discussion Questions Related To Assisted Suicide
What is the cultural and historic meaning of *killing?*
In Biblical times, did people believe that God killed?
Is there a general denial of the responsibility that accompanies the enormous technologic power we have developed over life and death?
Are we afraid we are *playing God?*
Is loss of dignity and loss of self as significant in the desire to die as unbearable pain?
For individuals in favor of euthanasia, is it related to an inability to tolerate or witness the suffering of others?
Is the Hippocratic oath, grounded in allegiance to Greek gods and selectively practiced, relevant to decisions about euthanasia?
What would be appropriate safeguards from misuse, neither too restrictive nor too liberal?
What nursing actions do you consider assisted suicide?

RESEARCH QUESTIONS

How does religiosity influence coping and grief resolution?
What are the phenomenologic aspects of dying at various ages: 65, 75, 85, and so forth? What is the significance of the variations? Similar studies are needed that are related to the particular type of death.
Do patterns of grief of elders differ depending on whether the person is spouse, sibling, or child?
What are the variables that influence elders to die at home?
What percentage of hospice patients are over age 65, and what are the conditions of their terminal illness?
When do elders usually complete an AD?
What are the nurses' interpretations of assisted dying versus euthanasia?
How do long-term care facilities cope with the dying elder?
How do nurses foresee their role if assisted suicide is legalized?

REFERENCES

American Nurses' Association: *Code for nurses with interpretative statements,* Kansas City, MO, 1985, The Association.
American Nurses' Association: *Standards and scope of hospice nursing practice,* Kansas City, MO, 1987, The Association.
American Nurses' Association: *Position statement on nursing care and do-not-resuscitate decisions,* Washington, DC, 1992, The Association.
Arbuckle NW, deVries B: The long-term effects of late life spousal and parental bereavement on personal functioning, *Gerontologist* 35(5):637, 1995.
Bernabi R et al: Management of pain in elderly patients with cancer, *Journal of American Medical Association* 279:1877, 1998.
Berrio MW, Levesque ME: Advance directives: most patients don't have one. Do yours? *Am J Nurs* 96(8):25, 1996.
Botwinick J et al: Predicting death from behavioral test performance, *J Gerontol* 33:(6)755, 1978.
Bowlby J: Process of mourning, *Int J Psychoanal* 42:317, 1961.
Brabant S, Forsyth CJ, Melanon C: Grieving men: thoughts, feelings and behaviors following deaths of wives, *Hosp J—Physical, Psychosocial, and Pastoral Care of the Dying* 8(4): 33, 1992.
Canavan K: ANA advises nurses not to participate in assisted suicide, *Am Nurs* 28(4):8, 1996.
Carr AC et al: Object-loss and somatic symptom formation. In Schoenberg B et al, editors: *Loss and grief: psychological management in medical practice,* New York, 1970, Columbia University Press.
Carter SL: Rush to a lethal judgment, *Time Magazine,* July 2, 1996.
Cartwright A: Is religion a help around the time of death? *Public Health* 105(1):79, 1991.
Caserta MS, Lund DA: Intrapersonal resources and the effectiveness of self-help groups for bereaved older adults, *Gerontologist* 33(5):619, 1993.
Chronicle News Services: Judge reins in Ashcroft on assisted suicide, *San Francisco Chronicle,* April 18, 2002.
Cohen E: Durable powers of attorney: an overview, *Aging Connection* 8(2):8, 1987.
Coolican MB et al: Education about death, dying, and bereavement in nursing programs, *Nurs Educ* 19(6):38, 1994.
Corr CA: Coping with dying: lessons that we should and should not learn from the work of Elisabeth Kübler-Ross, *Death Stud* 17(1):69, 1993.
Corr CA: A task-based approach to coping with dying. In DeSpelder LA, Strickland AL, editors: *The pathway ahead,* Mountainview, CA, 1995, Mayfield Publishing Company.
Corr CA, Nabe CM, Corr DM: *Death and dying, life and living,* ed 3, Stamford City, CT, 2000, Wadsworth.
Danis M et al: A prospective study of advance directives for life-sustaining care, *N Engl J Med* 324:882, 1991.
Delong MF: Caring for the elderly. V. Managing end of life issues, *NURSEweek* 8(9):4, 1995.
Depaola SJ et al: Death concern and attitudes toward the elderly in nursing home personnel, *Death Stud* 16(6):537, 1992.
DeSpelder LA, Strickland AL: *The pathway ahead: readings in death and dying,* Mountainview, CA, 1995, Mayfield Publishing Company.
DeSpelder LA, Strickland AL: *The last dance: encountering death and dying,* ed 4, Mountainview, CA, 1996, Mayfield Publishing Company.

Dessonville CL, Thompson LW, Gallagher D: The role of anticipatory bereavement in the adjustment to widowhood in the elderly, *Gerontologist* 23:309 (special issue), 1983.

Doka KJ: Disenfranchized grief. In Doka KJ, editor: *Disenfranchized grief: recognizing hidden sorrow,* Lexington, MA, 1989, Lexington Books.

Doka KJ: The spiritual crisis of bereavement. In Doka KJ, Morgan JD, editors: *Death and spirituality,* Amityville, NY, 1993, Baywood Publishing Company.

Douglas R, Brown HN: Patients' attitudes toward advance directives, *Journal of Nursing Scholarship* 34(1):61, 2002, Sigma Theta Tau International.

Eastman P: Dying at home not a priority for patients and families, *Caring for the Ages* 2(2):1, 2001.

Emanuel LL, Emanuel EJ: The medical directive: a new comprehensive advance care document, *JAMA* 261:3288, 1989.

Emanuel LL et al: Advance directives for medical care: a case of greater use, *N Engl J Med* 324:889, 1991.

Engel G: Grief and grieving, *Am J Nurs* 64:93, 1967.

Erikson E: *Childhood and society,* New York, 1963, WW Norton.

Fine PG: Chronic pain in long-term care: assessment, management, and improvement of quality indicators, Elder Care Summit Conference, San Francisco, April 25, 2002.

Foley KM: Death in America: a new dynamic for an old reality—the national debate, *Aging Today* 17(1):7, 1996.

Forbes SB: Hope: an essential human need in the elderly, *J Gerontol Nurs* 20(6):5, 1994.

Futterman EH, Hoffman I, Sabshin M: Parental anticipatory mourning. In Schoenberg B et al, editors: *Psychosocial aspects of terminal care,* New York, 1970, Columbia University Press.

Gass K: Coping strategies of widows, *J Gerontol Nurs* 13(8):29, 1987.

Gilfix M: Legal planning is essential for Alzheimer's victims, *Senior Spectrum* 6(12):5, 1987.

Glaser B, Strauss A: *Awareness of dying,* Chicago, 1963, AVC.

Godow S: Death and dying: a natural connection? *Generations* 11:15, 1987.

Goodman M et al: Cultural differences among elderly women in coping with the death of an adult child, *J Gerontol* 46(6):S321, 1991.

Gray VR: Dealing with dying, *Nursing '73* 3:27, 1976.

Habel M: Advance directives, a long way to go, *NurseWeek* 4(22):21, Oct. 22, 2001.

Harper BC: *Death: the coping mechanisms of the health professional,* Greenville, SC, 1977, Southeastern University Press.

Havens GAD: Differences in execution/nonexecution of advance directives by community dwelling, *Research in Nursing & Health* 23(4):319, August 2000.

Hendin H: The psychiatrist. In Wilkes P, editor: The next pro-lifers, *New York Times Magazine,* July 21, 1996.

Herth K: Relationship of hope, coping styles, concurrent losses and setting of grief resolution in the elderly widow(er), *Res Nurs Health* 13:109, 1990.

Hess PA: Loss, grief, and dying. In Beare P, Myers J, editors: *Adult health nursing,* ed 3, St Louis, 1998, Mosby.

Hohmann N, Kiyak H: *Social gerontology,* Boston, 1996, Allyn and Bacon Co.

Hopmeyer E, Werk A: A comparative study of family bereavement groups, *Death Studies* 18:243, 1994.

Horacek BJ: Toward a more viable model of grieving and consequences for older persons, *Death Stud* 15(5):459, 1991.

Huang ZB, Ahronheim JC: Nutrition and hydration in terminally ill patients: an update, *Clin Geriatr Med* 16(2):313, 2000.

Keleman S: Stages of dying, *Voices* 10:46, 1974.

Kelly JD: Grief: re-forming life's story, *J Palliat Care* 8(2):33, 1992.

Krohn B: When death is near, helping families cope, *Geriatr Nurs* 19(5):276, 1998.

Kübler-Ross E: *On death and dying,* New York, 1969, MacMillan.

Kuebler S, McKinnon S: Dehydration. In Kuebler KK, Berry PH, Heidrich DE, editors: *End-of-life care: clinical practice guidelines*, Philadelphia, PA, 2002, WB Saunders.

Lee BC, Brody R: *Compassion in dying, presentation at commonwealth club,* San Francisco, CA, March 6, 2002.

Lentzner HR et al: The quality of life in the year before death, *Am J Public Health* 82(8):1093, 1992.

Liaschenko J, Drought T: Euthanasia: pro and con, *Calif Nurs* 89(1):1, 1993.

Lindeman E: Symptomatology and management of acute grief, *Am J Psychiatr* 101:141, 1944.

Lindley DB: Process of dying: defining characteristics, *Cancer Nurs* 14(6):328, 1991.

Lund DA, Caserta MD, Dimond MF: Gender differences through two years of bereavement among the elderly, *Gerontologist* 26(3):314, 1986.

MacKay S: Durable power of attorney for health care. Is DPAHC the best advance directive for patients residing in long-term care facilities? *Geriatr Nurs* 13(2):99, 1992.

Martin TL, Doka KJ: Masculine grief. In Doka KJ, editor: *Living with grief after sudden loss: suicide, homicide, accident, heart attack, stroke,* Washington, DC, 1996, Hospice Foundation of America.

Martin TL, Doka KJ: Revisiting masculine grief. In Doka KJ, Davidson JD, editors: *Living with grief: who are we, how we grieve,* Washington, DC, 1998, Hospice Foundation of America.

Martocchio BC: *Living while dying*, Bowie, MD, 1982, RJ Brady Co.

McCaffery M, Pasero C: *Pain: clinical manual for nursing practice,* ed 2, St Louis, 1999, Mosby.

Meier DE et al: Marked improvement in recognition and completion of health care proxies: a randomized controlled trial of counseling by hospital patient representatives, *Arch Intern Med* 156(11):1227, 1996.

Messinger TJ: A gentle and easy death: from ancient Greece to beyond Cruzan—toward a reasoned legal response to the societal dilemma of euthanasia, *Denver University Law Review* 71(1):229, 1993.

Mezey M: Geriatric nursing standard of practice protocol: advance directives—nurses helping to protect patient rights, *Geriatr Nurs* 17(5):204, 1996.

Mezey M, Ramsey GC, Mitty E: Making the PSDA work for the elderly, *Generations* 18(4):13, 1994.

Mezey MD et al: Why hospital patients do and do not execute an advance directive, *Nurs Outlook* 48:165, 2000.

Mickley JR, Soeken K, Belcher A: Spiritual well-being, religiousness and hope among women with breast cancer, *Image J Nurs Sch* 24(4):267, 1992.

Minogue B: *Bioethics: a committee approach,* Boston, 1996, Jones and Bartlett Publishers.

Mittleman M: Taking grief to heart, *Harvard Health Letter* 21(8):8, 1996.

Morrison RS: Barriers to completion of health care proxies: an examination of ethnic differences, *Archives of Internal Medicine* 158(12):2439, 1998.

Morrison RS, Meier DE: Physician-assisted dying: fashioning public policy with an absence of data, *Generations* 18(4):48, 1994.

Moyers W: Healing and the mind, WNET public television, February, 1992.

Murphy P: In Caravan K: ANA advises nurses not to participate in assisted suicide, *Amer Nurs* 8, June 1996.

O'Hara PA et al: Patient death in a long-term care hospital: a study of the effect on nursing staff, *J Gerontol Nurs* 22(8):27, 1996.

O'Keefe M: The Dutch way of dying, *San Francisco Sunday Examiner,* February 19, 1995.

Parkman C: Using advance directives: part 2, *NURSEweek* 9(12):10, 1996.

Parks CM: *Bereavement,* New York, 1972, Tavistock.

Parks CM, Weiss RS: *Recovery from bereavement,* New York, 1983, Basic Books.

Pattison EM: The experience of dying, *Am J Psychother* 21:32, 1967.

Pietruszka FM: Management of bereavement in the elderly, *Phys Assist* 16(4):31, 1992.

Rando TA: *Grief, dying and death,* Champaign, IL, 1984, Research Press.

Raphael B: *Anatomy of bereavement,* New York, 1983, Basic Books.

Rees WD, Lukin SG: The mortality of bereavement, *BMJ* 4:13, 1967.

Retsinas J: A theoretical reassessment of the applicability of Kübler-Ross's stages of dying, *Death Stud* 12:207, 1988.

Richter J: Support: a resource during crisis of mate loss, *J Gerontol Nurs* 13(11):18, 1987.

Rigdon I, Clayton B, Dimond M: Toward a theory of helplessness for the elderly bereaved: an invitation to a new life, *Adv Nurs Sci* 9(2):32, 1987.

Rubin SS: The two-track model of bereavement: overview, retrospective and prospective, *Death Stud* 23:681, 1999.

Schmitt L: The right to choose: capacity study of demented residents in nursing homes (executive summary), Chicago, 1996, Franciscan Sisters of the Poor Hospital Systems.

Schreck IR: Commentary on grieving men: thoughts, feelings, and behavior following death of wives, *ONS Nursing Scan Oncol* 2(4):1, 1993.

Sedler RA: The constitution and hastening inevitable death, *Hasting Cent Rep* 23(5):20, 1993.

Siegel JM, Kuykendall DH: Loss, widowhood, and psychological distress among the elderly, *J Consult Clin Psychol* 58(5):519, 1990.

Sisneros J: *Language change as a function of growth after loss,* compiled for N112, San Francisco, 1994, San Francisco State University School of Nursing.

Steele L: Risk factor profile for bereaved spouses, *Death Stud* 16(5):387, 1992.

Steinhauser KE et al: Factors considered important at the end of life by patients, family, physicians, and other care givers, *JAMA* 284(19):2476, Nov 15, 2000.

Stroebe M et al: Broken hearts or broken bonds: love and death in historical perspective, *Am Psychol* 47(10)1205, 1992.

Stroebe M, Schut H: The dual process model of coping with bereavement: rational and description, *Death Stud* 23:197, 1999.

Thomas V: Hospice nursing: reaping the rewards, dealing with the stress, *Geriatr Nurs* 4:22, 1983.

Ulrich LK: The challenge of hospice care, *Bull Am Protestant Hosp Assoc* 21:6, 1978.

U.S. Bureau of the Census, *Statistical abstract of the United States: 1998,* ed. 118, Washington DC, 1998, U.S. Department of Commerce, Economic and Statistics Administration.

U.S. Bureau of the Census: *Statistical abstract of the United States: 2001,* ed 121, Washington, DC, 2001, U.S. Department of Commerce, Economic and Statistics Administration.

Verhovek SW: Oregon releases statistics on assisted-suicide cases, *San Francisco Chronicle,* February 7, 2000.

Watson W, Maxwell RJ: Elements of the social structure of dying. In Watson W, Maxwell RJ, editors: *Human aging and dying: study in sociocultural gerontology,* New York, 1977, St Martin's Press.

Weenolsen P: *The art of dying,* New York, 1996, St Martin's Press.

White KR, Coyne PJ, Patel UB: Are nurses adequately prepared for end-of-life care? *J Nurs Sch* 33(2):147, 2001.

White N, Cunningham WR: Is terminal drop pervasive or specific? *J Gerontol* 43(6):141, 1988.

Wilkes P: The next pro-lifers, *New York Times Magazine*, July 21, 1996.

Worden JW: *Grief counseling and grief therapy: a handbook for mental health practitioners,* ed 2, New York, 1991, Springer.

Zilberfein F: Coping with death: anticipatory grief and bereavement, *Generations* xxxiii(1):69, 1999.

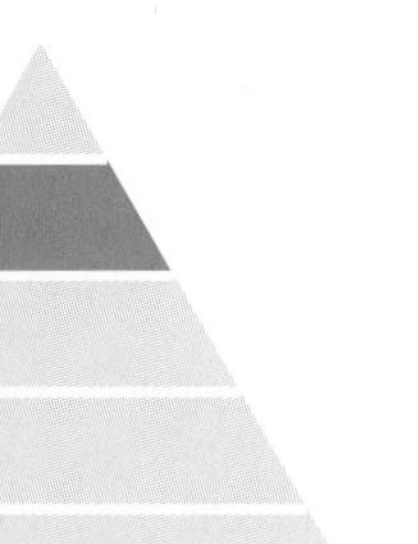

APPENDIX 24-A

The Medical Directive

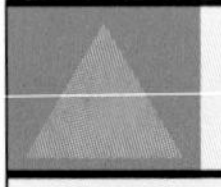

The Medical Directive

Introduction

As part of a person's right to self-determination, every adult may accept or refuse any recommended medical treatment. This decision is relatively easy when people are well and can speak. Unfortunately, during serious illness, individuals are often unconscious or otherwise unable to communicate their wishes—at the very time when many critical decisions need to be made.

The Medical Directive allows you to record your wishes regarding various types of medical treatments in several representative situations so that your desires can be respected. The Directive also lets you appoint a proxy, someone to make medical decisions in your place if you should become unable to make them on your own.

The Medical Directive comes into effect only if you become incompetent (unable to make decisions and too sick to have wishes). You can change the Directive at any time until then. As long as you are competent, you should discuss your care with your physician.

Completing the Form

You should, if possible, complete the form in the context of a discussion with your physician. Ideally, this discussion should occur in the presence of your proxy. This discussion also lets your physician and your proxy know what you think about these decisions, and it provides you and your physician with the opportunity to give or clarify relevant personal or medical information. You may also wish to discuss the issues with your family, friends, or religious mentor.

The Medical Directive contains six illness situations that include incompetence. For each situation, you consider possible interventions and goals of medical care. Situation A is permanent coma; B is near death; C is with weeks to live, both in and out of consciousness; D is extreme dementia; E is a situation you describe; and F is temporary inability to make decisions.

For each scenario, you identify your general goals for care and specific intervention choices. The interventions are divided into six groups: (1) cardiopulmonary resuscitation or major surgery; (2) mechanical breathing or dialysis; (3) blood transfusions or blood products; (4) artificial nutrition and hydration; (5) simple diagnostic tests or antibiotics; and (6) pain medications, even if they dull consciousness and indirectly shorten life. Most of these treatments are described briefly. If you have further questions, consult your physician.

Your wishes for treatment options (I want this treatment; I want this treatment tried, but stopped if no clear improvement is evident; I am undecided; I do not want this treatment) should be indicated. If you choose a trial of treatment, you should understand that this choice indicates that you want the treatment withdrawn if your physician and proxy believe that the attempt has become futile.

The PERSONAL STATEMENT section allows you to explain your choices and say anything you wish to people who may make decisions for you concerning the limits of your life and the goals of intervention. For example, in situation B, if you wish to define "uncertain chance" with numerical probability, you may do so here.

Next, you may express your preferences concerning organ donation. Do you wish to donate your body or some or all of your organs after your death? If so, for what purpose or purposes and to which physician or institution? If not, this choice should also be indicated in the appropriate box.

In the final section, you may designate one or more proxies, who would be asked to make choices under circumstances in which your wishes are unclear. You can indicate whether the decisions of the proxy should override your wishes if differences exist. Additionally, should you name more than one proxy, you can state who is to have the final say if disagreement exists. Your proxy must understand that this role usually involves making judgments that you would have made for yourself, had you been able—and making them by the criteria you have outlined. Proxy decisions should ideally be made in discussion with your family, friends, and physician.

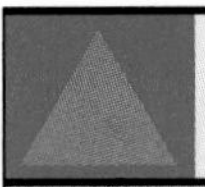

The Medical Directive—cont'd

What to Do with the Form

Once you have completed the form, you and two adult witnesses (other than your proxy) who have no interest in your estate need to sign and date it.

Many states have legislation covering documents of this sort. To determine the laws in your state, you should call the state attorney general's office or consult an attorney. If your state has a statutory document, you may wish to use the Medical Directive and append it to this form.

You should give a copy of the completed document to your physician. His or her signature is desirable but not mandatory. The Directive should be placed in your medical records and flagged so that anyone who might be involved in your care can be aware of its presence. Your proxy, a family member, a friend, or any combination should also have a copy. In addition, you may want to carry a wallet card noting that you have such a document and where it can be found.

My Medical Directive

This Medical Directive shall stand as a guide to my wishes regarding medical treatments in the event that illness should make me unable to communicate them directly. I make this Directive, being 18 years or more of age, of sound mind, and appreciating the consequences of my decisions

SITUATION A

If I am in a coma or a persistent vegetative state and, in the opinion of my physician and two consultants, have no known hope of regaining awareness and higher mental functions no matter what is done, then my goals and specific wishes—if medically reasonable—for this and any additional illnesses would be:

- ☐ Prolong life; treat everything
- ☐ Attempt to cure, but reevaluate often
- ☐ Limit to less invasive and less burdensome interventions
- ☐ Provide comfort care only
- ☐ Other (*please specify*):

SITUATION B

If I near death and in a coma, and, in the opinion of my physician and two consultants, have a small but uncertain chance of regaining higher mental functions, a somewhat greater chance of surviving with permanent mental and physical disability, and a much greater chance of not recovering at all, then my goals and specific wishes—if medically reasonable—for this and any additional illness would be:

- ☐ Prolong life; treat everything
- ☐ Attempt to cure, but reevaluate often
- ☐ Limit to less invasive and less burdensome interventions
- ☐ Provide comfort card only
- ☐ Other (*please specify*):

SITUATION C

If I have a terminal illness with weeks to live, any my mind is not working well enough to make decisions for myself, but I am sometimes awake and seem to have feelings, then my goals and specific wishes—if medically reasonable—for this and any additional illness would be:

*In this state, prior wishes need to be balanced with a best guess about your current feelings. The proxy and physician have to make this judgment for you.

- ☐ Prolong life; treat everything
- ☐ Attempt to cure, but reevaluate often
- ☐ Limit to less invasive and less burdensome interventions
- ☐ Provide comfort card only
- ☐ Other (*please specify*):

SITUATION D

If I have brain damage or some brain disease that in the opinion of my physician and two consultants cannot be reversed and that makes me unable to think or have feelings, *but I have no terminal illness*, then my goals and specific wishes—if medically reasonable—for this and additional illness would be:

- ☐ Prolong life; treat everything
- ☐ Attempt to cure, but reevaluate often
- ☐ Limit to less invasive and less burdensome interventions
- ☐ Provide comfort card only
- ☐ Other (*please specify*):

SITUATION E

If I...

(Describe a situation that is important to you and/or your doctor believes you should consider in view of your current medical situation):

- ☐ Prolong life; treat everything
- ☐ Attempt to cure, but reevaluate often
- ☐ Limit to less invasive and less burdensome interventions
- ☐ Provide comfort card only
- ☐ Other (*please specify*):

SITUATION F

If I am in my current state of health (describe briefly: __and then have an illness that, in the opinion of my physician and two consultants, is life threatening but reversible, and I am temporarily unable to make decisions, then my goals and specific wishes—if medically reasonable—would be:

- ☐ Prolong life; treat everything
- ☐ Attempt to cure, but reevaluate often
- ☐ Limit to less invasive and less burdensome interventions
- ☐ Provide comfort card only
- ☐ Other (*please specify*):

Please check appropriate boxes:	A: I want.	A: I want treatment tried. If no clear improvement, stop.	A: I am undecided.	A: I do not want.	B: I want.	B: I want treatment tried. If no clear improvement, stop.	B: I am undecided.	B: I do not want.	C: I want.	C: I want treatment tried. If no clear improvement, stop.	C: I am undecided.	C: I do not want.
1. Cardiopulmonary resuscitation (chest compressions, drugs, electric shocks, and artificial breathing aimed at reviving a person who is on the point of dying).		*Not applicable*				*Not applicable*				*Not applicable*		
2. Major surgery (for example, removing the gallbladder or part of the colon).		*Not applicable*				*Not applicable*				*Not applicable*		
3. Mechanical breathing (respiration by machine, through a tube in the throat).												
4. Dialysis (cleaning the blood by machine or by fluid passed through the belly).												
5. Blood transfusions or blood products.		*Not applicable*				*Not applicable*				*Not applicable*		
6. Artificial nutrition and hydration (given through a tube in a vein or in the stomach).												
7. Simple diagnostic tests (for example, blood tests or x-rays).		*Not applicable*				*Not applicable*				*Not applicable*		
8. Antibiotics (drugs used to fight infection).		*Not applicable*				*Not applicable*				*Not applicable*		
9. Pain medications, even if they dull consciousness and indirectly shorten my life.		*Not applicable*				*Not applicable*				*Not applicable*		

Please check appropriate boxes:	D: I want.	D: I want treatment tried. If no clear improvement, stop.	D: I am undecided.	D: I do not want.	E: I want.	E: I want treatment tried. If no clear improvement, stop.	E: I am undecided.	E: I do not want.	F: I want.	F: I want treatment tried. If no clear improvement, stop.	F: I am undecided.	F: I do not want.
1. Cardiopulmonary resuscitation (chest compressions, drugs, electric shocks, and artificial breathing aimed at reviving a person who is on the point of dying).		*Not applicable*				*Not applicable*				*Not applicable*		
2. Major surgery (for example, removing the gallbladder or part of the colon).		*Not applicable*				*Not applicable*				*Not applicable*		
3. Mechanical breathing (respiration by machine, through a tube in the throat).												
4. Dialysis (cleaning the blood by machine or by fluid passed through the belly).												
5. Blood transfusions or blood products.		*Not applicable*				*Not applicable*				*Not applicable*		
6. Artificial nutrition and hydration (given through a tube in a vein or in the stomach).												
7. Simple diagnostic tests (for example, blood tests or x-rays).		*Not applicable*				*Not applicable*				*Not applicable*		
8. Antibiotics (drugs used to fight infection).		*Not applicable*				*Not applicable*				*Not applicable*		
9. Pain medications, even if they dull consciousness and indirectly shorten my life.		*Not applicable*				*Not applicable*				*Not applicable*		

Health Care Proxy

I appoint as my proxy decision-maker(s):
Name and Address ______________________________
and (optional)
Name and Address ______________________________

I direct my proxy to make health care decisions based on his or her assessment of my personal wishes. If my personal desires are unknown, my proxy is to make health care decisions based on his or her best guess as to my wishes. My proxy shall have the authority to make all health care decisions for me, including decisions about life-sustaining treatment, if I am unable to make them myself. My proxy's authority becomes effective if my attending physician determines in writing that I lack the capacity to make or to communicate health care decisions. My proxy is then to have the same authority to make health care decisions as I would if I had the capacity to make them, EXCEPT *(list the limitations, if any, you wish to place on your proxy's authority)*:

I wish my written preference to be applied as exactly as possible/with flexibility according to my proxy's judgment. *(Delete as appropriate.)*

Should any disagreement exist between the wishes I have indicated in this document and the decisions favored by my above-named proxy, I wish my proxy to have authority over my written statements/I wish my written statements to bind my proxy. *(Delete as appropriate.)*

If I have appointed more than one proxy and disagreement exists between their wishes, ______________ shall have final authority.

Signed:
Signature ______________ Printed Name ______________
Address ______________ Date ______________

Witness:
Signature ______________ Printed Name ______________
Address ______________ Date ______________

Witness:
Signature ______________ Printed Name ______________
Address ______________ Date ______________

Physician (optional):
I am ______________'s physician. I have seen this advance care document and have had an opportunity to discuss his or her preferences regarding medical interventions at the end of life. If ______________ becomes incompetent, I understand that it is my duty to interpret and implement the preferences contained in this document so as to fulfill his or her wishes.

Signed:
Signature ______________ Printed Name ______________
Address ______________ Date ______________

Organ Donation

☐ I hereby make this anatomic gift to take effect after my death:

I give
- ☐ my body
- ☐ any needed organs or parts
- ☐ the following parts ______________

to
- ☐ the following person or institution ______________
- ☐ the physician in attendance at my death
- ☐ the hospital in which I die
- ☐ the following physician, hospital storage bank, or other medical institution: ______________

for
- ☐ any purpose authorized by law
- ☐ therapy of another person
- ☐ medical education
- ☐ transplantation
- ☐ research

☐ I do not wish to make any anatomic gift from my body.

Continued

Health Care Proxy—cont'd

My Personal Statement (use another page if necessary)

Please mention anything that would be important for your physician and your proxy to know. In particular, try to answer the following questions: (1) What medical conditions, if any, would make living so unpleasant that you would want life-sustaining treatment withheld? (Intractable pain? Irreversible mental damage? Inability to share love? Dependence on others? Another condition you would regard as intolerable?). (2) Under what medical circumstances would you want to stop interventions that might already have been started? (3) Why do you choose what you choose?

If any difference exists between my preferences detailed in the illness situations and those understood from my goals or from my personal statement, I wish my treatment selections/my goals/my personal statement *(please delete as appropriate)* to be given greater weight.

When I am dying, I would like—if my proxy and my health care team think it is reasonable—to be cared for:

☐ At home or in a hospice ☐ In a hospital
☐ In a nursing home ☐ *Other (please specify)*

Signed ______________________________

Date ______________________________

Witness ______________________________

Date ______________________________

Witness ______________________________

Date ______________________________

APPENDIX 24-B

Durable Power of Attorney

CMA California Medical Association

ADVANCE HEALTH CARE DIRECTIVE
Including Power of Attorney for Health Care Decisions
California Probate Code Sections 4600-4805

MY HEALTH CARE WISHES

This form lets you give instructions about your future health care. It also lets you name someone to make decisions for you if you can't make your own decisions. It's best if you fill out the whole form, but, as long as it is signed, dated and witnessed or notarized properly, you may choose only to appoint an agent (section 1) or provide health care instructions (section 3). If there is anything in this form you do not understand, read the booklet that comes with this form and the italicized instructions on the form, or ask your physician, other health care professional or an attorney for help. You may also review additional information and instructions concerning advance health care directives on the California Medical Association's website, ***www.cmanet.org****. Internet access is available at your local public library.*

1. APPOINTMENT OF HEALTH CARE AGENT

❑ **Option 1.** I, ______________________________, wish to appoint a health care agent.
(*Print* ***your*** *full name and date of birth*)

Fill in below the name and contact information of the person(s) (your agent and alternate agent(s)) you wish to make health care decisions for you if you are unable to make them for yourself. You may appoint alternate agents in case your first appointed agent is not willing, able or reasonably available to make these decisions when asked to do so.

Your agent may ***not*** *be:*

A. Your primary treating health care provider.
B. An operator of a community care or residential care facility where you receive care.
C. An employee of the health care institution or community or residential care facility where you receive care, unless your agent is related to you or is one of your co-workers.

If you choose to name an agent, you should discuss your wishes with that person and give that person a copy of this form. You should make sure that this person understands your wishes and this responsibility and is willing to accept it.

OR

❑ **Option 2.** I, ______________________________, do not wish to appoint an agent at this time.
(*Print* ***your*** *full name and date of birth*)

If you choose not to name an agent, initial the box above, print your name on the line in the space provided, draw a line through the rest of this page, then continue to Section 3.

I hereby appoint as my agent to make health care decisions for me:

Name ______________________________
(*agent's name*)

Address ______________________________
(*street address, city, state, zip code*)

Home Phone (____)__________ Work Phone (____)__________

Cell phone/Pager (____)__________ Fax (____)__________ e-mail __________

I understand this appointment will continue unless I revoke it as explained in Section 5.

If I revoke my agent's authority or if my agent is not reasonably available, able or willing to make health care decisions for me, I appoint the following person(s) to do so, listed in the order they should be asked:

OPTIONAL: 1st alternate agent: Name ______________________ e-mail __________

Address ______________________ Home phone (____)__________
(*street address, city, state, zip code*)

Work Phone (____)__________ Cell phone/Pager (____)__________ Fax (____)__________

OPTIONAL: 2nd alternate agent: Name ______________________ e-mail __________

Address ______________________ Home phone (____)__________
(*street address, city, state, zip code*)

Work Phone (____)__________ Cell phone/Pager (____)__________ Fax (____)__________

Continued

2. AUTHORITY OFAGENT

Your agent must make health care decisions that are consistent with the instructions in this document and your known desires. ***It is important that you discuss your health care desires with the person(s) you appoint as your health care agent, and with your doctor(s).*** *If your wishes are not known, your agent must make health care decisions that your agent believes to be in your best interest, considering your personal values to the extent they are known.*

If my primary physician finds that I cannot make my own health care decisions, I grant my agent full power and authority to make those decisions for me, subject to any health care instructions set forth below. My agent will have the right to:

A. Consent, refuse consent, or withdraw consent to any medical care or services, such as tests, drugs, surgery, or consultations for any physical or mental condition. This includes the provision, withholding or withdrawal of artificial nutrition and hydration (feeding by tube or vein) and all other forms of health care, including cardiopulmonary resuscitation (CPR).
B. Choose or reject my physician, other health care professionals or health care facilities.
C. Receive and consent to the release of medical information.
D. Donate organs or tissues, authorize an autopsy and dispose of my body, unless I have said something different in a contract with a funeral home, in my will, or by some other written method.

I understand that, by law, my agent may not consent to committing me to or placing me in a mental health treatment facility, or to convulsive treatment, psychosurgery, sterilization or abortion.

OPTIONAL: I want my agent's authority to make health care decisions for me to start now, **even though I am still able to make them for myself.** I understand and authorize this statement as proved by my signature____.

3. HEALTH CARE INSTRUCTIONS

You may, but are not required to, state your desires about the goals and types of medical care you do or do not want, including your desires concerning life support if you are seriously ill. If your wishes are not known, your agent must make health care decisions for you that your agent believes to be in your best interest, considering your personal values. ***If you do not wish to provide specific, written health care instructions, draw a line through this Section.***

The following are statements about the use of life-support treatments. Life-support or life-sustaining treatments are any medical procedures, devices or medications used to keep you alive. Life-support treatments may include: medical devices put in you to help you breathe; food and fluid supplied artificially by medical device (feeding tube); cardiopulmonary resuscitation (CPR); major surgery; blood transfusions; kidney dialysis; and antibiotics.

Sign either of the following general statements about life-support treatments if one accurately reflects your desires. If you wish to modify or add to either statement or to write your own statement instead, you may do so in the space provided or on a separate sheet(s) of paper which you must date and sign and attach to this form.

OPTIONAL: The statement I have signed below is to apply if I am suffering from a terminal condition from which death is expected in a matter of months, or if I am suffering from an irreversible condition that renders me unable to make decisions for myself, and life-support treatments are needed to keep me alive.

A. I request that all treatments other than those needed to keep me comfortable be discontinued or withheld and my physician(s) allows me to die as gently as possible. I understand and authorize this statement as proved by my signature________________________________.

OR

B. I want my life to be prolonged as long as possible within the limits of generally accepted health care standards. I understand and authorize this statement as proved by my signature___________________________.

OPTIONAL: Other or additional statements of medical treatment desires and limitations:________________

____

For additional Advance Health Care Directive options, go to the California Medical Association's website at ***www.cmanet.org.***

OPTIONAL: I have added ______ page(s) of specific health care instructions to this directive, each of which is signed and dated on the same day I signed this directive.

4. ORGAN AND TISSUE DONATION

I wish to be an organ donor. I understand and authorize this statement as proved by my signature____.

I have indicated this on ❑ my driver's license and/or ❑ an attached page.

*If you **do not** wish to be an organ donor, draw a line through this Section 4 and initial it.*

For additional information concerning organ and tissue donation, go to the California Medical Association website at www.cmanet.org.

5. PRIOR DIRECTIVES REVOKED

I revoke any prior Power of Attorney for Health Care or Natural Death Act Declaration.

You may revoke any part of or this entire Advance Health Care Directive at any time. To revoke the appointment of an agent, you must inform your treating health care provider personally or in writing. Completing a new California Medical Association Advance Health Care Directive will revoke all previous directives. If you revoke a prior directive, notify every person, physician, hospital, clinic, or care facility that has a copy of your prior directive and give them a copy of your new directive, if you execute one.

6. DATE AND SIGNATURE OF PRINCIPAL

I sign my name to and acknowledge this Advance Health Care Directive:

______________________	______________________	______________________
(signature of principal)	*(date of birth)*	*(date of signing)*

7. STATEMENT OF WITNESSES

*This Advance Health Care Directive will not be valid unless it is either (1) signed by two qualified adult witnesses who are present when you sign or acknowledge your signature or (2) acknowledged before a notary public in California. If you use witnesses rather than a notary public, the law **prohibits using the following as witnesses:** (1) the persons you have appointed as your agent or alternate agent(s); (2) your health care provider or an employee of your health care provider; or (3) an operator or employee of an operator of a community care facility or residential care facility for the elderly. Additionally, at least one of the witnesses **cannot** be related to you by blood, marriage or adoption, or be named in your will, or by operation of law be entitled to any portion of your estate upon your death.*

Special Rules for Skilled Nursing Facility Residents

If you are a patient in a skilled nursing facility, you must have a patient advocate or ombudsman sign as a witness and sign the Statement of Patient Advocate or Ombudsman. (See following page.) You must also have a second qualified witness sign below or have this document acknowledged before a notary public.

I declare under penalty of perjury under the laws of California (1) that the individual who signed or acknowledged this Advance Health Care Directive is personally known to me, or that the individual's identity was proven to me by convincing evidence (*see next page), (2) that the individual signed or acknowledged this Advance Health Care Directive in my presence, (3) that the individual appears to be of sound mind and under no duress, fraud, or undue influence, (4) that I am not a person appointed as agent by this Advance Health Care Directive, and (5) I am not the individual's health care provider nor an employee of that health care provider, nor an operator or employee of an operator of a community care facility or a residential care facility for the elderly.

First Witness: ______________________________ ______________________
(date) *(name printed)* *(signature)*

Residence Address: ____

Second Witness: ______________________________ ______________________
(date) *(name printed)* *(signature)*

Residence Address: ____

AT LEAST ONE OF THE ABOVE WITNESSES MUST ALSO SIGN THE FOLLOWING DECLARATION:

I further declare under penalty of perjury under the laws of California that I am not related to the individual executing this Advance Health Care Directive by blood, marriage, or adoption, and, to the best of my knowledge I am not entitled to any part of the individual's estate upon his or her death under a will now existing or by operation of law.

Date: ________________ Signature: ________________________________

Continued

FOR SKILLED NURSING FACILITIES: STATEMENT OF PATIENT ADVOCATE OR OMBUDSMAN

If you are a patient in a skilled nursing facility, a patient advocate or ombudsman must sign the Statement of Witnesses above, and must also sign the following declaration.

I further declare under penalty of perjury under these laws of California that I am a patient advocate or ombudsman as designated by the State Department of Aging and am serving as a witness as required by Probate Code 4675.

Name/Title Printed ______________________________ Signature: ________________________________

Date: __________ Address: ____

8. CERTIFICATE OF ACKNOWLEDGMENT OF NOTARY PUBLIC

Acknowledgment before a notary public is not required if two qualified witnesses have signed on page 3. If you are a patient in a skilled nursing facility, you must have a patient advocate or ombudsman sign the Statement of Witnesses on page 3 and the Statement of Patient Advocate or Ombudsman above, even if you also have this form notarized.

State of California }
} ss.
County of ______________________ }

On this ____________, before me, ____,
(Date) *(Name and Title of Officer)*

personally appeared ____,
(Name(s) of Signer(s))

personally known to me (or proved to me on the basis of satisfactory evidence) to be the person(s) whose name(s) is/are subscribed to the within instrument and acknowledged to me that he/she/they executed the same in his/her/their authorized capacity(ies), and that by his/her/their signature(s) on the instrument the person(s), or the entity upon behalf of which the person(s) acted, executed the instrument.

WITNESS my hand and official seal.

____
(Signature of Notary Public) **Notary Seal**

9. COPIES

My agent and others may use copies of this document as though they were originals.

Your agent may need this document immediately in case of an emergency. You should keep the completed original and give copies of the completed original to (1) your agent and alternate agents, (2) your physician(s), (3) members of your family and others who might be called in the event of a medical emergency, and (4) any hospital or other health facility where you receive treatment. Instruct your agent(s), family, and friends to provide a copy of your directive to your physician(s) or emergency medical personnel on request.

Additional forms can be purchased from:
CMA Publications, P.O. Box 7690, San Francisco, CA 94120-7690
Phone: 1-800-882-1CMA • Fax: (415) 882-5195 • Internet: www.cmanet.org

***EVIDENCE OF IDENTITY:** The following forms of identification are satisfactory evidence of identity: a California driver's license or identification card or U.S. passport that is current or has been issued within five years, or any of the following if the document is current or has been issued within 5 years, contains a photograph and description of the person named on it, is signed by the person, and bears a serial or other identifying number: a foreign passport that has been stamped by the U.S. Immigration and Naturalization Service; a driver's license issued by another state or by an authorized Canadian or Mexican agency; an identification card issued by another state or by any branch of the U.S. armed forces, or for an inmate in custody, an inmate identification card issued by the Department of Corrections. If the principal is a patient in a skilled nursing facility, a patient advocate or ombudsman may rely on the representations of family members or the administrator or staff of the facility as convincing evidence of identity if the patient advocate or ombudsman believes that the representations provide a reasonable basis for determining the identity of the principal.

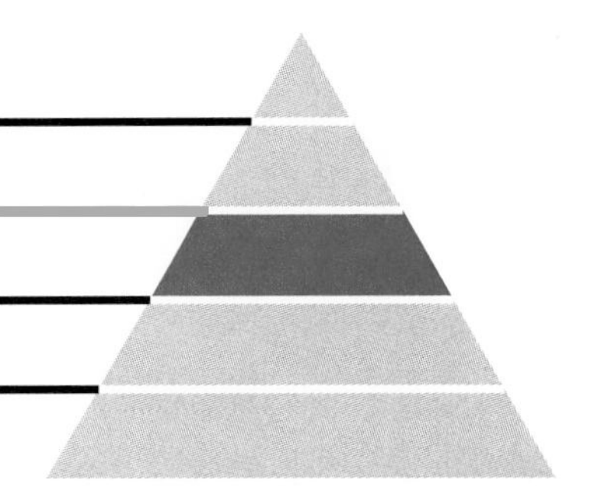

APPENDIX 24-C

Living Will Declaration

INSTRUCTIONS

PRINT THE DATE

PRINT YOUR NAME

PRINT THE NAME, HOME ADDRESS AND TELEPHONE NUMBER OF YOUR SURROGATE

PRINT NAME, HOME ADDRESS AND TELEPHONE NUMBER OF YOUR ALTERNATE SURROGATE

ADD PERSONAL INSTRUCTIONS (IF ANY)

SIGN THE DOCUMENT

WITNESSING PROCEDURE

TWO WITNESSES MUST SIGN AND PRINT THEIR ADDRESSES

Florida Living Will

Declaration made this ________________ day of ____________, 19________.

I, ______________________________, willfully and voluntarily make known my desire that my dying not be artificially prolonged under the circumstances set forth below, and I do hereby declare:

If at any time I have a terminal condition and if my attending or treating physician and another consulting physician have determined that there is no medical probability of my recovery from such condition, I direct that life-prolonging procedures be witheld or withdrawn when the application of such procedures would serve only to prolong artificially the process of dying, and that I be permitted to die naturally with only the administration of medication or the performance of any medical procedure deemed necessary to provide me with comfort care or to alleviate pain.

It is my intention that this declaration be honored by my family and physician as the final expression of my legal right to refuse medical or surgical treatment and to accept the consequences for such refusal.

In the event that I have been determined to be unable to provide express and informed consent regarding the witholding, withdrawal, or continuation of life-prolonging procedures, I wish to designate, as my surrogate to carry out the provisions of this declaration:

Name: ______________________________

Address: ______________________________

Zip code: ______________________________

Phone: ______________________________

I wish to designate the following person as my alternate surrogate, to carry out the provisions of this declaration should my surrogate be unwilling or unable to act on my behalf:

Name: ______________________________

Address: ______________________________

Zip code: ______________________________

Phone: ______________________________

Additional instructions (optional):

I understand the full import of this declaration, and I am emotionally and mentally competent to make this declaration.

Signed:

Witness 1: ______________________________

Signed: ______________________________

Address: ______________________________

Witness 2: ______________________________

Signed: ______________________________

Address: ______________________________

Courtesy Choice in Dying, Inc.

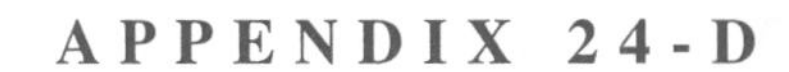

APPENDIX 24-D

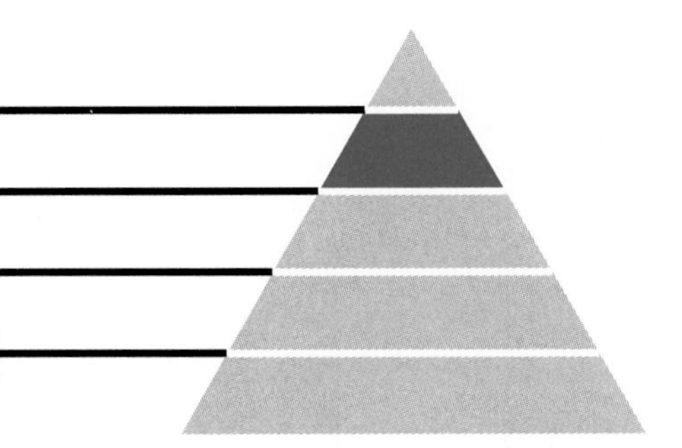

Definitions and Equivalent Language Examples for Key Issues

Issue	Working definition	Examples
Proxy	Person designated to make surrogate decisions Designation of proxy may be for limited or broad purposes.	Personal representative Agent Surrogate
Personal instructions	Designation of any specific desires about treatment Provision for care or limitation on medical care	Other wishes Special provisions
General life sustaining	Treatment without which the patient will die, excluding artificial nutrition and hydration	Life-prolonging treatment Death-delaying treatment Mechanical respiration
Terminal illness	Incurable condition from which no recovery is possible, to a reasonable degree of medical certainty, and death is likely to occur within a relatively short time	Incurable or terminal condition
Artificial sustenance	Provision of food and water through a tube or intravenous line	Artificial nourishment and tube feeding
Persistent vegetative state	Condition expected to last permanently, without improvement, and in which thought,sensation, purposeful action, social interaction, and awareness of self are absent	Permanently unconscious Comatose with no reasonable expectation of regaining consciousness
Advanced illness, dementia	Irreversible end-stage condition characterized by severe permanent deterioration and dependency	Severe dementia End-stage condition

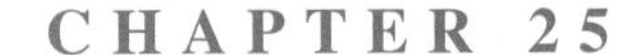
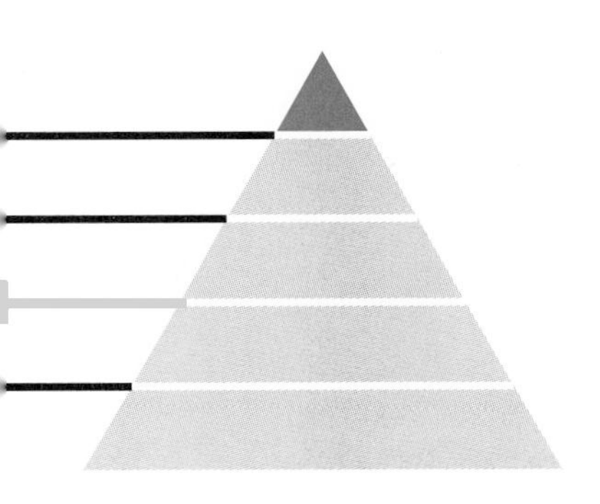

CHAPTER 25

Self-Actualization, Spirituality, and Transcendence

Priscilla Ebersole

A student learns

Well, I always went to church with my parents when I was a child, but it was really boring. Now, I sometimes go with my Grandmother to make her happy. I see how important it is to her, and I wonder if it will be important to me when I get really old. I'm just too busy right now.

Lori, age 22

An elder speaks

This is a real problem! I have three children and don't want them to squabble over my things when I'm gone. I would like it if they would each choose something special that would remind them of me, but every time I bring it up they cut me off and won't talk about it. I know there will be a big fight over the piano!

Mabel, age 74

LEARNING OBJECTIVES

After completing this chapter, the reader will be able to:

1. Provide a comprehensive definition of self-actualization and identify several qualities to be expected in self-actualized elders.
2. Describe several learning opportunities that are available to elders and the special characteristics and growth factors predominant in each.
3. Discuss the nursing role in relation to the self-actualization of elders.
4. Describe several evidences of transcendence as experienced by the aged.
5. Specify several types of creative self-expression, including those that are less often visible to the public.
6. Relate particular interventions geared to the individual who is feeling spiritually distressed.
7. Define the concept of *legacy* and name several types of legacies and what the nurse can do to facilitate their expression.

Self-actualization, spirituality, and transcendence are vague, ambiguous terms that mean whatever the theorist thinks. These expressions also serve as umbrella terms for other conditions and situations that will be addressed throughout this chapter. A great deal of overlap exists in these terms, but we have attempted to tease out the meanings for the reader, knowing that the perception of the reader will cast a particular interpretation that we may not have thought or intended. These conditions are ineffable, within the awareness of the individual but often inexpressible. We have used Maslow as our guide in comprehending self-actualization, as well as Jung and many others, in grasping at transcendence. Spirituality embodies religion, faith, and beliefs that sustain individuals through the vicissitudes of life. Why, if these concepts are so obscure, do we include them as the final chapter in a text for nurses working with elders? Because these concepts are the life tasks of aging, seldom fully approached earlier. Concerns of the young are to become established as adults; middle-aged are overwhelmed with the requirements of success and survival. Ferreting out the reason for being, existence, and the meaning of life are the concerns of elders.

Nurses will likely see numerous aged who are apparently not seeking any of these esoteric states of existence and have never tried to cultivate their deepest *inner nature* (Maslow,

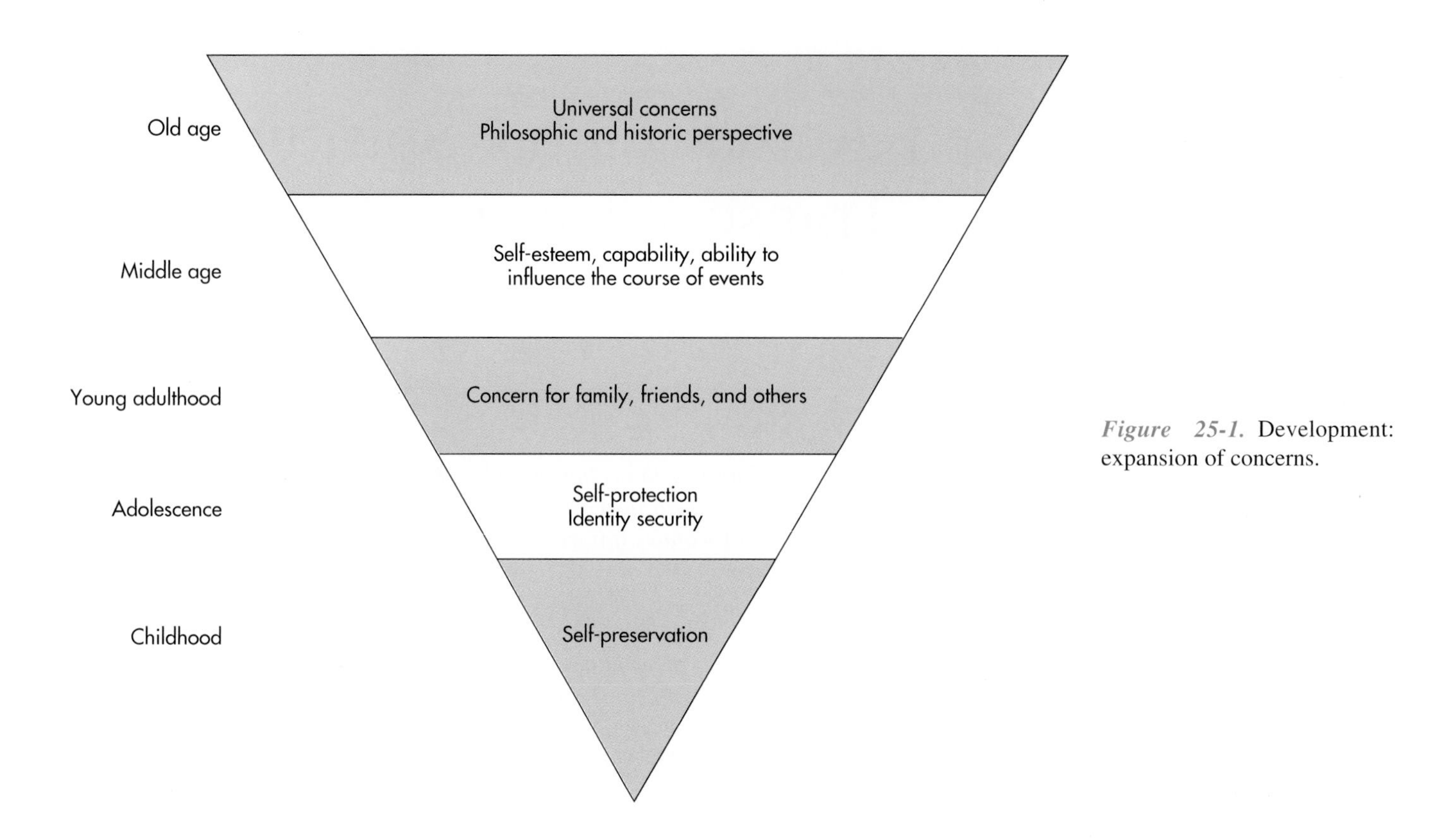

Figure 25-1. Development: expansion of concerns.

1970). We live in a mechanistic, scientifically based culture in which cultivation of immeasurable states of being have not been necessarily highly regarded, or regarded at all. The dramatic increase in the population of the aged has been considered a problem to be solved in an era of *dwindling resources*. Attempting to sort, dissect, and classify everything is a hazard of our society. In all of human efforts for several millennia, we have not been able to grasp or dissect the soul. Therefore, with effrontery and apologies, we will devote this last chapter to just that! I have many times approached this subject incorrectly by asking individuals what it is like to be old. Now that I am old, *what it is like* seems too concrete. What is the meaning of this stage of life? Every nurse must ask this question of his or her older clients, friends, and parents. Do not ask on your way out the door. For many people, this notion will take some pondering; for some, it will open the door of their later lives just a crack; others will be enlightened and will teach you a great deal.

SELF-ACTUALIZATION

Self-actualization is the highest expression of one's individual potential and implies inner motivation that has been freed to express the most unique self or the "authentic person" (Maslow, 1959, p. 3). The crux of self-actualization is defining life in such a way as to allow room for continual discovery of self. Self-actualization is an evolution of maturity and emotions that many writers have identified in one way or another. We have chosen Maslow's model because it moves one forward in continual self-development toward the most unique possibilities. Maslow's model can be viewed as a development model, a need model, and an evolutionary humanistic model that within existential psychology is investigated through phenomenology. This idea, simply stated, means human potential is unknown and unknowable, but our present understanding is based on analysis of individual experiences, always unique to that person. A child's first need is to be given food, shelter, safety, security, and love. An adult, who has moved to sufficient levels of maturity to give to the child, fulfills this need. In adolescence, the focus on self reaches narcissistic proportions, and development is powered by the need to be accepted. As one experiences love outside the family, goals enlarge. A pyramidal model of need appears to convey a narrowing, rising principle. True human development might be viewed as an inverted triangle. We might conceptualize energy that is focused in an intense, narrow manner on lower level needs, becoming less focused and intense as one moves upward in maturity. The inverted pyramid concept shows development as a process of enlarging concerns (Figure 25-1). At the top level, universal and world concerns and ethics transcend self, family, community, and nation.

Anywhere along the developmental continuum, concerns may again become constricted. A self-actualized person may,

Many of the thoughts in this chapter cannot be attributed to a single or multiple sources because they are the conglomerate of numerous studies over the years. When possible, citations to specific theorists and researchers are given.

under threat of illness, become self-centered and narrow. The task of nursing is to assist these individuals in achieving their highest potential within their present situation, "maximizing the potential of which an individual is capable within the environment where functioning occurs" (Hemstrom, 2000, p. 42).

McLeod (2001) interviewed Sue Bender regarding her spiritual trilogy, *Plain and Simple, Everyday Sacred,* and, most recently, *The Daring That Starts From Within.* Bender's thesis in all of these works is that we are constrained by self-judgment, past memories, and future expectations. The need to be and look good to others may stifle the real person who can emerge with *daring* to face our self-imposed limits and be who we are. Bender's message is particularly relevant to aging individuals in that she challenges herself and others to accept our *limping* selves, with the assurance that the body is a healer and teacher if we remain in the present and approach ourselves with a caring spirit and body awareness. Bender challenges us to not to become a smaller person with age but to grow new habits of accepting who we are.

A critical consideration in developing self-actualization is an underlying sense of mastery and a sense of coherence in the life situation. This effort depends to a large extent on individual attributes, as well as self-esteem. Informal social support is essential for most people, though some relatively isolated individuals have such a strong sense of self that they reach a satisfactory self-actualized state with few supports (Forbes, 2001). In this unit, we hope to expose the nurse to the myriad evidences of self-actualization in old age and suggest ways in which the nurse can assist older people in seeking their own unique way of living and growing. The focus is on nursing actions that may encourage elders to seek new possibilities within themselves. Holistic health practices, examined in depth in Chapter 3, are somewhat relevant to self-actualization because they are the first step in acknowledging one's active participation in becoming truly whole. (For additional thoughts on wellness and self-actualization, see the wellness paradigm in Chapter 3.)

Characteristics of the Self-Actualized

In old age, threats to self-esteem are strong if value is measured only by attainment, containment, power, and influence. Ethics, values, humor, courage, altruism, and integrity flourish in people who continue to grow toward self-actualization. Numerous other attributions can be mentioned. We will focus only on those qualities that seem most pertinent to the aged that health care professionals are serving (Box 25-1).

Courage. Courage is the quality of mind or spirit that enables a person to conquer fear and despair in the face of difficulty, danger, pain, or uncertainty. We believe that facing a long, painful, and restricted existence requires the highest level of courage. An old man, with diabetes, amputations, and failing vision, sits in his room at the retirement home, looking out the window for hours each day, for weeks, months, and years. This is courage. An old lady crippled with arthritis attends her ailing spouse, who no longer recognizes her. This is courage.

When asking old people how they keep going day by day, various answers are given. No one has ever said to me, "It is because I am courageous." Old people need to be told. A gold star can be given to people who have lived and survived the long battle of a mediocre existence. In current vernacular, mediocre means *ordinary*. These individuals are not ordinary. The origins of the word mediocre translate to "halfway up a stony mountain" (Merriam-Webster, 1974, p. 274). Many elders are enduring the climb up a stony mountain, and they are the epitome of courage. Memorials are made for people who die in battle, but few monuments are raised to those who courageously wake every morning with no great purpose or challenge to push them out of bed. Nonetheless, these individuals endure the seemingly purposeless, monotonous hours and somehow find meaning. Believing that the aged are unable to be self-actualized unless they are energetic, healthy, and wealthy is a mistake. The capacity of the spirit to find meaning in existence is often remarkable. Nurses may ask, "What sustains you in your present situation?"

Altruism. A high degree of helping behaviors is present in many aged. The very old will remember the Great Depression and the altruism that kept people physically and spiritually alive. Neighbor helped neighbor long before the government came to the rescue. Apparently, a sense of meaning in life is strongly tied to survival and is derived from the

Box 25-1 Traits of Self-Actualized People

- Time competent: The person uses past and future to live more fully in the present.
- Inner directed: The person's source of direction depends on internal forces more than on others.
- Flexible: The person can react situationally, without unreasonable restrictions.
- Sensitive to self: The person is responsive to his or her own feelings.
- Spontaneous: The person is able and willing to be self.
- Values self: The person accepts and demonstrates strengths as a person.
- Accepts self: The person approves of self, in spite of weaknesses or deficiencies.
- Positively views others: The person sees both the bad and the good in others as essentially good and constructive.
- Positively views life: The person sees the opposites of life as meaningfully related.
- Acceptance of aggressiveness: The person is able to accept own feelings of anger and aggressiveness.
- Capable of intimate contact: The person is able to develop warm interpersonal relationships with others.

conviction of, in some way, being needed by others. Many nurses are in the field because of altruistic motives and can understand the importance. This idea might be discussed with the elder.

Volunteering often involves new role development and endeavors that expand one's awareness. When volunteer services are considered as a means of personal enrichment and an expression of altruism, it is important for the elder to augment some latent interest areas and launch into pursuits perhaps unavailable earlier because of time constraints or other commitments. Nurses may question elders about latent interests and talents that they may want to cultivate. Volunteer activities are discussed in Chapter 18.

Humor. Metcalf (1993) explains humor: originating in the Latin root *humor,* meaning *fluid and flexible,* able to flow around and wear away obstacles. In the same way that water sustains our life and well being, humor sustains our mental well being. Cousins (1979) and many other researchers have recognized the importance of humor in recovery from illness. The physiologic effects of humor stimulate production of catecholamines and hormones and increase pain tolerance by releasing endorphins.

Elders often initiate humor, and in our seriousness, we may overlook the dry wit or, worse, perceive it as confusion. The aged are not a humorless group and frequently laugh at themselves. Objections to jokes about old age seem to emanate from the young far more than the old. Perhaps the old, from the vantage point of a lifetime, can more clearly see human predicaments. Ego transcendence (Peck, 1955) allows one to step back and view the self and situation without the intensity and despair of the egocentric individual.

Continuous Moral Development. The moral development of mankind, on an individual and collective basis, has been of interest to philosophers and religious leaders throughout history. The driving forces of morality are love (Plato) and intellect (Aristotle).

Kohlberg's refinements of his original theories have focused on the evidence, derived from autobiographies, that in maturity, transformations of moral outlook take place. Kohlberg posited old age as a seventh stage of moral development that goes beyond reasoning and reaches awareness of one's relative participation in universal morality. This stage of moral development involves identification with a more enduring moral perspective than that of one's own life span (Kohlberg and Power, 1981). This effort involves moral expansion and the exemplary impact of the fully developing elder on the following generations, born and unborn. We have come to believe that at present these exemplary lives may be the most important function of elders as we decry the honor and recognition given to individuals who seem to have little integrity or reliability. Each individual carries a mass of motivations and desires. Some people are stunted, and some will flourish. Youngsters must have models of honorable, truthful, and honest elders if we hope to cultivate these qualities in society and human experience.

Self-Renewal

Self-renewal is an ongoing process that ideally continues through adult life as one becomes self-actualized (Hudson, 1999). According to Hudson, self-renewal involves:

Commitment to beliefs
Connecting to the world
Times of solitude
Episodic breaks from responsibility
Contact with the natural world
Creative self-expression
Adaptation to changes
Learning from down times

Travel. Travel is a route many elders take to achieve knowledge while simultaneously increasing pleasure and renewal through new experiences. The self-actualization in travel often occurs as one becomes immersed in another culture and sees facets of the human experience through an unfamiliar lens.

The number of traveling elders is a reflection of the increased affluence and energy of the aged of today. Estimates suggest that individuals over 55 years of age take over 20% of all trips in the United States (Hudson and Rich, 1993).

Intergenerational travel seems to be increasing, with many elders traveling with grandchildren. The Grandtravel Agency and Elderhostel offer vacations specially designed for grandparents and grandchildren *(www.elderhostel.org).*

For people who have a strong desire to travel, and to seek new lands and scenes, many opportunities are available, if they are physically and economically able. The Senior Travel Exchange Program gives elders the opportunity to travel to other nations, develop friendships, and really get to know the people. These travelers are organized into groups of 20 to 25 elders, and trips are very economical. Travelers stay in the homes of locals, and at a later time, the hosts and guests reverse roles when the original hosts travel to the United States (Leitner and Leitner, 1996).

For elderly who are less affluent and content to stay closer to home territory, many organized low-cost tours explore unusual sites near one's area. The American Bed and Breakfast Association *(www.abba.com)* can provide information regarding providers nationwide who belong to the organization and offer inexpensive lodging and breakfast. These providers also give information to elders who wish to establish a bed and breakfast.

The personal effects of travel are as variable as the individuals and the places they select to see. Nursing involvement will be most useful in addressing potential problems and assisting elders in planning ahead for contingencies. Pets must be placed appropriately, house-sitting services are sometimes necessary, and physical limitations must be considered. The following questions should be asked and resolved before departing:

- Whom will you contact in an emergency? Is this person's phone number in your billfold? Is your blood type also noted?

- What health care and travel insurance coverage do you have? Is the coverage adequate for unforeseen illness? Do you have sufficient medications, hearing aid batteries, and extra eyeglasses?
- What immunizations will you need, and where can you obtain them?
- Do you have a safe place on your body for money?
- From where are you obtaining prior information about the places you intend to go?
- Are the areas you wish to see accessible in terms of your mobility and energy?
- Do you desire accommodations similar to those provided by locals or Western-type hotels?
- What is the usual weather during the time you will be visiting?

Changes in water, altitude, and climate can produce distressing reactions. Individuals must allow themselves time to adjust to the changed conditions, and using only bottled water would be wise.

People often find travel after retirement a vehicle for learning and growing. Careful planning will make travel safer and more enjoyable. Suggestions for travel are summarized in Box 25-2.

Box 25-2 Travel Tips for Elders

- Many organizations offer special group rates and tours planned for elders.
- Travel agencies can give information about reduced rates for charter flights or about less popular travel months. Choose the off-season to avoid crowds and to get best rates.
- Some air carriers have reduced rates for the aged or handicapped.
- Many countries offer special rates to older travelers. Information should be obtained from the tourist bureau of the countries on the itinerary.
- Social Security benefits continue indefinitely.
- Medicare coverage does not extend outside the United States and its territories; however, many European countries have national health services that are extended to travelers. Supplementary health insurance is a good idea.
- Passports should be applied for well in advance if birth certificates are not readily available. Visas are required for many countries.
- Immunizations are required to travel in certain countries. Check with the U.S. Public Health Service.
- Take a medical travel kit containing sufficient medication for any chronic condition; first aid equipment; medications for diarrhea, dyspepsia, and nausea; an extra pair of eyeglasses; and records of medication problems, allergies, and blood type.
- Take extras of equipment needed, such as hearing aid batteries, eyeglasses, braces, and orthopedic shoes.

Learning and Growing in Later Life

Opportunities for elders to learn are available in many formal and informal modes: self-teaching, college attendance, participation in seminars and conferences, public television programs, videotapes, courses via telecommunications, and countless other modes. The Internet has become one of the major vehicles of learning for the aged. Part of the nurse's function is to be informed and assist an elder in finding the learning mode and setting that is appropriate to his or her need or desire (Figure 25-2).

In most universities, older people are taking classes of all types. Fees are usually lower for individuals over 60 years of age, and elders may choose to work toward a degree and complete all assignments or audit classes just for enrichment and enjoyment. Many opportunities are also available for distance learning and external degrees.

On-campus classrooms provide the aged with an opportunity to share their perspective from a long-range view and for youth to interject theirs of immediacy and energy. The results are increased positive attitude toward the aged among the youth and elevated self-esteem in the elders who compete and achieve academic success, as well as increased understanding of the concerns of young adults.

Convenience, accessibility, scheduling of classes, and the opportunity to audit if desired are important to the aged. Many colleges now offer courses on television or the Internet that are inexpensive, fully accredited, and available to elders with impaired mobility or lower energy levels. Community colleges frequently offer weekend courses to familiarize residents with local areas of interest or special projects.

Elderhostel. The Elderhostel program, an adult education program originally based on the youth hostel concept, was originated by Marty Knowlton in 1974 at the University of New Hampshire and now offers a wide variety of programs around the world, in addition to those in the United States and Canada. Elderhostel offers opportunities for service, as well as learning. In addition, the program has recently added a discussion board to its well-established website *(www.elderhostel.org)* (Elderhostel, 2003).

Elderhostel is a nonprofit international program that provides low-cost room and board and specially designed classes for elders on college campuses, conference centers, state and national parks, museums, theaters, environmental outdoor education centers, and other sites. The program mails its catalogs to over one half million people, and each year nearly 300,000 people over age 55 or who have a spouse over age 55 participate in this phenomenally successful educational program for older adults. About one half of people who participate in the Elderhostel program live in dormitories and eat in college dining halls while taking brief noncredit college courses taught by regular faculty members or specialists in a particular field.

The national Elderhostel concept is a response to the awareness that the elderly want to continue learning and contributing in their later years. Some scholarships are offered for

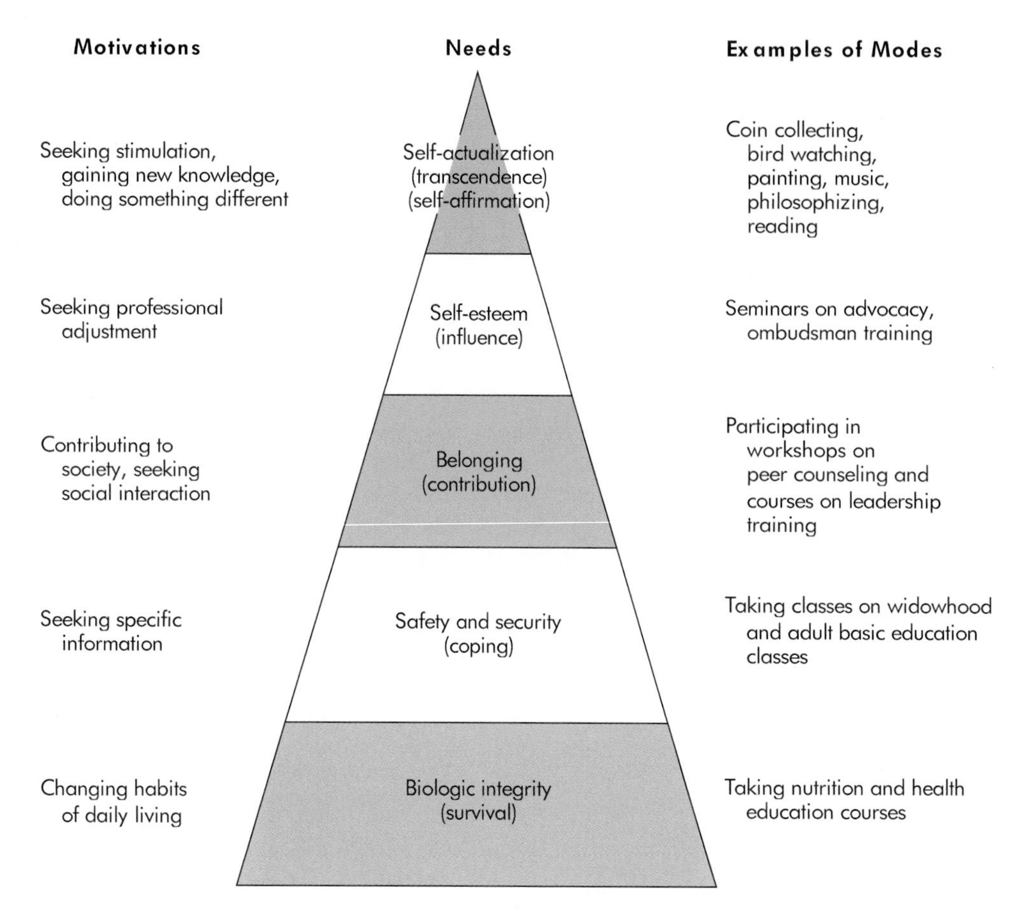

Figure 25-2. Learning and growing in later life. (Developed by Priscilla Ebersole.)

programs within the United States. Some of the reasons for attending Elderhostel are (1) change (opportunity to go somewhere or do something different), (2) time (short time frame for learning), (3) cost (low fixed cost), (4) courses (suitable course content), (5) absence of evaluation (no tests or homework), and (6) learning (opportunities to develop new interests and reexplore old ones). Programs of special interest include hiking and biking trips, historic houses, folk colleges, and study cruises. The opportunities for study address almost every interest one can imagine. Classes, taught by academics, specialists, and local experts, cover a broad range of subjects, such as jazz, art, religion, astronomy, history, and mythology. Older citizens who may wish intellectual stimulation and personal enrichment should be encouraged to investigate these programs. We encourage nurses to become aware of programs offered for elders in their community.

Education for Elders with Special Needs

Homebound Elderly. Education has become accessible to many homebound individuals through public television, teleconferencing, the Internet, and radio. Public libraries throughout the United States provide videotapes and audiotapes to the confined elderly. Many current methods are available for implementing educational outreach programs. With increasingly adaptable telecommunications technology and cost reductions, these opportunities are becoming common.

Reading for Self-Development. Bond and Miller (1987) call reading an ageless activity and find that institutionalized elders often much prefer the individual, passive involvement in reading to the group activities that are planned for them. Group reading and discussion can also be enjoyable, as demonstrated in the Great Books discussion groups that meet routinely in many libraries. Suffice it to say that when an array of books is available, many aged find them sustaining. Books extend boundaries imposed by physical limitations, allow exploration into untouched arenas of thought, and enrich the individual. For many elders, reading has been a major pleasure throughout life and, common as it seems, should not be underestimated as a form of self-discovery and actualization.

Many libraries across the country have developed creative programs to serve elders. Some of these programs include talking books for the blind, large-print books and magazines, mail delivery to the homebound, low-vision reading aids, 24-hour audio reader service through a closed-circuit radio station (through the University of Kansas), kits designed to provoke reminiscing, and one-to-one reading service in several languages. To provide these services, facilities rely on intergenerational projects through schools, grants, gifts, bequests, volunteers, and closeout book sales.

Peer Teaching and Learning

Peer teaching projects have served as a means to allow individuals to share their expertise while meeting the academic interests of retired people. These programs may be the first step in launching individuals into the pursuit of higher education that may have been closed to them earlier. In our diverse culture, peer teaching is an ideal way of including individuals who may not have the academic credentials or cultural comfort to pursue conventionally structured subjects.

To keep costs low, elderly individuals are enrolled as students but also teach some classes in which they are knowledgeable. Retired professionals sometimes teach courses in their particular area of expertise as a volunteer activity. In some classes, students set their own objectives, and a coordinator is chosen to find appropriate resources and instructors. Class members may prepare special topics and lead class discussions, which, in addition to inquiry, is a Socratic method of learning. The success of these programs is attributed to low cost, accessibility, hours, and location adapted to elders' needs, as well as using older individuals as instructors.

Learning and the Humanities. A great revival of interest has occurred in the humanities in what is considered the postmodern phase of our social culture. New Age phenomena are not of interest only to youth. The study of the humanities in old age may enlarge horizons, transcend limitations, and strengthen the connection between old age and wisdom. The old have always been involved in the dialogue of humanities and history as they become vitally interested in the exploration of life's meanings. The epic of a generation can be elaborated with the wisdom of those who lived it, and we find more and more individuals involved in seeking the wisdom and life experience of the old in numerous ways.

The tie between the humanities and life history becomes even clearer when we recognize the significance of the aged in the progression of culture through the ages of time. For a time, interest in the *storytelling* function of elders appeared small, because the printed and electronic media were accessible to almost everyone. However, this interest has been revived in a new appreciation of the personal interpretation of myths, legends, and experience. These interpretations also comprise the collective legacy discussed later in the chapter. The National Council on Aging (NCOA, 1993), with a grant from the National Endowment for the Humanities, has developed a method to capture the elusive threads of human experience that the aged hold. Program themes are developed around local history, family, the land, particular eras in history, work life, immigrant experience, and other topics. Information for individuals who are interested in starting such a program can be obtained from NCOA *(www.ncoa.org)*.

COLLECTIVE ACTUALIZATION

The collective power of self-actualized older people has already brought about many changes in society. Power is a term describing the capacity of an individual or group to accomplish something, to take command, to exert authority, and to influence. The self-actualized aged are powerful and confident. Power is the gateway to resources and recognition.

The age-equality movement, older citizens returning to school, and the revolution of older people in movements such as the Gray Panthers have produced major changes in the status and recognition of the aged. Gray Panthers recognize that issues of aging are not narrow or exclusive but rather are representative of human rights for people of all ages.

Kuhn (1979), founder of the Gray Panthers, died April 22, 1995 at the age of 89, but her beliefs and followers survive. Kuhn perceived that the issues confronting older people are not those of self-interest, but rather, as "elders of the tribe," the old should seek "survival of the tribe" (Kuhn, 1979, p. 3). Kuhn outlined steps by which old people can be advocates of the public interest:

- Identify and document the social issue, problem, or need. Providers delivering services to individuals should record cases, instances of critical need, scope, extent of deprivation, alienation, and that which needs to be changed.
- Bring together the victims of discrimination, abuse, and oppression to discuss their problems, understand their situation, and examine the interaction between personal need and public response.
- Raise the consciousness of victims, and educate them about the societal aspects, roots, and causes of their dilemmas.
- Organize victims to develop support groups for mutual support and empowerment, to confront oppressors, and to find local support from established bodies and agencies (insiders!).
- Map strategies for action, including new models for dealing with particular issues, legislative initiatives, court action, and forming coalitions of groups with similar problems.
- Go public: organize a rally with posters, speeches, marches to public places where public officials, interested people, agency heads, and boards can become aware and be held accountable. Go before television cameras with street theater. Go to press with well-prepared press releases.
- Present testimony in public hearings: set up telegram, telephone campaigns pressing for redress and change.
- Take stock of your advances or setbacks, evaluate results, and consider the next steps.
- Report back to groups for their information and encouragement. Keep communication open with members and coalitions.
- Draft legislation or prepare for legal action in the courts. Marshal arguments, collect *cases,* including *horror stories,* and evoke interest.
- Celebrate victories, even the small ones. Coverage in the press and on television may be significant to successes. Even failures should be recognized and evaluated.
- Regroup to fight on with increased knowledge, broader impact, and enlarged constituencies!

Although Kuhn is gone, others, such as Harry Moody of the International Longevity Center-USA (2002), continue to build on her ideals. The thoughts of these individuals challenge the old to reach beyond themselves. Realistically, the plights of the young, the poor, the ill, and single mothers with children are presently of greater concern than the lack of opportunity for the mass of well aged. However, a lag clearly exists between the capacities of long-lived people and opportunities for them to challenge these capacities.

Politics and Power

The aged are a powerful political group. Older voters generally recognize their power, as do politicians. Elders can be counted on to vote, but their voting behaviors demonstrate their diversity. Aside from issues of Medicare and Social Security, elders do not form strong voting blocks because they are individualistic. However, any politician who wishes to remain in office must gently manipulate sacrosanct programs such as Social Security and Medicare. Older voters are often more concerned about a candidate's character and experience than about party affiliation.

Nurses attuned to the political concerns of elders will find that these concerns are numerous and include:

- Comprehensive health care in rural areas
- Available mental health services
- Supports for their caregivers
- Affordable medications
- Transportation adapted to their needs
- Better training and screening of service providers
- Concern about the shortage of nurses

CREATIVITY

Creativity is a bridge between the growing self and the transcending of self. Creativity may be the transit mechanism between self-actualization (the reaching of one's highest potential) and the step beyond, to transcend the limitations of ego (Table 25-1). Creativity is risking a leap across the chasm of the known to reach the unknown. The creative act emerges from the consolidation of energies of thought, feelings, and imagination. The stages of creativity are preparation, frustration, incubation, illumination, and elaboration. Elders excel in illumination and elaboration.

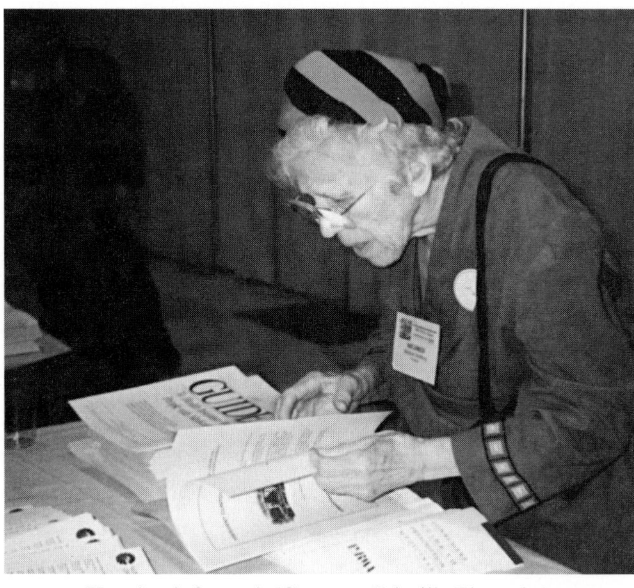

Keeping informed. (Courtesy Priscilla Ebersole.)

Products of creativity are less important than creative attitudes. Curiosity, inquisitiveness, wonderment, puzzlement, and craving for understanding are creative attitudes. Much of the natural creative imagination of childhood is subdued by enculturation. In old age, some people seem able to break free of excessive enculturation and again express their free spirit when practical matters no longer demand their sole attention.

Creativity is often considered in terms of the arts, literature, and music. A truly self-actualized person may express creativity in any activity. Breaking through the habitual or traditional mode into authentic expression of self is creativity, whether it is through cooking, cleaning, planting, or teaching.

Catherine was self-actualized and creative to the extent possible. Her physical constraints were enormous: she had no material assets,

Table 25-1 Interrelationships of Central Concepts of Flow, Creativity, and Watson's Theory of Human Care

Commonalities of flow experiences	Components of creativity/play	Goals of Watson's theory of human care
Growth, meaning		
Contributes of growth of the self	Leads to learning and evolution; expands one's field of action	Mental-spiritual growth for self-others
Reintegration; empowerment		
Promotes ordering of experience	Creative process relates us to context and environment	Finding meaning in one's own existence
Self-esteem		
Returns control to the individual	Freedom to explore without rules or restrictions	Discovering inner power and control
Transcendence		
Selfless state of absorption yields altered sense of time	Delight and enjoyment in the present moment/ suspension of time	Potentiating instances of self-transcendence and healing

From Sterritt PF, Pokorney ME: Art activities for patients with Alzheimer's and related disorders, *Geriatr Nurs* 15(3):155, 1994.

her range of activity was limited to her small cubicle in a skilled nursing facility, and her body was frail. However, her spirit was strong, and she knew and used her potential.

Catherine's creativity was expressed at each meal when she rearranged, mixed, and added to her food. She carefully chopped a pickle and sprinkled it on her cottage cheese and added a little honey to her applesauce. Each meal was a small adventure.

Several friends would visit regularly and bring Catherine small items she enjoyed. They could always count on being entertained with creatively embroidered tales of the past. The gifts they brought were always used in extraordinary ways. A scarf might be tied around her head. Powder, perfume, books, and other things would be bartered for favors from staff members or given as gifts. Her radio brought news of the day interspersed with classical music.

Catherine created a milieu in which she enjoyed life and maintained her self-esteem. That she was self-actualized was never in doubt. Her artistry overflowed in myriad small gestures. On her birthday, hospital volunteers presented her with a felt hanging. She stripped off its gigantic red heart and yellow daisy. The words "enjoy life" were all that remained on the forest-green felt (Figure 25-3).

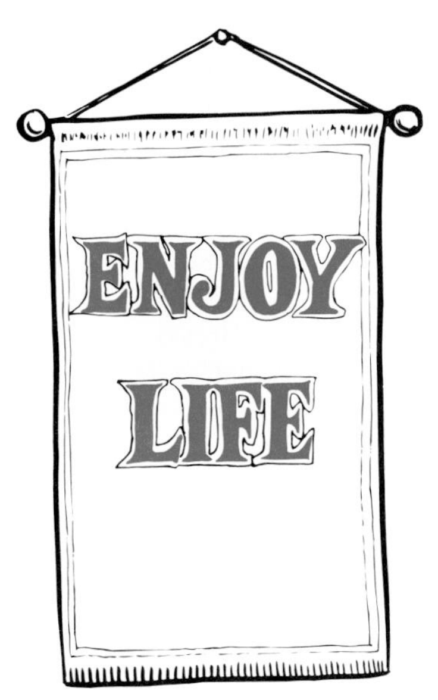

Figure 25-3. Enjoy life. (Illustrated by Joseph Pierre.)

Creative Arts for the Elderly

Maximizing the use of self in the later years in unique ways might be termed creative self-actualization. Many individuals will need the stimulus of an interested person to uncover latent interests and talents. Other people will need encouragement to try new avenues of self-expression—some will be fitting for them and others not. Several ideas are presented here for nurses working with the aged who may need an introduction to creative use of leisure time.

Many aspects of the developmental needs of the aged are met by artistic expressions. Among these achievements are (1) conflict resolution, (2) clarification of thoughts and feelings, (3) creation of balance and an inner order, (4) a sense of being in control of the external world, (5) creation of something positive from defeating experiences or in the face of paralyzing depression, (6) artistic communication as an integral part of human experience, and (7) the sustenance of human integrity. Each person has a private, symbolic, feeling world that can be brought out by certain expressive activities.

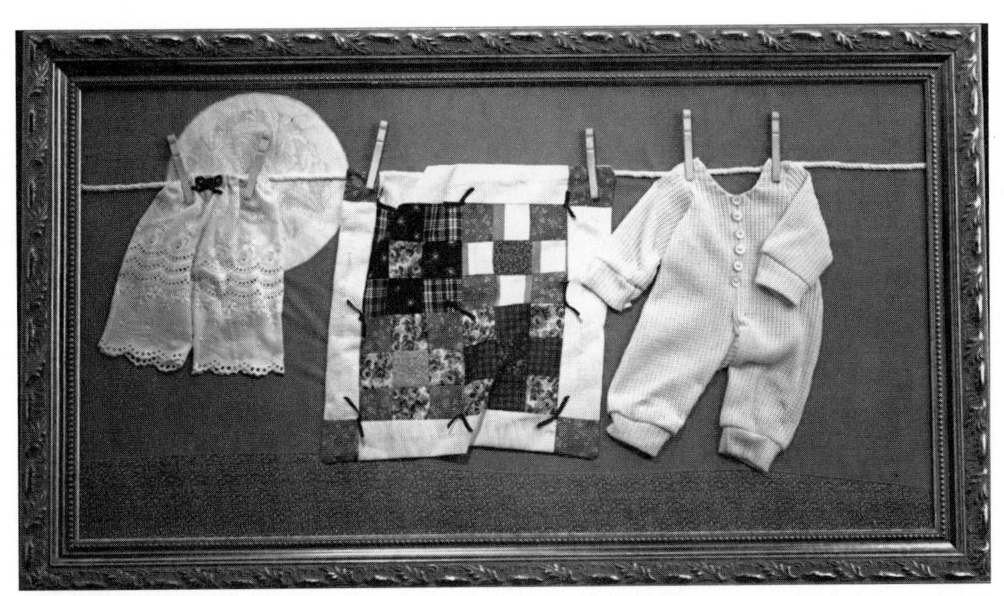

This tactile art has garments hanging from a clothesline. The clothespins can be manipulated and removed. Each garment can be taken down from the piece and reapplied. Items such as the quilt add visual interest, texture, and tactile stimulation for patients. (Courtesy ArtLine, Ltd.)

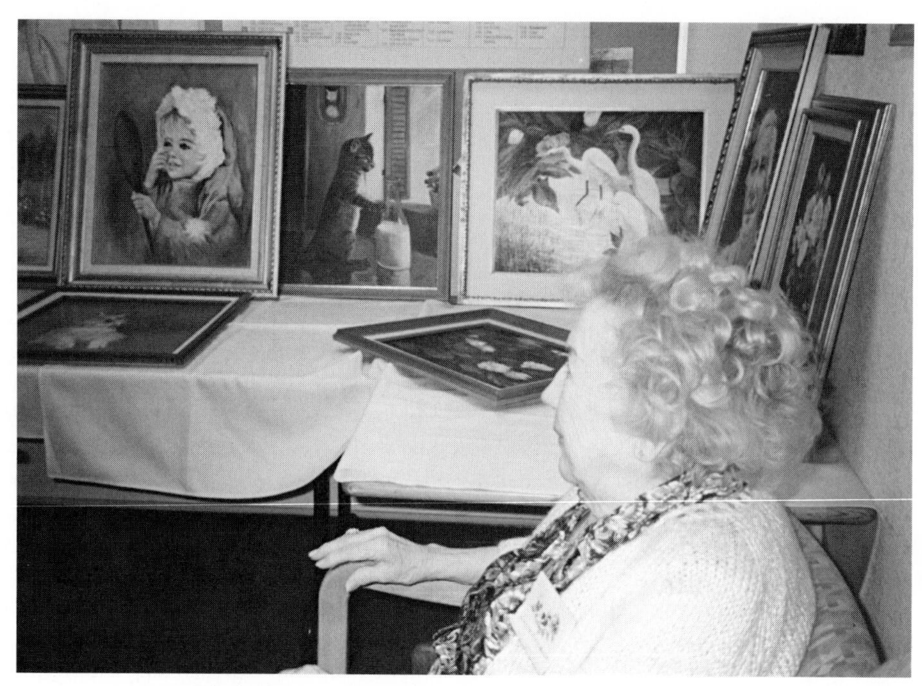

Displaying creative works. (Courtesy Priscilla Ebersole.)

The creative process is any activity in which the unconscious can be expressed in an integrated unique manner. To accomplish this task, an atmosphere of trust is essential. Trust is attained through rules, structure, and acceptance of all efforts without approval or disapproval. When this atmosphere is provided, creative expressions begin to occur. At that time, the facilitator needs to relax rules and structure and cultivate individualistic expressions. Useful concepts and guidelines for people who wish to involve the elderly in creative artistic expressions are noted in Boxes 25-3 and 25-4.

Activities may need to be modified for some elders because of sensory deficits or fatigue. Consider the following when an activity is not enjoyable or successful:

- Shift the expected outcome to meet individual or group needs.
- Modify equipment and supplies to make the activity easier.
- Provide intermittent rest and relaxation periods frequently.
- Deep breathing can be useful, both physiologically and psychologically.
- Partner or small group activities are usually less stressful than individual expectations.

Box 25-3 How to Begin Involving Older Adults in the Arts

Develop program ideas using older adults as advisors.
Plan specific ways that older adults can participate.
Survey Office of Aging, senior centers, nursing homes, adult day care centers, and community-dwelling elders regarding their needs, sources of talent, and possible contributions.
Contact local resource people who may be of assistance.
Consider access issues such as cost, transportation, and time of day.
Seek local and national funding.
Publicize.
Orient elders who are interested in participating.
Provide incentives for participating: awards, receptions, and refreshments.

Creative Arts and Theater

Endowment grants are available to ensure the continued contributions of elders as artists, teachers, mentors, students, volunteers, patrons, and consumers of the arts. Some of the programming grants have in the past supported drama groups, storytelling, dance, and singing. These activities are designed for aged people of all levels of ability; some are teachers and mentors, some are entertainers, some are participants, purely for the joy of living. Hillary Rodham Clinton said, "Some of our most powerful works of art have been produced by older Americans by hands that have engaged in years of hard work, eyes that have witnessed decades of change, and hearts that have felt a lifetime of emotions. Our whole society benefits when older Americans use their talents and experiences to become involved in the arts as creators, teachers, mentors, volunteers and audiences" (Sherman, 1996, p. 1).

McDonald (1996) reports the rapid emergence of numerous senior adult theater groups that have been flourishing because of national conferences, as well as increased awareness of and interaction among the various groups. A particular boost occurred when these older adults met

Box 25-4 Ideas for Developing Creative Abilities

Art

Using oil pastels, create a drawing that represents self, or select three colors you like and three colors you dislike, using all six colors to create a self-portrait.

Draw a representation of your world.

Create a collage or mobile out of an assortment of materials and pictures that can represent subjects such as the self, part of self you like or dislike, the family, etc.

In small groups, use clay to create an *art piece* or a statement.

Music

Play a variety of music; focus discussion on imagery and any feelings that the music evokes.

Discuss, or have clients bring in, music that elicits feelings of sadness, happiness, etc.

Show a picture (can be cut from a magazine) and ask members to see if they can imagine the sounds that might go with the picture.

Express self or group through dance and movement to selected music.

Movement

Create a movement to fit the way you are feeling while introducing self to group.

Have members stand and initiate a slow swaying motion (good exercise with which to end the group session).

Have members mirror each other's movements, such as hands or the entire body, creating a duet.

Imagery

Use guided fantasies and imagery to facilitate stress reduction and relaxation, awareness, the power of one's own healing capability, and self-expression through symbols and symbolisms.

Writing

Encourage journals or diaries; set a group time available to write and share ideas.

In small groups, create a *group poem.*

Read selected poems or stories as a group, then share reactions and feelings from the readings.

Create a *book* to be distributed to group consisting of a collection of members' writings.

in a mini-conference of the arts held during the White House Conference on Aging in 1995.

Creative Expression through Music, Poetry, and Dance. Rhythms infiltrate life on every level from individual cellular functions to the constantly expanding and contracting universe. Unseen and unfelt oscillating waves surround us. Felt waves—pulsating, vibrating, and undulating—stimulate us. These waves are intrinsic to existence and may somewhat explain the healing power of music, poetry, and repetitive movement. Life itself is an ongoing dance. One is reminded that the Polynesians express themselves beautifully with hand and body movements. In many countries today, song, dance, and poetic history flow as naturally as breath and are inextricably interwoven in daily existence.

Music. Music is a familiar and universal experience. Even the tone-deaf person expresses himself or herself in rhythmic patterns. Tonal or rhythmic music can be an inward experience or an outward expression. As such, music is adaptable to each individual. Deanna Edwards (1977) was one of the first nurses to use music to assist the ill and the dying in coping with and transcending their physical limitations. Many nurses have used music in myriad ways since that time.

Music therapy is an individual music program prescribed by a professional music therapist to bring about desirable changes in behavior. The self-determined use of music as a means of enjoyment and personal expression can be achieved by listening, meditating, improvising, relaxing, moving to music, creative dancing, composing, learning new songs, studying music history, rhythmic patterning, mastering an instrument, building an instrument, or in any other manner an individual chooses to adapt music toward self-fulfillment.

Nurses who want to use music as a springboard for client self-development must first find out the interests and talents of the client. One old man improvised lyrics to old tunes, expressing himself poetically. An old lady pleaded for some Baroque chamber music to ease her pain. A very regressed old man came alive when he was handed a banjo. Another aged man restored valuable violins and played them lovingly before returning them to their owners. An aged blind man taught pipe organ to university students and played the organ for chapel services. All of these instances were means of using music toward self-fulfillment.

Music can be a comforting, structured expression, a therapeutic tool, or it can provide the opportunity for creative and imaginative self-expression. Even the most mentally impaired individuals will often respond to music.

Poetry. Music and poetic expression are similar in rhythmic beauty. Traditionally, poetry has been judged and categorized by its rhythmic meter; however, modern poetry may have style and quality without a categorical rhythm. Old people enjoy the traditional patterns, rhyming qualities, and free verse. Many people who never thought of themselves as poets have discovered a talent for poetic expression.

Koch (1977) wrote a delightful book explaining the way he began poetry groups with elderly individuals who did not think of themselves as poets. Matsumoto (1978) modified Koch's techniques and applied them with the aged in senior centers, day-care centers, and residential housing complexes. Following are several ways to use poetry creatively:

1. Translate poetry if an aged person speaks or reads a second language.
2. Recite poetry individually and in groups.
3. Memorize poetry.

4. React to a poem.
5. Listen to poetry recorded or recited by poets in the community.
6. Create a group poem.
7. Copy favorite poems (to develop handwriting or calligraphy skills).
8. Illustrate a poem.
9. Sing a poem, setting it to familiar music.
10. Investigate and discuss children's poetry.
11. Discuss a contemporary poem.
12. Make a poetry notebook.
13. Compose nonsense or humorous poetry.
14. Make a literary analysis of a poem.
15. Rewrite a poem (start with a famous first line and then improvise).
16. Write a poem about a favorite object.
17. Create or read Haiku.
18. Find poetry from various cultures and identify themes and differences.
19. Listen for the meter in a poem; illustrate it with hand movements.
20. Find a favorite poem and discuss its appeal for you.
21. Try choral reading of poetry in small groups.

RECREATION

Recreation is akin to creation. The wisdom of regularly scheduled periods of recreation and recuperation following creative acts can be traced to early Jewish writings and the creation story. If God needed time to rest and recuperate, we certainly do. Inherent in creative acts is time for renewal, time for recreation. Burnout and boredom are companions of monotony and shorten the perceived life span by emptiness and vanished time. A change of scene or companions may be exhilarating. Retreats from routine to periods of recreation are important as are retreats following intensive efforts.

An important point to remember is that the lower four levels of need must be met to some degree before one is ready for recreation and creative acts. The individual struggling with feelings of insecurity needs predictable routines. Nurses need to assess readiness (in terms of needs met) for challenge, change, and creative expression. Many intricate plans for recreation and creative expression fail because (1) the individual is focusing energy on meeting needs at a more basic level or (2) the individual has not been consulted about his or her particular interests or talents.

Mass activities often provide a sense of belonging, body integration, and better function, but they do not necessarily supply self-esteem or the opportunity for self-actualization. Self-esteem grows out of individual accomplishments and personal recognition. Self-actualization flows from confidence and a milieu in which self-expression is cultivated and valued.

To facilitate a milieu conducive to revitalizing recreation, the following suggestions may be helpful:

1. Assess individual level of needs met.
2. Provide activities structured to meet needs of people who are dealing with the first three levels.
3. Explore individual needs, talents, interests, vocations, and hobbies to promote self-esteem and self-actualization.
4. Encourage individual activities and projects. Group activities are most appropriate in meeting the need for belonging and gaining group esteem. Self-esteem may arise from group esteem but remains dependent on the group until one gains the capacity of self-validation.
5. Provide materials and a milieu in which one may try new means of self-expression.

Leitner and Leitner (1996) provide an extensive list of resources that may be helpful in generating activities and obtaining donated items and volunteer assistance to provide stimulation and opportunities for elders in institutional or community settings (Box 25-5).

Leisure

Leisure is a time of relaxation when one is free of duties, the time to *smell the roses*. Real leisure is relatively self-determined and psychologically pleasant. Leisure may or may not result in a product or enhanced skill. Some leisure time will provide opportunities for recreation, personal growth, and service to others. Leisure may be (1) stimulating or restful, (2) expressive or instrumental, (3) active or passive, and (4)

Box 25-5 Resources that Can Enhance Recreational Activities and Programs

Local florists may present a flower show or provide a flower-arranging activity.
Police and fire departments may give safety presentations.
Local ministers may lead Bible readings and discussions.
Craft suppliers can give demonstrations.
Local pharmacist may give a talk on medication use.
Clothing stores can sponsor a fashion show.
Bakeries may give a demonstration of pastry decoration.
Beauty supply houses may give makeup demonstrations.
Travel agencies may present slide shows.
Librarians may institute great book discussions or other activities.
Students from community colleges may provide numerous educational events and activities.
Garden clubs or horticultural groups may provide gardening classes.
Collector's clubs may talk about collecting stamps, antiques, coins, memorabilia.
Historical societies may give tours to historic places of interest.
Whenever possible, events should be planned as field trips to the sites of the locals involved because trips add elements of additional interest, stimulation, and involvement in the community at large.

introverted or extroverted. The types of leisure chosen reflect something of an individual's value system and time orientation. Leisure time is an idea tied to relative affluence, industrialization, and technologic development that frees the individual from onerous and time-consuming tasks.

With changing retirement patterns, more comprehensive retirement benefits, flexible work hours, employee decision-making related to work schedules, healthier lifestyles, and the gradual lengthening of work life, intermittent and frequent leisure times will be needed for people who continue to work into late old age. Chapter 18 discusses retirement. For many elders, leisure time must be structured and held fast as more and more elders, in this electronic age, work from their homes, either to supplement income or for professional reasons. In these cases, setting aside some inviolable leisure time is important. The several conceptual models of leisure include the following:

- *Humanistic*: A celebration of life, an end in itself
- *Therapeutic*: An instrument of control and healing
- *Quantitative*: Uncommitted time after work is done
- *Institutional*: Segments of time committed to various interests—religious, marital, educational, or political
- *Epistemologic*: Activities that provide meanings and aesthetic appreciation
- *Assumptive*: Activities based on affirmation, legend, and folklore (past oriented)
- *Analytic*: To understand, question, and experiment (present oriented)
- *Aesthetic*: Transformative, involves creative action, and reordering ideas, objects, social institutions and organizations (future oriented)

Exercise, walking, and swimming are the most common activities of people 65 years and older. Cooper and colleagues (2001) report on health barriers that interfere with exercise for elders. This area must be a concern of nurses when considering the benefits of leisure and exercise. Creative nursing care calls for identifying or designing activities that are possible, comfortable, and renewing. For example, Tai Chi has become popular with elders because it interjects humor, relaxation, and control into movement.

Various types of leisure in which a person is engaged is based on need fulfillment. Other factors influencing leisure patterns are social networks, age, time, work role, health, income, location, and family situation. Some senior centers and day-care programs provide leisure activities that are suitable for physically and mentally impaired individuals.

Natural World

Spiritual stimulation and stress relief may be important aspects of contact with the natural landscape. In a survey of articles from June 2001 through March 2002, Irvine and Warber (2002) investigated studies of the significance of the natural world to biopsychosocial and spiritual well being. From their survey of the literature, the authors concluded that contact with the natural world:

Lessened physiologic effects of stress
Improved attentional attributes
Lessened frequency of aggressive behavior
Increased feelings of interconnectedness with others and the universe

Irvine and Warber suggest that these data indicate that the natural world is a vital part of well being and that we should approach public health as incorporating the preservation of natural resources and designing natural environments for human use.

Wilderness areas are not accessible to all older individuals, but some opportunities for contact with nature should be made for those so inclined. The revitalization that occurs for many people at the seashore or in the mountains may become more important in the later years. Carson (1970) believed that this access will become increasingly important to each cohort of aged as open space is reduced. One ancient man in San Francisco took a daily trip to the beach. As a sailor from the rugged coast of Norway, contact with the sea remained essential to him. Old people often feel a special intimacy toward plant and animal life. Laura walked in the woods each day, and each new sprout or flower she noticed was viewed as a personal reward from a bountiful nature. She felt very much a part of it all. One elderly lady took an intensive course to become a docent at the marine reserve. She now guides small groups of elders through the tide pools where they learn the myriad varieties of tiny sea life, often overlooked.

The institutionalized benefit from a horticultural program allows elders to cultivate their own small plot and watch the growth of their plants (Bassen and Baltazar, 1997). Some of the many possible activities are listed in Box 25-6.

Senior adult camping has been organized and sponsored by several groups. Benefits include sensory stimulation for individuals with some impairments, refreshing of memories of earlier times, renewal of confidence in physical abilities,

Box 25-6 Activity Ideas for a Horticulture Program

Drying plants and flowers
Pressing flower and plant arrangements
Arranging flowers
Making terrariums
Window box gardening
Tub gardening
Boxed herb gardens
Hanging baskets
Forcing bulbs
Vegetable garden plots
Flower garden plots
Hydroponics
Selling annual plants and flowers
Developing hybrids
Presenting flower arrangements to elders confined to bed

and spiritual elevation. The esthetics of dew on grass, the smell of water on willows, the clear views of the heavens at night all bring one closer to union with the earth and our origins. Many people use these opportunities for photography. Elders particularly respond to bird walks, horticulture walks, and other opportunities to learn more about the environment around them. The American Camping Association *(www.acacamps.org)* offers several camping experiences especially designed for seniors, as does Elderhostel *(www.elderhostel.org)*.

Area agencies on aging are designated in each state to provide senior centers and information about local recreational programs for the aging. These resources have been a great boon for the aged. The arts, trips, classes, activities, and assistance of numerous varieties are available. Some of the more innovative programs include teleconferencing programs for homebound elders, Internet computer contact through "Senior Net," and interactive television programs. Planning successful programs must reflect the local needs and culture. Area offices can be located through the U.S. Department of Health and Human Services. Nonfederal affiliated programs can be located through city and county park and recreational facilities. In addition, several national organizations promote recreational and sports opportunities specifically designed for seniors.

Bringing Young and Old Together

Recognizing the developmental significance of contact between the generations, many plans and projects have flourished in attempts to bring them together. Some institutions have included children in their milieu in various ways:

- As residents (children with profound retardation or severe neurologic disabilities); elders rock, stroke and cuddle these children, providing stimulation for both.
- As a service to employees (day-care centers for children of employees); elders sometimes assist in the care and special programs for the children, such as reading stories or teaching basic skills (tying shoes, telling time).
- In adopt-a-grandparent programs: one child affiliates with one institutionalized person with periodic visits, cards, and inclusion of grandparent in some special family events.

As community health nurses, exploring potential intergenerational experiences within your community may be rewarding. Although we recommend intergenerational contact, when desired by the aged, certain pitfalls must be considered. The very young energetic child must be taken in small doses, or the elder is likely to be exhausted, and the benefits will decrease in direct relation to uninterrupted time together. In intergenerational programs, young people need consistent supervision, support, and training in the developmental aspects of old age. Similarly, elders will need the assurance of assistance when needed.

Martee developed skits to present to schoolchildren that convey aging concepts in a humorous and positive manner. Genevieve interested a high school social studies class in exploring the students' genealogy. Whole families were soon contacting her for assistance in searching out their family history. Arthur revived his interest in music and developed a "kitchen band" of primary school children to entertain local groups and senior citizens.

An interesting program has been reported (Schulman, 1996) in which a school district in Kansas was short of teachers and the community had a high proportion of elders. The solution was to bring the two together. The elders provided living history experiences for the children, tutored those who needed extra help, worked as classroom aides and music education assistants, and functioned in many other ways to enrich the school experience for children. Both the youngsters and the elders were so enthusiastic about the program it has now been expanded to include connections with the park system, the library, and local church groups.

Teaching and assisting youngsters in other ways seems to fill many needs for some elders who find the experience personally gratifying. Some volunteer activities evolve into income-generating businesses or skills.

NURSING AND SELF-ACTUALIZATION

In this unit, we have considered what aging can be and that the last years can truly actualize the most unique capacities of aged individuals. Human potential movements are springing up throughout the United States like mushrooms and may be just as unpredictable. Nurses might caution people not to make a commitment until the credibility of a group has been established. The trend, however, is heartening because it indicates a general belief that humanity has much yet to learn about the capacity for self-actualization.

Our functions as health care workers who value self-actualization are (1) to continually spur our clients to ask, "What is possible and suitable for me?" and (2) to assist them in finding appropriate resources and, when needed, assist in implementing activities toward self-actualization. The nature of self-actualization is self-determination and direction. Nurses are ancillary to the process but may be needed to stir the beginnings of the search. In doing so, we may move forward with our own search.

Self-actualization implies that one actualizes the potential of self through various mechanisms. We have mentioned only a few of these mechanisms in a somewhat cursory manner, knowing that these individually instituted actions have a force of their own and that once activated goes far beyond the professionals' involvement. Activities such as yoga, focused meditation, the discipline of karate, and other forms of centered concentration are segued into spirituality and transcendence.

SPIRITUALITY

Spirituality is a rather indescribable need that drives individuals throughout life to seek meaning and purpose in their existence. We recognize that our readers will see great overlap and fuzzy boundaries between transcendence and spirituality. Spirituality is difficult to define, though many people have tried. Moberg (1996), one of the major contributors to our understanding of spirituality and aging, defines spirituality as the "totality of man's inner resources, the ultimate concerns around which all other values are focused, the central philosophy of life that guides conduct, and the meaning-giving center of human life which influences all individual and social behavior" (p. 2). Thibault and colleagues (1991) state, "Spirituality refers to the manner in which a person integrates three domains—knowledge or belief system, inner life experiences, and exterior life and institutional activities in support of these beliefs" (p. 29). Meraviglia (1999) describes spirituality as "a connectedness with oneself, others, nature, or God" (p. 18). Spiritual well being is defined as "the affirmation of life in a relationship with God, self, community, and environment that nurtures and celebrates wholeness" (National Interfaith Coalition on Aging, 1975, p. 1).

MacKinley (2001) used a spiritual inventory to determine spiritual health among a group of Londoners and to determine generic *spiritual tasks*. These tasks, MacKinley posits, are transcending disabilities, searching for final meanings, achieving intimacy with God and others, and finding hope. MacKinley finds that elders have a wide range of images of God, are interested in prayer and liturgy, value reminiscence and life-review, and find humor and comfort in their spirituality.

The spiritual path leads one into self-discovery, self-acceptance, affirmation of self-love, and a connection with all others that are brought about by loving the most unlovable aspects of self and of others. Religious beliefs and church participation are often the avenues of spiritual expression, but they are not necessarily interchangeable. For some people, formalized religion helps them feel fulfilled. At the deepest level of spirituality, a profound connection exists with all living things, the universal awareness of which Jung was cognizant (Freke and Gandy, 2001). Even though we have learned to clone, isolate particles of DNA, and alter the structure of most living things, the mystery of life itself cannot be comprehended. True spirituality endeavors to make the world a better place, often in small daily acts or in a larger sense. The enormity of the actions and where they occur are not as significant as the love that produces them.

Some people see the essence of aging as a spiritual journey in which one connects with the transcendent self and the route of spiritual growth (Berggren-Thomas and Griggs, 1995). The nursing role is not to intervene but to accompany along the path and be fully present with the individual.

The spiritual aspect transcends the physical and psychosocial to reach the deepest individual capacity for love, hope, and meaning. The spiritual person can rise above that which is humanly expected in a situation. For example, a dying elder in great pain to whom I was attending said to me, "This is so hard for you." That he was able to see beyond himself at that time was difficult to believe.

Study of Spirituality and Aging

Life satisfaction, happiness, morale, and health have all been studied in relation to religion and spiritual expression. Although successful aging has been studied in numerous ways, Crowther and colleagues (2002) contend that spirituality must be considered a significant factor. Rowe and Kahn's (1998) prevalent model of successful aging includes active engagement in life, minimal risk and disability, and the maximum physical and mental abilities. Crowther and colleagues maintain that positive spirituality must be the fourth element of the model and is interrelated with all of the others.

Gerontologists are appreciative of the significance of religion and spirituality in the adaptational capacity of elders. However, spirituality has not achieved the central focus it merits in the study of aging. At the 1971 White House Conference on Aging, spiritual well being was an aspect of aging that was deemed significant enough for a section focus. At the 1995 White House Conference on Aging, 45 conference resolutions were adopted; none of these addressed spirituality directly, but all supported the fundamental needs of elders that form the foundation for health, economic security, and life satisfaction.

In the last few years, we have seen a *revival* of interest in philosophy, religion, and spirituality. The movement is more than a New Age fad, but spiritual studies are elusive and not adaptable to elegant research design. Nonetheless, these topics are emerging as an insistent need long sacrificed to the god of science. Henderson (1996) calls the movement a spiritual renaissance that has captured the interest of professionals. This description has certainly been observed in the last 5 years given that the focus of conferences of the American Society on Aging and the Gerontology Society of America (previously the bastion of medical research) have had spiritual overtones in a great majority of the symposia and presentations.

Benner (1994) discusses the emergence of interest among nurses in interpretive phenomenology that opens the possibility of studying meanings as individually defined. Interpretive phenomenology is a way of looking at human experience through the interpretation of the individual who is experiencing the events. Interpretive phenomenology is looking at the whole of experience and the way in which it makes sense to that person. Meanings, commitments, and concerns cannot be encompassed in ordinary scientific research calculations. The particular science of interpretation is dubbed hermeneutics; thus one reads of hermeneutic phenomenology, the method by which experience is interpreted and then analyzed. From an accumulation of many interpretations from numerous individuals, new understanding of the human experience can emerge. This concept is the essence of this chapter.

van Manen (1990) suggests research guidelines for hermeneutic phenomenologic research:

- Commit to an area of serious interest.
- Investigate experience as it is lived rather than through a conceptualized pattern.

- Reflect on the essential themes that characterize the phenomena.
- Describe the phenomena through writing and rewriting.
- Examine the parts and the whole.

One might say that historic research at its best or biography at its best displays evidence of hermeneutic phenomenologic examination.

Religion

Throughout history and in all cultures, sacraments, symbols, and metaphor have been used to recognize, organize, and understand human experience. The myths, allegories, and traditions of religious expression have occurred with all cultures in all of recorded time and are useful as a means to ensure connectedness with the miraculous.

The religious impulse, as conceptualized by Maslow (1970), resides within each person and in its highest fulfillment integrates the life experience rather than splitting life into the sacred and the profane. Maslow believes that the organizational and ritual aspects of religion can be expressions of meaning or become empty gestures when one separates self from the source of spirituality. Jung proposed the presence in humans of a natural religious energy. Jung believed that religion unites the inner and outer man in equal degree (Fordham, 1966). No completely rational approach can accomplish this task, but art, dreams, fantasies, and other intuitive expressions, steeped in logic, may assist the person in reaching into the soul and becoming whole. One can touch religious energies within and outside of formalized religion in many ways. We have seen evidence of this embedded desire for religious expression in the eagerness with which many people grasp cults and "isms" of all kinds, some with destructive rather than constructive beliefs and outcomes.

For some people, formalized religion helps them to feel fulfilled. As an elder sees the curtain slowly closing on the last act, he or she may have a pressing need to talk about philosophy and spiritual development. A need may exist for private time for prayer, meditation, and reflection. Nurses may neglect to explore this issue with elders because religion may not seem the high priority. The client should be assured that religious longings and rituals are important and that opportunities will be made available as desired (Hermann, 2000).

Nurses may interpret a patient's spiritual needs in terms of religious affiliation, rites, and rituals, but religion is only one aspect of spirituality, and it may or may not fill an individual's spiritual needs. Spiritual needs are much broader and more personal than any particular religious persuasion. Nurses may not lead individuals to soul growth and acceptance when facing illness and disability but may have the privilege of accompanying them on the journey. Reflection, feedback, comfort, and affirmation are all a part of being with the elder, providing the supports that release energy for spiritual seeking. The importance of the spiritual to an individual's well being, hopeful attitudes, and will to live are of increasing interest to nurses and other professionals.

Ramsey observes that true spirituality cannot be institutionalized because it is a lifetime sacred search. Although some mystical moments do occur, the mundane aspects of existence take on deeper meanings. Ramsey transcended self and became a part of a greater whole. Another insight that is important to recognize is that a *spiritually mature* person is not necessarily happy or content. "If faith is a relationship, with God and with other people, then days of distance and doubt are part of the rhythm of the spiritually intimate life ..." (Ramsey, 2001, p. 62).

Ramsey (2001) sees the religious community as providing an opportunity for intimacy through the rituals and sense of connectedness with the invisible members of the religious community.

A personal experience with a group of evangelical missionaries emphasized this connectedness to the invisible and to the world community of like-minded individuals. Each morning, a devotional session included a prayer for a certain missionary family noted in the denomination booklet. Around the world, all members and missionaries of that particular faith were sending prayers for the one select missionary noted in the devotional booklet. Many of these missionaries were in remote and isolated stations around the world. A powerful sense of connectedness was found in this daily ritual.

Ramsey (2001) writes of developing a religious life in response to her father's death and the need to say a kaddish (a prayer) and to make a connection with his religion. In the process, Ramsey discovered her own spirituality and a "religious chain of belonging" that has deepened and made significant the events in her life.

Spirituality, as defined by Ramsey (2001), refers to "a direct, lived experience of inner searching that also involves a dynamic, animated relationship with a sacred reality" (p. 60). Spirituality is a very sacred and intimate search that cannot be ordered or interpreted by another person.

Religion and Health. In early societies, religion and health care were tightly interwoven, and the priesthood controlled both. As scientific method changed the practice of medicine, health and spirituality grew apart, though the residue of the priesthood remains in the practice of medicine.

Evidence suggests that religion and spirituality still hold a strong connection to physical and mental health (Mackenzie et al, 2000). In a small qualitative study in two continuing care retirement communities, the researchers found that most of these older adults believed in the power of prayer in healing and that a higher power constantly guides, protects, and supports them. Residents also believe that God works through physicians, medicine, loving friends, and helpful strangers.

Kennedy and colleagues (1996) found that religious preference and practice were inversely related to depressive symptoms for religious people who were able to attend services of their faith. Individuals who were unable to attend services, particularly those of the Catholic and Jewish faith, had a greater prevalence of depression.

Religious doubt also had deleterious effects on elders studied by Krause and colleagues (1999). These researchers found among a national sample of Presbyterians that doubt was associated with psychologic distress and diminished feelings of well being. However, one often goes through periods of doubt in the transcendent process. Listening and avoiding platitudes is important, recognizing that this time of development is crucial.

According to one study, reported by Kleyman (2002), certain forms of religious struggle are linked to an increased risk of death among elderly men and women. People who believed that God had abandoned them, those who questioned God's love, and those who felt that the devil had made them ill were at an increased likelihood of dying (Box 25-7).

Signs of spiritual distress include doubt, despair, guilt, boredom, ennui, and anger at God (see Box 25-4). Interventions may involve calling clergy; sharing spiritual readings, poems, and music; obtaining religious articles such as the Bible or a rosary; or praying.

Box 25-7 Assessing and Intervening in Spiritual Distress

Assessment

Brief history:
- Losses
- Challenged belief, value system
- Separation from religious and cultural ties
- Death
- Personal and family disasters

Symptoms (defining characteristics) such as the following:
- Unmet needs
- Threats to self
- Change in environment, health status, self-concept, etc.
- Questioning meaning of own existence
- Depression
- Feeling of hopelessness, abandonment, fear

Assessment of the cause of spiritual distress
- Depletion anxiety
- Helplessness, hopelessness
- Perceived powerlessness
- Medication reaction
- Hormonal imbalances

Interventions

Create a therapeutic environment.
Assess the support system.
Assess past methods of decreasing distress (e.g., prayer, imagery, healing, memories-reminiscence therapy, medication, relaxation).
Determine environmental changes needed to enhance function.
Assess and assist implementation of coping mechanisms.
Refer to clergy.
Evaluate effects of nursing interventions.
Activate and evaluate appropriate community referrals.
Use techniques to assist client and family in reducing spiritual distress.

Physicians, as well as nurses, should routinely inquire about religious and spiritual beliefs. This inquiry should not just be considered only when it appears the person may not survive. Ehman and colleagues (1999), in a study of 177 ambulatory adult patients in a pulmonary clinic, found that more than one half of the participants described themselves as religious, and 90% believed that prayer might influence recovery from illness. Forty five percent of the respondents said that their beliefs influence the health decisions they make, and 94% of those agreed that they should be asked about these beliefs. Two thirds of the respondents would welcome questions regarding their religious beliefs.

George (2002) addressed links between religion and health. In reviewing research in this domain, the author identified dimensions of religious experience as including frequency of church attendance, time given to personal devotions such as prayer and readings, use of religious beliefs to address life problems, and extent to which religious beliefs influence lifestyle. Research (Ellison, Levin, 1998; George et al, 2000) shows that regular participation in religious services is associated with a lower prevalence of physical illness and increased longevity. Religious services have also shown therapeutic effects as improved recovery from illness and decreased functional limitations in chronic disabilities. The immediate question is whether the sample of elders involved in church is skewed toward healthy, ambulatory individuals. Considering all such variables, George found that strong relationships remain between religious participation and positive health outcomes. Part of this relationship may be attributed to the importance of the rich social, ethical, and the reciprocal nature of religious involvement, as well as the healthier life styles that many religions promote (Idler, 2002). Koenig and Brooks (2002) note that the benefits of religion involve a source of hope and meaning, a code of ethics, and a reliable source of social interaction and support. The authors further contend that because religious organizations have historically provided for the poor, sick and elderly, policies are needed that support the combined efforts of churches and health care providers in a more integrated manner.

Parish nursing. Parish nursing is one such effort that has expanded enormously in the last decade. From the handful practicing in 1990, currently, 7000 parish nurses are practicing in a variety of roles in every state (Deaconess Parish Nurse Ministries, 2002). Religious communities and hospitals working together might provide for the preventive and health maintenance needs of many frail elders, as well as their spiritual needs.

Parish nursing has found a niche in the care of elders and has begun to flourish in the last decade. Many models of parish nursing have been developed, but the underlying motivation is to address and blend the maintenance of physical and spiritual health to the satisfaction of parishioners. Weis and Schank

(2000) found, among over 400 subjects, that health-seeking behavior was the primary reason for seeing the parish nurse for services, but unidentified needs were equal motivators. A very small number of people expressed spiritual distress (7% under 80 years and 5% over 80 years of age). The most frequent nursing interventions were active listening, emotional support, and spiritual support. Touching and nursing presence were also valued.

Nurses who are involved in religious organizations can be advocates for increasing the attention given to the health needs of the aged. Nurses may even spearhead particular services to the aged, such as peer counseling, health screening activities, day care, home visitation programs, and respite for families. *Parish nurses* are becoming visible nationwide as churches and hospitals join forces to provide health maintenance and monitoring activities for parishioners (Schank, Weis, Matheus, 1996).

Homebound elders and religious connections. Powers (1996) notes that at the time elders need spiritual connections the most, these connections may break down. The spiritual nourishment that comes from being an integral part of a congregation of like-minded individuals is diminished when an elder becomes homebound and can no longer attend services or observe comforting rituals. Some individuals deeply need the connection with others and to participate in meaningful ways in the activities of the church.

According to Reverend Elwood Spackman, interviewed by Powers, roles can be devised that meet these needs for the elders who are unable to attend services. Spackman suggests that these individuals be given names of parishioners with particular prayer requests and those needing telephone reassurance. Parish newsletters and tapes of sermons can be provided to isolated elders, as well as visits from youthful members of the church. Spackman also suggests that family members may be encouraged to create meaningful rituals that can be observed at home.

Some parishioners find televised church services comforting, including participating in the singing. Singing is seldom considered as a transcendent mechanism, though participating in song and dance renews the spirit and takes one beyond self into the higher human attributes.

Wesley Woods Geriatric Center in Atlanta, Georgia, reports a program designed to maintain a sense of spiritual community for homebound elders who are no longer able to attend services (Powers, 1996). For elders who throughout their life maintained strong ties with a church community, the sense of loss when unable to attend services can be acute. Not only the ritual has been lost, but also the fellowship. Some of the suggestions for maintaining ties are to provide tapes of services, involve youth groups in home visitations, develop prayer circles in which homebound members not only are included in the prayers of others, but also have several individuals for whom to pray, thus keeping spiritual linkages strong. Family members can be encouraged to set aside a special time in which all members join in hymns, Bible reading, and watching a televised sermon. Important rituals may also be included as the individuals' desire. These ideas are actually resurrections of those practiced several generations ago when families lived in isolated areas.

Wesley Woods undoubtedly has a predominantly Protestant, Methodist approach to religious needs, even though it is interdenominational in practice. That elders be connected with their preferred spiritual roots and rituals is extremely important, whether Protestant, Jewish, Buddhist, Shinto, or any of the numerous religions in our multicultural society. Additional discussions of cultural differences are found in Chapter 19.

Striepe, a parish nurse coordinator in Spencer, Iowa, gives these suggestions for approaching spirituality with a homebound elder (Powers, 1996, p. 13):

"How do you feel spiritually?"
"How satisfied are you with your spiritual health?"
"When do you feel most connected to God?"
"What helps you feel connected?"
"Have you had an intense spiritual experience that dramatically changed your relationship with God?"
"What gives you joy?"
"Would you be interested in visits with young people from your congregation?"

Interfaith volunteers. Communities nationwide have organized interfaith volunteer services to provide in-home services for isolated frail elders. Many of these efforts have been organized and supported by the Robert Wood Johnson Foundation.

Healing. The evolution of the word *heal* from the Old Norse usage, through Old and Medieval English and its German derivations (Partridge, 1959), gives a fuller sense of the meaning of the word, which has largely been lost in present-day tendencies to equate heal with cure and cure with eradication of physical disease. Cure sometimes inexplicably occurs, but it is not our health care emphasis. The words hail, heil, be whole, be healthy, and be well all underlie the word heal. These words were originally used in greeting another and to convey blessings and the desire for communion (intimate fellowship and rapport). Clearly, the desire for interaction was integral to hailing (healing). Similarly, in departures, *good-bye* was a contraction of the original "God be with you." My old friend, Catherine, always said, "Go with God," when I would leave her.

This somewhat esoteric examination of word origins is meant only to convey the larger meaning of the word *heal*. Underpinning this whole text is our conviction that wholeness in person, holiness, and healing are possibilities, regardless of tissue and organ disturbances or the wear and tear of living. "Going with God," in whatever sense one conceives of God, is our meaning when we talk of healing.

Healing as a religious activity has been neglected for so long that we have almost forgotten that in antiquity priests and healers wore the same hat. Two nurses in Toronto, Canada, thought the time was right to again look at spiritual healing (MacLennan and Tsai, 1995). The nurses began with questions about whether nurses were concerned about spiritual needs, and if so, were they applying concepts related to spirituality in nursing practice. What was found was that nurses tended to avoid dealing with spiritual needs because they believed the subject was too personal. How can one begin to discuss spiritual matters?

- Ask the individual his or her source of strength and hope.
- Ask if the individual sees any connection between physical health and spiritual beliefs.
- Discuss sources of spiritual strength throughout life.

Healing often occurs in the search for the meaning of untoward events and most particularly when in true communion with another. Healing emanating from the mind or soul is an ancient method that has been neglected and even denigrated by the scientific community. Recently, medicine and nursing have been receptive to the idea that prayer may heal and restore well being (American Association of Critical Care Nurses, 1995; MacLennan, Tsai, 1995). Finally, the amazing power of the mind is being recognized as essential to the healing process.

Creative Health Care

Belief is often stronger than any medicine known and more effective than any treatment. The normal body processes can be transcended. Although we would not advocate instilling unfounded expectations, we would hope nurses would openly share with clients the limits of our knowledge and the unknown potential that lies within. We can then say to an ill or dying person, "There is much within the human body and spirit we don't understand. Almost anything is possible. Holding onto one's own hopes and beliefs will undoubtedly affect the course of illness and recovery."

The Academy of Parapsychology and Medicine (1975) states several fundamental beliefs that encompass an enlarged view of the treatment of disease and potential for health:

- That man is a multidimensional being whose experience and ultimate purpose are inextricably and meaningfully related and that meaning is made manifest in patterns of health and disease
- That medicine must adopt a new view of man, one that recognizes the unity of body, mind, and spirit, and the importance of the interrelationship of these dimensions in health and disease
- That all physical and mental disease is directive experience in human development and that they must be viewed as a manifestation of conditions existing on subtler levels—whether mental, emotional, or spiritual
- That the treatment of disease must be directed to the whole man and that no lasting healing of the physical body can be achieved where the mental, emotional, and spiritual elements have been untouched
- That no condition or disease in the human body exists that cannot be successfully treated if a means is discovered for treating on the appropriate level

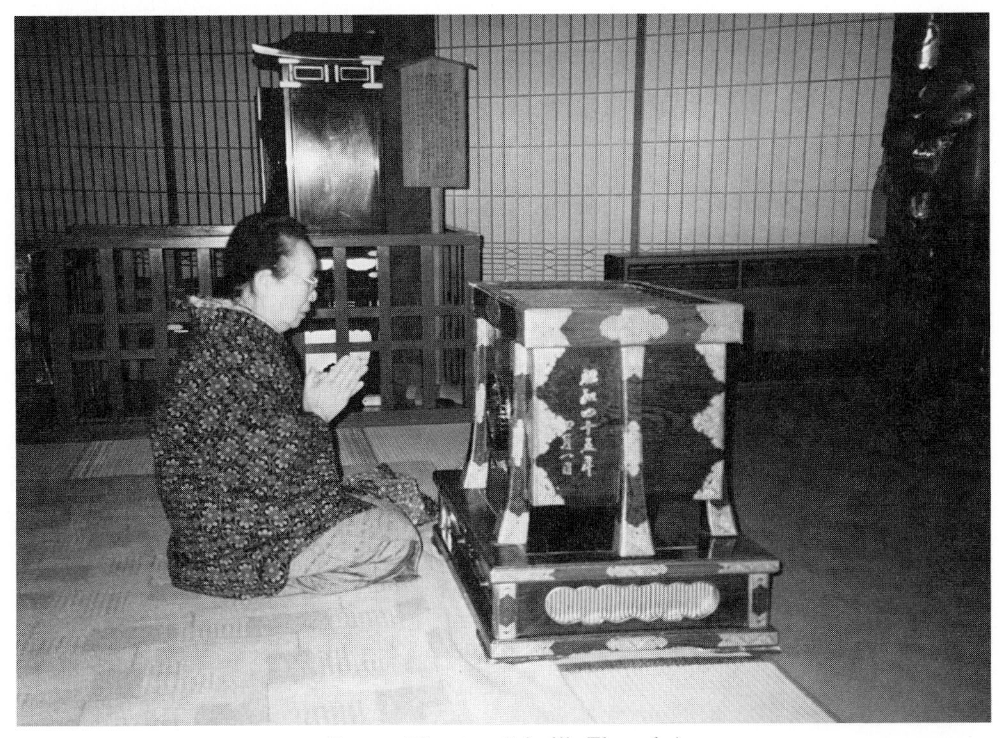

Prayer. (Courtesy Priscilla Ebersole.)

Bill Moyers, a widely known journalist, has recently joined the large cadre of people, scientists, and mystics, who believe in the healing power of the mind.

Nurses may introduce the discussion with elders and explore experiences they have had with extraordinary events that stirred the subconscious or paranormal powers within themselves. The nurse's receptivity and caring are essential components of the healing process, which releases the forces of self-healing.

Healing may be experienced in many ways. The result may or may not be the eradication of a disease but always brings about the integration of a condition or situation into a sense of wholeness, wellness, and greater understanding. To do so, "we will need a rapprochement between ancient wisdom and modern science, between mystery and mastery" (Cole, 1992, p. 17). Stoll (1979) espouses the interrelatedness of forgiveness, love, and trust in achieving health and wholeness (Figure 25-4). We would emphasize the importance of self-forgiveness and hope.

Nursing Assessment and Intervention to Encourage Spiritual Well Being

Hungelmann and colleagues (1996) have developed an assessment tool that provides a way of establishing the diagnosis of spirituality that emphasizes strengths, as well as possible spiritual distress (Figure 25-5).

The scale is multidimensional and includes factors that affect psychologic and physical welfare. The authors identify four areas of nursing intervention: affirmation through listening and discovering the gift and identifying need; therapeutic communication as a vehicle for identifying strengths, as well as pain; reminiscing that encourages the emergence of the life story; and referral to clergy or another health professional when desire or need is indicated.

How do these areas relate to geriatric nurses? First is the awareness of one's own spirit, then, knowing that caring for an aging body is the least of work with the elderly. Recognizing the primacy of the spirit is necessary. Some very spiritual individuals are unable to articulate their knowing; do not negate that aspect of an individual's experience because it is not expressed verbally. Realizing that biopsychosocial aspects of aging are all shards of the spirit will integrate every aspect of your work in geriatric nursing.

TRANSCENDENCE

Transcendence is the high-level emotional response to religious and spiritual life and finds expression in numerous rituals and modes of cosmic consciousness. Rituals provide a means of connecting with everyone through the ages who have observed like rituals. These modes of thinking and feeling are sometimes unfamiliar to individuals who are immersed in the necessary materialistic concerns of young adulthood, yet moments do occur throughout life when one is deeply aware of being part of a larger scheme. Although some of this chapter

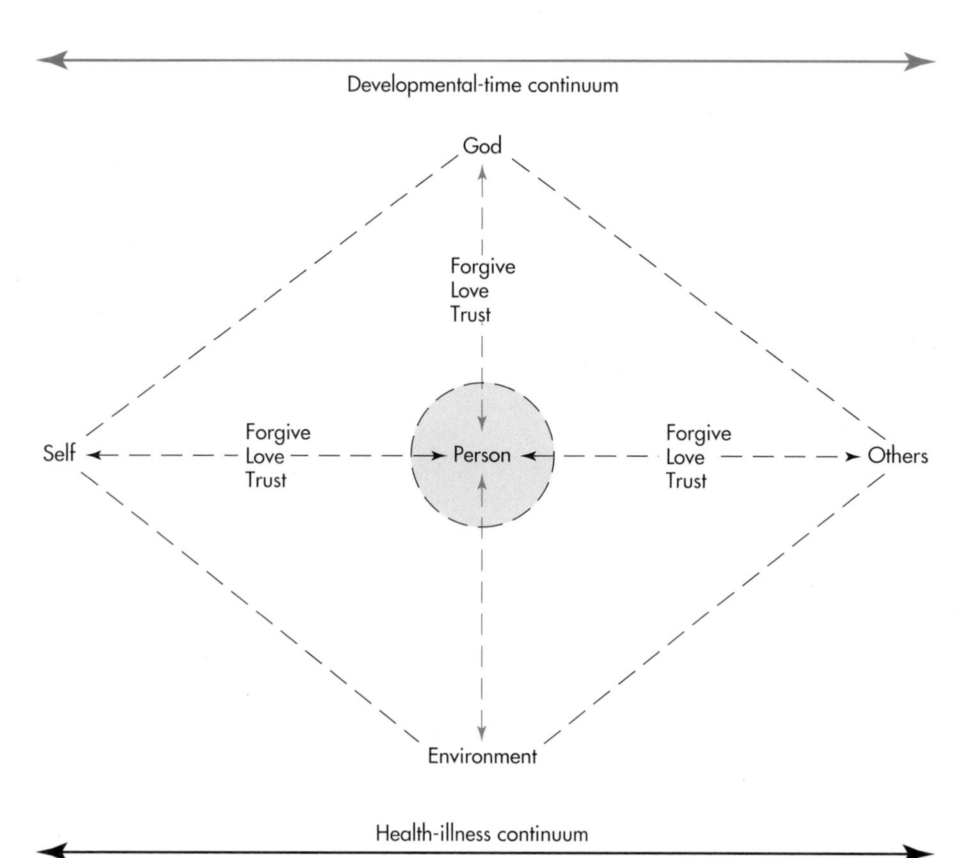

Figure 25-4. Stoll's model of spiritual interrelatedness via forgiveness, love, and trust, resulting in meaning, purpose, and hope in life. (Redrawn from Frisch NC, Kelley J: *Healing life's crises: a guide for nurses,* Albany, NY, 1996, Delmar.)

DIRECTIONS: Please circle the choice that best describes how much you agree with each statement. Circle only one answer for each statement. There is no right or wrong answer.

	Strongly Agree	Moderately Agree	Agree	Disagree	Moderately Disagree	Strongly Disagree
1. Prayer is an important part of my life.	SA	MA	A	D	MD	SD
2. I believe I have spiritual well-being.	SA	MA	A	D	MD	SD
3. As I grow older, I find myself more tolerant of others' beliefs.	SA	MA	A	D	MD	SD
4. I find meaning and purpose in my life.	SA	MA	A	D	MD	SD
5. I feel there is a close relationship between my spiritual beliefs and what I do.	SA	MA	A	D	MD	SD
6. I believe in an afterlife.	SA	MA	A	D	MD	SD
7. When I am sick I have less spiritual well-being.	SA	MA	A	D	MD	SD
8. I believe in a supreme power.	SA	MA	A	D	MD	SD
9. I am able to receive and give love to others.	SA	MA	A	D	MD	SD
10. I am satisfied with my life.	SA	MA	A	D	MD	SD
11. I set goals for myself.	SA	MA	A	D	MD	SD
12. God has little meaning in my life.	SA	MA	A	D	MD	SD
13. I am satisfied with the way I am using my abilities.	SA	MA	A	D	MD	SD
14. Prayer does not help me in making decisions.	SA	MA	A	D	MD	SD
15. I am able to appreciate differences in others.	SA	MA	A	D	MD	SD
16. I am pretty well put together.	SA	MA	A	D	MD	SD
17. I prefer that others make decisions for me.	SA	MA	A	D	MD	SD
18. I find it hard to forgive others.	SA	MA	A	D	MD	SD
19. I accept my life situations.	SA	MA	A	D	MD	SD
20. Belief in a supreme being has no part in my life.	SA	MA	A	D	MD	SD
21. I cannot accept change in my life.	SA	MA	A	D	MD	SD

From Hungelmann J, Kenkel-Rossi E, Klassen L, Stollenwerk R: Marquette University College of Nursing, 1987, Milwaukee, Wisconsin (Copyright).

Figure 25-5. Jarel Spiritual Well-Being Scale. *Continued*

may be obscure, it is the springboard for learning to appreciate the full life cycle. The privilege of briefly walking alongside an elder on the last great journey can be truly inspiring.

Transcending is roused by the desire to go beyond the self as delimited by the material and the concrete aspects of living, to expand self-boundaries and life perspectives. Transcending embodies aspects of belonging, connecting, giving life, holding commitments, struggling with and surrendering ego, turning inward, and becoming free (Forbes, 1994). Creative thought and actions are vehicles of both self-actualization and self-transcendence, the bridge to universal expression and existence. Self-transcendence is generally expressed in five modes: creative work, religious beliefs, children, identification with nature, and mystical experiences (Reed, 1991). This segment of the chapter deals with various mechanisms by which one transcends the purely physical limitations of existence.

Self-transcendence is thought to be a developmental process that forestalls depression in middle age and aging (Ellerman and Reed, 2001). Using Reed's Self-Transcendence Scale, Ellerman and Reed revealed significant gender differences and increasing levels of self-transcendence in the aging process. The way one perceives the passage of time, experiences extensions of the self, and copes with the sure knowledge that death is inevitable may be the ultimate victory or defeat.

Some people may use asceticism, self-denial, and rigorous rituals to reach the peaks of human experience; many others find more prosaic approaches just as effective. The thesis of Maslow's writings is that mystic, sacred, and transcendent experiences frequently arise from the ordinary elements of one's life (Maslow, 1970). Planting and harvesting, one of the most persistent interests of elders, is the "substance of

JAREL SPIRITUAL WELL-BEING SCALE

Factor I Faith/Belief Dimension

(Scoring: SA = 6 SD = 1)
Item 1 _______
Item 2 _______
Item 3 _______
Item 4 _______
Item 5 _______
Item 6 _______
Item 8 _______ Subscore _______

Factor II Life/Self Responsibility

(Reverse Scoring: SA 1 SD 6)
Item 7 _______
Item 12 _______
Item 14 _______
Item 17 _______
Item 18 _______
Item 20 _______
Item 21 _______ Subscore _______

Factor III Life Satisfaction/Self Actualization

(Scoring: SA 6 SD 1)
Item 9 _______
Item 10 _______
Item 11 _______
Item 13 _______
Item 15 _______
Item 16 _______
Item 19 _______ Subscore _______ Total score _______

Figure 25-5. Cont'd.

things hoped for, the evidence of things not seen" (Hebrews 11:1). Gardening, reading, holding an infant, dealing with loss, and numerous other normal events have elements of mystery.

With each death of a loved one, throughout life, one is reborn to a slightly altered state. When deaths of significant others abound in the later years, elders must be given opportunity to express how they personally have been altered by the loss. We can speculate that with each personal loss, one moves slightly closer to the universal and away from the individual until, toward the end, one feels an affiliation with all living things, animal, plant, and mineral. Some of the old have achieved a state of existence that transcends the limits of the failing body.

An 86-year-old widow seemed to blend with her world of plants, birds, and flowers. Each new blossom or birdcall excited her as she mused in her small apartment and garden. Her conversation was sprinkled with minute discoveries, each of which thrilled her. She became so close to nature that some people thought her eccentric. In her last years of life, her interest in the living and growing things consumed her. Hours were spent gazing at leaves, grass, ants, and twigs. The cycles of nature seemed to become a part of her being as she experienced her own limited existence. She was found dead in her apartment one morning. It was then learned that her breasts were eroded with cancer. She had not gone to a physician and had never given evidence of pain; rather a sense of mild euphoria filled her last months.

Chidester (1990), a professor of religion, organized transcendence into segments that resemble anthropologic studies: the primal, the Eastern, and the Western. All segments evolved out of the human necessity to make meaning of the major events in life and to develop rituals by which to support the transitions, birth and death being the central issues. Symbolic death and rebirth form the essence of transcendent rituals and in one form or another are common to all transcendent mechanisms. As the world continually shrinks and peoples of the world intermingle, few purely classic examples of any one transcendent system exist. As jeans, colas, and T-shirts have infiltrated the world, so have the predominant ways of dealing with the exigencies of life. Among the enlightened elders with whom we have worked, it often seems as if elements of primitive animism, Eastern cyclic death-rebirth, and Western universal love have all been observed.

Briefly, primal transcendence describes the way in which native peoples achieved meaning and structure primarily through natural phenomena. The elements, the natural occurrences, were interpreted as the source of help or harm. Dreams and animals were deified and became the channels to the supernatural. In some groups, the spirits of the dead were thought to reside in animals or to return to earth through the birth of a child. Natural objects, animals or birds, were the emblems of particular groups, containing their spirits and distinguishing features.

Eastern transcendence in the overall sense, with many variations, embodies reverence for life, ancestors, balance, and order. Liberation from passions, disorder, and lack of discipline form the foundations of spiritual growth and transcendence of the purely physical. Many mechanisms are used to achieve this state of peace and enlightenment. Westerners have observed and employed some of these mechanisms and are in awe of individuals who have achieved mastery. Gerontologists often cite the Eastern respect for the aged and ancestors as a more cultural phenomenon than a spiritual necessity.

Western modes of transcendence have been fraught with the struggle between good and evil, the separation of mind and body, the Cartesian duality of which Benner (1994) writes. Each life event is judged as it is integrated; personal responsibility is highly valued, and one can expect no help from ancestors or atavistic aids to achieve a transcendent state of universal love. Cause and effect are in linear motion. Transcending evil to reach eternal bliss or attain rewards after death is an overriding expectation of many people.

Gerotranscendence

Tornstam (1994, 1996) theorizes that human aging brings about a general potential for what he terms gerotranscendence, a shift in perspective from the material world to the cosmic and, concurrent with that, an increasing life satisfaction. Tornstam found, in a survey of 912 Danish elders, that shifts in cosmic awareness and ego transcendence were accompanied by satisfaction and a lesser need for social activity. The higher the level of transcendence, the more internal were the sources of satisfaction.

This satisfaction is qualitatively different than disengagement (Cumming and Henry, 1961) or the achievement of ego integrity (Erikson, 1950). Disengagement or activity is of little significance in this transformation. There is not an either-or duality but a more profound, all-pervasive change in perspective. Gerotranscendence is conceptualized as a metamorphosis, an alteration in conception of time, space, life, death, and self. Tornstam says, "Simply put, gerotranscendence is a shift in metaperspective, from a mid-life materialistic and rational vision to a more cosmic and transcendent one, accompanied by an increase in life satisfaction" (Tornstam, 1996, p. 38).

Indices of gerotranscendence are summarized in Box 25-8. Gerotranscendence is thought to be a gradual and ongoing shift that is generated by the normal processes of living, sometimes hastened by serious personal disruptions. In prior studies (1994), Tornstam found, when studying Swedish citizens between ages 15 and 80, that loneliness decreased with every consecutive age group, and time alone became more valued.

Tornstam believes that many theories of aging arise from the personal values of rather young gerontologists and their wishes about what reality ought to be. These imposed expectations and other elements in our culture may inhibit or prohibit the full possibilities of old age.

Wadensten and Carlsson (2001) wondered if nurses recognized signs of gerotranscendence and how they were interpreted. In their study, nurses did recognize these signs (declining interest in social activity, alterations in perspectives of time, space, life and death, increased life satisfaction) occurring in many old people but saw them as evidence of aging or pathologic conditions rather than a natural developmental process of transcendence. However, given that this study was conducted in a nursing home in Sweden, the conclusions are limited. An additional study conducted by Raes and Marcoen (2001) in Belgium found that a gerotranscendence scale developed by Tornstam showed that individuals who had experienced recent crises had higher scores on the Transcendent Connection subscale. Apparently, specific attributes of gerotranscendence need to be articulated more clearly if nurses, and others, are to identify the process.

Time Transcendence

Life as experienced ordinarily involves the chronologic passage of time. Some types of conscious experience alter our

Box 25-8 Characteristics of Individuals with a High Degree of Gerotranscendence

Have high degrees of life satisfaction
Engage in self-controlled social activity
Experience satisfaction with self-selected social activities
Social activities not essential to their well-being
Midlife patterns and ideals no longer prime motivators
Demonstrate complex and active coping patterns
Have greater need for solitary philosophizing
May appear withdrawn when engaged in inner development
Have accelerated development of gerotranscendence fomented by life crises
Feel shifts in perception of reality

Data from gerotranscendence theory development of Lars Tornstam.

time perception, but the unconscious destroys time. Therefore the release of the unconscious transcends the limitations of time that conscious life experience generally imposes on us. If we conquer time, we conquer annihilation and the dimensions of time that lie within the mind. Recognizing the importance of time perception, particularly in old age, is a fertile field to explore more fully. Influences on time perception include age; imminent death, level of activity, emotional state, outlook on the future, and the value attached to time. Conclusions from studies of the aged generally support the view that elders perceive time as passing quickly and favor the past over the present or the future.

Sexuality as a Transcendent Mechanism

Sublimation, or reaching the sublime realization of sexuality, requires a connection with the spiritual beginnings of sexual acts. "In both sex and religion there is the common mystic element which is the essence of both ecstasies" (Goldberg, 1958, p. 8). For thousands of years, procreation, fertility, and sex were celebrated as integral to religious rites (Goldberg, 1958). Sex and sexuality can be expressions of great spirituality, the great mystery of the universe and continuous replenishment. Sex is the source of life itself, but on an individual level, it can be as mechanical or mystical as one believes it to be.

As relevant to aging, one might inquire, "What are your thoughts about sexuality at this stage of your life?" Most elders dismiss the topic rather quickly, "Oh, that is no longer important" or "It is physically too taxing." However, one lady who I consider enlightened said, "It is a definite presence in all of life, even in later life." She understands that sex is much more than a mechanical act; it is the supreme mystery. Further discussion of sexuality is found in Chapter 17.

Altered Mind States

In every society and every age, humans have sought spiritual enlightenment through altered mind states by using substances, rituals, and deprivations. An inherent need seems apparent in almost every culture to incorporate methods of seeking some enlightenment outside the common daily experience. Some of these exceptional experiences are treasured, and some are feared. The ritual use of peyote by the Southwest Indians, sake by the Japanese, isolation and deprivation by some of the Northwest Native tribes, withdrawal into nirvana by East Indians, and mind-altering drugs by the flower children are only a few of the most obvious of these methods. These examples simply exemplify some of the routes individuals take to move out of the common thought modes that may keep them trapped in the mundane levels of existence.

Mystical experiences seem to strengthen the immune system in that spontaneous remissions of illness sometimes seem to result from moods and altered perceptions, sometimes in a religious manner or with psychedelic drugs. Roberts advances the idea that mystical experiences boost the immune system (Roberts, 1999).

For some people, mind states are altered without using a particular substance or mechanism. These altered mind states may be frightening. Professionals may validate the experiences and assist the person in achieving a coping style that balances the internal reality with the demands of daily living. In the following discussion of some of these situations, examples and suggestions are given for facilitating acceptance and valuing these extraordinary occurrences.

Peak Experiences. A peak experience is when one momentarily transcends self through love, wisdom, insight, worship, commitment, or creativity. These experiences are the extraordinary events in one's life that clearly demonstrate self-actualization and personal authenticity. Peak experience is the time when restrictive boundaries seem to vanish, and one feels more aware, more complete, more ecstatic, or more concerned for others. Peak experiences include many modes of transcending one's ordinary limitations. Spiritual and paranormal experiences, creative acts, courage, and humor may all produce peak experiences. Levin (1993) defines these mystical experiences as including déjà vu, clairvoyance, and other occurrences in which the self-perceptions reach beyond the ordinary limits. These mechanisms move humans beyond the boundaries of visible, concrete reality and toward a wholly integrated *self.* The self, as conceptualized by Jung, means the supreme oneness of being: integration of aspects of self that are generative and destructive, light and dark, conscious and unconscious, male and female. The ability to embrace the possibility of every potential behavior as native to self instills compassion and a sense of oneness with the world. Keeping oneself open to transcendence involves finding the places in which such experiences can break through: soul-stirring concerts, sunrises, sunsets, or raging storms on mountaintops (Kimble, 1993). Each individual seeks states of being in which he or she feels part of a larger whole.

Parapsychologic Phenomena. Some older people may have experienced unusual events such as telepathic messages, predictive dreams, premonitions, out-of-body experiences, or poltergeist activity. These individuals may be reluctant to share these experiences unless the listener maintains an accepting attitude. Some people will find it important that they can share these paranormal experiences that may have made them feel abnormal or bizarre. Some individuals who do not appear to be psychotic experience such events. If they have sought professional help, these people may have become frustrated, given that our present understanding of these events is limited. These individuals are most often thought to be psychotic. Even people with lifelong psychotic disorders may experience valid parapsychologic events. Therapists open to the limits of their knowledge will offer validation, support, and reassurance and refer the individual to organizations studying such phenomena. The patterning of such events and the relationships to stresses, illness, accidents, and personality components are of interest. Many people who experience these phenomena develop a great sense of alienation or attempt to deny the experiences.

George had the sense that he was floating above the scene of an accident. He heard a commotion and even moaning that emanated from a body, though he had no sense of it being his body or of making a sound. He saw his body being carefully lifted onto the stretcher and put in the ambulance. No pain or distress was evident. Slowly, it seemed, George reentered his body, and by the time they arrived at the hospital, he was very aware. Expressing the out-of-body experiences that sometimes occur is particularly difficult. It seems as if one's essence disengages from the body, and, psychiatrically, this experience would be labeled as an episode of depersonalization.

Harriet had a prophetic dream about her son-in-law (who was a logger) that was so vivid that she was unable to go back to sleep. She *knew* he would be crushed by a falling tree the following day and begged him not to go into the woods. No doubt existed in her mind. It was as if the event had occurred for her before it occurred in reality, as it did, the next afternoon. Harriet, at 101 years of age, still vividly retrained the awe and the memory.

Freida *knew* the moment her grandmother died, though the family was not notified until the next day.

These stories are only some of the examples we have heard of extraordinary occurrences for which we have no explanation. However, nurses must become aware that many elders have experienced some of these events.

A nurse may initiate a revealing conversation by saying, "There are many things going on in this universe that we do not understand. Have you ever experienced something that there was no logical explanation for, such as a premonition?" "Were you frightened by it?" "Did you tell anyone?" "How did you explain it to yourself?" Such conversations can be enlightening and also renew an individual's awareness of the unknown possibilities existing in all situations.

Near-Death Experience. From antiquity to the present, near-death experiences (NDE) have been reported that have given insight into the experience of death itself. Individuals who have survived tell us what it is like to ostensibly return from the dead. Feelings of peace, tranquility, and unconditional love were described. Some people do not wish to return but believe they must. The urge to express these transcendental experiences is often strong but is mixed with fears of being considered crazy. The health care provider must realize that these experiences may have profound significance and lasting impact on the individual who has experienced them.

Though most NDEs report great peace and a reluctance to return, Joe was in his home relaxing in reverie, following which he went to bed and began meditating. He experienced a terrorizing psychic trauma in which he had a profound realization of his own death, "Since I could not know this tremendous thing and remain among the living, I assumed that I was dying. Yet, I was thinking rather calmly, 'So, this is what it's like!' I always knew I would die someday—so, this is what it's like. After a crescendo of effort, it felt as if my heart burst, and I was dropping through eternity. I knew I was dead, and I knew it would be forever. I wished it could only be for a million years or so, but I knew that it would never end. I concentrated on remembering the last details of my life, and then, suddenly I returned, inexplicably, to my body, lying in bed, still thinking I was dead. Then, I tried moving a finger. It worked. I spoke to my wife, and she answered. Her credulity was strained, however, when I told her that I had died and returned to life. No need to go on. I had experienced death and infinity, in my mind, and it blew my fuses" (Pierre, 1999).

To elicit a discussion of an NDE, you might ask, "Do you recall any unusual feelings or perceptions during any critical episode you have survived?" Suggestions for dealing with people who have experienced these remarkable events include the following:

1. Be receptive and nonjudgmental when listening to an account of the event.
2. Reassure the individual that although these experiences are not common, they have been reported, and they are not evidences of psychoses.
3. Recognize the emotional impact this experience may have on the individual, and explore the meaning attached to it.
4. Anticipate anger from some people who felt compelled to come back from the NDE.
5. Realize that, as in any major crisis, the individual may become obsessed with the experience and repeat it over and over whenever a willing or unwilling listener is present.
6. Explore your own biases and keep an open mind to the unknown aspects of our universe.

We know so little of the human limits, the mystical and the universal. Let us keep ourselves open to the unknown and the immeasurable.

Hallucinations and Visions. Hallucinations and visions have great meaning for some people. These experiences differ from ordinary fantasies in that the individual believes the origin is external. History has given us many examples of such events: Saint Paul's confrontation with God, the voices heard by Joan of Arc, and the vision of the Virgin at Lourdes. These phenomena are sometimes collectively witnessed. Most of these experiences seem to have some religious or ethereal motif and are mentioned because they are poorly understood and often judged a psychotic symptom or a miracle. Religious old people sometimes report visions of angels or other heavenly emissaries. Most often, these individuals see a person who has died and may feel comforted.

Meditation. Many types and rituals of meditation have flourished in Western societies in the last two decades. Some methods of mediation have been used for thousands of years in Eastern cultures. Whatever the method, the goal is to quiet the mind and center oneself. When the mind slows, the body relaxes, and less oxygen and nutrients are needed. In addition, meditation has been found to yield the following benefits (Bloomfield, 1975):

- Increased measured intelligence
- Increased short-term and long-term recall
- Decreased anxiety, depression, and irritability
- Greater perceived self-actualization (realization of potential)
- Better mind-body coordination
- Increased perceptual awareness

- Normalization of blood pressure
- Relief from insomnia
- Normalization of weight

These benefits are all significant to aged people; the fact that we see the polar opposites of these benefits so frequently attests to the stress level of many older citizens, which might be reduced through meditation.

Effective meditation requires approximately 20 minutes of focusing on a sound, a thought, or an image. Practicing two or more times daily will bring calmness, better health, and higher energy levels in its wake. Although meditation can be accomplished in any setting, a place with few distractions is helpful. People who meditate with consistency often begin to be aware of a transcendent state of being. Although meditation has unique meanings for each person, some common dynamics that tend toward transcendence exist:

- It is noncompetitive.
- It integrates body-mind function.
- It is not dependent on others.
- It taps into beliefs about oneself.
- There is always room for improvement.
- You are in control.
- You cannot fail.

Nurses may introduce the values of meditation to the aged and serve as guides in the beginnings of such activities. Chanting psalms, reciting poetry by rote, praying, saying the Rosary, practicing yoga, and playing a musical instrument are all mechanisms of release and renewal that may bring one into higher states of awareness.

Dreams—Personal and Collective. Jung's view of the work of dreams is most appropriate in a gerontology text. Jung believed that dreams promote growth and individuation and that they are sources of informative and creative power. Jung saw the goal of the last half of life as reconciliation of one's various repressions to become a whole person by using dreams, myths, and symbols. To discover the hidden and embrace the unconscious is the process of individuation and transcendence, which may occupy one intensely after midlife. To explore the hidden, one may analyze dreams. Dreams are the window of the unconscious.

Jung believed each person was able to best analyze and interpret his or her own dreams by meditating on them and examining them in great detail. To understand the meaning, several steps are employed. Establish the context of the present life situation, then examine each image or symbol carefully for all the possible meanings. Jung suggests a series of dreams may be a most satisfactory basis for interpretation, because important images occur repeatedly in dreams.

Following is an example of a dream an old woman had following the death of her roommate. "I have dreamed of her every night since she died. She sometimes sings to me, and she is waiting for me on an island and says she won't go on without me. She's holding a big bowl of soup." We talked about the dream, about death, and about the fear of dying alone. She spoke of how her roommate knew she enjoyed soup and was never able to get a bowl of hot soup in the nursing home. She also mentioned that her roommate had been deaf. The dream seemed to give her assurance that she would not be alone in death (a compensatory aspect of the dream because so many do die alone) and that physical limitations were conquered through death (the singing of her deaf roommate). In a symbolic sense, the soup might mean nourishment, love, a blending, an offering, or it might be from the present context of her life in which she seldom got the soup she so enjoyed. The old woman died 2 weeks after her roommate. Jung might call this a *prospective* dream because it prepared her for a future place and time.

Ron had a vivid dream a few months before he died in which he was planting corn in sequential plots on neatly terraced hillsides to be sure they would always be ripening and ready for his family. He was a very providential man, and the dream was prophetic of his death in one sense and a summary of his life in another.

Dreams provide access to the unconscious of the individual or the collective unconscious. The individual may express desires, conflicts, fears, prophecies, hidden aspects of personality, compensation, or modifications of recent or distant experiences. To fully use dream material for self-transcendence, the concept of collective unconscious must be explored. Jung (1961) viewed the collective unconscious as composed of archetypal images or symbols, which include powerful, collectively carried, instinctual reactions:

- *Anima*: Feminine principle
- *Animus*: Masculine principle
- *Wise old man*: King, hero, medicine man, savior
- *Great mother*: Infinite love, understanding, help, protection, tyranny over the dependent

Dreams that connect one with the collective unconscious may be very vivid, seem highly significant, and include surprising or incomprehensible symbols that seem to have no relationship to the dreamer's life. Jung believed that these dreams are especially significant in transcending the personal and deepening one's experience by connection with remote people through symbols significant to many. We believe nurses should express interest in the dreams of their aged clients and explore meanings with them. Sharing a dream is a revealing and intimate activity.

Dombeck (1995) reports a dream-sharing group in which *dream telling* is a mechanism for increasing spiritual awareness. The session has been found to be a healing experience for victims of abuse, disadvantaged youths, and prisoners. No efforts at dream interpretation were made but only to explore feelings, commonalties with others, and speculations about personal meanings.

We did not find reports of such activity with elders but believe it might be very illuminating. We would be particularly interested in recurring dreams and the meaning for the elder. Dream research seems a fruitful area of study with elders, presently being studied by Moody (2003).

In fantasies and daydreams, there seems to be a thinning of the psychic membrane between conscious, directed thought, and the stream of *consciousness* or unconscious that presses through the conscious so easily in old age. The barrier thins, just as the skin thins. The barrier between conscious and unconscious becomes friable.

Most studies indicate a decreasing importance and intensity of daydreams and fantasies in old age. However, we must remember cohort effects and realize that people born 75 years ago were culturally conditioned in a way that put little importance on dreams and fantasies. We might assist the aged to value their self-exploratory activities by giving credence to them.

Memories might well be included with dreams and fantasies because they become so intertwined in the later years. The conscious and unconscious seem to merge in a more holistic manner when the very old move backward and forward in time with ease, weaving recurrent dreams, hopes, and fantasies into their memories. We often mistakenly label this fluidity as confusion or inaccuracy if we hold strict boundaries and a segmented personal reality. We might take lessons from the old who have learned to make peace with their multiple realities.

Hypnosis. Throughout the history of medicine, hypnosis has appeared again and again as a means of healing, yet it has not gained a respected status or large following. Although the eclectic psychiatrists today have largely abandoned hypnosis and free association, most are aware that the mind has more power over illness and health than the physician. The ingredient of interpersonal trust enhances hypnotic responsiveness. The aged subjected to minimum stimulation over long periods are thought to be susceptible to hypnotic suggestion. Some drugs also increase suggestibility; however, the ability for intense concentration seems to be a prerequisite of hypnotic trance.

Confusion and Transcendence. Nursing literature and gerontologic studies approach the issue of confusion in the elderly as a problem. Confusion often becomes a problem for the individual in negotiating the milieu and for health care providers who have certain expectations of the realities of effective functioning. However, we propose another way of assessing and dealing with confusion. What is the human need addressed by the confusion? A better time? A more comfortable place? More loving people? Attention? In our observations, we have noted the following positive effects of confusion in certain individuals:

1. Individuals are largely unaware of biologic disturbances and the betrayal of their bodies as they mentally roam in spiritual territories.
2. Some people find security and safety in imagining that they are in a familiar place. We encountered a specific example of this situation in an elderly man who thought he was in a bordello and spent much of his time searching for *the girls.* This episode was indicative of a need for safety and sexual expression.
3. We often find people who augment their need for belonging when they imagine nurses to be cousins, granddaughters, or other significant people from their past. Some individuals talk at length to invisible companions.
4. The attempts to order others about and the insistence on obscure demands or enigmatic activities are a means of compensating for an erosion of self-esteem and power.

However, we have been most impressed by the value of delirium when one is dying. The snatches of reality (as consensually defined) are often interspersed with extended periods of other worldliness in which the individual is clearly in a transcendent level of consciousness. Distortions become symbols of meaning, ceremonies occur, and dream consciousness invades the wakeful states, producing occult meanings. Conversations occur with people long gone as the individual makes peace with those he or she loved. A feeling of people beckoning and waiting *on the other side* often occurs.

One ordinarily thinks of transcendent experiences as accompanied by a supreme mind state or a moment of extreme clarity. The following is an example of a *confused* elder in a transcendent state:

> Jay was lingering on earth, strongly willing himself to *whip the cancer.* Each day, he struggled slowly, with assistance, to his chair in the living room where he kept up the pretense of ordinary living, joking, and chatting with visiting friends and family. When Jay returned to his bedroom and the rented hospital bed, he would intermittently lapse into delirious states. In these altered states of consciousness, his mind would leave the mundane affairs of the household, and he would be mentally inaccessible to people with him. He carried on long conversations with people from the past—challenging, answering, forgiving, and setting things right. Jay often spoke in symbols and enigmatic phrases. His mind seemed to leap with equal ease to the distant past and the unknown future. He spoke with the family members who had preceded him in death and discussed his coming. Most interestingly, he participated in death ceremonies with the Cheyenne Indians and went through the litany of Christ on the cross. In his lucid periods, as judged by his awareness of daily events, he still spoke of beating the cancer. Within 6 weeks he died.

From this and similar experiences, we suggest nurses begin to assess more astutely the meaning of confusion and the need that it may be satisfying. Clearly, in many instances, certain episodes of confusion may be the individual's manner of meeting a felt need (Figure 25-6).

There is much we do not yet understand about the dynamics of confusion. This lack of knowledge is frequently thought to arise from brain dysfunction and certainly often does in the mechanistic sense. It may also be that the mind is indeed an essence of itself that moves toward the resolution of

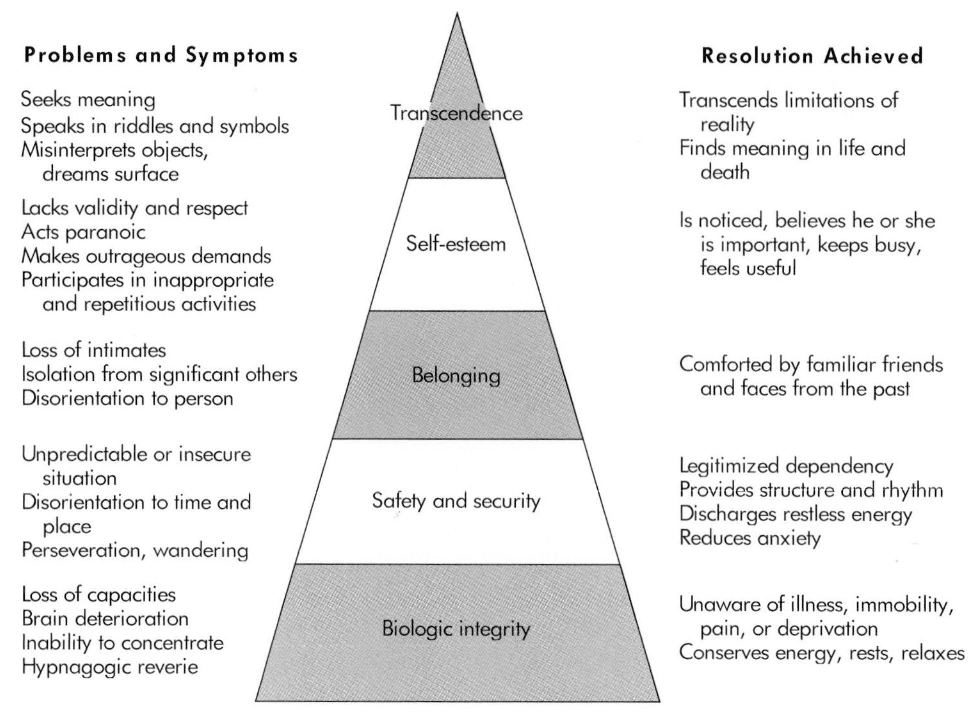

Figure 25-6. Needs met through confusional states. (Developed by Priscilla Ebersole.)

psychosocial needs and cosmic consciousness during confusional states.

Hope as a Transcendent Mechanism

A definition of hope, based on extensive study and analysis, is provided by Morse and Doberneck (1995): "Hope is a response to a threat that results in the setting of a desired goal; the awareness of the cost of not achieving the goal; the planning to make the goal a reality; the assessment, selection and use of all internal and external resources and supports that will assist in achieving the goal; and the reevaluation and revision of the plan while enduring, working and striving to reach the desired goal" (p. 284). Hope is the belief in the future and the expectation of fulfillment. Hope is the anchor that sustains life in the most difficult times and in the face of doubts and ennui. Some level of hope must be maintained to survive and to die in peace. Hope embodies desires and expectations and the limitless possibilities of humans in all times and places—present, past, and future. For many an elder, hope is a major means of coping, and those who lose hope lose the capacity and desire for survival.

O'Connor (1996) enumerates the critical aspects of hope: (1) the presence of an inner human energy, (2) positive expectations for the future, (3) motivation for action, and (4) formulations of meaningful, realistic goals. The author further states that a person without hope has no goals or expectations for the future. All practicing nurses have observed how a small goal or hope for the future can sustain an elder. The grandson's graduation from college, the daughter's return from her travels, even a birthday may keep an elder alive until the event is safely fulfilled.

Hope is much more than magical thinking. Components of hope as delineated by Morse and Doberneck (1995) include the following:

- Recognition of a predicament or threat
- Realistic assessment of the severity and implications
- Determining various methods of resolution or ways out of dilemma
- Recognizing negative outcomes that may occur and preparing to deal with them
- Remaining realistically optimistic about outcomes
- Assessing conditions and resources that may influence outcomes
- Seeking supportive relationships and realistic tangible supports
- Evaluating progress toward goals and revision as necessary
- Having the determination to endure

These components resemble any problem-solving process, with the added element of the deep belief that problems can be solved and that one can endure and learn from the outcome if it is less perfect than hoped.

Nurses may not recognize the small things they do, routinely and preconsciously, to impart hope. Grooming conveys a quiet belief that it matters; pain relief and comfort measures reinforce the recognition of an individual's needs and confirm the value of that individual. Nurses may foster hope by:

1. Presenting honestly the limits of human knowledge
2. Determining significant aspects of the individual's life
3. Identifying important goals not yet reached
4. Involving significant others in plans
5. Exploring beliefs and values of the elder

The nurse serves as a sounding board as the elder sorts through these important elements of survival.

Transcendence in Illness

Serious illnesses influence how one perceives the meaning of life. A distinct shift in goals, relationships, and values often occurs among people who have survived life-threatening episodes. A heightened awareness may occur of beauty and of caring relationships, but a long period of emotional "splinting" may be necessary while recovering from the psychic wound of body betrayal. Newman (1994) contends that disease can be a manifestation of health as one confronts the crisis and as it reveals special meanings.

Steeves and Kahn (1987) found from their work in hospice care that certain conditions facilitate the search for meaning in illness, noting the following:

- Suffering must be bearable and not all-consuming if one is to find meaning in the experience.
- A person must have access to and be capable of perceiving objects in the environment. Even a small window on the world may be sufficient to match the limited energy one has to attend.
- One must have time that is free of interruption and a place of solitude to experience meaning.
- Clean, comfortable surroundings and freedom from constant responsibility and decision-making free the soul to search for meaning.
- An open, accepting atmosphere in which to discuss meanings with others is important.

The following nursing actions may facilitate the search for meaning in suffering:

1. Make opportunities for the person to talk.
2. Ask how they have experienced the changes.
3. Accept the process as it unfolds, including anger and bitterness that may accompany the search.
4. Listen and facilitate expression of feelings about life and death.
5. Recognize and confirm any evidence of a rebirth of a sense of beauty. The patient may often share a *peak experience* if he or she is made comfortable enough to do so.
6. Lead discussion groups for recovering patients, knowing that, for many people, enlightenment is a lonely process.
7. Seek the meaning to self while learning from the elders with whom we are privileged to walk for however brief the time.

Accompanying someone in their grief and quest for meaning in painful events is a privilege nurses are often given. This spiritual intimacy means being willing to suffer with another, and both the nurse and the client will reap the benefits. One of the great rewards of working with older clients is observing and participating as they turn suffering into a spiritual event.

Sister Rosemary Donley (1991) defines the nursing role in the spiritual search of suffering individuals as compassionate accompaniment, meaning entering into another's reality and quietly, attentively sharing the experience. "Nurses need to be with people who suffer, to give meaning to the reality of suffering, and, in so far as possible, to remove suffering and its causes. Here lies the spiritual dimensions of health care" (Donley, 1991, p. 180). The challenge is to find meaning and some purpose in the affliction that, unchallenged, entwines and chokes identity. Holstein and Cole (1996) say, "Thus, part of the 'work' of chronic illness is to tell a new story about the self that integrates the illness into the ongoing story" (p. 18).

The pain that often accompanies chronic illness adds another dimension to the self that must be addressed and given meaning. We do not concur with people who say, "You must learn to live with it." We believe pain relief, to the greatest extent possible, is necessary to release the mind and soul from the grip of intractable pain. Additional discussion of pain can be found in Chapters 8 and 9.

Meaning is derived from cultural ideals, images, and metaphors (Holstein and Cole, 1996). Little tolerance can be found in the Eurocentric culture for dependency, help-seeking, inactivity, and indecision. For the most part, aspects of a declining life are "culturally construed as personal and medical failures, devoid of social or cosmic meaning" (Cole, 1994, pp. 4-5).

Suicide as Transcendence

Buchanan and colleagues (1995) found that, among the elders that they surveyed, the notion of death as a means to rise beyond morbid life conditions was seen as an option. The wish to die may be a transcendent phenomenon at certain times with some elders. Long ago, Robert Murphy, in a *Pendle Hill* (the Friends' Publishing House) pamphlet, wrote about transcendent suicide, although he did not classify it as such. Simply stated, Murphy saw suicide as a declaration of hope and an affirmation of personal strength, an individual acting out the statement, "I simply refuse to live in this way. There must be more to life."

Great strength and protest can be found in suicidal thoughts and gestures, and these qualities must become the focus of therapeutic efforts. The individual may be seeking to transcend the limits experienced by the present self. As always, the nurse may learn much by truly listening and providing affirmation of an individual's strength and courage. The desire for assisted suicide and the topic of suicide in general is discussed in Chapters 14 and 24. Our point here is to affirm that suicide can be a search for transcendence through death.

Oregon's 1997 Death with Dignity Act legalizes physician-assisted suicide. Although 78% of the 91 Oregonions who died were enrolled in hospice, little is known about the way in which the hospice practitioners were affected. The recent study by Ganzini and colleagues (2002) showed that appreciable differences were not found between people who were requesting assisted suicide and other hospice enrollees. The most important reason for the request, cited by these patients, was to control the circumstances of their death. Wide variance of opinion exists about the morality of suicide.

Nursing Interventions

When focusing on the supreme needs of an individual—those for transcending the usual limits of life experience—nursing interventions may become obscure. Finding meaning in life is a uniquely individual task and does not occur quickly or through the efforts of another. Young, attentive nurses often find the aged leading the way toward development of the spirit. We can provide a milieu of acceptance, openness, and validation. These attitudes come from our own awareness of the importance of the inner person and our willingness to accede to its supremacy. This view means we cannot always measure coping by visible evidence, nor can we be the arbiters of meaning. For the aged who are reaching for transcendence through a higher level of consciousness, courses and workshops are offered throughout the United States. The goals are integrative—the connection of the finite and the infinite, mortality and immortality, matter and spirit, physics and metaphysics, humans and God.

LEGACIES

A legacy is one's tangible and intangible assets that are transferred to another and may be treasured as a symbol of immortality. The purpose of legacies is to supersede death. Courage, wisdom, and insights that we perceive in our elders become part of their legacy (Wyatt-Brown, 1996). Not only the giver, but also the receiver is essential to the concept of legacy; reciprocity is also essential (Kivnick, 1996).

The search for meaning and immortality seem to be the basic motivations for leaving a legacy. Extending one's authentic self to others can be an important activity in the last years. Throughout life, shared experiences provide satisfaction, but in the last years this exchange allows one to gain a clearer perspective on how his or her movement on earth has had impact.

Old people must be encouraged to identify that which they would like to leave and who they wish the recipients to be. This process has interpersonal significance and prepares one to leave the world with a sense of meaning. A legacy can provide a transcendent feeling of continuation and tangible or intangible ties with survivors. Although we have not studied bonding with elders, it seems the shared authenticity is the glue that binds us together. Legacies are the evidence of this process.

Interestingly, *Generations,* the publication of the American Society on Aging, devoted an entire issue to the consideration of legacies (volume 20, issue 3, 1996). Most of the issue was focused on legacies of health systems, economic policies, entitlements, and the transmission of wealth and burden. These aspects are certainly significant, and many elders and others now wonder what legacy of debt and conflict we are leaving for generations to follow. Our main focus is not on the impact of policy on legacies, though these are significant in transfers of wealth and require expert assistance.

Legacies are manifold and may range from memories that will live on in the mind of others to bequeathed fortunes. Box 25-9 is a partial list of legacies. The list is as diverse as individual contributions to humanity. Erikson's seventh stage of man identifies the generative function as the main concern of the adult years and the last stage (eighth) as that of reviewing with integrity or despair that which one has accomplished. Legacies are generative and are identified and shared best as one approaches the end of life. This activity reinforces integrity.

Autobiographies and Life Histories

Oral histories are an approach to immortality. As long as one's story is told, one remains alive in the minds of others. Doers leave their products and live through them. Powerful figures are remembered in fame and infamy. The quiet, unobtrusive person survives in the memory of intimates and in family anecdotes. Everyone has a life story. The quest for immortality grew out of words—the human ability to articulate meaning and personality to others. Without words, experience would contain no past or future. The short span of one's days would amount to only a series of sensory impressions, not even rising to the perceptual level, because perceptions are formed through internalized concepts and words spoken to the self.

Autobiographies and recorded memoirs can serve a transcendent purpose for people who are alone—and for many who are not. Nurses can encourage older people to write, talk, or express in other ways the meaning of their lives. The human

Box 25-9 Example of Legacies

Oral histories
Autobiographies
Shared memories
Taught skills
Works of art and music
Publications
Human organ donations
Endowments
Objects of significance
Written histories
Tangible or intangible assets
Personal characteristics such as courage or integrity
Bestowed talents
Traditions and myths perpetuated
Philanthropic causes
Progeny children and grandchildren
Methods of coping
Unique thought: Darwin, Einstein, Freud, and others

experience and the poignant anecdotes bind people together and validate the uniqueness of each brief journey in this level of awareness and the assurance that one will not be forgotten. Dying patients can express and order their memories through audiotapes that are then bequeathed to families if the aged person desires. Sharing one's personal story creates bonds of empathy, illustrates a point, conveys some of the deep wisdom that we all contain, and connects us with our deepest human consciousness.

These stories are influenced by gender, culture, history, social class and context, race, and ethnicity (Schuster, 1996; Harrienger, 1996). All facets come together to form a unique, never-to-be-reproduced individual legend. In addition, stories from a grandparent will bring to life historic periods that have previously seemed sterile (Kivnick, 1996). Reaching across generations in this way decreases self-absorption and releases "grand-generativity" that incorporates care for the present and concern for the future (Kivnick, 1993, p. 13).

Creating a Life History. Birren (Kleyman, 2000) says "Guided autobiography is a nontherapy. It's life centered, not problem-centered like psychotherapy." In an interview by Paul Kleyman he quoted Malcolm Cowley from *The View from Eighty,* "Our lives that seemed a random and monotonous series of incidents are something more than that. Each of them has a plot" (p. 11).

Becoming whole requires one to integrate all of life's remembered experience into the self-concept in a way that sustains or enhances self-esteem. Numerous geriatric nurses have used reminiscence, individually and in groups, as a therapeutic strategy to achieve these goals. Because it is such a natural function of many elders, reminiscence is one of the simplest and most enriching for elder and nurse. Life-review, the recall of *not me* life events, is painful and is the real psychotherapeutic work of reminiscing. Rigorously controlled studies of its effects, however, are seriously lacking, and the few that exist are often contradictory. Haight (1992) (a nurse) has been the foremost researcher in the measurable aspects of reminiscing and continues to work in that field to illuminate the process. Haight is also the organizer and driving force of the *International Reminiscence and Life Review Organization.* Possibilities grow out of life history. One's life history is a product of multiple histories that shift and change with the passage of time and development of maturity. Examining the peaks and valleys in one's life facilitates understanding. When both inner and outer structures are changed, reorganization becomes possible. The period of disequilibrium is necessary for growth. (See Chapter 22 for additional discussion.) Periods of stability, crisis, and joy are necessary. Some theorists believe that the spacing of these elements is critical to the possibility for continued growth.

Life history and reminiscence for older learners in classroom settings is useful in many ways. The reminiscing of elders who attend classes in adult education or community college programs may reveal connections between early-life and present interest in education. For many individuals, attending classes is a return to an interrupted education or a youthful intention that had waited 50 or more years for fulfillment. Elders often recall a latent interest, a parent's hope, or a teacher's appraisal. Almost all older students can connect their current educational experience with the past. Taped interviews that focus on childhood and early experiences in school can be intriguing; encourage details and elaboration. Cully and colleagues (2001) found in their study of 76 healthy elders that those who were depressed often reminisced of unpleasant memories, and the authors speculate that reminiscence treatment (life-review) may be therapeutic for them. An entire issue of *Dimensions* (the quarterly newsletter of the Mental Health and Aging Network of the American Society on Aging, volume 7, issue 3, 2000) was devoted to reminiscence and life-review, addressing concepts such as therapeutic and cultural practices, use of reminiscence with demented individuals, life-review groups for older women, and reminiscence as celebrating the legacy at the end of life. Grudzen and Soltys (2000) state, "It is only when people who have loved and cared for us reach the end of life that we see the full gift we have received from them. By leaving us their reminiscences, their spirits can continue in our lives as a living memorial" (p. 8).

Reminiscence of places in which one has lived, drawing these, and reexperiencing the effect of events attached to place are all significant to stability of self. The social and physical settings of remembered episodes are potent. Chaudbury (1996) expresses place as the "container of lived experience." Developing a residential life history may have unexpected benefits in revealing surroundings significant to individuality and attachment. During these activities, the awareness of self as continually growing and learning can be affirmed.

Creation of Self through Journaling. Through the personal journal, one can, in thoughtful reflection, discover meaning and patterns in daily events. The self becomes a coherent story with successive revisions as old events are reread and perceived in new contexts. Dellasega (2001) used reflective writing to assist troubled individuals in self-discovery, strengthening identity and self-esteem.

The journals of elders provide rich descriptions of the interior lives of the authors. May Sarton (1984) and Florida Scott-Maxwell (1968) are two of the most well-known authors. The study of these journals and of the journals of less well-known and less articulate elders assists nurses in understanding the inner experience of the aged and, perhaps, their own.

Historic Linkages and Roots. Elders who link their lives with their participation in historic events may seek a secure place in the stream of generations that will transcend the limitations of the brief mortal existence. Thorsheim and Roberts (1995) found that shared reminiscing enhanced the capacity of elders to see the uniqueness of others while simultaneously seeing unknown aspects of self. Through shared history, shared reminiscing strengthened cohort linkages with others.

Even the events one would think devastating often leave one with a sense of participation in a grander plan. Recent efforts to record World War II memoirs ("the good war," the "patriotic" war) has become a preoccupation of several authors because these old veterans are fast fading away. These veterans share their thoughts about war and combat and the important effects on their later development. This activity may provide some closure for them and understanding for us.

Historic events rated most significant included wars, space exploration, changes in transportation, the civil rights movement, assassinations, and the development of the nuclear age. Martin and colleagues (1996) were able to categorize these significant events as recent micro events (personal and present occurrences), distant micro events (personal childhood events that left an emotional residual), recent macro events (world economic, political, and environmental occurrences), and distant macro events (major markers of world events, such as wars, depressions, and so forth). Events that were considered most potent by the very old were distant macro events and recent micro events. These findings stir questions regarding effects of early events on adult identity formation and constriction of concerns as energy is depleted in advanced old age.

Seeking one's roots is going beyond the self to reach preceding generations. In a graveyard in New England, a simple hand-cut marker has held a message for 200 years, "Vishna Miller, 1782-1797." Who were you, Vishna? Where did your mystical name originate? How did you die when just beginning to live? You, my remote ancestor, begin to breathe life. The search for me begins anew. Genealogy is more than a hobby of the old; it is the means to reach back to those who have gone before. Journals, old letters, autobiographies, photos, cemeteries, and treasured objects carry me back to communicate with my forbears. I hear and see myself in them. I more clearly see my charge to the future.

Margery Kemp, born in 1373, an illiterate healer, dictated her memoirs to a priest near the end of her life. Though married and the mother of 14 children, Kemp left them and traveled alone from England, throughout Europe, and to the Holy Land (Collis, 1964). Would this journey not stir the longings of anyone named Kemp? Much of genealogy is carried on to seek one's connections in the stream of time, as well as to preserve the legacy of the past.

Collective Legacies. Each person is a link in the chain of generations (Erikson, 1963) and as such may identify with generational accomplishments. An old man may think of himself as a significant part of a generation that survived the Great Depression. A middle-aged man may identify with the generation that walked on the moon. The years of youthful idealism are impressed in one's memory by the political or ideologic climate of the time. This time is the stage when one searches for a fit in the larger society.

The importance of collective legacies to nurses lies in how they use this knowledge. For instance, the nurse may ask, "Who were the great men of your time?" "Which ones were important to you?" "What events of your generation changed the world?" "What were the most important events you experienced?" Mentioning certain historic events and asking about individual reactions is sometimes helpful.

Childless individuals are becoming more prevalent with each passing generation, and they must find a way to outlive the self through a legacy. Many people choose a *social* legacy (Rubinstein, 1996). Florence Nightingale would be one such person, with the grand legacy she left to nurses.

Legacies Expressed through Other People. One's legacy can be expressed in many ways through the development of others in a teaching or learning situation or through mentorships, patronage, shared talents, organ donations, and genetic transmission. Some creative works and research are legacies left to successive generations for continued modification and growth (Philip, 1995). In other words, one's legacy may be a product of his or her own brought to fruition through someone else who may also become an intermediary to later developments. Thus people and generations are tied in sequential progress. Some examples may illustrate this type of legacy.

An aged man cried as he talked of his grandson's talent as a violinist. Both the man and his grandson shared their love for violin, and the grandfather believed that he had genetically and personally contributed to his grandson's development as an accomplished musician.

A professor emeritus spoke of visiting his son in a distant state and hearing him expound ideas that had been partially developed by the professor and his father before him.

Great-aunt Laura worried about preserving the environment for future generations, so she took young children on nature walks to stimulate their interest in birds, plants, and animals. She also donated land for a natural park. Years later, her grandnephew became a park ranger and passed on the knowledge he had learned from her.

People who amass a fortune and allocate certain funds for endowment of artists, scientific projects, and intellectual exploration are counting on others to complete their legacy.

The following are suggestions for assisting elders to identify and develop their legacy:

1. Find out lifelong interests.
2. Establish a method of recording.
3. Identify recipients—either generally or specifically.
4. Record the legacy.
5. Distribute the legacy as planned.
6. Provide for systematic feedback of results to the older person.

A legacy that can be converted into some tangible form can be gratifying to the aged, ensuring that it will not be readily dismissed or forgotten. The following vehicles can convey legacies:

- Summation of life work
- Photograph albums, scrapbooks
- Written memoir
- Taped memoirs (video or audio)
- Artistic representations
- Memory gardens
- Mementos

- Genealogies
- Recorded pilgrimages

Living Legacies

Many old people wish to donate their bodies to science or donate body parts for transplant. This mechanism is a means to transcend death. Parts of the body keep another person alive, or, in the case of certain diseases, the deceased body may provide important information leading to preventive or restorative techniques in the future. Donation of body parts in old age may not be encouraged because they are often less viable than those from younger people. Nonetheless, old bodies are welcome for use as cadavers. People who are interested in providing such a legacy should be encouraged to call the nearest university biomedical center and obtain more information. The nurse then has a postmortem obligation to the client to assist in carrying out his or her wishes.

Keating (1996) identifies the generational transfer of a farm as a living legacy. Although not an organ donation, the transfer certainly represents a living donation. In the days of primogeniture, generational transfer was a simple affair though not necessarily satisfactory. Now, the process is more complex. A study conducted in Canada, New Zealand, and the United States showed that keeping the farm intact and in the family was a high priority (Keating, 1996). A successful resolution included keeping all family members content and maintaining a viable farm operation (Stalker, McGregor, and Rock, 1996). This task was accomplished successfully when all family members were involved in the planning early on, and various aspects of the farm management were turned over to the children who were best able to manage them. In other cases, encumbrances on the farm or fluctuating market values imposed inequities on various siblings. Most parents attempted to compensate nonsuccessor children in some way.

Property and Assets. Wealth may be viewed as a means toward power more often than transcendence; therefore, old people are often reluctant to disperse material goods before their death. Some elders use the future legacy as a means to exert power and control over offspring. One man said, "So long as I have that bankroll, they've got to treat me with respect" (Lustbader, 1996). The power to exert influence, to punish, and to reward is often bound up in an anticipated estate distribution.

Many old people die each year leaving inheritances with no will or specified beneficiaries. These assets are then retained in county and state treasuries until someone successfully substantiates a claim to them.

Families often consider wills a taboo subject and refuse to discuss them but on distribution may be sorely disappointed. When older people leave large gifts to *unnatural* or *unworthy* legatees, the will is often challenged by children or other relatives (Frolik, 1996).

Estates can be planned in certain ways that are decidedly advantageous for the planner, as well as the recipient, in terms of control, avoidance of lengthy probate proceedings, and taxation. Because the laws are complex and ever changing, using the services of an estate planner would be advisable (see Chapter 15). The nurse's responsibility regarding wills may be limited to advising older people to obtain legal counsel while they are healthy and competent and plan how they would like to distribute their worldly goods.

Knowledge. We carry thought legacies, without conscious awareness, of individuals, such as Ban Zhao*, Sappho†, Lao-Tzu‡, Hippocrates§, St. Augustine‖, James Madison¶, Nightingale#, Darwin, Helen Hunt Jackson**, Einstein, Freud, and others who underlie many of our thoughts and actions. Erik Homberg Erikson, one of the respected thinkers of our time, is just one of many formulators of human thought constructs who left numerous published works for future generations and has markedly influenced the understanding of life span development in our era. Erikson's legacy and that of many others continue with modifications and reinterpretations. As has been said in many ways before, we build on the thought and works of those who have preceded us. In a sense, all creative thinkers and teachers leave their legacy in their students and devotees.

Personal possessions. Possessions carry more meaning as time passes; individuals change, but the possession remains much the same. A possession is a way of symbolically hanging on to individuals who are gone or times that are past. For some people, keeping personal possessions is a means of hanging on to the self that is changing with time. Cherished possessions passed on through several generations may have achieved meaning through the close family member to whom they belonged (Tobin, 1996). One's personally significant items become highly charged with memories and meaning, and transferring them to friends and kin can be a tender experience. Personal possessions should never be dispersed without the individual's knowledge. Because of the uncertainty of late life lucidity, these issues should be discussed early with older individuals.

People who are approaching death must be given the opportunity to distribute their important belongings appropriately to those who they believe will also cherish them. Nurses may encourage elders to plan the distribution of their significant items carefully. Deciding when and how best these posses-

---

*Ban Zhao, Chinese astronomer, mathematician, and poet, circa 115 AD.

†Sappho, Greek educator and priestess of the feminine love cult, circa 610 BC.

‡Lao-Tzu, Chinese founder of Taoism, circa 575 BC.

§Hippocrates, Greek father of medicine, circa 425 BC.

‖St. Augustine, Christian theologian, circa 400 AD.

¶James Madison, father of the US Constitution, circa 1775 AD.

#Florence Nightingale, mother of organized nursing, circa 1860 AD.

**Helen Hunt Jackson, author, defender of Native Americans, their rights, and intermarriage, circa 1884 AD.

sions should be given is often difficult. Some people choose to distribute possessions before dying. In these cases, nurses often need to help family members accept these gifts, appreciating the meaning and recognizing the significance.

Certain questions allow the aged person to consider a legacy if he or she is ready to do so; for example:

- What is the meaning to you of your life experience right now?
- Have you ever thought of writing an autobiography?
- If you were able to leave something to the younger generation, what would it be?
- Have you ever thought of the impact your generation has had on the world?
- What has been most meaningful in your life?
- What possessions have special meaning for you? Who else is interested in them?
- Do you see some of your genetic traits emerging in your grandchildren?

These suggestions should stimulate ideas for spontaneous statements, which are revealing in an interpersonal context.

SELF-ACTUALIZATION, TRANSCENDENCE, LEGACIES, AND NURSING

"The responsibility of the nurse is not to make people well, or to prevent their getting sick, but to assist people to recognize the power that is within them to move to higher levels of consciousness" (Newman, 1994, p. xv). In this chapter, we have dealt with methods of expanding one's limited existence by developing the authentic self, transcendent self, spiritual self and several mechanisms used to establish immortality through a legacy. These areas often become major issues in the latter part of life, and the nurse will find it a revealing, absorbing, and challenging task to be a part of this effort. An important point to remember is that some people may avoid any such interest or concern, particularly when angry, in pain, or denying their own mortality. Nurses need not push the individual to accomplish this task but should be available to assist the person and family members.

The basic mysteries of life elude scientific researchers, yet they are the essence of existence with meaning. Remembering, feeling, dreaming, worshipping, and grasping one's connection to the universe are the realities of the human spirit. Being old is not the centrality of the self—spirit is. Spirit synthesizes the total personality and provides integration, energizing force, and immortality.

Human Needs and Wellness Diagnoses

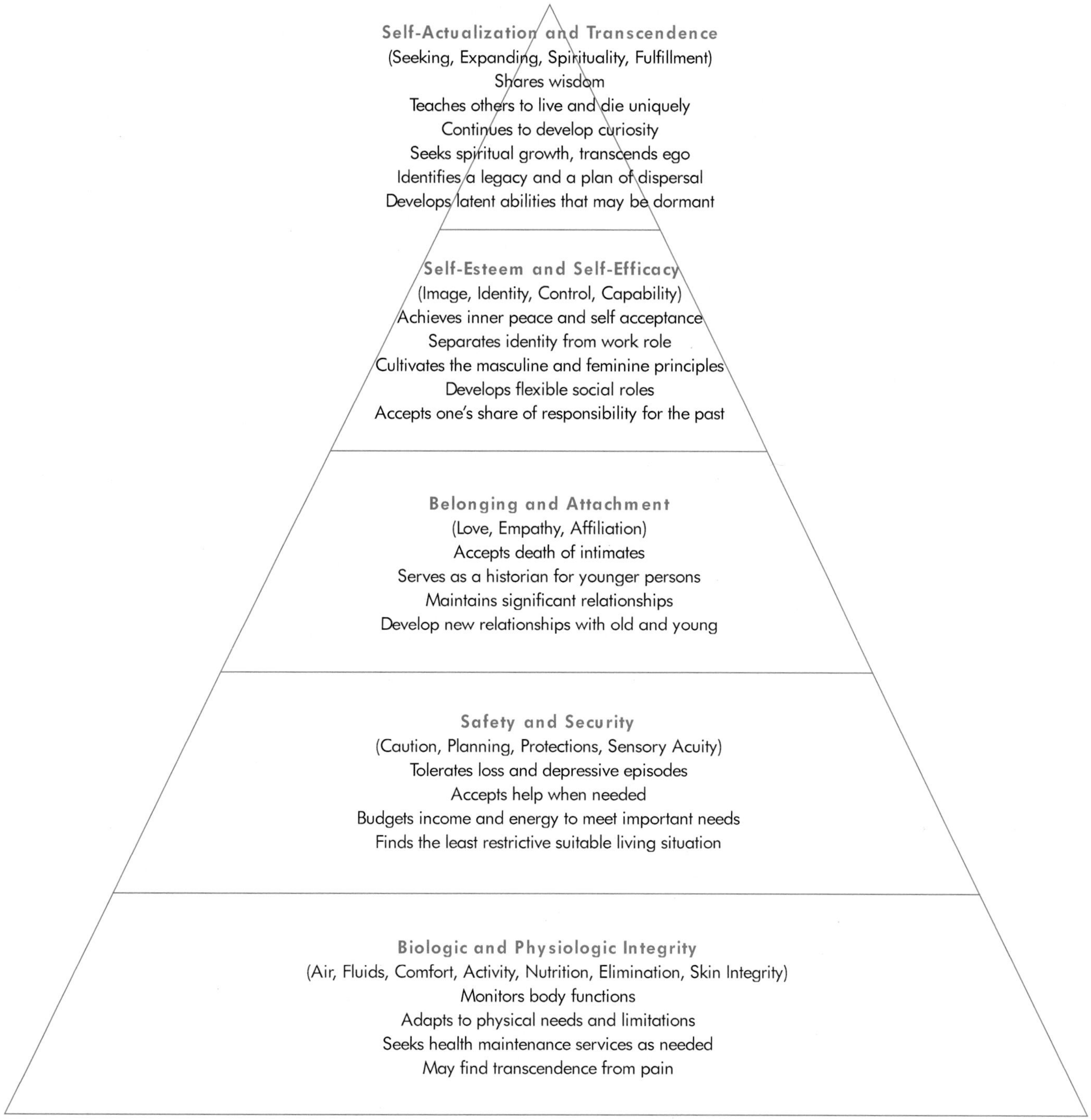

Self-Actualization and Transcendence
(Seeking, Expanding, Spirituality, Fulfillment)
Shares wisdom
Teaches others to live and die uniquely
Continues to develop curiosity
Seeks spiritual growth, transcends ego
Identifies a legacy and a plan of dispersal
Develops latent abilities that may be dormant

Self-Esteem and Self-Efficacy
(Image, Identity, Control, Capability)
Achieves inner peace and self acceptance
Separates identity from work role
Cultivates the masculine and feminine principles
Develops flexible social roles
Accepts one's share of responsibility for the past

Belonging and Attachment
(Love, Empathy, Affiliation)
Accepts death of intimates
Serves as a historian for younger persons
Maintains significant relationships
Develop new relationships with old and young

Safety and Security
(Caution, Planning, Protections, Sensory Acuity)
Tolerates loss and depressive episodes
Accepts help when needed
Budgets income and energy to meet important needs
Finds the least restrictive suitable living situation

Biologic and Physiologic Integrity
(Air, Fluids, Comfort, Activity, Nutrition, Elimination, Skin Integrity)
Monitors body functions
Adapts to physical needs and limitations
Seeks health maintenance services as needed
May find transcendence from pain

These are not all the possible wellness diagnoses that may be identified. The above are examples of nursing diagnoses that should be considered when planning care for the older adult.

KEY CONCEPTS

- Self-actualization is a process of developing one's most authentic self. Maslow thought of self-actualization as the pinnacle of human development.
- Self-actualized individuals embody qualities of courage, humor, high moral development, and seeking to learn more about themselves and others.
- Opportunities for pursuing interests will assist individuals in developing latent talents, expressing their creativity, and rising beyond daily concerns.
- Groups working toward societal humanitarian advancement may accomplish collective actualization.
- Creativity emanates from people who are self-actualized and may be expressed in mundane activities, as well as the arts, music, theater and literature.
- Transcending the material and physical limitations of existence through ritual and spiritual means is an especially important aspect of aging.
- Gerotranscendence is a theory, proposed by Tornstam, that implies a natural shift in concerns that occurs in the aging process. Elders are thought to spend more time in reflection, less on materialistic concerns, and to find more satisfaction in life. This effort is an attempt to define aging not by the standards of young and middle adulthood but as having distinctive characteristics of its own.
- Peak experiences are the times during which one seems to rise above the ordinary and participate in the mystical.
- Illnesses that occur have the potential for altering one's fundamental beliefs and hopes. Nurses must give elders the opportunity to discuss the meanings of an illness. Some people find that these experiences bring new insights; others are angry. Empathic nurses will provide a sounding board while the elder makes sense of an illness within a satisfactory framework.
- Spiritual healing has ancient religious roots, but scientists are now recognizing and accepting the power of the mind in restoring health and, if not restoring health, enhancing one's ability to cope.
- Although many do not attend churches, elders have a high level of interest in the spiritual and religious elements of life.
- Nurses need not neglect discussing spirituality with elders. Elders will respond only if it has significance for them.
- Life satisfaction, happiness, morale, and health are related in some ways to beliefs, hope, and motivation that may be derived from a spiritual awareness.
- Dreams and fantasies are avenues to the subliminal life and often yield insights to the elder who is in search of meanings.
- NDE are remarkably consistent in producing a sense of profound peace for most people, though some have found them terrorizing. More study is needed in this area.

▲ CASE STUDY

Melba had no children but numerous nieces and nephews, though she did not feel particularly close to any of them. She had been a nursing instructor at a community college and had enjoyed her students but had not developed a sustained relationship with any of them after they had completed her courses. At her level of nursing education, the opportunity for mentorship was lacking, though she had occasionally taken students under her wing and arranged special experiences that they particularly desired. Because she had taught several courses each year, Melba never really developed a strong affiliation to a specialty but considered herself a pediatric nurse. She had not made any major contributions to the field in terms of research or publications; a few reviews, continuing education workshops, and some nursing newsletters had really been the extent of her work outside of that which was required. Melba's husband died in 1988, and she had felt very much alone since that time, especially after her retirement 3 years ago. Before her husband's death, Melba had been too busy to think about the ultimate meaning of all her years of teaching and wifely activities. With time on her hands, she began to wonder what it all meant. Had she done anything meaningful? Had she really made a difference in anything or in anyone's life? Was anyone going to remember her in any special way? So many questions were making her morose. She had never been a religious person, though her husband had been a devoted Catholic. He had believed that God had a purpose for him in life, and though he was not always able to understand what it might be, he seemed to have a sense of satisfaction. She began to wonder if she should go to church ... would that make her feel less depressed?

One Sunday morning, Melba had decided to attend her neighborhood Catholic church, but on her way out she slipped on the icy walkway and sustained Colles' fractures on both wrists. After a brief emergency room visit for assessment, immobilization of the wrists, and medications, Melba was sent back home with an order for home health and social service assessment on the following day. Of course, she had extreme difficulty managing the most basic self-care while keeping her wrists immobilized and was very dejected. When the home health nurse arrived the next morning, to Melba's amazement, it was a former student who had graduated 4 years previously. Melba was more chagrined than pleased and greeted her with, "Oh, I hate to have you see me so helpless. I've been feeling so useless and, now with these wrists, I am totally useless." If you were the home health nurse, how would you begin working with Melba, knowing that your visits would be limited to just a few?

Based on the case study, develop a nursing care plan using the following procedure:*

---

*Students are advised to refer to their nursing diagnosis text and identify possible or potential problems.

List the client's comments that provide subjective data.
List information that provides objective data.
From these data, identify and state, using accepted format, two nursing diagnoses you determine are most significant to this client at this time.
Determine and state the outcome criteria for each diagnosis. These criteria must reflect some alleviation of the problem identified in the nursing diagnosis and must be stated in concrete and measurable terms.
Plan and state one or more interventions for each diagnosed problem. Provide specific documentation of sources used to determine appropriate intervention.
Plan at least one intervention that incorporates the client's existing strengths.
Evaluate success of intervention. Interventions must correlate directly with the stated outcome criteria to measure the outcome success.

STUDY QUESTIONS/ACTIVITIES

Discuss the meanings and the thoughts triggered by the student and elder's viewpoints as expressed at the beginning of the chapter. How do they vary from your own experience?

RESEARCH QUESTIONS

Kane (1996) suggests the following aspects of legacies that need to be studied:

How do elders balance their own present needs against estate planning?
Who makes out wills and when?
How do bequests relate to gifts given during one's lifetime?
Is the perpetuation of one's name an important aspect of a legacy?
What are the motivating differences between gifts during life and those after one's death?
How do recipients view the adequacy of their legacy?
These important questions might be suggested for nursing research.

REFERENCES

Academy of Parapsychology and Medicine: First National Congress on Integrative Health, Tucson, Arizona, October 1975.

American Association of Critical Care Nurses (AACN): Prayer and medicine: do they mix? *AACN News,* February 1995.

Bassen S, Baltazar B: Flowers, flowers everywhere: creative horticulture programming at the Hebrew Home for the Aged, *Geriatr Nurs* 18(2):53, 1997.

Benner P: *Interpretive phenomenology: embodiment, caring and ethics in health and illness,* Thousand Oaks, Calif, 1994, Sage.

Berggren-Thomas P, Griggs MJ: Spirituality in aging: spiritual need or spiritual journey, *J Gerontol Nurs* 21(3):5, 1995.

Bloomfield H: *Discovering inner energy and overcoming stress,* New York, 1975, Dell.

Bond C, Miller M: Reading: the ageless activity, *Geriatr Nurs* 8(4):910, 1987.

Buchanan D, Farran C, Clark D: Suicidal thought and self-transcendence in older adults, *J Psychosoc Nurs* 33(10):31, 1995.

Carson D: Natural landscape as meaningful space for the aged. In Pastalan L, Carson D, editors: *Spatial behavior of older people,* Ann Arbor, Mich, 1970, University of Michigan.

Chaudbury H: *Self and reminiscence of place: toward a theory of re-discovering selfhood in place-based reminiscence for people with dementia.* Paper presented at the meeting of the Gerontological Society of America, Washington, DC, November 19, 1996.

Chidester D: *Patterns of transcendence: religion, death and dying,* Belmont, Calif, 1990, Wadsworth Publishing.

Cole T: The humanities and aging: an overview. In Cole T, Van Tassel D, Kastenbaum R, editors: *Handbook of aging and the humanities,* New York, 1994, Springer.

Cole TR: The aging spirit: ageism and the journey of life in America, *Aging Today* 13(4):17, 1992.

Collis L: *Memoirs of a medieval woman: the life and times of Margery Kemp,* New York, 1964, Harper and Row.

Cooper KN et al: Health barriers to walking for exercise in elderly primary care, *Geriatr Nurs* 22(5):258, 2001.

Cousins N: *Anatomy of an illness,* New York, 1979, WW Norton.

Crowther MR et al: Rowe and Kahn's model of successful aging revisited: positive spirituality—the forgotten factor, *Gerontologist* 42(5):613, 2002.

Cully JA, LaVoie D, Gfeller JD: Reminiscence, personality, and psychological functioning in older adults, *Gerontologist* 41(1):89, 2001.

Cumming E, Henry WE: *Growing old: the process of disengagement,* New York, 1961, Basic Books.

Deaconess Parish Nurse Ministries: Frequently Asked Questions, July 1, 2002. Available at *www.parishnurses.org/faq.phtml*

Dellasega CA: Using structured writing experiences to promote mental health, *J Psychosoc Nurs* 39(2):15, 2001.

Dombeck M-TB: Dream telling: a means of spiritual awareness, *Holist Nurs Pract* 9(2):37, 1995.

Donley R: Spiritual dimensions of health care: nursing's mission, *Nurs Health Care* 12(4):178, 1991.

Edwards D: Presentation at American Nurses' Association Gerontological Nurses Conference, St Paul, Minn, April 1977.

Ehman JW et al: Do patients want physicians to inquire about their spiritual or religious beliefs if they become gravely ill? *Arch Intern Med* 159(15):1803, 1999.

Elderhostel: *Elderhostel international catalog: 2003,* Boston, 2003, Elderhostel.

Ellerman CR, Reed PG: Self-transcendence and depression in middle-age adults, *West J Nurs Res* 23(7):698, 2001.

Ellison CG, Levin JS: The religion-health connection: evidence, theory and future directions, *Health Educ Behav* 25:700, 1998.

Erikson EH: *Childhood and society,* New York, 1950, WW Norton.

Erikson EH: *Childhood and society,* ed 2, New York, 1963, WW Norton.

Forbes DA: Enhancing mastery and sense of coherence: important determinants of health in older adults, *Geriatr Nurs* 22(1):29, 2001.

Forbes EJ: Spirituality, aging, and the community-dwelling caregiver and care recipient, *Geriatr Nurs* 16(6):297, 1994.

Fordham F: *An introduction to Jung's psychology,* New York, 1966, Penguin Books.

Freke T, Gandy P: *Jesus and the lost goddess: the secret teachings of the original Christians,* New York, 2001, Three Rivers Press.

Frolik LA: Legacies of possessions: passing property at death, *Generations* 20(3):9, 1996.

Ganzini L et al: Experiences of Oregon nurses and social workers with hospice patients who requested assistance with suicide, *N Engl J Med* 347(8):582, 2002.

George LK: The links between religion and health: are they real? *Public Policy Aging Rep* 12(4):1, 2002.

George LK et al: Spirituality and health: what we know and what we need to know, *J Soc Clin Psychol* 19:102, 2000.

Goldberg BZ: *The sacred fire: the story of sex in religion,* New York, 1958, University Books.

Grudzen M, Soltys FG: Reminiscence at end of life: celebrating a living legacy, *Dimensions* 7(3):4,5,8, 2000.

Haight B: Long term effects of a structured life review process, *J Gerontol* 47(5):P312, 1992.

Harrienger M: Writing a life: the composing of grace. Paper presented at the meeting of the Gerontological Society of America, Washington, DC, November 19, 1996.

Hebrews 11:1, *Holy Bible,* Chicago, 1964, John A Dickson.

Hemstrom MM: Wellness. In Fitzpatrick JJ et al, editors: *Geriatric nursing research digest,* New York, 2000, Springer.

Henderson R: The spirituality 'renaissance': professional interest grows, *Aging Today* 17(2):11, 1996.

Hermann C: A guide to the spiritual needs of elderly cancer patients, *Geriatr Nurs* 21(6):324, 2000.

Holstein MB, Cole TR: Reflections on age, meaning, and chronic illness, *J Identity Health* 1(1):7, 1996.

Hudson F: *The adult years: mastering the art of self-renewal,* San Francisco, 1999, Jossey-Bass.

Hudson SD, Rich SM: Group travel programs: a creative way to meet the leisure needs of older adults, *J Phys Educ Recreation Dance* 64(4):38, 1993.

Hungelmann J et al: Focus on spiritual well-being: harmonious interconnectedness of mind-body-spirit—use of the Jarel Spiritual Well-Being Scale, *Geriatr Nurs* 17(6):262, 1996.

Idler EL: The many causal pathways linking religion to health, *Public Policy Aging Rep* 12(4):7, 2002.

Irvine KN, Warber SL: Greening health care: practicing as if the natural environment really mattered, *Altern Ther Health Med* 8(5):76, 2002.

Jung C: *Memories, dreams, reflections,* translated by Jaffe A, editor, New York, 1961, Random House.

Kane RA: Toward understanding legacy: a wish list, *Generations* 20(3): 92, 1996.

Keating NC: Legacy, aging and succession in farm families, *Generations* 20(3):61, 1996.

Kennedy GJ et al: The relation of religious preference and practice to depressive symptoms among 1855, *J Gerontol* 51B(6):P301, 1996.

Kimble M: A personal journey of aging: the spiritual dimension, *Generations* 17(2):27, 1993.

Kivnick HQ: Everyday mental health: a guide to assessing life strengths, *Generations* 17(1):13, 1993.

Kivnick HQ: Remembering and being remembered: the reciprocity of psychosocial legacy, *Generations* 20(3):49, 1996.

Kleyman P: Did the devil do it? Study links mortality, religious struggle, *Aging Today* 23(5):6, 2002.

Kleyman P: Life stories: a "nontherapy" for elders and their families, *Aging Today* 21(4):9,11, 2000.

Koch K: *I never told anybody,* New York, 1977, Random House.

Koenig HG, Brooks RG: Religion, health and aging: implications for practice and public policy, *Public Policy Aging Rep* 12(4):13, 2002.

Kohlberg L, Power C: Moral development, religious thinking and the question of a seventh stage. In Kohlberg L, editor: *The philosophy of moral development,* vol I, San Francisco, 1981, Harper and Row.

Krause N et al: Aging, religious doubt and psychological well being, *Gerontologist* 39(5):525, 1999.

Kuhn M: Advocacy in this new age, *Aging* 3:297, Jul/Aug 1979.

Leitner MJ, Leitner SF: *Leisure in later life,* ed 2 New York, 1996, Haworth Press.

Levin JS: Age differences in mystical experience, *Gerontologist* 33(4):507, 1993.

Lustbader W: Conflict, emotion and power surrounding legacy, *Generations* 20(3):54, 1996.

Mackenzie ER et al: Spiritual support and psychological well-being: older adults' perceptions of the religion and health connection, *Altern Ther Health Med* 6(6):37, 2000.

MacKinley E: *The spiritual dimension of aging,* London, 2001, Jessica Kingsley Publishers.

MacLennan S, Tsai S: A nursing perspective on spiritual healing, *Perspectives* 19(1):9, 1995.

Martin P et al: Significant events in the lives of the oldest old. Paper presented at the meeting of the Gerontological Society of America, Washington, DC, November 20, 1996.

Maslow A: Creativity in self-actualizing people. In Anderson H, editor: *Creativity and its cultivator,* New York, 1959, Harper and Row.

Maslow A: *Religions, values and peak-experiences,* New York, 1970, Viking Press.

Matsumoto M: Class presentation in the Gerontological Certificate Program, Division of Continuing Education, San Francisco State University, San Francisco, 1978.

McDonald A: The changing scope of senior adult theater, *Aging Today* 17(6):18, 1996.

McLeod BW: The aging spirit: Sue Bender's stretching lessons extends spiritual reach, *Aging Today* 22(4):17, 2001.

Meraviglia M: Critical analysis of spirituality: its empirical indicators, *J Holist Nurs* 17:18, 1999.

Merriam-Webster: *Merriam-Webster dictionary,* New York, 1974, Simon & Schuster.

Metcalf CW: *Lighten up,* Niles, Ill, 1993, Nightingale Conant, (audiotapes).

Moberg DO: Religion in gerontology: from benign neglect to belated respect, *Gerontologist* 36(2):264, 1996.

Moody HR: Oceans for the second half of life: *Human values in aging* Newsletter Apr 1, 2003, UPDATE, 2002. Available at *hrmoody@yahoo.com*

Morse JM, Doberneck B: Delineating the concept of hope, *Image J Nurs Sch* 27(4):277, 1995.

National Council on Aging (NCOA): *Senior centers: 50 years of progress—1943-1993,* Washington, DC, 1993, NCOA.

National Interfaith Coalition on Aging: *Spiritual well-being,* Washington, DC, 1975, National Interfaith Coalition on Aging.

Newman MA: *Health as expanding consciousness,* ed 2, New York, 1994, National League for Nursing Press.

O'Connor P: Hope: a concept for home care nursing, *Home Care Provider* 1(4):175, 1996.
Partridge E: *Origins: a short etymological dictionary of modern English,* New York, 1959, Macmillan.
Peck R: Psychological developments in the second half of life. In Anderson J, editor: *Psychological aspects of aging,* Washington, DC, 1955, American Psychological Association.
Philip CE: Lifelines, *J Aging Stud* 9(4):265, 1995.
Pierre JH: *The road to Damascus: our journey through eternity,* ed 2, New York, 1999, to Excel.
Powers M: Homebound elders still need spiritual connections, *Aging Today* 17(5):13, 1996.
Raes F, Marcoen A: Gerotranscendence in the second half of life, *Tijdschr Gerontol Geriatr* 32(4):150, 2001.
Ramsey JL: Spiritual intimacy in later life: implications for clinical practice, *Generations* 25(2):59, 2001.
Reed PG: Toward a nursing theory of self-transcendence: deductive reformulation using developmental theories, *Adv Nurs Sci* 13(4):64, 1991.
Roberts TB: Do entheogen-induced mystical experiences boost the immune system? Psychedelics, peak experiences, and wellness, *Adv Mind Body Med* 15(2):139, 1999.
Rowe JW, Kahn RL: *Successful aging,* New York, 1998, Pantheon–Random House.
Rubenstein RL: Childlessness, legacy, and generativity, *Generations* 20(3):58-61, 1996.
Sarton M: *At seventy: a journal,* New York, 1984, WW Norton.
Schank MJ, Weis D, Matheus R: Parish nursing: ministry of healing, *Geriatr Nurs* 17(1):11, 1996.
Schulman K: Older Kansas volunteers go back to school, *Aging Today* 17(5):19, 1996.
Schuster E: *Transformative functions of life writing.* Paper presented at the meeting of the Gerontological Society of America, Washington, DC, November 19, 1996.
Scott-Maxwell F: *The measure of my days,* New York, 1968, Alfred A Knopf.
Sherman J: The arts and older Americans, monographs: National Assembly of Local Arts Agencies, *Americans for the Arts* 5(8):1, 1996.
Stalker N, McGregor J, Rock G: *From one generation to the next: successful farm transfer from the perspectives of retiring and successor farm family members.* Report to the Rural Education Development Association. Edmonton, Alberta, Canada, 1996.
Steeves R, Kahn D: Experience of meaning in suffering, *Image J Nurs Sch* 19(3):114, 1987.
Stoll R: Guidelines for spiritual assessment, *AJN* 79(9):1574, 1979.
Thibault JM, Ellor JW, Netting FE: Conceptual framework for assessing the spiritual functioning and fulfillment of older adults in long-term care settings, *J Religious Gerontol* 7(4):29, 1991.
Thorsheim HI, Roberts B: Finding common ground and mutual social support through reminiscing and telling one's story. In Haight BK, Webster JD, editors: *The art and science of reminiscing: theory, research, methods and applications,* Washington, DC, 1995, Taylor and Francis.
Tobin S: Cherished possessions: the meaning of things, *Generations* 20(3):46, 1996.
Tornstam L: Gerotranscendence: a theoretical and empirical exploration. In Thomas LE, Eisenhandler SA, editors: *Aging and the religious dimension,* Westport, CT, 1994, Greenwood Publishing Group.
Tornstam L: Gerotranscendence: a theory about maturing into old age, *J Aging Identity* 1(1):37, 1996.
van Manen M: *Researching lived experience: human science for an action sensitive pedagogy,* Ontario, Canada, 1990, Althouse.
Wadensten B, Carlsson M: A qualitative study of nursing staff members' interpretations of signs of gerotranscendence, *J Adv Nurs* 36(5):635, 2001.
Weis D, Schank MJ: Use of a taxonomy to describe parish nursing practice with older adults, *Geriatr Nurs* 21(3):125, 2000.
Wyatt-Brown AM: The literary legacies: continuity and change, *Generations* 20(3):65, 1996.

Name Index

D

E

L

M

Subject Index

Page numbers followed by *b*, *f*, or *t* refer to boxes, figures, or tables, respectively.

T